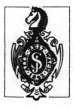

Springer-Verlag France S.A.R.L

Cancer Treatment
An Update

Edited by :

P. Banzet, J.F. Holland, D. Khayat, M. Weil

Springer-Verlag France S.A.R.L

Professeur P. Banzet
Hôpital Saint-Louis
1, avenue Vellefaux
75475 Paris Cedex 10, France

Professor J.F. Holland
The Mount Sinai Medical Center
1 G. Levy Place
New York
NY 10029-6574, USA

Professeur D. Khayat
Service d'Oncologie Médicale
Hôpital Pitié-Salpêtrière
Pavillon Jacquart
47, boulevard de l'Hôpital
75651 Paris Cedex 13, France

Docteur M. Weil
Hôpital Pitié-Salpêtrière
Pavillon Jacquart
47, boulevard de l'Hôpital
75651 Paris Cedex 13, France

Important note : Medicine is an ever-changing science undergoing continual development. Research and clinical experience are continually expanding our knowledge, in particular our knowledge of proper treatment and drug therapy. Insofar as this book mentions any dosage or application, readers may rest assured that the authors, editors and publishers have made every effort to ensure that such references are in accordance with the state of knowledge at the time of production of the book. Nevertheless this does not involve, imply, or express any guarantee or responsibility on the part of the publishers in respect of any dosage instructions and forms of application stated in the book. Every user is requested to examine carefully the manufacturers' leaflets accompanying each drug and to check, if necessary in consultation with a physician or specialist, whether the dosage schedules mentioned therein or the contraindications stated by the manufacturers differ from the statements made in the present book. Such examination is particularly important with drugs that are either rarely used or have been newly released on the market. Every dosage schedule or every form of application used is entirely at the user's own risk and responsibility. The authors and publishers request every user to report to the publishers any discrepancies or inaccuracies noticed.

Some of the product names, patents and registered designs referred to in this book are in fact registered trademarks or proprietary names even though specific reference to this fact is not always made in the text. Therefore, the appearance of a name without designation as proprietary is not to be construed as a representation by the publisher that it is in the public domain.

All translation, reproduction and adaptation rights reserved for all countries.

The law of March 11, 1957 forbids copies or reproductions intended for collective use. Any representation, partial or integral reproduction made by any process whatsoever without the consent of the autor or his executors is illicit and constitues a fraud dealt with by Articles 425 and following of the Penal Code.

© Springer-Verlag France 1994
Originally published by Springer-Verlag France Paris in 1994.
Softcover reprint of the hardcover 1st edition 1994

ISBN 978-2-8178-0767-6   ISBN 978-2-8178-0765-2 (eBook)
DOI 10.1007/978-2-8178-0765-2

Contents

Foreword XXI

Educational lectures

The pathogenesis of human cancer metastasis, I.J. Fidler 3
The role of molecular genetics in medical oncology, E.J. Freireich .. 7
Cell line-based screening for new anticancer drugs, B.A. Chabner, J.N. Weinstein, K.D. Paull, M.R. Grever 10
Anti-EGF receptor monoclonal antibodies as potential anti-cancer therapy, J. Mendelsohn 17
Clinical relevance of drug resistance : Where do we stand now and where are we going to ?, S.C. Linn, G. Giaccone, H.M. Pinedo 19
Mobilization, purification and ex vivo expansion of human peripheral blood progenitor cells, W. Brugger, R. Mertelsmann, L. Kanz 24
Fluoropyrimidine cancer chronotherapy, W.J.M. Hrushesky, F.O. Cope 29
Chemo-immunotherapy of metastatic malignant melanoma. The Salpetriere Hospital (SOMPS) experience, D. Khayat, E. Antoine, O. Rixe, J.M. Tourani, E. Vuillemin, Ch. Borel, A. Benhammouda, L. Thill, C. Franks, G. Auclerc, M. Weil, Cl. Soubrane, P. Banzet 40
Concomitant chemoradiotherapy for solid tumors, E.E. Vokes, R. Stupp 47
Current status of therapy for small cell carcinoma of the lung, D.C. Ihde 50
Systemic treatment of bladder cancer, L.Y. Dirix, A.T. van Oosterom 55
Metastatic breast cancer : current management options and future directions, G. Hortobagyi 62
Present and future prospects for the chemotherapy of gliomas, V. Levin 66
Neo-Adjuvant chemotherapy in breast cancer. Study of 477 evaluable patients with primary breast cancers treated between 1980 and 1992, M. Weil, G. Auclerc, Ch. Borel, F. Baillet, A. Thomas, Cl. Soubrane, M. Housset, D. Nizri, O. Rixe, E. Antoine, E. Vuillemin, D. Khayat 70
Osteogenic sarcoma : a 15-year experience in treating 287 patients with preoperative chemotherapy, G. Rosen, S. Lowenbraun, C. Forscher .. 79
Cell cycle regulation and the chemosensitivity of cancer cells, K.W. Kohn, P.M. O'Connor 85
Reversal of multidrug resistance of hematologic malignancies with chemosensitizers : laboratory and clinical studies, S.E. Salmon, T.P. Miller, A.F. List, T.M. Grogan, W.S. Dalton 90
Practical approach to bladder cancer, L. Denis 98

Breast cancer

Primary chemotherapy for breast cancer : response to preoperative chemotherapy as prognostic factor, G.N. Hortobagyi, A.U. Buzdar, D. Frye, S.E. Singletary, F.A. Holmes, F. Ames, M.D. McNeese, R.L. Theriault 105

Breast cancer, cytoprognostic grades and proliferative activity (DNA ploidy, S phase) MA de Maublanc 110

Primary chemotherapy in the individualized non-mutilating treatment of breast cancer, R. Poisson, S. Legault, R. Guévin 114

Neo-Adjuvant chemotherapy in 100 patients with locally advanced carcinoma of the breast, B. Coudert, P. Gabez, C. Lamaille, C. De Gislain, F. Mayer, P. Fargeot 120

Surgical aspects of the conservative treatment of large size breast cancer after primary chemotherapy, S. Zurrida, M. Greco, V. Galimberti, U. Veronesi 123

Efficacy of a chemotherapy regimen combining Vinorelbine, Epirubicine and Methotrexate (VEM) in locally advanced and metastatic breast cancer, J. Van Praagh, N. Martineau, V. Feillel, H. Curé, E. Bélembaogo, M.A. Ravoux, J. Fleury, C. Deloche, R. Plagne, P. Chollet 127

Recurrent breast carcinoma after conservative treatment : MRI features and pathologic correlation, T.-H. Dao, F. Campana, A. Fourquet, M. Laurent, B. Asselain, A. Rahmouni 131

Intensive chemotherapy for inflammatory breast cancer : how much clinical value ?, B. Chevallier, C. Couteau, D. Atlan, V. Chatikhine, Y. Graic, J.-P. Julien, A. Kunlin, P. Bastit, C. Veyret, J. D'Anjou . 135

A Phase II study of 2-weekly high-dose Epirubicin with r-met-hu G-CSF in advanced breast cancer, G. Fountzilas, D. Skarlos, T. Giannakakis, A. Athanasiades, D. Bafaloukos, J. Protopsaltis, M. Beer, N. Pavlidis, P. Kosmidis 146

Cyclophosphamide, Novantrone, Fluorouracil (CNF) + G-CSF Neo-Adjuvant chemotherapy in operable breast cancer, V. Lorusso, M. De Lena, M. Brandi, S. Longo, F. Berardi, A. Catino, M.G. Sapia, G. Simone, F. Marzullo, A. Racanelli, F. Schittulli 150

Adjuvant chemohormonal therapy with Cyclophosphamide, Doxorubicin and 5-Fluorouracil (CAF) with or without medroxyprogesterone acetate (MPA) in node-positive breast cancer patients, P. Hupperets, J. Wils, L. Volovics, L. Schouten, M. Fickers, H. Bron, H. Schouten, J. Jager, J. Smeets, J. de Jong, G. Blijham 155

Follow-up results of an ECOG study of adjuvant therapy in postmenopausal women with breast cancer, H.C. Falkson, R. Gray, W.H. Wolberg, G. Falkson 160

Long-term efficacy and late sequelae of Doxorubicin-containing adjuvant therapy for breast cancer : MD Anderson Cancer Center studies, A. Buz-

Contents

dar, G. Hortobagyi, S. Kau, F. Holmes, G. Fraschini, R. Theriault, M. McNeese, S. Singletary 163

Taxol in metastatic breast cancer : the MD Anderson Cancer Center experience, F.A. Holmes, V. Valero, R. Walters, R. Theriault, D. Booser, A. Buzdar, H. Gibbs, D. Frye, K. Young, G. Hortobagyi 167

Taxol plus recombinant human granulocyte colony stimulating factor as salvage chemotherapy for metastatic breast cancer, A.D. Seidman, B.S. Reichman, J.P.A Crown, T.-J. Yao, V. Currie, T.B. Hakes, C.A. Hudis, T.A. Gilewski, P. Forsythe, J. Lepore, L. Marks, M. Souhrada, N. Onetto, S. Arbuck, L. Norton 172

Head and neck cancer

A model for chemosentivity testing using in vitro MTT assay on a human squamous carcinoma tongue cell line, W.K. Walter King, P.K. Lam, K.C. Arthur Li 179

Head and neck cancer treatment : present status and future direction, M. Al-Sarraf 185

Chemotherapy (CT) followed by radiotherapy (RT) vs. RT alone in patients with resected and negative margins squamous cell carninoma of the head and neck : Phase III Intergroup Study, M. Al-Sarraf, C.B. Scott, K. Ahmad, J.G. Schwade, D. Schuller, G.E. Laramore, J. Jacobs 191

Neo-Adjuvant infusion Cisplatin, 5-FU and high-dose leucovorin for squamous cell carcinoma of the head and neck (SCCHN) : high rates of complete response (CR) and definitive radiotherapy as primary site management, J. Clark, A. Dreyfuss, P. Busse, C. Norris Jr, J. Lucarini, R. Rossi, J. Andersen, D. Casey, E. Frei III 196

Primary (Neo-Adjuvant) combined modality therapy in the management of locally advanced squamous cell carcinoma of the head and neck, G. Mantovani, E. Proto, L. Contini, S. Littera, L. Curreli, F. Cossu, P. Puxeddu, G.S. Del Giacco 201

A Phase II trial of induction Cisplatin, 5-FU, Leucovorin and Interferon-α-2B (PFL-α) followed by concurrent Hydroxyurea, 5-FU and radiation for Stage IV squamous cell cancers of the head and neck (HNC), M.S. Kies, D.J. Haraf, B. Mittal, I. Athanasiadis, M. Kozloff, J. McEvilly, R. Mick, W. Moran, W. Panje, H. Pelzer, T.D. Sheehan, R. Weichselbaum, B. Wenig, E.E. Vokes 207

Induction chemotherapy with Cisplatin (P), 5-Fluorouracil (FU) and Folinic Acid (FA) in locally advanced head and neck cancer, E. Fonseca, J.-J. Cruz, J. Garcia, A. Panadero, P. Sanchez, A. Gomez, G. Martin, M.-J. Garcia, J.-C. Vallejo 211

A randomized study of CDDP and 5-FU as Neo-Adjuvant chemotherapy in head and neck cancer : an interim analysis, M. Martin, L. Vergnes, Lelièvre, P. Michel-Langlet, C. Peytral, J.-J. Mazeron, E. Malaurie, R. Peynegre 214

Concomitant chemoradiotherapy in locally advanced head and neck cancers : a prospective study of 68 patients, S. Walter, C. Hennequin, M.D. Brette, P. Leblanc, P.Y. Cheriff-Cheikh, M. Espie, J.-P. Monteil, M. Marty, C. Maylin 219

Epidermal growth factor receptor in upper aerodigestive tract cancer, J.-L. Formento, M. Francoual, O. Dassonville, J. Santini, A. Ramaioli, G. Milano, M. Schneider, F. Demard 225

Concomitant α-Interferon and chemotherapy in advanced squamous cell carcinoma of the head and neck, M. Benasso, M. Merlano, F. Blengio, M. Cavallari, R. Rosso, S. Toma 234

Thymidylate synthase activity and Folate levels in head and neck squamous cell carcinomas, O. Parise Jr, F. Janot, B. Luboinski, M.-A. Verjus, A. Gouyette, G.-G. Cabot 237

Long term nephrotoxicity of Cisplatinum (CDDP) in man, Y. Bahmed, M. Déchaux, V. Bassot, D. Brasnu, C. Kindermans, H. Laccourreye, C. Sachs 243

Prognostic factors in head and neck cancer patients included in a program of Neo-Adjuvant chemotherapy and radical radiotherapy, J. Castillo, F. Gomez, R. Guerrero, P. Sanchez, I. Martin Lopez, J. Cueto, J.-L. Garcia Puche 248

Induction chemotherapy for larynx preservation in laryngeal and hypopharyngeal cancers, F. Demard, M. Schneider, O. Dassonville, P. Chauvel, A. Thyss, J. Santini 251

A pilot study of vinorelbine on a weekly schedule in recurrent and/or metastatic squamous cell carcinoma of the head and neck, V. Gebbia, A. Testa, R. Valenza, G. Zerillo, S. Restivo, F. Ingria, G. Cannata, N. Borsellino, N. Gebbia 257

Concomitant radiotherapy and Cisplatin in head and neck cancer : a pilot study, P. Olmi, C. Fallai, C. Chiostrini 260

Ifosfamide/Mesna plus Carboplatin as Neo-Adjuvant therapy for stage I-III head and neck cancer. Preliminary report, M. Bruno 263

Role of Ifosfamide, Cisplatinum (IC) combination in the metastatic neck nodes, V.-R. Pai, D.-M. Parikh, A.T. Mazumdar, R.S. Rao 267

Clinical pharmacokinetics of Pure 1 Folinic Acid and Fluorouracil during a phase I-II trial of Fluorouracil biomodulation in head and neck cancer patients. Preliminary data, M.C. Étienne, G. Milano, M. Schneider, A. Thyss, O. Dassonville, M. Bardon, T. Guillot, F. Demard 274

Long-term follow-up of the patients with recurrent or advanced head and neck cancer who received chemotherapy for palliation, Y. Inuyama .. 280

Intensified concomitant chemoradiotherapy for poor prognosis head and neck cancer, E.E. Vokes, D.J. Haraf, W. Moran, B. Wenig, D. Brachman, S. Rubin, J.-M. McEvilly, P. Luckett, W.-R. Panje, R.-R. Weichselbaum 283

Contents

Response to chemotherapy of ulcerative lymphoma of the midface, J. Cabane, Cl. Grange, G. Lamas, B. Meyer, P. Godeau, J.-C. Imbert... 288

A multicentric study of the GETTEC (Groupe d'Études des Tumeurs de la Tête et du Cou) about 408 clinically complete responders after Neo-Adjuvant chemotherapy for head and neck carcinomas, P. Chauvel, J.-L. Lefèbvre, B. Luboinski, G. Kantor, M. Bolla, G. Andry, J. Brugère, J.-J. Pessey, F. Demard.................... 291

Chemotherapy of undifferentiated thyroid cancer (UCT) and sarcoma of the thyroid gland (ST), F. Kober, A. Heiss, B. Neugebauer, R. Roka 295

Retinoid chemoprevention of aerodigestive carcinogenesis, W.-K. Hong, S.-M. Lippman, S.-E. Benner, J.-S. Lee................... 298

Definite radiation and concomitant Cisplatin administration in locally advanced head and neck cancer, G. Fountzilas, D. Skarlos, P. Kosmidis, E. Samantas, J. Tzitzikas, P. Makrantonakis, P. Pantelakos, A. Nicolaou, H. Bacoyiannis, M. Sinodinou, P. Papaspyrou, C. Banis, A. Vritsios, J. Daniilidis.................... 303

Improved survival of patients with advanced squamous cell carcinoma of the head and neck with alternating chemotherapy and radiotherapy, M. Benasso, R. Corvó, M. Cavallari, G. Sanguineti, G. Margarino, R. Rosso, V. Vitale, M. Merlano and members of affiliated institutions 307

Treatment of patients with cancer of the head and neck or esophagus with carboplatin, 5-FU, Interferon-α and interleukin-2, O. Schlappack, A. Hainz, P. Berghammer, M. Grasl, M. Kautzky, G. Kment, W. Dobrowsky, C. Dittrich.................... 311

Surgical considerations in the treatment of well-differentiated thyroid cancer, I. Roisman, V. Barak, D. Sapir, A. Bitterman, N. Livni, J. Honigman, Z. Gimmon, J. Manny, A.L. Durst................ 315

Lung cancer

Intensive chemotherapy with recombinant-human granulocyte-macrophage colony stimulating factor (r-hu-gm-csf) for small cell lung cancer (sclc) : a pilot study, C. Besana, E. Bucci, A. Borri, G. Di Lucca, S. Tognella, M. Tresoldi, M. Marcatti, C. Corti, G. Citterio, F. Inversi, C. Rugarli 319

Sequential high-dose chemotherapy with r-metHu-G-CSF (Filgrastim) and infusion of peripheral blood progenitor cells (PBPC) in patients with small cell lung cancer (SCLC). A feasibility study, S. Leyvraz, N. Ketterer, J.Ph. Grob, Ph. Schneider, P. Vuichard, V. von Fliedner, F. Lejeune. 322

Cisplatinum and 5-Fluorouracil in small cell lung cancer, J.F. Morere, A. Duran, F. Tcherakian, C. Boaziz, J.P. Battesti, L. Israël, J.L. Breau 328

Phase I-II study of oral Etoposide and modulation of drug resistance with ketoconazole in small cell lung cancer, D. Dalley, B. Brigham .. 331

Angiogenesis : a novel target for Adjuvant chemotherapy in locally advanced non-small cell lung cancer, P. Macchiarini, G. Fontanini, E. Dulmet, V. de Montpreville, A. Chapelier, B. Lenot, J. Cerrina, F. Le Roy Ladurie, P. Dartevelle 336

A statistical model for investigating Adjuvant chemotherapy in T1N0M0 non-small cell lung cancer, J.M. Hardin, P. Macchiarini, K.P. Singh 343

A combination chemotherapy with Ifosfamide (I), Cisplatin (P) and Etoposide (E) for advanced non-small cell lung cancer (NSCLC), G. Martin, M.J. Garcia, J.J. Cruz, A. Gómez, A. Panadero, E. Fonseca, P. Sánchez, P. Soria, J. Garcia, J.C. Vallejo 348

Mitomycin, Ifosfamide and Platin (MIP) in advanced and disseminated non-small cell lung cancer (NSCLC), P.J. Souquet, C. Bohas, T. Zenone, E. Michaud, M.T. el Khoury, P. Romestaing, J.P. Bernard 351

Phase III randomized study of Neo-Adjuvant chemotherapy surgery in non-small cell lung cancer (NSCLC) preliminary results, A. Depierre, B. Milleron, Cl. Chastang, B. Lebeau, P. Terrioux, E. Quoix, D. Moro, G. Miech, N. Paillot, J.L. Breton, H. Danicot, J.N. Lombard, J. Clavier, E. Lemarie, P. Jacoulet 354

Vinorelbine, 5-Fluorouracil, Folinic acid and Cisplatin in non-small cell lung cancer : Vindesine for Vinorelbine ? H. de Cremoux, I. Monnet, N. Azli, S. Voisin, P. Ruffié, L. Vergnes, J. Huet, J.C. Saltiel, J.P. Armand, E. Cvitkovic, ATTIT 357

Preoperative chemotherapy in non-small cell lung cancer (NSCLC) - A pilot study, J.R. Fischer, C. Manegold, D. Branscheid, I. Vogt-Moykopf, P. Drings 362

Neo-Adjuvant Cisplatin and Etoposide for stage IIIA (clinical N2) non-small cell lung cancer, S. Darwish, V. Minotti, R. Rossetti, G. Ciccarese, L. Crinò, P. Fiaschini, U. Mercati, E. Maranzano, P. Latini, M. Tonato 366

Concomitant chemoradiotherapy with Cisplatin dose escalation as palliative therapy for advanced malignancies of the chest, C. Lee Drinkard, J. Daniel Haraf, C. Philip Hoffman, M. Harvey Golomb, K. Mark Ferguson, J. Nicholas Vogelzang, E. Everett Vokes 370

Concomitant chemoradiotherapy for inoperable non-small cell carcinoma of the lung : results of continuous infusion Cisplatin in 85 patients, F. Reboul, P. Vincent, B. Chauvet, Y. Brewer, C. Felix Faure, M. Taulelle 375

Late results of Neo-Adjuvant chemoradiotherapy for primary inoperable non-small cell lung cancer, J.L. Rebischung, J.M. Vannetzel, P. Dartevelle 377

Gastro-intestinal tumors

Conservative treatment of esophagus cancer concomitant chemoradiotherapy treatment. First results of a 143 patients serial, J.H. Jacob, A. Roussel, J.M. Ollivier, J.Ph. Izard, J.C. Vernhes 383

Induction chemotherapy, surgery and concomitant chemoradiotherapy for

carcinoma of the esophagus, P.C. Hoffman, M.K. Ferguson, D.J. Haraf, L.C. Drinkard, H.M. Golomb, E.E. Vokes 386

Superiority of combined chemoradiotherapy to radiotherapy alone in patients with esophageal cancers. An intergroup study, M. Al-Sarraf, K. Martz, A. Herskovic, L. Leichman, J.S. Brindle, V.K. Vaitkevicius, J. Cooper, R. Byhardt, L. Davis, B. Emami 389

Neo-Adjuvant chemoradiotherapy for advanced gastric cancer : a pilot study with angiotensin II induced drug delivery system, K. Sugiyama, H. Sato, M. Hoshi, M. Urushiyama, K. Ishizuka, R. Kanamaru 393

Combination of 5-FU, Leucovorin and Cisplatin (CDDP) : an efficient low-toxic chemotherapy in advanced gastric adenocarcinoma, M. Ychou, Y. Fedkovic, A. Christopoulou, B. Saint-Aubert, Ph. Rouanet, C. Astre, H. Pujol 396

Adjuvant chemotherapy and radiotherapy in liver transplantation for primary hepatocellular carcicoma : a feasibility study, J.-Y. Pierga, P. Pied-bois, D. Cherqui, C. Duvoux, A. Ramouni, J.-M. Métreau, D. Mathieu, M. Julien, D. Dhumeaux, P.-L. Fagniez, J.-P. Le Bourgeois 399

Intensive weekly chemotherapy for advanced gastric cancer using 5-Fluorouracil, Cisplatin, Epirubicin, 6S-Leucovorin and Granulocyte-colony stimulating factor, S. Cascinu, A. Fedeli, S. Luzi Fedeli, G. Catalano 405

Neo-Adjuvant chemotherapy for inoperable gastric cancer via local and general delivery routes (FLEP Therapy), T. Nakajima, S. Ishihara, H. Motohashi, Y. Kitamura, Y. Nakajima, M. Fujii, A. Tokunaga, K. Matai, H. Anzai, M. Nishi 411

Gastric cancer — a place for preoperative induction regional chemotherapy, B.Y. D.W. Storey, P.J. Gallagher, R.C. Waugh, F.O. Stephens 414

α-2b-Interferon (IFN) plus chemotherapy in inoperable biliary-tract carcinoma, preliminary data, G. Frasci, M. Monaco, L. Cremone, U. Sapio, F. Faiella, G. Persico 419

A phase II study of weekly 48 hours infusion with high-dose Fluorouracil (FU) in colorectal cancer, E. Aranda, E. Diáz-Rubio, C. Camps, C. Fernández-Marto, A. Carrato, A. Antón, A Cervantes, J.J. Cruz-Hernández, A. Tres, J. Belón, J. Sánchez, M. Garciá-Paredes 422

Phase II trial of Fluorouracil, Leucovorin and Interferon-α, R.M. Bukowski, V. Gibson, S. Murthy, D. McLain, T. Olencki, G.T. Budd 428

Continuous simultaneous intra-arterial and intravenous therapy of liver metastases of colorectal carcinoma. Results of a prospective randomized study, F. Safi, K.H. Link, H.G. Beger 433

D-Verapamil and Adriamycin in the treatment of advanced colorectal cancer, W. Scheithauer, G. Kornek, S. Globitz, M. Raderer, T. Schenk, C.H. Müller, C.H. Tetzner 441

Perioperative multimodal treatment of locally advanced rectal cancer.

Results of a pilot study, P. Schöffski, H.R. Raab, I. Wildfang, C.H. Köhne-Wömpner, J.H. Karstens, R. Pichlmayr, H.J. Schmoll .. 444

Gynecologic cancer

Neo-Adjuvant chemotherapy for advanced ovarian cancer, Y. Shimizu, S. Umezawa, N. Takeshima, T. Kato, K. Hasumi.................. 453

Hyperfractionation using weekly Cisplatin, Cyclophosphamide and Adriamycin (CAP) in advanced epithelial tumors of the ovary, K. Tonkin, L. Levin... 460

Adjuvant treatment of ovarian carcinoma, I.B. Vergote, C.G. Tropé, L.N. De Vos, J. Kærn, W.M. Abeler, M. Winderen, E.O. Pettersen 464

Cyclophosphamide (CTX) and high-dose 4-Epidoxorubicin (EPI) in advanced ovarian cancer (OC) treatment, G. Cartei, M. Signor, E. Vigevani, M. Giovannoni, A. Sibau, G. Clocchiatti, M. Mansutti............ 469

High-dose chemotherapy (HDC) and autologous bone marrow transplant (ABMT) in 39 advanced ovarian cancers : long-term results, A. Legros, H. Curé, J. Fleury, F. Suzanne, J. Dauplat, Ph. Chollet, R. Plagne 473

Concomitant chemotherapy and radiotherapy in the treatment of advanced cervix carcinomas, M. Resbeut, M. Noirclerc, G. Gravis, Cl. d'Ercole, P. Pechikoff, G. Houvenaeghel, J.R. Delpero, J.L. Blache, P. Viens 476

Adjuvant chemotherapies for small cell carcinoma of the uterine cervix, T.C. Chang, H.C. Chang, C.H. Lai, S. Hsueh, S.F. Huang, H.K. Chang, Y.K. Soong... 479

Neo-Adjuvant M-VAC (Methotrexate, Vinblastine, Doxorubicin, Cisplatin) chemotherapy for locally advanced or metastatic cervical and vaginal cancer, G.R. Garton, T.O. Wilson, L.C. Hartmann, H.J. Long, K.C. Podratz.. 482

A phase II trial of Neo-Adjuvant chemotherapy (CT) with Ifosfamide (I), Mesna and Cisplatinum (C) in stage IIA-IIIB cervical cancer, A. Erazo, L. Torrecillas, G. Cervantes, B. Ortega....................... 485

Bleomycin, Ifosfamide and Carboplatin in advanced uterine cervix carcinoma : preliminary results, C. Louvet, S. Moreau, A. de Gramont, C. Varette, B. Demuynck, K. Beerblock, L. Marpeau, D. Zylberait, A. Pigné, D. Soubrane, M. Krulik................................. 488

Urological and germinal tumors

Surveillance in stage I non-seminomatous germ cell tumors of the testis (NSGCTT). Experience at the Instituto Nacional de Cancerología of México, J.W. Zinser, R. Gaona, A. Mendoza, O. Ocampo, H. Domínguez, L. Vicencio... 495

Combination chemotherapy with Etoposide, Cisplatin, Bleomycin and Cyclophosphamide for advanced metastatic non-seminomatous germ cell tumors, A. Gerl, C. Clemm, M. Hentrich, R. Hartenstein, P. Kohl, W. Wilmanns 499

Extented resection after primary chemotherapy for residual malignant non-seminomatous germ cell tumors of the mediastinum : is it worthwhile ? P. Macchiarini, E. Dulmet, V. de Montpreville, A. Chapelier, B. Lenot, J. Cerrina, P. Dartevelle 503

The prediction of treatment outcomes in non-seminomatous extragonadal germ cell tumors (NSEGCT) by using different criteria of « poor » and « good » risk, F. Gutierrez Delgado, A. Garin, S. Tjulandin, M. Ramirez Mendoza, A. Khlebnov 510

Advanced seminoma treated with chemotherapy (CT), J.W. Zinser, R. Gaona, A. Mendoza, O. Ocampo, H. Domínguez-Malagón, E. Gómez, L. Vicencio 513

Concomitant 5-FU-CDDP and bifractioned split course radiation therapy for invasive bladder cancer, C. Maulard, M. Housset, Y. Chrétien, S. Delanian, F. Colardelle, J.P. Hallez, B. Dufour, F. Baillet 516

Neo-Adjuvant treatment for locally advanced bladder cancer : a randomized prospective clinical trial, A. Pellegrini, E. Cortesi, N. Gioacchini, E. Ballatori, R.A. Virdis 520

Ultrastructural and clinical study of the urothelium after Interferon-α-2b treatment, P. Stravoravdi, J. Belivanis, Th. Dimopoulos, J. Hatzigiannis, M. Polyzonis 523

Chemoradiotherapy in locally advanced bladder cancer : Neo-Adjuvant and definitive treatment, L. Canobbio, F. Boccardo, A. Curotto, M. Pace, D. Guarneri, A. Rubagotti, M. Venturini, M. Orsatti, V. Vitale, M. Schenone, M. Cussoto, C. Pegoraro, G.B. Traverso, G. Salvia, G. Martorana, L. Giuliani 527

Interferon-α (IFN-α) combined with 5-Fluorouracil (5-FU) is an active regimen in metastatic renal cell cancer, A. Sella, L. Finn, R. Amato, C. Logothetis 535

Comparative efficacy of hormonal therapy used alone or in combination for treatment of prostatic carcinoma, W. Mulloy 540

Etoposide in treatment of hormone refractory advanced carcinoma of the prostate, M.D. Firouz Daneshgari, E. David Crawford, B.A. Suzan, A. Majeski 542

Sequential therapy with recombinant Interleukin-2 (rIL-2) and α-Interferon (IFN) for advanced renal cell cancer (rcc) : a preliminary report, C. Besana, E. Bucci, A. Borri, A. Schoenheit, G. Citterio, P. Matteucci, S. Tognella, C. Baiocchi, G. Landonio, E. Ghislandi, C. Rugarli 548

No advantage for the use of an early high-dose chemotherapy with autologous bone marrow transplantation in first-line treatment of poor risk non-seminomatous germ cell tumors, H. Curé, J.P. Droz, J.L. Pico, P. Biron, P. Kerbrat, C. Chevreau, J.F. Héron, B. Chevallier, P. Fargeot, J. Bouzy, A. Kramar, and the Urologic Group of the French Cancer Centers Federation 551

Bone and soft tissue sarcomas

Initial experience with autologous transplantation of 7 days noncryopreserved peripheral blood stem cells, mobilized with G-CSF, in rhabdomyosarcoma, P. Sobrevilla-Calvo, E. Reynoso-Gomez, J. de la Garza-Salazar... 557

High-dose chemotherapy with granulocyte colony-stimulating factor in advanced and/or metastatic soft tissue sarcomas, S. Toma, R. Palumbo, U. Folco, G. Canavese, E. Aitini, E. Cantoni, M. Vincenti, R. Rosso 561

Treatment of osteosarcoma with Cisplatin and Doxorubicin either as Adjuvant or Neo-Adjuvant chemotherapy, J.W. Zinser, N. Castañeda, A. Alfeirán, E. Maafs, M. Durán, G. Flores, R. Gaona, L. Vicencio 565

The role of preoperative and Adjuvant chemotherapy in the treatment on non rhabdomyosarcoma soft tissue sarcoma in children and adolescents, U. Gross-Wieltsch, M. Morgan, E. Koscielniak, J. Treuner ... 568

Escalating doses of Epirubicin in combination with Ifosfamide and GM-CSF in previously untreated soft tissue sarcoma patients ; a phase I-II study, S. Frustaci, A. Buonadonna, D. Favaro, M. Santarosa, F. Latini, S. Lamon, E. Galligioni, S. Monfardini....................... 573

Primary chemotherapy in malignant fibrous histiocytoma of bone - Updated UTMD Anderson Cancer Center Experience, S.R. Patel, T. Armen, C.H. Carrasco, A.K. Raymond, A.G. Ayala, J.A. Murray, S.P. Chawla, R.S. Benjamin... 577

Concomitant radiation-Doxorubicin administration in locally advanced and/or metastatic soft tissue sarcomas, S. Toma, R. Palumbo, A. Grimaldi, S. Barra, G. Canavese, B. Castagneto, C. Frola, E. Aitini, R. Rosso 581

Malignant melanomas and cerebral tumors

Chemotherapy as a first treatment for malignant primary CNS non-Hodgkin's lymphoma of the central nervous system (PCNSL), A. Boiardi, A. Silvani, A. Salmaggi, S. Valentini, A. Allegranza, G. Broggi 587

Effect of six retinoids and retinoic acid catabolic inhibitor liarozole on two glioblastoma cell lines, and in vivo experience in malignant brain tumor patients, M.E. Westarp, M.P. Westarp, W. Bollag, J. Bruynseels, H. Biesalski, N. Grossmann, H.H. Kornhuber 590

Phase II trial with BCNU plus α-2B-Interferon in patients with recurrent high-grade gliomas, A. Brandes, P. Zampieri, A. Rigon, E. Scelzi, P.L. Zorat, A. Rotilio, P. Amistà, A. Paccagnella, M.V. Fiorentino 599

Carboplatin combined with Carmustine and Etoposide in the treatment

of glioblastoma (GBM) patients, A. Boiardi, A. Silvani, S. Valentini, A. Salmaggi, M. Botturi, M. Farinotti, C. Giorgi 604

Phase II trial of Cystemustine, a new nitrosourea, as second-line treatment of malignant gliomas, A. Tisserant, R. Plagne, H. Roché, A. Adenis, P. Fargeot, N. Guiochet, P. Cattan, Y. Krakowsky, M.A. Lentz, P. Fumoleau, B. Chevallier, P. Chollet 607

Age effect on the survival of patients with glioblastoma and anaplastic astrocytoma, J. Hildebrand, The EORTC Brain Tumour Group 612

Concurrent radiochemotherapy in high-grade glioma, A. Brandes, P. Zampieri, A. Rigon, E. Scelzi, M. Pignatarox, F. Berti, A. Rotilio, A. Padoan, P. Amistà, A. Paccagnella, M.V. Fiorentino 616

Interferon-α-2b + fotemustine in disseminated malignant melanoma, L. Kowalzick, P. Mohr, M. Weichenthal, H. Langenbahn, D.K. Hossfeld, E.W. Breitbart 620

Tamoxifen-augmented biochemotherapy (Interferon-α-2b, Tamoxifen, BCNU, CDDP, DTIC) for malignant melanoma, H. Voigt, R. Claßen, J. Ramaker 623

Locoregional treatment

Chemofiltration for locally advanced cancer, M. Inbar, M. Gutman, S. Chaitchik, J.M. Klausner 631

Treatment optimization guidelines for hyperthermic antiblastic limb perfusion, M. Pace, L. Millanta, A. Galli, A. Bellacci 635

5-FU + Folinic Acid (FA, Rescuvolin®) i.a., 5-FU + FA i.v., 5-FUDR i.a., or 5-FUDR i.a. + i.v. for treatment of non-resectable colorectal liver mestastases ? K.H. Link, E.D. Kreuser, F. Safi, A. Schalhorn, E. Schmoll, J. Pillasch, H.G. Beger 639

Hepatic arterial chemotherapy (HAI) for unresectable liver metastases from gastrointestinal cancer, F. Musca, R. Esposito, G. Toma 649

The treatment of presacral recurrences of rectal cancer by the use of locoregional pelvic chemotherapy. A discussion of these methods as a Neo-Adjuvant time in locally advanced rectal tumors, P. Manivit, R. Polo, D. Tabary, M. Nabet, M. Polo, B. Rubini, P.N. Chipponi, J.M. Fromaget, M. Untereiner 652

Repeated chemo-occlusion with Degradable Starch Microspheres (DSM) — Enhanced drug uptake and regional efficacy in the treatment of primary and secondary liver tumors, B. Nilsson, C.J. Johansson, B. Bunke, T. Taguchi 658

Antitumor efficacy of intraperitoneal hyperthermochemotherapy combined with aggressive surgery for patients with advanced gastric cancer, S. Fujimoto, M. Takahashi, K. Kobayashi, T. Mutou, M. Kure, H. Masaoka, H. Ohkubo 665

Intraperitoneal hyperthermic chemoperfusion in patients with peritoneal carcinomatosis and malignant ascites, F. Kober, B. Neugebauer, A. Heiss, R. Roka 669

Intra-aortic infusion chemotherapy in advanced penile carcinoma, M.C. Sheen, H.M. Sheu, C.Y. CHai, C.H. Huang, Y.W. Wang 672

Psychosocial issues in cancer

The influence of both surgery and Adjuvant chemotherapy on breast cancer women quality of life, O. Caffo, G. Ambrosini, S. Agugiaro, C. Eccher, S. Maluta 677

Psychological side effects induced by Interleukin-2/α-Interferon : clinical observations, biological correlations, M.J. Smith, R. Mouawad, E. Vuillemin, A. Benhammouda, C. Soubrane, D. Khayat 681

Quality of life in advanced colorectal cancer, G. Francini, R. Petrioli, A. Aquino, S. Marsili, S. Bruni, L. Lorenzini, S. Mancini, M. Lorenzi, G. Marzocca, F. Tani, S. Armenio, G. Tanzini, F. Cetta, F. Silvetrini, C. Stacci, M. Nardini, I. d'Errico 691

Advance directives in the intensive care unit of a tertiary cancer center, M.S. Ewer, J. Taubert, M.K. Ali, ... 695

Do cancer related pain problems exist in France ? L. Brasseur, F. Larue, M. Dubiez, S. Colleau, C. Cleeland 699

Intravenous granisetron-simple, safe and effective single-dose. Administration for control of chemotherapy induced nausea and vomiting, S.G. Dilly 702

Control of refractory nausea and vomiting with adjuvant propofol during cancer chemotherapy, A. Borgeat, O.H.G. Wilder-Smith, K. Rifat, M. Forni 705

Liposomal Daunorubicin treatment increases quality of life in HIV-associated Kaposi's Sarcoma, C.A. Presant, M. Scolaro, P. Kennedy, D.W. Blayney, B. Flanagan, J. Lisak, J. Presant 707

Biology and clinical pharmacology

Comparison of 12 multidrug-resistance modulating agents in a model of doxorubicin-resistant rat glioblastoma cells in vitro, J. Robert, S. Huet, S. Bennis, C. Chapey 713

Differential formation, repair and tolerance of Cisplatin-induced DNA damage in two human small cell lung carcinoma cell lines, B.T. Hill, S.A. Shellard 720

Identification of a distinctive multiple drug resistance phenotype in tumour cells following in vitro exposure to X-irradiation, B.T. Hill, R.H.D. Whelan, S. McClean 723

Functional activity of P-glycoprotein localized in subcellular structures

Contents

and reversal of multidrug resistance (MDR), G. Toffoli, L. Tumiotto, M.G. Dall'Arche, C. Cernigoi, M. Boiocchi 726

New strategy for the production of monoclonal antibodies to external portion of the P-glycoprotein, M. Pagé, X. Yang, P. Roby, R. Paradis, N. Berkova 730

Myeloperoxidase is involved in Vincristine resistance in human myeloblastic leukemia, D. Schlaifer, M.R. Cooper, M. Attal, A.O. Sartor, J.B. Trepel, C. Muller, G. Laurent, C.E. Myers 736

A new multidrug resistance modulating agent S 9788 : preliminary report of the phase clinical trial in combination with Vincristine, D. Khayat, A. Benhammouda, M. Weil, E. Vuillemin, G. Bastian, E. Antoine, O. Rixe, G. Auclerc, C. Lucas, M. Sarkany, J.-P. Bizzari 740

Effect of Pentoxifylline, ethacrynic acid and O^6-benzyl-guanine as resistance modifiers to alkylating agents in haematological malignancies, M.R. Müller, L. Schlenger, Chr. Boogen, M.R. Nowrousian, S. Seeber 745

Structural alterations of human topoisomerase IIα responsible for drug-resistance, DNA-binding and nuclear localization, F. Boege, F. Gieseler, P. Meyer 749

Measurement of human tumor pharmacokinetics in vivo noninvasively by 19-F magnetic resonance spectroscopy predicts clinical 5-FU sensitivity and resistance, C.A. Presant, W. Wolf, V. Waluch, R. Brechner, C. Wiseman, D.W. Blayney, P. Kennedy 757

Immunoregulation by tumor necrosis factor α (TNF) : an opportunity for therapeutic intervention ? E. Mihich, D. Maccubbin, S. Pocchiari, S. Ujházy, S. Verstovšek, M.J. Ehrke 759

Tumor necrosis factor alpha : its relationship with clinical data, J.J. Bosco Lopez, M. Escobar, P. Gallurt, P. Rodriguez, A. Lorenzo, A. Morán, A. Senra, J. Millán 765

The antiproliferative effect of lymphoblastoid α interferon and its ability to re-induce or amplify major histocompatibility complex antigen expression on human renal carcinoma cells in culture, R.L. Angus, C.M.P. Collins, M.O. Symes 770

Is there any predictive factor of the clinical response to IL-2 therapy in metastatic malignant melanoma ? Cl. Soubrane, R. Mouawad, M. Ichen, J. Suissa, E. Vuillemin, Ch. Borel, A. Benhammouda, M. Weil, D. Khayat 774

How IL-2 can affect melanoma cells, S. Plaisance, A. Alileche, E. Rubinstein, D. Han, B. Azzarone, C. Jasmin 779

Potentiation of 5-Fluorouracil-[6RS]leucovorin cytotoxicity by recombinant human Interferon-α2A in colon carcinoma cells, J.A. Houghton, D.A. Adkins, P.J. Houghton 785

Evidence for a role of immunosuppression in the pathogenesis of small cell lung cancer, J.R. Fischer, M. Schindel, N. Stein, H. Lahm, H. Gallati, P. Drings, P.H. Krammer 789

p53 expression in human soft tissue sarcomas. Correlation with biological

aggressiveness, G. Toffoli, T. Perin, C. Doglioni, S. Frustaci, A. Buonadonna, A. de Paoli, C. Cernigoi, L. Tumiotto, M.G. Dall'Arche, M. Boiocchi 794

Synergistic cytotoxicity as an endpoint for the development of rational chemotherapeutic. Drug combinations, J.L. Abbruzzese, P. Frost 798

5-Fluorouracil may have different mechanisms of action depending on the dose schedule : clinical implications, C. Aschele, A. Sobrero, A. Guglielmi, A. Mori, L. Tixi, E. Bolli, R. Rosso, J.R. Bertino 804

Clinical studies of CPT-11 in Japan, T. Taguchi 809

Evaluation of CPT-11 against human xenografts of colon adenocarcinoma and childhood sarcomas, P.J. Houghton, J.A. Hougthon 813

Microencapsulation, Tamoxifen analogues, and in vivo microscopy for tumor targeting, D. Yang, S. Wallace, L.-R. Kuang, C. Li, A. Cherif, Z. Kan, P. McCuskey, K.C. Wright 817

A new generation of Doxorubicin-loaded liposomes with improved localization in tumors : preclinical and clinical studies, A. Gabizon, B. Uziely, B. Kaufman, T. Safra, R. Catane, Y. Barenholz 820

Degradable starch microspheres increase the cytostatic effect of the bioreductive drug RSU-1069 (aziridine 2-nitroimidazole) at arterial administration in rats with a liver carcinoma, U. Stenram, G. Roos 823

Therapeutic use of polyspecific mab-labelled liposomes as carriers for radioisotopes and drugs, G. Rombi, F. Cossu, G. Melis, V. Anedda, A. Facchini 826

An in vitro model for neutrophil-mediated damage to tumour vasculature : effects of a novel anti-cancer agent, J.C. Murray, K.A. Smith, M. Bastaki, K.B. Wilson 833

Stimulation of tumor growth in-vitro and in-vivo by Suramin in an experimental model, M. Julieron, L. Ramirez, M. Bonnay, G. Vassal, A. Gavoille, D. Piron, D. Gandia, L. Mir, J.-N. Munck 838

Phase I-II trial of Seraspenide (AcSDKP) : a supressor of myelopoiesis protects against chemotherapy myelotoxicity (version 10 february 1993), P. Carde, E. Gonçalves, F. Isnard, E. Deschamps de Paillette, C. Chastang, N. Mathieu-Tubiana, E. Vuillemin, V. Delwail, O. Corbion, A. Vekhoff, J.-M. Ferrero, E. Garcia-Giralt, J.-F. Gimonet, A.M. Stoppa, E. Leger-Picherit, J.-P. Monpezat, E. Fadel, C. Domenge, F. Guilhot, F. Thomas, D. Khayat, A. Monnier, R. Zittoun, B. Brun, D. Maraninchi, J.-N. Munck, F. Beaujan, M. Guigon, E. Frindel, A. Najman, M. Tubiana 843

A review on the use of sheep epidermal squamous cell carcinoma to evaluate intra-arterial infusion chemotherapy, G.J.S. Harker, F.O. Stephens 850

Cellular and pharmacokinetic factors which influence genotoxicity of topoisomerase II inhibiting drugs in human leukemia cells, F. Gieseler, V. Nüßler, F. Boege, D. Biller, P. Meyer, W. Willmanns, K. Wilms 855

Clinical application of gene transfer in oncology : preliminary results of a French study, Y. Merrouche, C. Bain, G. Clapisson, S. Negrier, B. Coronel, A. Mercatello, J.-F. Moskovtchenko, B. Mœn, T. Philip, M.C. Favrot 861

Effects of Vitamin-A on the oestrogen dependant breast carcinoma cell line ZR75-1, P.G. Horgan, J. O'Donoghue, J. Byrne, C. Phelan, H.F. Given 865

Measurement of the early level of mdr1 gene expression is a predictive marker of tumour response in breast cancer patients treated by Neo-Adjuvant chemotherapy, J.Y. Pierga, S. Chevillard, P. Pouillart, Ph. Vielh 871

Hematologic effects of recombinant human Interleukin-6 (rhIL-6) in sarcoma patients receiving maid chemotherapy : phase I trial, R.M. Bukowski, R. Isaacs, M. Gordon, G.D. Demetri, B. Amuels, D.C. Young, S. Samuel, D. McLain, D. Levitt... 875

Role of G-CFS and GM-CSF in the treatment of febrile neutropenia induced by chemotherapy ; preliminary results of a randomized trial, F. Rivera, J.I. Mayordomo, M.T. Díaz-Puente, M.P. Lianes, M. López-Brea, E. López, L. Paz-Ares, S. Alonso, H. Cortés-Funes 880

First line chemotherapy for patients with multiple myeloma with vad regimen followed by consolidation with high-dose chemoradiotherapy with peripheral stem cells autograft (PSCA) : the experience of IGR center, P. Brault, E. Gilles, A. Ibrahim, F. Beaujean, S. Jimenz, G. Tertian, M. Hayat, J.H. Bourhis, J.L. Pico 885

Author's index... 889

Foreword

This book gathers the educational lectures and the texts of the main presentations given at the 4th International Congress on Anticancer Chemotherapy which took place in February 1993 in Paris and was attended by 5 000 oncologists from all continents, physicians, students and nurses. This book aspires to give update of the most scientific and clinical aspects of modern oncology.

It aims also at showing the prospects that are opened by the rapid progress of cancer biology. The editors are grateful to the authors whose scholarship defines the quality of the book.

Educational lectures

The pathogenesis of human cancer metastasis

IJ Fidler

Cancer is a collection of malignancies with each cancer of each organ consisting of numerous subsets. This biologic and clinical heterogeneity is probably due to the different etiologies, origins, and selection pressures. Despite this heterogeneity, all malignant neoplasms have a uniform characteristic: the ability to invade host tissues and produce metastases. Clinical observations of cancer patients and studies with experimental rodent tumors have revealed that certain tumors produce metastasis to specific organs independent of vascular anatomy, rate of blood flow, and number of tumor cells delivered to each organ. The distribution and fate of hematogeneously disseminated, radiolabelled tumor cells in experimental rodent systems amply demonstrate that tumor cells reach the microvasculature of many organs. Extravasation into the organ parenchyma and proliferation in the organ parenchyma of tumor cells occur in only some organs. Therefore, the presence of viable tumor cells in a particular organ does not always predict that metastases will develop [1].

The search for the mechanisms that regulate the pattern of metastasis began in 1889 when Stephen Paget, MD, FRCS, questioned « what is it that decides what organs shall suffer in a case of disseminated cancer » ? [2]. Paget's inquiry was motivated by the discrepancy between blood flow and relative frequency of metastases in different organs. He examined the autopsy records of 735 women who died of breast cancer and concluded that their pattern of metastases was predictable. He also drew attention to the frequency of ovarian metastases and to the different incidences of skeletal metastases from different primary tumors. Paget concluded that certain favored tumor cells (the « seed ») had a specific affinity for growth in the milieu provided by certain organs (the « soil »). Metastasis resulted only when the « seed and soil » were compatible [2].

A modern definition of this hypothesis consists of three principles. First, neoplasms are heterogeneous for biologic and metastatic properties [3]. Second, the process of metastasis consists of a series of linked, sequential steps that must be completed by tumor cells if metastases are to develop [4]. Thus, metastatic cells must succeed in invasion, embolization, survival in the circulation, arrest in a distant capillary bed, and extravasation into and multiplication in organ parenchyma. Although some of the steps in this process contain stochastic elements, as a whole, metastasis is selective and favors the survival and growth of a few subpopulations of cells that preexist within the parent neoplasm [5]. Metastases can have a clonal origin and different metastases can originate from the proliferation of different single cells [6]. Third, the outcome of metastasis depends on the interaction of metastatic cells with different organ environments. Patterns of organ-specific metastasis are prevalent in many human cancers independent of blood flow and initial arrest, a phenomenon

---

Department of Cell Biology, The University of Texas MD Anderson Cancer Center, Houston, Texas, USA

well demonstrated in autochthonous human tumors in patients with peritoneovenous shunts. Organ-specific metastases have also been demonstrated in a variety of experimental tumor systems [7].

One interesting model demonstrating organ-specific metastasis was recently described in mice injected with syngeneic tumor cells into the internal carotid artery simulating the hematogenous spread of tumor emboli to the brain. We found a remarkable difference between two murine melanomas in patterns of brain metastasis ; the K-1735 melanoma syngeneic to C3H mice produced lesions only in the brain parenchyma, whereas the B16 melanoma syngeneic to C57BL/6 mice produced only meningeal growths. These results demonstrate specificity for metastatic growth in different regions within a single organ and were not correlated with site distribution analysis of radiolabelled cells. Rather, the different sites of tumor growth involved interactions between the metastatic cells and the organ environment, possibly in terms of specific interaction with endothelial cells and responses to local stimulatory or inhibitory growth factors [8].

Data such as these raise the question : does metastasis result from the ability of tumor cells to evade host defenses (including inhibitory growth control mechanisms) or does metastasis occur because metastatic cells usurp homeostatic mechanisms ? Recent evidence support the latter possibility.

We have shown that the implantation of human cancer cells derived from surgical specimens into anatomically correct (orthotopic) sites of nude mice can be used to ascertain their metastatic potential. For example, the implantation of human renal carcinoma cells into the kidney of nude mice, but not into other organs, produces metastases to the lung of recipient mice [9]. Human colorectal carcinoma cells obtained from surgical specimens and implanted either into the spleen or cecum of nude mice (but not into other organs) produce hepatic and lymph node metastases [10]. Human prostate carcinoma cells implanted into the prostate of nude mice (but not the subcutis) grow and produce lymph node, lung, and bone metastases [11]. For melanomas, however, the intradermal-subcutaneous implantation site is adequate [12]. Clonal analysis of a human renal carcinoma, colon carcinomas, and melanomas has revealed that these tumors are indeed heterogeneous for metastatic properties, an observation made only after orthotopic implantation [13].

All of the aforementioned studies indicate that growth in a specific organ's environment is selective and that the environment per se influences this process. While it is clear that vascularity and local immunity can facilitate or retard tumor growth, we have concentrated our efforts on understanding how metastatic tumor cells usurp physiologic growth factors produced by an organ environment to potentiate their growth at specific metastatic sites. Factors that control the processes of organ repair and/or regeneration are known to be organ-specific. For example, subsequent to a >50 % hepatectomy, the liver undergoes rapid cell division termed « regeneration ». In a hepatectomized mouse, however, no similar cell division can be found in the kidneys. In contrast, the mouse kidney compensates for unilateral nephrectomy by hypertrophy and hyperplasia, whereas the liver does not regenerate after nephrectomy.

We carried out transplantation experiments on human colon carcinomas and human renal cell carcinomas in nude mice that have subsequently been subjected to either nephrectomy, hepatectomy, or abdominal surgery (as a trauma control). The results were intriguing. Human colon carcinoma cells implanted s.c. demonstrated accelerated growth in partially hepatectomized mice but not in nephrectomized mice. Human renal cell carcinoma cells established as micrometastases in the lung of nude mice underwent a significant growth acceleration subsequent to unilateral nephrectomy but not hepatectomy. These results indicate that metastatic cells can respond to physiological signals associated with organ repair, i.e., homeostasis. Tumor cells that either originate from or have an affinity for growth in this particular organ can respond to these signals [1].

Host growth factors (autocrine or paracrine) that control the processes of organ repair are known to be organ-specific. During liver regeneration, it is common to find factors in the circulation that stimulate DNA synthesis in hepatic tissue. These include TGF-α and hepatocyte growth factor (HGF). We have found that all human colon cancer cells capable of growing in the liver parenchyma of nude mice (Dukes' stage D) express a high number of functional receptors for TGF-α (EGF-R) and HGF (c-met) as compared with cells with low metastatic potential (Dukes' stage B). The more malignant the colon cancer cells, the more cell surface EGF-R. Since EGF-R levels also correlate with advance stage disease of human non-small cell lung cancer, gastric cancer, and bladder cancer, the results suggest a physiological significance of inappropriate expression of the EGF-R tyrosine kinase in abnormal cell growth control. Thus, the production of liver-specific metastasis results from the proliferation of tumor cells expressing growth factor receptors for tissue-specific paracrine factors involved in homeostasis [14].

The organ microenvironment can also influence the response of metastases to chemotherapy. It is not uncommon to observe the regression of cancer metastases in one organ and their continued growth in other sites after systemic chemotherapy. Since the orthotopic implantation of cancer cells influences their metastatic properties in nude mice, we wished to determine whether different organ microenvironment can also influence response of cancer metastases to systemic chemotherapy. The highly metastatic murine colon cancer cell line CT-26 was injected intravenously, into the cecal wall, the spleen, and the subcutis of syngeneic BALB/c mice. Doxorubicin (DOX) at 10 mg/kg or saline (control) was injected intravenously on days 7 and 14 after tumor cell injection. The *in vivo* response of tumors growing in the lung, cecum, liver, spleen, and subcutaneous (s.c.) sites as well as the *in vitro* DOX sensitivity of cell lines established from lung, liver, and s.c. tumors were compared. Colon cancers growing s.c. or in the spleen were more sensitive to DOX than tumors growing in the cecal wall, liver, or lung of nude mice. The differences in response to DOX between s.c. tumors (sensitive) and lung or liver tumors (resistant) were not due to the selection of cell populations with different sensitivity to DOX or DOX distribution. Levels of protein kinase C activity varied among the lines. The expression of the multidrug resistance-associated P-glycoprotein as determined by flow cytometric analysis of tumor cells harvested from lesions in different organs correlated inversely with their sensitivity to DOX. The increased level of P-glycoprotein was associated with overexpression of mdr1 mRNA.

Hence, the organ environment influenced the level of mdr1 mRNA and P-glycoprotein expression in colon carcinoma cells and thereby their response to DOX [15].

In conclusion, metastasis is a highly selective process that is regulated by many interdependent mechanisms. This conclusion offers some optimism. Belief that certain rules regulate metastasis implies that the elucidation and understanding of these rules will lead to better therapeutic intervention and improvements in the way oncologists deal with cancer metastasis.

References

1. Fidler IJ (1990) Critical factors in the biology of human cancer metastasis : Twenty-eighth GHA. Clowes Memorial Award Lecture. Cancer Res 50 : 6130-6138
2. Paget S (1889) The distribution of secondary growths in cancer of the breast. Lancet 1 : 571-573
3. Fidler IJ, Hart IR (1982) Biological diversity in metastatic neoplasms : Origins and implications. Science (Washington, DC) 217 : 998-1003
4. Poste G, Fidler IJ (1979) The pathogenesis of cancer metastasis. Nature (Lond) 283 : 139-146
5. Fidler IJ, Kripke ML (1977) Metastasis results from pre-existing variant cells within a malignant tumor. Science (Washington, DC) 197 : 893-895
6. Fidler IJ, Talmadge JE (1986) Evidence that intravenously derived murine pulmonary metastases can originate from the expansion of a single tumor cell. Cancer Res 46 : 5167-5171
7. Weiss L (1987) Principles of Metastasis. Academic Press, Orlando
8. Schackert G, Fidler IJ (1988) Site-specific metastasis of mouse melanomas and a fibrosarcoma in the brain or the meninges of syngeneic animals. Cancer Res 48 : 3478-3483
9. Naito S, von Eschenbach AC, Giavazzi R, Fidler IJ (1986) Growth and metastasis of tumor cells isolated from a human renal cell carcinoma implanted into different organs of nude mice. Cancer Res 46 : 4109-4115
10. Morikawa K, Walker SM, Nakajima M, Pathak S, Jessup JM, Fidler IJ (1988) Influence of organ environment on the growth, selection, and metastasis of human colon carcinoma cells in nude mice. Cancer Res 48 : 6863-6871
11. Stephenson RA, Dinney CPN, Gohji K, Ordonez NG, Killion JJ, Fidler IJ (1992) Metastatic model for human prostate cancer using orthotopic implantation in nude mice. J Natl Cancer Inst 84 : 951-957
12. Cornil I, Man MS, Fernandez B, Kerbel RS (1989) Enhanced tumorigenicity, melanogenesis, and metastasis of a human malignant melanoma observed after subdermal implantation in nude mice. J Natl Cancer Inst 81 : 938-944
13. Fidler IJ (1986) Rationale and methods for the use of nude mice to study the biology and therapy of human cancer metastasis. Cancer Metastasis Rev 5 : 29-49
14. Radinsky R, Fidler IJ (1992) Regulation of tumor cell growth at organ-specific metastasis. In vivo 6 : 325-332
15. Wilmanns C, Fan D, O'Brian CA, Bucana CD, Fidler IJ (1992) Orthotopic and ectopic organ environments differentially influence the sensitivity of murine colon carcinoma cells to Doxorubicin and 5-Fluorouracil. Int J Cancer 52 : 98-104

The role of molecular genetics in medical oncology

EJ Freireich

Molecular genetics is a powerful new tool for detection, diagnosis, evaluation of treatment, and understanding of the biology of malignant disease. The first malignant disease to be characterized by a specific cytogenetic aneuploid abnormality was chronic myelogenous leukemia (CML) which was first recognized in 1962 as an abnormal shortening of the long arm of either chromosome 21 or 22, the smallest chromosomes in the human genome. This cytogenetic abnormality was subsequently shown to represent not a loss of genetic material, but a pseudodiploid aneuploidy with a reciprocal translocation of chromosomal material from the long arms of chromosome 9 and 22. The discovery that the abl oncogene was located at the breakpoint on chromosome 9 allowed the molecular geneticists to identify the genetic material adjacent to the translocated material from chromosome 9 and because the breakpoint on chromosome 22 was variable but restricted to a small region, it was named the breakpoint cluster region (BCR). The BCR/abl gene has been found exclusively in leukemic cells from patients with CML. The somatic cells of the host are not involved and at least to date, every individual that has been found to have this gene has also had the disease CML. Approximately 15 % of CML patients lack the Philadelphia chromosome on cytogenetics. However, approximately half of these patients can be shown to have the BCR/abl neogene present as a masked translocation. The importance of this is that these patients have a natural history and response to therapy which is identical to patients who have the Philadelphia chromosome. Thus, the BCR/abl identified by the procedure of Southern blotting has become a fundamental component of the diagnostic criteria for the disease CML.

Successful treatment for the disease CML was first described in the early 1950's with the use of alkylating agents. Such therapy could result in complete clinical and hematological remissions. Correction of massive splenomegaly, anemia, leukocytosis, and thrombocythemia was associated with return to completely normal health. Astonishingly, the observation of complete clinical and hematological remissions was not associated with significant prolongation of life, rather there was for approximately 85 % of alkylating agent treated patients with CML conversion to an acute blastic phase which had a high morbidity and mortality. With the discovery of the Philadelphia chromosome, the biological basis for this soon became clear. Virtually all of the patients that respond to alkylating agents with complete clinical and hematological remission still have the persistent genetic abnormality. This indicates that the abnormal gene is the biologically significant factor and transformed the treatment objective for this disease. The observation that interferon and, in some instances intensive combination chemotherapy, can result in suppression of the Philadelphia chromosome cytogenetic aneuploidy with return of normal diploid

---

The University of Texas, MD Anderson Cancer Center, Houston, Texas 77030, USA

metaphases to a proportion of these patients has provided a new therapeutic objective for this disease. It is clear that patients who have major reduction, that is, more than 70 % reduction, in the BCR/abl gene with return of diploid hematopoiesis have significantly improved survival and a substantially reduced frequency of conversion to the blastic phase. The observation that allogeneic transplantation can result in substantial disease free survival is also associated with elimination of the BCR/abl gene. Thus, the new objective of treatment effects of CML is control, or elimination of the BCR/abl gene.

Cytogenetics and molecular genetic techniques involving Southern blotting are sensitive to detect approximately 5 % of residual aneuploid cells in CML. However, by applying the reverse transcriptase to RNA transcripts in CML patients, and then applying the polymerase chain reaction to the cDNA derived there from, greatly enhances the sensitivity for detection of residual BCR/abl gene transcripts. Studies to date indicate that patients who have complete molecular genetic remissions resulting from interferon, in virtually every instance have detectable transcripts of the neogene in their peripheral blood cells. In contrast, a significant number of patients who have been treated with allogeneic transplant show complete disappearance of the gene suggesting eradication of the disease.

The BCR/abl gene is not only transcribed but translated and a unique protein is the result of this genetic change. Techniques for detection of the protein product of this gene have been developed and show promise for improving sensitivity for detecting this abnormal gene product. With improving techniques of molecular genetics improved understanding of the biology of CML have resulted and it offers the potential and screening for early detection of the disease in addition to being useful in diagnosis and in the evaluation of treatment.

While CML has played a leading role in the development of molecular genetic techniques for studying malignant disease, many more recent examples indicate that such techniques will be useful for virtually all of oncology. In the case of acute myeloblastic leukemia, approximately 55 % of patients have cytogenetic aneuploidies which have prognostic significance as it relates to the natural history of their disease and to response to therapy. Moreover, it has been shown that patients who achieve complete clinical and hematological remission generally also have complete cytogenetic and molecular genetic remission. However, it has recently been shown that persistence of an aneuploid metaphase in patients otherwise in complete hematological remission is predictive of relapse and therefore, indicates the presence of residual disease. This has stimulated studies to developing more sensitive genetic techniques, such as fluorescent *in situ* hybridization and application of the polymerase chain reaction to detection of residual disease. In the case of acute promyelocytic leukemia, characterized by a reciprocal translocation between chromosomes 15 and 17, a polymerase chain reaction test has already been devised. In the case of acute myeloblastic leukemia, FAB m-2, containing reciprocal translocation between chromosome 8 and chromosome 21, a similar polymerase chain reaction has been developed and the breakpoint has been cloned and sequenced. The inversion 16 aneuploidy is susceptible to detection by fluorescent *in situ* hybridization techniques. These three specific cytogenetic aneuploidies constitute between

15-20 % of patients with acute myeloblastic leukemia, but they represent an important subset since these diseases are extremely sensitive to currently available chemotherapy and they have the highest frequency of long-term disease free survival. Thus the techniques for detection of residual disease become extremely important for these diagnoses.

In addition to neogenes which result from chromosomal translocation which are described above there can result an overexpression of normal genes which result from translocation of the gene to a site adjacent to the promoters of immunoglobulin gene production such as occurs in the Burkitt's lymphoma. Here the myc gene is overexpressed and undoubtedly contributes to the highly malignant nature of this disease. In the case of the nodular lymphomas, the translocation of the bcl-2 gene to an immunoglobulin site results in overexpression of bcl-2 and this results in prolongation of the survival of the highly differentiated lymphoid cells as a result of interferring with the natural death process of apoptosis.

Finally, the important new area of tumor suppressor genes is having a major impact on medical oncology. Alterations of the retinoblastoma gene and the p-53 gene which can suppress proliferation are both associated with a high degree of malignancy in many different tumors. These powerful tools already play a major role in the practice of medical oncology and their importance will undoubtedly continue to grow in the future.

References

1. Freireich EJ, Cork A, Stass SA, McCredie KB, Keating MJ, Estey EH, Kantarjian HM, Trujillo JM (1992) Cytogenetics for detection of minimal residual disease in acute myeloblastic leukemia. Leukemia 6 : 500-505
2. Chang K-S, Wang G, Freireich EJ, Daly M, Naylor SL, Trujillo JM, Stass SA (1992) Specific expression of the annexin VIII gene in acute promyelocytic leukemia. Blood 79 : 1802-1810
3. Lee M-S, Kantarjian H, Talpaz M, Freireich EJ, Deisseroth A, Trujillo JM, Stass SA (1992) Detection of minimal residual disease by polymerase chain reaction in Philadelphia chromosome-positive chronic myelogenous leukemia following interferon therapy. Blood 79 : 1920-1923
4. Kantarjian HM, Talpaz M, Keating MJ, Estey EH, O'Brien S, Beran M, McCredie KB, Gutterman JU, Freireich EJ (1991) Intensive chemotherapy induction followed by interferon-α maintenance in patients with Philadelphia chromosome-positive chronic myelogeneous leukemia. Cancer 68 : 1201-1207
5. Freireich EJ, Kantarjian H (eds) (1991) Therapy of Hematopoietic Neoplasia. Marcel Dekker Inc, New York
6. Freireich EJ, Lemak N (1991) Milestones in Leukemia Research and Therapy. Johns Hopkins University Press, Baltimore, Maryland
7. Freireich EJ, Marmont AM, McCulloch EA, Rees JKH, Reizenstein P, Wiernik PH (1990) New Approaches to the Treatment of Leukemia. In : Freireich EJ (ed). Springer-Verlag, Berlin

Cell line-based screening for new anticancer drugs

BA Chabner, JN Weinstein, KD Paull, MR Grever

Since 1955, the National Cancer Institute (USA, NCI) has actively sought to identify new anticancer agents through screening. Through the first three decades of that effort, up to 40,000 new chemical entities per year were tested against a variety of murine tumors, primarily lymphocytic leukemias, resulting in the discovery of a number of useful agents, including BCNU and hydroxyurea [1]. Other clinically useful compounds, including Taxol, Fludarabine phosphate and Deoxycoformycin, were confirmed to be active agents *in vivo* in the screen following their discovery as cytotoxic agents in *in vitro* assays. However, the failure of the screen to discover new entities with significant activity in solid malignancies prompted a reevaluation and redirection of drug discovery efforts in 1985. With the aid of the Board of Scientific Counselors of the Division of Cancer Treatment and the extramural community of researchers, we undertook a major change in screening strategy at that time [2]. The first step taken was to dramatically increase support for academic and industry-based drug discovery efforts through research project grants. Second, it was decided to establish a new primary NCI screen with the following features :
 1. The initial screening would be conducted *in vitro*, thus eliminating the expense and controversy of large-scale screening in animals.
 2. It would employ human solid tumor cell lines, based on the hypothesis that human solid tumors have a different, and unique, biology as compared to murine leukemias.
 3. It would be highly automated, thus reducing the expense and increasing the potential through-put of the screen.
 Each of these features is incorporated in the 60-cell-line panel currently employed by the Division of Cancer Treatment. Full-scale screening of approximately 26,000 synthetic compounds has been completed since April 1990 [3]. In addition, thousands of crude natural-product extracts have also been screened.
 In setting up an *in vitro* primary screen, it is realized that there are significant disadvantages as compared to *in vivo* screening, including the lack of an activation system for compounds that require metabolic transformation outside the tumor to an active form. In fact, few of the currently useful anticancer drugs require extratumoral activation, and most of these are alkylating agents such as cyclophosphamide, procarbazine and DTIC. We were willing to forego the discovery of such compounds in return for the convenience and logic of a cell line screen. A second disadvantage is the absence of a therapeutic index, that is, an assessment of the relative toxicity for malignant as compared to normal tissues. However, since the *in vitro* screen is intended to be simply a first step in the evaluation process, the therapeutic index would be established by subsequent *in vivo* testing, a requirement for preclinical development.

Division of Cancer Treatment, National Cancer Institute, NIH, Bethesda, Maryland 20892, USA

Crucial to the success of a drug screening program is the source of compounds that enter the screen. Prior to 1985, most compounds tested by NCI came from industry and represented new synthetic chemical entities. For a number of reasons, we chose to emphasize natural products in the cell line screen. The general experience of drug screening operations for cancer drugs has been that the rate of positives is considerably higher among natural products, averaging 1 to 2 percent of extracts tested, while synthetics yield a much lower rate of positives [1]. The natural products tend to represent highly unique structural classes that could not or would not be rationally synthesized, and tend to have a broader variety of biological properties; for example, a compound such as the marine animal (bryozoan) product bryostatin cause induction of differentiation [4], stimulation of growth-factor pathways [5], or interactions with the immune system [6]. Finally, the source of natural products in the biosphere is rapidly disappearing; this may be the last opportunity to collect and test many such compounds. Thus the cell line screen was coupled to a major investment in the collection and testing of biological materials derived from plants, marine animals and fermentation. These same materials enter the NCI drug screen for AIDS antiviral activity as well.

Since formally initiating the cancer drug cell line screen in 1990, NCI staff have introduced a number of innovations in methodology of testing as well as in analysis of results. Automated assays of cell number based on dye reduction (the MTT and XTT assays [7]) and on protein content [8, 9] (the sulforhodamine B assay) have been developed and are now widely used in cell culture studies in biomedical research. A mean graph analysis depicts the relative sensitivity of the various cell lines, grouped according to disease category, as shown in Figure 1. This format allows the identification of compounds or extracts that display inhibitory activity for specific categories of disease, as shown in Figure 1. More complex computer-based analyses of the screening results include the following:

1. A COMPARE program that searches for compounds displaying a pattern of activity matching the profile of a lead compound [10]. For example, when the microtubule binding compound taxol was entered as the lead, a number of unique natural products were identified that had very similar patterns of activity in the cell line screen, including the dolostatins [11] and halochondrin [12], both of which subsequently proved to have potent effects on microtubule formation and which represent unique chemical entities of considerable interest for chemotherapy.

2. A neural network analysis that allows identification of the mechanism of action of a new compound, based on the pattern of cell line response [13]. If compounds with known mechanisms of action are used to train the network, then unknowns can be classified into the major categories of action (alkylating agent, DNA synthesis inhibitor, topoisomerase II inhibitor, etc.) and compounds with unique mechanisms of action can be identified. Obviously, the latter compounds are of greatest interest. Neural networks, such as that shown in Figure 2, differ from conventional computer programs in that they learn from examples rather than being programmed to get the right answer. Information is encoded in the strenght of the network's « synaptic » connections, and even highly complex interactions between input variables can be

```
TGI  MEAN GRAPH OF NSC 106408    9211EM14
                            3    2    1    0    1    2    3
Leukemia
  CCRF-CEM       > -4.00
  HL-60(TB)      > -4.00
  K-562          > -4.00
  MOLT-4         > -4.00
  RPMI-8226      > -4.00
  SR             > -4.00
Non-Small Cell Lung Cancer
  EKVX           > -4.00
  HOP-62         < -8.00
  HOP-92           -7.48
  NCI-H23          -7.26
  NCI-H322M        -5.25
  NCI-H460         -4.85
  NCI-H522         -7.23
Colon Cancer
  COLO 205         -7.46
  HCT-116        > -4.00
  HCT-15         > -4.00
  HT29             -6.77
  KM12           > -4.00
  SW-620           -4.84
CNS Cancer
  SF-268           -6.59
  SF-295         > -4.00
  SF-539         < -8.00
  SNB-19           -4.71
  SNB-75         < -8.00
  U251             -4.93
Melanoma
  LOX IMVI       > -4.00
  MALME-3M         -7.87
  M14              -7.37
  SK-MEL-2       < -8.00
  SK-MEL-28        -7.49
  SK-MEL-5       < -8.00
  UACC-257         -7.35
  UACC-62        < -8.00
Ovarian Cancer
  OVCAR-4          -7.11
  OVCAR-5        > -4.00
  OVCAR-8          -4.97
  SK-OV-3          -4.09
Renal Cancer
  ACHN           > -4.00
  SN12C            -4.49
  TK-10          > -4.00
  UO-31            -7.13
Prostate Cancer
  PC-3             -5.55
Breast Cancer
  MCF7           > -4.00
  MCF7/ADR-RES   < -8.00
  MDA-MB-231/ATC < -8.00
  MDA-N            -7.78
  BT-549         < -8.00
  T-47D          > -4.00
                            3    2    1    0    1    2    3
```

Fig. 1. A neural network used to classify agents in the NCI cancer drug screening program by mechanism of action. Each input number represents a measure of the relative potency of a compound for one particular cell line out of the 60. As indicated by 1's for the appropriate « actual » categories, chlorambucil is an alkylating agent and methotrexate is an RNA/DNA antimetabolite (more specifically, an antifol). To train the network, such compounds of known mechanism are presented iteratively. Weights associated with the synaptic connections are changed progressively according to a learning rule until the output pattern for each agent comes to resemble as closely as possible the « actual » category pattern of 1's and 0'. Solid and dashed interconnections schematically represent differing weights in the trained network. Clearly, the network does very well for the two drugs shown. Topo I and II, topoisomerase I and II inhibitors, respectively ; RNA/DNA, RNA/DNA antimetabolites ; DNA, DNA antimetabolites ; alkyl, alkylating agents (Modified from ref. [13], see that reference for details)

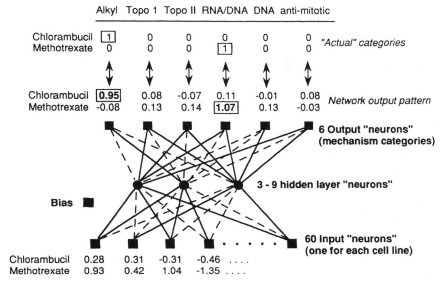

Fig. 2. Shown above is a graph depicting the effect of a new chemical entity, anthramycin 11-methyl ester, on cell lines in the NCI screen. Cells were exposed to a range of drug concentrations for 48 hours, and growth inhibition was determined by comparison with the growth of control cultures. Data are plotted by setting the « O » point as the mean inhibitory concentration for all cell lines tested, lines to the left of « O » representing more resistant cells, and lines to the right more sensitive cells. Distances from the « O » line are represented in log units, and the 50 % inhibitory concentration (in molar concentration) for each cell line is indicated to the left of the bar. Note the disease specificity for breast cancer, melanoma, and non-small cell lung cancer and the high degree of resistance among leukemic cell lines

Table 1. Prediction of mechanism category from cancer drug screen data using a neural network with seven hidden layer « neurons ». numbers Italic are correct predictions. R/D indicates RNA/DNA antimetabolites ; DNA indicates DNA antimetabolites (modified from [13])

Actual Category	Predicted Category						
	Alkyl 1	Topo I 2	Topo II 3	R/D 4	DNA 5	Antimitotic 6	None 7
1. Alkylating	*33*		2				
2. Topoisomerase I		*35*					
3. Topoisomerase II	1		*18*				
4. RNA/DNA	1		1	*17*		1	
5. DNA	1		1	1	*12*	1	
6. Antimitotic	1	1				*14*	

Correct predictions : 129 (91.5 %), incorrect predictions : 12 (8.5 %)

recognized. Table 1 shows the results obtained from one particular network, which correctly predicted the categories of mechanism of action of 129 out of 141 agents that it had not seen during the training process. We are currently using neural networks (in combination with other statistical pattern recognition techniques) for a number of other tasks in drug discovery and development [14] : to classify agents by molecular structure ; to correlate patterns of activity with specific aspects of molecular structure ; to correlate activity with molecular targets ; and ultimately to predict patterns of clinical efficacy.

3. Analysis of patterns of drug resistance. Thus far the cell lines have been characterized with respect to their expression of the *mdr-1* [15, 16] phenotype and the expression of the guanine 0-6 alkyl transferase [17]. Response to agents known to be affected by these resistance mechanisms correlates well with expression of these factors. It is hoped that this information with allow the staff to identify new agents that are not susceptible to known mechanisms of resistance, as, for example, topoisomerase II inhibitors that are not affected by multidrug resistance (MDR). Secondly, it may be possible to identify compounds that are substrates for the MDR efflux pump (selectively inactive in MDR-type cells) and therefore potentially effective as MDR-reversing agents.

4. Molecular characterization of the cell lines with respect to oncogene expression, suppressor gene expression, and growth factor dependence, which may allow a search for compounds that target these key molecular lesions in transformed cells. Our initial efforts will be directed toward determining the expression of the *ras*, her 2/neu and *myc* family of oncogenes, as well as *RB* and *p53* suppressor genes. With this information in hand, it should be possible to ask the screen to identify compounds or extracts uniquely active in cells that possess these molecular changes.

5. Computer analysis of the unique information forthcoming from each cell line in the panel, thus allowing the elimination of redundant or non-informative lines. This analysis has been done in the past year based on the first two years of screening experience, and has allowed the introduction of a new breast cancer panel of cell lines, a high-priority area of treatment research.

Our current criteria for selecting agents for further evaluation *in vivo*, and ultimately for clinical trial, require further refinement and experience. Essentially we are looking for agents that show disease specificity, uniqueness of structure and mechanism of action, potency, and ultimately selectivity for malignant cells. An additional factor in choosing an agent for clinical development, often neglected in the theoretical discussions of cancer drug discovery, is an adequate supply ; many of the natural products that have interesting activities are exceedingly difficult to synthesize or to isolate in sufficient quantity. Along with progress in drug screening, the field of cancer drug discovery needs the help and participation of innovative natural-product chemists who are willing to accept the challenge of isolating, characterizing and synthesizing difficult molecules such as taxol [18] and camptothecin [19].

The challenges of cancer drug discovery touch every field of biomedical research, from the biologists, who unravel the molecular lesions of cancer and thus identify new targets for drug development, to the medicinal chemists and pharmacologists, who devise ways of inhibiting these aberrant pathways. The cell line screening system will afford each of these parties a convenient and informative mechanism for applying their ideas and talents to the problem of cancer treatment.

Acknowledgements. The authors wish to thank Michael Boyd, Robert Shoemaker, Anne Monks, Nick Scudiero and their colleagues for their devoted work in making the cell line screen a reality.

References

1. Driscoll J (1984) The preclinical new drug research program of the National Cancer Institute. Cancer Treat Rep 68 : 63-76
2. Chabner BA (1990) In defense of cell line screening. J Natl Cancer Inst 82 : 1083-1085
3. Grever MR, Schepartz SA, Chabner BA (1992) The National Cancer Institute : cancer drug discovery and development program. Sem Oncol 19 (6) : 622-638
4. Al-Katib A, Mohammad RM, Dan M, Hussein ME, Akhtar A, Pettit GR, Sensenbrenner LL (1993) Bryostatin 1-induced hairy cell features on chronic lymphocytic leukemia cells in vitro. Exp Hematol 21 : 61-65
5. Sharkis SJ, Jones RJ, Bellis ML, Demetri GD, Griffin JD, Civin C, May WS (1990) The action of bryostatin on normal human hematopoietic progenitors is mediated by accessory cell release of growth factors. Blood 76 : 716-720
6. Esa AH, Boto WO, Adler WH, May WS, Hess AD (1990) Activation of T-cells by bryostatins : induction of the IL-2 receptor gene transcription and down-modulation of surface receptors. Int J Immunopharmacol 12 : 481-490
7. Scudiero DA, Shoemaker RH, Paull KD, Monks A, Thierry S et al (1988) Evaluation of a soluble tetrazolium/formazan assay for cell growth and drug sensitivity in culture using human and other tumor cell lines. Cancer Res 48 : 4827-4833
8. Shekan P, Storeng R, Scudiero D et al (1990) New colorimetric cytotoxicity assay for anticancer drug screening. J Natl Cancer Inst 82 : 1107-1112
9. Monks A, Scudiero D, Skehan P, Shoemaker R et al (1991) Feasibility of a high-flux anticancer drug screen using a diverse panel of cultured human tumor cell lines. J Natl Cancer Inst 83 : 756-766
10. Paull KD, Shoemaker RH, Hodes L et al (1989) Display and analysis of patterns of differential activity of drugs against human tumor cell lines : development of mean graph and COMPARE algorithm. J Natl Cancer Inst 81 : 1088-1092
11. Bai R, Pettit GR, Hamel E (1990) Dolastatin 10, a powerful cytostatic peptide derived from a marine animal. Inhibition of tubulin polymerization mediated through the vinca alkaloid binding domain. Biochem Pharmacol 39 : 1941-1949
12. Bai RL, Paull KD, Herald CL et al (1991) Halichondrin B and Homohalichondrin B, marine natural products binding in the vinca domain of tubulin : discovery of tubulin-based mechanism of action by analysis of differential cytotoxicity data. J Biol Chem 266 : 15882-15889
13. Weinstein JN, Kohn KW, Grever MR et al (1992) Neural computing in cancer drug development : predicting mechanism of action. Science 258 : 447-451
14. Weinstein JN, Rubintein LV, Koutsoukos AD et al (1993) Neural networks in the discovery of new treatments for cancer and AIDS. Symp of World Congress on Neural Networks (in press)
15. Alvarez M, Paull K, Monks A, Hose C, Weinstein J, Grever M, Lee JS, Bates S,

Fojo T (1993) Expression of *mdr-1* in the 60 cell lines of the NCI's new drug-screen : a tool to identify novel P-glycoprotein substrates and antagonists. Proc Am Assoc Cancer Res (abstr) (in press)

16. Wu Lo, Smythe AM, Stinson SF, Mullendore LA, Monks A et al (1992) Multidrug-resistant phenotype of disease-oriented panels of human tumor cell lines used for anticancer drug screening. Cancer Res 52 : 3029-3034
17. Shoemaker RH, Smythe AM, Lin W et al (1992) 06-Methylguanine DNA methyltransferase (MGMT) mRNA levels and *in vitro* sensitivity of human tumor cell lines to alkylating agents. Proc Am Assoc Cancer Res 33 : 403 (abstr)
18. Wani MC, Taylor HL, Wall ME, Coggon P, McPhail AT (1971) Plant antitumor agents. VI. The isolation and structure of Iaxol, a novel antileukemic and antitumor agent from Taxus brevifolia. J Am Chem Soc 93 : 2325-2327
19. Wall ME, Wani MC, Cook CE, Palmer KH, McPhail AT, Sim GA (1966) Plant antitumor agents. I. The isolation and structure of camptothecin, a novel alkaloidal leukemia and tumor inhibitor from Camptotheca accuminata. J Am Chem Soc 88 : 3888-3890

Anti-EGF receptor monoclonal antibodies as potential anti-cancer therapy

J Mendelsohn

The long-range goal of this laboratory is to explore the role of growth factors and receptors for growth factors in regulating the proliferation of malignant cells. A distinctive feature of our approach is an hypothesis that monoclonal antibodies (mAbs) that block the binding of growth factors to their receptors might be effective antitumor agents. Our current studies focus upon epidermal growth factor (EGF) and its receptor, which are of special interest because of three recent discoveries. First, many tumor cells appear to secrete transforming growth factor alpha (TGF-α), which can bind to the EGF receptor and produce autoregulation of proliferation through an « autocrine » pathway. Second, the v-erb B oncogene codes for a truncated version of the EGF receptor, which implicates the gene for the EGF receptor as a proto-oncogene. Third, it has been found that many human tumor cells express high levels of EGF receptors on their plasma membranes, and high expressers have a poorer prognosis.

We have produced a panel of mAbs against the EGF receptor. Two of these, 225 IgG1 and 528 IgG2A, bind to the EGF receptor with affinity comparable to the natural ligand, compete with EGF binding, precipitate the receptor, and block EGF-induced tyrosine kinase activation. The antireceptor mAbs can directly inhibit the proliferation of cells bearing high numbers of EGF receptors, both in culture and in xenografts, presumably by blocking access to autostimulation by TGF-α. This has been demonstrated with cell lines from carcinomas of the skin, lung, colon, breast, and kidney. Recent collaborative studies have demonstrated that the antibodies also can inhibit proliferation of nonmalignant breast cell lines as well as adenomatous colon cell lines bearing normal numbers of EGF receptors, when these cells (which can produce TGF-α) are cultured in serum-free medium. These results provide evidence for the widespread existence of autocrine-stimulatory pathways utilizing the EGF receptor. Furthermore, experiments in our laboratory have demonstrated that TGF-α produced and secreted in an autocrine fashion directly stimulates A431 cells by activating receptors on the exterior surface of the cells, and does not act by intracellular binding of ligand to receptor.

To investigate the therapeutic potential of anti-EGF receptor mAbs, we have explored the efficacy and pharmacokinetics of treatment with MAb and with F(ab')$_2$ in xenografted mice. Successful inhibition of tumor growth was demonstrated. A new approach is combination treatment with anti-EGF receptor mAb plus a chemotherapeutic agent. Studies with Adriamycin plus MAb in cell culture and in xenografts, have demonstrated synergistic antitumor activity. The combination treatment successfully eliminated well-established

---

Winthrop Rockefeller Chair in Medical Oncology, Department of Medicine, Memorial Sloan-Kettering Cancer Center

xenografts (400 mm³). Similar findings were obtained with cisplatin plus anti-EGF receptor MAb. We are exploring the mechanism of this interaction. We believe that activated tyrosine kinase-dependent signal transduction pathways may be needed to repair drug-induced cell damage and to avoid programmed cell death (apoptosis).

Phase I clinical trials with 225 IgG1 anti-EGF receptor mAb have been completed in patients with squamous carcinoma of the lung. This tumor was chosen because numerous studies have demonstrated increased expression of EGF receptors. The initial trial examined the toxicity of an anti-EGF receptor antibody and explored the capacity of 111-indium-labelled antibody to image the sites of tumor involvement in these patients. In this study, we demonstrated that 225 IgG1 can be administered without toxicity to patients in doses as high as 120 mg, which produce saturating serum concentrations of antibody for longer than three days. At doses higher than 20 mg, 111-indium-labelled immunoconjugates produced imaging of tumors in these patients and also identified all metastatic sites > 1 cm in diameter that were detected by x-rays and CT scans. Liver uptake of mAb was also prominent. Future studies will explore the therapeutic responses to exposure to repeated doses of human-murine chimeric 225 mAb for prolonged periods, and to combination therapy with antireceptor mAb plus a chemotherapeutic agent.

References

1. Kawamoto T, Sato JD, Le A, Polikoff J, Sato GH, Mendelsohn J (1983) Growth stimulation of A431 cells by EGF : Identification of high affinity receptors for epidermal growth factor by an antireceptor monoclonal antibody. Proc Natl Acad Sci (USA) 80 : 1337-1341
2. Gill GN, Kawamoto T, Cochet C, Le A, Sato JD, Masui H, MacLeod CL, Mendelsohn J (1984) Monoclonal anti-epidermal growth factor receptor antibodies which are inhibitors of epidermal growth factor binding and antagonists of epidermal growth factor-stimulated tyrosine protein kinase activity. J Biol Chem 259 : 7755-7760
3. Masui H, Kawamoto T, Sato JD, Wolf B, Sato GH, Mendelsohn J (1984) Growth inhibition of human tumor cells in athymic mice by anti-EGF receptor monoclonal antibodies. Cancer Res 44 : 1002-1007
4. Goldenberg A, Masui H, Divgi C, Kamrath H, Pentlow K, Mendelsohn J (1989) EGF receptor overexpression and localization of nude mice xenografts using ^{111}indium labelled anti-EGF receptor monoclonal antibody. J Natl Ca Inst 81 : 1616-1625
5. Sunada H, Yu P, Peacock JS, Mendelsohn J (1990) Modulation of tyrosine serine and threonine phosphorylation and intracellular processing of the epidermal growth factor by antireceptor monoclonal antibody. J Cell Physiol 142 : 284-292
6. Divgi C, Welt C, Kris M, Real FX, Yeh SDJ, Gralla R, Merchant B, Schweighart S, Unger M, Larson SM, Mendelsohn J (1991) Phase I and imaging trial of indium-111 labelled anti-EGF receptor monoclonal antibody 225 in patients with squamous cell lung carcinoma. J Natl Ca Inst 83 : 97-104
7. Van de Vijver M, Kumar R, Mendelsohn J (1991) Ligand-induced activation of A431 cell EGF receptors occurs primarily by an autocrine pathway that acts upon receptors on the surface rather than intracellularly. J Biol Chem 266 : 7503-7508

Clinical relevance of drug resistance: Where do we stand now and where are we going to?

SC Linn, G Giaccone, HM Pinedo*

While chemotherapy can cure several tumours even in advanced stages, like testicular cancer, several cancers of childhood and some haematological malignancies, and can prolong survival in a number of other malignancies, relapse is often inevitable in the majority of patients due to the occurrence of drug resistance to a broad variety of antineoplastic agents [1]. Drug resistance can be intrinsic or acquired. The former refers to tumours which are initially unresponsive to chemotherapy. Acquired drug resistance develops in a responsive tumour during treatment.

Theoretical aspects of drug resistance

« Temporary » and intrinsic drug resistance [2]

Since the seventies research on drug resistance has focussed more and more on biochemical strategies of the tumour cell to survive the attack of cytotoxic drugs (cellular drug resistance). Other factors, however, may make a tumour resistant, e.g. an inadequate treatment schedule. Poor drug absorption, poor tumour vascularisation, high intratumoral interstitial pressure or an unfavourable tumour pH may be overcome by another route of administration, a higher drug dosage, a longer treatment duration or a more suitable drug (or combination of drugs). Drug interactions, though rarely, may also be the cause of a lack of response to chemotherapy. Furthermore intrinsic resistance may be due to a low growth fraction of the tumour, or to a localisation at a pharmacological sanctuary (brain, testis, etc.).

Biochemical mechanisms of acquired drug resistance [3]

Knowledge on biochemical mechanisms of drug resistance has been achieved through the extensive study of tumour cell lines growing in tissue culture. Cell lines have been made resistant by step-wise selection with increasing doses of antineoplastic agents and the mechanisms developed to determine resistance have been investigated.

The development of drug resistance in tumour cell lines most likely results from genetic alterations, mutations, which are thought to occur in one out of 10^6 cell divisions [4]. This rate can be increased by mutagenic agents, including many cytotoxic drugs. When a tumour becomes clinically detectable,

---

Free University Hospital, Department of Medical Oncology, De Boelelaan 1117, 1081 HV Amsterdam and * The Netherlands Cancer Institute, Amsterdam, The Netherlands

it consists of at least 10^9 cells and contains a great deal of heterogeneity [3]. The eradication of this mixture of mutant tumour cells is usually more successfully obtained by a combination of different anticancer drugs, as monotherapy will more easily select for the resistant mutants.

Several biochemical mechanisms obtaining drug resistance have been described, like a decreased drug uptake or an increased drug efflux ; an enhanced drug inactivation or a decreased drug activation ; an increased repair of drug induced damage. Furthermore a proportional decreased formation of drug-target complexes can cause drug resistance, which can be due to a decrease or overproduction of a target enzyme, to production of an altered target enzyme with less affinity for the drug, to an increased level of normal substrate which determines competition with the drug for the target enzyme or to a decrease in the production of essential co-substrates necessary for the formation of the drug-target complex.

Drug resistance to different classes of antineoplastic agents.

Resistance to alkylating agents and Cisplatin [3]

Not much is known on the possible mechanisms underlying resistance to alkylating agents and Cisplatin. The different classes of alkylating agents show cross-resistance only to a limited extent *in vitro*. A possible explanation for this phenomenon may be that different types of alkylating drugs appear to enter cells by different routes. O^6-Methylation of guanine appears to be the major lesion induced in tumours by methylating cytotoxic drugs, like Dacarbazine (DTIC) and the nitrosoureas. It is known that O^6-Methyltransferase, an enzyme involved in DNA repair, can remove this methyl group from guanine. It has been shown that overproduction of the methyl transferase can lead to resistance to nitrosoureas in tumour cell lines and this observation has partly been confirmed by transfection experiments. Another association has been found between Cisplatin resistance and increased levels of Dihydrofolate reductase (DHFR) and thymidylate synthase (TS). However, transfection experiments are still awaited. Glutathione (GSH) and Glutathione-S transferase (GST) mediated drug resistance are still poorly understood.

Resistance to drugs interfering with nucleotide biosynthesis [4]

This group of drugs can be divided into two subgroups ; one group of drugs interfering with Purine and Pyrimidine synthesis, like 6-Mercaptopurine (6-MP), 6-Thioguanine (6TG) and PALA and a second group of drugs interfering with normal nucleotide biosynthesis, like 5-Fluorouracil (5-FU) and Cytarabine (ara-C). Methotrexate (MTX) belongs to both groups, as it inhibits both Purine ring biosynthesis as synthesis of Deoxythymidine monophosphate (dTMP).

At present six different mechanisms causing MTX resistance *in vitro* have been described [3]. Of these a decreased uptake of MTX via the high-affinity carrier system for reduced folates and an increased production of normal Dehydrofolate reductase (DHFR), the target enzyme for MTX, are the most often encountered mechanisms. Amplification of the DHFR gene in clinical samples has been observed in chronic myeloid leukaemia, acute myelocytic leukaemia and ovarian cancer. Increased nucleoside salvage has also been described as a MTX resistance mechanism with clinical interest. An increased Thymidine and Purine nucleoside uptake circumvents the need for the almost completely blocked DHFR by MTX. As Dipyridamole can block the nucleoside uptake, a clinical trial combining MTX and Dipyridamole has been initiated.

The Pyrimidine analogue 5-FU is converted into 5-Fluoro-Deoxyuridine monophosphate (FdUMP) and binding of FdUMP with the folate cofactor Methylene-Tetrahydrofolate (CH2THF) to TS in a ternary complex causes inhibition of TS. TS is an essential enzyme for biosynthesis of dTMP, while dTMP is a nucleotide necessary for DNA synthesis. In clinical samples the degree of TS inhibition correlates well with tumor response [5]. Six different mechanisms of resistance to 5-FU have been described in cell lines, of which at least two seem to be important in clinical samples [5, 6] : *a)* lowered levels of Tetetrahydrofolate cofactor required for TS function and *b)* increased levels of TS. The addition of Leucovorin (CH2THF) to 5-FU enhances cytotoxicity of 5-FU *in vitro* and this has been confirmed in clinical trials in colorectal cancer. *In vitro* it has been shown that an increase in TS levels can be prevented by the addition of interferon-α (IFN-α). The clinical relevance of the combination of 5-FU and IFN-α is being investigated.

P-glycoprotein (P-gp) mediated multidrug resistance (MDR) [3, 7]

P-gp, a glycoprotein of 170 kD present in the plasma membrane of tumor cells, acts *in vitro* as an energy dependent drug efflux pump for a broad variety of natural product anticancer drugs (e.g. Anthracyclines, Epipodophyllotoxins, *Vinca* alkaloids, Actinomycin-D, Colchicine, Taxol). P-gp mediated MDR is characterised by a decreased MDR drug accumulation, an increased drug efflux and, at least for Anthracyclines, an altered intracellular distribution. Furthermore the MDR phenotype can be reversed *in vitro* by several resistance modifying agents (RMAs) (e.g. Verapamil).

P-gp is expressed in several normal human tissues and although a detoxifying function, a role in Cortisol, Aldosterone and Bilirubin transport and a role in regulating epithelial cell volume have been proposed.

Increased P-gp expression after chemotherapy has been reported in neuroblastoma, sarcoma, breast cancer, ovarian cancer, nephroblastoma and several hematological malignancies, while an association between P-gp expression and worse prognosis has been described in neuroblastoma, sarcoma and some hematological malignancies. P-gp expression is generally high in tumors originating from tissues normally expressing P-gp.

Several investigators tried to reverse MDR in patients with refractory malignancy, with the use of RMAs. Miller et al (1991) [8] reported 13/18 responses including 5 CR in drug resistant lymphoma patients (Hodgkin's disease and low — and intermediate-grade NHL) to CVAD in combination with Verapamil. P-gp assessment revealed 5 responses out of 7 Pgp+ tumors and 2 responses out of 4 P-gp — tumors. It is difficult to establish whether presence of P-gp in tumor cells in this kind of studies might have influenced response to treatment. The lack of response of some P-gp positive tumors might be caused by additional resistance mechanisms. Furthermore, responses observed in P-gp negative tumors might be due to P-gp expression below the detection level of the assay used. Although higher sensitivity can be obtained with the use of bulk tissue techniques coupled with PCR amplification steps, information on heterogeneity of cells within the tumor is lost with these techniques.

A significant problem with the employment of RMA, like Verapamil, is the substantial (cardio)toxicity ensuing at doses of drug required to build up plasma concentrations which are able to revert resistance in *in vitro* systems. However, plasma levels adequate for MDR reversal can be obtained in humans with Cyclosporin-A, Bepridil and Quinidine, and adequate tumor tissue levels have been achieved for Bepridil and Quinidine. Despite these results, clinical trials with RMAs in solid tumors have been unrewarding so far.

Properly designed clinical studies will help to improve insight in attempts to revert resistance in refractory malignancies. The use of less toxic RMA, in combination with extensive investigation of the expression of P-gp in patients' tumor tissues and pharmacokinetic interactions between RMAs and cytotoxic agents, will shed new light onto the real impact of our basic understanding of P-gp mediated MDR in clinical practice.

Non-Pgp mediated multidrug resistance [3, 7]

Non-Pgp mediated MDR has been observed in various cell lines exhibiting the same drug resistance pattern as P-gp MDR cell lines, while not expressing P-gp. The clinical relevance of non-Pgp mediated MDR is at present unknown.

Topoisomerase II mediated multidrug resistance [3, 9]

Topo II mediated MDR involves crossresistance to drugs which have topoisomerase II as a common cellular target. Except for the *Vinca* alkaloids, colchicine and Gramicidin-D, topo II MDR drugs are the same as those involved in P-gp mediated MDR. Decreased cytotoxicity of these drugs was correlated with a reduced topo II level both *in vitro* and *in vivo*. Besides resistance induced by reduction in the cellular target enzyme, mutations can take place resulting in an altered topo II protein with less affinity for the drug. The role of topo II in clinical MDR is currently being investigated.

References

1. Pinedo HM, Longo D, Chabner B, eds (1991) Cancer Chemotherapy and Biological Response Modifiers, Annual 12. Elsevier Science Publishers, Amsterdam
2. De Vita VT Jr (1990) The problem of resistance ; keynote address. In : Mihich E (ed) Drug resistance : mechanisms and reversal. John Libbey CIC, Rome, pp 7-27
3. Borst P (1991) Genetic mechanisms of drug resistance. A review. Reviews in Oncology 4 (in Acta Oncologica 30) : 87105
4. Allegra CJ, Grem, JL, Chu E, Johnston P, Chao Yeh G, Chabner BA (1990) An-

timetabolites. In : Pinedo HM (ed) Cancer Chemotherapy. The EORTC Cancer Chemotherapy Annual n° 12
5. Peters GJ, Van der Wilt, CL, Van Groeningen CJ et al (1990) Development of 5-Fluorouracil-Leucovorin combinations. In : Pinedo HM, Rustum YM (eds) Leucovorin modulation of fluoropyrimidines : a new frontier in cancer chemotherapy. International Congress and Symposium Series, n° 158. Royal Society of Medicine Services Ltd., London, pp 21-35
6. Pinedo HM, Peters GJ (1988) Fluorouracil : Biochemistry and pharmacology. J Clin Oncol 6 : 1653-1664
7. Van Kalken CK, Pinedo HM, Giaccone G (1991) Multidrug resistance from the clinical point of view. Eur J Cancer 27 : 1481-1486
8. Miller TP, Grogan TM, Dalton WS et al (1991) P-Glycoprotein expression in malignant lymphoma and reversal of clinical drug resistance with chemotherapy plus high-dose Verapamil. J Clin Oncol 9 : 17-24
9. Giaccone G, Gazdar AF, Beck H et al (1992) Multidrug sensitivity phenotype of human lung cancer cells associated with topoisomerase II expression. Cancer Res 52 : 1666-1674

Mobilization, purification and ex vivo expansion of human peripheral blood progenitor cells

W Brugger, R Mertelsmann, L Kanz

Peripheral blood progenitor cells (PBPCs) have been used with increasing frequency for autografting following high-dose chemotherapy [1]. Successful transplantation of PBPCs with complete and sustained engraftment has been shown in a variety of disorders, including ANLL, lymphoma, neuroblastoma, breast cancer, and other solid tumors [1-8]. When compared with autologous bone marrow transplantation, the advantages of this modality include a more rapid restoration of neutrophils and platelets, the possibility of autografting when bone marrow aspiration is hampered by tumor cell infiltration, fibrosis or hypoplasia following radio-/chemotherapy, and the possibility of reduced contamination with malignant cells in disseminated cancer [9]. The actual level of malignant cell contamination, however, is a matter of debate [10] as well as the exact number of mononuclear cells, CFU-GM colonies or $CD34^+$ cells which have to be transplanted in order to allow a complete and sustained hematopoietic reconstitution [11, 12].

This paper shortly summarizes our own results on stem cell recruitment by different growth factors following standard-dose chemotherapy as well as data on peripheral blood progenitor cell purification and *ex vivo* expansion.

Recruitment of PBPCs

Several methods for the mobilization of PBPCs have been described. Chemotherapy-induced mobilization occurs during the recovery phase after bone marrow hypoplasia, such as cyclophosphamide treatment [13-15]. Hematopoietic growth factors (e.g. G- or GM-CSF) give alone also expand the pool of circulating progenitors [16-19]. This effect is further induced by combining chemotherapy with growth factors such as GM-CSF [8, 17, 21, 23] or G-CSF [20, 26].

At our institution, we investigated the requirements that have to be met to combine standard-dose chemotherapy with the mobilization of PBPCs by different hematopoietic growth factors. The rationale for this approach was to treat patients with standard-dose VP16, Ifosfamide, and Cis-platinum (VIP regimen) for remission induction and at the same time to recruit PBPCs. Therefore, we applied VIP chemotherapy (VP16 500 mg/m^2, Ifosfamide 4,000 mg/m^2, Cisplatin 50 mg/m^2) to a total of 91 patients with solid tumors in order to investigate stem cell mobilization by different growth factors, i.e. G-CSF (n = 40), GM-CSF (n = 18) or the combined sequential administra-

Albert-Ludwigs University Medical Center, Department of Hematology and Oncology, 7800 Freiburg, Germany

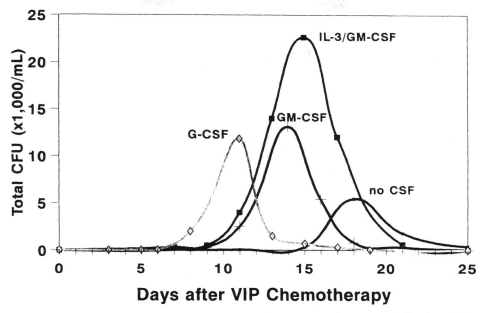

Fig. 1. Kinetic of PBPC recruitment by different growth factors following VIP chemotherapy. Data are presented as total number of clonogenic progenitor cells per mL blood for G-CSF, GM-CSF, or IL-3/GM-CSF treated patients. Control patients were treated without CSF

tion of IL-3 and GM-CSF (n = 18). 15 control patients were treated without growth factors following standard-dose VIP chemotherapy.

The application of different growth factors resulted in a differential induction of PBPCs with peak levels being reached at different time points after VIP chemotherapy (Fig. 1) [22-26]. The combined IL-3/GM-CSF administration resulted in the highest number of progenitor cells with a median of 10,490 CFU-GM/ml blood (range 1,000-24,300) 10,600 BFU-E/ml blood (range 3,870-24,300), 840 CFU-GEMM/ml blood (range 160-2,070), and 600 CFU-Meg/ml blood. The number of CD34$^+$ cells, however, did not differ between the G-CSF, GM-CSF, or IL-3/GM-CSF treated patients (median of 450,000 CD34$^+$ cells/ml blood), suggesting that IL-3/GM-CSF induced CD34$^+$ cells have the highest clonogenic capacity *in vitro*. The biological significance of this finding, however, remains to be demonstrated.

Dual color flow cytometry analyses of mobilized CD34$^+$ cells revealed that the majority of CD34$^+$ cells co-express CD33, CD38 or HLA-DR molecules. However, between 10 and 30 % of CD34$^+$ cells lack the co-expression of CD33, CD38 or HLA-DR antigens, indicating that these cells might comprise early hematopoietic stem cells.

The recruitment of PBPCs was strongly dependent on the prior treatment status. In previously untreated patients, highest numbers of CD34$^+$ cells as well as clonogenic progenitor cells were mobilized. In mildly to moderately pretreated patients (less than 6 chemotherapy cycles), however, significantly less precursor cells could be mobilized. In very intensively pretreated patients, i.e.

patients who have had radiotherapy to more than 20 % bone marrow in addition to more than 6 chemotherapy cycles, only very low numbers of PBPCs with a median of less than 20 CD34$^+$ cells/μL blood could be recruited. These findings argue for the collection of PBPCs early during the treatment of the disease.

When compared to published data, our data document that standard-dose VIP chemotherapy plus IL-3/GM-CSF treatment allows to recruit circulating progenitors in numbers comparable to data published with high-dose Cyclophosphamide + GM-CSF [21]. In addition, we were able to detect not only myeloid and erythroid progenitors but also significant numbers of circulating multipotential as well as megakaryocytic progenitor cells [22]. Moreover, with the use of the standard-dose VIP regimen, there has been no severe thrombocytopenia, which would impede leukapheresis at the time of maximal levels of progenitor cells.

High-dose chemotherapy supported by VIP + G-CSF recruited peripheral blood progenitor cells

So far, VIP chemotherapy + G-CSF primed PBPCs were collected in 24 patients eligible for dose-intensification. One single 2 hour leukapheresis at the time of peak levels of progenitor cells yielded sufficient numbers of PBPCs for autografting (1.6 $\times$ 10^8 mononuclear cells/kg ; 5.4 $\times$ 10^6 CD34$^+$ cells/kg ; 1.2 $\times$ 10^5 CFU-GM/kg). Up to now, PBPCs were retransfused into 15 patients after high-dose VIP chemotherapy with cumulative doses of 1.5 g/m^2 VP16, 12 g/m^2 Ifosfamide, and 150 mg/m^2 Cisplatin. Recovery data of all patients treated with (n = 8) or without (n = 7) PBPC-support revealed a significant reduction in the duration of neutropenia as well as thrombocytopenia in patients with PBPC support as compared to patients who were treated with growth factors alone [25, 26]. Phase II/III studies in patients with chemosensitive tumors or lymphomas are ongoing at our institution to demonstrate the clinical efficacy of such an approach.

Purification and *ex vivo* expansion of peripheral blood progenitor cells

To provide sufficient numbers of PBPCs for repetitive use in high-dose chemotherapy, we investigated the ability of hematopoietic growth factor combinations to expand PBPCs *ex vivo*. VIP chemotherapy + G-CSF recruited CD34$^+$ cells from 18 patients were enriched with an avidin-biotin immunoadsorption column (kindly provided by R.J. Berenson, CellPro, Bothell, WA, USA) to a purity of more than 85 % CD34$^+$ cells and cultured in suspension up to 28 days. A combination of 5 growth factors including stem cell factor (SCF), erythropoietin (EPO), Interleukin-1β (IL-1), IL-3, and IL-6 was identified as the optimal combination for the expansion of clonogenic progenitors. Proliferation peaked at day 12-14 with a mean 190-fold increase (range 46-930) of clonogenic cells (CFU-GM, BFU-E, CFU-GEMM). The number of CFU-GEMM increased

250 fold as compared to pre-expansion values. Moreover, $CD34^+/Lin^-$ ($CD34^+/HLA\text{-}DR^-$; $CD34^+/CD38^-$) cells as well as mafosfamide-resistant $CD34^+$ cells (4-HC resistant cells) increased dramatically during *ex vivo* culture. Interferon-gamma synergized with the 5-Factor combination (1.5 fold increase in clonogenic cells), whereas the addition of G-CSF or GM-CSF decreased the number of clonogenic cells. Large-scale expansion of $CD34^+$ cells in autologous plasma supplemented with the 5-Factor combination resulted in an equivalent expansion. These data indicate that PBPCs from cancer patients can be successfully expanded *ex vivo*. Moreover, our data suggest the feasibility of large-scale expansion, starting from small numbers of $CD34^+$ cells. The number of cells generated *ex vivo* might be sufficient for use in high-dose chemotherapy, possibly obviating the need for aphereses procedures.

References

1. Kessinger A, Armitage JO (1991) The evolving role of autologous peripheral stem cell transplantation following high-dose chemotherapy for malignancies. Blood 77 : 211-213
2. Körbling M, Holle R, Haas R, Knauf W, Dörken B, Ho AD, Kuse R, Pralle H, Fliedner TM, Hunstein W (1990) Autologous blood stem-cell transplantation in patients with advanced Hodgkin's disease and prior radiation to the pelvic site. J Clin Oncol 8 : 978-985
3. Kessinger A, Armitage JO, Smith DM, Landmark JD, Bierman PJ, Weisenburger DD (1989) High-dose therapy and autologous peripheral blood stem cell transplantation for patients with lymphoma. Blood 74 : 1260-1266
4. Körbling M, Dörken B, Ho AD et al (1986) Autologous transplantation of blood-derived hematopoietic stem cells after myeloablative therapy in a patient with Burkitt's lymphoma. Blood 72 : 529-532
5. Juttner CA, To LB, Ho JQK et al (1988) Early lympho-hematopoietic recovery after autografting using peripheral blood stem cells in acute non-lymphoblastic leukemia. Transplant Proc 20 : 40
6. Sheridan WP, Begley CG, Juttner C, Szer J, To LB, Maher D, McGrath KM, Morstyn G, Fox RM (1992) Effect of peripheral-blood progenitor cells mobilised by filgrastim (G-CSF) on platelet recovery after high-dose chemotherapy. Lancet i : 640
7. Siena S, Bregni M, Brando B, Belli N, Ravagnani F, Gondola L, Stern AC, Landsdorp PM, Bonadonna G, Gianni AM (1991) Flow cytometry for clinical estimation of circulating hematopoietic progenitors for autologous transplantation in cancer patients. Blood 77 : 400-406
8. Elias AD, Ayash L, Anderson C, Hund M, Wheller C, Schwartz G, Telpler I, Mazanet R, Lynch C, Pap S, Pelaez J, Reich E, Critchlow J, Demetri G, Bibbo J, Schnipper L, Griffin JD, Frei E, Antman H (1992) Mobilization of peripheral blood progenitor cells by chemotherapy and granulocyte-macrophage colony-stimulating factor for hematologic support after high-dose intensification in breast cancer. Blood 79 : 3036-3042
9. To LB, Russel J, Moore S, Juttner CA (1987) Residual leukemia cannot be detected in very early remission peripheral blood stem cell collections in acute non-lymphoblastic leukemia. Leuk Res 11 : 327
10. Moss TJ, Sandes DG, Lasky LC, Bostrom B (1990) Contamination of peripheral blood stem cell harvests by circulating neuroblastoma cells. Blood 75 : 1879-1883
11. Lasky LC, Ash RC, Kersey JH, Zanjani ED, McCullough J (1982) Collection of pluripotential hematopoietic stem cells by cytapheresis. Blood 59 : 822

12. Juttner CA, To LB, Haylock DN, Cyson PG, Thorp D, Dart GW, Ho JQK, Horvath N, Bardy P (1989) Autologous blood stem cell transplantation. Transplant Proc 21 : 2929
13. Richman CM, Weiner RS, Yankee RA (1976) Increase in circulating stem cells following chemotherapy in man. Blood 47 : 1031
14. Abrams RA, McCormack, Bowles C, Deisseroth AB (1981) Cyclophosphamide treatment expands the circulating haemopoietic stem cell pool in dogs. J Clin Invest 67 : 1392
15. To LB, Shepperd M, Haylock DN, Dyson PG, Charles P, Thorp L, Dale BM, Dart GW, Roberts MM, Sage RE (1989) Single high doses of cyclophosphamide enable the collection of high numbers of haemopoietic stem cells from the peripheral blood. Exp Hematol 18 : 442
16. Haas R, Ho AD, Bredthauer U, Cayeux S, Egerer G, Knauf W, Hunstein W (1990) Successful autologous transplantation of blood stem cells mobilized with rhGM-CSF. Exp Hematol 18 : 94
17. Socinski MA, Cannistra SA, Elias A, Antman KH, Schnipper L, Griffin JD (1988) GM-CSF expands the circulating haemopoietic progenitor cell compartment in man. Lancet ii : 1194-1200
18. Villeval JL, Dührsen U, Morstyn G, Metcalf D (1990) Effect of recombinant human GM-CSF on progenitor cells in patients with advanced malignancies. Br J Hematol 74 : 36
19. Dührsen U, Villeval JL, Boyd J, Kannourakis G, Morstyn G, Metcalf D (1988) Effects of recombinant human G-CSF on hematopoietic progenitor cells in cancer patients. Blood 72 : 2074
20. Pettengell R, Demuynck H, Testa NG, Dexter TM (1992) The engraftment capacity of peripheral blood progenitor cells mobilized with chemotherapy ± G-CSF. Int J Cell Clon 10 : 59-61
21. Gianni AM, Siena S, Bregni M, Tarella C, Stern AC, Pileri A, Bonadonna G (1989) Granulocyte-macrophage colony-stimulating factor to harvest circulating haemopoietic stem cells for autotransplantation. Lancet ii : 580-585
22. Kanz L, Brugger W, Bross KJ, Frisch J, Schulz G, Mertelsmann R (1991) IL-3 $^+$ GM-CSF induced mobilization of myeloid, erythroid, multilineage as well as megakaryocytic progenitor cells following polychemotherapy in cancer patients. Blood 78 : 1222 (abstr)
23. Brugger W, Bross J, Frisch J, Dern P, Weber B, Mertelsmann R, Kanz L (1992) Mobilization of PBPCs by sequential administration of IL-3 and GM-CSF following polychemotherapy with etoposide, Ifosfamide and Cisplatin. Blood 79 : 1193-1200
24. Kanz L, Brugger W, Bross J, Mertelsmann R (1992) Correlation analyses between CD34 $^+$ cells and clonogenic progenitors mobilized into the peripheral blood by IL-3 $^+$ GM-CSF following polychemotherapy in cancer patients. Int J Cell Cloning 10 : 68-70
25. Brugger W, Frisch J, Schulz G, Mertelsmann R, Kanz L (1992) Sequential administration of IL-3 and GM-CSF following standard-dose combination chemotherapy with Etoposide, Ifosfamide and Cisplatin. J Clin Oncol 10 : 1193-1200
26. Brugger W, Birken R, Bertz H, Hecht T, Pressler, Frisch J, Schulz G, Mertelsmann R, Kanz L (1993) Peripheral blood progenitor cells mobilized by chemotherapy plus G-CSF accelerate both neutrophil and platelet recovery after high-dose VP16, Ifosfamide, and Cisplatin. Br J Hematol (in press)
27. Brugger W, Möcklin W, Heimfeld S, Berenson RJ, Mertelsmann R, Kanz L (1993) Ex vivo expansion of enriched peripheral blood CD34 $^+$ progenitor cells by stem cell factor, interleukin-1β, Interleukin-6, Interleukin-3, Interferon-gamma, and Erythropoietin. Blood (in press)

Fluoropyrimidine cancer chronotherapy

WJM Hrushesky*, FO Cope**

Background

In 1972, a paper appeared in *Science* which reported that the arrangement within a given day of 3-hourly doses of Cytosine arabinoside (Ara-C) had a profound effect on the survival rate of mice inoculated with L-1210 leukemia cells [1]. This study was built on extensive prior work demonstrating that all Ara-C toxicities are markedly dependent on the time, in the day/night cycle, at which the drug is administered [2]. Together, the experiments showed unequivocally that, in mice, the timing of Ara-C administration predictably modulates its therapeutic index.

Surprisingly, nearly twenty years later, this simple hypothesis has still not been extended to clinical trials for human leukemia, even though the mainstay treatment for the most common deadly acute leukemias has remained Ara-C, used at higher and higher dose intensity with greater and greater toxicity [3]. In the meantime, it has been shown that all anthracyclines, which are generally coupled with Ara-C to treat the non-lymphocytic leukemias, also exhibit a pronounced circadian time dependency in their pharmacology, toxicology and efficacy in mice and in humans [4-6]. Furthermore, many combination chemotherapy studies, done in follow-up to the initial Ara-C study, have demonstrated that the addition of a second or third drug to the regimen seldom interferes with the enhancement in therapeutic index resulting from circadian optimization of each drug [7].

A personal background of clinical experience with high-dose cytoxan in G.W. Santos' pioneering bone marrow transplant unit and with ultra-high-dose intensity chemotherapy for small-cell lung cancer as a member of the National Cancer Institute (NCI) solid tumor service, made it impossible for me to ignore the likely clinical import of diminishing the toxicity and increasing the efficacy of the drugs available to us by any means, including optimal circadian timing. In Minnesota, we began a series of studies in rodents that led to the circadian optimization of the Doxorubicin/Cisplatin combination [8]. NCI-sponsored randomized clinical studies then revealed that each and every Doxorubicin and Cisplatin toxicity is largely dependent upon the circadian timing of these agents in human beings [4, 9]. In patients with widespread ovarian cancer, optimal circadian drug timing resulted in safer administration of higher doses of drug and, in turn, a 4-fold improvement in the 5-year survival rate of women with advanced ovarian cancer [10]. These clinical studies have also remained largely ignored.

More recently, a shift in patient accrual and the availability of program-

---

* Professor of Medicine and Microbiology/Immunobiology, Albany Medical College of Union University Volweiler Laureate, Stratton VA Medical Center, ** Ross Laboratories Medical Department

mable, implantable drug-delivery devices have pointed us toward studies of the time dependency of Fluoropyrimidine pharmacology, toxicology and efficacy. As with Cytosine arabinoside, Doxorubicin/Cisplatin and other anticancer agents, the Fluoropyrimidine story began with rodent experimentation. Studies with mice in the early 1980's revealed that the LD_{50} of 5-Fluorouracil (5-FU), a mainstay of solid tumor treatment, is markedly and reproducibly higher when given in the sleep span [11, 12]. Peters confirmed this early work and extended it to show that both nonspecific 5-FU toxicity and toxicity toward a murine colon carcinoma are each dependent on circadian timing [13].

Fluoropyrimidine chronotherapy

The programmable automatic delivery systems initially available for clinical cancer treatment were of small volume, and thus required highly concentrated drug. In anticipation of new clinical chronobiologic chemotherapy studies, Fluorodeoxyuridine (FUDR), a more highly concentratable Fluoropyrimidine, was studied in mice and rats. Chronotoxicology studies of intravenous and intraperitoneal bolus FUDR administration in mice revealed that the safest time for this drug was several hours earlier in the day than for 5-FU [14]. The highest LD_{50} (lowest toxicity) occurred reproducibly late in the daily activity span. FUDR has an extremely short half-life, and hence must be administered by constant infusion. Extensive continuous infusion studies performed upon Fisher 344 rats afflicted with the Fluoropyrimidine-sensitive 13762-NT adenocarcinoma revealed that continuous infusions weighted in the late activity and usual sleep span are reproducibly far less toxic and significantly more effective than constant-rate infusions or infusions that delivered peak levels of the drug at other times during the day [15].

With this preclinical information, we initiated a series of randomized clinical studies to investigate whether the systemic or intrahepatic toxicities of FUDR can be lessened and the dose intensity safely increased by administering the drug late in the cancer patient's usual daily activity span [16]. So far, we have shown that optimal drug timing offers a clinical advantage for systemic FUDR infusion in patients with metastatic renal cell cancer [17]; and for intrahepatic FUDR infusion in colorectal cancer patients with liver metastases [18]. Moreover, Lévi has demonstrated a clinical advantage to shaping 5-FU infusion (to peak at 4 am) in patients with widespread colorectal cancer [19].

We and other investigators have begun to attempt to define why the mechanisms that underlie the circadian time dependency of fluoropyrimidine toxicity and anticancer activity. Of potential importance is the way drugs are handled by the organs primarily responsible for catabolism or excretion (drug pharmacology), the way drugs are handled by the targets of toxicity (biochemical pharmacology) and, correlatively, the cell-cycle phase of the target cells at the time of drug exposure (circadian cytokinetics). Figure 1 demonstrates the circadian time dependency of FUDR continuous infusion in tumor bearing rats (left panel) and in patients with metastatic renal cell carcinoma.

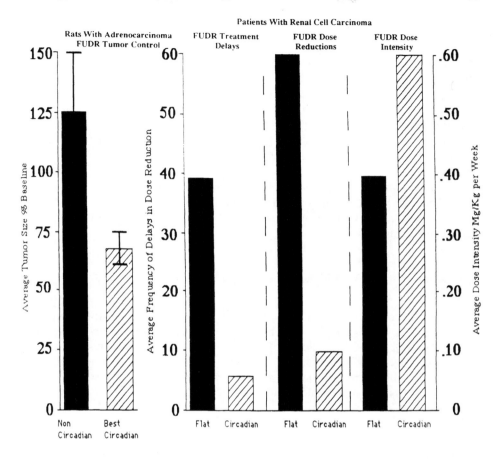

Fig. 1. This figure contrasts the circadian schedule dependency of FUDR induced tumor control in a rat tumor model system (left panel) with the circadian schedule dependency of FUDR measures of toxicity in human patients. Each member of these groups of rats and cancer patients was randomized to receive the identical dose of infusional FUDR chemotherapy. In one group, rats or patients received continuous constant rate infusion *(black)* or infusions peaking late in each daily activity span and early in the usual daily sleep span. In the schedules, 68 % of each day's dose was given during these 6 hours, 15 % in each abutting daily quadrant and 2 % of each daily dose was given near daily arising. In the rat, toxicity of FUDR was affected by the circadian shape of the infusion (data not shown) and tumor shrinkage was enhanced by optimal circadian FUDR infusion shape (left panel). In cancer patients, toxicity was markedly diminished by optimal timing (data not shown). This circadian toxicity dependence resulted in 8 times more frequent treatment delays and 6 times more frequent dose reductions than if flat infusion was employed. This also resulted in being able to safely increase the average dose intensity by circadian infusion by at least 50 % (from 0.4 to 0.65 mg/kg/week of FUDR), data from Roemeling and Hrushesky (1989) J Clin Oncol 7 : 1710-1719

5-FU chronopharmacokinetics

The circadian-dependent pharmacology of continuous, constant-rate 5-FU infusion, as measured by rhythmic fluctuations in plasma levels of the drug throughout the day was first demonstrated by Petit et al [20] and later by Harris et al [21]. Each group noted marked variations in pharmacokinetics at different times of the day, although the timing of peak FU levels differed between the two groups of patients. The difference may be related to the fact that the patients in the first study received Cisplatin at fixed time of day prior to each 5 day 5-FU infusion, whereas the patients in the second study received only 5-FU and for much longer spans. Nonetheless, both papers clearly demonstrate that there are large, within-study and cross-subject-reproducible differences in plasma levels of 5-FU at different times of day during a continuous, constant-rate drug infusion.

Circadian fluoropyrimidine biochemical pharmacology

Work by Tuchman [22] and, later, by Diasio et al [23] demonstrated the importance of Dihydropyrimidine dehydrogenase (DPD) as the rate-limiting enzyme involved in the breakdown of 5-FU to non-toxic metabolites. When human peripheral blood mononuclear cells were isolated around the clock in seven subjects, Tuchman found that DPD levels were much higher just after usual sleep onset than at other times of the day [24]. In their recent elegant *ex vivo* rat liver perfusion study, Harris et al demonstrate unequivocally that 5-FU clearance and metabolism by the liver are critically circadian-stage dependent. Eight times as much 5-FU was extracted per unit time from perfused rat livers removed in mid to late sleep compared to those removed in mid activity [25]. Tuchman's data showing that the levels of human mononuclear DPD [24] peak during sleep are consistent with the results of the perfusion experiments in rodents. In aggregate, these data suggest that a prominent circadian rhythm in DPD activity exhibited by both organs of metabolism as well as by cells more peripheral to 5-FU catabolism, may be responsible, at least in part, for the circadian dependence of 5-FU toxicity in rodents and humans and perhaps also for the circadian dependence of its anticancer efficacy documented in rodent models and, more recently, suggested by work with cancer patients.

The circadian pharmacology and biochemical pharmacology of FUDR are less clearly established than those of 5-FU, in part, because the former drug is administered in much lower milligram amounts and requires much more sensitive analytical methods. This picture is also complicated by the fact that these two Fluoropyrimidines are interconvertible. In preliminary experiments, von Roemeling has observed a 2-fold circadian difference in the convertibility of FUDR to 5-FU, indicating that FUDR pharmacodynamics may depend upon the circadian DPD rhythms at some times of the day but not others [26]. The activities of other enzymes of important in the activation of FUDR to FDUMP (i.e., Diehydrouracil dehydrogenase, Uridine phosphorylase and Thymidine phosphorylase) have each been shown to be subject to circadian rhythms in mouse liver [27], however, assessment of the exact contribution of these enzymes to the crisp, high amplitude circadian rhythm in FUDR toxicity and efficacy requires further work in murine and human systems. Together, these preclinical and clinical results with Fluoropyrimidine indicate that circadian time structure in the organs of catabolism and excretion and the biochemical enzyme activity rhythms in normal or malignant target cells may each be critically important in determining the optimal time of day for bolus drug administration or the optimal circadian shape of continuous infusion Fluoropyrimidine therapy. Because the metabolic processes necessary to catabolize these two closely related drugs are different yet related and the intracellular targets are overlapping but to some extent distinct, the two agents when given by bolus have distinct optimal circadian timings that are nearly a third of a day apart [14]. However, all therapeutic strategies which focus the Fluoropyrimidine upon thymidylate synthase result in an optimal time of day in the first half of the daily sleep span. These strategies include the use of FUDR which is metabolically closer to FDUMP than 5-FU ; the longterm infusion of 5-FU also pushes more of the drug toward FDUMP and less toward incorporation into RNA resulting in greater TS inhibition ; adding Leukovorin to 5-FU also increases Fluoropyrimidine induced TS inhibition by stabilizing the FDUMP/TS complex. The fact that each of these three therapeutic maneuvers which result in an optimal circadian timing located in the first half of the daily sleep span and focus on TS blockade indicates TS blockade may be least effectively achieved in normal gut tissue at this time of day and that this fact results in less gut damage from the Fluoropyrimidine which is given in the first half of the daily sleep span.

Normal tissue circadian cytokinetic coordination

In addition to the circadian patterns of crucial enzyme activities, circadian patterns of cytokinetic activity in malignant and nonmalignant tissues damaged by Fluoropyrimidines may be of equal importance in explaining the circadian pharmacodynamics. Both 5-FU and FUDR are most active against dividing cells undergoing DNA synthesis. DNA synthesis in all tissues studied throughout the circadian cycle is nonrandomly distributed throughout the day [28]. Depending on dose and duration of infusion, the gut, skin and bone marrow are the primary targets of Fluoropyrimidine toxicity. Human skin [29], bone marrow [30, 31] and human colorectal mucosa have each been found to exhibit marked circadian rhythms in DNA synthesis [32]. When FUDR is infused such that lower levels are delivered during early morning hours, the clinical toxicity is markedly diminished and dose intensity can be safely elevated. In humans, the dose-limiting target of FUDR infusional toxicity is the colorectal mucosa. Serial biopsies of rectal mucosa every three hours for 24 hours from 24 human volunteers in both the fed and fasted states reveal that there is much greater *in vitro* uptake of ^{3}H-thymidine (presumably reflecting DNA synthesis) in colonic epithelial cells removed during the early morning hours (4 hours

Fig. 2. *The top panel* of this figure illustrates the experimentally determined circadian rhythmic patterns of the activities of 3 key enzymes in fluoropyrimidine metabolism. Dihydropyridine dehydrogenase (DPD) catabolizes 5-Fluorouracil (5-FU) to noncytotoxic metabolites; thymidine phosphorylase (TP) converts 5-FU to its nucleotide fluorodeoxyuridine (FUDR); thymidine kinase (TK) converts FUDR to fluordeoxyuridyl monophosphate FDUMP which binds to thymidylate synthase (TS) blocking DNA synthesis by starving the cell for thymidine. DPD activity peaks about midnight; TP activity does not vary during the day; TK activity peaks around noon. *The middle panel* demonstrates the result of these rhythmic enzyme activities upon the pharmacokinetics of constant rate 5-FU infusion (5-FU levels) and the final activation product FDUMP. DPD removes 5-FU rhythmically during the

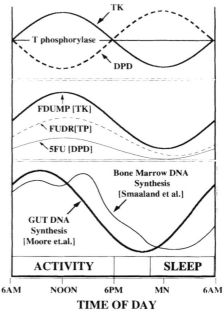

day making much more 5-FU available in the early daytime hours, TP converts 5-FU to FUDR at a constant rate but the higher substrate levels in the morning result in higher FUDR levels in the morning. TK activity is higher in the morning converting more of the higher levels of FUDR to FDUMP at that time of day. *The bottom panel* illustrates the experimentally determined circadian patterns of gut and bone marrow DNA synthesis in human beings. Much more DNA synthesis is ongoing at the time of day associated with highest FDUMP levels. This coincidence of enzyme activities and tissue DNA synthesis results in the experimentally observed amplitude circadian rhythm in susceptibility to 5-FU. Giving a zero order 5-FU infusion results in non zero order and very unfavorable pharmacodynamics from the perspective of toxicity to normal tissues. Changing the circadian pattern of the infusion so that most of the daily continuous infusion that is given in the evening would completely change the resultant pharmacokinetics and pharmacodynamics to a much more favorable toxic therapeutic profile

prior to usual awakening) than later in the day and evening [33]. This circadian-stage coincidence of minimal ^{3}H-thymidine uptake and minimal FUDR toxicity in colon epithelial cells is intriguing and warrants further study.

Continuous 5-FU constant rate infusion

The top panel of Figure 2 depicts the circadian time structures of the activities of certain key enzymes relevant to Fluoropyrimidine cytotoxic effects. This figure also relates the implications of these rhythms to Fluoropyrimidine metabolism during a continuous infusion of 5-FU at a constant (zero order) rate. Thymidine phosphorylase is an important enzyme in the conversion of 5-FU to FUDR. This enzyme activity remains constant throughout the day. This results in a constant rate conversion of 5-FU to FUDR. Dihydropyridine dehydrogenase activity which catabolizes 5-FU is, however, rhythmic throughout each day. The waning of DPD activity during the daily activity span results in an accumulation of 5-FU during the day. The endogenous circadian increase in DPD activity during the evening results in a daily lowering 5-FU concentrations during the evening. This enzyme activity rhythm results in a waxing and waning of the 5-FU available for activation to FUDR by Thymidine phosphorylase. The effective concentration of FUDR (which is subsequently converted to FDUMP) is therefore higher during the morning hours when less FU has been removed resulting in a more efficient conversion of FU to FUDR even though the activity of the enzyme that makes this conversion is not changing during the day. The activity of Thymidine kinase which converts FUDR to FDUMP, which in turn binds to and inactivates Thymidylate synthase and thereby blocks DNA synthesis is not constant throughout the day. This enzyme has far greater activity in the morning hours when levels of 5-FU and thereby FUDR are highest. This Thymidine kinase circadian rhythmic activity results in an even greater amplitude in daily FDUMP availability. The middle panel demonstrates the effects that these circadian patterns of enzyme activity have upon the concentrations of Fluoropyrimidine and its active metabolite during a constant rate continuous infusion of 5-FU. The amount of target enzyme (Thymidylate synthase) activity also covaries with the DNA synthetic capacity of the tissue. Thymidylate synthase is in fact only in critical supply during the process of DNA synthesis. The bottom panel of Figure 2 demonstrates the experimentally determined circadian pattern of DNA synthetic activity in the two human tissues which are most prominently damaged by Fluoropyrimidines. DNA synthetic activity in human gut mucosa and human bone marrow cycles prominently within each day. Much more DNA synthesis occurs in the morning, during the first half of the daily activity span. The daily timing of high DNA synthesis activity in both of these critical tissues occurs at the time of day when DPD levels are lowest and T are highest ; therefore the time of day associated with highest 5-FU, FUDR and FDUMP levels. This timing coincides with time of day of highest DNA synthesis and the time of day associated with the greatest need for Thymidylate synthase activity. These coincidences mean that a zero order FU infusion results in a high amplitude circadian rhythm in the active compound FDUMP. This peak daily FDUMP availability happens at the time of day associated with the highest daily DNA synthesis and therefore the time of day of the greatest need for Thymidylate synthase activity in gut and bone marrow and the time of day of highest tissue susceptibility. Changing the 5-FU infusion shape to give more drug in the evening hours and less in the morning hours would be expected, for the same reasons, to result in predictably less interference with gut and bone marrow DNA synthesis and less normal tissue toxicity.

Tumor circadian cytokinetic dynamics

Few data are available to evaluate whether spontaneous human malignancies are cytokinetically coordinated on the circadian time scale. The most thorough evaluation of this difficult question has been accomplished in patients with ovarian cancer. Braly, levecz et al sampled cells washed from the peritoneal cavities of a large number of women, every 2-4 hours, for up to four days. Using sophisticated Cytofluorometric techniques, these investigators found circadian coordination of the proportion of both malignant epithelial and nonmalignant mesothelial cells synthesizing DNA ; that is, a higher proportion of malignant cells were actively synthesizing DNA in the morning hours while a higher proportion of nonmalignant cells synthesizing DNA in the morning hours while a higher proportion of nonmalignant cells were engaged in DNA synthesis in the evening hours [34]. In another study, a smaller number of patients with non-Hodgkin's lymphoma underwent thin needle aspiration of tumor masses every four hours for a minimum of 24 hours. Although no clear population circadian rhythm in the proportion of cytofluorometrically determined S-phase cells has been found, some individuals were found to exhibit large time-dependent differences with peak activities clustering in the early morning hours of the day [35]. Serial biopsies of tumor and normal skin in one of our patients with widespread cutaneous epidermoid carcinoma revealed high amplitude circadian rhythms in mitotic index of her tumor cell population with the same phase as her normal skin. Mitotic indices of tumor and normal tissues were identical at the times of daily lowest values, whereas tumor cell mitoses were many-fold more frequent at times in the day associated with the usual highest daily mitotic activity (W.J.M. Hrushesky, E. Haus, D. Lanning, unpubl.). These limited data suggest that the cytokinetic activity of tumor tissues is likely to be coordinated in circadian time and that there may well be windows in circadian time when cell-cycle-stage specific attacks on these cells may be more or less effective.

Taken together, the preclinical and clinical data defining optimum timings of 5-FU and FUDR are compelling. The time-dependent differences in toxic/therapeutic ratios of these drugs are substantial and we are now beginning to understand the biochemical and cellular mechanisms that contribute to these differences.

Implications for clinical trial and cytotoxic drug discovery and drug development

A complete understanding of circadian control mechanisms should not be a prerequisite for incorporation of these ideas into clinical trials. It is clear that many advances in the chemotherapeutic control of human malignancy have been gained without a sophisticated understanding of the mechanisms of action of each drug in effective chemotherapy regimens. In my view, our present knowledge of circadian pharmacology is sufficient to enable us not only to optimize the effectiveness of the chemotherapeutic agents currently in use but perhaps also to expand the repertoire of effective anticancer agents. It is daunting to realize that the scores of anticancer drugs discovered in murine screens and subsequently rejected in phase I trials because of unacceptably high toxicity were recommended for clinical study on the basis of murine toxicology and efficacy studies performed during the animals' usual sleep span and were later rejected clinically on the basis of studies routinely performed during the activity span of cancer patients.

The future

As newer therapeutic approaches are developed with growth factors and other genetically engineered proteins, temporal questions become ever more important. We have already found, for example, that the $_{50}$ for tumor necrosis factor varies one log and its curative efficacy varies some 7-fold, depending on what time of day it is administered [36]; that recombinant human erythropoeitin increases reticulocyte response 10-fold if it is given at an optimal circadian stage [37]; and that recombinant human Interleukin-2 either doubles splenocyte (putative) natural killer (NK) cell number or fails to increase it, depending on whether it is given during the rest or activity phase of the murine circadian cycle [38]. More importantly, perhaps, IL-2 circadian timing has been repeatedly shown to be responsible for reproducible tumor growth enhancement if given at certain times of day. The identical dose and schedule at an opposite time of day is associated with reproducible tumor shrinkage [39]. A wide variety and rapidly growing number of programmable drug delivery strategies are being perfected and applied to the practical challenges of circadian-optimized treatment [40]. We can no longer afford to deny either the existence or the importance of the circadian time structure of living organisms if we are to optimally apply both established and new technologies to effective cancer therapy.

References

1. Haus E, Halberg F, Scheving LE, Cardoso S, uhl JFW, Sothern R, Shiotsuka RN, Hwang DS, Pauly JE (1972) Increased tolerance of leukemic mice to arabinolsyl cytosine with schedule adjusted to circadian system. Science 177 : 80-82
2. Scheving LE, Haus E, Kuhl JFW et al (1976) Close reproduction by different laboratories of characteristics of circadian rhythm in 1-β-D-arabinofuranosylcytosine. Cancer Res 36 : 1133-1137
3. Freireich E (1987) Ara-C : A Twenty Year Update. J Clin Oncol 5 (4) : 523-524
4. Hrushesky WJM (1985) Circadian timing of cancer chemotherapy. Science 228 : 73-75
5. Levi F, Mechkouri M, Roulon A, Bailleul F, Lemaigre G, Reinberg A, Mathe G (1985) Circadian rhythm in tolerance of mice for the new anthracycline analog 4'-0-Tetrahydropyranyl Adriamycin (THP). Eur J Cancer Clin Oncol 21 : 1245-1251
6. Mormont MC, Roemeling Rv, Sothern RB, Berestka JS, Langevin TR, Hrushesky WJM (1988) Circadian rhythm and seasonal dependence in tolerance of mice to 4'-Epi-Doxorubicin. Invest New Drugs 6 : 273-283
7. Scheving LE, Burns ER, Pauly JE et al (1977) Survival and care of leukemic mice after circadian optimization of treatment with cyclophosphamide and 1-β-D-Arabinofuranosylcytosine. Cancer Res 37 : 3648-3655
8. Sothern RB, Levi F, Haus E, Halberg F, Hrushesky WJM (1988) Doxorubicin-cisplatin control of a murine plasmacytoma depends upon circadian stage of treatment. J Natl Cancer Inst 80 : 1232-1237

9. Hrushesky WJM (1983) The clinical application of chronobiology to oncology. Am J Anat 168 : 519-542
10. Hrushesky WJM, Roemeling Rv, Sothern RB (1989) Circadian chronotherapy : from animal experiments to human cancer chemotherapy. In : Lemmer B (ed) Chronopharmacology : Cellular and Biochemical Interactions. Marcel Dekker, New York/Basel, pp 439-473
11. Popovic P, Popovic V, Baughman J (1982) Circadian rhythm and 5-Fluorouracil toxicity in C3H mice. Biomed Therm 25 : 185-187
12. Burns ER, Beland SS (1984) Effect of biological time on the determination of the LD_{50} of 5-Fluorouracil in mice. Pharmacol 28 : 296-300
13. Peters GJ, Van Dijk J, Nadal JC, Van Groeningen CJ, Lankelma J, Pinedo HM (1987) Diurnal variation in the therapeutic efficacy of 5-Fluorouracil against murine colon cancer. In Vivo 1 : 113-118
14. Gonzalez JL, Sothern RB, Thatcher G, Nguyen N, Hrushesky WJM (1989) Substantial difference in timing of murine circadian susceptibility to 5-Fluorouracil and FUDR. Proc AACR (abstr), 2452
15. Roemeling Rv, Hrushesky WJM (1990) Circadian FUDR infusion pattern determines its therapeutic index. J Natl Cancer Inst 82 : 386-393
16. Roemeling Rv, Hrushesky WJM (1990) The advantage of circadian shaping of Fluoropyrimidine infusions. In : Lokich JL (ed) Cancer Chemotherapy by Infusion, Volume 2. Precept Press, Chicago
17. Hrushesky WJM, Roemeling Rv, Lanning RM, Rabatin JT (1990) Circadian shaped infusions of FUDR for progressive metastatic renal cell carcinoma. J Clin Oncol 8 : 1504-1513
18. Wesen C, Roemeling Rv, Lanning R, Grage T, Olson G, Hrushesky WJM (1992) Circadian modification of intra-arterial FUDR infusion rate reduces its toxicity and permits higher dose intensity. J Infus Chemo 2 (2) : 89-93
19. Levi F, Soussan A, Adam R, Caussanel JP, Metzger G, Misset JL, Descorps-Decleres, Kustlinger F, Lorphelin D, Jasmin C, Bismuth H, Reinberg A, Mathe G (1989) Programmable-in-time pumps for chronotherapy of patients with colorectal cancer with 5-day circadian-modulated venous infusion of 5-Fluorouracil (CVI-5FUra). Proc ASCO (abstr) 429
20. Petit E, Milano G, Levi F, Thyss A, Bailleul F, Schneider M (1988) Circadian rhythm-varying plasma concentration of 5-Fluorouracil during a five-day continuous venous infusion at a constant rate in cancer patients. Cancer Res 48 : 1676-1679
21. Harris BE, Song R, Soong SJ, Diasio RB (1990) Relationship between Dihydropyrimidine dehydrogenase activity and plasma 5-Fluorouracil levels with evidence for circadian variation of enzyme activity and plasma drug levels in cancer patients receiving 5-Fluorouracil by protracted continuous infusion. Cancer Res 50 : 197-201
22. Tuchman M, Stoeckeler JS, Kiang DT, O'Dea RF, Ramnaraine ML, Mirkin BL Familial Pyrimidinemia and Pyrimidinuria associated with severe Fluorouracil toxicity. N Engl J Med 313 : 245-249
23. Diasio RB, Beavers TL, Carpenter JT (1988) Familial deficiency of Dihydropyrimidine dehydrogenase biochemical basis for familial Pyrimidinemia and severe 5-Fluorouracil-induced toxicity. J Clin Invest 81 : 47-51
24. Tuchman M, Roemeling Rv, Lanning R, Sothern RB, Hrushesky WJM (1988) Sources of variability of Dihydropyrimidine dehydrogenase (DPD) activity in human blood mononuclear cells. In : Reinberg A, Smolensky M, Labrecque G (eds) Annual Review of Chronopharmacology, volume 5. Pergamon Press, New York, pp 399-402
25. Harris BE, Song R, Soong SJ, Diasio RB (1989) Circadian variation of 5-Fluorouracil catabolism in isolated perfused rat liver. Cancer Res 49 : 6610-6614

26. Roemeling Rv, Fukuda E, Fudin J, Mormont MC, Sothern R, Hrushesky WJM (1989) Are FUDR pharmacokinetics circadian stage dependent ? Proc AACR (abstr) 2345
27. El Kouni MH, Naguib FMN, Cha S (1989) Circadian rhythm of Dihydrouracil dehydrogenase (DHUDase), Uridine phosphorylase (UrdPase), and Thymidine phosphorylase (dThdPase) in mouse liver. FASEB J 3 : A397
28. Scheving LE, Tsai TH, Feuers RJ, Scheving LA (1989) Cellular mechanisms involved in the action of anticancer drugs. In : Lemmer B (ed) Chronopharmacology : Cellular and Biochemical Interactions. Marcel Dekker, New York, pp 317-369
29. Scheving LE Mitotic activity in the human epidermis (1959) The Anatomical Record 135 : 7-19
30. Mauer AM (1965) Diurnal variation of proliferative activity in the human bone marrow. Blood 26 : 1-7
31. Smaaland R, Sletvold O, Bjerknes R, Lote, Laerum OD (1987) Circadian variations of cell cycle distribution in human bone marrow. Chronobiologia 14 : 239
32. Buchi N, Rubin NJ, Moore JG (1989) Circadian cellular proliferation in human rectal mucosa. In : Reinberg A, Smolensly M, Labrecque G (eds) Annual Review of Chronopharmacology, volume 5. Pergamon Press, Oxford, p 355
33. Buchi N, Moore JG, Hrushesky WJM, Sothern RB, Rubin NH (1991) Circadian rhythm of cellular proliferation in the human rectal mucosa. Gastroenterology 101 : 410-415
34. Klevecz RR, Shymko RM, Blumenfeld D, Braly PS (1987) Circadian gating of S phase in human ovarian cancer. Cancer Res 47 : 6267-6271
35. Smaaland R, Lote K, Laerum OD, Vokac Z (1989) A circadian study of cell cycle distribution in non-Hodgkin lymphomas. In : Reinberg A, Smolensky M, Labrecque G (eds) Annual Review of Chronopharmacology, volume 5. Pergamon Press, Oxford, p 383
36. Langevin T, Young J, Walker K, Roemeling Rv, Nygaard S, Hrushesky WJM (1987) The toxicity of tumor necrosis factor (TNF) is reproducibly different at specific times of the day. Proc AACR 28 (abstr) 281
37. Wood PA, Sanchez S, Hrushesky WJM (1991) Evidence for circadian dependency of recombinant human erythropoietin (rhEPO) response in the mouse. In : Hrushesky WJM, Langer R, Theeuwes F (eds) Temporal Control of Drug Delivery. Ann NY Acad Sci 618 : 619-622
38. Roemeling Rv, Salzer M, Connerty M, DeMaria L, Wood PA, Portuese E, Sanchez S, DeConti, R, Chikkappa G, Pasquale D, Ferro T, Hrushesky WJM (1990) Circadian IL-2 bioactivity in mouse spleen and bone-marrow. Proc AACR (abstr) 1571]
39. Sanchez S, Hrushesky WJM, Wood PA, Vyzula R (1993) Host-tumor balance depends upon IL-2 circadian timing, AACR, Orlando, FL, May 19-22 [submitted abstr]
40. Hrushesky WJM (1988) The rationale for non-zero-order drug delivery using automatic, computer-based drug delivery systems (chronotherapy). J Biol Response Modifiers. 6 : 587-598

Abstract. *Circadian variation in drug metabolism and tissue sensitivity to drugs impacts their activity and toxicity. A growing body of data suggests that therapy may be improved and toxicity reduced, by administering antineoplastic agents at carefully selected times of the day. This article briefly reviews molecular, cellular and organismic time keeping mechanisms as well as cytokinetic, pharmacokinetic and pharmacodynamic data, which support the predictable and exploitable nonlinear dynamic relationship between dose and effect that occurs each day.*

Chemo-immunotherapy of metastatic malignant melanoma The Salpetriere Hospital (SOMPS) experience

D Khayat*, E Antoine*, O Rixe*, JM Tourani**, E Vuillemin*, Ch Borel*, A Benhammouda*, L Thill***, C Franks****, G Auclerc*, M Weil*, Cl Soubrane*, P Banzet*****

Chemotherapy as well as immunotherapy seem today to have reached a plateau in Melanoma, with objective response rates between 10 to 25 % for the best studied single agents like Dacarbazine, Nitrosoureas, Interleukine-2 and Interferons. Although long lasting and complete responses have been obtained in those studies, clinical benefit is still achieved only in a minority of patients. More successful strategies are necessary for the systemic treatment of metastatic malignant melanoma.

Table 1. CDDP combinations in melanoma patients

Investigators	Chemotherapeutic regimens	No pts	% CR	% PR	% RR
Del Prete (1984) [6]	CDDP/DTIC/BCNU/TAM	20	20	35	55
McClay (1987) [15]	CDDP/DTIC/BCNU/TAM	20	0	50	50
(1989) [16]	CDDP/DTIC/BCNU	20	5	5	10
(1989) [16]	CDDP/DTIC/BCNU + TAM	21	9.5	43	52.5
Adlakha (1990) [1]	CDDP/DTIC/BCNU + TAM	20	5	35	40
Murren (1991) [18]	CDDP HD/DTCI	22	14	18	32
Stephens (1991) [25]	CDDP HD/DTIC	30	0	17	17
Buzaid (1991) [5]	CDDP HD/DTIC + TAM	23	9	4	13
Glover (1987) [10]	CDDP HD + WR2721	36	0	53	53
Avril (1992) [3]	CDDP HD + WR2721	21	15	20	35

A number of combination chemotherapy regimens has been reported to have higher response rates than single agent therapy and recently the introduction of cisplatinum has resulted in some promising regimens (Table 1). However role of combination chemotherapy is still controversial because of the lack of prospective trials directly demonstrating an increase in response rate and in

---

* Medical Oncology Department, Salpetriere Hospital Paris, France,
** Medical Oncology Department, Laennec Hospital Paris, France,
*** Roche France Laboratory, Neuilly-sur-Seine, France,
**** Eurocetus BV, Amsterdam, The Netherlands,
***** Surgery Department, Saint-Louis Hospital, Paris, France

median survival over use of DTIC alone. Median duration of response of several three or four-drug regimens ranges between 6 and 9 months and median survival appears not to be substantially better than DTIC alone. Biological therapies and particularly interferons and Interleukine-2 have been intensively studied during the past decade. Overall response rate for IFNs in melanoma ranges 12 % to 18 % with some disease control for long time in few patient, however optimal schedule and doses for IFNs in melanoma patients remain unclear. Results from phase II trials using I-L2 (with or without LAK cells) have shown a reproducible anti melanoma activity with objective responses in the 10 % to 30 % range using a variety of doses and schedules combinations. Median duration of response is about 6 to 8 months but some responses, even in visceral metastatic sites, have been extremely durable extending over 3 years. Although synergistically in preclinical models, combination of IL-2 and IFN in clinical trials have produced disappointing result with response rates ranging from 20 to 30 % (Table 2). In an attempt to enhance response rate, complete response rate and duration of response, some investigators have combined cytotoxics drugs and cytokines.

Table 2. IL-2 and IFN in advanced melanoma

	Evaluable patients	CR	PR	RR	%
Rosenberg (1989) [22-23]	39	3	10	12	33
Lee (1989) [13]	16	1	3	4	25
Atzpodiem [2]	8	0	1	1	12
Mittelmann (1990) [17]	14	0	0	0	0
Bergman (1990)	15	0	3	3	27
Goey (1990) [11]	35	0	10	10	28
Stahel (1990)	10	0	2	2	20
Whitehead (1990)	14	0	0	0	0

Preclinical data support the concept of combining cytokine and cytotoxic drugs to enhance synergistically their antiproliferative activity. Chemotherapy may potentiate immunotherapy not only by cytoreduction but also by functioning as a biomodulator with multiple levels of possible interactions like vascularisation, blood flow, alteration in the cellular drugs uptake, modulation of drug target enzymes, membrane fluidity, antigen stabilisation and immunologic responsiveness.

Although molecular mechanisms underlying these interactions should be more clearly defined, synergistic interactions between cytokines and cytotoxic agents seem to be sequence and schedule dependent.

First studies have combined IL-2 (with or without LAK) or IFNs and the best single chemotherapeutic agent, DTIC, in various doses and schedules.

However, reported results from published studies failed to indicate an improvement as compared to single agent used alone with response rates range 22 to 33 % (Table 3).

Table 3. DTIC and IL-2 in advanced melanoma

	Regimen	Evaluable patients	RR (%)
Shiloni (1989) [24]	DTIC/IL-2 (CI)	27	22
Stoter (1989) [26]	DTIC/IL-2 (CI)	33	22
Dillman (1990) [8]	DTIC/IL-2 + LAK	27	26
Papadopoulos (1990) [19]	DTIC/IL-2 bolus	30	33
Flaherty (1990) [9]	DTIC/IL-2 bolus	32	22
Flaherty (1990)	DTIC/IL-2 bolus	15	0

Table 4. CDDP based chemo-immunocombination in metastatic melanoma

Investigators	Regimen	No pts	CR (%)	PR	RR (%)	MDR	MS
Blair (1991) [4]	CDDP d. 1 DTIC d. 1, D. 12-16/d. 19-23 IL-2 bolus d. 12, d. 16/d. 19, d. 23	28	5 (18)	7	43	—	10
Demchak (1991) [7]	CDDP HD, d. 33, d. 54 IL-2 bolus d. 1-5, d. 15-19	27	3 (11)	7	37	4	—
Hamblin (1992) [12]	CDDP d. 1 DTIC d. 1 IL-2 CI d. 12-17/d. 20-25 IFN sc	12	3 (25)	7	83	—	—
Richard (1992) [21]	CDDP d. 1-3/d. 22-25 BCNU d. 1, DTIC d. 1-3 TAM p.o. 2xd.x6 weeks IL-2 bolus d. 4-8/d. 17-21 IFN sc d. 4-8/d. 17-21	74	11 (15)	29	57	9.1	14
Legha (1992) [14]	CDDP-DTIC VLB IL-2 CI alternating IFN	30	6 (20)	11	56	5	—
Khayat (1992)	CDDP d. 0 IL-2 d. 3-d. 6/d. 17-d. 21 IFN sc tiw/week	39	5 (13)	16	54	6	10

Although cisplatyl at doses $\leqslant 100$ mg/m^2 produces responte rates of less than 15 % when used as single agent, preclinical data suggest a potential synergism or at least additivity when combined with IL-2 and/or Interferon. Recently, clinical trials combining Cisplatyl containing regimens with IL-2 alone or associated with IFN have been reported. Interesting response rates, range 37 % to 83 % have been completed but most results are preliminary and toxicities in some studies, particularly those combining multiple agents, were greater than expected (Table 4).

On the same hand, our experience at the Salpetriere Hospital in Paris with chemo-immunotherapy regimens seems very promising and we report here the high response rate and long-term remissions of metatastic malignant melanoma treated by CDDP-r IL-2 and α-IFN suggesting, as expected, a true synergism being able to increase the therapeutic index.

Since February 91, 61 eligible patients with progressive metastatic malignant melanoma were entered into two consecutive chemo-immunotherapeutic trials. From 02/91 to 04/92, 39 evaluable patients have been treated with two monthly induction cycles of : Cisplatyl (CDDP) 100 mg/m^2 on day 1, rIL-2 18-MUI/m^2/d by 24 hours intraveinous infusion on day 3-6 and 17-21, and simultaneous subcutaneous INF-9 MUI three times weekly. In order to try to increase the response rate (RR) Tamoxifen (TAM) was added to the same dose and schedule regimen of CDDP-IL-2-IFN and was given from day − 4 to day + 5 at each CDDP administration. Since 04/92, 22 patients were included and 4 patients are too early to be evaluated.

Response rates were similar in the two studies with responses obtained both on visceral {(TAM + : 7/18 (39 %) ; TAM- : 11/18 (41 %)] or non visceral metastatic sites {(TAM + : 16/22 (73 %) ; TAM- : 11/18 (52 %)}. We confirm here on 55 evaluable patients the high activity of CDDP-IL-2-INF combination (RR $\geqslant$ 50 %) suggesting a potential synergism between CDDP and IL-2-INF, and the ability of this type of combination to induce responses in heavily chemotherapy-pretreated patients. Although these regimens could be given safely (no life-threatening toxicity), TAM increased significantly the haemotological toxicity without enhancing neither the response rate nor complete response rate. However, in no case, an ICU supportive care was required.

It is noteworthy to indicate that median survival of responders from the date of entry onto the study in our first uncontrolled trial was 13.5 months (2-21.5+) which is 4 months longer than the usual overall survival of melanoma patients (9 months) from the time of recurrence of disease. Since most patients entered the study after receiving other forms of treatment, their survival from the time of first recurrence was certainly longer than reported.

Although promising, because of their interesting efficacy/toxicity ratio, and in view of the fact that neither compound given as a monotherapy or bitherapy has shown equivalent efficacy, our results need to be confirmed in a larger scale study. Furthermore, several important questions remain to be answered : What is the role of r-IL2 in these results ? Are there ways to increase the complete response rate ?

While pilot studies with different maintenance treatment or combined Tamoxifen or Nitrosourea help in addressing some of these questions, a larger multicenter study is to be started in the very near future comparing

Table 5.

	Without TAM (n = 39)	With TAM (n = 18)
Median age	44 (21-68)	42 (23-65)
ECOG PS	0 (0-2)	0 (0-2)
Nb of metastatic sites		
< 2	24 (61 %)	15 (68 %)
> 2	15 (39 %)	7 (32 %)
Visceral/non visceral	18 (46 %)/21 (54 %)	9 (41 %)/13 (59 %)
Prior treatment with chemotherapy	33 (85 %)	20 (91 %)
Follow-up (week)	42 (16-95)	22 (8-36)
Toxicity (gr. III-IV) : n (%)		
Anemia	15 (38)	10 (55)
Neutropenia	14 (35)	8 (45)
Thrombopenia	10 (26)	8 (45)
Renal toxicity	2 (5)	4 (17)
Hypotension	17 (43)	11 (61)
Infectious episodes	1 (2.5 %)	11 (61)
Thyroid dysfunction	13 (41)	6 (33)
Vitiligo	5 (13)	2 (11)
Dose-intensity		
TAM	—	0.95
CDDP	0.89	0.85
IL-2	0.84	0.83
IFN	0.47	0.60
Response rate		
OR	21 (54 %) (95 % CI : 38-70)	9 (50 %) (95 % CI : 26-76)
CR	5 (13 %)	2 (11 %)
Resp. duration (months)		
CR	3, 3, 16+, 17+, 20+	1, 5+, 2
PR	5 (2.5-16+)	2+, 2+, 3+, 4.5, 4.5+, 6+, 9+
Med. survival (months)	10.5 (2-21.5)	not reached

rIL-2-CDDP-α-IFN to CDDP-α-IFN that may definitely indicate the value of rIL-2 in combination chemoimmunotherapy for metastatic malignant melanoma.

Chemo-immunotherapy represents today a new clinical concept of therapy with biomodulation of anticancer drug agents which warrants further evaluation.

References

1. Adlakha A, Robinson WA, Gonzalez R et al (1989) Combination chemotherapy and Tamoxifen in the treatment of dissemiated malignant Melanoma (abstr). Presented at the 2nd International Conference on Melanoma, Venice, Italy, october
2. Atzpodiem MJ, Korfer A, Franks CR et al (1990) home therapy with recombinant Interleukin-2 and Interferon-2β in advanced human malignancies. Lancet 335 : 1509-1512
3. Avril MF, Bonneterre J, Cupissol D et al (1992) Fotemustine plus Dacarbazine for Malignant Melanoma. Eur J Cancer 28 A (11) : 1807-1811
4. Blair S, Flaherty L, Valdivieso M et al (1991) Comparison of high-dose Interleukin-2 with combined chemotherapy low-dose IL-2 in metastatic malignant melanoma. Proc Am Soc Clin Oncol 10 : 2940 (abstr 1031)
5. Buzaid AC, Murren JR, Durivage HJ (1991) High-dose Cisplatin with Dacarbazine and Tamoxifen in the treatment of Metastatic Melanoma. Cancer 68 : 1238-1241
6. Del Pretre SA, Maurer LH, O'Donnell J, Forcier RJ, Le Marbre P (1984) Combination chemotherapy with Cisplatin, Carcmustine, Dacarbazine and Tamoxifen in metastatic melanoma. Cancer Treat Rep 68 : 1403-1405
7. Demchak PA, Mier JW, Robert NJ et al (1991) Interleukin-2 and high-dose Cisplatin in patients with metastatic melanoma. A pilot study. J Clin Oncol 9 : 1821-1830
8. Dillman RO (1990) Recombinant Interleukin-2 and adoptive immunotherapy alternated with Dacarbazine therapy in melanoma. N Natl Cancer Inst 82 : 1345-1349
9. Flaherty LE, Redman BG, Chabot GG et al (1990) A phase I-II study of Dacarbazine in combination with out patient Interleukin-2 in Metastatic Malignant Melanoma. Cancer 65 : 2471-2477
10. Glover D, Glick JH, Weiler C, Fox K, Guerry D (1987) WR-2721 and high-dose Cisplatin : an active combination in the treatment of metastatic melanoma. J Clin Oncol 5 : 574-578
11. Goey SK, Monson JRT, Stahe LRA et al (1990) A multicenter study of human recombinant Interleukin-2 and α2a interferon in metastatic melanoma. Proc Am Soc Clin Oncol 9 : 185 (abstr)
12. Hamblin TJ, Davies B, Sadullah S et al (1991) A phase 2 study of the treatment of metastatic malignant melanoma with a combination of Dacarbazine, Cisplatin, Interleukin 2 and α-Interferon. Proc Am Soc Clin Oncol 10 : 294 (abstr 1029)
13. Lee H, Talpaz M, Rothberg JM et al (1989) Concomitant administration of recombinant human Interleukine-2 and recombinant Interferon-α-2A in cancer patients : a phase I study. J Clin Oncol 7 : 1726-1732
14. Legha S, Plager C, Ring S, et al (1992) A phase 2 study of biochemotherapy using Interleukin 2 + Interferon α-2A in combination with Cisplatin, Vinblastin and DTIC in patients with metastatic melanoma. Proc Am Soc Clin Oncol 11 : 343, (abstr 1179)
15. McClay EF, Mastragelo MJ, Bellet RE, Berd D (1987) Combination chemo/hormonal therapy in the treatment of Malignant Melanoma Cancer Treat Rep 71 : 465-469
16. McClay EF, Mastrangelo MJ, Bellet RE et al (1989) An effective chemo/hormonal therapy regimen for the treatment of disseminated Malignant Melanoma. Proc Am Soc Clin Oncol 8 : 282 (abstr 1098)
17. Mittelman A, Huberman M, Fallon B, et al (1989) Phase I study of recombinant Interleukin-2 (IL-2-R) and recombinant human Interferon-α (IFN-Roche) in patients with melanoma, renal cell carcinoma, colorectal carcinoma and malignant B-cell disease. Proc Am Soc Clin Oncol 8 : 179 (abstr 696)

18. Murren JR, De Rosa W, Durivage HJ, Davis C, Makuch R, Portlock CS (1991) High-dose Cisplatin plus DTIC in the treatment of metastatic. Cancer 67 : 1514-1517
19. Papadopoulos NEJ, Howard JG, Murray JL et al (1990) Phase II DTIC and Interleukin 2 (IL-2) Trial for metastatic malignant melanoma. Proc Am Soc Clin Oncol 9 : 277 (abstr 1072)
20. Richards JM (1991) Sequential chemo-immunotherapy for metastatic melanoma. Sem Oncol 18 : 5 : 91-95 (suppl 7)
21. Richards JM, Metha N, Ramming et al (1992) Sequential chemo-immunotherapy in the treatment of metastatic melanoma. J Clin Oncol 10 : 1338-1343
22. Rosenberg SA, Lotze MT, Yang JC et al (1989) Combination therapy with Interleukin-2 and Interferon-α for the treatment of patients with advanced cancers. J Clin Oncol 7 : 1863-1874
23. Rosenberg SA, Packard BS, Aebersold PM, et al (1989) Experience with the use of high-dose Interleukin-2 in the treatment of 652 cancer patients. Ann Surg 210 : 474
24. Shiloni E, Poullart P, Janssen J et al (1989) Sequential Dacarbazine chemotherapy followed by recombinant Interleukin-2 in Metastatic Melanoma. A pilot multicentre phase I-II study. Eur J Cancer Clin Oncol 25 : 45-49 (suppl 3)
25. Steffens TA, Bajorin DF, Chapman PB et al (1991) A phase II trial of high-dose Cisplatin and Dacarbazine : lack of efficacy of high-dose, Cisplatin-based therapy for Metastatic Melanoma. Cancer 68 : 1230-1237
26. Stoter G, Shiloni E, Aamdal S et al (1989) Sequential administration of recombinant human Interleukin-2 and Dacarbazine in Metastatic Melanoma. A Multicentre phase II study. Eur J Cancer Clin Oncol 25, 3 : 41-43

Concomitant chemoradiotherapy for solid tumors

EE Vokes, R Stupp

The treatment of locoregionally advanced solid tumors has been hampered by the inability of currently available therapy modalities to eradicate all tumors cells. This applies to surgery and radiation therapy, which frequently are able to control the bulk of locoregional disease but ultimately do not prevent locoregional recurrence. Similarly, chemotherapy can at times induce locoregional tumor shrinkage, but is unable to successfully eradicate macroscopic disease. On the other hand, chemotherapy can, at least in some tumor types, eradicate micrometastatic systemic disease. In addition, chemotherapy might be able to improve locoregional control rates of surgery and/or radiotherapy if given in sequence or concurrently. Based on this background, combined modality programs have been investigated intensively. For many years, research has focused predominantly on the sequential use of combined modality regimens, i.e., neoadjuvant or adjuvant chemotherapy. At present, concomitant chemoradiotherapy is increasingly being viewed as a potentially more successful combination of multiple treatment modalities.

The simultaneous use of chemotherapy and radiation is based on the assumption that radiation augmented by chemotherapy will successfully treat locoregional disease, and chemotherapy will eradicate systemic micrometastases. It is also hoped that the toxicities of the two modalities will be non-overlapping, although in practice this has rarely been achieved [1]. Chemotherapy can increase the efficacy of radiation through a number of possible mechanisms which have been studied intensively in the laboratory. For example, chemotherapy and radiation may be active against different subpopulations of tumors cells, i.e., rapidly proliferating cells in the S-phase of the cell cycle are more radiation resistant but might respond to a number of antimetabolite drugs. Similarly, hypoxic cells have been shown to be less responsive to radiation therapy than well oxygenated cells but might respond to bioreductive alkylating agents. Another potentially important mechanism of interaction is the inhibition of potentially lethal or sublethal radiation damage repair. This has been shown to apply to several drugs including hydroxyurea and cisplatin [1].

Clinically, concomitant chemoradiotherapy has been studied in most common solid tumors [1, 2]. In locoregionally advanced head and neck cancer, improved disease-free survival has been shown with single agent Bleomycin, Mitomycin-C, Methotrexate and Cisplatin [3, 4]. One trial employing bolus intravenous 5-FU also demonstrated improved overall survival. More aggressive combination chemotherapy regimens administered concomitantly with radiotherapy are currently under investigation. Recently, a randomized trial comparing combination chemotherapy with Cisplatin, 5-FU administered in rapid alternation with radiotherapy versus radiotherapy alone (to a higher total radiation dose) demonstrated improved disease-free and overall survival for patients

University of Chicago, Department of Medicine

treated with the combination [5]. Additional phase II and phase III studies are currently in progress and, hopefully, will succeed at solidifying the evidence that concomitant chemoradiotherapy may lead to improved treatment outcome in locoregionally advanced head and neck cancer.

Esophageal cancer is another frequently studied tumor type. Here, too, a recent study conducted by the Radiation Therapy Oncology Group in the United States demonstrated improved overall survival through the use of Cisplatin, 5-FU and simultaneous radiation therapy compared with radiotherapy alone in patients with locoregionally advanced disease. This occurred as a function of both, improved locoregional and systemic tumor control [6].

In locoregionally advanced non-small cell lung cancer, most patients eventually die of systemic metastases. Therefore, this disease in particular will require active chemotherapy if overall survival is to improve. However, randomized studies investigating the use of concomitant chemoradiotherapy to date have focused on single agent chemotherapy. Since single agent chemotherapy in non-small cell lung cancer is fairly inactive, these studies by definition aim at a fairly small increase in survival or disease-free survival rates through improved locoregional control. Studies testing hydroxyurea, ACNU (a nitrosourea) and two studies testing Ciplastin as a single agent have all failed to show any improvement in outcome. However, a recent study conducted by the EORTC comparing radiation alone to radiation with weekly Cisplatin to radiation with daily doses of Cisplatin succeeded at showing an improved survival in patients treated with daily Cisplatin and radiotherapy compared to radiotherapy alone. As expected, this improved survival occurred as a function of improved locoregional control in Cisplatin-treated patients [7, 8].

Randomized trials in cervical cancer, pancreatic cancer and malignant gliomas have also indicated improved survival in patients treated with concomitant chemoradiotherapy compared with radiotherapy alone.

While much work needs to be done, these studies support the continued intensive investigation of concomitant chemoradiotherapy in practice. Such studies should be conducted in a careful prospective manner with the goal of identifying additional single agents with a possible role in this setting (e.g., Taxol, Taxotere, and the Camptothecin analogues) as well as novel combinations.

References

1. Vokes EE, Weichselbaum RR (1990) Concomitant chemoradiotherapy : Rationale and clinical experience in patients with solid tumors. J Clin Oncol 8 : 911-934
2. Vokes EE (1993) The interaction of chemotherapy and radiation. Semin Oncol (in press)
3. Vokes EE, Haraf DJ, Weichselbaum RR et al (1992) Perspectives on combination chemotherapy with concomitant radiotherapy for poor prognosis head and neck cancer. Semin Oncol 19 (suppl 11) : 47-56
4. Vokes EE, Weichselbaum RR, Lippman S, Hong WK (1993) Head and Neck Cancer. N Engl J Med 328 : 184-194
5. Merlano M, Vitale V, Rosso R, Benasso M et al (1992) Treatment of advanced squamous-cell carcinoma of the head and neck with alternating chemotherapy and radiotherapy. N Engl J Med 327 : 1115-1121

6. Herskovic A, Martz K, Al-Sarraf M et al (1992) Combined chemotherapy and radiotherapy compared with radiotherapy alone in patients with cancer of the esophagus. N Engl J Med 326 : 1593-1598
7. Haraf DJ, Devine S, Ihde DC, Vokes EE (1992) The evolving role of systemic therapy in carcinoma of the lung. Semin Oncol 19 (suppl 11) : 72-87
8. Vokes EE, Haraf DJ, Hoffman PC et al (1993) Concomitant chemoradiotherapy for non-small cell lung cancer. Lung Cancer (in press)

Current status of therapy for small cell carcinoma of the lung

DC Ihde

The therapeutic approach to small cell carcinoma of the lung (SCLC), which comprises about 25 % of lung cancer cases in the USA, differs markedly from the management of the other cell types of pulmonary carcinoma. Since SCLC is disseminated at the time of diagnosis in most patients and is sensitive to cytotoxic drugs, combination chemotherapy forms the backbone of treatment for this disease. Despite often impressive responses to chemotherapy in newly diagnosed SCLC, however, few physicians dispute that only very modest improvements in treatment occurred over the past decade.

Modern principles of treatment for SCLC have been established for close to two decades [Minna, 1989]. They include : 1) review of the diagnostic pathologic material with an experienced pulmonary pathologist ; 2) determination of the extent of tumor spread to identify sites of disease which can be used to assess response, establish the patient's prognosis, and, in some patients with more localized cancer, to select therapy ; 3) assessment of the patient's ability to tolerate aggressive combination chemotherapy ; 4) administration of a two- to four-drug regimen of proven efficacy ; 5) the capacity to provide meticulous supportive care, particularly for complications of myelosuppression ; 6) discontinuation of chemotherapy in stable responding patients after a defined interval ; and 7) consideration of cranial irradiation for prevention of brain metastases in complete responders to treatment.

New therapeutic approaches during the 1980s and older treatments whose utility was more precisely clarified include 1) development of less toxic chemotherapy regimens that do not sacrifice therapeutic effects ; 2) documentation that the addition of chest irradiation to chemotherapy in limited-stage patients enhances survival, with better definition of optimal drugs and radiation schedules to be incorporated in combined modality therapy ; 3) reappraisal of the role of surgical resection ; and 4) recognition that few useful chemotherapeutic agents were being introduced and diversification of methods for selection of new drugs for clinical evaluation.

Etoposide/Cisplatin (EP) is the most prominent example of a chemotherapy program with a better therapeutic index. EP has activity in SCLC patients whose tumors progressed following Cyclophosphamide/Doxorubicin/Vincristine (CAV) [Evans, 1985 ; Porter, 1985], improves survival when added to CAV in some randomized trials [Evans, 1987 ; Einhorn, 1988], and appears to produce maximal antitumor effects at doses associated with only very modest myelosuppression [Ihde, 1991]. In prospective controlled studies, the hematologic toxicity of EP is significantly less than that of CAV [Fukuoka, 1991 ; Roth, 1992]. In extensive-stage patients, CAV, EP, and alternation of these

National Cancer Institute and Uniformed Services University of the Health Sciences, Bethesda, MD 20892, USA

two drug regimens yield equivalent survival [Fukuoka, 1991 ; Roth, 1992], but there may be a survival advantage to adding EP to CAV in limited-stage patients [Einhorn, 1988 ; Fukuoka, 1991].

Uncontrolled data [Feld, 1984], now confirmed by several randomized studies [Spiro, 1989 ; Ettinger, 1990 ; Splinter, 1988] have shown that administration of chemotherapy for more than 4-6 months in responding patients does not improve survival, although duration of first remission may be prolonged. Furthermore, maintenance treatment increases toxicity and may reduce chances of palliation with salvage chemotherapy [Evans, 1985 ; Porter, 1985 ; Batist, 1986]. Elimination of prolonged maintenance chemotherapy obviously improves the therapeutic index of treatment. Finally, newer studies of administration of single-agent chemotherapy, particularly of Etoposide or Teniposide in elderly patients [Bork, 1991 ; Carney, 1990] have yielded surprisingly impressive therapeutic results. Whether survival is compromised is not yet certain, but single-agent treatment clearly represents an effective, less toxic option for patients at risk of severe side effects from chemotherapy. Such an approach cannot be recommended for fully ambulatory patients with limited-stage cancer, in whom there is a small chance of cure with standard treatment [Minna, 1989].

Mature results from several large randomized studies [Bunn, 1987 ; Perry, 1987 ; Perez, 1984] and a meta-analysis have demonstrated that chest irradiation in limited-stage SCLC, although associated with increased morbidity and some excess mortality, yields modestly better survival when given in conjunction with chemotherapy. In the meta-analysis of 13 randomized trials, the addition of thoracic radiotherapy to combination chemotherapy yielded a 14 % decrease in rate of mortality and a 5.4 % absolute improvement in 3-year survival [Pignon, 1992]. Sequential combined modality therapy, in which chemotherapy is temporarily discontinued for the administration of irradiation, produces relatively little hematologic, pulmonary, and esophageal toxicity. However, more toxic concurrent chemoradiotherapy or alternating combined modality regimens, in which chemotherapy is not delayed while split-course irradiation is delivered, were administered in most controlled trials demonstrating enhanced survival. Recent uncontrolled studies suggest EP can be given concurrently with irradiation with less toxicity than other drug regimens [McCracken, 1990], and that delivery of chest irradiation in twice daily fractions may also lead to superior results [Turrisi, 1990 ; Johnson, 1991].

The documentation that rare SCLC patients can be cured with surgical resection alone [Shields, 1982] and frequent recurrence at the primary tumor site after chemoradiotherapy has led to renewed interest in the role of surgery. Limited-stage patients who receive chemoradiotherapy after surgical resection have demonstrably better prognosis than such patients given similar treatment without prior surgery [Friess, 1985 ; Shepherd, 1988], but the extent to which the surgical resection contributes to these better results is uncertain. This subject is not a suitable topic for a controlled clinical trial, since many otherwise surgically resectable patients are discovered to have SCLC only at thoracotomy. Recent studies have focused on attempting surgical resection only after maximal response to chemotherapy is achieved. Some patients have no evidence of cancer in the surgical specimen [Williams, 1987], but elucidating whether survival is improved by this strategy is fraught with difficulty and will almost certainly require results from randomized clinical trials. Early results of the first such large trial investigating this issue do not appear promising [Lad, 1991].

Thoracic radiotherapy and surgical resection can have only a restricted impact on survival in SCLC, however, since the overwhelming cause of death even in limited-stage patients is failure to control distant metastatic tumor. More effective systemic treatments, presumably new chemotherapeutic agents, will be needed to address this problem successfully. A recent randomized trial suggests that survival of carefully selected previously untreated extensive-stage patients is not compromised by initial therapy with an investigational agent, provided standard combination chemotherapy is administered at the first sign of lack of response [Ettinger, 1992]. This finding should encourage study of promising new and previously untested drugs in newly diagnosed extensive-stage patients and may optimize the chances of identifying superior agents. The more standard approach of testing new agents only in SCLC patients who have failed combination chemotherapy can identify useful agents only if the response rate demanded of an active drug is relaxed, unless testing is confined to patients who develop tumor progression only after a period of at least several months off chemotherapy [Grant, 1992].

Our group has shown that *in vitro* drug sensitivity of cell lines established from SCLC patients prior to therapy is highly correlated with clinical response to chemotherapy [Gazdar, 1990]. Drug testing results have been less helpful in choosing the most effective chemotherapy program for an individual patient, probably because the sensitivity to each agent tested is associated with sensitivity to most other agents [Gazdar, 1990 ; Tsai, 1990]. Cell lines established directly from patients without any *in vitro* selection may be more useful in evaluating potential mechanisms responsible for the development of clinical drug resistance, for example the expression of the P-170 glycoprotein product of the human multidrug resistance gene [Lai, 1989], and in screening for new chemotherapeutic agents. The National Cancer Institute (USA) has recently incorporated tumor cell lines derived from lung and other human cancers into its screening process [Monks, 1991].

References

Batist G, Carney DN, Cowan et al (1986) Etoposide (VP-16) and Cisplatin in previously treated small-cell lung cancer. J Clin Oncol 4 : 982-986

Bork E, Ersboll J, Dombersky P et al (1991) Teniposide and Etoposide in previously untreated small-cell lung cancer. J Clin Oncol 9 : 1627-1631

Bunn PA, Lichter AS, Makuch RW et al (1987) Chemotherapy alone or chemotherapy with chest radiation therapy in limited stage small cell lung cancer. Ann Intern Med 106 : 655-662

Carney DN, Grogan L, Smit EF et al (1990) Single-agent oral Etoposide for elderly small cell lung cancer patients. Sem Oncol 17 (suppl 2) : 49-53

Einhorn LH, Crawford J, Birch R et al (1988) Cisplatin plus Etoposide consolidation following Cyclophosphamide, Doxorubicin, and Vincristine in limited small-cell lung cancer. J Clin Oncol 6 : 451-456

Ettinger DS, Finkelstein DM, Abeloff MD et al (1990) A randomized comparison of standard chemotherapy versus alternating chemotherapy and maintenance versus no maintenance therapy for extensive stage small-cell lung cancer. J Clin Oncol 8 : 230-240

Ettinger DS, Finkelstein DM, Abeloff MD et al (1992) Justification for evaluating new anticancer drugs in selected untreated patients with extensive-stage small-cell lung cancer. J Natl Cancer Inst 84 : 1077-1084

Evans WK, Osoba D, Feld R et al (1985) Etoposide (VP-16) and Cisplatin : An effective treatment for relapse of small-cell lung cancer. J Clin Oncol 3 : 65-71

Evans WK, Feld R, Murray N et al (1987) Superiority of alternating non-cross-resistant chemotherapy in extensive small cell lung cancer. Ann Intern Med 107 : 451-458

Feld R, Evans WK, DeBoer G et al (1984) Combined modality induction therapy without maintenance chemotherapy for small cell carcinoma of the lung. J Clin Oncol 2 : 294-304

Friess GG, McCracken JD, Troxell ML et al (1985) Effect of initial resection of small-cell carcinoma of the lung. J Clin Oncol 3 : 964-968

Fukuoka M, Furuse K, Saijo N et al (1991) Randomized trial of Cyclophosphamide, Doxorubicin, and Vincristine versus Cisplatin and Etoposide versus alternation of these regimens in small-cell lung cancer. J Natl Cancer Inst 83 : 855-861

Gazdar AF, Steinberg SM, Russell EK et al (1990) Correlation of in vitro drug-sensitivity testing results with response to chemotherapy and survival in extensive stage small cell lung cancer. J Natl Cancer Inst 82 : 117-124

Grant SC, Gralla RJ, Kris MG et al (1992) Single agent chemotherapy trials in small-cell lung cancer, 1970-1990. J Clin Oncol 10 : 484-498

Ihde DC, Mulshine JL, Kramer BS et al (1991) Randomized trial of high vs. standard dose Etoposide (VP-16) and Cisplatin in extensive stage small cell lung cancer (abstr). Proc Am Soc Clin Oncol 10 : 240

Johnson BE, Salem C, Nesbitt J et al (1991) Limited stage small cell lung cancer treated with concurrent BID chest radiotherapy and Etoposide/Cisplatin followed by chemotherapy selected by in vitro drug sensitivity testing (abstr). Proc Am Soc Clin Oncol 10 : 240

Lad T, Thomas P, Piantadosi S (1991) Surgical resection of small cell lung cancer : A prospective randomized evaluation (abstr). Proc Am Soc Clin Oncol 10 : 244

Lai SL, Goldstein LJ, Gottesman MM et al (1989) MDR-1 gene expression in lung cancer. J Natl Cancer Inst 81 : 1144-1150

McCracken JD, Janaki LM, Crowley JJ et al (1990) Concurrent chemotherapy/radiotherapy for limited small cell lung carcinoma. J Clin Oncol 8 : 892-898

Minna JD, Pass H, Glatstein E et al (1989) Cancer of the lung. In : DeVita VT, Hellman S, Rosenberg SA (eds) Cancer : Principles and Practice of Oncology, 3rd Ed. JB Lippincott, Philadelphia, p 591

Monks A, Scudiero D, Skehan P et al (1991) Feasibility of a high-flux anticancer drug screen using a diverse panel of cultured human tumor cell lines. J Natl Cancer Inst 83 : 757-766

Perez CA, Einhorn L, Oldham RK et al (1984) Randomized trial of radiotherapy to the thorax in limited small-cell carcinoma of the lung treated with multiagent chemotherapy and elective brain irradiation. J Clin Oncol 2 : 1200-1208

Perry MC, Eaton WL, Propert KJ et al (1987) Chemotherapy with or without radiation therapy in limited small-cell carcinoma of the lung. N Engl J Med 316 : 912-918

Pignon JP, Arriagada R, Ihde DC et al (1992) A meta-analysis of thoracic radiotherapy for small-cell lung cancer. N Engl J Med 327 : 1618-1624

Porter LL, Johnson DH, Hainsworth JD et al (1985) Cisplatin and Etoposide combination chemotherapy for refractory small cell carcinoma of the lung. Cancer Treat Rep 69 : 479-481

Roth BJ, Johnson DH, Einhorn LH et al (1992) Randomized study of Cyclophosphamide, Doxorubicin, and Vincristine versus Etoposide and Cisplatin versus alternation of these two regimens in extensive small-cell lung cancer. J Clin Oncol 10 : 282-291

Shepherd FA, Evans W, Feld R et al (1988) Adjuvant chemotherapy following surgical resection for small cell carcinoma of the lung. J Clin Oncol 6 : 832-838

Shields TW, Higgins GA, Matthews MJ et al (1982) Surgical resection in the management of small cell carcinoma of the lung. J Thorac Cardiovasc Surg 84 : 481-488

Spiro SG, Souhami RL, Geddes DM et al (1989) Duration of chemotherapy in small cell lung cancer. Br J Cancer 59 : 578-583

Splinter TAW (1988) Induction vs. induction plus maintenance chemotherapy in small cell lung cancer (abstr). Proc Am Soc Clin Oncol 7 : 202

Tsai CM, Ihde DC, Kadoyama C et al (1990) Correlation of in vitro drug sensitivity testing of long-term small cell lung cancer cell lines with response and survival. Eur J Cancer 26 : 1148-1152

Turrisi AT, Glover DJ (1990) Thoracic radiotherapy variables : Influence on local control in small cell lung cancer limited disease. Int J Radiat Oncol Biol Phys 19 : 1473-1479

Williams CJ, McMillan I, Lea R et al (1987) Surgery after initial chemotherapy for localized small cell carcinoma of the lung. J Clin Oncol 5 : 1579-1588

Systemic treatment of bladder cancer

LY Dirix, AT van Oosterom

Although bladder cancer is the fifth most common cancer in the Western world, it is only seventh in the ranking of cancer related mortality. This is due to its presentation as a superficial disease in up 80-90 % of new cases. Only 10 % and 30 %, respectively, of Tis and T1 cancers will actually develop into invasive disease. The majority of patients that die of bladder cancer will have muscle invasive disease at presentation.

Cancer of the bladder is primarily a disease of older white men, with a male/female ratio of 3 : 1 to 4 : 1. Both incidence and mortality rates increase with age. Nearly 70 % of cases occur in men over 65 years of age. The often associated other medical conditions of this age group have be taken into account when combined modality treatment programs are being designed. The stage of disease at diagnosis increases also with age, with the lowest stage of disease at presentation being diagnosed in young white females.

From recent epidemiological data there seems to be an increase in incidence and a decrease in mortality during the 1970s and 1980s. These data should however be interpreted with caution, as the increase in incidence is mainly due to an increase in localized disease.

The survival data on non-invasive bladder cancer are excellent with 5-year disease specific survival of nearly 90 %, for invasive disease this figure drops to less than 50 % regardless of which local treatment strategy is being applied.

Molecular biology of invasive TCC

As the majority of patients with superficial bladder cancer never develop invasive disease, a great deal of attention has been directed at the identification of factors, both at the histological and at the cellular level, that would predict for the transition of superficial to invasive and/or metastatic disease.

A crude way of identifying genetic alterations in a tumour is the measurement of DNA content with flow cytometry. This allows for the measurement of the ploidy state of a particular tumour. In most studies the percentage of tumours being aneuploid increases with increasing stage and grade of the tumour and these correlations are excellent. However, aneuploid or diploid invasive carcinomas share a similar prognosis and in one series of 22 patients with invasive carcinomas with lymph node metastases, 8 cases had diploid primary tumours and 6 of these even had diploid metastases [1]. These and other studies lead to the conclusion that ploidy measurements in bladder carcinoma have only limited significance in the clinical decision making process in patients with invasive tumours.

Department of Medical Oncology, University Hospital Antwerp, Wilrijkstraat 10, 2650 Edegem, Belgium

A more direct manner of assessing genetic alterations is the chromosomal analysis of a tumour by karyotyping [2]. These investigations have shown non-random changes in chromosomes 1, 7, 9, 11, 15 and 17 [2, 5, 9, 15]. In an attempt to identify early genetic changes Hopman et al investigated 24 low-grade, diploid tumours with *in situ* hybridization [9]. The most important finding of this study was the detection of monosomy 9 in 9 out of 24 cases, suggesting that loss of chromosome 9 could be an early event in the development of bladder cancer.

With recombinant DNA markers a more detailed analysis of genetic changes can be detected by analysing restriction fragment length polymorphism. These studies confirmed changes in chromosomes 9q, 11p and 17p. In one study a 9q deletion was detected in more than half of all tumours examined, both superficial and invasive, corroborating this deletion as a possible early event in bladder oncogenesis [15].

Mutations of the cellular K-, H- and N-ras genes have been observed in many different human cancers. The cellular Harvey ras oncogene, c-H-ras was first isolated from bladder carcinoma cell lines EJ and T24 by transfection of NIH/3T3 fibroblasts. In bladder carcinomas only mutations in H-ras but not of K- and N-ras have thusfar been identified. Although initial studies have reported that some 10 % of investigated bladder tumours had mutations of H-ras, others reported much higher frequencies. In a study by Knowles et al 152 bladder tumours were examined by single-strand conformation polymorfism and restriction fragment polymorphism for mutations of the H-ras gene [10]. The frequency of H-ras mutations was low in this study, 6 % of all examined tumours. No correlation was found between absence or presence of H-ras mutations and tumour grade or stage.

The p53 gene is a tumour suppressor gene located on chromosome 17p. The gene product is a 53-kd nuclear protein and is supposed to have a controlling function on the transcription of growth inhibitory genes [22]. In bladder cancer, as in most other human malignancies, mutations in this gene have been identified in a majority of cases. In 43 T1, i.e. non-invasive, bladder tumours nuclear overexpression of p53 was sought for with an immunohistochemical technique [16]. In this study p53 overexpression in non-invasive bladder tumours correlates with a higher probability to develop into invasive disease. It is also suggestive for a relative early role of chromosome 17 mutations in the multistep oncogenesis of transitional cell carcinoma (TCC).

Recent studies have also investigated the role of the erb gene family in TCC. The human proto-oncogene c-erbB-1 is located on chromosome 7 and normally encodes for the epidermal growth factor receptor (EGFr). The epidermal growth factor (EGF) is found in high concentrations in urine and the EGFr is normally present in the basal layers of the normal urothelium. A study investigating amplification of the erbB-1 gene in bladder cancer, could demonstrate this in only 1 out of 31 tumours. Neal et al studied 101 bladder tumours with an immunohistochemical technique for the presence of the EGFr [14]. Nearly half of all tumours were positive for EFGr, with increasing percentage of positivity occurring with increasing stage and increasing grade of the tumours. Importantly in patients with Tis and T1 disease, EGFr positivity was associated with multiplicity, recurrence rate and time to recurrence. In this group of 52 patients with non-invasive disease, progression to a higher tumour stage or development of metastases occurred in 11 patients. These were 9 out of 13 with EGFr-positive tumours and 2/39 EGFr-negative tumours. How the expression of EGFr could contribute to early progression is still not clear, but possible interactions with other growth factors such as transforming growth factor alfa (TGF-α) may be significant and could contribute in the emergence of an invasive phenotype leading to extracellular matrix (ECM) degradation.

Another member of the erb gene family is the human proto-oncogene c-erbB-2 located on chromosome 17. This gene encodes for a protein similar, but distinct from the EGFr. Several studies have shown increased expression of the erbB-2 gene product in TCC and correlations have found with tumour grade.

These and other exciting findings will eventually lead to a more complete understanding of the biology of TCC leading to a more individualised treatment strategy.

Tumor staging of TTC

Tumor staging systems are used in order to help physicians make optimal treatment choices for their patients and to help in the comparison of treatment results in different centers with different modalities. This means that clinical assessment is both dependent on the clinician's experience and on the quality of the techniques used in making the tumour staging. The pathological staging system pTNM is a very reliable method and accurately reflects prognosis. Clinical T1 invades the lamina propria but not beyond and is the same as stage A in the Jewett-Marshall-Strong system. Clinical stages T2-T4 correspond to B and C categories in the J-M-S system. A T2 tumour invades no deeper than the superficial half of the muscle wall, a T3a tumour invades into the outer half of the muscle wall but does not penetrate it. A T3b tumour invades into the perivesical fat. All T4 tumours have extended into neighboring organs, with T4a tumours invading into either the prostate, the vagina or the uterus and T4b tumours invading the bone pelvis, the rectum or the abdominal wall. The N stage is always Nx unless surgical exploration has been performed.

The clinical TNM system is much less accurate with both overstaging but even more frequently understaging occurring. This is of particular importance when comparing of results of patients treated with surgery or other treatment modalities.

The role of chemotherapy in the treatment of TCC

The necessity for systemic treatment of invasive transitional cell carcinoma is evident knowing that nearly half of the patients presenting with muscle-invasive disease will die from metastatic disease within the first 5 years. Several drugs have been shown to possess significant activity against metastatic TCC.

The most active agent remains at present Cisplatin (CDDP) with a single agent response rate of 20 % to 30 %. In most studies Cisplatin was given in dosages ranging from 50 to 120 mg/m^2, without arguments for a dose or schedule dependency of Cisplatin in this disease. Several randomized trials have investigated the role of adding a second drug to Cisplatin, and all of these failed to demonstrate superiority of the two drug combination over single agent Cisplatin. Soloway et al added 750 mg/m^2 Cyclophosphamide to 70 mg/m^2 Cisplatin with no difference in response rate, number of complete response or survival [7]. The study by Hillcoat et al compared Cisplatin 80 mg/m^2 with the same dosage of CDDP in combination with Methotrexate 50 mg/m^2 twice every 4 weeks [8]. This study also failed to demonstrate benefit of the combination. In other phase II studies the CDDP-MTX combination proved very active [20].

Methotrexate however is considered to be the other most active agent against this disease. In several studies a response rate of 25 % to 30 % is reported. No data exist to suggest that higher doses of MTX are superior to the commonly used dose of 30 to 40 mg/m^2. No data are available comparing single agent CDDP with MTX.

Other agents with significant single agent activity include Doxorubicin, Vinblastin, Mitomycin, Cyclophosphamide and possibly also for 5-Fluorouracil.

From these disease-oriented phase II studies some important conclusions can be drawn. First of all the anatomical location of the primary tumour is of no influence on the chemosensitivity, second that even in metastatic disease complete and durable responses, although rare with single agent treatment, do occur and that the bladder primary is very chemosensitive and that response rate of metastatic deposits is site specific, with bone and liver lesions being less responsive [4].

Combination chemotherapy led to a variety of different schemes but most of those failed to result in superior response rates or survival rates in comparison with single agent Cisplatin.

As mentioned previously the addition of Cyclophosphamide to CDDP was not superior to CDDP and the same holds true for the combination of CDDP with MTX versus single agent CDDP in randomized studies. This last study showed a, statiscally not significant, higher response rate for CM versus C and again a not significant improvement in survival, be it that the β error for this study is large [8]. In a randomized trial from the Southeastern Cancer Study Group compared CDDP with CAP (Cyclophosphamide, Doxorubicin, Cisplatin) in 91 patients without a significant difference for both arms in response rate, response duation or survival [21]. Another frequently used regimen is the CMV combination consisting of Methotrexate 30 mg/m^2 and Vinblastine 4 mg/m^2 on days 1 and 8, and CDDP 100 mg/m^2 on day 2 [7]. With this regimen a response rate of 56 % was reported including a 28 % complete response rate in a study on 50 patients. This regimen never underwent direct comparison with CDDP in a randomized trial, as such it can not placed in comparison to the current optimal chemotherapy.

The M-VAC regimen consists of Methotrexate 30 mg/m^2, Vinblastine (V) 3 mg/m^2, Doxorubicin 30 mg/m^2 and CDDP 70 mg/m^2 and on days 15 and 22, the MTX and V are repeated if hematological toxicity allows. With this regimen a response rate of 72 % was reported in study on 121 evaluable patients with a CR rate of 36 % and a median survival of the CR patients exceeding 38 months [18]. Interestingly, and underscoring the impact of this regimen on the natural history of the disease, 16 % of the responders developed brain metastasis, half of whom had no systemic relapse at the time of progression. The M-VAC regimen was compared in a randomized phase III study to single agent CDDP and the combination showed superior response rate and survival figures [11]. In another randomized phase III study M-VAC underwent comparison with the CISCA regimen (Cyclophosphamide 650 mg/m^2, Doxorubicin 50 mg/m^2 and Cisplatin 100 mg/m^2) in 110 patients with metastatic urothelial tumours [12]. In these study M-VAC again was superior both with respect to response rate as with respect to overall survival.

The experience with the M-VAC regimen is now considerable and while its activity is being confirmed, it is judged to be a toxic regimen with frequent dose reductions or even omissions of days 15 and 22 [3, 18].

The introduction of colony-stimulating factors of the type of G- or GM-CSF has led to several trials in the treatment of metastatic transitional cell carcinoma with M-VAC or dose escalated versions of the regimen. First Gabrilove et al showed that by giving G-CSF on days 4 through 11 in the conventional M-VAC regimen all patients were able to receive the planned dose-intensity, and a significant reduction of infections and days on antibiotics [6]. Remarkable was also the finding of a significantly reduced incidence of mucositis in the G-CSF treated patients.

The study by Logothetis et al reported on the use of escalated M-VAC with GM-CSF support in 32 patients refractory to standard M-VAC [13]. In this escalated regimen MTX dose was left unchanged, V was up to 4 mg/m^2, Doxorubicin 60 mg/m^2, CDDP 100 mg/m^2 and GM-CSF was given at a dose 250 µg/m^2 from days 3 through 13. A response rate of 40 % was obtained with seven patients (23 %) achieving a CR.

The study by Sternberg et al used a modified M-VAC schedule with a cycle length of 2 weeks and thereby increasing dose intensity, giving MTX at 30 mg/m^2, V 3 mg/m^2, Doxorubicin 30 mg/m^2 and CDDP 70 mg/m^2 together with GM-CSF at a dose of 250 µg/m^2 from days 4 through 10 [19]. In the second part of this study a dose escalation was done with MTX at 35 mg, V at 3.5 mg, dox at 35 mg and CDDP at 80 mg all per meter square body surface area. Again in this study the high response rate, including 32 % complete responders, was confirmed. The second dose level however, proved too toxic with excessive thrombocytopenia.

These studies confirm the chemosensitivity of transitional cell carcinoma and suggest a dose response relationship for Doxorubicin and Cisplatin. Whether these new approaches will have an impact on survival has to be awaitened. Further development of dose-escalated regimens with multi-lineage growth factors and the modulation of chemotherapy with biological response modifiers such as leukocyte interferon are promising new developments.

References

1. Baladement RA, O'Toole RV, Keyhan-Rofagha S et al (1992) Flow cytometric analysis of primary and metastatic bladder cancer. J Urol 143 : 912-916
2. Badu VR, Lutz MD, Miles BJ et al (1987) Tumor behaviour in transitional cell carcinoma of the bladder in relation to chromosomal markers and histopathology. Cancer Res 47 : 6800-6805
3. Boutan-Laroze A, Mahjoubi M, Droz JP et al (1991) M-VAC for advanced carcinoma of the bladder. Eur J Cancer 27 : 1690-1694
4. Dirix LY, Van Oosterom AT (1991) Neoadjuvant and adjuvant therapy for invasive bladder tumours. Eur J Cancer 27 : 326-330
5. Fearon ER, Feinberg AP, Hamilton SH (1985) Loss of genes on the short arm of chromosome 11 in bladder cancer. Nature 318 : 377-380
6. Gabrilove JL, Jakubowski A, Scher H et al (1988) Effect of granulocyte colony-stimulating factor on neutropenia and associated morbidity due to chemotherapy for transitional cell carcinoma of the urothelium. N Engl J Med 318 : 1414-1422
7. Harker WG, Meyers FJ, Frehia FS et al (1985) Cisplatin, Methotrexate, and Vinblastine (CMV) : an effective regimen for metastatic transitional cell carcinoma of the urinary tract : a Northern California Oncology Group study. J Clin Oncol 3 : 1463-1470
8. Hilcoat BL, Raghavan D, Mattews J et al (1989) A randomized trial of Cisplatin versus Cisplatin plus methotrexate in advanced cancer of the urothelial tract. J Clin Oncol 7 : 706-709
9. Hopman AHN, Moesker O, Smeets W et al (1991) Numerical chromosome 1, 7, 9 and 11 aberrations in bladder cancer detected by in situ hybridization. Cancer Res 51 : 644-651
10. Knowles MA, Williamson M (1993) Mutation of H-ras is infrequent in bladder cancer : confirmation by single-strand conformation polymorphism analysis, designed restriction fragment length polymorphisms, and direct sequencing. Cancer Res 53 : 133-139
11. Loehrer PJ, Einhorn LH, Elsin PJ et al (1992) A randomized comparison of Cisplatin alone or in combination with Methotrexate, Vinblastine, and Doxorubicin in patients with metastatic urothelial carcinoma : a cooperative group study. J Clin Oncol 10 : 1066-1073
12. Logothethis CJ, Dexeus FH, Finn L et al (1990) A prospective randomized trial comparing MVAC with CISCA chemotherapy for patients with metastatic urothelial tumors. J Clin Oncol 8 : 1050-1055
13. Logothethis CL, Dexeus FH, Sella A et al (1990) Escalated therapy for refractory urothelial tumors : Methotrexate-Vinblastine-Doxorubicin-Cisplatin plus unglycosylated recombinant human granulocyte-macrophage colony-stimulating factor. J Natl Cancer Inst 82 : 667-672
14. Neal DE, Sharples L, Smith et al (1990) The epidermal growth factor receptor and the prognosis of bladder cancer. Cancer 65 : 1619-1625
15. Olumi AF, Tsai YC, Nichols PW et al (1990) Allellic loss of chromosomes 17p distinguishes high grade from low grade transitional cell carcinomas of the bladder. Cancer Res 50 : 7081-7083
16. Sarkis AS, Dalbagni G, Cordon-Cardo C, Zhang Z-F, Fair WR, Herr HW, Reuter VE (1993) Nuclear overexpression of p53 protein in transitional cell bladder carcinoma : a marker for disease progression. J Natl Cancer Inst 85 : 53-59
17. Soloway MS, Einstein A, Corder MP et al (1983) A comparison of Cisplatin and Cyclophosphamide in advanced urothelial cancer. Cancer 52 : 767-772

18. Sternberg CN, Yagoda A, Scher HI et al (1989) Methotrexate, Vinblastine, Doxorubicin, and Cisplatin for advanced transitional cell carcinoma of the urothelium. Cancer 64 : 2448-2458
19. Sternberg CN, De Mulder PHM, van Oosterom AT et al Escalated M-VAC chemotherapy and recombinant human granulocyte-macrophage colony stimulating factor (GM-CSF) in patients with advanced urothelial tract tumours. Ann Oncol 4
20. Stoter G, Splinter TAW, Child JA et al (1987) Combination chemotherapy with Cisplatin and Methotrexate in advanced transitional cell cancer of the bladder. J Urol 137 : 663-667
21. Troner M, Birch R, Omura GA, Williams S (1987) Phase III comparison of Cisplatin alone versus Cisplatin, Doxorubicin and Cyclophosphamide in the treatment of bladder (urothelial) cancer : a Southeastern Cancer Study Group trial. J Urol 137 : 660-662
22. Vogelstein B, Kinzler KW (1992) p 53 Function and dysfunction. Cell 70 : 523-526

Metastatic breast cancer : current management options and future directions

G Hortobagyi

Although fewer than 10 % of patients are initially diagnosed with distant metastasis, most patients who present with Stage II or III primary breast cancer, and many of those who present with Stage I, eventually develop distant metastatic disease. The natural history of metastatic breast cancer is quite heterogenous, with some patients demonstrating a rapid and precipitous dissemination and death from multiorgan failure within a year of the first evidence of distant disease, while others live in apparent symbiosis with their neoplasm, alternating periods of slow progression and stability for many years. Older clinical reports have shown that even in the absence of effective systemic treatment, a small fraction of patients survive for 10, 15, and even longer years [1].

To treat metastatic breast cancer optimally, the physician resorts to multiple modalities of therapy. Systemic treatments have a predominant role in the management of this stage of breast cancer, while surgery and palliative radiotherapy have a limited, but important role for specific localized problems. Approximately one-third of breast cancers maintains hormone dependence. This subgroup can be identified empirically by clinical characteristics, or by the presence of steroid hormone receptors (estrogen and progesterone receptors). Patients with hormone-dependent metastatic breast cancer benefit from hormonal treatment [2]. Previously popular major surgical ablative therapies (adrenalectomy, hypophysectomy) have been discarded in favor of synthetic antiestrogens, aromatase inhibitors, LHRH analogues, and progestins. In unselected groups of breast cancer patients, any of these hormonal approaches produces major objective remissions in approximately 30 % of patients : when treatment is limited to patients with estrogen-receptor positive disease, the response rate may exceed 50 %, and in subgroups of patients with very high content of estrogen-receptor ($>$ 100 fm/mg protein), may be even higher. There is no evidence that combinations of hormonal therapies are more effective than single agent hormone treatments. However, it is well known that after a response to a first hormonal therapy, when progressive disease appears, changing to a second, but different hormone therapy (for instance from an antiestrogen to a progestin) might induce a second high quality response. Thus, some patients benefit from two or three, and sometimes even four sequential hormonal therapies. This may result in adequate tumor control for several years.

Most patients with metastatic breast cancer do not benefit from hormone therapy. Furthermore, those who do eventually will require chemotherapy because their tumors lose their hormone dependence. For all these patients, chemotherapy is today the treatment of choice [3]. Metastatic breast cancer is moderately sensitive to many individual cytotoxic agents. However, single

---

Department of Breast and Gynecologic Medical Oncology, The University of Texas MD Anderson Cancer Center, 1515 Holcombe Boulevard, Box 56, Houston, Texas 77030, USA

agent chemotherapy produces objective responses in only 20-30 % of patients with the notable exception of the anthracyclines, and some of the newer cytotoxic agents mentioned below. In addition, responses after single agent therapy are shortlasting, and complete remissions are exceptional. Several effective combinations have evolved. The most commonly used consist of Cyclophosphamide, Methotrexate, and Fluorouracil (CMF), or Cyclophosphamide, Doxorubicin, or Epirubicin and 5-Fluorouracil (CAF, FAC, or FEC). In general terms, it is accepted that the anthracycline-containing regimens are more effective in producing objective remissions, and these objective remissions last a few months longer than those obtained with alternative therapies. These combinations also produce somewhat more toxicity, especially alopecia. Response rates with combination chemotherapy vary from 40-80 %, depending on patient selection, dose intensity of the regimen, and the criteria used for evaluation of response. Response duration varies from 7-12 months, being longer for patients who achieve a complete remission (15-18 months). The median surival after combination chemotherapy varies from 15-24 months, again being longer for patients with high quality objective regressions, and shorter for patients with progressive disease. Complete remissions occur in 10-20 % of patients only ; however, a small percentage of these patients (< 10 %) survive within an unmaintained complete remission for periods that may exceed 10-15 years [4].

Over the last 10 years, dose intensification has been identified as a major variable in the efficacy of cytotoxic chemotherapy [5]. Several small randomized trials have confirmed the results of preclinical experiments and demonstrated that higher dose intensity often (but not always) results in higher remission rate, and in the case of combination chemotherapy, a prolonged response duration and survival. Most of these trials were performed without the benefit of hematopoietic growth factor support, or autologous stem cell reinfusion. More recently, the appearance of effective hematopoietic support to counteract the severe myelosuppressive toxicity of high-dose chemotherapy allowed the administration of cytotoxic therapy at much higher doses and dose intensity. Thus, doses that exceeded standard dose by a factor of 4 to 20, have been administered to patients with metastatic breast cancer. When high-dose single agent chemotherapy is administered to patients with refractory metastatic breast cancer, higher than expected overall response rate (approximately 50 %) is achieved ; however, complete responses are rare, remission duration is short (3 months on average), and no survival benefit is detected. High-dose combination chemotherapy for refractory metastatic breast cancer produces a higher overall response rate and a creditable complete remission rate (20 %), both of which are in excess of what one would expect from standard dose salvage chemotherapy. However, long-term remissions are seldom achieved, and the morbidity and mortality of these regimens is substantial. When high-dose combination chemotherapy is used as front-line chemotherapy, overall response rates approach 100 % and complete remission rates reach almost 50 %. Remission durations after one or two high-dose chemotherapy cycles are similar to those achieved with a longer duration of standard dose chemotherapy, and some centers have reported that 10-20 % of patients so treated remain in complete remission two and three years after the administration of therapy. A more recent approach uses high-dose chemotherapy as consolidation of objective remissions obtained by standard dose therapy. A somewhat higher complete remission rate is obtained by this combined modality therapy, but the survival benefit (if any) remains to be demonstrated. Prospective randomized trials are being conducted to assess the relative benefits and toxicity of these regimens compared to standard dose chemotherapy.

The last three years have witnessed the appearance of several new and exciting cytotoxic agents with demonstrated antitumor efficacy against metastatic breast cancer [6]. The taxanes (Taxol and Taxotere) have been evaluated more extensively than some of the others. In previously untreated, or minimally treated metastatic breast cancer, these agents produce objective responses in 50-60 % of patients, including some with clear-cut resistance to anthracyclines, previously the gold standards for the treatment of this tumor [7]. Currently the taxanes are being incorporated into combination chemotherapy, and Phase III trials to assess their role in the treatment of breast cancer are in progress. Vinorelbine, a new vinca alkaloid, has also shown efficacy in the range of 40 % in patients with untreated metastatic breast cancer, and between 20-30 % in patients with refractory metastatic disease. Amonafide has demonstrated more modest activity (a 20 % response rate in untreated metastatic breast cancer). The anthrapyrazoles have shown highly promising activity in limited Phase II trials. The camptothecin analogues (topotecan, CPT-11), have shown a high degree of activity *in vitro*, although clinical trials in breast cancer have not been completed. The development of these various exciting new cytotoxic agents will certainly affect our approaches to chemotherapy of breast cancer within the next several years.

There are still other interesting developments. New technology has lead to the development of monoclonal antibodies [8]. While antibodies alone have not shown major antitumor efficacy, it is expected that they may function as vehicles for more specific (and therefore less toxic) cytotoxic therapy when conjugated with standard cytotoxic agents, radiosotopes, or natural toxins. Similar approaches are being developed with the use of growth factors, growth factor receptors, liposomes, and steroid hormonal agents. These approaches to therapy are relatively new, and technical obstacles have slowed their development. However, multiple Phase I-Phase II clinical trials are on course, and we expect their results with interest.

Finally, the initial steps have been taken for the evaluation of genetic therapies in metastatic breast and other cancers. Antisense therapy, and other forms of genetic modification, are being developed to modulate the expression of specific proteins, to control or reverse the activation of specific genetic segments, or to replace specific tumor suppressor genetic messages. Although serious technical obstacles exist to take these exciting conceptual approaches to the clinic, the initial steps of clinical development are already in process.

Although treatable, metastatic breast cancer has been quite resistant to major modifications of its natural history by currently available treatments. We provide substantial and effective palliation for most patients, but the effect of our current treatments over survival is modest at best. The exciting new therapies described above are expected to add to our therapeutic armamentarium, and change both the efficacy and toxicity of the regimens to treat this disease.

References

1. Bloom HJB, Richardson WW, Harries EJ (1962) Natural history of untreated breast cancer (1805-1933) Comparison of untreated and treated cases according to histological grade of malignancy. Br Med J 2 : 213-221
2. Buzdar AU (1990) Current status of endoctrine treatment of carcinoma of the breast. Sem Surg Oncol 6 : 77-82
3. Henderson IC (1991) Principles in the management of metastatic disease. In : Haris JR, Helman S, Henderson IC et al (eds) Breast diseases. 2nd Ed, JB Lippincott, Philadelphia, pp 547-677
4. Hortobagyi GN, Frye D, Buzdar AU et al (1988) Complete remissions in metastatic breast cancer : A thirteen year follow-up report. Proc 24th Annual Meeting Am Soc Clin Oncol 7 : 37 (abst 143)
5. Hortobagyi GN (1990) The importance of dose-response in cytotoxic therapy for breast cancer. In : Henderson IC, Borden EC (eds) Advances in breast cancer treatment, Mediscript, London, pp 47-69
6. Hortobagyi GN (1992) Overview of new treatments for breast cancer. Breast Cancer Res Treat 21 : 3-13
7. Holmes FA, Walters RS, Theriault RL et al (1991) Phase II Trial of taxol, an active drug in the treatment of metastatic breast cancer. J Natl Cancer Inst 83 : 1797-1805
8. Waldmann TA (1991) Monoclonal antibodies in diagnosis and therapy. Science 252 : 1657-1662

Present and future prospects for the chemotherapy of gliomas

V Levin

That there has been « littleprogress in the treatment of malignant gliomas » has almost become a cliche in oncology, yet from the past quarter century of effort we have learned a great deal about those empiric covariates that influence survival and have increased the quality and length of survival for some tumors. It has been shown that outcome (survival) for supratentorial gliomas is related to the following covariates : tumor histology and grade, labelling index, age at diagnosis, performance status, post-operative residual tumor volume, and the type and extent of radiation and chemotherapy.

Histologically, glioms are comprised of astrocytomas, oligodendrogliomas, ependymomas, or mixed tumors. Tumor proliferation can be quantitated by the Bromodeoxyuridine (BrdU) or the Ki-67 antibody labelling index (LI). The largest studies using BrdU LI have shown that a LI of < 1 % carried a 90 % 3 year survival probability while the astrocytoma designation only a 70 % 3 year survival (Hoshino et al, 1989).

Age at diagnosis not only is coupled with the occurrence of specific tumor subtypes, but also, within a subtype, strongly influences survival. For instance, the diagnosis of astrocytoma can be made between the ages of approximately 1 year of age through the seventh decade, yet tumor related survival decreases markedly with age. Five-year survival remains approximately 70 % through age 24 but falls to 10 % between 65-74 years. This is also reflected, as expected, in relatively poor radiotherapy (RT) and chemotherapy responses in those over approximately 60 years of age at the time of diagnosis. Paradoxically, survival for patients with brainstem gliomas is directly related to age at onset with those > 18 years surviving longer than children (Edwards et al, 1989).

A balance between bulk resection and surgical morbidity must always be sought with the survival scale tilting toward greatest bulk resection. Bulk resection can alleviate some symptoms and signs of tumor and increased intracranial pressure. From three different studies that encompassed astrocytoma through glioblastoma multiforme, the conclusions are similar : significant survival benefits appear greatest with resections in excess of 70-75 % of tumor leaving a residual tumor volume of 3-4 cc (Levin et al, 1980 ; Ammirati et al, 1987 ; Wood et al, 1988). Better performance status following surgery is also likely to lead to longer survival, although this has not been directly addressed in glioma patients.

Given the apparent limits of RT efficacy, drugs have been used to enhance the tumoricidal effects of RT. The hypoxic-cell sensitizers have not lived up to earlier experimental promise. Those agents that potentiate toxic cell damage

---

University of Texas MD Anderson Cancer Center, 1515 Holcombe Boulevard, Box 100, Houston, Texas 77030, USA

such as hydroxyurea and the halopyrimidines have shown more clinical promise, but still require additional study.

Where does chemotherapy stand today ? Studies of the Brain Tumor Cooperative Group failed to show any clear advantage of any adjuvant chemotherapy over single agent BCNU (Walker et al, 1980 ; Shapiro et al, 1989 ; Deutsch et al, 1989). Studies from the NCOG, however, did show a two-fold increase in survival for anaplastic gliomas receiving CCNU, Procarbazine, and Vincristine (PCV) over BCNU alone (Levin et al, 1990). Studies of Jermeic also showed that, post-RT, a combination of CCNU, Procarbazine, and Vincristine (mPCV) to be much to superior to VM-26 and CCNU (Jeremic et al, 1992). A study conducted by the Northern California Oncology Group that closed November 1987 showed that 96 hour infusions of BUdR given during each week of comparable benefits for anaplastic glioma patients but no activity in glioblastoma patients (Phillips et al, 1991 ; Levin et al, in preparation).

For recurrent and progressive tumors, phase II chemotherapy studies demonstrate combined response and disease stabilization in up to 50 % of GM patients with median times to progression (MTP) of 16-27 weeks ; for AG rates of 20-95 % and MTP of 16-47 weeks have been reported (Levin et al, 1989). In all cases palliation is the end result with virtually no or only occasional long-term survivors. Typically, however, some patients appear to benefit from several different sequential therapies attaining cumulatively long survival, whereas others with comparable sized tumors of the same histology fail quickly and never demonstrate any benefit from therapy. Among the new agents investigated, Eflornithine (Levin et al, 1992) appears the most active with nearly 50 % of AA attaining an MTP of nearly 1 year. As far as drug combinations go, the combination of 6-Thioguanine, Procarbazine, Dibromodulcitol, CCNU, 5-Fluorouracil, and Hydroxyurea appears one of the most active (Levin & Prados, 1992).

Biologics such as the interferons (α and β) have been used as single agents with some benefit. In a multi-institutional study of 67 patients who received Interferon-β, response and stable disease rates of 50 % were achieved for both GM and AG tumors for a short MTP of 16-18 weeks (Yung et al, 1991).

Anecdotal reports indicate that oligodendrogliomas are response to a number of different chemotherapies, although the largest series of similarly treated patients are those receiving PCV (Cairncross et al, 1988). In most ways, however, these patient behave similar to those with astrocytoma or anaplastic astrocytomas.

The literature for chemotherapy for ependymomas is even less defined. Small series suggest activity of BCNU, Dibromodulcitol, and, possibly, Etoposide. The typical course of these patients is to have multiple surgeries, several forms of chemotherapy, and reirradiation to slow tumor growth. Because of their involvement of the spinal axis and 4th ventricle, evaluating chemotherapy benefit was difficult prior to MRI.

Brainstem gliomas are primarily astrocytomas. Surgery, because of location, rarely offers lasting benefit. RT has benefit, but long-term survivors are uncommon. Median survival less than 1 year is the norm. Recently hyperfractionated RT has been used increasing the total dose to 72 Gy with an approximate 50 % increase in survival (Edwards et al, 1989). Newer studies utilizing 78 Gy do not appear more beneficial. Chemotherapy is palliative providing, at recurrence, up to 6 months of progression free survival in 50 % of patients.

Cerebellar gliomas differ from cerebral gliomas in that more cerebellar tumors are low-grade and frequently surgical resection alone or with RT can lead to long-term survival. What will be « *tomorrow's chemotherapies* » ? Given current knowledge, one must conclude that chemotherapy, broadly defined to include cytotoxic agents as we know them today as well as pharmacologic doses of natural and modified cytokines will continue to be palliative for gliomas. To reach the next level, chemotherapies will be directed against unique cellular or nuclear targets that are specific for the malignant phenotype. Targets may be specific DNA sequences or proteins that are important in embryogenesis but serve little if any function in mature organisms. Drug approaches likely to be important will be 1) antisense oligonucleotide and triplex approaches, 2) specific DNA sequence blockers (reactors), 3) specific protein (enzyme) inhibitors, and 4) retroviral initiated gene therapies.

References

Ammirati M et al (1987) Effect of the extend of surgical resection on survival and quality of life in patients with supratentorial glioblastomas and anaplastic astrocytomas. Neurosurg 21 : 201-206

Cairncross JG, MacDonald DR (1988) Successful chemotherapy for recurrent malignant oligodendroglioma. Ann Neurol 23 : 360-364

Deutsch M, Green SB, Strike TA et al (1989) Results of a randomized trial comparing BCNU plus radiotherapy, Streptozotocin plus radiotherapy, BCNU plus hyperfractionated radiotherapy, and BCNU following Misonidazole plus radiotherapy in the post-operative treatment of malignant glioma. Int J Radiat Oncol Biol Phys 16 : 1389-1396

Edwards MS et al (1989) Hyperfractionated radiation therapy for brain-stem glioma : A phase I-II trial. J Neurosurg 70 : 691-700

Hoshino T et al (1989) Prognostic implications of the bromodeoxyuridine labelling index of human gliomas. J Neurosurg 71 : 335-341

Jeremic B, Jovanovic D, Djuric LJ et al (1992) Advantage of post-radiotherapy chemotherapy with CCNU, Procarbazine, and Vincristine (mPCV) over chemotherapy with VM-26 and CCNU for malignant gliomas. J Chemotherapy 4 : 123-126

Levin VA, Sheline GE, Gutin PH (1989) Neoplasms of the central nervous system. In : DeVita VT, Jr, Hellman S, Rosenberg SA (eds) Cancer. Principles and Practice of Oncology. 3rd Edition, JB Lippincott, Philadelphia, pp 1557-1579

Levin VA et al (1980) Prognostic significance of the pretreatment CT scan on time to progression for patients with malignant gliomas. J Neurosurg 52 : 642-647

Levin VA, Silver P, Hannigan J et al (1990) Superiority of post-radiotherapy adjuvant chemotherapy with CCNU, Procarbazine, and Vincristine (PCV) over BCNU for anaplastic gliomas : NCOG 6G61 final report. Int J Radiat Oncol Biol Phys 18 : 321-324

Levin VA, Prados MD, Yung WA et al (1992) Treatment of recurrent gliomas with Eflornithine, J Natl Cancer Inst 84 : 1432-1437

Levin VA, Prados MD (1993) Treatment of recurrent gliomas and metastatic brain tumors with a polydrug protocol designed to combat nitrosourea resistance. J Clin Oncol 10 : 766-771

Shapiro WR, Green SB, Burger PC et al (1989) Randomized trial for three chemotherapy regimens and two radiotherapy regimens in post-operative treatment of malignant glioma. Brain Tumor Coop Group Trail 8001. J Neurosurg 71 : 1-9

Walker MD, Green SN, Byar DP et al (1980) Randomized comparisons of radiotherapy and nitrosoureas for malignant glioma after surgery. N Engl J Med 303 : 1323-1329

Wood JR, Green SB, Shapiro WR (1988) The prognostic importance of tumor size in malignant gliomas : a computed tomographic scan study by the Brain Tumor Coop Group. J Clin Oncol 6 : 338-343

Neo-Adjuvant chemotherapy in breast cancer
Study of 477 evaluable patients with primary breast cancers treated between 1980 and 1992

M Weil, G Auclerc, Ch Borel, F Baillet, A Thomas,
Cl Soubrane, M Housset, D Nizri, O Rixe, E Antoine,
E Vuillemin, D Khayat

Neo-Adjuvant chemotherapy in breast cancer means that chemotherapy is used as the first therapeutic tool and that the locoregional treatment is considered as an adjuvant. The term has been contested and others were proposed, but induction treatment is too specific for the first chemotherapy combination used in leukemia to achieve complete remission. Primary treatment does not encompass the consolidation phase which belongs to our strategy so that even if it is not quite satisfactory we keep the term Neo-Adjuvant which has been coined in the seventies by E. Frei for head and neck cancers.

I — This strategy was proposed by Claude Jacquillat [1] who refused thus the separation between non-operable advanced breast cancer for whom some authors have already proposed initial chemotherapy and operable breast cancer for whom his proposals were considered by some collegues, still ruled by the science of a previous area as almost scandalous :
Which were the justifications of Claude Jacquillat ?
He was aware of B. Fisher's data on the significance of regional lymph node involvement which is the indicator of biological relationship between host and tumor and which is not the instigator of distant disease [2]. As an hematologist, he was already familiar with interrelationship between the blood and lymphatic systems.
He was aware of Skipper's experimental data on the relationship between tumor burden and curability [3].
He was aware of the Goldie Coldman model which indicates that as a tumor cell population increases, there is an ever expanding number of drug resistant phenotypic variants arising due to spontaneous somatic mutations, which become then more difficult to eradicate [4].
He was aware of the experiments of Fisher demonstrating that after removal of a primary tumor, an increase in the labelling index of distant tumor focus occurs resulting in an increase in tumor size and hence in the number of resistant cells [5].
He was aware of course of the poor long term prognosis of breast cancer treated by surgery alone and he was familiar with the pioneer studies of perioperative chemotherapy initiated by Niessen Meyer [6] and by Fisher [7] in the

---

SOMPS Salpetriere Hospital, 47 bd de l'Hopital, 75013 Paris, France

late sixties. Very short perioperative treatment improves by 20 % long term survival. Its delay according to Niessen Meyer abrogates its benefit. He was of course aware [8] of the studies indicating the benefit of treating node negative patients since the major reproach he was addressed was to inflict unnecessary systemic treatments to good prognosis patients by ignoring their axillary node histology. Thus, as far as the systemic disease is concerned for chemotherapy onset, the earlier seems to be the better.

Two other advantages are expected from Neo-Adjuvant chemotherapy : to increase breast preservation by downstaging large tumors and to assess the effectiveness of the chemotherapy combination by measuring tumor regression. We shall indicate our personal experience and we shall compare our results to other studies.

II — The SOMPS studies : 10 years results in 477 patients with non metastatic breast cancer

A — Material and methods

477 evaluable patients entered two consecutive protocols : 250 patients were treated between 1980 and 1986 by protocol 03 SR 80 mean follow 77 months (1-147) and 227 patients since 1986 by protocol 02 SR 86 mean follow 39 months (4-78). Patients with tumors less than 1 cm and/or requiring surgical biopsies for diagnosis and patients over 75 years of age were non eligible.

Table 1. Patients characteristics according to stage

Stages	Protocol 03 SR 80 (250 pts) No pts (%)	Protocol 02 SR 86 (227 pts) No pts (%)	Total (477 pts) No pts (%)
I	19 (8)	30 (13)	49 (10)
IIa	86 (34)	80 (35)	166 (35)
IIb	51 (20)	59 (26)	110 (23)
IIIa	36 (14)	25 (11)	61 (13)
IIIb	58 (23)	33 (15)	91 (19)

Table 1 indicates the distribution of TNM stages. These protocols have been described previously [9] [10] [11] and have major similarities and minor differences. In both of them, diagnosis is insured by fine needle aspiration which allows cytopronostic grading (CPI), hormone receptors studies, cathepsine determination, flow cytometry measure. Induction phase consists in the combination of VLb, Thiotepa, Methotrexate, 5-FU and Adriamycine given according to a weekly and thereafter a bimonthly schedule in order to insure maximal tolerated dose intensity. Locoregional treatment in both protocols consists in teleradiotherapy (4,500 CGy within 5 weeks or 2,300 CGy in 4 sessions) combined to a boost by wire implants of iridium 192.

In both protocols, consolidation duration depends on pronostic parameters. There are differences in patients stratification that includes cell differenciation in addition to tumor size and clinical lymphnodes in the second protocol.

Adriamycine which was restricted to poor prognosis patients in the first protocol was given to all patients except group I in the second one (T1No CPI 1).

Tamoxifen was given to all premenopausal and postmenopausal women in the second protocol (in the 1st protocol, it was planned to give it to all menopausal women and to randomize its administration in pre-menopausal women).

In the second protocol, a rescue protocol combining Cisplatinum, Etoposide, 5-Fu and alternatively Mitomycin and Adriamycine was planned for poor responders (less than 50 % tumor regression after 3 doses).

B — Results

Before radiotherapy, we observed 61 % partial remission (PR) and 30 % complete (CCR) (Table 2) clinical remission in the first protocol, 44 % PR and 44 % CCR in the second protocol. Among 20 poor responders, the rescue protocol induced 10 PR and 2 CR. Induction results were influenced by tumor size ($P < 0,004$) CR being more frequent in small tumors and by cell differenciation $P < 0,02$, CR being less frequent in well differentiated tumors (25 % CCR in CPI versus 45 % in CPI 3) (Table 2).

Table 2. Induction results in 477 patients

Protocols	Number patients	% RC	% RP	Total responders	
03 SR 80	250	30	61	91	
02 SR 86	227	44	44	88	
Size					
T1	56	59	34	93	
T2	197	35	57	92	
T3	133	30	58	88	
T4	91	34	50	84	< 0.004
CPI					
Grade 1	80	25	65	90	
Grade 2	209	36	54	90	
Grade 3	103	45	40	85	< 0.02

Table 3. Distribution of relapses according to tumor size 03 SR 80 + 02 SR 86

	No pts	Metastasis	Local or Local + metastasis	% actuarial 5 years local relapses
T1	54	3	2	6
T2	191	19	24	12
T3	127	30	12	10
T4	90	23	17	25

Table 4. 5 years and 8 years actuarial DFS according to various parameters

	No pts	No/relapses	% 5 years actuarial DFS (number at risk)	% 8 years actuarial DFS (number at risk)
TNM				
St. I	49	5	91 (19)	83 (5)
II A	166	28	84 (85)	74 (18)
IIB	110	31	69 (43)	58 (10)
IIIA	61	29	48 (18)	45 (3)
IIIB	91	42	52 (32)	44 (13)
				$p < 0.0001$
Grade				
CP1	80	13	90 (43)	69 (9)
CP2	208	57	69 (78)	62 (19)
CP3	103	35	62 (36)	55 (9)
				$p < 0.006$
Initial responses to chemotherapy				
< 50 %	50	18	54 (9)	46 (3)
50 < R < 100	255	80	71 (128)	60 (35)
100 %	172	37	73 (59)	71 (11)
				$p < 0.04$

These results should not surprise us; well differentiated tumor have low phase S and Remvikos [12] and others did demonstrate the relationship between cell proliferation fraction and sensitivity to chemotherapy.

After radiotherapy, all patients except four of them achieved complete clinical remission. Despite the large tumor size of the majority of our patients the cosmetic results that were graded according to Danoff's classification were excellent or good in 85 % patients. The local control was relatively good as shown on Table 3 that indicates the distribution of relapses according to tumor size. The 8 years actuarial rate of breast preservation is 94 %.

5 years and 8 years DFS according to TNM stages are shown on Table 4.

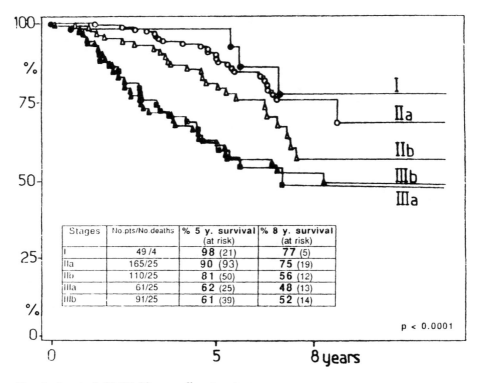

Fig. 1. Survival 03 SR 80 according to stage

In our experience, prognosis of stage IIIB was not significantly worse than that of III A which is different from the experience of most authors. 5 years and 8 years DFS according to CPI and according to tumor regression are represented on the same table. They show that despite their decreased sensitivity to chemotherapy, CPI 1 patients have the best prognosis. In these well differentiated patients, slow responders may actually have the best prognosis.

Despite the lack of significance of tumor regression in well differentiated tumors, tumor regression remains a significant prognostic parameter. But in our experience there is no significant difference between complete clinical remission and partial remission which proves that clinical examination does not allow CR to be identified.

104 patients died among whom there were 100 metastatic deaths and 4 unrelated deaths (1 early leukemia, 2 traffic accidents, 1 fulminant glioblastoma).

Survival according to stage is shown on Figure 1. As shown on Table 5, the multifactorial analysis according to Cox model confirms that tumor size, clinical lymphnodes, cell differentiation (CPI) and tumor regression are significant and independant indicators parameter for survival.

Table 5. Multifactorial analysis (Cox) for survival 03 SR 80 and 02 SR 86

Variable	Coefficient	P. value	Exp. (coeff.)
T	0.3748	< 0.0001	1.4547
N	0.3944	0.012	1.4835
CPI	0.9029	0.004	2.4669
Response	0.5491	0.042	0.5775

T = T1, T2, T3
N = N0, N1, N2
CPI Cox = CPI, CPI and 3
Responses = R < 50 % ; 50 % < R < 99 % ; 100 %

III — Other published studies

Most published studies at this time concern mostly so called locally advanced breast cancer. Their comparison is difficult because the population is not always described in term of TNM classification, the definition of non-operable breast cancer depending on many factors. The inclusion of inflammatory breast cancer varies from study to study as well as the definition of inflammatory breast cancer requiring or not histologic assessment. On the whole, the rate of response is high, around 80 %. The rate of CCR varies from 17 % to 50 %. The rate of PCR when it is indicated is about 70 % of CCR. For most authors there is significant difference between stage IIIB with about 30 % 3 years survival and stage IIIA with median survival over 5 years.

There is a tendancy for better results in patients who had surgery rather than radiotherapy as locoregional treatment but the modalities of radiotherapy are never indicated. Some results are reported on Table 6.

In early forms of breast cancer, reports are much more rare. In a non randomized study, Blelembaogo and AI [17] treated 101 patients with breast cancer over 3 cm, or situated in the central area of the nipple (20 cases) or with bulky suspicious lymphnodes in the axillar (44 pts). These patients would have been candidates to mastectomy. After 6 cycles CFVA or CMFVA, 30 CCR were treated by exclusive radiotherapy, 44 were treated by tumorectomy and radiotherapy and only 15 mastectomies were performed no data on long term reports.

In the Milan study [18] preoperative chemotherapy was administrated recently to 157 patients who would have been candidate to mastectomy because the largest diameter of their tumor was > or = to 3 cm. In 127 patients, tumor shrinkage allowed breast conservation. Quite recently in a randomized study dealing with 414 premenopausal patients Scholl and AI [19], after a median follow up of 46 months observed a significant difference in survival in favour of the Neo-Adjuvant arm. In this study indicating 65 % responses to chemotherapy, a significant advantage was observed in good responders. Ragaz randomized patients between immediate mastectomy and mastectomy fol-

Table 6. Preoperative chemotherapy in stage III breast cancer

Authors	Nb of pts	Stage	Chemotherapy regression	Local treatment	DFS	Survival
Swain [13]	51	IIIA	90 %	Surgery	Median not reached for IIIA	
		IIIB	(52 %) CCR among whom 71 % PCR		30 months for IIIB (median follow up 16 months)	
Hortobagyi [14]	174	IIIA (48 pts)	87 % (17 % CCR)	Radiotherapy till 1981 Mastectomy thereafter	5 DFS 71 % for IIIA 33 % for IIIB	
		IIIB (126 pts) non inflammatory				
Valagussa [15]	277	IIIA-IIIB non inflammatory		Radiotherapy (198) Surgery (79)	10 years DFS 14 % 10 years DFS 22 %	10 years S (26 %) 10 years S (28 %)
Chauvergne [16]	270	non operable	80 %	Radiotherapy for C.R. Surgery for other pts	NA	5 years S 60 % for responders 0 for non responders

lowing one single dose of CMF and observed no significant differences, which is not really surprising [20].

IV — Discussion

More than 12 years after the activation of our first protocol, we may discuss our achievements and our failures.

— That Neo-Adjuvant chemotherapy increases the rate of breast preservation cannot be disputed anymore. We observed this phenomenom by achieving 94 % breast preservation but other authors with less important breast preservation rate observed the same advantage.

— That Neo-Adjuvant chemotherapy preserves an important and independant predictive parameter by allowing to measure tumor regression is shown by the multifactorial analysis that we have performed. Other authors found also a significant advantage in survival for good responders. In well differentiated tumors, this parameter is not predictive because of kinetic resistance.

In terms of DFS and of survival, the 5 years and the 8 years results that we report here are encouraging. However, to assert their superiority over surgery and adjuvant treatment would have required a randomized study. The results of the NSABP study are waited for with much expectation.

Thus we think that in palpable infiltrative tumors, the concept of Neo-Adjuvant treatment is valid but it should incorporate new drugs, revertant of resistance, repeated intensifications with the support of cytokines and of stem cells in high risk patients. In the near future, manipulation of growth factors and of immunological responses and perhaps even gene manipultion should be contemplated. At the same time, all efforts should be aimed at detecting breast cancer earlier and even at clinically occult stage and at preventing in patients at risk especially in those with benign mastopathy the occurrence of infiltrative breast cancer.

References

1. Jacquillat Cl, Baillet F, Auclerc G, Maylin Cl, Weil M (1982) Initial chemotherapy + conservative radiotherapy in stages I, II and III breast cancer in Proceedings of the 13th International Cancer Congress, Seattle, Washington
2. Fisher B, Fisher ER (1966) Transmigration of lymphnodes by tumor cells. Sciences (Washington DC) 152 : 1397-1398
3. Skipper HE (1971) Kinetics of tumor cell growth and implication for therapy. Cancer (Philadelphia) 28 : 1479-1499
4. Goldic JH, Coldman AI (1979) A mathematical model for relating the drug sensitivity of tumors to their spontaneous mutation rate. Cancer Treatment Report 69 : 1727-1733
5. Gundus N, Fisher B, Safter EA (1979) Effect of surgical removal on the growth and kinetics of residual tumor. Cancer Res 39 : 3861-3865
6. Niessen Meyer R, Kjellgren K, Malmiok, Mansson B, Morin (1978) Surgical adjuvant chemotherapy : result on one short course with Cyclophosphamide after mastectomy for breast cancer. Cancer 41 : 2088-2098

7. Fisher B, Carbone P, Economou SG et al (1975) Phenylalanine mustard (LPAN) in the management of primary breast cancer : a report of early findings. N Engl J Med 292 : 117-122
8. National Institute of Health consensus Development Conference Statement Treatment of early stage breast cancer (1990) Bethesda MD. Natl Inst Health June : 18-21
9. Jacquillat Cl, Baillet F, Weil M et al (1988) Results of a conservative treatment combining induction (Neo-Adjuvant) and consolidation chemotherapy, hormonotherapy and irradiation in 98 patients with locally advanced breast cancer (IIIA-IIIB). Cancer 61 : 1977-1982
10. Jacquillat Cl, Weil M, Baillet M et al (1990) Results of Neo-Adjuvant chemotherapy and radiation therapy in the breast conserving treatment of 250 patients with all stages of infiltrative breast cancer. Cancer 66 : 119-129
11. Jacquillat Cl, Weil M, Auclerc G et al (1991) Ten years of breast preserving management in infiltrative breast cancer results in 412 patients treated by Neo-Adjuvant Chemotherapy and radiotherapy with or without hormonotherapy. In : Banzet P, Holland JF, Khayat D, Weil M (eds) Proceedings of the 3rd International Congress on Neo-Adjuvant Chemotherapy. Springer-Verlag, Paris, pp. 126-136
12. Remvikos Y, Beuzebac P, Zajdela A et al (1989) Correlation of pretreatment proliferative activity of breast cancer with the response to cytotoxic chemotherapy. J Nat Cancer Inst 81 : 1383-1387
13. Swain S, Bagley C, Findley P, Lippman M (1986) Neo-Adjuvant therapy of locally advanced breast cancer in Proceeding of the 1st International Congress on Neo-Adjuvant chemotherapy. In : Jacquillat Cl, Weil M, Khayat D (eds) Colloque INSERM/John Libbey Eurotext 137 : 243-252
14. Hortobagyi GN, Blumonsclein GR, Spanos W et al (1983) Multimodality treatment of locoregionally advanced breast cancer. Cancer 51 : 763-68
15. Valugussa P, Zambetti M, Zucali R, Bonadonna G (1988) Locally advanced breast cancer : ten year results after combined treatment in Proceedings of the 2nd International Congress on Neo-Adjuvant chemotherapy. In : Jacquillat Cl, Weil M, Khayat D (eds) Colloque INSERM John Libbey Eurotext 169 : 123-127
16. Chauvergne I, Durand M, Mauriac L et al (1988) Traitement combiné de 270 cancers mammaires localement étendus : résultats d'un programme thérapeutique contrôlé in Proceedings of the 2nd International Congress on Neo-Adjuvant chemotherapy. In : Jacquillat Cl, Weil M, Khayat D (eds) Colloque INSERM, John Libbey Eurotext 169 : 225-230
17. Belembaogo E, Vernis M, Chollet P et al (1991) Neo-Adjuvant chemotherapy in 101 non inflammatory breast cancers : treatment results. In : Banzet P, Holland JF, Khayat D, Weil M (eds) Proceedings of the 3rd International Congress on Neo-Adjuvant chemotherapy. Springer-Verlag, Paris, pp. 154-158
18. Bonadonna G, Veronesi U, Brambilla C et al (1990) Primary chemotherapy to avoid mastectomy in tumors with diameters of three centimeters and more. J Natl Cancer Inst 82 : 1539-1545
19. Scholl SM, Asselain B, Beuzabac P et al (1993) Improved survival rate following first line chemotherapy in operable breast cancer. 4 years results of a randomized trial. 4th International Congress on Anticancer Chemotherapy, Paris (abstr 27)
20. Ragaz J, Bavid B, Rebbeck P et al (1991) Early results of the British Columbia breast cancer preoperative (Neo-Adjuvant) chemotherapy trial. In : Banzet P, Holland JF, Khayat D, Weil M (eds) Proceedings of the 3rd International Congress on Neo-Adjuvant chemotherapy. Springer-Verlag, Paris, pp. 154-158

Osteogenic sarcoma : a 15-year experience in treating 287 patients with preoperative chemotherapy

G Rosen, S Lowenbraun, C Forscher

With the introduction of the T-7 chemotherapy regimen in 1976, all patients with primary osteogenic sarcoma were treated with preoperative chemotherapy [1]. The T-7 regimen also marked the commencement of the use of high-dose Methotrexate (HDMTX) at the doses of 12 gm/m^2 for young children and 8 gm/m^2 for adults. The T-7 regimen used HDMTX with Leucovorin rescue, the combination of Bleomycin, Cyclophosphamide, and Dactinomycin (BCD), and Adriamycin as a single agent, given at the dose of 90 mg/m^2 over two days.

Early data showed that patients who had a complete histologic response to preoperative chemotherapy had an excellent prognosis, whereas patients who had only a partial histologic response to preoperative chemotherapy were at risk for relapse. When Cisplatinum was introduced as an effective agent in osteogenic sarcoma, the T-7 regimen was modified to give six courses of Cisplatinum (120 mg/m^2) combined with Adriamycin (60 mg/m^2) administered postoperatively to patients that did not have a good histologic response to preoperative T-7 chemotherapy. This regimen was named « T-10 »[2] ». However, giving Cisplatinum combined with Adriamycin to patients that did not have a complete histologic response to preoperative chemotherapy did not significantly increase such patients' survival at five or 10 year follow-up.

In 1981, the next regimen (T-12) was designed to reduce the total amount of chemotherapy given to patients who had a complete response to preoperative chemotherapy. Complete response was an indication of excellent prognosis, and perhaps these patients did not need prolonged treatment with both HDMTX and Adriamycin (which, at the time, had been reported to have high incidence of late cardiac effects). The T-12 regimen gave HDMTX with Leucovorin rescue and the BCD combination preoperatively. Patients who had a complete histologic response to preoperative chemotherapy received only one more BCD treatment and just two more HDMTX treatments postoperatively. Patients who did not have a complete histologic response received 6 Cisplatinum and Adriamycin combination chemotherapy treatments postoperatively [3].

For the first time, relapses were seen on the T-12 regimen in patients that were complete responders. We were also concerned that the complete response rate to the T-12 regimen was slightly lower than to the T-10 regimen (44 % vs 49 %).

In an attempt to increase the complete response rate to preoperative chemotherapy, the T-14 regimen replaced the preoperative and postoperative BCD chemotherapy with the combination of Cisplatinum and Adriamycin. However, early results of the T-14 regimen failed to demonstrate an increased

---

The Cedars-Sinai Comprehensive Cancer Center, 8700 Beverly Boulevard, Los Angeles, California 90048, USA

complete response rate in patients undergoing preoperative chemotherapy. The T-14 regimen was thus modified twice, once by adding Bleomycin to the Adriamycin/Cisplatinum combination chemotherapy regimen. This produced more mucositis, and there was no apparent increase in the complete response rate. In a second modification of the T-14 regimen, Mitomycin-C was added to the Adriamycin/Cisplatinum combination. This led to prolonged thrombocytopenia and delays in treatment that resulted in a decrease in patients having a complete response to preoperative chemotherapy.

In 1991, with the definition of high-dose Ifosfamide (14 gm/m^2) as effective in the treatment of metastatic osteogenic sarcoma, we replaced one of the Cisplatinum/Adriamycin preoperative treatments in the T-14 regimen with two high-dose Ifosfamide treatments. This regimen was termed « T-19 ». Another modification included the complete elimination of HDMTX if there was no apparent clinical, biochemical, or imaging response of the primary tumor following the first two HDMTX treatments. This regimen was stopped after only 8 patients were treated. Two of 6 patients that had a complete response, had the elimination of HDMTX (that did not appear to be active in their primary tumor). Both patients relapsed with pulmonary metastases within a very short time of discontinuing therapy (3 and 6 months). We had never witnessed such a phenomenon in patients who had a complete response to preoperative chemotherapy. At this point, we also realized that the overall survival of patients treated on the T-12 and T-14 regimens were not as good as that obtained with the earlier versions of T-7 and T-10 regimens, where patients had more HDMTX, single-agent high-dose Adriamycin and BCD chemotherapy.

Patients

Of the 287 patients, 53 were treated on the T-7 regimen, 116 on the T-10 regimen, 78 on the T-12 regimen, 32 on the T-14 regimen, and only 8 patients on the T-19 regimen (Table 1). Patients included were those who had a primary extremity osteogenic sarcoma, had no evidence of pulmonary or bone metastasis, had no prior chemotherapy, had primary surgery performed either at Memorial Sloan-Kettering Cancer Center or UCLA, and had chemotherapy administered by the authors at Memorial Sloan-ettering Cancer Center (NY) or Cedars-Sinai Comprehensive Cancer Center (Los Angeles).

Table 1. Osteosarcoma survival

Protocol	# pts (%)*	5 yr dfs
T-7	53 (19)	83 %
T-10	116 (42)	80 %
T-12	78 (27)	65 %
T-14	32 (11)	75 % (3 yr)

Osteogenic sarcoma

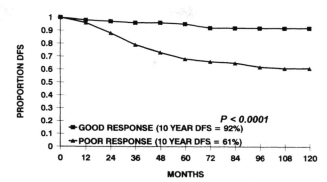

Fig. 1. Osteosarcoma survival response to chemotherapy

Results

The 5-year disease-free survivals (DFS) of the T-7, T-10, T-12, and T-14 regimens are listed in Table 1. Figure 1 shows the DFS of all 287 patients, categorized by response to preoperative chemotherapy. It is still highly significant that a complete response is still the best prognostic factor, leading to a 10-year DFS of 92 %, as compared to 61 % for the poor responders (P < 0.0001). Also significant is that the complete histologic response rate for the T-7 regimen was 75 %, as compared to 49 % for T-10, 44 % for T-12, and 60 % for T-14. The 10-year DFS for children 10 years of age or less was 89 %, which was significantly better (P < 0.01) than the 10-year DFS for patients 11-21 years of age (72 %), 21-30 years of age (74 %) and adults older than 30 years of age (64 %). Analysis of the total amounts of HDMTX, Adriamycin and Cisplatinum given to patients on the various chemotherapy regimens is enumerated in Figures 2 and 3. In Figure 2, the DFS in patients having only a partial response to preoperative chemotherapy has not improved beyond the rate of roughly 65 % obtained in the T-10 chemotherapy regimen. The T-7 regimen had only a 43 % 5-year DFS for poor responders, but that only represented 13 out of 53 patients treated on that regimen. Note also that the addition of large amounts of Cisplatinum and Adriamycin in the subsequent regimens could not raise the DFS rate above the 66 % obtained on the T-10 regimen.

Of the complete responders (Fig. 3), the T-7 regimen had the highest DFS rate of 94 %, followed by 92 % for the T-10 regimen. All of the patients who were complete responders on these regimens who relapsed, did so very late in the course of their disease. Complete responders on the T-12 regimen had only an 83 % DFS, which was similar to that obtained in the T-14 regimen (where BCD was replaced with the combination of Adriamycin and Cisplatinum). On the T-19 regimen, complete responders (6 patients) had only a 66 % 2-year DFS because of the early relapse of two patients who had HDMTX eliminated from their chemotherapy course (due to a lack of apparent early response).

We now use a new regimen (T-20). It increases the total amount of HDMTX as well as single-agent Adriamycin (100 gm/m^2) given to patients to try to recreate the good results for complete responders obtained on those early regimens. Also, patients who do not have a complete response to preoperative

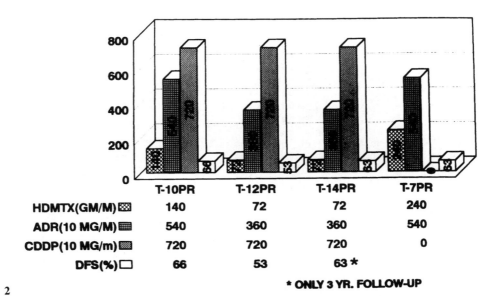

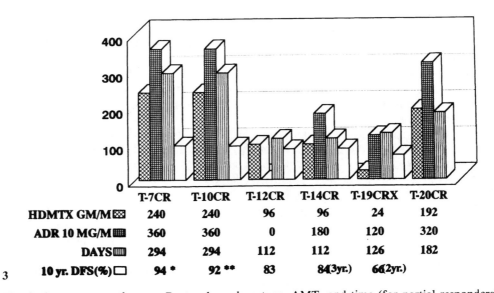

Fig. 2. Osteosarcoma therapy. Protocol vs. drug type, AMT, and time (for partial responders)

Fig. 3. Osteosarcoma therapy. Protocol vs. drug type, AMT, and time (complete responders)

chemotherapy on the new T-20 regimen do not have HDMTX eliminated postoperatively, but are given more HDMTX at a higher dose for the reasons to follow.

Discussion

Our interpretation of the above data leads us to the following conclusions.

High-dose Methotrexate is the most important drug in analyzing survival. This conclusion is bolstered by the fact that young children $\leq$ 10 years old had a much worse prognosis without chemotherapy, or with earlier regimens (T-4) where the dose of HDMTX was not increased to 12 gm/m^2. The fact that they had a significantly superior 10-year DFS on the regimens discussed above is attributed to the higher dose of HDMTX than that given to older patients. We also attribute the better results of the T-7 regimen (i.e., the 75 % complete histologic response rate to preoperative chemotherapy) to the fact that many patients on the T-7 regimen had their dose of Methotrexate escalated if they did not have a clinical response to the first four HDMTX treatments, or if they had 24 hour Methotrexate levels that were below 1×10^5 molar. It was our clinical impression that patients who had higher 24-hour levels (and had urine output restricted during the first 24 hours to achieve those higher levels), seemed to do better. Statistically, we were never able to prove this with the pharmacokinetic data that we collected. It may be that 6-hour Methotrexate levels are more predictive of effective plasma levels that lead to a better response in osteogenic sarcoma, as has been recently reported [4]. We did not do 6-hour Methotrexate levels in our patients.

In the T-12 regimen, the reduction in the number of HDMTX treatments and the dose of Adriamycin led to both lower complete histologic response rates and overall 10-year DFS rates. The large amount of Cisplatinum and Adriamycin given to the partial responders to preoperative chemotherapy may have raised their DFS rate from somewhere around 40 % as seen in the T-7 regimen to approximately 65 %. However, this is still not good enough for that group of patients.

It is now our feeling that HDMTX should be given to all patients (both children and adults) at the dose of 12 gm/m^2. High-dose Ifosfamide and Cisplatinum combined with Adriamycin might still be used in the chemotherapy regimen but should not replace HDMTX or compromise the utilization of HDMTX in these regimens. Patients who have a partial response to chemotherapy should still be given the same chemotherapy with HDMTX. However, in those patients, we now raise the dose of HDMTX to 15 gm/m^2 and continue chemotherapy for a longer time than we do in the complete responders. The complete responders to our new T-20 regimen will still get substantial amounts of HDMTX, Adriamycin (given as a single agent at the dose of 100 mg/m^2 given over 2 days), high-dose Ifosfamide, and the combination of Cisplatinum and Adriamycin. To accomplish this, we have utilized not only G-CSF to prevent severe neutropenia, but continue with HDMTX two weeks following other myelosuppressive chemotherapies, even if the patient is still neutropenic.

It is our hope that the return to a greater utilization of HDMTX will give us the same high cure rate (> 90 %) seen in our earlier regimens. We also hope that the escalation of the dose of HDMTX for the poor responders might be the key to increasing their survival. To date, this has not been possible with the use of other seemingly more active agents in place of HDMTX.

References

1. Rosen G, Marcove R, Caparros B et al (1979) Primary osteogenic sarcoma : the rationale for preoperative chemotherapy and delayed surgery. Cancer 43 (6) : 2163-2177
2. Rosen G, Caparros B, Huvos A et al (1982) Preoperative chemotherapy for osteogenic sarcoma : selection of postoperative adjuvant chemotherapy based upon the response of the primary tumor to preoperative chemotherapy. Cancer 49 (6) : 1221-1230
3. Rosen G (1985) Preoperative (Neo-Adjuvant) chemotherapy for osteogenic sarcoma : a ten-year experience. Orthopedics 8 (5) : 659-664
4. Delepine N, Delepine G, Desbois J (1991) A monocentric therapy study : an approach to optimize the results of the treatment of osteosarcoma by protocols based upon HDMTX, associated with systematic conservative surgery. In : Humphrey G (ed) Osteosarcoma in children and young adults. Kluwer Academic Publishers, Boston, p 327

Abtract. This manuscript reviews the experience in the treatment of 287 patients with primary osteogenic sarcoma of an extremity at the Memorial Sloan-Kettering Cancer Center in New York (1976-1983) and the Cedars-Sinai Comprehensive Cancer Center in Los Angeles (1984-1992).

Cell cycle regulation and the chemosensitivity of cancer cells

KW Kohn, PM O'Connor

Recent advances in our understanding of cell cycle regulation suggest the possibility that successful chemotherapy may often depend on the presence of cell cycle control defects in the responding tumor cells. These control defects may arise, directly or indirectly, from functional abnormalities in proto-oncogenes or tumor suppressor genes that are common in clinical tumors. This paper will outline some aspects of cell cycle regulation — as currently understood in this rapidly advancing field — that may affect drug sensitivity and that might become the basis for a new approach to cancer chemotherapy.

The view that the regulatory defects that cause partially uncontrolled growth in tumors could also enhance drug sensitivity is an attractive notion, because it implies a cytotoxic mechanism that tumor cells may not easily evade. The essential concept is diagrammed in Figure 1. Carcinogenesis may begin when mutation alters the function of one or more proto-oncogenes or tumor suppressor genes. This impairs growth control of the neoplastic cell because (we assume) it impairs cell cycle regulation. Cell cycle events occurring at the wrong time due to defective regulation can produce chromosome instability and increase the likelihood of further alterations in oncogene function (reviewed by Hartwell 1992). This cycle of events may be the basis of tumor progression. The issue that concerns us here however is how cell cycle control defects might be the basis of chemotherapeutic responses. The normal control system prevents the initiation of a critical cell cycle event, such as mitosis, before the completion of a critical preceding event, such as DNA replication (reviewed by Murray 1992). When defective control prematurely allows a critical event to initiate too early, and if the disparity of events is large enough, then cell would die. For example, inhibition of DNA synthesis by an S-phase specific drug normally prevents initiation of mitosis and limits continued cell enlargement. Impairment of this control would obviously enhance drug sensitivity. Cell cycle control systems also monitor DNA damage, and defects in this monitoring could be responsible for the sensitivity of tumors to alkylating agents or topoisomerase blocking drugs.

The development of chemotherapeutic stratagems based on these concepts could entail the following steps : (1) elucidate the mechanisms of cell cycle control ; (2) identify defective control steps in cancer ; (3) identify non-toxic agents to modulate particular control steps that may be defective in certain tumors ; (4) utilize cell cycle manipulation to design selective cytotoxicity protocols.

Laboratory of Molecular Pharmacology, Developmental Therapeutics Program, Division of Cancer Treatment, National Cancer Institute, Bethesda, MD (USA)

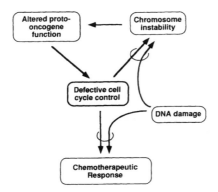

Fig. 1. General scheme showing how carcinogenesis and chemotherapeutic responsiveness may have a common basis in defective cell cycle control

G2 → M checkpoint

The cell cycle control step about which we presently know the most is the G2 → M transition (Fig. 2). This step is implicated in the action of a variety of drugs such as Cisplatin (Sorenson et al 1990) or Etoposide (Lock 1992), both of which cause cells to become arrested in G2, presumably because of damage to DNA, either directly or via topoisomerase II. The final common pathway for the initiation of mitotic events in eukaryotes from yeast to man is the cyclin-activated cdc2 kinase which phosphorylates several key proteins and brings about chromosome condensation, nuclear membrane breakdown and mitotic spindle assembly (Murray 1992). The cdc2 protein is present throughout the cell cycle and becomes associated with cyclin B which is synthesized during S phase. The cyclin B-cdc2 complex is thus prepared earlier in S phase to be used later for the G2 → M transition. Premature initiation of mitosis is prevented by phosphorylation of the cdc2 in the complex at tyr-15 and thr-14, which inhibits the kinase.

The premature initiation of mitotic events in cells that are still in S is familiar in the premature chromosome condensation caused by fusion with a mitotic cell. Chromosome condensation during S phase also occurs in temperature-sensitive tsBN2 hamster cells when the temperature is raised to non-permissive levels, and this is caused by loss of function of the RCC1 gene product which was thereby identified as a « regulator of chromosome condensation » (Seki et al 1992). Although the details of RCC1 function are not yet known, recent evidence indicates that it goes via the final common pathway of the cdc2 kinase.

The final determinant of the G2 → M transition then is a switch from preactive phosphorylated cyclin B-cdc2 to its active dephosphorylated form. The removal of the phosphates from the tyr-15 and thr-14 positions of cdc2 is accomplished by the phosphatase, cdc25C (Fig. 2). Cdc25C has been implicated in the functioning of RCC1 (Seki et al 1992). The activated form of cdc25C is multiply phosphorylated, and current evidence indicates that these phosphates are put on by the active cyclin B-cdc2 kinase, thus seeming to form a positive feedback loop (Hoffmann et al 1993).

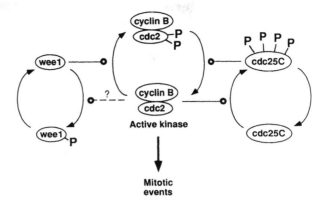

Fig. 2. Switching network through which the G2 → M transition may be controlled

The other side of the control switch is a kinase that phosphorylates cdc2 at tyr-15 and thr-14 so as to maintain it in the inactive state. This kinase may be the mammalian homolog of the yeast wee1 gene product, which is probably itself inactivated by phosphorylation and activated by dephosphorylation (Fig. 2). The cyclin B-cdc2 switch mechanism thus seems to contain 3 phosphorylation dephosphorylation couples that are interconnected in a rather symmetrical pattern (Fig. 2). There are several possible ways in which this switch might be controlled, and these will hopefully become elucidated in the very near future.

Effects of HN2 on cell cycle progression

We have been studying the regulation of the cyclin B-cdc2 switch in cells that undergo G2 arrest following treatment with nitrogen mustard (HN2). Cells synchronized in early S by double aphidicolin block were treated with a modestly cytotoxic dose of HN2 for 30 min, as a consequence of which the cells become accumulated, 10-12 hours later, in G2. We find that the dephosphorylation that normally activates cdc2 does not take place under these circumstances. Therefore the HN2-induced block is not directly at the step where active complex would phosphorylate the effector proteins of mitosis (O'Connor et al 1992, 1993). Moreover, the hyperphosphorylation of cdc25 also does not take place (unpublished data). We are now looking at the wee1 kinase to see whether its expected inactivation is also blocked. Since the system appears to be an integrated switch, an effect at any one point may toggle the entire configuration.

We have also examined the behavior of cyclin A and its associated cdk2 kinase (O'Connor et al 1993). This kinase complex normally reaches maximum activity during S phase, a few hours earlier than cyclin B-cdc2. Contrary to the block of the kinase activity associated with cyclin B, the kinase activity associated with cyclin A increases as HN2-treated cells accumulate in G2 (O'Connor et al 1993). The significance of this finding is not clear, because we do not yet know how the cyclin A associated kinases interacts with the cyclin B system. An additional complication is that, besides activating cdk2, cyclin A also associates with cdc2 during the G2 → M transition (O'Connor et al 1993). The G2 arrest caused by HN2 seems to occur at a point following the activation of cyclin A-cdk2 kinase, but prior to activation of the cyclin B-cdc2 and cyclin A-cdc2 kinases.

Effects of pentoxifylline

As a known inhibitor of G2 arrest in cells that have been treated with DNA damaging agents (Fingert et al 1986), we examined the effects of pentoxifylline. Addition of pentoxifylline following the HN2 treatment diminished the G2 delay and at the same time prevented the HN2-induced changes in the behavior of cyclin B and cyclin A associated kinase activities (O'Connor et al 1993). The effect of pentoxifylline however was not confined to the G2 delay: the drug also allowed S-phase cells to initiate mitosis prematurely in a progressive stochastic process extending over many hours.

The HN2 treatment not only delayed cells in G2, but also caused a prolongation of S phase. This prolongation was reversed by pentoxifylline, suggesting that it may not be due directly to a slowing of replication forks by DNA damage, but rather may involve effects on the control of replicon initiation. A monitoring mechanism may be implicated which shuts down replicon initiation in S phase cells in the presence of DNA damage, and which appears to be defective in ataxia-telangiectasia cells.

G1 → S checkpoint

The most common genomic abnormality in human cancer is in the p53 tumor suppressor gene which, when mutated, may interfere with the function of its normal allele. Loss or perturbation of normal p53 function causes genomic instability due to interference with the control of the G1 → S transition (reviewed by Hartwell 1992). p53 normally may function as a monitor of conditions that could be deleterious if cells were to commit to DNA replication (see reviews by Lane 1992 and by Vogelstein & Kinzler 1992). Tumor cells having defective p53 function may be relatively autonomous in their progress from G1 into S. It may therefore be possible pharmacologically to arrest normal cells in G1 while tumor cells continue into S where they would be susceptible to S-phase specific drugs. We are presently studying possible pharmacologic means of taking advantage of defective p53 function to enhance cytotoxicity.

Concluding remarks

It is often said that cancer chemotherapy is limited primarily by intrinsic or acquired drug resistance. Prior to the issue of drug resistance, however, one must consider the question of why cancer cells may sometimes be selectively drug sensitive. The recent work discussed here suggests that selective drug sensitivity may often be due to metabolic regulatory defects. Regulatory defects in cancer cells would arise from altered function of proto-oncogenes or tumor suppressor genes, some of which influence cell cycle control. A future direction for improved cancer chemotherapy would entail the characterization of regulatory defects existing in individual patients' tumors and the selection of treatment strategies designed to take advantage of the particular defects.

References

Fingert HJ, Chang JD, Pardee AB (1986) Cytotoxic, cell cycle, and chromosomal effects of methylxanthines in human tumor cells treated with alkylating agents. Cancer Res 46 : 2463-2467

Hartwell L (1992) Defects in a cell cycle checkpoint may be responsible for the genomic instability of cancer cells. Cell 71 : 542-546

Hoffmann I, Clarke PR, Jesus Marcote M, Karsenti E, Draetta G (1993) Phosphorylation and activation of human cdc25C by cdc2-cyclin B and its involvement in the self-amplification of MPF at mitosis. EMBO J 12 (in press)

Lane DP (1992) p53, guardian of the genome. Nature 358 : 15-16

Murray AW (1992) Creative blocks : cell-cycle checkpoints and feedback controls. Nature 359 : 599-604

O'Connor PM, Ferris D, White GA, Pines J, Hunter T, Longo DL, Kohn W (1992) Relationships between cdc2 kinase, DNA crosslinking and cell cycle perturbations induced by nitrogen mustard. Cell Growth Diff 3 : 43-52

O'Connor PM, Ferris D, Pagano M, Draetta G, Pines J, Hunter T, Longo DL, Kohn W (1993) G2 delay induced by nitrogen mustard in human cells affects cyclin A/cdk2 and cyclin B1/cdc2-kinase complexes differently. J Biol Chem (in press)

O'Connor PM, Kohn W (1992) A fundamental role for cell cycle regulation in the chemosensitivity of cancer cells ? Sem Cancer Biol 3 : 409-416

Seki T, Yamashita K, Nishitani H, Takagi T, Russell P, Nishimoto T (1992) Chromosome condensation caused by loss of RCC1 function requires the cdc25C protein that is located in the cytoplasm. Molec Biol Cell 3 : 1373-1388

Sorenson CM, Barry MA, Eastman A (1990) Analysis of events associated with cell cycle arrest at G2 phase and cell death induced by Cisplatin. J Natl Cancer Inst 82 : 749-756

Vogelstein B, Kinzler W (1992) p53 function and dysfunction. Cell 70 : 523-526

Reversal of multidrug resistance in hematologic malignancies with chemosensitizers: laboratory and clinical studies

SE Salmon, TP Miller, AF List, TM Grogan, WS Dalton

There has been much recent progress in the understanding of molecular mechanisms of resistance of cancer cells to chemotherapeutic agents. Knowledge of these mechanisms has provided the basis for rational approaches to overcoming or reversing drug resistance and thereby making cancer chemotherapy more effective. *In vitro* studies with tumor cell lines carried out by Ling in the mid-1970's suggested that prolonged exposure of the cells to one compound (e.g. Colchicine) could give rise to a multidrug resistant phenotype, with cross resistance to a series of structurally quite different compounds (Ling, 1975). Importantly, Ling's group established that cell lines exhibiting this form of multidrug resistance (MDR), overexpressed a 170kd Glycoprotein termed the « P- glycoprotein »(P-gp) on tumor cell membranes. Mechanistic studies have established that P-gp functions as a drug-efflux pump, capable of actively transporting a variety of structurally diverse anticancer drugs out of the tumor cell (Beck et al 1979 ; Gerlach et al 1986 ; Ling, 1975 ; Riordan and Ling, 1979). Included in this heterogeneous group of heterocyclic compounds effluxed by P-gp are antitumor antibiotics such as the anthracyclines, mitomycins and actinomycins, and plant alkaloids such as the vincas and the podophyllotoxins. The mechanism of drug resistance associated with MDR expression is considered related to the inability to achieve adequate intracellular cytotoxic drug concentrations. Freshtumor biopsy specimens have been studied for MDR1 gene expression using northern or western blots, the polymerase chain reaction or immunohistochemical or flow cytometry detection methods. In some tumor types (e.g. renal and colon cancer), MDR expression has been observed prior to any treatment (Fojo et al 1987a ; Fojo et al 1987b). Increased expression of MDR in human tumors is not associated with gene amplification but rather appears to result from altered gene regulation. In some types of cancer, pretreatment samples are generally negative for P-gp. However, MDR expression appears to develop after chemotherapy (Dalton et al 1989a ; Dalton et al 1989b ; Grogan et al 1992).

At the same time that the MDR phenomenon was being characterized, Tsuruo and co-workers observed in a murine leukemia/lymphoma model which acquired vinca alkaloid resistance *in vivo* could be reversed by administration of the vinca alkaloid plus the calcium channel blocker, Verapamil (Tsuruo et al 1982 ; Tsuruo et al 1984). Subsequently it was established that drug resistance

---

From the Section of Hematology/Oncology, Arizona Cancer Center and the Departments of Medicine, Pathology and Pharmacology, University of Arizona College of Medicine, Tucson, Arizona 85724, USA

in this model was due to P-gp expression. At this point it became clear that there was opportunity to develop a new class of drugs which can be considered as « chemosensitizers », with specificity for circumventing the MDR mechanism of resistance to anticancer drugs. Studies using photoaffinity labelling with tritiated Azidopine established that Verapamil and other chemosensitizers blocked the binding of vinca alkaloids or anthracyclines to acceptor sites on the P-gp molecule (Cornwell et al 1986 ; Cornwell et al 1987 ; Beck et al 1984). This type of blockade of P-gp function *in vitro* appears to represent competitive inhibition of the pump mechanism. Of interest, a variety of chemosensitizers have now been identified in *in vitro* culture systems. These agents are structurally diverse and include some anti-arrythmics such as Verapamil, Quinidine and Amiodarone, but also other agents such as Trifluperazine, Quinine (the stereoisomer of Quinidine), Medroxyprogesterone and Cyclosporine (Tsuruo et al 1984b ; Ganapathi and Grabowski ; 1983, Slater et al 1986). In a recent observation, we've also found evidence for *in vitro* synergism of Quinine and Verapamil (Lehnert et al 1991). In addition to the MDR mechanism described above, there have been reports of alternative mechanisms for multi-agent drug resistance wherein P-gp expression is not increased but increases in drug efflux occur nonetheless (Harker et al 1989). In this report, we will focus particularly on reviewing our recent clinically oriented studies of P-glycoprotein and the effects of chemosensitizers in hematologic malignancies which we have carried out at the Arizona Cancer Center.

Clinical trials of chemosensitizers in myeloma, lymphoma and acute leukemia

Clinical studies on reversal of MDR at the Arizona Cancer Center with chemosensitizers evolved from laboratory studies in which Dalton and his colleagues characterized a Doxorubicin-resistant human multiple myeloma cell line and found it to express P-gp (Dalton et al 1986). In this model, Doxorubicin-resistance in this line was readily reversed *in vitro* by using Verapamil as a chemosensitizer. A clinical protocol was then devised wherein high doses of Verapamil were administered simultaneously with an intravenous infusion of Vincristine and Doxorubicin (Adriamycin) along with oral Dexamethasone. The latter three drugs had previously been used in this combination as « VAD » by Barlogie and co-workers for second-line therapy in patients with multiple myeloma who were alkylating agent resistant (Barlogie et al 1984). In our initial pilot study we treated myeloma patients who had also become resistant to VAD with the combination of VAD/Verapamil and found it capable of reinducing remission in some of these refractory patients (Dalton et al 1989a). In that study, one refractory lymphoma patient was also treated and also regained remission. Thereafter, we continued to focus our clinical efforts on hematologic malignancies, which may be considered to be the clinical equivalent of the murine leukemia-lymphoma model of Tsuruo et al Subsequently we have conducted larger phase II clinical evaluations of VAD/Verapamil in myeloma (Salmon et al 1991), and VAD plus Cyclophosphamide (CVAD/

Verapamil) in patients with malignant lymphoma (Miller et al 1990). These studies confirmed and extended our earlier pilot findings and more firmly established that Verapamil could be used as a chemosensitizer for drug resistant patients, especially for those patients whose tumor biopsies were P-gp positive. Survival from the start of Verapamil-containing regimens was significantly better for responders than for non-responders. The dose-limiting toxicity of Verapamil in these studies was cardiac (hypotension and heart block), but these toxicities were transient and resolved when Verapamil administration was reduced or terminated (Pennock et al 1991). Nonetheless, in these initial studies, hospitalization in a cardiac monitoring unit was required during Verapamil administration. Because of the toxicity observed at the required doses of Verapamil, we considered this drug to provide proof of concept by a first generation agent, and this increased our interest in using alternative agents with higher potency and less toxicity. Cyclosporine A (CSA) appeared particularly promising based on *in vitro* studies carried out by our group and others (Lehnert et al 1993 submitted). For example, the use of CSA as a chemosensitizer was explored by our group in a phase I-II clinical trial of drug resistant forms of acute leukemia (List et al 1992). In this phase I-II study, patients received sequential high-dose Cytosine Arabinoside for 5 days followed by 3 days of continuous infusion Daunorubicin in combination with CSA. After administration of Cytosine Arabinoside, the patients first received a loading dose of CSA followed by continuous infusion of CSA plus daunorubicin. This regimen, proved to be less toxic than Verapamil and was devoid of cardiac toxicity. The duration of myelosuppression was increased by the addition of CSA, and patients also developed dose-related hyperbilirubinemia as a transient effect of CSA. Overall response rates (CR's plus PR's) in these studies are summarized in Table I. An analogous study using VAD/CSA for multiple myeloma was recently reported by a European group (Sonneveld et al 1992), providing further indication that CSA may prove to be a clinically useful chemosensitizer.

Table 1. Results of Recent Arizona Cancer Center clinical Trials Using Chemosensitizers in Drug-Resistant Myeloma, Lymphoma and Acute Leukemia

Tumor Type	Sensitizer*	No pts	No Responsive (%)	Reference
Myeloma	V	22	5 (23)	Salmon et al 1991
Lymphoma	V	18	13 (73)**	Miller et al 1991
Leukemia	C	42	26 (69)***	List et al 1992

* V = Verapamil, C = Cyclosporin-A
** 5 lymphoma patients (26 %) achieved complete remissions
*** 26 leukemia patients (62 %) achieved complete remissions

A subset of patients in our chemosensitizer studies were tested for P-gp expression in tumor biopsies prior to therapy. Our evaluation of MDR expression was first conducted using immunohistochemical methods incorporating the C219 and JSB1 monoclonal antibodies to P-gp (Grogan et al 1991). Using this method, we have only rarely observed P-gp expression in previously untreated myeloma or lymphoma patients, whereas it was observed in a significantly greater proportion of patients in relapse from prior chemotherapy. Moreover, in myeloma, P-gp expression could be correlated directly with the total prior dose of Doxorubicin and/or Vincristine received by the patient (Grogan et al 1993). In some of our studies, P-gp expression was also confirmed by RNA slot-blot analysis, and most recently, in acute leukemia, a quantitative PCR reaction (Futscher et al 1992) was also employed for some patients. Unlike the situation in myeloma and lymphoma, patients with drug resistant forms of acute leukemia often expressed P-gp on their leukemic cells prior to receiving chemotherapy (List et al 1992). Precise immunohistochemical localization is essential to demonstrate cell type-specific localization of P-gp expression, and this cannot be currently achieved with molecular techniques such as northern analysis or PCR. In our therapeutic studies with chemosensitizers, there is a trend towards relationship between P-gp expression and responsiveness to chemotherapy plus chemosensitizers in myeloma and lymphoma, but not in acute leukemia (Table II). Larger scale studies (including randomized trials) of chemosensitizers are currently underway in multiple myeloma, non-Hodgkin's lymphoma and acute leukemia in the Southwest Oncology Group.

Table 2. Relationship of Expression of P-glycoprotein and Response to Chemotherapy Plus Chemosensitizer in Patients with Drug-Resistant Lymphoma, Myeloma or Acute Leukemia

Tumor Type	No pts responding*		Reference
	P-gp – (%)	P-gp + (%)	
Multiple Myeloma	0/5 (0)	4/10 (40)	Salmon et al 1991
Malignant Lymphoma	2/4 (50)	5/7 (72)	Miller et al 1991
Acute Leukemia	8/10 (80)	18/23 (78)	List et al 1992

* Partial or complete remission

In related laboratory studies of fresh tumor biopsies from patients with myeloma, lymphoma and breast cancer, we found a correlation between *in vitro* resistance to Doxorubicin and P-gp expression (Salmon et al 1989b). In more recent *in vitro* evaluations of bone marrow aspirates from refractory myeloma patients, we also found a correlation between *in vitro* drug resistance to Doxorubicin and/or Vincristine and the ability of Verapamil to chemosensitize myeloma cells to the cytotoxic effects of these drugs (Salmon et al 1991). In the acute leukemia setting, using a quantitative PCR reaction, relapse from a cytosine Arabinoside/Daunomycin/CSA regimen was associated with a significant decrease in MDR1 expression (List et al 1992), suggesting that an alternative subclone of leukemic cells was « selected out » by the use of the chemosensitizer. This phenomenon warrants further laboratory and clinical investigation.

Discussion

Given our findings and those of others in the hematologic malignancies, we believe that further explorations of chemosensitizers are warranted not only in hematologic malignancies, but also in solid tumors in which P-glycoprotein has been implicated as a drug resistance mechanism. Unfortunately, the ability to obtain tumor biopsy specimens from solid tumors is often more difficult, an thereby making it harder to correlate P-gp expression with the effects of chemosensitizers. New agents including analogs of the « first generation chemosensitizers are indicated. For example, with respect to Verapamil, the clinical formulation is comprised of a racemic mixture of S and R-Verapamil. While the cardiac effects of this clinical formulation are primarily due to S-Verapamil, in the laboratory, both the R and S isomers individually can block P-gp function (Keilhauer C et al 1989). Accordingly, have initiated a phase I study of R-Verapamil as a potential second generation chemosensitizer. Similar studies are now underway also at other centers including the National Cancer Institute. The non-immunosuppressive CSA analog PSC833 exhibits potent chemosensitizing activity preclinically in an *in vivo* model (Boesch et al 1991), and has recently been advanced to phase I clinical trials. A variety of other compounds are currently undergoing clinical evaluation in various centers based on preclinical evidence for chemosensitization. Such extrapolations are often based on *in vitro* effects of the agent in standard tissue culture conditions. We believe that before such agents are advanced to clinical trials, it is important to establish that the chemosensitizing-effects on MDR cells can be observed in the presence of high-serum concentration and/or *in vivo* in murine tumor models. This is because standard *in vitro* tissue culture conditions can be quite misleading for drugs which are highly protein-bound. Such agents (e.g. Trifluperazine and Amioderone) may show substantial chemosensitizing effects in the presence of 10 % serum, but be virtually inactive in the presence of 100 % serum (Lehnert et al 1990). In our own program, a SCID mouse model for P-gp expressing and γ light chain excreting human myeloma 8226 (Doxorubicin resistant) has been developed (Bellamy et al 1993a). Most recently, this model has been applied to evaluate the effects of chemosensitizers on reversing MDR (Bellamy et al 1993b). It seems likely that once the precise molecular mechanism for chemosensitizer and drug interaction with P-gp is determined (e.g. with X-ray crystallography), better chemosensitizers may be developed using molecular modeling and other rationally based drug-development techniques. While there are clearly many other mechanisms by which cancer cells develop resistance to anticancer drugs, it is also clear from our studies that P-gp-mediated MDR represents a clinically relevant mechanism of drug resistance in the hematologic malignancies. Based on our initial observations directed towards overcoming MDR in the clinic, there is every reason to think that the future for drug development in this area is very bright, and that during the coming decade, investigators will have a variety of new chemosensitizers available for clinical investigation. Another approach to dealing with relative drug resistance involves the use of higher doses of chemotherapy such as used with autologous bone marrow stem cell support. We anticipate that the high-dose chemotherapy approach and the use of chemosensitizers may also converge in the future. We also speculate that a major future role for chemosensitizers may be identified by incorporating them into initial chemotherapy for previously untreated patients with tumor types known to acquire MDR after drug exposure.

Acknowledgements. *These studies were supported in part by grants CA-17094, CA-23074, and CA-43043 from the National Institutes of Health, DHHS, Bethesda, Md 20205 and a grant from the Arizona Chronic Disease Research Commission (8277-000000-1-0-YR-9301). We also thank our clinical and laboratory colleagues at the Arizona Cancer Center for their participation in these studies.*

References

Barlogie B, Smith L, Alexanian R (1984) Effective treatment of advanced multiple myeloma refractory to alkylating agents. New Engl J Med 310 : 1353-1356
Beck WT, Mueller TJ, Tanzer LR (1979) Altered surface membrane glycoproteins in vinca alkaloid resistant leukemic lymphoblasts. Cancer Res 39 : 2070-2076
Beck WT (1984) Cellular pharmacology of vinca alkaloid resistance and its circumvention. Adv Enz Reg 22 : 207-227
Bellamy W, Odeleye A, Finley P et al (1993a) An in vivo model of human multidrug resistant multiple myeloma in SCID mice. Am J Pathol 142 : 3
Bellamy W, Odeleye A, Finley P et al (1993b) An in vivo model of chemosensitization of multidrug resistant human myeloma cell line in SCID mice. Proc Am Assoc Cancer Res (in press)
Boesch D, Gaveriaux C, Jachez B et al (1991) In vivo circumvention of P-glycoprotein mediated multidrug resistance of tumor cells with SDZ PSC 833. Cancer Res 51 : 4226-4233
Cornwell MM, Safa AR, Felsted RL et al (1986) Membrane vesicles from multidrug resistant human cancer cells contain a specific 150-170 kDa protein detected by photoaffinity labelling. Proc Natl Acad Sci USA 83 : 3847-3850
Cornwell MM, Pastan I, Gottesman MM (1987) Certain calcium channel blockers bind specifically to multidrug resistant B carcinoma membrane vesicles and inhibit binding to P-glycoprotein. J Biol Chem 262 : 2166-2170
Dalton WS, Durie BGM, Alberts DS et al (1986) Characterization of a new drug resistant human myeloma cell line which expresses P-glycoprotein. Cancer Res 46 : 5125-5130
Dalton WS, Grogan TM, Durie BGM et al (1989a) Drug resistance in multiple myeloma and non-Hodgkin's lymphoma : Detection of P-glycoprotein and potential circumvention by addition of Verapamil to chemotherapy. J Clin Oncol 7 (4) : 415-424
Dalton WS, Grogan TM, Rybski JA et al (1989b) Immunohistochemical detection and quantitation of P-glycoprotein in multiple drug-resistant human myeloma cells : Association with level of drug resistance and drug accumulation. Blood 73 (3) : 747-752
Durie BGM, Dalton, WS (1988) Reversal of drug-resistance in multiple myeloma with Verapamil. Br J Haematol 68 : 203-206
Fojo AT, Ueda K, Slamon DJ et al (1987a) Expression of a multidrug resistant gene in human tumors and tissues. Proc Natl Acad Sci 84 : 265-269
Fojo AT, Shen DW, Mickley LA et al (1987b) Intrinsic drug resistance in human kid-

ney cancer is associated with expression of a human multidrug resistance gene. J Clin Oncol 5 : 1922-1927

Futscher BW, Blake LL, Grogan TM et al (1992) Submitted for publication

Ganapathi R, Grabowski D (1983) Enhancement of sensitivity to Adriamycin in resistant P388 leukemia by the Calmodulin inhibitor Trifluoperazine. Cancer Res 43 : 3696-3699

Gerlach JH, Kartner N, Bell DR et al (1986) Multidrug resistance. Cancer Surveys 5 : 25-46

Goldstein LJ, Fojo AT, Ueda K et al (1990) Expression of the Multidrug Resistance, MDR1, Gene in Neuroblastomas. J Clin Onc 8 (1) : 128-136

Grogan T, Dalton WS, Rybski J et al (1990) Optimization of immunocytochemical P-glycoprotein assessment in multidrug resistant plasma cell myeloma using three antibodies. Lab Invest 62 : 815-824

Grogan TM, Spier CM, Salmon SE et al (1993) P-glycoprotein expression in human plasma cell myeloma : correlation with prior chemotherapy. Blood 81 : 490-495

Harker WG, Slade DL, Dalton WS et al (1989) Multidrug resistance in mitoxantrone-selected HL-60 leukemia cells in the absence of P-glycoprotein overexpression. Cancer Res 49 : 4541-4549

Keilhauer C, Emling F, Rachbach M et al (1989) The use of R-Verapamil (R-VPM) is superior to racemic VPM in breaking multidrug resistance (MDR) of malignant cells. Proc Am Assoc Cancer Res 30 : 503

Lehnert M, Dalton WWS, Roe D, Emerson S, Salmon SE (1991) Synergistic inhibition by Verapamil and Quinine of P-glycoprotein-mediated multidrug resistance in a human myeloma cell line model. Blood 77 : 348-354

Lehnert M, Kunke K, Dalton WS, Roe D, Dorr RT, Salmon SE (1990) *In vivo* concentration of serum proteins significantly inhibits P-glycoprotein-mediated drug resistance by some chemosensitizers. Proc Am Assoc Cancer Res 31 : 2250

Ling V (1975) Drug resistance and membrane alterations in mutants of mammalian cells. Can J Genetics Cytol 17 : 503-515

List AF, Spier CM, Greer JP et al (1992) Biochemical modulation of Anthracycline resistance in acute leukemia with Cyclosporin-A. Proc Am Soc Clin Oncol 11 : 264

Miller TP, Grogan TM, Dalton WS et al (1991) P-glycoprotein expression in malignant lymphoma and reversal of clinical drug resistance with chemotherapy plus high-dose Verapamil. J Clin Oncol 9 : 17-24

Pennock GD, Dalton WS, Roeske WR et al (1991) J Natl Cancer Inst 83 : 105-110

Riordan JR, Ling V (1979) Genetic and biochemical characterization of multidrug resistance. Pharmacol Therapeutics 18 : 51-75

Salmon SE, Dalton WS, Grogan TM et al (1991) Multidrug-resistant myeloma : laboratory and clinical effects of Verapamil as a chemosensitizer. Blood 78 : 44-50

Salmon SE, Grogan TM, Miller TP, Dalton WS (1979b) Prediction of Doxorubicin resistance in vitro in myeloma, lymphoma and breast cancer in P-glycoprotein staining. J Natl Cancer Inst 81 (9) : 696-701

Slater L, Sweet P, Stupecky M et al (1986) Cyclosporin-A reverses vincristine and daunorubicin resistance in acute lymphatic leukemia in vitro. J Clin Invest 77 : 1405-1408

Sonneveld P, Durie BGM, Lokhorst HM et al (1992) Modulation of multidrug-resistant multiple myeloma by Cyclosporin. Lancet 340 : 255-259

Tsuruo T, Iida H, Tsukagoshi S, Sakurai Y (1982). Increased accumulation of Vincristine and adriamycin in drug resistant P388 tumor cells following incubation with calcium antagonists and calmodulin inhibitors. Cancer Res 42 : 4730

Tsuruo T, Iida H, itatani Y et al (1984) Effects of Quinidine and related compounds on cytotoxicity and cellular accumulation of Vincristine and Adriamycin in drug resistant tumor cells. Cancer Res 44 : 4303-4307

Abstract. In vitro *studies with tumor cell lines as well as* in vivo *murine models have indicated that acquired multidrug resistance (MDR) associated with P-glycoprotein expression can be reversed using « chemosensitizers » capable of competitively inhibiting the P-glycoprotein cell membrane efflux pump. In studies at the Arizona Cancer Center, we have combined laboratory studies identifying the P-glycoprotein with clinical studies of chemosensitizers in hematologic malignancies including multiple myeloma, malignant lymphoma and acute leukemia. In our therapeutic studies, Verapamil combined with chemotherapy has been used successfully to reverse multi-drug resistance in patients with lymphoma or myeloma in relapse from chemotherapy alone. For patients with acute leukemia, Cyclosporine was used as the chemosensitizer, and it appeared to be an active chemosensitizer which was less toxic than Verapamil. For both myeloma and lymphoma, resistance was clinically reversed somewhat more frequently in patients whose tumors expressed P-glycoprotein, but this was not the case in acute leukemia. In myeloma, P-glycoprotein expression could be correlated with prior clinical exposure to Doxorubicin and/or Vincristine in a dose-related fashion. In* vitro *studies with fresh myeloma bone marrows established that Verapamil enhanced drug sensitivity of myeloma cells to Doxorubicin and Vincristine of intrinsically drug-resistant cells but not of drug sensitive tumor cells. These laboratory and clinical studies suggest that chemosensitizers may play an increasing role in the treatment of multidrug resistant human tumors and support the development of more effective and less toxic chemosensitizers.*

Practical approach to bladder cancer

L Denis

Bladder cancer ranks as the tenth cancer in incidence in worldwide statistics. However, a great number of the reported cases are of the squamous type, especially in countries where bilharzia infestation is endemic. This calls for a general information and prevention program in these countries.

On the contrary, bladder cancer is mainly of the transitional cell type (TCC) in the industrialized world and is the fourth most important cancer in males and the fifth in estimated cancer death in the US statistics of the American Cancer Society in 1993 [1]. The European statistics match these figures [2].

Etiology — Prevention

The fact that the great majority of TCC is found in the bladder points to the urine and its metabolites as the source of the multiple initiators and promoters of TCC. A number of agents are identified and smoking is a known risk factor. The long induction time and the multistage process of development makes the identification of the weaker agents cumbersome but the list is growing. The focus of the Europe against cancer program on acquired diseases in the working environment will boost the necessary epidemiological studies.

Preventive screening of the urine for haematuria and cytology is already standard in the petrochemical industry in a number of countries.

Histopathology — Diagnosis — Staging

TCC is a heterogeneous disease with 2 main pathways of development. Two thirds of the TCC are papillary in nature and develop from normal or hyperplastic epithelium while the other third presents as solid tumor. The usual cells of the papillary form are of low cytological atypia and it is quite normal that cytology fails to diagnose these tumors. This is not a great clinical problem since the majority are superficial and their clinical importance lies in the problem of recurrence, bleeding and infection. Maximal 10 % of these tumors, most of a well differentiated grade, ever progress or metastasize. This is very different for the solid form of TCC which is always invasive and of a more anaplastic grade. Higher stages of disease are common at the time of the initial diagnosis. Most of these tumors metastasize within a year of deep muscle invasion, an incurable disease, which requires that invasive bladder cancer should be treated as a systemic disease [3].

Dept of Urology, A.Z. Middelheim, Antwerp, Belgium

Practical approach to bladder cancer

DIAGNOSTIC WORK-UP SUSPECTED BLADDER CANCER

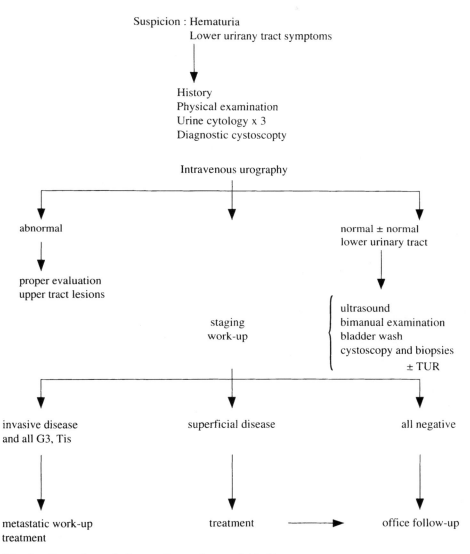

Fig. 1. Algorythm of diagnostic work-up of bladder cancer

A different form of the disease is carcinoma *in situ*, a flat lesion that looks superficial but by its grade 3 cells by definition acts as a biological active disease. Its presence next to papillary tumors means a worse prognosis. The examination of urine cytology in perfect conditions (fresh specimen, qualified lab) is vital to the treatment of bladder cancer. Beware of a resected specimen of grade I TCC and a positive cytology. A search for the missing tumor is absolutely indicated.

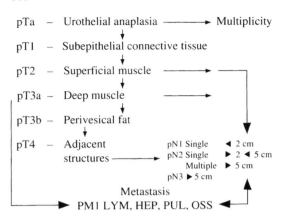

Fig. 2. Pathological (p) classification of bladder cancer. pTis may be concomitant to all T. Regional lymph node invasion pN1-3 and pM1 LYM (extraregional lymph nodes), HEP (lung), PUL (lung) and OSS (bone) should be evaluated as lethal disease

The diagnosis of the exophytic tumors is based on the specimen obtained by transurethral resection. Biopsies of the resected portion, of the neighbouring tissue, and of the distant bladder mucosa as well as of the prostate are no luxury. The final diagnosis has to correlate the visual, histological and cytological findings.

The clinical diagnosis is usually made by the visual inspection of the bladder with a flexible cystoscope. This procedure is easy to perform and requires no anaesthesia. It is indicated in all forms of painless haematuria, microscopic haematuria and irritative voiding as well as in deformities presented by imaging of the urinary tract.

The final diagnosis includes the staging of the tumor (T) by definition and meticulous care in the description of the lesions, the number of specimens taken by biopsy and the inclusion of bladder muscle in the last specimen are a prerequisite for a proper treatment. An algorythm for the diagnosis of bladder cancer and the pathological classification for the TNM system are presented in Figures 1 and 2 [4, 5]. Invasive tumors are followed by a search for positive nodes (N) or metastases (M). The extent of disease directs the treatment. Some forms of superficial disease with invasion of the subepithelial connective tissue and higher grades pose a serious threat to the patient and should be classified for aggressive therapy. On the other hand, some forms of cancer *in situ* react quite well to intravesical treatment. The remaining problem in staging is the detection of the nodal staging and the unavoidable understaging of the invasive tumors which runs up to 40 % in the best of hands [6].

Natural history — Prognostic factors

Superficial bladder cancer is labelled as a polychronotopic disease meaning that it recurs frequently on different time slots in other places of the bladder. Synchronous tumors of the upper tract and of the prostate are found in approximately 5 % of the patients. Invasive bladder cancer with deep muscle invasion have positive regional nodes in 1/3 of the cases. Few patients survive if left untreated and half of the patients survive 5 years after radical treatment.

The prognosis of superficial bladder cancer is so good that substitute endpoints have been proposed to evaluate treatment. A multivariate analysis of the EORTC trials revealed prior recurrence, grade and number and location of the tumors to be the 3 main prognostic factors [7].

Linked to the prognostic factors are the response criteria which in term define the endpoints. Complete response is defined as visible absence of the tumor, negative biopsies of the tissues left after treatment and a negative cytology. The universally accepted endpoint is the recurrence rate during a follow-up period. The prognostic factor in invasive tumor is the extent and grade of disease. Additional factors are related to the patient as haemoglobin and performance status that characterize the host and his resistance to biological aggression. Aneuploidy, placental, protein production and genotypic indicators characterize the biological aggression of the tumor.

Treatment of superficial bladder cancer

The diagnosis by transurethral resection includes primary treatment. By experience we know that single TaG1 lesions deserve no other treatment and only careful follow-up is recommended.

Multiple tumors with higher grades tend to recur and intravesical instillation of chemotherapeutic or immunological agents is now the mainstay of treatment. A number of active agents have been identified but Mitomycin-C (MMC), 4 Epirubicin (EPR) and the immunostimulator BCG are effective in chemoresection of marker lesions in phase II studies or in the definitive treatment of cancer *in situ*. Despite a lack of pharmacological information on agent penetration and a subsequent lack of scientific established dosage intravesical chemotherapy/immunotherapy is now standard treatment in cancer *in situ*. Different schemes are applied but induction and maintenance treatment emerge as standard. Complications of BCG instillations are frequent and can be serious. Newer clinical research focuses on KW-2149, a derivative of MMC, and the use of the interferons and interleukin 6 as active agents. The successful and vital use of this agents has been a boost to their application in chemoprophylaxis which is now accepted treatment in patients with multiple recurrences at high risk for new occurrence or recurrence.

Treatment of invasive bladder cancer

The optimal treatment is not known at the moment but multimodality treatment including surgery, radiotherapy and systemic chemotherapy are actual treatment and await proper indications.

Surgery is, of course, still a leading therapy as a single modality of treatment and cystectomy resulted in excellent up to 70 % 5 year survival in early invasive treatment as T1 and T2 disease. Radiotherapy has been shown to be effective in sterilizing bladders after complete resection of tumors of a papillary nature. The combination of surgery and radiotherapy studied in depth brought no definitive advantage to the individual patient [8]. The technique of radical surgery became routine in expert hands [9] and all efforts are now directed at the creation of a substitute bladder utilizing bowel as a reservoir.

The development of effective chemotherapy in advanced measurable TCC opened new avenues of treatment. There is now hope that induction chemotherapy usually Cisplatin, Methotrexate, Vinblastine and the haematopoietic agents, offers a chance for bladder preservation by partial cystectomy in selected cases [10] or by combining with radiotherapy [11]. The small numbers and the limited follow-up of 4 years require caution while we wait for the results of the proper phase III trials. Invasive bladder cancer has to be treated in the framework of a multidisciplinary approach.

References

1. Boring CC, Squires TS, Tong T (1993) Cancer statistics, 1993. CA Cancer J Clin 43 : 7-26
2. Möller Jensen O, Estève J, Möller H, Renard H (1990) Cancer in the European Community and its Member States. EJC 26 (11/12) : 1167-1256
3. Prout GRJr, Griffin PP, Shipley WU (1979) Bladder carcinoma as a systemic disease. Cancer 43 : 2532-2539
4. Niijima T, Denis L, Pontes E, Alfthan O, Akaza H, Jaeger N, Kotake T, Ohi Y, Fujime M (1986) Diagnostic work-up. In : Denis L, Niijima T, Prout GJr, Schröder FH (eds) Developments in bladder cancer. Alan R Liss Inc, New York, p 211
5. Hermanek P, Sobin LH (1992) TNM classification of malignant tumours. Fourth revised edition. Springer-Verlag, London
6. Pagano F, Bassi P, Galetti TP, Meneghini A, Milani C, Artibani W, Garbeglio A (1991) Results of contemporary radical cystectomy for invasive bladder cancer : a clinicopathological study with an emphasis on the inadequacy of the tumor, nodes and metastases classification. J Urol 145 : 45-50.
7. Sylvester R (1985) The analysis of results in prophylactic superficial bladder cancer studies. In : Schröder FH, Richards B (eds) Superficial bladder tumors. Alan R Liss Inc, New York, p 3
8. Slack NH, Prout GRJr (1980) The heterogeneity of invasive bladder carcinoma and different responses to treatment. J Urol 123 : 644-652
9. Skinner EC, Lieskovsky G, Skinner DG (1990) The technique of radical cystectomy. AUA Updata Series Lesson 7 (Volume IX) : 50-55
10. Denis L, Bouffioux C, Kurth KH, Debruyne F, Sylvester R, De Pauw M, Members of the EORTC Urological Group (1987) Current status of intravesical chemotherapy trials in the EORTC Urological Group. An overview. Cancer Chemother Pharmacol 20 : 67-71
11. Shipley WU et al (1988) Combined chemotherapy and radiation therapy in the treatment of patients with muscle invasive bladder carcinoma following transurethral surgery : an update of bladder sparing effort. Radiat Oncol Biol Phys 15 : 132

Breast cancer

Primary chemotherapy for breast cancer : response to preoperative chemotherapy as prognostic factor

GN Hortobagyi, AU Buzdar, D Frye, SE Singletary, FA Holmes, F Ames, MD McNeese, RL Theriault

Preoperative (or neoadjuvant) chemotherapy, followed by the appropriate local regional treatment (either surgery or radiotherapy, or both) has become the preferred treatment for locally advanced and inflammatory breast carcinoma [1]. Primary chemotherapy has been shown to produce major objective regression of the primary lesion and regional lymph node metastasis in the majority of patients. In addition, downstaging of the primary lesion offers the possibility to treat the breast with a subtotal mastectomy, and, therefore, breast conservation. It is unclear at this point, whether preoperative chemotherapy offers a survival benefit in the context of multimodal treatment over the postoperative administration of adjuvant chemotherapy. Our first protocol of primary chemotherapy suggested that response to this treatment correlated with long-term disease-free and overall survival [2]. The clinical trial reported here was designed to confirm the prognostic implication of response to preoperative chemotherapy, and to determine whether a response to preoperative chemotherapy could be the basis for the selection of postoperative systemic treatments. More specifically, we wanted to determine whether the addition of a non-cross-resistant combination of cytotoxic agents after optimal local/regional treatment to patients with suboptimal response to preoperative chemotherapy would result in an improvement in disease-free and overall survival.

Patients and methods

Patients with Stage II, IIIA and IIIB primary breast cancer were eligible for treatment on this combined modality therapy. Patients with Stage IV breast cancer with metastases limited to the ipsilateral supraclavicular or subclavicular lymph node region were also eligible. After histological or cytological documentation of primary breast carcinoma, patients underwent an extensive evaluation of metastatic spread that included a complete history and physical examination, a complete blood count, a multiparameter biochemical profile (SMA-12), a carcinoembryonic antigen level, chest X-ray, radionuclide bone scan, and liver imaging by CT scan or abdominal ultrasound. In addition, all patients underwent a bilateral xeromammogram and bilateral breast and regional ultrasound examination. Once distant metastases were thus excluded, and a written informed consent obtained, a central venous catheter was inserted, and

---

The University of Texas MD Anderson Cancer Center, 1515 Holcombe Boulevard, Box 56, Houston, Texas 77030, USA

combination chemotherapy was initiated with the VACP regimen as shown on Table 1. Cycles of chemotherapy were administered at 21-day intervals. In the absence of neutropenic fever or documented infection, the doses of Doxorubicin and Cyclophosphamide were escalated for the second and third cycle, to optimize dose intensity. After the completion of the third cycle of combination chemotherapy, a metastatic staging evaluation was repeated. In the absence of any evidence of response to preoperative chemotherapy, patients had a total mastectomy followed by a non-cross-resistant combination (VbMF, see Table 1) for five cycles, also repeated at 21-day intervals. If the tumors were inoperable, radiation therapy preceded mastectomy. In the presence of a partial or complete regression of the tumor after preoperative chemotherapy, a total mastectomy was performed. If after the hispathologic evaluation, there was no evidence of disease, or residual tumor added up to < 1 cm^3 of viable neoplasm, the same regimen used for preoperative chemotherapy (VACP) was administered for five additional cycles, followed by radiation therapy to the chest wall and regional lymphatics. For patients with > 1 cm^3 of residual tumor, after appropriate stratification for initial stage, response to therapy and hormone-receptor status, postoperative adjuvant therapy was randomly selected to be five cycles of VACP, or five cycles of VbMF, each followed, in turn, by radiation therapy (Table 2). This design guaranteed that patients with poor response would be treated with an alternative therapy, and that patients with an excellent response to preoperative chemotherapy, whom in our earlier experience had a good long-term prognosis, would not be exposed to the potential risks of changing a successful treatment. The total duration of this combined modality therapy varied from 43 to 52 weeks.

Table 1. Chemotherapy program

Drug	VACP Dose in mg/m^2	Route	Days
Vincristine	1.5 2.0)	IV	1
Adriamycin	60-75	IV × CI	1-3
Cyclophosphamide	600-750	IV	1
Prednisone	40 (total)	PO	1-5

Drug	VbMF Dose in mg/m^2	Route	Days
Vinblastine	1.5	IV × CI	1-4
Methotrexate	120	IV	1
5-FU	1.000	IV	2
Folinic acid	8 × 6	PO	1-2

Between 1985-1989, 200 patients were entered on this trial. Five were ineligible and two were inevaluable ; 193 patients were evaluable for toxicity and response to therapy.

Table 2. Study design biopsy and staging

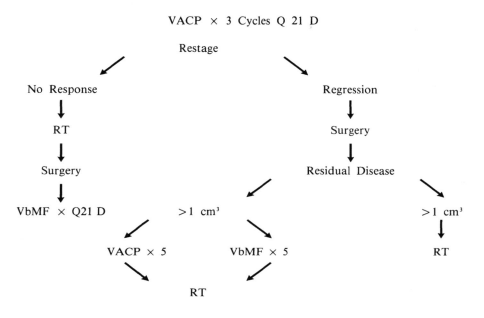

Table 3. 85-01 Patient characteristics

No of patients entered	200
No inevaluable	7
No evaluable	193
Median age in years :	49
(range)	(15-75)
Premenopausal	98
Postmenopausal	95
Estrogen receptor status :	
Positive	70 (36 %)
Negative	67 (35 %)
Unknown	56 (29 %)
Clinical stage :	
IIA	2 (1 %)
IIB	34 (18 %)
IIIA	64 (33 %)
IIIB	80 (41 %)
IV (limited)	13 (7 %)

The median age of these patients was 49 years (range = 15-75 years) ; 98 patients were premenopausal. The distribution of estrogen-receptor status and clinical stage in the evaluable group is shown on Table 3. During active treatment, a complete blood count and multiparameter biochemical survey were repeated at each visit, while a chest X-ray and bone scan were performed every 3-4 months. After completion of all therapy, the blood count, biochemical survey, chest X-ray, and bone scan were performed at 4-6 month intervals, and a contralateral mammogram, once a year for the first five years; thereafter, all these tests, with the exception of the bone scan, were performed yearly.

A Chi square was used to detect differences between randomized subgroups, and a Kaplan and Meier method was used for disease-free, and overall survival curves.

Results

At the time of this analysis, the median follow-up time for these studies is 48 months (range 26-92 months). On the 193 evaluable patients, there have been 23 (12 %) local or regional recurrences, and 66 (34 %) distant metastases. Thirty-four patients (34) (18 %) achieved a complete remission, while 127 (66 %) achieved a partial remission, for an overall major remission rate of 83 %. After preoperative chemotherapy and the appropriate local/regional treatment, 190 patients were rendered disease-free (complete remission), while three patients still harbored residual disease. Following the originally designed treatment strategy, 106 patients were stratified, and randomly assigned to postoperative VACP or VbMF. The median time to progression for the entire group was 68 months, and the median duration of survival has not been reached. At five years, 53 % of the patients are projected to be recurrence-free, and 66 %, alive. Eighty-eight percent (88 %) of patients remain free of local/regional recurrence.

Analysis of disease-free and overall survival by response to preoperative chemotherapy confirmed our previous findings: the projected 5-year disease-free survival rates for patients who achieved a CR, PR, or anything less than a PR, were 79 %, 52 %, and 27 %, respectively. The correlation of response to preoperative chemotherapy with overall survival paralleled the figures given in the previous sentence. The two groups randomized to postoperative VACP or VbMF showed similar disease-free and overall survival curves. While visually the group treated with VbMF had a higher disease-free (47 % v.s. 45 %) and overall survival rates (72 % v.s. 56 %), the differences between the groups did not approach statistical significance.

Discussion

This prospective randomized trial demonstrated and confirmed that preoperative chemotherapy is a highly effective strategy, that produces major downstaging for over two-thirds of patients with locally advanced primary breast cancer. In addition, this prospective study confirmed the close correlation between response to preoperative chemotherapy and outcome, as measured by disease-free and overall survival. Although it could be argued that response to chemotherapy only identifies patients with a better prognosis, applying the landmark method obviates this criticism without changing the outcome of the analysis [3].

There was no difference in outcome after the use of VACP or VbMF for postoperative adjuvant chemotherapy. In view of the slight separation of the curves in favor of the VbMF regimen, this lack of statistically significant difference could be interpreted as inadequate sample size, or the result of an incomplete lack of cross-resistance between the two regimens. The exclusion of non-responders from the randomization may have precluded the finding of a substantial difference ; however, we felt that randomizing non-responders to continuing the same regimen would be unethical.

The confirmation of the close correlation between response to preoperative chemotherapy and outcome suggests to us that additional trials should be performed with non-cross resistant regimens for remission consolidation, to improve disease-free and overall survival. This strategy has successful precedents in the treatment of osteogenic sarcoma, and the acute leukemias. However, our experience indicates that more effective cross-over regimens, and a considerably larger sample size will be needed to confirm this hypothesis, and complete a successful trial. Dose-intensive regimens with hematopoietic support are currently being explored to assess their efficacy for remission consolidation in patients with high-risk primary breast cancer.

References

1. Hortobagyi GN, Buzdar AU (1991) Locally advanced breast cancer : A review including the MD Anderson experience. In : Raga H, Ariel IM (eds) High-risk breast cancer, Springer-Verlag, Berlin, pp. 382-415
2. Hortobagyi GN, Ames FC, Buzdar AU, et al (1988) Management of stage III primary breast cancer with primary chemotherapy, surgery, and radiation therapy. Cancer 62 : 2507-2516
3. Anderson JR, Cain KC, Gelber RD (1983) Analysis of survival by tumor response. J Clin Oncol 1 : 710-719

Breast cancer, cytoprognostic grades and proliferative activity (DNA ploidy, S phase)

MA de Maublanc

Increase of breast cancer diagnosis especially of T1 tumors (over 60 % in 1990), decrease of N+ cancers (65 % in 1970, 45 % in 1990), the fact that we know that 30 % patients with N− cancers will metastase within 5 years after the diagnosis do modify indeed our appreciation of classical prognostic factors and especially of the importance of lymphnode involvement. The histoprognostic grade described by Scarff-Bloom and Richardson (SBR) keeps its value despite the large proportion of SBRII which have no specific predictive value [1]. Le Doussal and al [2] showed that SBR (modified SBR) influenced metastasis free survival of N-patients and allowed to recognize low risk and high risk categories.

The low risk group includes all grade I patients and 50 % grade II patients. The high risk group includes all grade III and 50 % grade II. Since 1981 [3,4] we perform fine needle aspirations and we determined cytopronostic grades which are comparable to SBR : grade II are separated into grade II− and grade II+.

The aims of this study are to analyse the correlation between grades and other prognostic factors, namely DNA ploidy, S phase, oestrogen and progesteron receptors and to justify regrouping grade I with grade II- and grade II+ with grade III.

Patients and methods

Between 12/91 and 7/92, we performed 140 CP 20 cases were eliminated (metastasis, relapses, 3 non gradable carcinoma, 2 metaplasic carcinoma) 120 cases are evaluable indicating the diagnosis of infiltrative duct carcinoma, the cytoprognostic grade, the hormone receptors level, the results of flow cytometry (DNA, ploidy, S phase).

All CP were performed by us using $6/10^e$-23 gauge fine needle, without aspiration according to a technic that was already described [5].

The diagnosis of carcinoma was established according to the OMS classification of breast cancer [6].

The cytoprognostic grade is determined in reference to the SBR, according to an already described technic [3, 4] and divides grade II [6, 7] into grade II − [6] and grade II+ [7]. Hormone receptors are measured on the same CP by immunocytochemistry (kit Abbott) and are rated as negative, positive and in percent of marked cells.

ADN ploidy and S phase are studied by flow cytometry and are figured

Centre de Cytopathologie Clinique, 87 rue Daguerre, 75014 Paris by histograms. S phase is rated as low < 4 %, intermediate (between 4 % and 8 %) and high (> 8 %) [7].

Results

All CP indicate the formal diagnosis of carcinoma and in 116 cases of duct carcinoma. The distribution of the cytoprognostic grades is the following grade I 27 (22.5 %), grade II- 35 (29.2), grade II+ 28 (23.3 %) grade III 30 (25 %). As in other series, grade II represents the majority of cases (52.5 % Table I).

Table 1. Prognostic grades. Histology = SBR and cytology = CP

Grades	SBR		CP		
	IGR*	CRH**			
	n = 267	n = 1262	n = 358	n = 152	n = 120
I	19 %	11 to 14 %	21.7 %	19 %	21.8 %
II	58 %	55 to 57 %	54.9 %	53 %	54 %
III	22.8 %	29 to 34 %	23.3 %	28 %	23.3 %

* : Institut Gustave Roussy - Villejuif (France)
** : Centre René Huguenin - St Cloud (France)

ADN ploidy

By convention, for tumor cells, it is the first DNA peak, the lowest one that is retained. Interpretable histograms were obtained in 119 cases with 30 diploid (25 %) and 89 aneuploid (75 %) among which 14 were multiploid. In grade I, the peak is diploid or paradiploid, in grade II − the peak is diploid or paradiploid with a few tetraploid peaks. In grade II +, the peaks are paradiploid or aneuploid (typical of carcinomas) and in grade III there are more aneuploid peaks. There are no much difference between grade I and II − on one hand and between grade III and grade II + on the other hand. There is a sharp distinction between grades II − and II +.

S phase calculated from histograms

S phase could be calculated in 84 % cases (97/120) the number of low S phase varies from 95.6 % in grade I to 4.3 % in grade III and the number of high S phase (0 % in grade I) reaches 52 % in grade III (Table 2). Mean values increase progressively and significantly from grade I (1.922) to grade II (8.129) including grade II − (3.793) and grade II + (5.404).

All standart deviations between grades are significant at 95 % and there is a sharp distinction between II − and II +.

Table 2. S phase and prognostic grades. 97 cytopunctures of breast carcinomas

Risk of metastasis	Grades	S phase		
		Low < 4 %	Moderate	High > 8 %
Low	I : n = 23	95.6 %	4.3 %	0 %
	II : n = 28	75 %	14.3 %	10.7 %
High	II+ : n = 23	26 %	60.8 %	13 %
	III : n = 23	26 %	43.5 %	52.1 %
Total	97	51.5 %	29.9 %	18.5 %

Hormone receptors

E and P receptors positivity is correlated to grades with a significant difference between II (Er+ 88.5 %, Pr+ 85.7 %) and II+ (Er+ 60.7 %, Pr 39.3 %). DNA ploidy, S phase and Er and Pr are also correlated (Table 3).

Table 3. ADN ploidy - S phase and hormonal receptors 98 cytopunctures of breast carcinomas

	ER+ (%)	PR+ (%)	ER- (%)	PR- (%)
Diploid	92	79	8	21
Aneuploid	65	54	35	46
S. Ph : mean	2.8	2.7	7.1	6.2
S. Ph : diploid	1.7	1.6	3.0	2.6
S. Ph : aneuploid	3.8	3.6	7.6	7.1
significant differences over 1 %				

Conclusion

Diagnostic and prognostic data (CPI, grades, hormone receptors, proliferative activity) provided by CP are reliable, reproducible and do show significant correlations between them. Separating grade II into II− and II+ and regrouping patients into low risk and high risk groups for metastasis appears thus to be justified in order to optimize therapeutic decision. The proliferative activity as a prognostic parameter may help therapeutic decision and according to some authors [7] it may predict response to chemotherapy.

References

1. Bloom HJ, Richardson WW (1957) Histological grading and prognosis in breast cancer : a study of 1409 cases of which 359 have been followed for 15 years. Br J Cancer 11 : 359-377

2. Le Doussal V, Tubiana-Hulin M, Friedman S, Hacene K, Spyratos F, Brunet M (1989) Prognostic value of histologic grade nuclear components of Scarff-Bloom-Richardson (SBR). An improve score modification based on a multivariate analysis of 1262 invasive ductal breast carcinomas. Cancer 64 : 1914-1921
3. De Maublanc MA, Zajdela A (1981) Actualités de la cytologie mammaire par ponction aspiration. Evaluation des moyens de diagnostic du cancer du sein. JMT Conseil, Paris : 143-151
4. De Maublanc MA, Remvikos Y, Collet JF, Lesec G (1992) Cytoponctions des cancers du sein et facteurs de pronostic. Cah Oncol 1 : 113-123
5. De Maublanc MA, Briffod M (7-1989) Cytodiagnostic en pathologie mammaire. Encycl Med Chir (Paris-France), Sein 810, F10, 7 p
6. Scarff W, Torloni H (1981). Type histologique des tumeurs du sein. Classification histologique internationale des tumeurs. N° 2, 2ᵉEdt, OMS, Genève
7. Remvikos Y, Beuzeboc P, Zajdela A, Voillemot N, Magdelenat H, Pouillart P (1990) Correlation of pretreatment proliferative activity of breast cancer with the response to cytotoxic chemotherapy. J Natl Cancer Inst 81 : 1383-1387

Abstract. 120 breast carcinoma which had been diagnosed by fine needle aspiration were stratified into prognostic grades of increased severity I, II−, II+, III in reference to histopronostic grades SBR. Grade II which are most frequent (> 50 %) were separated into II− and II+. The proliferative activity (DNA ploidy and S phase) was studied by flow cytometry in each case and was rated as low < 4 %, intermediate > 4 % < 8 % and high > 8 %. The correlations between grades and proliferative activity were studied. The mean values increase progressively and significantly from grade I (1.922) to grade III (1.129) that of grade II− being 3.793 and that of II+ being 5.404. All deviations (Fisher, PLDS) are significant at 95 %. The sharp distinction between II− and II+ justifies regrouping grade I and II− into a low risk group and II+ and III into a high risk group to optimise therapeutic decision by suppressing intermediate groups which have no prognostic significance.

Primary chemotherapy in the individualized non-mutilating treatment of breast cancer

R Poisson, S Legault, R Guévin

Primary chemotherapy is not well known nor recognized as a good local treatment of breast cancer because it is used mainly to destroy micrometastases at distance, (the same applies to anti-hormonal agents) [2-12-13]. Although different and not really comparable to radiotherapy or surgery, it is increasingly improving both at the systemic and local levels. We have observed that many women with inflammatory breast carcinoma and/or locally advanced breast cancer experienced a dramatic clinical tumour volume reduction after primary chemotherapy [1-7-10], so much so that the cancerocidal radiotherapy given in second line in the high responder patients might eliminate the need for surgery, in a good subset of them. However, for smaller lesions or less advanced cases, except for the French school of Jacquillat [8-9], fewer studies have been performed along these lines. Not all breast tumours respond to primary chemotherapy in the same fashion, on account of their great heterogeneity. In our experience, the high primary chemotherapy responder patients are more inclined to also respond well to radiotherapy and conversely. In poor or mediocre responder patients, a tumorectomy or a wide local excision can handle the situation more quickly. In that respect, a certain flexibility is mandatory.

Based on this background, the purpose of this pilot study is to find out, whether the same principles also applies in more favorable and smaller tumors. Is primary chemotherapy followed by either cancerocidal radiotherapy, if an excellent response has been obtained, or by surgery and then radiotherapy for the stable or poorer responders, better than a rigid uniform treatment for everyone ? At least as far as breast preservation is concerned.

As far as survival, if a cancer is controlled locally, one way or the other [3-4], why should survival be affected ? It is very unlikely that primary chemotherapy would adversely affect survival, on the contrary it may to some extent improve survival ; so why be reluctant to use it ?

It can always be argued that without any axillary dissection to provide a good staging, it is difficult to adjust the systemic treatment ! Node negative (N−) patients have a better prognosis than patients with positive nodes (N+). However, in the past, N− breast cancer patients have been under-estimated as far as mortality at 10 and 15 years. Cancer of the breast is a systemic disease and except for very small tumors of less than 1cm in diameter or some very special forms of somewhat larger tumors, this great emphasis on whether breast cancers are N+ or N− is a moot one [11]. Both pre-menopausal [5] and post-menopausal N− patients [6] benefit from systemic chemotherapy. Whether they should be treated differently in a systemic way is open to discussion.

Service of Surgical Oncology and Hemato-oncology, St-Luc Hospital, University of Montreal, 1058 St-Denis, Montreal, Quebec, Canada

We think it would be naive to expect dramatic improvements in disease-free survival or survival with primary chemotherapy, because unfortunately, in spite of the numerous theoretical advantages, multiple drug resistances does come into play.

On the other hand, the close sequential use of primary chemotherapy and radiation therapy, working in a synergistic fashion, should more successfully treat locoregional disease [14], with or without limited surgery (depending on the heterogeneity of the tumors), and spare the breast in most of the cases even in tumors greater than 5 cm in diameter, with good cosmesis.

Material and method

Since early 1991 we have treated 139 operable breast cancers, first by intraveinous chemotherapy consisting of Adriamycin 60 mg/m^2 and Cyclophosphamide 600 mg/m^2, for 4 cycles at 3 weeks interval. Pre-treatment evaluation consisted of a physical examination, complete blood cells count, biochemistry profil, chest X-rays, bone scan and abdominal ultrasound. All patients had a proven fine needle aspiration biopsy, not only for the exact diagnosis but also to obtain the nuclear grade and the receptors by immuno assay, ER-ica and PgR-ica. A new mammography is obtained to further objectivate the exact percentage of remission of the tumors.

This group of 139 patients consisted of : 28 patients T1, 49 : T2 and 62 : T3 tumours. The median age was 45 (range 28-65), 65 % were pre-menopausal. The median follow-up is 18 months.

During primary chemotherapy, the various clinical measurements of the tumor volume were carefully recorded at each cycle. In general, good responders, responded quickly. Although, by and large, young women with nuclear grade III, tumour with negative or low ER-ica were usually responding better. However, the best *in vivo* sensitivity test is to use chemotherapy in the first line of treatment and observe. (In case of distant failure, the quality of this response may help in selecting patients for autologous bone marrow transplant.) No axillary dissection was performed, unless suspicious nodes were still palpable.

A)

In case of complete clinical response (CR) or in almost complete clinical response (response > 75 % of the tumor volume) we began 3 weeks later a cancerocidal radiotherapy of a minimum 50 Gy was administered 10 Gy per week in daily increments of 2 Gy per day for 5 days per week for 5 weeks, followed by an external beam boost of 15 Gy to the quadrant involved, for a total of 65 Gray. Only 3 were treated by interstitial brachytherapy. No surgery was used in these cases. Furthermore, for patients who had suspicious nodes proven positive with FNA, or the ones with primary tumor of more than 5 cm, a consolidation course of chemotherapy with CMF for 3 months was given 2 weeks after the radiotherapy, thinking that 2 1/2 months of induction chemotherapy might not be enough for these more advanced cases. This sequential chemo-radiotherapy, chemotherapy, might very well be a potentially more sucessful combination of multiple treatment modalities. All patients passed 50 received Tamoxifen 10 mg bid, and also the younger ones with strongly positive ER-ica.

B)

For the patients who have poorly responded to primary chemotherapy one should keep an open mind regarding the proven value of a tumorectomy. When we did not obtain a partial response of more than 75 %, or in stable cases, a tumorectomy or a wide local excision was performed with clear margins (margins taken on the patient's side at each cardinal point in the surgical field rather than on the surgical specimen). No inside breast reconstruction, no prosthesis, no drainage were used. A low axillary dissection was done if nodes were still palpable. This surgical excision was done in a very traumatic fashion with a great deal of asepsis. If infection or delay in the wound healing occurs, it may become very annoying because it may take a long time to heal, delaying radiotherapy etc and compromise cosmesis. Post-operative radiotherapy was started 3 to 4 weeks later. A minimum of 50 Gy is administered without boost or bolus unless a margin happened to be positive. The systemic treatment is the same as in the previous group. All patients passed 50 received Tamoxifen 10 mg bid, and also the younger ones with strongly positive ER-ica.

Results

The down staging has been spectacular and is not always tumor size dependant. We have observed 32 % of complete clinical responses (Table 1).

We have 48 % of partial clinical responses. None of these have shown a complete response on the mammography control 2-3 weeks post-chemotherapy. We are obliged to subdivide these partial responses into 20 % of almost complete response, that is to say more than 75 % of the tumor has responded. We have 26 % of partial response from 50 % to 75 % of the tumor volume. These were also treated by surgery in second line.

We have 18.6 % of the patients stable and 2 patients showed progression. As shown on Table 2, 54 % of the patients did not require any surgery.

Axillary dissection was performed, only when suspicious nodes were still palpable that is to say in only 10 % of the cases. Only 7 total mastectomies were required. So far we did observe 5 distant metastases and 2 deaths. Although it is much too soon to rejoice, we have seen only 2 local recurrences so far.

As far as toxicity, some degree of hematological toxicity was almost constant. However, it was well tolerated, sometimes with the help of growth factors. Gastro-intestinal symptoms have been much less severe as compared to the same chemotherapy of a few years ago, thanks to the use of new antiemetic drugs. Complete alopecia was the rule.

Table 1. Results of primary chemotherapy on 139 patients

	No of pts	%
Complete response (CR)	45	32
Partial response (PR)	67	48
— PR of more than 75 %	31	22
— PR of 50 % to 75 %	36	25
Stable	25	18.3
Progression	2	1.7

Table 2. Local treatment post-primary chemotherapy

		No of pts	%
1.	Cancericidal radiotherapy (65 Gy) (no surgery) for GR and PR > 75 %	76	54
2.	Tumorectomy for PR < 75 % + 50 Gy to the breast and axilla	50	35
3.	Tumorectomy + axillary dissection + 50 Gy to the breast only	6	4
4.	Modified radical mastectomy (no radiotherapy)	7	5
Total number of Patients		139	

The cosmetic results have been excellent in 70 % of the cases even for big tumours, good in 20 %, and poor in 10 %. So far, we have not seen any post-radiotherapy skin sequelea like telangiectasia. We have no post-treatment arm oedema, no shoulder ankylosis ; in other words, much less functional disorders than when we used to do routine axillary dissection.

Discussion and conclusions

In many instances, reduction of tumour mass offer the prospect of converting an otherwise inoperable into an operable and potentially curable lesion, or transforming radiotherapy from a palliative procedure to a potentially curative treatment [8-9]. An overall rigid protocol could negate the potential opportunity that primary chemotherapy afford for more flexible individualized treatment as far as radiotherapy and/or surgery is concerned. It is now possible to shrink tumors a great deal in 50 % of the cases and to provide control of the primary breast cancer with radiotherapy alone for those patients responding well to primary chemotherapy. If and when surgery is required, a selective non mutilating treatment is possible in 95 % of the cases, even for the tumors initially much greater than 5 cm in diameter [1]. Although not really proven, we do have the distinct impression, based on our large previous experience, that primary chemotherapy seems to decrease local recurrences, at least as compared to when we used to do the non-mutilating surgical treatment first. Chemotherapy and radiotherapy work better concomitantly or almost concomitantly on well oxygenated cells [14]. Chemotherapy can induce locoregional tumor shrinkage but not permanently, unless followed by radiotherapy or surgery, the tumor recurs. This is what we see at distance. Most of our patients' failures are due to multiple distant metastases, in sites where of course, no radiotherapy was given. For some fractions of the tumours primary chemotherapy is the treatment of choice and is a good local treatment but it has to be combined with other therapeutic modalities afterwards. Too many oncologists considered chemotherapy as a systemic treatment only ; yet, not only it shrinks tumors a great deal but also increases the efficacy of radiation and of local surgery, when given as the first line of treatment.

Prospective, controlled and randomized studies are certainly the best way to obtain reliable data and results, especially as far as survival. On the other hand they may take a long time to be performed and are not always possible in real life. Furthermore, when one sees the spectacular results of primary chemotherapy on the down staging and how efficient cancerocidal radiotherapy acts, one can't helped wondering why surgery still continues to be performed as the first line of treatment, at least for T2, T3 tumors... Not only does it helps to save the breast most of the time with or without surgery but, as far as survival, again it seems to be just as good if not slightly better. Surgery should not be condemned, at least not in the near future, for drug resistant tumors or for the small tumours which are more easily handled surgically.

Nowadays, with a greater expertise with needle aspirations stereotaxis, fine needle biopsies and better mammographies, it is possible to know, most of the time if a tumor has not completely been sterilized or is recurring. If the patients are followed closely enough, one can easily change one's opinion and switch to a salvage tumorectomy. With the improvement in chemotherapy, like the possible use of Taxol combined with Adriamycin, what is expressed here is likely to become even more appropriate in the very near future. The same applies for primary hormonotherapy in older women, with the advances in the field of newer anti-oestrogenic agents.

Primary chemotherapy appears to be the way of the future. There is nothing to lose, everything to gain, especially in this fascinating field of breast preservation. Women certainly deserve better than in the past...

Improvement in survival will more likely come from successful attempts to revert drug resistance in refractory malignancies, better hormonotherapy and chemotherapeutic agents, or new approaches in regulating the up and down mechanisms of the multiple growth factors modulation involved in tumorogenesis. A better understanding of modern molecular biology and molecular genetics are more likely to give the breakthrough, someday...

So far, we have been trying to repair the engine without knowing completely how it works. In a few percentage of the cases, we are increasingly lucky.

References

1. Bonadonna G, Veronesi U, Bramvilla C et al. Primary chemotherapy to avoid mastectomy in tumours with diameters of three centimeters or more. J Natl Cancer Inst 82 : 1539-1545
2. Early Breast Cancer Trialist's collaborative Group (1988) Effects of adjuvant Tamoxifen and cytoxic therapy on mortality in early breast cancer : an overview of 61 randomized trials among 28,896 women. N Engl J Med 319 : 1681-1692
3. Fisher B, Bauer M, Margolese R, Poisson R, Pilch Y, Redmond C, Fisher E, Wolmark N et al (1985) Five-year results on a randomized clinical trial comparing total mastectomy and segmental mastectomy with or without radiation in the treatment of breast cancer. N Engl J Med 312 : 665-673
4. Fisher B, Redmond C, Poisson R, Margolese R, Wolmark N, Wickerham L, Fisher E, Deutsch M et al (1989) Eight-year results of a randomized clinical trial comparing total mastectomy and lumpectomy with or without irradiation in the treatment of breast cancer. N Engl J Med 320 : 822-828
5. Fisher B, Redmond C, Dimitrov NV, Bowman D, Legault-Poisson S et al (1989) A randomized clinical trials evaluating sequential Methotrexate and Fluorouracil in the treatment of patients with node negative breast cancer who have estrogen receptor negative tumors. N Engl J Med 320 : 473-478
6. Fisher B, Constantino J, Redmond C, Poisson R, Bowman D, Couture J et al (1989) A randomized clinical trials evaluating Tamoxifen in the treatment of patients with node-negative breast cancer who have estrogen-receptor-positive tumors. N Engl J Med 320 : 479-484
7. Hortobagyi GN, Ames FC, Buzdar AU et al (1988) Management of stage III primary breast cancer with primary chemotherapy, surgery and radiation therapy. Cancer 62 : 2507-2516
8. Jacquillat Cl, Weil M, Auclair G, Auclerc MF, Khayat D, Baillet F (1987) Neo-Adjuvant chemotherapy in the conservative management of breast cancer : A study of 205 patients. In : Salmon SE (ed) Adjuvant Therapy of Cancer, vol 5. Grune and Stratton, New York, p. 403
9. Jacquillat Cl, Weil M, Baillet F, Borel CH, Auclerc G et al (1990) Results of Neo-adjuvant chemotherapy and radiation therapy in the breast conserving treatment of 250 patients with all stages of infiltrative breast cancer. Cancer 66 : 129
10. Lippman MR, Swain SM, Egan EF et al (1988) Neo-Adjuvant chemotherapy in the combined modality approach of locally advanced non-metastatic breast cancer. In : Jacquillat Cl, Weil M, Khayat D (eds) Neo-Adjuvant chemotherapy. John Libbey Eurotext, Paris, p. 225
11. Mansour EG, Gray R, Shatila AH et al (1989) Efficacy of adjuvant chemotherapy in high risk node negative breast cancer. N Engl J Med 320 : 485-490
12. Papaioannou AN (1981) Preoperative chemotherapy for operable solid tumors. Eur J Cancer 17 : 263-269
13. Ragaz J, Band PR, Goldie JH (1986) Preoperative (neo-adjuvant) chemotherapy. Recent results in cancer Res 103 : 1-160
14. Vokes EE, Weischselbaum RR (1990) Concomitant chemoradiotherapy : Rational and clinical experience in patients with solid tumors. J Clin Oncol 8 : 911-934

Neo-Adjuvant chemotherapy in 100 patients with locally advanced carcinoma of the breast

B Coudert, P Gabez, C Lamaille, C De Gislain, F Mayer, P Fargeot

Materials and methods

From the 1st June 1975 to 1st March 1990 a hundred patients with locally advanced carcinoma of the breast were treated with Neo-Adjuvant chemotherapy. The mean age of our group was 50.7 years (median 49 years, range 23-71 years). 60 % of the patients were non or pre-menopaused while 40 % were menopaused. 87 % of the tumors could be classified T3 or T4 while only 13 % were T2. The clinical nodal status was N1 for 70 % of the patients, N2 for 6 % and N3 for 7 %. 89 % were classified stage IIIA or IIIB. All patients had a negative metastatic staging. Clinical inflammation of the tumor was evaluated and classified PEV0 in 16 patients, PEV1 in 51, PEV2 in 26 and PEV3 in 7. Histopathology was undifferentiated carcinoma in 77 % of the cases. Histologic grading was SBRI for 8 patients, SBRII for 42 and SBRIII for 13. The oestrogen and progesterone receptors were totally negative in 28 patients, both present in 26 patients and only one positive receptor could be detected in 22 patients. 44 patients (1975-1981) received the AVM1 protocol every 4 weeks : Adriamycin (50 mg/m^2, IV, J1), Vincristine (1 mg/m^2 IV, J2), Methotrexate (7,5 mg/m^2 SC, J3-J4-J5). 34 patients (1982-1987) received the weekly AVM2 protocol : Adriamycin (13 mg/m^2, IV, J1), Vindesine (2 mg/m^2 IV, J1), Methotrexate (6 mg/m^2 SC, J2). 22 patients (1987-1990) received the NVM protocol : Mitoxantrone (13 mg/m^2, IV, J1), Vindesine (2 mg/m^2 IV, J2), Methotrexate (6 mg/m^2 SC, J3-J4-J5). The patients received a mean of 4 sequences of chemotherapy (range 2 to 10 sequences). Neo-Adjuvant chemotherapy lasted 14 weeks (3 to 40 weeks). An hormonotherapy was associated with chemotherapy for 26 patients (Tamoxifen 15, Castration 6, both Tamoxifen and Castration 4, Norfor 1). An other Neo-Adjuvant protocol was associated in 14 patients.

Results

We noted hematologic toxicity in 32 % of the patients (grade 3 and 4 in 3 and 1 patient), digestive toxicity in 35 % (grade 1-2), alopecia in 32 %, grade 1 cardiologic or neurologic toxicity in respectively 1 and 8 patients.

Clinical response of the tumor was E0-E1 (stabilization or progression) for 21 patients and E2 (Response < 50 %) for 19. An objective response was obtained in 59 patients (CR : 6, PR : 53). There was no difference in the objective response rates between the 3 protocols. Menopaused status, age over 50,

---

Centre GF Leclerc, 1 rue du Pr Marion, 21034 Dijon. Dir : Pr J Guerrin

presence of positive hormone receptors influenced favorably the tumor response. Inflammation of the tumor or histologic grading did not correlate with tumor response. Adjunctive hormonal therapy did not increase objective response rate (48 % v.s. 57 %). Three cycles of chemotherapy obtained lower responses rate (39 %) than more than 3 (60 %). 7 patients undergone conservative surgery while 82 had a mammectomy. Histologic evaluation showed tumor necrosis and persisting invasive carcinoma in respectively 25 % and 94 % of the tumors. Lymphatic embolism was noted in 63 % of the cases. Invaded nodes were absent in 12 % of the cases, < 3 in 31 % and > 3 in 57 %. 85 patients had post surgical irradiation. Adjuvant chemotherapy was started in 83 patients while adjuvant hormonotherapy was initiated for 27.

Disease free survival was 81 %, 61 %, 53 %, 46 % and 40 % at respectively 1, 2, 3, 4 and 5 years. Actuarial survival (AS) was 94 %, 75 %, 66 %, 62 % and 59 % at respectively 1, 2, 3, 4 and 5 years. There was no significant difference in the disease free survival and actuarial survival rates between the 3 protocols. The 5 years AS was favorably influenced by objective tumor response (AS : 70 % v.s. 38 %) and the positive hormone receptors (AS : 71 % v.s. 41 %) but was detrimentally influenced by initial inflammatory status (AS : PEV0 = 100 %, PEV1 = 65 %, PEV2 − 3 = 38 %) or post surgical nodal status (AS N − = 100 %, N + 1 − 3 = 75 %, N + > 3 = 47 %).

Discussion

One of the main characteristic of our series was the major prevalence of stages IIIA and IIIB with T3 or T4 tumors that might have been initially considered as improper for surgery. Despite this, 89 % of our population undergone carcinologically complete surgery. This result has been obtained without significant toxicity and primary chemotherapy did not have a detrimental influence on the loco-regional treatment.

The clinical response to our primary chemotherapy reached 78 % with 59 % objective response. Because of the size of the tumors, this result was lower than in others series containing very often smaller tumors (T1 or T2). Jacquillat in 1984, 1986, 1988 has obtained between 80 and 91 % of objective response [1, 2, 3]. Nevertheless we obtained a similar result to Chauvergne who treated a comparative population with a similar protocol [4]. Also Schwartz obtained 71 % response better than 25 % in stage III breast cancer [5]. The 5 % complete histologic response of our group had to be compared to the 10 % obtained by Hortobagyi [6] or Kemeny [7].

As other groups working in the same area [6, 8], we found that initial size of the tumor, inflammatory clinical signs, clinical or post surgical nodal status, hormone receptors status and response of the tumor to primary chemotherapy represented significant prognostic factors for our patients. The exact role of primary chemotherapy as compared to adjuvant chemotherapy remains to be assessed in a multicentre randomized study.

Currently, to improve our results of primary chemotherapy in breast cancer with initial bad prognosis factors, we initiated a new study of reinforced primary chemotherapy with support of granulocyte colony stimulating factor to allow a sufficient Neo-Adjuvant dose-intensity. This new attitude is proposed to any T1, T2 tumor with positive clinical or radiological nodal disease or to any T3, T4 tumor.

References

1. Jacquillat C, Baillet F, Auclerc G et al (1984) Chimiothérapie précédent le traitement locorégional avec extension des indications du traitement conservateur. Bull Cancer 71 : 354-360
2. Jacquillat C, Weil M, Auclerc G et al (1986) Neo-Adjuvant chemotherapy in the conservative management of breast cancer, Study of 143 patients. Recent Results in Cancer Research 103 : 113-119
3. Jacquillat C, Baillet F, Weil M et al (1988) Results of a conservative treatment combining induction (Neo-Adjuvant) and consolidation chemotherapy, hormonotherapy and external and interstitial irradiation in 98 patients with locally advanced breast cancer (IIIA and IIIB). Cancer 61 : 1977-1982
4. Chauvergne J, Durand M, Hoerni B et al (1979) La chimiothérapie d'induction dans les cancers du sein à haut risque. Bull Cancer 66 : 9-16
5. Schwartz GF, Carter SL and Panico J (1992) Induction chemotherapy prior to definitive treatment improves outcome in stage III carcinoma of the breast. In : Banzet P et al (eds) Neo-Adjuvant chemotherapy. Springer-Verlag, Paris, p. 117
6. Hortobagyi GN, Singletary SE, Buzdar AU et al (1992) Primary chemotherapy for breast cancer, MD Anderson experience. In : Banzet P (ed) Neo-Adjuvant chemotherapy. Springer-Verlag, Paris, p 146
7. Kemeny F, Vadrot J, D'Hubert E et al (1991) Evaluation histologique et radioclinique de l'effet de la chimiothérapie première sur les cancers non inflammatoires du sein à propos de 56 observations. Third International congress on Neo-Adjuvant chemotherapy, Paris
8. Gardin G, Conte PF, Pronzato P et al (1992) Induction chemotherapy in locally advanced breast cancer, prognostic variables affecting results. In : Banzet P (ed) Neo-Adjuvant chemotherapy. Springer-Verlag, Paris, p 196

Abstract. Primary chemotherapy was introduced as an experimental approach for the treatment of locally advanced breast cancer. The aims of Neo-Adjuvant chemotherapy were the downstage of the tumors to facilitate the loco-regional treatment, the evaluation of the tumor response to chemotherapy and the control of the micrometastases. We retrospectively analyzed our results obtained in a hundred patients. Future directions are exposed.

Surgical aspects of the conservative treatment of large size breast cancer after primary chemotherapy

S Zurrida, M Greco, V Galimberti, U Veronesi

Primary or Neo-Adjuvant chemotherapy is to be understood as antineoplastic pharmacological treatment carried out prior to loco-regional treatment in an attempt to [1] render the tumor amenable to radical surgical control when it is locally advanced ; [2] bring a systemic therapy into play, at an early stage, against micrometastatic disease ; [3] permit conservative surgery where the initial dimensions of the tumor would normally required a demolitive or mutilatory intervention.

Primary chemotherapy was first used in cases of local advanced breast cancer (T3b, T4) : medical treatment was employed before loco-regional therapy in order to rapidly reduce the size of the tumor and consent safe surgery or radiotherapy [1].

Two further developments led to the wider use of Neo-Adjuvant chemotherapy in the earlier stages of breast cancer : the first was the fact that survival in patients with small size breast cancer did not depend on whether they were treated by mastectomy or conservative surgery (quadrantectomy or tumorectomy), and the second that modern antineoplastic agents are more efficacious [2-5].

A study of the use of hormonal or chemotherapy to obtain the maximum possible tumor regression began in the second half of the 1980s at the Royal Marsden Hospital in London. Its aim was to test the feasibility of substituting conservative surgery for mastectomy in women so treated [6]. Other studies soon followed, and the common denominator was the idea of being able to offer a greater number of women with operable breast cancer the choice of conserving their breasts [7, 8].

In the study carried out at the Istituto Nazionale Tumori, Milano, 89 % of patients with breast cancers ⩾ 3 cm in diameter underwent quadrantectomies after being treated with various Neo-Adjuvant chemotherapy regimes, as reported by Bonadonna et al [9].

The present work discusses the problems that confront the surgeon when operating on women who have undergone these neoadjuvant treatments. In particular it is concerned with the type of surgical treatment to be adopted, the extent of the resection, and other problems arising in these cases : clinical evaluation of the extent of tumor regression, identification of the exact site of the tumor when it is no longer palpable, evaluation of the resection margins and the efficacy of the treatment.

Istituto Nazionale Tumori, via G Venezian, 1, 20133 Milan, Italy

Discussion of case series

Patients eligible for the study, which began in January 1988, were those with breast carcinoma of radiological diameter ⩾3 cm and age less than 65. Complete staging consisted of mammography, chest X-ray, bone scan, liver ultrasound and cardiological assessment.

A total of 227 patients were enrolled ; 150 (66 %) were premenopausal at diagnosis and 77 (34 %) were postmenopausal ; median age was 49 years. After determination of malignancy (incisional biopsy, fine needle aspiration, trucut), receptor status, ploidy and cell kinetics, they underwent primary chemotherapy prior to surgical treatment. One of 5 different chemotherapeutic regimes was administered.

Three weeks after the last chemotherapeutic cycle had been administred, the patients were re-evaluated clinically and mammographically and were then ready for surgery. If, both clinically and in the X-ray the mass had reduced sufficiently in size to consent safe conservative surgery, a classic quadrantectomy was performed. The proportion of patients whose breasts were conserved, was the same for all chemotherapeutic regimes.

The primary tumor regressed in 177 patients and it was found that the larger the initial size, the less likely it would shrink to the size considered compatible with conservative treatment. In nearly all cases where the initial diameter was ⩽ 5 cm conservative treatment proved possible (Table 1).

Table 1. Percentage of tumors whose maximum diameter after primary chemotherapy reduced to less than 3 cm

		Initial T (cm) 3.0-5.0	> 5.0
No of patients (Total 220)		183	37
T at surgery	< 3 cm	87 %	62 %
	not measurable	11.5 %	13.5 %
No of complete remission after chemotherapy		8	0
Quadrantectomy		95 %	73 %

Surgical technique

The operation began with a losenge-shaped cutaneous incision including the biopsy scar or the tatoo marks made before chemotherapy. And continued with resection of the tumor and a wide margin of surrounding mammary parenchyma down to the muscular fascia of the pectoralis major. When the quadrant had been removed, the macroscopic dimensions of the residual tumor were determined intraoperatively.

If microcalcifications in association with the cancer were noted in the mammogram taken at the beginning of treatment, the specimen was sent for radiological evaluation to ascertain that all had been removed.

Samples from the margins of the quadrant were examined histologically to exclude the presence of residual carcinoma and non visible in situ components. Even when no residual tumor was discernible, the two above mentioned controls were always carried out ; furthermore the extent of the quadrantectomy, as indicated by the tatoo marks was always respected in such cases. The resection margins should not be so limited as to carry a risk of local recurrence and not so wide as to deform the breast and thus neutralize the object of the treatment. A difficulty often arises here because the tumor mass may have become soft to palpation and difficult to detect due to destruction of part of the tumor. In such cases in particular, as well as noting the dimensions of the tatoo, the surgeon must bear in mind the mammographic dimension of the tumor and the resection margin must respect this.

If the macroscopic dimensions of the residual tumor were too large to satisfy the indication for a safe conservative result, or not all the microcalcifications (when initially present) had been removed, or the resection margins were positive, a Patey mastectomy was performed. Fifteen quadrantectomies were performed on tumors greater than the 3 cm diameter taken as the limit above which conservation of the breast was not indicated. In these cases the ratio between tumor size and breast volume was such as to assure a quadrantectomy with sufficiently large margins in healthy glandular tissue.

Axillary dissection was performed next. This was continuous or discontinuous depending on the site of the primary, and the presumed aesthetic outcome. All three levels were always removed and tagged with metal disks to identify them. The vascular nervous tract associated with the dorsal muscle and the long thoracic nerve (Bell's nerve) were always identified and conserved. Whenever possible the pectoralis minor was also conserved but this depended on whether level II lymphnodes were palpated and suspected.

In quadrantectomies the next stage is reconstruction of the breast. In most cases this is achieved by drawing together the resection margins. Two or three sutures are usually sufficient and should be placed so as to avoid permanent skin retraction. Where tissue loss is relatively great it is useful to detach part of the mammary parenchyma from the muscular fascia, and sometimes from the overlying skin, with the fingers. This mobilizes the gland and avoids deformation.

Radiotherapy was given in all cases undergoing conservative treatment, starting 3 to 6 weeks after the operation. The required dose of 50 Gy was administered in 5 weekly sections ; in the 6th week an overdose was given to an approximately 12 x 8 cm field around the tumor bed using X-rays or 10 MeV electrons.

With a median follow up of 30 months from the initiation of primary chemotherapy, it is too early to draw conclusions about disease free survival and survival.

It is concluded that conservative breast surgery followed by radiotherapy is an eminently feasible treatment for large tumors when primary chemotherapy reduces tumor size. It is emphasized however that the final decision as to which surgery should be performed must be taken in the operating room, after assessment of objective tumor size in relation to breast size, and evaluation of all the variables discussed here.

The results of this study change the classic indication for mastectomy and offer the possibility of breast conservation to those women with larger tumors who wish to preserve the integrity of their bodies.

References

1. Valagussa P, Zambetti M, Bonadonna G, et al (1990) Prognosis factors in locally advanced non-inflammatory breast cancer. Long term results following primary chemotherapy. Breast Cancer Res Treat 15 : 137-147
2. Veronesi U, Costa A, Saccozzi R (1986) Surgical technique of breast quadrantectomy and axillary dissection. In : Strombeck JO, Rosato FE (eds) Surgery of the breast. Diagnosis and treatment of breast disease. Thieme Verlag, Stuttgart, pp. 127-131
3. Veronesi U, Salvadori B, Luini A, et al (1990) Conservative treatment of early breast cancer. Ann Surg 211 (3) : 250-259
4. Fisher B, Redmond C, Poisson R, et al (1989) Eight year results of a randomized trial comparing total mastectomy and lumpectomy with or without irradiation in the treatment of breast cancer. N Eng J Med 320 : 820-828
5. Pierguin B, Huart J, Raynal M, et al (1991) Conservative treatment for breast cancer - long term results (15 years). Radiother Oncol 20 : 16-23
6. Mansi JI, Smith IE, Walsh G, et al (1989) Primary medical therapy for operable breast cancer. Eur J Cancer Clin Oncol 25 (11) : 1623-1627
7. Jacquillat C, Weil M, Baillet F, et al (1990) Results of Neo-Adjuvant chemotherapy and radiation therapy in breast-conserving treatment of 250 patients with all stages of infiltrative breast cancer. Cancer 66 : 119-129
8. Bolembaogo E, Feillel V, Chollet P, et al (1990) Neo-Adjuvant chemotherapy in 126 operable breast cancers. Eur J Cancer 28A, 4/6 : 896-900
9. Bonadonna G, Veronesi U, Brambilla C, et al (1990) Primary chemotherapy to avoid mastectomy in tumors of three centimeters or more. J Natl Cancer Inst 82 : 1539-1545

Efficacy of a chemotherapy regimen combining Vinorelbine, Epirubicine and Methotrexate (VEM) in locally advanced and metastatic breast cancer

I Van Praagh, N Martineau, V Feillel, H Curé, E Bélembaogo, MA Ravoux, J Fleury, C Deloche, R Plagne, P Chollet

A recent phase II study [1] has shown a high response rate of 50 % with Vinorelbine in metastatic breast cancer. It seemed logical to combine this new compound with the well tolerated and effective drugs Epirubicine and Methotrexate (respective response rate of 45 % and 20 %). A weekly (day 1 & 8) administration of Vinorelbine was performed as proposed in the phase II study ; Epirubicine and Methotrexate were also infused at day 1 and 8 to decrease toxicity. In metastatic relapse, our aim was to increase complete response rate (CR) ; and in Neo-Adjuvant situation, aims were to obtain maximal tumor's reduction to avoid modified radical mastectomy (MRM) and increase of clinical and pathological response rates.

Patients and methods

Patients

From March 1991 to January 1993, 36 females were treated in our institute ; 17 in metastatic relapse, of mean age 61 years (45-76), all with menopausal status. Metastatic sites were 10 bones, 9 liver, 3 nodes, 2 pleural and 1 skin. All had at least one non-squeletal measurable target. The whole population was pretreated in adjuvant situation with anthracyclins, 8 patients had received Tamoxifen. Mean delay of relapse was 68.8 months (11-252). 19 patients, of mean age 51 years (34-70) had a Neo-Adjuvant treatment for tumors > 3 cm in diameter or situated in the central area of the nipple ; 10 were premenopausal and 9 postmenopausal. The initial staging included clinical examination, bilateral mammography and echography, cyto and/or histological diagnosis by cytology and surecut needle. Absence of metastasis was proven by chest X-ray, liver biology and echography, bone scintigraphy and tumor's markers. TNM : 1 Tx, 14 T2, 3 T3, 1 T4 (with a mean T of 37 mm) ; 6 N0, 10 N1, 3 N2 (2 had cutaneous attraction and 6 tumors situated in the central area). Pathology : 16 invasive ductal and 1 invasive lobular carcinomas. SBR grade : I : 4, II : 6, III : 6 and Modified SBR grade : 2 : 6, 3 : 4, 4 : 6, 5 : 1. Hormonal receptors : RE+RP+ : 2, RE+ RP− : 5, RE−RP+ : 3, RE−RP− : 7. Flow cytometry : aneuploid population : 12 and S phase > 5 % : 12.

Centre Jean Perrin and Inserm U 71, rue Montalembert, BP 392, 63011 Clermont-Ferrand Cedex, France

Methods

The following treatment scheme was used every 28 days : d1 and d8 Vinorelbine (V) 25 mg/sq.m, Epirubicine 35 mg/sq.m and Methotrexate 20 mg/sq.m. In metastatic relapse, 111 cycles were infused (6.5 per person) with a satisfying dose-intensity of average V : 480 mg (74 mg/cycle), of E : 655 mg (100 mg/cycle), of M : 373 mg (57 mg/cycle). In Neo-Adjuvant treatment, 114 cycles were infused (6 patient) and fair dose-intensity was also observed ; V : 486 mg (86 mg/cycle), E : 661 mg (110 mg/cycle), M : 399 mg (66 mg/cycle).

Assessment of responses

For metastatic disease clinical examination was performed every month and paraclinical assessment on targets every 3 months. For Neo-Adjuvant treatment, measurement (clinic, mammographic and echographic) was done at the beginning of the 4th and at the end of the 6th cycle. After 6 cycles, surgical treatment, or at least tumorectomy occured even if a complete response was reached.

Results

Tolerance

Haematological tolerance was acceptable. Toxicity was higher for metastatic patients probably because of a lesser performance status and of previous chemotherapy. However no hospitalisation for febrile aplasia and no toxic death was registered. Drugs doses had to be decreased in only 3 cases.

% of cycles	WHO grade		
	Leucocytes	Neutrophils	Platelets
Metastatic	8 % grade 3 20 % grade 4	8 % grade 3 20 % grade 4	100 % grade 0-1
Neo-adjuvant	10 % grade 3 10 % grade 4	10 % grade 3 10 % grade 4	100 % grade 0-1

Other toxicities : in about 80 % of cases, were represented by grade 3-4 alopecia and venous toxicity was noted in 30 % of cases.

Responses

In metastatic situation, we observed 1 CR, 9 PR, 3 SD and 4 PD (59 % of major responses). 3 patients died of their metastatic evolution. In Neo-Adjuvant situation, response was estimated according 3 clinical methods :

	After 3 cycles				After 6 cycles			
	CR	PR	MR	SD	CR	PR	MR	SD
Clinical	4	9	5	1	6	9	4	0
Echographic	3	7	7	2	4	9	6	0
Mammographic	2	5	6	6	4	5	5	5

After surgery, we obtained 3 pathological CR and in 2 cases only isolated neoplasic cells. Then, 79 % of clinical major responses were reached with 30 % CCR and 16 % pCR. Neo-Adjuvant chemotherapy allowed conservative surgery in 94 % of cases (16/17). Because of extended intraductal carcinoma, the semaining patient was submitted to MRM.

Discussion and conclusions

In metastatic disease, this regimen can be compared with the well-known regimen FAC in terms of response. In Neo-Adjuvant treatment, the 3 methods gave a high response rate, comparable with our previous study with AVCF. Echographic responses were found to be intermediate between clinical and mammographic results [2]. Special emphasis should be drawn on the 5 excellent histological results (3 complete, 2 isolated remaining cells) as generally these results are less than 10 % of cases in induction breast cancer chemotherapy [3]. This encouraging results have to be confirmed by larger series and after a longer follow up.

References

1. Fumoleau P et al (1990) Phase II trial with Navelbine in advanced breast cancer. Preliminary results. Asco 9 (1) : Abst 76. French Epirubicin Study Group (1988) A prospective randomized phase III trial comparing combination chemotherapy with Cyclophosphamide, Fluorouracil, and either Doxorubicin or Epirubicin. J Clin Oncol 6 : 679-688
2. Anderson EDC, Forrest APM, Hawkins RA, Anderson TJ, Leonard RCF, Chetty U (1991) Primary systemic therapy for operable breast cancer. Br J Cancer 63 : 561-566
3. Mansi JL, Smith IE, Walsh G, et al (1989) Primary medical therapy for operable breast cancer. Eur J Cancer Oncol 25 : 1623-1627
4. DeVita VT Jr (1990) Primary chemotherapy can avoid mastectomy, but there is more to it than that. J Natl Cancer Inst 82 : 1522-1524
5. Jacquillat C, Weil M, Baillet F, et al (1990) Results of Neo-Adjuvant chemotherapy and radiation therapy in the breast-conserving treatment of 250 patients with all stages of infiltrative breast cancer. Cancer 66 : 119-129
6. Jacquillat C, Baillet F, Auclerc G, et al (1984) Cancer du sein. Chimiothérapie précédant le traitement loco-régional avec extension des indications du traitement conservateur. Bull Cancer 7 (suppl 1) : 5

7. Bonadonna G, Veronesi U, Brambilla C, et al (1990) Primary chemotherapy to avoid mastectomy in tumors with diameters of 3 centimeters or more. J Natl Cancer Inst 19 : 539-545
8. Mauriac L (1990) Chimiothérapie première des cancers du sein opérables. Étude randomisée. Bull Cancer 77 (suppl 1) : 47-53
9. Bélembaogo E, Feillel V, Chollet P, et al (1992) Neo-Adjuvant chemotherapy in 126 operable breast cancers. Eur J Cancer 28 : 896-900 (2)
10. Feldmann LD and al (1986) Pathological assessment of response to induction chemotherapy in breast cancer. Cancer Research 46 : 2578-2581

Recurrent breast carcinoma after conservative treatment : MRI features and pathologic correlation

TH Dao, F Campana, A Fourquet, M Laurent, B Asselain, A Rahmouni

Early detection of recurrent breast carcinoma treated conservatively may be a diagnostic challenge when patients have undergone prior breast irradiation, either alone or in combination with surgery, chemotherapy or hormone therapy. Post-treatment follow-up is often difficult as post-radiation changes may mimic or obscure recurrent tumors on clinical examination or mammography. In fact these techniques are known as limited for differentiating fibrotic lesions and tumorous tissue, and repeated biopsies are often required. Previous reports have shown promising results with magnetic resonance (MR) imaging in differentiating these conditions with Gadolinium enhanced-sequences, with partial results in the follow-up of irradiated breast [1-3].

In our experience, MR imaging of the breast is a valuable problem-solving technique in these difficult cases by differentiating fibrotic post-treatment lesions from recurrent tumors [4]. The particular aspect of recurrent breast carcinoma on MRI is presented and correlated with pathological specimen.

Materials and method

Patients

92 patients were prospectively examined with MR imaging between November 1990 and October 1992. All these patients were treated conservatively for previous breast cancer. Radiation therapy was the sole local treatment in 70 cases, associated or not with adjuvant hormonal therapy or chemotherapy ; radiation therapy was associated to limited surgery in 22 cases. 3 patients were treated conservatively by a combination of different treatments including tumorectomy, radiotherapy and insertion of a breast prosthesis.

All the patients were suspected to have a recurrent tumor on clinical examination or on mammography, and were refered to MRI in a mean delay time of 3 years (1-13 years) after completion of radiation therapy . All the patients were scheduled for guided-biopsy of breast abnormalities in the days following MR imaging examination. Cinical-radiological follow-up over a period of 12-18 months (mean 15 months) was done in all patients. In case of biopsy-proven recurrence, mastectomy was performed with pathological examination of the resected specimen.

Departments of Radiology, Radiotherapy, Pathology and Biostatistic, Institut Curie, 26 rue d'Ulm, 75005 Paris

MRI technique

MR Imaging was performed in all patients on a 0.5T magnet (MR Max, GE-CGR, Milwaukee) using a breast coil provided by the manufacturer. Patients were placed in the prone position with the affected breast centered in a 15 cm diameter surface coil.

The same sequences were performed in all patients and included T1 (TR : 400 ms, TE : 25 ms, 1 excitation) and T2 (TR : 2000 ms, TE : 60-120 ms, 1 excitation) spin-echo sequences, and a short time inversion-recovery (STIR) sequence (TR : 2000 ms, TI : 110 ms, TE : 25 ms, 1 excitation). This STIR sequence was obtained in order to nullify the fat signal and has been described to increase the contrast of malignant tissue [5]. Dynamic Gadolinium enhanced T1-weighted sequences were then performed in order to study the hemokinetics of the suspected lesions. Soustraction of post and precontrast images was also performed in an attempt to increase the sensitivity of the method. The total MR examination required less than 40 minutes.

MR images analysis

A quantitative analysis of MR images was performed on T1 images, before and after injection of Gadolinium : multiple measurements of signal intensity were performed at different points of the suspected lesion, on all pre and postcontrast SET1 images. Curves of signal intensity over time were established from these measurements. Statistical analysis was performed with a Student t-test and ROC curves [6] were generated from measurements before and after injection in order to indicate how well the intensity of enhancement of the lesion can distinguish the two groups (fibrosis/recurrence).

Results

19 cases of recurrent carcinoma were diagnosed on MRI because early and significant contrast-enhancement after bolus injection of Gadolinium. These diagnoses were confirmed in 17 patients by biopsies performed after the MRI examination and by the histological examination performed on the mastectomy specimen. In two cases, dynamic-enhanced MRI concluded to recurrent breast carcinoma : fine needle aspiration of suspected lesions found no malignant cells and the patients refused surgical biopsy. However, clinical follow-up of these patients demonstrate a recurrent tumor in one patient 6 months later. One case was a false negative result with an inflammatory recurrent tumor 8 months after MR examination.

In all recurrent cases, MR imaging with dynamic Gadolinium enhanced sequences demonstrated areas of early increased signal intensity within the first minutes after bolus injection. Signal intensity of localized fibrosis varied differently with the time from recurrences, demonstrating no significant contrast enhancement after injection.

Table 1. Demographic and Clinical Characteristics of All Patients

Characteristic	Patients (n = 51)
Karnofsky Performance Status (median, range)	70 (60-90)
Age (years) (median, range)	47 (26-73)
Sites of metastases (%)	
Lymph node	43
Cutaneous/soft tissue	47
Lung	45
Liver	33
Bone	47
Multiple organ-system sites	86
Prior Stage IV chemotherapy regimens (median, range)	3 (2-6)
Prior high dose chemotherapy (%)	14
Prior radiotherapy - Stg IV disease (%)	67

Table 2. Response by prior anthracycline/anthracenedione (A/A) sensitivity*

	Response/evaluable pts	Response Proportion (95 % confidence intvl)
A/A Refractory	5/22	22.7 % (5-40)
A/A Sensitive	6/27	22.2 % (7-38)
A/A Stable	2/2	

* Resistant = recurrent disease < 12 months after completing anthracycline-containing adjuvant chemotherapy, or lack of intervening response to anthracycline in the setting of advanced disease. Sensitive = recurrent disease > 12 months after completing anthracycline-containing adjuvant chemotherapy, or history of an intervening response while receiving anthracycline for advanced disease.

3 patterns of contrast-enhancement of the suspected lesions can be described : 1- homogeneous and diffuse, 2- homogeneous and partial, 3- heterogeneous. MR findings were correlated with microscopic analysis of the tumors.

Discussion

The late or chronic phase of radiation changes is related to development of late fibrosis, and is usually stable by 12 months after completed radiation therapy [7]. All the patients in our series were examined 1 year-13 years after completion of radiation therapy, and MRI changes related to early post-radiation fibrosis were considered to have disappeared. The signal intensity of late fibrosis is known to be low on SE T1 and T2 weighted sequences, reflecting decreased vascularity, no edema and presence of mature connective tissue [8].

T2 and STIR sequences were not contributive in our series in differentiating fibrosis from tumor recurrences because delineation of the lesions is often difficult. However, after bolus injection of Gadolinium, dynamic MR imaging clearly demonstrated different enhancement patterns of suspected lesions : 1) early enhancement corresponded, in all our cases, to recurrent breast carcinoma, 2) weakly enhanced areas corresponded to late non vascularized fibrotic tissue and sterilized lesions.

In most patients with recurrences, with our protocol and system, the peak of enhancement was obtained at 3 minutes after contrast injection with a 100 % accuracy for a cut-off level of enhancement equal to 1.3. Therefore, imaging at 3 minutes after contrast injection appears as the optimal time for diagnosis of recurrences versus post-radiation changes.

Conclusion

MR imaging of the breast with dynamic gadolinium-enhanced sequences is a valuable technique by permitting the differentiation of late post-radiation changes from recurrent carcinoma when patients have undergone prior breast irradiation. MRI is a complement to other imaging modalities in these difficult cases when there is a clinical or mammographic suspicion : in dense breasts, in the presence of a prosthesis, in the presence of post-treatment fibrosis. This distinction is of clinical importance and should be useful in the management and follow-up of patients who have received a breast-conserving treatment.

References

1. Heywang SH, Wolf A, Pruss E, Hilbertz T, Eiermann W, Permanetter W (1989) MR Imaging of the Breast with Gd-DTPA : Use and Limitations. Radiology 171 : 95-103
2. Kaiser WA, Zeitler E (1989) MR Imaging of the Breast : Fast Imaging Sequences with and without Gd-DTPA. Preliminary Observations. Radiology 170 : 681-686
3. Dao TH, Campana F, Fourquet A, Rahmouni A (1991) Tumor recurrence versus fibrosis in breast carcinoma treated by radiation therapy : differentiation with dynamic Gadolinium enhanced MR imaging. RSNA Chicago
4. Dao TH, Rahmouni A, Campana F, Laurent M, Asselain B, Fourquet A (1993) Tumor recurrence versus fibrosis in the irradiated breast : differentiation with dynamic Gadolinium enhanced MR imaging. Radiology, in press
5. Metz CE (1978) Basic principles of ROC analysis. Sem Nucl Med, vol VIII, 4 : 283-298
6. Zobel BB, Patrizio G, Confalone D, D'Archivio C, Passariello R (1989) MR STIR imaging versus spin-echo imaging of the breast : lesion characterization. RSNA : 1078
7. Ebner F, Kressel HY, Mintz MC et al (1988) Tumor Recurrence versus Fibrosis in the Female Pelvis : Differentiation with MR Imaging at 1.5 T. Radiology 166 : 333-340
8. Saryan LA, Hollis DP, Economou JS, Eggleston JC (1974) Nuclear magnetic resonance studies of cancer. IV. Correlation of water content with tissue relaxation times. J Natl Cancer Inst 52 : 599-602

Intensive chemotherapy for inflammatory breast cancer: how much clinical value?

B Chevallier, C Couteau*, D Atlan*, V Chatikhine*, Y Graic**,
JP Julien***, A Kunlin***, P Bastit*, C Veyret*, J D'Anjou****

Inflammatory adenocarcinoma of the breast is a rare disease with severe prognostic implications due to an almost constant metastatic evolution. Its definition is mainly clinical [11]: enlargement, tenderness, firmness, redness of the breast with usually no fever. With either surgery or radiotherapy alone or the use of combination surgery and radiotherapy, less than 5 % of patients will survive at 5 years [2, 30]. A combined modality approach including chemotherapy is at the present time admitted worldwide [14, 30]. This strategy has led to a significant improvement in survival, with 30 to 50 % of the patients surviving beyond 5 years [30]. Achievement of a mastectomy specimen free of residual macroscopic tumor after induction chemotherapy has been shown to be an excellent indicator of a prolonged disease free and overall survival [8]. Unfortunately, this situation accounts for less than 20 % of the patients [7, 16, 21, 23, 29-33]. One area of research is to increase survival by the search of more efficient induction chemotherapy regimens yielding a higher histologic response rate. More aggressive cytotoxic regimens using the concept of dose efficacy can be tested for this goal.

We present here the results of combined modality approach used in 227 IBC patients. Different induction chemotherapy regimen were used aiming 1) to improve the response rate, 2) to obtain the best loco-regional control of the disease, 3) to increase overall survival and disease free survival of these patients.

Patients and methods

The 227 patients retained for this analysis represent 4 % of the newly diagnosed invasive non metastatic adenocarcinomas of the breast between January 1977 and August 1992. All of them meet the following criterias: histologically proven invasive adenocarcinoma of one breast, inflammatory signs (erythema + « peau d'orange » + increase of the local heat) involving at least one third of the breast (T4d of the 1988 UICC classification), no history of previous malignancy, no prior specific treatment, serum bilirubin $\leqslant$ 35 μmol/l, serum creatinine $\leqslant$ 130 μmol/l. A positive skin biopsy was not mandatory for the diagnosis since we considered as others [7, 9, 14, 19, 30] that inflammato-

---

* Service d'Oncologie Médicale, ** Service de Radiothérapie, *** Service de Chirurgie, *** Service d'Anatomo-pathologie, Centre H. Becquerel, 76038 Rouen

ry breast cancer is a clinical diagnosis rather than a pathologic definition. 133 patients included in the second study and the third study had a skin biopsy performed at the time of initial diagnosis. Cases with previous history of breast cancer, bilateral breast cancer, prior history of heart failure or with an history of another malignant tumor were not kept for this analysis. This excludes also advanced breast cancer such as scirrous or ulcerated cancers and also rapidly progressing breast cancers without inflammatory signs. Since January 1977, every patient had a pretreatment check-up including history and physical examination, bilateral mammographies, chest X-ray, bone scan, liver echography or CT scan, EKG and echocardiography or radionuclide cardiac scan (since 1983), complete blood count, standard biological tests, carcinoembryonic antigen (until 1986), CA 15.3 (since 1987). Estrogen and progesterone receptors were measured at time of initial diagnosis according to the coal-dextran technique for the patients of the second and third study.

Assessment of tumor response was performed at least every 2 cycles with clinical examination and mammographies. All baseline investigations were repeated at the end of the treatment.

Follow-up was every 3 months the first year, bi-annual for the next 4 years and once a year thereafter, with clinical examination, chest X-ray and biochemical screen. Mammographies were performed once a year. Loco-regional or controlateral relapses were confirmed by biopsy or unequivocal radiological evidence.

Treatment modalities

The patients of each of the 3 groups were treated with a combined modality approach. Induction chemotherapy was always given first for an average of 4 cycles (range : 2-8). Loco-regional treatment consisted of radiotherapy or surgery. Radiotherapy as exclusive loco-regional treatment employed Cobalt 60 and delivered 60 grays to the tumor, the whole breast and the axilla, 50 grays to the internal mammary chain and 46 grays to the supraclavicular area. Ten Grays per week were given in 5 fractions. 4-6 weeks after the first irradiation, a 20 grays boost was given to the breast tumoral remainders. No chemotherapy was administered during radiotherapy. Surgery consisted in every cases of a modified radical mastectomy with homolateral axillary clearance. No conservative surgery was performed. Maintenance chemotherapy was administered only if induction chemotherapy obtained at least a partial response and used the same schedule as induction chemotherapy for an average of 4 cycles (Range : 0-12). No standard protocol was adopted in the treatment of loco-regional or distant recurrences : patients were given the most suitable therapy for their state.

Between 1977 and 1992 modifications in the treatment program have been made in 3 steps.

First study

In January 1977, induction chemotherapy was introduced at the Centre H. Becquerel before loco-regional treatment. This induction chemotherapy consisted either in CMF (n = 22 ; until April 1979) or AVCF thereafter (n = 42) (Table 1) given for 3 cycles. Retreatment was decided at day 28 if platelets were > 100 000/mm^3 and PNN > 2000/mm^3. Loco-regional treatment consisted in every cases in exclusive radiotherapy. Surgery was only employed as a salvage treatment in case of loco-regional relapse after radiotherapy (n = 8). Maintenance chemotherapy was the same than induction chemotherapy for 8 cycles. From January 1977 to June 1983 64 patients have been included in this study [4].

Table 1. Chemotherapy schedules employed in the 3 consecutive series

Chemotherapy regimen	Days	Drugs and dosage	Number of patients
CMF (ref. n° 4)	1 and 8	5-Fluorouracil 600 mg/m^2*	
	1 and 8	Methotrexate 40 mg/m^2*	22
	1 to 7	Cyclophosphamide 150 mg/m^2	
AVCF (ref. n° 4)	1	Doxorubicin 30 mg/m^2*	
	2	Vincristin 1.4 mg/m^2 (Max = 2 mg)*	63
	3 to 6	Cyclophosphamide 300 mg/m^2*	
	3 to 6	and 5-Fluorouracil 400 mg/m^2*	
VAC (ref. n° 20)	1 to 4	Vindesin 1 mg/m^2*	
	1 to 3	Doxorubicin 15 mg/m^2*	23
	1 to 3	Cyclophosphamide 200 mg/m^2*	
FAC	1	Doxorubicin 50 mg/m^2*	
	1	5-Fluorouracil 500 mg/m^2*	39
	1	Cyclophosphamide 500 mg/m^2*	
FEC-HD (ref. n° 5)	1 to 4	5-Fluorouracil 750 mg/m^2 (CIVI)	
	2 to 4	Epirubicin 35 mg/m^2*	80
	2 to 4	Cyclophosphamide 400 mg/m^2*	
FEC 75 (adjuvant)	1	Epirubicin 75 mg/m^2*	
	1	5-Fluorouracil 500 mg/m^2*	80
	1	Cyclophosphamide 500 mg/m^2*	
		Total =	227

Legend : CIVI : Continuous IV infusion
* : Bolus IV infusion

Second study

From July 1983 to December 1987, 83 patients have been included in this second study. Because of the poor results in loco regional control with high incidence of intramammary remainders and loco-regional relapses observed in the first study [4], we decided to test the value of surgery as loco-regional treatment. This was done only for the patients with no supra clavicular lymph node involvement achieving at least a good partial response with disappearance of erythema after induction chemotherapy. This chemotherapy was more intensive as compared to that of the first study. It consisted either of AVCF (n = 21) FAC (n = 39) or VAC (n = 23) [20] (Table 1). 2-6 cycles were given (average = 4 cycles). One patient received 8 cycles. Policy for retreatment at Day 28 for the patients treated with AVCF was the same than in the first study. The same blood count criteria were used for the patients treated with FAC or VAC but retreatment was planned to be at day 21 instead of day 28.

Twenty-three patients had either supra clavicular lymph node involvement or achieved stabilization or progressive disease after induction therapy and received exclusive radiotherapy for loco-regional treatment.

Sixty patients without supra clavicular lymph node involvement and who achieved at least a partial response after Neo-Adjuvant chemotherapy were either operated on (n = 38) or received exclusive radiotherapy (n = 22). This choice was not randomized but left to the clinician and patient choice. No adjuvant radiotherapy was given in case of surgery.

Maintenance chemotherapy was the same as induction chemotherapy for 4 cycles.

Third study

From January 1988 to August 1992, 80 patients entered this study aiming at finding a more aggressive cytotoxic induction regimen [5]. Estrogenic recruitment was introduced in the combination given the impressive results obtained by other teams [6, 31]. High response rates had been reported with continuous 5-FU infusion in pretreated metastatic breast cancer [13] and this was the reason why we incorporated this drug with this particular modality of administration in our induction regimen. Sixteen patients received G-CSF, 5 μg/kg from day 6 to day 15 within the framework of a multicentric trial testing the value of G-CSF versus placebo in the reduction of neutropenia in IBC patients treated with FEC-HD induction chemotherapy.

Induction chemotherapy with FEC-HD lasted 4 cycles. Retreatment at day 21 was decided if the platelets were > 75000/mm^3 and PNN > 1500/mm^3. Loco-regional treatment policy was the same as in the second study. However all the patients without supra clavicular involvement who achieved at least a partial response after induction therapy were proposed surgery. Seven refused and received radiotherapy. Adjuvant chemotherapy consisted in 4 cycles of FEC 75 (Table 1). Adjuvant radiotherapy was given after Adjuvant chemotherapy to the patients who underwent surgery.

Statistical analysis

Results were last updated in December 1992. Overall response rates were estimated at the end of induction chemotherapy, taking into account both the breast tumor, the lymph nodes and the inflammatory signs, using the WHO criterias [24]. Disease-free survival was defined as the time elapsed between date of remission and date of first relapse wherever this relapse might be. We choose the date of remission to be the date of surgery or the date of last day of radiotherapy. Overall survival was the time separating date of initial diagnosis and date of last known to be alive/or date of death, whatever might be the cause of death. The survival curves have been established according to the Kaplan and Meier method [17]. The degree of signification between the curves (p) was calculated using the Log rank test [22]. Percentage differentials were tested by application of the Chi-2 test.

Results

The main characteristics of the patients are shown in Tab. 2. Median follow up for the whole population is 39.5 months (Range : 3-197).

The objective response rate (RR) between CMF and AVCF in study I was not statistically different (RR = 50 % ± 22 % versus 58.5 % ± 15.5 % ; p = 0.46). The same was observed between AVCF, FAC and VAC in study II (RR = 71.5 % ± 17.5 % versus 74 % ± 13 % versus 74 % ± 16 % respectively ; p = 0.96). This prompted us to pool the patients of study I and those of study II and to analyse and compare the results of the patients included in the first, the second and the third study, whatever the induction chemotherapy might be. The objective response rate (CR + PR) was 53.1 % in the first study, 73.5 % in the second one and 88.75 % in the third study. The difference is statistically significant between the first and the second study (p = 0.028), between the second and the third study (p = 0.019) and between the first and the third study (p = 0.0004). Hematologic and non hematologic side effects were greater in the third study than in the second and also greater in the second study than in the first.

Median, 5 year and 10 year disease free or overall survival results appear in Tab. 4, in Figs. 1, 2. Metastase free survival curves appear in Fig. 3.

Discussion

This paper summarises an experience from one center of combined modality approach of unilateral non metastatic inflammatory breast cancer. Comparison between our 3 studies conducted within 15 years have been made. We know that caution should be kept because of the historical comparisons we made. However, inflammatory breast cancer is a rare disease and historical controls remain our best approach. No randomized trial have been published so far in this field.

Table 2. Main characteristics of the patients

Factor studied	First study	Second study	Third study
Number of patients	64	83	80
Age at initial diagnosis	49.4	49.3	50
Average (range)	(25-76)	(24-76)	(29-68)
Menopausal status at initial diagnosis			
— Pre	33	53	40
— Post	31	30	40
Clinical size of the tumor (mm)	85.5	70.9	68.7
Average (range)	(30-160)	(30-120)	(0-150)
Mammographic size of the tumor (mm)	62.1	50.7	45.2
Average (range)	(25-150)	(15-100)	(0-95)
Extent of inflammatory signs			
— Limited	35	56	47
— Diffuse	29	27	33
Clinical lymph node involvement			
— N0	5	13	15
— N1b	40	52	54
— N2	11	10	6
— Supra clavicular	8	8	5
Histopathological grading			
— 1	2	7	11
— 2	14	27	44
— 3	10	14	12
— Not done	38	35	13
ER			
Average (range)	NA	18.1 (1-825)	24 (1-465)
PR	NA	10.0 (1-275)	16.2 (1-275)
Cutaneous Biopsy			
— Negative	—	41	47
— Positive	—	18	27
— Not done	64	24	6

NA : Not available. ER : Estrogen receptor. PR : Progesterone receptor

Table 3. Overall response rates observed after induction chemotherapy

| Response observed | First study | | Second study | | | Third study |
	CMF	AVCF	FAC	VAC	AVCF	FEC-HD
CR	2	2	4	2	0	50
PR	9	23	25	15	15	21
SD	10	11	9	5	6	8
PD	1	6	1	1	0	1
Total	22	42	39	23	21	80

CR : Complete response. PR : Partial response. SD : Stable disease. PD : Progressive disease

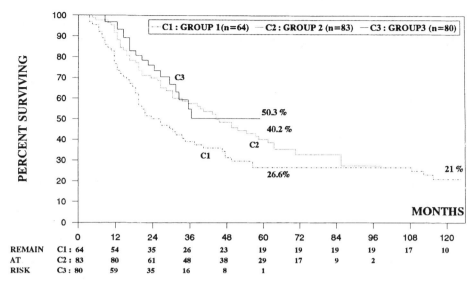

Fig. 1. Overall survival

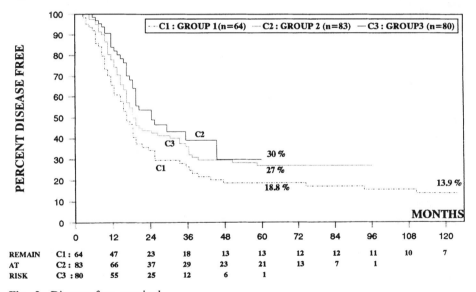

Fig. 2. Disease free survival

The patients included in these 3 studies are superimposable to those reported in other series of inflammatory breast cancer [7-10, 16, 21, 23, 27-33]. All other advanced breast cancers were excluded from this study. A positive skin biopsy was not mandatory as an inclusion criteria since the diagnosis of inflammatory breast cancer can accurately be made by clinical examination only [7, 9, 11, 14, 19, 30]. However for those patients who underwent a skin biopsy at the time of initial diagnosis, no difference in disease free survival or in overall survival could be pointed out when a dermal lymphatic involvement was noted or not.

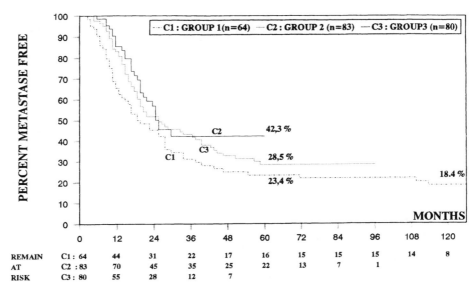

Fig. 3. Metastase free survival

Table 4. Results on disease free and overall survival

	Overall survival			Disease free survival		
	Median	5 years	10 years	Median	5 years	10 years
Overall	39.3 months	39.5 %	24 %	19.3 months	30 %	20 %
Study 1	25 months	26.6 %	21 %	16.7 months	18.8 %	13.9 %
Study 2	45.9 months	40.2 %	NA	19 months	27 %	NA
Study 3	37.9 months	50.3 %	NA	25 months	39.3 %	NA

Legend : NA : Not available

The treatment chosen for the first study is a very classical one and has been applied similarly by other teams worldwide with similar results [3, 25-28, 30]. The use of surgery for loco-regional treatment is more controversial in inflammatory breast cancer. This has however been applied less often by other teams and the results already published compare with ours [1, 6, 8, 12, 16, 21, 23, 25, 29, 30, 32].

Very few teams have introduced intensive induction chemotherapy in the treatment of inflammatory breast cancer as we did in our third study [10, 30]. The therapeutic schedule we choose for this induction chemotherapy had never been reported previously.

The overall response rate observed was better in the third study than in the second one, and better in the second study than in the first one. This is statistically significant. High-dose chemotherapy regimen seems thus to be correlated with better response rate. Although these are not randomized studies, the results seem to point out a strong correlation between intensity of induction chemotherapy and tumor response. This could be an additional evidence of the relationship between dose and efficacy to response rates in breast cancer as stated by Hryniuk et al [15]. Considering the response rate only, more seems to be better. However this higher response rate was obtained at the expense of an increasing toxicity from study I to study II and from study II to study III.

In spite of the better response rate observed in study II and III compared to study I, we did not observe a major dramatic difference in the median disease free survival or overall survival of the patients treated in these 3 studies. A slight advantage was seen for disease free survival only for the patients of the 3rd study compared to the patients of the first study. No plateauing of the curves has been seen. These results are therefore disappointing since they seem to indicate that overall survival and disease free survival are not dramatically affected by the better responses observed with intensive chemotherapy. Considering survival, intensive chemotherapy seems of little clinical value and « more is perhaps not better ».

Similar disappointing results have been reported for chemosensitive solid tumors such as small cell lung cancer [18]. One possible explanation for the disappointing results we observed is that in our 3rd study, estrogenic recruitment could have stimulated a tumoral resistant clone thus debasing the results on overall and disease free survival. However such a conclusion on this hypothesis has not been retained by other teams [6, 31]. We believe that the superiority of intensive induction chemotherapy over classical regimen would be tested in a prospective randomized manner to test the impact of such treatment on overall survival and disease free survival.

References

1. Calderoli H, De Manzini N, Keiling R (1988) Role of chemotherapy in acute breast cancer : analysis of 41 cases. Int Surg 73 : 112-115
2. Camp E (1976) Inflammatory carcinoma of the breast : The case for conservatism. J Surg 131 : 583-586
3. Chauvergne J, Durand M, Dilhuydy MH, Hoerni B, Germain T, Lagarde C (1981) Traitement des cancers du sein inflammatoires : étude contrôlée d'un programme d'association thérapeutique. Rev Fr Gyn Obst 76 : 227-235
4. Chevallier B, Asselain B, Kunlin A, Veyret C, Bastit PH, Graic Y (1987) Inflammatory breast cancer : determination of prognostic factors by univariate and multivariate analysis. Cancer 60 : 897-902
5. Chevallier B, Roche H, Olivier JP, Hurteloup P (1990) Inflammatory breast cancer : intensive chemotherapy (FEC-HD) results in a high histologic complete response rate. Proc ASCO, 9, Abstr : 158
6. Conte PF, Alama A, Bertelli G, Canavese G, Carnino F, Catturich A, Di Marco E, Gardin G, Jacomuzzi A, Monzeglio C, Mossetti C, Nicolin A, Pronzato P, Rosso R (1987) Chemotherapy with estrogenic recruitment and surgery in locally advanced breast cancer : clinical and cytokinetic results. Int J Cancer 40 : 490-494
7. Fastenberg NA, Buzdar AU, Montague ED, Jessup JM, Martin RG, Hortobagyi GN, Blumenschein GR (1985) Management of inflammatory carcinoma of the breast : a combined modality approach. Am J Clin Oncol 8 : 134-141

8. Feldman LD, Hortobagyi GN, Buzdar AU, Ames FC, Blumenschein GR (1986) Pathological assessment of response to induction chemotherapy in breast cancer. Cancer Res 46 : 2578-2581
9. Fields J, Kuske R, Perez C, Fineberg B, Bartlett N (1989) Prognostic factors in inflammatory breast cancer : univariate and multivariate analysis. Cancer 63 : 1225-1232
10. Gissebrecht C, Lepage E, Extra JM, Espie M, Andolenko P, Morvan F, Ganem G, Bourstyn E, Marty M, Boiron M (1989) Cancer du sein : traitement intensif avec autogreffe de moelle osseuse. Bull Cancer 76 : 99-104
11. Haagensen CD (1971) Inflammatory carcinoma. In Disease of the breast. WB Saunders Company. Philadelphia, London, Toronto, 2nd, pp. 576-584
12. Hagelberg RS, Jolly PC, Anderson RP (1984) Role of surgery in the treatment of inflammatory breast carcinoma. Am J Surg 148 : 125-131
13. Hansen R, Quebbeman E, Beatty P, Ritch P, Anderson T, Jenkins D, Frick J, Ausman R (1987) Continuous 5-FU infusion in refractory carcinoma of the breast. Breast Cancer Res Treat 10 : 145-149
14. Hortobagyi GN, Buzdar AU (1986) Progress in inflammatory breast cancer : cause for cautious optimism. J Clin Oncol 4 : 1727-1729
15. Hryniuk WM, Figueredo A, Goodyear M (1987) Application of dose intensity to problems in chemotherapy of breast and colorectal cancer. Sem Oncol 14 : 3-11
16. Israel L, Breau JL, Morere JF (1986) Two years of high-dose Cyclophosphamide and 5-Fluorouracil followed by surgery after 3 months for acute inflammatory breast carcinomas. A phase II study of 25 cases with a median follow-up of 35 months. Cancer 57 : 24-28
17. Kaplan EL, Meier P (1957) Non parametric estimation from incomplete observation. J Am Statis Assist 53 : 457-471
18. Klasa RJ, Murray N, Coldman AJ (1991) Dose intensity meta analysis of chemotherapy regimens in small cell carcinoma of the lung. J Clin Oncol 9 : 499-508
19. Lucas FV, Perez-Mesa C (1978) Inflammatory carcinoma of the breast. Cancer 41 : 1595-1605
20. Malhaire JP, Chevallier B, Barral D, Genot JY, Goudie MJ, Kerbrat P, Gedoin D, Morice MF (1988) Inflammatory breast cancer : Neo-Adjuvant chemotherapy with Vindesin, Adriamycin and Cyclophosphamide. In : C Jacquillat, M Weil, D Khayat (eds) Neo-Adjuvant chemotherapy. Colloque INSERM/John Libbey Eurotext Ltd. 169, pp. 211-214
21. Maloisel F, Dufour D, Bergerat JP, Herbrecht R, Duclos B, Boilletot A, Giron C, Jaeck D, Aennel P, Jung G, Oberling F (1990) Results of initial Doxorubicin, 5-Fluorouracil and Cyclophosphamide combination chemotherapy for inflammatory carcinoma of the breast. Cancer 65 : 851-855
22. Mantel N (1966) Evaluation of survival data and two new rank order statistic arising in its consideration. Cancer Chem Rep 50 : 163-191
23. Mignot L, Espie M, Morvan F, De Roquancourt A, Belpomme D, Gorins A, Marty M (1984) Cancers du sein en poussée évolutive : expérience du Groupe Saint Louis Beaujon, à propos de 71 cas. Gynécologie 35 : 175-180
24. Miller A, Hoogstraten B, Staquet M, Winkler P (1981) Reporting results of cancer treatment. Cancer 47 : 207-214
25. Mourali N, Tabbane F, Muenz LR, Bahi J, Belhassen S, Kamaraju LS, Levine PH (1982) Preliminary results of primary systemic chemotherapy in association with surgery or radiotherapy in rapidly progressing breast cancer. Br J Cancer 45 : 367-374
26. Palangie T, Jouve M, Bretaudeau B, Garcia-Giralt E, Pouillart P (1985) Administration d'un protocole de chimiothérapie première dans le traitement des cancers

du sein. Exemple des cancers inflammatoires. In : J Lemerle (ed) Actualités Carcinologiques. Masson, Paris, pp. 176-191
27. Rouesse J, Friedman S, Mouriesse H, Sarrazin D, Spielmann M (1990) Therapeutic strategies in inflammatory breast carcinoma based on prognostic factors. Breast Cancer Res Treat 16 : 15-22
28. Rouesse J, Friedman S, Mouriesse H, Le Chevalier T, Arriagada R, Spielmann M, Papacharalambous A, May-Levin F (1986) Primary chemotherapy in the treatment of inflammatory breast carcinoma : a study of 230 cases from the Institut Gustave Roussy. J Clin Oncol 4 : 1765-1771
29. Schafer P, Alberto P, Forni M, Obradovic D, Pipard G, Krauer F (1987) Surgery as part of a combined modality approach for inflammatory breast carcinoma. Cancer 59 : 1063-1067
30. Swain SM, Lippman ME (1989) Treatment of patients with inflammatory breast cancer. In : V De Vita, S Hellman, S Rosenberg (eds) Important advances in Oncology. JB Lippincott Company, Philadelphia, pp. 129-150
31. Swain S, Sorace R, Bagley C, Danforth D, Bader J, Wesley M, Steinberg S, Lippman M (1987) Neo-Adjuvant chemotherapy in the combined modality approach of locally advanced non metastatic breast cancer. Cancer Res 47 : 3889-3894
32. Thons WW, McNeese MD, Fletcher GH, Buzdar AU, Singletary E, Oswald MJ (1990) Multimodal treatment for inflammatory breast cancer. Int J Rad Oncol Biol Phys 17 : 739-745
33. Wiseman C, Jessup JM, Smith TL, Hersh E, Bowen J, Blumenschein G (1982) Inflammatory breast cancer treated with surgery, chemotherapy and allogenic tumor cell/BCG immunotherapy. Cancer 49 : 1266-1271

Abstract. 277 patients with unilateral non metastatic inflammatory breast cancer (IBC) have been treated at the Centre H. Becquerel since January 1977 with combined modality approach : Neo-Adjuvant chemotherapy (Mean number of cycles = 4 ; Range : 2-6), followed by a loco-regional treatment (Radiotherapy = XRT or modified radical mastectomy = S), followed by Adjuvant chemotherapy. During this period, the types of chemotherapy and loco-regional treatment have been the following : Study I : 64 patients treated with CMF or AVCF and XRT (Cancer 1987, 60, 897-902) ; Study II : 83 patients, treated with either AVCF, FAC or VAC followed by S (n = 39) or XRT (n = 22) in case of complete or partial response, or followed by XRT (n = 22) in case of initial supraclavicular lymph node involvement or lack of response after chemotherapy ; Study III : 80 patients treated with FEC-HD ± Estrogenic recruitment (Proc. ASCO 1990, 9, 158) followed by S and XRT after Adjuvant chemotherapy (n = 59), or XRT (n = 21) according to the same policy than in study II. Median follow up is 39.5 months (Range : 3-197). Although objective response rates (= 53.1, 73.5 and 88.75 % for study I, II and III respectively) are statistically better in the 3rd study, this does not translate in a dramatical improvement in disease free survival (Median = 16.7, 19 and 25 months respectively for study I, II and III) or 5 year overall survival (26,6 %, 40,2 % and 50,3 % respectively for study I, II and III). Advantage on disease free survival or overall survival from intensive chemotherapy for IBC remains thus to be proven with appropriate randomized trials.

A Phase II study of 2-weekly high-dose Epirubicin with r-met-hu G-CSF in advanced breast cancer

G Fountzilas, D Skarlos, T Giannakakis, A Athanasiades,
D Bafaloukos, J Protopsaltis, M Beer, N Pavlidis, P Kosmidis

Precis

Forty-one patients with advanced breast cancer were treated with high-dose epirubicin every 2 weeks with r-met-hu G-CSF. This intensified regimen was highly active and well tolerated.

Introduction

Epiadriamycin (EPI) is one of the most active drugs in the treatment of advanced breast cancer and is probably less toxic than its parent compound. There are experimental [1] as well as clinical data [2] suggesting that anthracyclines have a steep dose-response curve and that small increases of the drug dose may be critical in order to obtain the maximal cytocidal effect.

Our group has tested in a phase II study the efficacy of high-dose (110 mg/m^2) EPI monotherapy in advanced breast cancer. However, the administration of high drug dose was accompanied often by serious myelotoxicity [3]. Thus, in a sequential phase II study we administered the same dose of EPI with prophylactic use of r-met-hu G-CSF. The actually administered average dose per unit time per patient amounted to 99.6 % of the dose prescribed by the protocol and the morbidity was mininal. Following that study we attempted to further intensify the EPI dose by delivering the same dose as in the previous studies but every 2 weeks instead of every 4 weeks with r-met-hu G-CSF support. In this report we present our preliminary results in using this intensified regimen in advanced breast cancer.

Patients and methods

From December '91 until October '92, 39 patients with distant metastases and 2 with locally advanced breast cancer were entered in this phase II study, conducted by the Hellenic Co-operative Oncology Group. Eligibility criteria included the presence of measurable or evaluable disease, a life expectancy of longer than 2 months, absence of active heart disease or infection, evidence of adequate bone marrow, renal and hepatic function and an informed con-

---

AHEPA Hospital, Aristote University, Thessaloniki, Macedonia, « Agii Anargiri » Cancer Hospital, Athens, « METAXA » Cancer Hospital, Piraeous, University of loannina, loannina, all in Greece

sent according to our Institutional policies. Patients who received mitoxantrone as adjuvant treatment were eligible providing that the relapse-free interval from the completion of adjuvant chemotherapy to recurrence was longer than 1 year. All patients were required to have a normal left ventricular ejection fraction and to have stopped any previous hormonotherapy or adjuvant chemotherapy for the 4 weeks preceding their entry in the study. Pretreatment evaluation included a complete medical history, clinical examination, EKG, CBC, complete biochemistry, chest X-ray, bone scan and CT as indicated. Median age of these 41 patients was 59 (range, 32-78) years and median performance status 0 (range, 0-3) of WHO scale. Median relapse-free interval from the date of surgery to tumor recurrence was 3 (range, 0-10) years. Previous treatment included Tamoxifen (21 patients), CMF chemotherapy [12], mitoxantrone-containing chemotherapy [6] and radiation [13]. Site distribution was as follows: local (in 10 patients), nodes [20], skin [3], bone [22], lung [13], liver [16] and CNS [2].

Tumor response was assessed after the completion of treatment using the WHO criteria. EPI was to be given at the clinic at a dose of 110 mg/m^2 as a short infusion. Treatment with r-met-hu G-CSF was started 24 hours after chemotherapy and was continued for 13 days. Each cycle was repeated every 14 days. Antiemetic therapy included either ondansetron or metochlopramide.

Results

Thirty-five patients completed all 6 cycles of chemotherapy, whereas 6 patients stopped treatment because either they refused to continue [3] or demonstrated tumor progression [3]. The actually administered mean dose per week per patient was 54 mg/m^2, amouting to 97.4 % of the dose prescribed by the protocol. The median average interval between treatment cycles was 14.3 (range, 13.7-48.5) days. Tumor response is evaluable to date in 37 patients. Of these, 7 demonstrated a complete response (CR), 16 a partial response (PR), while 10 had stable disease and 4 progressed during treatment.

The mean nadir WBC was $5.9 \times 10^9/l$ (range, 0.2-30) on day 14, and neutrophils 2.8/l (range, 0-6.1) on day 15 (Table 1). Seventeen patients had hematologic toxicity. Nausea/vomiting was noticed in 21 cases despite the use of ondansentron. Other toxicities are presented in Table 2.

Table 1. Hematologic toxicity

	Nadir values		
	median	range	day
Hemoglobin	10.5	7.4-14	36
WBC	5.9	0.2-30	14
Neutrophils	2.8	0.0-6.1	15
Platelets	188	53-330	31

Table 2. Non-hematologic toxicity

	Grade			
	1	2	3	4
Stomatitis	8 %	5 %		
Alopecia	5 %	19 %	60 %	
Nausea/Vomiting	31 %	19 %		
Infection	3 %		3 %	
Neurologic	5 %			
Fever	8 %			
Cardiac				3 %
Bone Pain	15 %			
Fatigue/Malaise	10 %			

WHO criteria

Discussion

The dose effect in conventional chemotherapy of breast cancer still remains a controversial issue. There are several published randomized studies which addressed the question whether higher than conventional doses of antracyclines have a significant impact on prolongation of survival of patients with advanced breast cancer [4-7]. Survival benefit was reported only in two of them [4, 7]. However, dose intensification of anthracyclines is usually accompanied by serious side effects, such as stomatitis and myelotoxicity. In our first phase II study with high-dose EPI every 3 weeks the median treatment interval per patient was 26 days and the median drug dose actually received per patient was 79 % of the protocol dose. With the concomitant use of r-met-hu G-CSF we were able in a sequential study to administer 27.4 mg/m^2/week, of EPI amouting to 99.6 of the dose prescribed by the protocol with minimal morbidity. However, even though the quality of life of our patients was improved as compared to the first study, an increase in the response rate was not evident. Only 2/42 (4.5 %) achieved a CR and 14 (33 %) a PR. In the present study we attempted to double dose intensity by reducing the interval between treatments from 4 to 2 weeks. Our preliminary analysis showed that treatment with high-dose EPI every 2 weeks is feasible and resulted in a significant increase of CR rate with manageable morbidity. Whether this increase is due to dose intensification or to patient selection in unclear. Therefore, in order to test the relationship of dose intensity with response rate and survival, our Group has initiated a prospective randomized phase III study, comparing 4-weekly versus 2-weekly high-dose EPI in patients with advanced breast cancer.

References

1. Fountzilas G, Inone S, Ohnuma T (1990) Schedule-dependent interaction of Cytarabine plus Doxorubicin or Cytarabine plus mitoxantrone in acute myelogenic leukemia cells in culture. Leukemia 4 : 321-324

2. Wheeler RH, Ensminger WD, Thrull JH et al (1982) High-dose Doxorubicin : An exploration of the dose-response curve. Cancer Treat Rev 66 : 493-498
3. Fountzilas G, Skarlos D, Pavlidis N et al (1991) High-dose Epirubicin as a single agent in the treatment of patients with advanced breast cancer. A Hellenic Cooperative Oncology Group Study. Tumori 77 : 232-236
4. Carmo-Pereira J, Costa FO, Henriques E et al (1987) A comparison of two doses of Adriamycin in the primary chemotherapy of disseminated breast carcinoma. Br J Cancer 56 : 471-473
5. Hortobagyi GN, Bodney GP, Buzdar AU et al (1987) Evaluation of high-dose versus standard FAC chemotherapy for advanced breast cancer in protected environment units : a prospective randomized study. J Clin Oncol 5 : 354-364
6. French Epirubicin Study Group (1991) A prospective randomized trial comparing Epirubicin monochemotherapy to two Fluorouracil, Cyclophosphamide, and Epirubicin regimens differing in Epirubicin dose in advanced breast cancer patients. J Clin Oncol 9 : 305-312
7. Habeshaw T, Paul J, Jones E et al (1991) Epirubicin at two dose levels with prednisone as treatment for advanced breast cancer : the results of a randomized trial. J Clin Oncol 9 : 295-304

Cyclophosphamide, Novantrone, Fluorouracil (CNF) + G-CSF Neo-Adjuvant chemotherapy in operable breast cancer

V Lorusso, M De Lena, M Brandi, S Longo, F Berardi, A Catino, MG Sapia, G Simone, F Marzullo, A Racanelli, F Schittulli

Chemotherapy as the primary treatment of breast cancer (Neo-Adjuvant chemotherapy) will become a common therapeutic option even in operable disease. In fact, it has been demonstrated that breast conserving surgery in women with small tumors (< 2 cm), can achieve results comparable to radical mastectomy [1, 2], and that in locally advanced disease, optimal results can be obtained by the multidisciplinary approach (chemotherapy, surgery, radiotherapy) [3, 4].

As a result of these previous studies, some authors have suggested that with primary chemotherapy, mastectomy for women with tumors larger than 3 centimeters, can be avoided [5, 6].

Nevertheless, a number of major drawbacks still exist for complete acceptance of Neo-Adjuvant chemotherapy :

1) the necessity to delay the surgical procedure for 2-3 months with consequential negative psychological effects on women ;

2) the reluctance of physicians to treat patients with chemotherapy when it could be spared ;

3) the toxicity often related to the aggressive chemotherapeutic approach.

The hematopoietic growth factors offer the opportunity to reduce hematological toxicity due to chemotherapy [7, 8, 9]. In particular, G-CSF (granulocyte colony stimulating factor) permits either to increase drug dosage or to shorten the interval between cycles (accelerated chemotherapy) [10, 11]. The latter would be particularly useful in Neo-Adjuvant chemotherapy in order to give maximum dose intensity in a short period, thus allowing tumor shrinkage without delaying surgical intervention. The aim of this study was to evaluate the activity and the toxicity of CNF (Cyclophosphamide, Novantrone, Fluorouracil) when administered in full doses plus G-CSF for three cycles with 14 day intervals, to patients with operable breast cancer not eligible for quadrantectomy.

Patients and methods

Since February 1992 26 patients with operable breast cancer (T2 > 3 cm-T3, NO-1b) not eligible for quadrantectomy, have been treated with Cyclophosphamide 600 mg/mq/iv, Novantrone 10 mg/mq/iv, Fluorouracil 600 g/mq/iv (CNF) every 14 days, plus G-CSF 4-5 ug s.c. on days 7 to 12.

Oncology Institute of Bari (Italy)

Eligibility criteria included cytological diagnosis of breast cancer (fine needle aspiration) ; tumor diameter clinically measured > 3 cm with or without axillary nodes (N0-N1b) ; age 18-70 years ; ECOG performance status 0-1 ; absence of pregnancy or distant metastases ; no previous or concomitant neoplasia in other sites ; informed consent.

Response and toxicity evaluation criteria were those suggested by WHO [12]. The plan of the study, after fine needle aspiration and detection by immuno cytochemical assay (ICA) of ER, PgR, Ki 67, P 170, P-53 and Neu, provided for 3 cycles of chemotherapy and subsequent clinical — mammographic reevaluation. If the clinical diameter of the tumor was reduced to less than 3 cm, quadrantectomy plus axillary node dissection (QT) was performed ; whereas a radical mastectomy (Mx) was effected for tumors larger than 3 cm. The post (QT) treatment included radiotherapy on the operated breast (50 Gy on the residual breast plus a boost of 10 Gy on the scar) and 4 cycles of the above chemotherapy at 3 week intervals (without G-CSF) irrespectively of the number of positive axillary nodes. For patients submitted to radical mastectomy an adjuvant chemotherapy with Adriamycin 75 mg/mq for 4 cycles (3 week intervals) was administered. Table 1 shows the main characteristics of 24/26 evaluable patients. Two patients refused to continue chemotherapy and were submitted to Mx just after the first cycle of chemotherapy in other institutions.

Table 1. Patient characteristics

Entered on study		26
Evaluable		24*
Median age (29-70)		46
Menopausal status		
	pre	16
	post	8
Clinical tumor diameter		
cm > 5		5
> 4 < 5		8
> 3 < 4		11
Number of chemotherapy presurgical cycles		
2 cycles		1
3 cycles		21
4 cycles		2

* 2 patients were not evaluable because they refused continuing neo-adjuvant treatment after 1st cycle

Results

Complete (CR) or partial response (PR) > 75 % was observed in 17/24 (71 %) cases and an additional PR > 50 % was obtained 5/24 patients (21 %) ; only 2/24 patients (8 %) showed no response to therapy. In spite of the excellent response to chemotherapy only 16/24 (67 %) patients were submitted to QT. In fact two out of the 8 remaining patients did not respond to chemotherapy,

4 patients (3 with initial tumor diameter > 5 cm) did not reach the threshold diameter of 3 cm in spite of good clinical response, and 2 patients were submitted to Mx instead of QT for geographical impossibility to receive radiotherapy. Table 2 summarizes the results with regard to initial tumor diameter.

Table 2. Results with regard to initial tumor diameter

Tumor diameter in cm	N pts	QT	MX	% QT/tot
>5	5	2	3	43
>4 <5	8	7	1	87.5
>3 <4	11	7	4*	64

* Two patients underwent mastectomy (MX) instead of quadrantectomy (QT) on clinical grounds

Toxicity was very manageable. Mild gastrointestinal side effects were observed with the administration of 16 mg of Ondansetron at the moment of drug delivery. Hematological toxicity was insignificant during Neo-Adjuvant chemotherapy due to the G-CSF support. Nevertheless, three patients showed prolonged leuko-thrombocytopenia during the post surgical treatment when chemotherapy and radiotherapy were administered concurrently. Moderate alopecia (GI-II) was also present in 75 % of patients while G-III alopecia (requiring wig) was observed in only 25 % of cases. It is important to note that the median time to deliver the 3 presurgical cycles was 30 days (range 26-32) and the median time to surgery (period from first cycle to surgery) was 45 days (range 27-58).

Discussion

The « ideal » regimen for Neo-Adjuvant chemotherapy should have : 1) high activity ; 2) time from first cycle to surgery as shortest as possible ; 3) low toxicity. In our opinion the regimen CNF is a reasonable candidate to this setting. In fact its activity is comparable to anthracycline containing regimens with a significantly lower toxicity [13, 14]. In a previous study with CNF (three week intervals) Lemaire et al [15] reported 61 % clinical remission with 50 % breast conservation. In another study with a more intensive regimen including also Vindesin (CNFV) Calais et al [15] achieved only 45.5 % objective remission with 42 % of patients submitted to conservative surgery. Nevertheless, the median tumor diameter which has been reported to be a critical factor in Neo-Adjuvant chemotherapy [6], was 5.2 cm (range 3.1-9.5) in the latter series.

In our study the percentage of breast conserving surgery is actually 67 % which is higher than those previously reported, but lower than the 90 % success rate reported by Bonadonna et al [6]. Nevertheless it is important to emphasize that in the Bonadonna's study only 18 % of patients had tumors larger than 5 cm. In fact, our regimen which is more intensive than other regimens previously used in Neo-Adjuvant chemotherapy, obtained 92 % clinical response ; therefore it is our opinion that a more accurate selection of patients eligible for this treatment could provide better results. Moreover, it is noteworthy that two patients with PR after CT were not submitted to QT only because of geographical reasons for subsequent radiotherapy. If these patients could have been submitted to QT, the percentage of breast conserving surgery in this study would have increased to 75 %.

In conclusion, these preliminary data suggest that CNF + G-CSF every 14 days is a safe and feasible regimen for Neo-Adjuvant chemotherapy. Further sutdies with increased dose intensity are warranted.

References

1. Veronesi U, Saccozzi R, Del Vecchio M et al (1981) Comparing radical mastectomy with quadrantectomy, axillary dissection, and radiotherapy in patients with small cancer of the breast. N Engl J Med 305 : 6-11
2. Fisher B, Bauer M, Margolese R et al (1985) Five-year results of a randomized clinical trial comparing total mastectomy and segmental mastectomy with or without radiation in the treatment of breast cancer. N Engl J Med 312 : 665-673
3. Valagussa P, Zambetti M, Bonadonna G, et al (1990) Prognostic factors in locally advanced non-inflammatory breast cancer. Long-term results following primary chemotherapy. Breast Cancer Res Treat 15 : 137-147
4. Hortobagyi GN, Blumenschein GR, Spanos W, et al (1983) Multimodal treatment of locoregionally advanced breast cancer. Cancer 51 : 763-768
5. Mansi JL, Smith IE, Walsh G, et al (1989) Primary medical therapy for operable breast cancer. Eur J Cancer Clin Oncol 25 : 1623-1627
6. Bonadonna G, Veronesi U, Brambilla C, et al (1990) Primary chemotherapy to avoid mastectomy in tumors with diameters of three centimeters or more. Vol 82, n° 19 : 1539-1545
7. Bronchud MH, Potter MR, Morgenstern G et al Dexter TM (1988) In vitro and in vivo analysis of the effects of recombinant human granulocyte colony-stimulating factor in patients. Br J Cancer 58 : 64-69
8. Morstyn G, Souza LM, Keech J et al (1988) Effect of granulocyte colony-stimulating factor on neutropenia induced by cytotoxic chemotherapy. Lancet i : 667-672
9. Morstyn G, Campbell L, Lieschke G et al (1989) Treatment of chemotherapy — induced neutropenia by subcutaneously administered granulocyte colony-stimulating factor with optimisation of dose and duration of therapy. J Clin Oncol 7 : 1554-1562
10. Bronchud MH, Howell A, Crowther D et al (1989) The use of granulocyte colony-stimulating factor to increase the intensity of treatment with Doxorubicin in patients with advanced breast and ovarian cancer. Br J Cancer 60 : 121-125
11. Berardi F, Tatulli C, Lorusso V et al (1992) Mitoxantrone plus G-CFS as a dose intensive therapy in « Salvage treatment » of advanced breast cancer. Ann Oncol 3 (suppl 5) Abstr 314 : 81
12. World Health Organization (1979) WHO handbook for reporting results of cancer treatment. Geneva : World Health Organization
13. Bennet JM, Muss HB, Doroshow JH et al (1988) A randomized multicenter trial comparing Mitoxantrone, Cyclophosphamide and Fluorouracil with Doxorubicin, Cyclophosphamide and Fluorouracil in the therapy of the metastatic breast carcinoma. J Clin Oncol 6 : 1611-1620

14. Periti P, Pannuti F, Robustelli della Cuna G, et al (1991) Combination chemotherapy with Cyclophosphamide, Fluorouracil and either Epirubicin or Mitoxantrone : A comparative randomized multicenter study in metastatic breast carcinoma. Cancer invest 9(3) : 249-255
15. Lemaire M, Closon M, Desaive C et al (1991) Short term preoperative chemotherapy with CNF in large primary breast tumors : a well tolerated down staging procedure and an in vivo assay of chemotherapy. Proceedings of Third International Congress on Neo-Adjuvant chemotherapy, Paris, abstr B 26 : 16
16. Calais G, Descamps P, Turgeon V, et al (1992) Primary chemotherapy to allow breast conserving treatment for locally advanced breast cancer. Is tumor chemosensitivity a prognostic factor ? Proc ASCO vol 11, abstr 28 : 50

Adjuvant chemohormonal therapy with Cyclophosphamide, Doxorubicin and 5-Fluorouracil (CAF) with or without medroxyprogesterone acetate (MPA) in node-positive breast cancer patients

P Hupperets *, J Wils, L Volovics, L Schouten, M Fickers, H Bron, H Schouten, J Jager, J Smeets, J de Jong, G Blijham

Meta-analysis on adjuvant chemotherapy studies revealed statistical significant benefit for premenopausal and also, although in a lesser extent, for postmenopausal breast cancer patients in terms of both DFS and OS [1]. Adjuvant hormonal treatment with Tamoxifen improves DFS in node+ breast cancer patients, but OS advantage is more difficult to demonstrate and in the meta-analysis OS reaches significance only in patients over 50 years of age. Adjuvant chemohormonal therapy (CMF-type chemotherapy in addition to 1 year of Tamoxifen) have yielded negative results [2-9] although sometimes showing some superiority of the combination in subgroups of patients for DFS [10, 11]. In 1982 we started an adjuvant chemohormonal study using different regimens. A Doxorubicin containing regimen was chosen because of better results of these regimens over CMF based combinations [12] and because of less influence of the number of positive nodes and menopausal status on the efficacy of adjuvant therapy [13]. MPA was chosen because of possible activity in estrogen receptor (ER) negative tumors [14, 15] and because of protective activity against chemotherapy induced bone marrow toxicity [16].

Patients and Methods

Pre and postmenopausal women younger than 71 years with histologically proven infiltrative breast cancer treated with a modified radical mastectomy or lumpectomy with postoperative breast irradiation (50,00 Gy to the total breast with a boost of 14,00 Gy to the operated region) having one or more histopathologically involved ipsilateral axillary lymph nodes were considered for entry in the protocol. Lumpectomy was performed in patients with primary tumors ≤ 3 cm. Patient characteristics are summarized in Table 1. All patients have been treated with Adjuvant chemotherapy. Randomization determined whether patients in addition received MPA or not.

The adjuvant therapy schedule is summarized in Table 2. Follow-up included a history and physical examination, blood counts, liver function tests, ESR, every 3 months, during the first 2 years, every 4 months in the third year, every 6 months in the fourth and the fifth year and every 12 months thereafter. Chest radiographs and mammography were performed every year.

Comprehensive Cancer Center Limburg, Maastricht, * Academic Hospital Maastricht, P.O. Box 5800, 6202 AZ Maastricht, The Netherlands

Table 1. Patient characteristics

	Treatment (CAF)			
	MPA−	(209)	MPA+	(199)
Characteristic	No	(%)	No	(%)
age premenopausal	113	(54 %)	123	(62 %)
postmenopausal	96	(46 %)	76	(38 %)
Weight (kg ⩾ 74 kg)	44	(21 %)	50	(25 %)
ER pos. (⩾ 10 fmol/mg prot.)	148	(71 %)	131	(66 %)
Tumor stage (AJCC classification)				
I	31	(15 %)	26	(13 %)
II A + B	144	(69 %)	147	(74 %)
IIIA	33	(16 %)	28	(14 %)
T1 (TNM class.)	54	(26 %)	64	(32 %)
T2	136	(65 %)	115	(58 %)
T3	19	(9 %)	20	(10 %)
Number of axillary nodes				
1-4	134	(65 %)	135	(68 %)
5-9	54	(26 %)	46	(23 %)
⩾ 10	19	(9 %)	18	(9 %)
% died from malignancy	56	(27 %)	48	(24 %)
other causes	21	(1 %)	20	(1 %)
% relapsed				
loco-regional*	23	(11 %)	22	(12 %)
metastatic	65	(31 %)	44	(22 %)
loco-regional + metastatic	12	(6 %)	10	(5 %)
chemotherapy dose reduction (0 %-10 %)	25	(12 %)	14	(7 %)

* Chest wall relapse after mastectomy or mammary relapse after lumpectomy and/or ipsilateral axillary lymph node metastases or ipsilateral supraclavicular lymph node metastases

Table 2. CAF-MPA regimen

C : Cyclophosphamide	500mg/m² i.v. day 1
A : Adriamycin (Doxorubicin)	40 mg/m² i.v. 1 hr infusion day 1
F : 5-Fluorouracil	500 mg/m² i.v. day 1 q 4 wks
MPA : medroxyprogesterone acetate day 1 through 28	
500 mg daily i.m.	
twice a week 500 mg i.m. for 5 months	
WBC <3.10⁹/1 and/or platelets ⩽ 100.10⁹/1 : 1 week postponement	

Results

There is a difference in DFS in favor of the MPA+ arm as far as all recurrences are concerned, 59 % v.s. 49 % at 5 years, but the difference is not statistically significant, p-value is 0.12 (RR of occurrence of all recurrences,

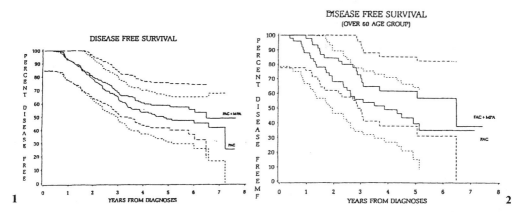

Fig. 1. Disease free survival (DFS) curves for both treatment arms for all types of relapses (locoregional, distant metastases and both types simultaneously) (p = 0.12). Dotted lines represent 95 % simultaneous confidence bounds.

Fig. 2. Disease free survival (DFS) curves for both treatment arms for all types of relapses in patients ⩾ 60 and ⩽ 70 years. Difference in favor of the FAC + MPA treatment arm (p = 0.06). Dotted lines represent 95 % simultaneous confidence bounds.

MPA+ v.s. MPA−, is 0.79 ; 95 % CI is 0.59-1.07) (Fig. 1). If the comparison is carried out in the subgroup of patients ⩾ 60 and ⩽ 70 years the two curves show a difference of 62 % v.s. 41 % at 5 years in favor of MPA+ arm (RR 0.57 ; 95 CI is 0.32-1.03) with a p-value of 0.06 (Fig. 2). This difference is even more marked for the occurrence of distant metastases in this age group (p = 0.02). No differences in DFS can be found within subgroups according to tumor size, steroid receptor value or number of positive nodes.

There is currently no significant OS benefit for the MPA+ arm. An estimate of RR (MPA+ v.s. MPA−) for cancer related death is 0.88. A 95 % CI is 0.60-1.30. There is a survival advantage for the MPA+ arm in elderly patients, statistically most significant in patients ⩾ 55 and ⩽ 70 years (p = 0.002) and pT1 patients (p = 0.045).

Toxicity of the treatment

In the MPA+ treatment group 18 (9 %) patients have discontinued MPA treatment. Six cycles of chemotherapy are administered to all patients. MPA related toxicity has been assessed by comparing CAF + MPA in CAF. The major side effects are shown in Table 3.

Discussion

Although no survival or disease-free survival difference for all treated patients is observed, the current trial has demonstrated a therapeutic benefit of MPA

Table 3. Major side effects occurring during treatment with each regimen (%)

Side Effect	CAF 209 No	(%)	CAF + MPA 199 No	(%)	p-value
Infiltrate in injected muscle			11	(6 %)	
Vomiting (gr. III, IV)	97	(46 %)	57	(28) %	< 0.001
Nausea (gr. III, IV)	106	(51 %)	68	(34 %)	< 0.001
Leucocyte nadir (III, IV)	42	(20 %)	22	(11 %)	= 0.003
Leucocyte count at 4 wks after treatment (II, III)	23	(11 %)	16	(8 %)	N.S.
Granulocytes nadir (III, IV)	38	(18 %)	40	(20 %	N.S.
Granulocytes at 4 wks (II, III)	25	(12 %)	18	(9 %)	N.S.
Platelets nadir (I, II)	2	(1 %)	2	(1 %)	
Platelets at 4 wks (I)	2	(1 %)	2	(1 %)	
Vaginal bleeding	0	(0 %)	30	(15 %)	
Weight gain (kg)	1.8		5.5		= 0.01

added to CAF in terms of OS in elderly patients. Only one trial studied a similar question and showed MPA adding efficacy to CMF treatment in patients over 50 years [17]. Combinations of Tamoxifen and chemotherapy, using 1 year of Tamoxifen showed negative results, whereas meta-analysis of trials with 2 years of treatment has shown a reduction in odds of recurrence with 7 % for patients < 50 years and 28 % for patients ⩾ 50 years of age. Direct comparisons between Tamoxifen and MPA in adjuvant treatment are not available but may be worthwhile to perform. The loco-regional failure rate in our study is 11-12 % after a m.f.u. of 42 months which is comparable to that reported in the literature [4, 7]. MPA does not appear to effect the occurrence of loco-regional relapse. The addition of Tamoxifen for 5 [7] or 1 year [4] did not improve loco-regional control over chemotherapy alone in both studies.

The beneficial effect of MPA in elderly patients can in part be explained by higher ER levels in this patient group. However, in our study ER content did not predict for MPA efficacy, and MPA was given over a short period of time that may be unfavorable to obtain a meaningful adjuvant effect through an endocrine mechanism. Another beneficial effect of MPA in this trial is bone marrow protection in particular amelioration of the leucocyte nadir. However, this did not lead to dose intensification and therefore is not the explanation for the difference in efficacy. In conclusion, this trial suggests a beneficial effect of MPA combined with chemotherapy on the occurrence of distant metastases in stage II breast cancer patients. Currently the trial does not show an OS advantage but the present trend in favor of the MPA + group may become significant after a longer follow-up period.

References

1. Anonymous (1992) Systemic treatment of early breast cancer by hormonal, cytotoxic or immune therapy. Early Breast Cancer Trialists' Collaborative Group. The Lancet 339 : 71-84
2. Hubay CA, Gordon NH, Crowe JP et al (1984) Antiestrogen-cytotoxic chemotherapy and bacillus Calmette-Guerin vaccination in stage II breast cancer : seventy-two months follow-up. Surgery 96 : 61-72
3. Mauriac L, Durand M, Chauvergne J et al (1988) Adjuvant trial for stage II receptor-positive breast cancer : CMF v.s. CMF plus Tamoxifen in a single center. Breast Cancer Research and Treatment 11 : 179-186
4. Ingle JN, Eversson LK, Wieland HS et al (1988) Randomized trial of observation versus adjuvant therapy with Cyclophosphamide, Fluorouracil, prednisone with or without Tamoxifen following mastectomy in postmenopausal women with node-positive breast cancer. J Clin Oncol 6 : 1388-1396
5. Ingle JN, Eversson LK, Wieland HS et al (1989) Randomized trial to evaluate the addition of Tamoxifen to Cyclophosphamide, 5-Fluorouracil, prednison adjuvant therapy in premenopausal women with node-positive breast cancer. Cancer 63 : 1257-1264
6. Taylor SG, Knuiman NW, Sleeper LA et al (1989) Six-year results of the Eastern Cooperative Oncology Group Trial of observation versus CMFP versus CMFPT in postmenopausal patients with node positive breast cancer. J Clin Oncol 7 : 879-889
7. Tormey DC, Gray R, Gilchrist K et al (1990) Adjuvant chemohormonal therapy with Cyclophosphamide, Methotrexate, 5-Fluorouracil and prednisone (CMFP) or CMFP plus Tamoxifen compared with CMF for premenopausal breast cancer patients. Cancer 65 : 200-206
8. Boccardo F, Rubagotti A, Bruzzi P et al (1990) Chemotherapy versus Tamoxifen versus chemotherapy plus Tamoxifen in node-positive, estrogen receptor-positive breast cancer patients : results of a multicentric Italian Study. J Clin Oncol 8 (8) : 1310-1320
9. Henderson IC (1990) Editorial. J Clin Oncol 8 : 1297-1300
10. Carbone PP (1990) Breast cancer adjuvant therapy. Cancer 66 : 1378-1386
11. Fisher B, Constantino J, Redmond C et al (1989) A randomized clinical trial evaluating Tamoxifen in the treatment of patients with node-negative breast cancer who have estrogen receptor-positive tumors. N Engl J Med 320 : 479-484
12. Bull JM (1978) A randomized compared trial of Adriamycin versus Methotrexate in combination drug therapy. Cancer 41 : 1649-1657
13. Buzdar AU (1978) Intensive postoperative chemo-immunotherapy for patients with stage II and III breast cancer. Cancer 41 : 1064-1075
14. Gundersen S, Kvinnsland S, Klepp O et al (1992) Chemotherapy with or without high-dose medroxyprogesterone acetate in oestrogen-receptor-negative advanced breast cancer. Eur J Cancer 28 : 390-394
15. Van Veelen H, Willemse P, Tjabbes T et al (1986) Oral high-dose medroxyprogesterone acetate versus Tamoxifen. Cancer 58 : 7-13
16. Gercovich FG (1981) Three consecutive multidisciplinary trials in advanced breast cancer. ASCO abstr 431
17. Focan C, Beauduin M, Salomon E et al (1990) Influence of age, node involvement and CMF chemotherapy on the outcome of early breast cancer treated with high dose medroxyprogesterone acetate (HD-MPA) as adjuvant hormonotherapy : 5-years results of a randomized trial. In : Salmon SE (ed) Adjuvant Therapy of Cander IV. WB Saunders Company, Philadelphia, pp. 319-329

Follow-up results of an ECOG study of adjuvant therapy in post-menopausal women with breast cancer

HC Falkson, R Gray, WH Wolberg, G Falkson

In 1982 the Eastern Cooperative Oncology Group started a prospectively controlled, randomized trial in postmenopausal women with operable node positive breast cancer. The aim of the study was to compare the adjuvant efficacy of 4 cycles versus 12 cycles of chemotherapy as well as to evaluate the effect of long-versus short-term Tamoxifen. This is the first study directly evaluating the importance of Tamoxifen duration in an adjuvant setting. In addition to investigating duration of adjuvant treatment, the study was also designed to investigate the impact of pretreatment patient characteristics, namely the number of involved nodes and the hormone receptor status of the tumor, on disease-free interval and disease recurrence.

Patients were randomized to one of 3 treatment arms : 4 cycles of Cyclophosphamide, Methotrexate, 5-Fluorouracil, Prednisone and Tamoxifen (CMFPT) or 12 cycles of CMFPT or 12 cycles of CMFPT plus continuous Tamoxifen for 5 years. In 1986 the study was modified to allow patients on CMFPT x 12 + continuous Tamoxifen to be rerandomized after completing 5 years of Tamoxifen to a second step, namely to continue with Tamoxifen for life or to stop therapy. Dosages and schedules were : Cyclophosphamide 100 mg/m^2 p.o. days 1-14 of each cycle as a single daily dose, Methotrexate 40 mg/m^2 i.v. day 1 and 8 of each cycle, 5-Fluorouracil 600 mg/m^2 i.v. day 1 and 8 of each cycle, Prednisone 40 mg/m^2 po days 1-14 of each cycle as a single daily dose and Tamoxifen 10 mg p.o. b.i.d. daily, continuously for the total duration of treatment. Patients were stratified for number of involved nodes and ER status.

A total of 962 women were entered on this prospectively controlled randomized trial. Appropriate informed consent was obtained from all patients. An eligibility review was performed prospectively by the study chairmen when each patient entered the study. Pathology review was done of the primary tumor as well as of the involved axillary lymph nodes. The median age of the women was 60 (27-80 years). There were 803 patients eligible with follow-up data. Patients were considered ineligible for the following reasons (some patients had more than one reason) : 5 women were premenopausal, 35 had tumors > 5 cm, 16 had skin or muscle infiltration and/or fixation, 13 had dermal lymphatic invasion, 3 had involved regional nodes other than the ipsilateral axillary nodes, 3 had metastatic disease, one patient had bilateral breast cancer, 4 had surgical procedures that were not within the protocol guidelines, in 5 the initial biopsy was done more than 4 weeks prior to the mastectomy, 7 were entered on study much later than the protocol requisite of 6 weeks, 4 had node-negative breast cancer, one had noninvasive breast cancer, in

---

University of Pretoria, South Africa, Dana-Farber Cancer Institute, Boston, MA 02115 and Wisconsin Clinical Cancer Center, Madison, WI 53792

8 pretreatment blood counts or chemistries were abnormal or not done, 10 had abnormal bone scans or chest X-rays, 2 had had prior treatment for breast cancer, 4 had previous or concomitant malignancies, 21 had diabetes mellitus and 24 had other concomitant diseases including heart disease, peptic ulcers, clotting problems, kidney disease and psychiatric disorders. Thirteen patients were excluded because they never started on therapy. There were 10 patients entered from an institution where there was some question of possibly fraudulent data submission in an FDA audit; by agreement with the NCI we are not using data from this institution for any purpose. Of the 803 analyzable patients 393 patients had 1-3 positive nodes and 410 had > 3 positive nodes. A value of equal or more than 10 fm/mg cytosol protein was considered ER positive, values less than 10 fm/mg were considered negative for this trial. Five hundred and sixty one patients had ER positive tumors and 242 had ER negative tumors.

We published preliminary results of this study in the Journal of Clinical Oncology [1]. Longer term results at a median follow-up of 6.8 years are now available.

Toxicity, during and after induction, was not statistically different in the 3 arms. Most commonly encountered side effects were hematologic, nausea and vomiting, and alopecia. Life-threatening toxicity occurred in 75 and lethal toxicity in 7 patients. Toxicities recorded in patients randomized on step 2 are not different for those on observation versus those on Tamoxifen for life. It has not been necessary to stop Tamoxifen in those randomized to long-term Tamoxifen. At this stage no increase in the incidence of uterine cancer has been seen.

Time to relapse is significantly longer for patients on CMFPT x 12 + continuous Tamoxifen than for CMFPT x 4 (p 0.002), the difference between CMFPT x 12 + continuous Tamoxifen and CMFPT x 12 is nearly significant (p 0.06). Differences between 4 or 12 cycles of CMFPT are not significant. Relapse free rates at 5 years are 66 % for CMFPT x 12 + continuous Tamoxifen; 58 % on CMFPT × 12 and 56 % on CMFPT x 4. Treatment differences in overall survival are not significant, the 5-year survival rate is 71 % for CMFPT x 12 + continuous Tamoxifen; 73 % for CMFPT x 12 and 72 % for CMFPT x 4. Since 16.5 % of randomized patients were excluded because of ineligibilities it was necessary to determine if the exclusions could have biased the comparisons in any way. Relapse free survival and overall survival curves are essentially the same for all randomized patients as those for eligible patients.

Hormone receptor status and number of involved nodes were significant prognostic parameters. Patients with ER-negative tumors and patients with > 3 positive axillary nodes had a significantly shorter time to treatment failure, the same correlation was found for survival.

Conclusion

(1) Neither the time to treatment failure, nor the survival, was significantly different for 4 or 12 cycles of CMFPT.

(2) Disease-free survival was significantly better with long-term Tamoxifen. However, this impact of long-term Tamoxifen was only seen on disease-free survival, treatment differences in overall survival was not different.

(3) Despite the improved disease free survival the life threatening and lethal toxicities that were associated with CMFPT are disturbing.

(4) Hormone receptor status and number of involved nodes remain important prognostic indicators both for disease free survival and overall survival.

This study was conducted by the Eastern Cooperative Oncology Group (Doug C Tormey, Chairman, CA 21115).

Reference

1. Falkson HC, Gray R, Wolberg WH, Gillchrist KW, Harris JE, Tormey DC, Falkson G (1990) Adjuvant trial of 12 cycles of CMFPT followed by observation or continuous Tamoxifen versus 4 cycles of CMFPT in postmenopausal women with breast cancer : An ECOG phase III study. J Clin Oncol 8 : 599-607

Long-term efficacy and late sequelae of Doxorubicin-containing adjuvant therapy for breast cancer : MD Anderson Cancer Center studies

A Buzdar, G Hortobagyi, S Kau, F Holmes, G Fraschini, R Theriault, M McNeese, S Singletary

Since 1974 at MD Anderson Cancer Center, Doxorubicin-containing regimens have been evaluated as adjuvant therapy in patients with node-positive breast cancer. In our initial studies, all patients had either stage II or III disease and were treated with adjuvant therapy following local therapy. The earlier results of these studies have been previously published [1-4]. The objective of this report is to present the long-term follow-up data on survival and late sequelae of the treatment.

Patients and methods

In four studies between 1974 and 1986, 1107 patients with stage II or III breast cancer were treated with adjuvant Fluorouracil, Doxorubicin, and Cyclophosphamide (FAC) with or without biological therapies. Details of the systemic therapies have been previously reported [1-4]. Briefly, in the first study (N = 222), after mastectomy and postoperative radiation therapy, patients received FAC plus non-specific immunotherapy with BCG at 4-week intervals ; after 300 mg/m² of Doxorubicin, patients were crossed over to maintenance therapy ; Methotrexate was substituted for Doxorubicin, and treatment was continued for a total of 2 years. In the second study (N = 238), all patients were randomly assigned to receive for non-specific immunotherapy with or without BCG in addition to FAC ; in the latter part of the study, patients who had not been irradiated prior to referral were also randomized to receive postoperative radiation therapy or not. The interval between the FAC cycles was reduced to 3 weeks. The duration of chemotherapy in this study was also 2 years. In the third study (N = 336), Vincristine and Prednisone were added to the FAC regimen. Total cumulative Doxorubicin dose was increased to 400 mg/m², except that patients with ⩽ 3 positive nodes received 300 mg/m². After completion of FAC chemotherapy, patients whose estrogen receptor status was positive or unknown were randomized to receive either Tamoxifen alone for 6 months or Tamoxifen with Methotrexate and Vinblastine administered sequentially. Total duration of therapy was 1 year. Estrogen receptor-negative patients received Methotrexate and Vinblastine sequentially. In the fourth study (N = 311), all patients received escalating doses of Doxorubicin and Cyclosphosphamide, and Doxorubicin was administered as a continous infusion

---

Department of Breast and Gynecologic Medical Oncology, The University of Texas, MD Anderson Cancer Center, 1515 Holcombe Blvd., Box 56, Houston, TX 77030, USA

over 72 hours through a central venous catheter. Total cumulative dose of Doxorubicin was increased to 430 mg/m^2, while total duration of chemotherapy was shortened to 18-21 weeks. All patients with estrogen receptor-positive or - unknown tumors also concomitantly received Tamoxifen for 1 year. After completion of chemotherapy, patients were randomized to receive biological therapy with partially purified leukocyte α-Interferon for 1 year or no further therapy.

Results of these studies were compared with those of a historical control group from our institution that consisted of 186 consecutive patients who received mastectomy plus postoperative radiation therapy but no adjuvant chemotherapy. This control group was compared with control patients in randomized trials at other institutions and was found to have similar overall and disease-free survival rates in comparable subgroups of patients [5]. Disease-free survival and overall survival curves were plotted by the methods of Kaplan-Meier, differences between groups were calculated based on the generalized Wilcoxon test, and two-tailed P values were utilized. Estimated reductions in mortality were based on the ratio of relative death rates in relevant FAC and control groups. Toxicities and incidence of second malignancies were tabulated by treatment for each study. The data were updated for each study through September 1992.

Results

At this time of analysis, the median follow-up periods for the four studies were 183 months for the first study, 155 for the second, 123 for the third, and 88 for the fourth. The estimated 5 and 10 year survival rates by stage and nodal status are shown in Table 1.

Table 1. Estimated 5- and 10-year survival rates in FAC studies

| | % 5-yr survival | | | | % 10-yr survival | | | | |
| | Study | | | | Study | | | | |
Subgroup	1	2	3	4	1	2	3	4*	P
Stage II	74	73	83	79	62	55	68	—	0.17
1-3 nodes	81	79	87	84	75	66	73	—	0.64
4-10 nodes	73	75	84	78	57	55	70	—	0.43
> 10 nodes	60	58	62	63	42	37	40	—	0.99
Stage III	54	58	59	64	37	34	47	—	0.41

* Ten year data not yet available

There were no significant differences in 5- and 10-year estimated disease-free or overall survival rates between comparable subgroups of patients in the four studies.

Table 2 shows overall reduction in mortality from adjuvant chemotherapy (all FAC studies combined) at 10 years compared with the historical control group.

Table 2. Estimated reduction in mortality at 10 years in FAC group compared with historical control group

Subgroup	% reduction in mortality
Total patients	44
Stage II	46
1-3 nodes	55
4-10 nodes	42
> 10 nodes	29
Age	
< 50 yr	61
≥ 50 yr	31
Stage III	34

The FAC regimen was effective in reducing the risk of death in each subgroup, but the most marked effect was observed in patients younger than 50 years and patients with fewer than four positive nodes.

In the control group, five (2.7 %) patients had congestive heart failure, whereas in the FAC group, eight (0.7 %) patients had congestive heart failure. In patients who received Doxorubicin by continuous infusion, the risk of congestive heart failure was lower than in patients who received Doxorubicin in a bolus doses. The 2 patients who received Doxorubicin by continuous infusion and had congestive heart failure both had pre-existing symptomatic cardiovascular disease prior to initiation of therapy.

The 10-year estimated incidence of second malignancies was 8.6 % (SE ± 2.8 %) in the control group and 6.5 % (± 1.1 %) in the FAC patients. The risk of second malignancy was therefore lower in the FAC patient population than in the control patients. The 10-year estimated risk of developing leukemia was 0.8 % (± 0.6 %) in the FAC group, 1.2 % (± 0.8 %) in the control group, and 2.1 % (± 0.8 %) in the FAC plus irradiation group. Although the estimated risk of developing leukemia was higher in the FAC plus irradiation group then in the control group and FAC alone group, the differences were not statistically significant (P = 0.08).

Discussion

Adjuvant FAC therapy has been established to reduce the risk of recurrence and improve survival in breast cancer patients following local therapy [1-4]. Long-term data in these studies illustrate that Doxorubicin-containing regimens are effective in reducing the risk of death in patients with stage II and III disease. A large number of patients with stage III disease and stage II disease with ≥ 10 positive nodes were treated in these studies, and more than > 37 % were alive beyond 10 years.

The data on late sequelae illustrate that Doxorubicin can be safely administered and that administering the drug by continuous infusion reduces the risk of cardiac dysfunction. The overall incidence of second malignancy was lower in the FAC patient population than in the historical control group, although slightly increased risk of leukemia was observed in the patients treated with chemotherapy and radiation therapy. However, the number of patients is too small to draw any definitive conclusions about leukemia risk. Continued observation is needed to define further the therapeutic benefit and late sequelae of these treatments.

References

1. Buzdar AU, Blumenschein GR, Gutterman JU et al (1979) Postoperative adjuvant chemotherapy with Fluorouracil, Doxorubicin, Cyclophosphamide, and BCG vaccine : A follow-up report. JAMA 242 : 1509-1513
2. Buzdar AU, Blumenschein GR, Smith TL et al (1984) Adjuvant chemotherapy with Fluorouracil, Doxorubicin, and Cyclophosphamide (FAC) with or without bacillus Calmette-Guerin and with or without irradiation inoperable breast cancer : A prospective randomized trial. Cancer 53 : 384-389
3. Buzdar AU, Hortobagyi GN, Smith TL et al (1988) Adjuvant therapy of breast cancer with or without additional treatment with alternate drugs. Cancer 62 : 2098-2104
4. Buzdar AU, Hortobagyi GN, Kau SW et al (1992) Adjuvant therapy with escalating doses of Doxorubicin and Cyclophosphamide with or without leukocyte α-Interferon for stage II or III breast cancer. J Clin Oncol 10 : 1540-1546
5. Moon TE, Jones SE, Bonadonna G et al (1987) Development and use of a natural history data base (NHBD) of breast cancer studies. Am J Clin Oncol 10 : 396-403

Taxol in metastatic breast cancer : the MD Anderson Cancer Center experience

FA Holmes, V Valero, R Walters, R Theriault, D Booser, A Buzdar, H Gibbs, D Frye, K Young, G Hortobagyi

We have performed three studies with taxol in metastatic breast cancer : a phase II trial in patients who had received only one prior chemotherapy regimen [1], an ongoing phase I trial of taxol with a fixed dose of Doxorubicin [2, 3], and an ongoing phase II trial in patients with either two or three or more chemotherapy regimens.

Phase II trial in patients with one prior regimen of chemotherapy (adjuvant or palliative)

Eligibility criteria were standard including measurable or evaluable disease and written informed consent. Pretreatment evaluations included standard laboratory evaluation, an electrocardiogram, and X-rays of chest, abdomen, and bones. Taxol was given over 24 hours at 250 mg/m^2 (200 mg/m^2 for patients who had experienced excessive myelosuppression with prior chemotherapy or prior irradiation to marrow-bearing bones) without hematopoietic growth factors. All patients received standard premedication with oral Dexamethasone 20 mg at 14 and 7 hours before taxol and intravenous Diphenhydramine 50 mg and Cimetidine 300 mg 1 hour before taxol. Taxol was given in hospital with routine monitoring of the vital signs every 4 hours but no cardiac monitoring. Treatments were repeated every 21 days if all toxic effects had resolved. The planned duration of treatment was for 6 months after maximum response or no change. Evaluations between treatments were : a complete blood count (CBC) with differential and platelet counts once or twice weekly, and liver and renal function tests before each subsequent treatment. Disease sites were evaluated after every 2 treatments until response was documented, then after every 3 to 4 treatments to confirm continued response. Standard criteria were used to determine response [4] ; all responses were confirmed by at least three reviewers. National Cancer Institute common toxicity criteria were utilized to grade toxic effects [5].

Twenty-five patients were enrolled and evaluable (Table 1). Six patients were Doxorubicin-resistant. Doxorubicin resistance was defined as relapse during palliative treatment for metastatic disease with a Doxorubicin-containing regimen either after an initial response or without any evidence of initial response, or relapse within 6 months of completing a Doxorubicin-based adjuvant treatment.

Results are shown in Table 2 ; 297 treatments were given, a median of 13

Department of Breast and Gynecologic Medical Oncology, UTMD Anderson Cancer Center-56, 1515 Holcombe Blvd, Houston, TX 77030, USA

per patient (range, 2-21). The median dose was 200 mg/m² (range, 130-250). Objective remissions were seen in 56 % of patients (12 % complete) ; 32 % had minor responses. Only 2 patients had no benefit from taxol. The median duration of response was 9 months (range, 3-19 months). The durations of response in the complete responders were 5, 15, and 19 months. The median overall survival, updated January 1993, was 24 months (range, 5-34+ months) ; 8 patients are alive.

Hematologic toxic effects consisted of grade 4 granulocytopenia with rare thrombocytopenia or anemia. The median lowest recorded granulocyte count for the first 3 treatments was 100-200/mm³ and occurred between days 7-16.

Nonhematologic toxic effects were mild and not dose-limiting with the exception of the unique side effects seen with taxol. Myalgias/arthralgias simulating the prodrome of influenza occurred 3-6 days after treatment in most patients and were relieved by mild analgesics except in 4 patients in whom they were dose-limiting. Acute neurotoxic effects, manifested as a tingling in the feet and fingertips within 24 hours of the taxol infusion, occurred and often merged into the myalgia syndrome. The chronic neurotoxic effect was a cumulative glove-and-stocking neuropathy associated with painful paresthesias, some diminution of fine motor skills, and loss of the deep tendon reflexes. These symptoms reversed or stabilized after doses were reduced. Although all patients experienced grade 4 granulocytopenia, only 6 % of all treatments were complicated by infection or fever. All patients experienced alopecia ; no anaphylactoid reactions were seen. Two other side effects were notable, although mild : 60 % of patients experienced diarrhea 24-48 hours after taxol that was easily controlled with oral antimotility agents. Second, 60 % of patients developed an erythroderma on the face (especially malar areas), anterior neck and chest in the sun-exposed areas 24 hours after Dexamethasone ; this is not related to taxol, but rather a known complication of high-dose steroids, and resolved spontaneously. Cardiac toxic effects were seen in only 4 patients. In 2 patients, the relationship to taxol was unclear. In 2 other patients, asymptomatic sinus bradycardia was observed.

Phase I trial of taxol with Doxorubicin as initial chemotherapy for metastases

We concluded taxol is active in metastatic breast cancer, and combination studies with Doxorubicin and Cyclophosphamide were indicated. The next study was a phase I trial of taxol with fixed doses of Doxorubicin as the initial chemotherapy for metastases. Eligibility criteria included normal cardiac ejection fraction, no underlying dysrhythmias as documented by a 24-hours Holter monitor, < 300 mg/m² Doxorubicin previously by rapid injection or < 400 mg/m² by 48 hours infusion as adjuvant therapy, and no evidence of Doxorubicin resistance.

Taxol was given over 24 hours followed by Doxorubicin over 48 hours with cardiac monitoring by telemetry and 72-hour Holter. Granulocyte colony stimulating factor (G-CSF, Amgen) 5 mcg/kg was given subcutaneously days

5-19. Treatments were repeated every 21 days. The planned schedule of doses (mg/m^2) was : Doxorubicin 60 with escalating doses of taxol 125, 150, 180, 210. The maximum tolerated dose (MTD) was defined as one dose level below the dose at which 3 to 6 patients who were started at that level developed grade 3 non-hematologic toxic effects or granulocytes < 500/mm^3 with fever or infection or granulocytes < 250/mm^3 for more than 5 days.

As of January 1993, 102 treatments were given. Only 10 patients (Table 1) were required to determine the MTD. Infection with or without stomatitis occurred in 3 patients at the initial dose level, so reduced dose-levels of taxol/Doxorubicin (mg/m^2) were created : 125/48, 100/48, 100/40, 90/36. The MTD (mg/m^2) in this schedule for taxol/doxorubicin was 125/48. Doses were reduced in 22 % of treatments because of stomatitis, fever, thrombocytopenia or a combination.

Table 1. Characteristics of patients treated on taxol trials at MD Anderson Cancer Center

Characteristic	1 prior CT	Tax-->Dox	Dox-->Tax	⩾3 prior CT
Number entered	25	10	21	21
Med. age, yrs	51	48	47	52
range	34-70	36-62	32-66	39-75
Med. Zubrod PS[1]	1	1	0	1
range	0-2	0-2	0-2	0-2
Med. disease-free,	18	20	18	25
mo, range	0-94	0-72	0-96	0-107
Prior Doxorubicin	23	3	5	25
Doxorubicin resistant	6	0	0	11
Dominant disease site				
soft tissue	6	1	0	3
bone	4	1	0	0
viscera	15	8	21	18
Med. no. sites	2	2	2	4
range	1-10	1-9	1-6	1-8

[1]Zubrod PS, Zubrod performance status ; CT, chemotherapy ; Med., median ; mo, months

Hematologic toxic effects included a median of grades 4, 3, and 1 granulocytopenia during treatments 1, 2, and 3, respectively, despite G-CSF. The median lowest recorded platelet counts (x 10^3/mm^3) in treatments 1, 2, 3, and 6 were 127, 88, 53, and 54 which occurred on days 8-15. Non-hematologic effects included grade 2 or 3 stomatitis in all patients (60 % of treatments), infection or fever in 80 % of patients (16 % of treatments), and total alopecia in all patients. No patient had an anaphylactoid reaction ; one patient had asymptomatic ventricular dysrhythmias during treatment 8 that never recurred during 6 additional treatments.

Objective responses were seen in 8 patients (95 % CI = 48-98 %) ; one was a complete remission. The median duration of response was 4 months (range, 3-13). The median duration of survival was 14 months (range, 8-17+). Four patients have died ; all patients had progressive disease.

We concluded : this combination was active, but complete remissions were rare and the durations of response were short. A phase I trial at the National Cancer Institute, using a 72-hours infusion schedule of both drugs, reported similar response rates and achieved doses that were 15-25 % higher [6]. We hypothesized a schedule-dependent interaction and repeated this trial but reversed the sequence of drug administration.

As of January 1993, 21 patients have received 187 treatments. Patients' characteristics are shown in Table 1. The MTD (mg/m^2) is Doxorubicin 60 with taxol 150 and was defined by infection and stomatitis. The toxic effects are similar with severe granulocytopenia seen initially despite G-CSF and progressive thrombocytopenia that diminishes as doses are reduced. The study continues with 11 patients receiving treatment. Of 18 evaluable patients, 50 % have objective remissions of which 6 % are complete (95 % CI = 26-74).

We concluded : higher doses can be given in the reverse schedule, but there is no increase in the response rate. A pharmacokinetic study of each sequence is ongoing.

Phase II trial in patients with multiple prior chemotherapy regimens

This trial is an ongoing phase II evaluation of taxol in patients with either 3 or more prior chemotherapy regimens or only 2 prior regimens. Patients are not eligible if more than 25 % of their bone marrow has been irradiated. The standard premedication precedes taxol 150 mg/m^2 given over 24 hours (135 mg/m^2 for patients with prior Mitomycin-C or irradiation). No G-CSF is used. Treatments are repeated every 21 days.

As of January 1993, 21 patients with 3 or more prior chemotherapy treatments have received 78 treatments ; 5 patients with 2 prior chemotherapy treatments have received 15 treatments. Patients' characteristics are shown in Table 1 ; preliminary responses, in Table 2. The median time to progress is 2+ months (range, 1-5+). Treatment of patients with only 2 prior chemotherapy regimens has just begun, but 4 of 5 treated patients show early evidence of response.

Table 2. Response rates in patients treated on taxol trials at MD Anderson Cancer Center

Response %	1 prior CT (N = 25)	Tax-->Dox (N = 10)	Dox-->Tax* (N = 18 eval)	≥3 prior CT* (N = 18 eval)
Complete (CR)	12	10	6	0
Patrial (PR)	44	70	44	33
Minor	32	10	44	11
No change	4	10	6	28
Progress	8	0	0	28
95 % CI for CR + PR	35-76	48-98	26-74	13-59

*studies are ongoing. Responses reported as of January 1993. eval, evaluable

We conclude that taxol is active in patients with metastatic breast cancer regardless of the extent of prior therapy. Although evidence is limited, there does not appear to be complete cross-resistance to Doxorubicin. Combination with Doxorubicin has not improved response rates nor increased the number of complete remissions. A schedule-dependent interaction may occur with doxorubicin and taxol when administered sequentially. Future studies will clarify this. Issues to be addressed in other studies : Is there a dose-response curve ? Is G-CSF necessary ? What is the best schedule of administration ? Is combination with Doxorubicin superior to dose-intense single agent therapy ? Are other drugs more suitable for combinations ?

References

1. Holmes FA, Walters RS, Theriault RL et al (1991) Phase II trial of taxol, an active drug in the treatment of metastatic breast cancer. J Natl Cancer Inst 83 : 1797-1805
2. Holmes FA, Frye D, Valero V et al (1992) Phase I study of taxol and Doxorubicin with G-CSF in patients without prior chemotherapy for metastatic breast cancer (Abstr 66). Proc Am Soc Clin Oncol 11 : 60
3. Holmes FA, Valero V, Walters RS et al (1992) The MD Anderson Cancer Center experience with taxol in metastatic breast cancer. Proceedings of the Second National Cancer Institute Workshop on Taxol and the Taxanes, Arlington, VA, September 23-24, 1992
4. Hayward JL, Rubens RD, Carbone PP et al (1977) Assessment of response to therapy in advanced breast cancer. Br J Cancer 35 : 292-298
5. Ajani JA, Welch SR, Raber MN et al (1990) Comprehensive criteria for assessing therapy-induced toxicity. Cancer Invest 8 : 147-159
6. Fisherman J, McCabe M, Hillig M et al (1992) Phase I study of taxol and Doxorubicin with G-CSF in previously untreated metastatic breast cancer (Abstr 54). Proc Am Soc Clin Oncol 11 : 57

Taxol plus recombinant human granulocyte colony stimulating factor as salvage chemotherapy for metastatic breast cancer

AD Seidman*, BS Reichman*, J PA Crown*, T-J Yao***, V Currie*, TB Hakes*, CA Hudis*, TA Gilewski*, P Forsythe**, J Lepore*, L Marks****, M Souhrada****, N Onetto****, S Arbuck*****, L Norton*

Clinical trial results in refractory ovarian carcinoma, and more recently in other human malignancies, have led taxol to be referred to as the most promising new chemotherapeutic agent of the decade. Distinct from other antimicrotubular agents, taxol's promotion of tubulin dimerization and stabilization against depolymerization is unique [1-3]. This cellular effect appears to result in growth inhibition and cell death.

Significant activity for taxol as initial chemotherapy in the treatment of metastatic breast cancer has been observed, with response proportions of approximately 60 % [4, 5]. The remarkable activity of taxol as first chemotherapy for metastatic breast cancer motivated the present study of the agent as salvage therapy in patients with refractory advanced disease who had received multiple prior chemotherapy regimens. Preliminary *in vitro* and *in vivo* studies have indicated the possibility of significant mdr-1 mediated cross-resistance between anthracyclines and taxol [6-8]. As all of the patients receiving taxol in this trial had prior anthracycline exposure, prospective identification of each patient's prior sensitivity to these agents was made for subsequent correlation with response to taxol. We here summarize the findings of this trial, with the caveat that response and toxicity assessment is still ongoing in 16 patients still actively receiving taxol on study.

Patients and methods

To be eligible, patients must have had received a minimum of 2 prior chemotherapy regimens for metastatic disease, including prior Anthracycline or anthracene-dione, either as adjuvant to surgery, for advanced disease, or in both settings. There were no restrictions on the extent or nature of prior

---

* Breast and Gynecological Cancer Medicine Service, Division of Solid Tumor Oncology, Department of Medicine, Memorial Sloan-Kettering Cancer Center, New York, New York 10021
** Department of Neurology, Memorial Sloan-Kettering Cancer Center, New York, New York 10021
*** Department of Biostatistics, Memorial Sloan-Kettering Cancer Center, New York, New York 10021
**** Bristol-Myers Squibb, Pharmaceutical Research Institute, Wallingford, Connecticut 06492-7660
***** National Cancer Institute, Medicine Branch, Bethesda, Maryland
Supported in part by NCI grants CA-09207-14 and 1-CM07311

hormonal therapy, on the cumulative anthracycline dose received, or on prior high-dose chemotherapy with hematopoietic support. Patients were allowed to have received radiation to no more than 30 % of marrow-bearing bone. Bi-dimensionally measurable disease was required ; radiographically measurable lytic bone lesions were acceptable in conjunction with radionuclide scans. Other inclusion criteria included : total white blood cell count > 3000 cells/mm^3, absolute granulocyte count (AGC) $\geqslant$ 1500 cells/mm^3, hemoglobin $\geqslant$ 8 gm/dL, platelet count $\geqslant$ 100,000 cells/mm^3, Serum creatinine $\leqslant$ 1.4 mg/dL, total bilirubin < 1.5 mg/dL, Serum calcium $\leqslant$ 10.5 mg/dL, Karnofsky performance status $\geqslant$ 60 %, and an anticipated survival of $\geqslant$ 12 weeks. Unstable or untreated central nervous system disease, carcinomatous meningitis, symptomatic lymphangitic pulmonary involvement, or history of serious cardiac arrhythmia were criteria for exclusion.

The starting dose of taxol was 200 mg/m^2 administered as a continuous 24 hours intravenous infusion every 21 days. To shorten the duration of neutropenia, the anticipated dose-limiting toxicity, recombinant human granulocyte colony stimulating factor (rhG-CSF ; Neupogen^{TM}, Amgen) was given at 5 μg/kg/day subcutaneously on days 3-10. To prevent hypersensitivity reactions, patients were premedicated with Dexamethasone, Cimetidine, and Diphenhydramine hydrochloride. Dose modification was planned based on toxicity encountered.

Fifty-one evaluable patients who had received a median of 3 (range 2-6) prior chemotherapy regimens for metastatic disease entered this trial between February and April 1992. Their characteristics indicate a significant tumor burden and extensive prior therapy (Table 1). All but 3 patients received Doxorubicin for stage IV disease ; of these 3 patients who received Mitoxantrone-based regimens for metastatic disease, 2 had previously received Doxorubicin-based adjuvant therapy.

Table 1. Demographic and clinical characteristics of all patients

Characteristics	Patients (n = 51)
Karnofsky performance status	
(median, range)	70 (60-90)
Age (years)	
(median, range)	47 (26-73)
Sites of metastases (%)	
Lymph node	43
Cutaneous/soft tissue	47
Lung	45
Liver	33
Bone	47
Multiple organ-system sites	86
Prior stage IV chemotherapy regimens	
(median, range)	3 (2-6)
Prior high dose chemotherapy (%)	14
Prior radiotherapy - Stg. IV disease (%)	67

Results

The median number of courses administered per patient was 6 (range 1-14); 16 patients remain on study. Objective partial responses were observed in 13 of 51 evaluable patients (25.5 %; 95 % C.I.: 14-37 %). Responses were observed in all sites of metastatic disease. Of note, responses were as likely in patients with prior Anthracycline-resistant disease as in those with Anthracycline sensitive-disease (Table 2). The median number days/cycle with AGC < 500 cells/mm^3 was 4. Febrile neutropenia resulting in hospitalization occurred in 24 of 312 cycles (8 %) in 9 of 51 patients (18 %). Twenty-four patients (47 %) required dose reductions: 11 to 180 mg/m^2, 11 to 150 mg/m^2, and 2 to 125 mg/m^2. Non-hematologic toxicity included generalized alopecia in all patients and, in most, mild myalgias, arthralgias, and peripheral neuropathy (> grade 2 in < 10 % of patients); no patients discontinued taxol secondary to neurotoxicity. Significant hypersensitivity reactions or cardiac toxicities were not observed.

Table 2. Response by prior anthracycline/anthracenedione (A/A) sensitivity*

	Responses/evaluable pts.	Response proportion (95 % confidence intvl)
A/A Refractory	5/22	22.7 % (5-40)
A/A Sensitive	6/27	22.2 % (7-38)
A/A Stable	2/2	

* Resistant = recurrent disease <12 months after completing anthracycline-containing adjuvant chemotherapy, or lack of intervening response to anthracycline in the setting of advanced disease. Sensitive = recurrent disease > 12 months after completing anthracycline-containing adjuvant chemotherapy, or history of an intervening response while receiving anthracycline for advanced disease.

Conclusions

Taxol is active as a single agent regimen when given as salvage therapy for patients with metastatic breast cancer, including those with Anthracycline-refractory disease. Adverse effects were tolerable in the majority of patients treated at this dose and schedule. With rhG-CSF administration, neutropenia was brief in these heavily pretreated patients. At least partial non-cross resistance is observed with respect to prior Anthracycline exposure; further investigation into potential non-mdr-1 mediated mechanisms of taxol resistance is warranted.

References

1. Schiff PB, Fant J, Horwitz SB (1979) Promotion of microtubule assembly in vitro by taxol. Nature 277 : 665-667
2. Manfredi JJ, Parness J, Horwitz SB (1982) Taxol binds to cellular microtubules. J Cell Biol 94 : 688-696
3. Kuman N (1981) Taxol-induced polymerization of purified tubulin. Mechanism of action. J Biol Chem 256 : 10435-10441
4. Holmes FA, Walters RS, Theriault RL et al (1991) Phase II trial of Taxol, an active drug in the treatment of metastatic breast cancer. J Natl Cancer Instit 83 : 1797-1805
5. Reichman BS, Seidman AD, Crown JPA et al (1993) Taxol and recombinant human granulocyte colony stimulating factor as initial chemotherapy for metastatic breast cancer. J Clin Oncol (in press)
6. Roy SN, Horwitz SB (1985) A phosphoglycoprotein associated with taxol resistance in J 774.2 cells. Cancer Res 45 : 3856-3863
7. Gupta RS (1985) Cross-resistance of Vinblastine — and taxol-resistant mutants of chinese hamster ovary cells to other anti-cancer drugs. Cancer Treat Rep 69 : 515-521
8. Wilson WH, Kang YK, Bryant G et al (1992) Phase I/II study of 96 hour infusional taxol in refractory lymphomas and breat cancer. Proc 2nd Natl Cancer Instit Workshop on Taxol and taxus, Alexandria, VA

Head and neck

A model for chemosentivity testing using in vitro MTT assay on a human squamous carcinoma tongue cell line

WK Walter King, PK Lam, KC Arthur Li

In recent years much work has focused on the development of an *in vitro* method for predicting the clinical chemosensitivity of human tumors accurately [1-5]. Because of its simplicity, accuracy, reproductivity, the MTT assay developed by Mosmann [4] has been extensively ultilized for chemosensitivity testing of human tumor cell lines [6-8]. We have recently established and characterized a human cell line PWH-SI derived from squamous carcinoma of tongue of a Chinese patient. This study was undertaken to evaluate the chemosensitivity of PWH-SI cell line to single and combination cytotoxic drugs using the MTT assay.

Materials and methods

The squamous carcinoma cell line, PWH-SI, established in our laboratory was derived from the metastatic lymph node of a forty-one years old Chinese female with squamous carninoma of tongue. The cell line was maintained in DMEM (Gibco), supplemented with 10 % FBS (Gibco) and cultured in a humidified incubactor at 37 °C with an atmosphere containaing 5 % CO_2 in air. Cell counts were performed using a haemocytometer and the concentration was adjusted to 7×10^5/ml. The doubling time of PWH-SI cell line during exponential growth was 28 hours.

MTT test was performed with $3-(4,5\text{-Dimethylthiazol-2-yl})-2,5$ Diphenyltetrazolium bromide (MTT) and DMSO, both from Sigma. 5-Fu and Cisplatin were provided by Roche and Nippon Kayaku, respectively. Adriamycin and Epirubicin were from Farmitalia. Carboplatin was from Bristol-Myers. Stock cytotoxic drugs were prepared in appropriate solvents to a concentration of 100 µg/ml for Cisplatin, Adriamycin and Epirubicin, 1 µg/ml for Carboplatin and 10 g/ml for 5-FU and stored at -20 °C.

The cytotoxic effects of different drug concentrations were assessed by the MTT test after 48 hours of exposure in 96-well incubating plates according to the method of Mosmann [4]. The growth inhibition rate was calculated as (1-O.D. test sample/O.D. control) $\times$ 100 %. In the experiment with combination drugs, the concentration of one drug was fixed at a concentration of ID_{30} (the drug concentration giving 30 % growth inhibition).

Department of Surgery, Prince of Wales Hospital, The Chinese University of Hong Kong, Hong Kong

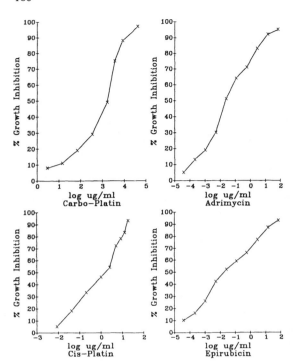

Fig. 1. The growth inhibition curves of Cisplatin, Carboplatin, Adriamycin and Epirubicin

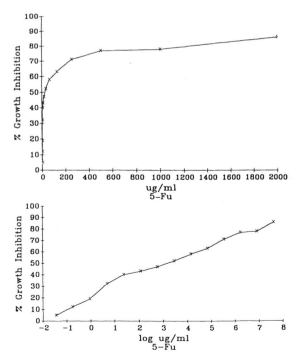

Fig. 2. The growth inhibition curve of 5-FU. An obvious resistent fraction was observed

Results

The squamous carcinoma cell line PWH-SI was sensitive to all of the cytotoxic single agents screened with their respective ID_{50} as follows: Cisplatin (1.26 µg/ml), Carboplatin (25.7 µg/ml), Adriamycin (0.2 µg/ml), Epirubicin (0.2 µ/ml) and 5-FU (30.8 µg/ml). There was no significant difference (p < 0.005) in the growth inhibitory effect of Adriamycin and Epirubicin as the growth inhibition curves overlapped each other (Fig. 1). To achieve equal levels of growth inhibition, the required dose of Carboplatin (ID_{50} 25.7 µg/ml) was approximately 20 times of that of Cisplatin (ID_{50} 1.26 µg/ml) (Fig. 1). There was an obvious resistance fraction in the 5-FU growth inhibition curve (Fig. 2).

In the experiment with combination cytotoxic drugs with the concentration of Carboplatin and Cisplatin fixed at their ID_{30} values, 12.5 µg/ml and 0.44 µg/ml respectively, only a mild additive inhibition effect with 5-FU was observed (Table 1). The additive index A.I., which is defined in this experiment as a ratio of the observed cytotoxicity of combination drugs to the calculated additive cytotoxicity of individual drugs, of Carboplatin and Cisplatin ranged from 0.69 – 0.81 and 0.73 – 0.86, respectively. However, either platin compounds plus Adriamycin demonstrated a stronger growth inhibition on PWH-SI cell line as reflected by a higher A.I. which approached 1.0 (Table 2). The difference in A.I. between either platin compounds plus 5-FU versus either platin compounds plus Adriamycin was statistically significant using Kruskal-Wallis test (P = 0.003).

Table 1. Growth inhibition by platin compounds and 5-FU expressed as Additive Index (A.I.)

Adriamycin dosage µg/ml	Adriamycin + Cisplatin* A.I.	Adriamycin + Carboplatin** A.I.
0.012	0.94	1.17
0.025	0.95	0.9
0.05	1.02	1.0
0.1	1.06	1.03
0.2	0.90	0.91
0.4	0.85	0.85
0.8	0.94	0.92

* Cisplatin dosage fixed at ID_{30} (0.44 µg/ml) ** Carboplatin dosage fixed at ID_{20} (12.5 µg/ml)

Additive Index $AI = \dfrac{a + b}{A + B}$, where a + b = observed % inhibition of combined drugs

A + B = The sum of % inhibition of single drug

Table 2. Growth inhibition by platin compounds and Adriamycin expressed as Additive Index (A.I.)

5-FU dosage µg/ml	5-FU + Cisplatin* A.I.	5-FU + Carboplatin** A.I.
0.23	0.86	0.80
0.46	0.79	0.71
0.925	0.94	0.69
1.85	0.79	0.71
3.95	0.81	0.66
7.80	0.82	0.71
15.60	0.84	0.75
31.25	0.82	0.74
62.50	0.85	0.80
125	0.84	0.81
250	0.78	0.75
500	0.74	0.72
1 000	0.78	0.73
2 000	0.73	0.71

* Cisplatin dosage fixed at ID_{30} (0.44 µg/ml), ** Carboplatin dosage fixed at ID_{30} (12.5 µg/ml)

Additive Index $AI = \dfrac{a + b}{A + B}$, where $a + b$ = Observed % Inhibition of combined drugs

$A + B$ = The sum of % inhibition of single drug

Discussion

In this study PWH-SI cell line was found to be sensitive to the cytotoxic effects of Cisplatin, Carboplatin, Adriamycin, Epirubicin and 5-FU at the concentrations tested. Schwachoffer [9] also studied the chemosensitivity of a human squamous carcinoma cell line of tongue, HN-1, grown as multi-cellular spheroids. He reported that Carboplatin was required at a concentration approximately 16 times that of Cisplatin in order to produce isoeffect levels of growth delay in spheroids. Similarly, our MTT assay on PWH-SI showed that the ID_{50} of Carboplatin was about 20 times that of Cisplatin. Because of reduced neurotoxicity and nephrotoxicity [10], Carboplatin, a second-generation platin analogue has been increasingly used as an alternative to Cisplatin [11]. Previous pharmacokinetic study has shown that high-dose Carboplatin is attainable in refractory cancer patients to achieve optimal responses although it is less cytotoxic than Cisplatin in terms of ID_{50} [12].

Unlike 5-FU, Adriamycin demonstrated a stronger additive effect in combination with either platin compounds. Adriamycin combined with especially Carboplatin produced significant additive effect against PWH-SI cell line.

Therefore, in this *in vitro* chemosensitivity screening model, Carboplatin combined with Adriamycin appeared to be a more effective chemotherapeutic regimen than the conventional combination therapy with Cisplatin and 5-FU [13]. This model for chemosentivity screening can be further developed to provide rapid screening of head and neck tumors so that effective cytotoxic agents may be used to improve the clinical results of chemotherapy.

References

1. Twentyman PR, Walk GA, Wright KA (1984) The response of tumor cells to radiation and cytotoxic drugs. A comparison of clonogenic and isotope uptake assays. Br J Cancer 50 : 625-631
2. Von Hoff DD, Forseth B, Warfel LE (1985) Use of a radiometric systme to screen for antineoplastic agents : Correlation with a human tumor cloning system. Cancer Res 45 : 4032-4038
3. Peng ZL, Perras JP, Sevin BV (1987) ATP-bioluminescence assay for evaluation of tumor chemosensitivity. Proc Am Assoc Cancer Res 28 : 427, abst 1694
4. Mosemann T (1983) Rapid colorimetic assay for cellular growth and survival : Application of proliferation and cytotoxicity assays. J Immunol Methods 65 : 55-63
5. Rotman B, Teplitz C, Dickinson K (1987) An in vitro chemosensitivity study of 128 individual human tumors. Proc Am Assoc Cancer Res 28 : 424, abst 1682
6. Wilson JK, Sargent JM, Elgie AW, Hill JG, Taylor CG (1990) A feasibility study of the MTT assay for chemosensitivity testing in ovarian malignancy. Br J Cancer 62 : 289-194
7. Chun Ming Tsai, Adi F Gazdar, Reury-Perng Perng, Barnetts Kramer (1991) Schedule-dependent in vitro combination effects of Methotrexate and 5-Fluorouracil in human tumor cell lines. Int J Cancer 47 : 401-407
8. Meijer C, Mulder NH, Hospers GAP, Vges DRA, De Vries EGE (1990) The role of glutathione in resistence to Cisplatin in a human small cell lung cancer cell line. Br J Cancer 62 : 72-77
9. Schwachoffer JHM, Crooijmans RPMA, Hoogenhout J, Kal HB, Theeuwes AGM (1990) Effectiveness of Cisplatin and Carboplatin in the Chemotherapy of Squamous Cell Carcinoma Grown as Multicellular Spheroids. Anticancer Research 10 : 805-812
10. Lelieveld P, Vijgh WJF van der, Veldhuizen RW, Velzen D van, Putten LM van, Atassi G, Danguy A (1984) Preclinical studies on toxicity, and antitumor activity and pharmacokinetics of cisplatin and three recentlydeveloped deriviatives. Eur J Cancer Clin Oncol 20 : 1087-1104
11. Harrap KR (1985) Preclinical studies identifying Carboplatin as a viable Cisplatin alternative. Cancer Treat Rev 12 : 21-33 (suppl A)
12. Eisenberg M van, Echo D, Aisener J (1989) Carboplatin : the experience in head and neck cancer. Sem Oncol 16 (suppl 5) : 34-41
13. Decker DA, Drelichman A, Jacobs J et al (1983) Adjuvant chemotherapy with Cis-diamminedichloroplatinum II and 120 hour 5-Fluorouracil in stage III and IV squamous cell carcinoma of the head and neck. Cancer 51 : 1353-1355

Abstract. *The chemosensitivity of a new cell line (PWH-SI) derived from a Chinese patient with squamous cell carcinoma of tongue was studied by an* in vitro *colorimetric MTT Assay. Adriamycin and Epirubicin were found to have an equivalent ID_{50} (i.e. the dose required to reduce cell survival by 50 %) of 0.20 g/ml. Carboplatin (ID_{50} of 25.7 µg/ml) was required at a concentration approximately 20 times more than that of Cisplatin (ID_{50} of 1.26 µg/ml). An obvious resistent fraction existed in the 5-Fluorouracil (5-FU) inhibition curve. Adriamycin combined with Cisplatin or Carboplatin showed more inhibitory effect against PWH-SI cell line than Cisplatin of Carboplatin combined with 5-FU. This model for chemosensitivity screening of single or combination cytotoxic agents holds promise for further development for clinical application.*

Head and neck cancer treatment: present status and future direction

M Al-Sarraf

The primary treatment for patients with localized squamous cell carcinoma of the head and neck has been surgery and/or radiotherapy. The results of therapy will depend on the clinical stage, and resectability of the disease.

Radiotherapy (RT) is used primarily in the treatment of patients with early stages (I and II) with excellent local control, and five year survival. If the cancer recur locally or regionally, these patients usually are evaluated for possible salvage surgery. Radiation therapy is also being used for patients with inoperable and/or unresectable stage III or IV tumor. Patients with persistent but resectable nodal disease may have surgery performed. The local control achieved with RT in these patients is up to 50 %, but the five year survival is less than 10 %, with the majority of the patients recurred or have persistent disease and are dead within 18 months.

Surgery is usually employed in patients with resectable stages III and IV cancer as the primary treatment. Most of these patients usually will receive adjuvant post-operative radiotherapy especially those with stage IV, nodal involvement, or patients with positive surgical margin(s). The overall results in these patients are poor, more than 60 % will recur loco-regionally in spite of the complete removal of all of the disease and the adjuvant RT. About 20 % of the patients will develop distant metastasis, and 70 % are dead within five years. Not all the remaining living patients (30 %) at five year, are free of disease.

Patients with M1 disease, those with loco-regional recurrence after and beyond definitive treatments, and in patients with persistent cancer, palliative systemic chemotherapy are usually given.

With the introduction of more active agents and combinations of chemotherapy like cisplatin combination, and better and safer combinations like Cisplatin and 5-Fluorouracil (5-FU) infusion, this led to the investigation of chemotherapy as part of combined modality therapy (CMT) in patients with stages III and IV cancer. In addressing the present status and future direction of the treatment of patients with head and neck cancer, we will concentrate primarily on the role of chemotherapy as part of the initial planned treatment of patients with locally advanced cancer.

Before discussing the possible role of chemotherapy as part of CMT, it is important to mention the prognostic factors and the timing of chemotherapy that may influence the results obtained.

Many prognostic factors will influence the survival of patients with locally advanced head and neck cancers that are treated with CMT. The most important of these factors are: performance status, site, resectability, margins of the resection, and stage of the disease. The most important part of the stage

---

Division of Hematology and Oncology, Wayne State University, Detroit, Michigan 48201, USA

is the degree and level of nodal involvement. Many of these factors will influence the response to chemotherapy when it is given prior to definitive treatments. Stage of the disease, and especially the nodal stage, again the most important factor. These factors will not only influence the overall response (complete + partial) to chemotherapy, but also the clinical and histological complete response (CR) to these agents. Many chemotherapy factors will influence the overall and complete response rates. These include single agent v.s. combination, type of chemotherapy, number of courses given, and the intensity of chemotherapy.

Timing and sequence of chemotherapy as part of the CMT, especially in patients with resectable stage III and IV cancer, is important factor that will influence the results of treatments. In the beginning, combination CT was investigated before (induction, Neo-Adjuvant, proto) definitive treatments, to study its effectiveness and possible side effects. At the present time the following timing of chemotherapies are being investigated :
1. Induction chemotherapy.
2. « Sandwich : chemotherapy (after surgery and before RT).
3. Adjuvant chemotherapy (post definitive treatments).
4. Concurrent chemo-radiotherapy :
   a. As total treatment,
   b. Post-operative,
   c. Pre-operative.
5. Combination of the above.

From the natural history of this disease, the majority of the failure are loco-regional, in spite of the definitive treatments or surgery and radiotherapy and the incidence of complete clearance post these treatments. It is important, as part of our strategy, to decrease the incidence of loco-regional failure and to prolong the incidence of local disease free progression. At the same time we should not neglect the possible 20 % incidence of distant metastasis that will influence the overall results of therapy in these patients. Based on these strategies it is most likely that we may need combination chemotherapy to be given alone and concomitantly with RT.

Induction chemotherapy

As mentioned above, with the introduction of Cisplatin combination in mid 1970s, many phase II trials were activated by local institutions and cooperative groups. The only purpose of these studies, were to investigate chemotherapy effectiveness (response rate), incidence of CR, chemotherapy induced toxicities, and other side effects associated with surgery and/or RT. In performing these trials, the factor that influenced overall and complete response rates to these chemotherapy were observed and reported. Some of these factors related to the chemotherapy type, courses and intensity. Many of these pilots, compared survival to matched historical control, and the majority reported a survival advantage in favor of the administration of chemotherapy. This led to activation of many randomized trials to test the efficacy of induction chemotherapy as part of combined modality treatment. In patients with resectable disease, two of these studies are well performed that deserve the discussion.

The first of these randomized trial is the NCI-Head and Neck Cancer Contract. Patients with stages III and IV were randomized to 1) Surgery (S) and post-operative RT, 2) one course of Cisplatin and Bleomycin, followed by S and RT, and 3) one course of Cisplatin alone. At the time of activation of this protocol the design and dose and courses of chemotherapy were considered the best of its time (1978). One course of Cisplatin and Bleomycin produced about 50 % overall response rate, and less than 5 % CR. As expected, this amount and possible type of chemotherapy did not change the survival of these patients as compared to standard treatments.

The second randomized protocol is the Southwest Oncology Group, in which patients randomized S + RT ± induction chemotherapy. Three courses of Cisplatin, Oncovin, Methotrexate, and Bleomycin were administered on an outpatients schedule. The study was negative in spite of overall response rate of 70 %, and CR of approximately 25 %. Although the incidence of distant metastasis was less for the patients treated with chemotherapy, it is our strong feeling that in resectable patients induction chemotherapy may not change the loco-regional control above what the surgeon will remove all the disease regardless of the response to these chemotherapy. This is one reason that leads us to study timing of chemotherapy as part of CMT. Table 1 summarized the results and achievements that were obtained and reported with the use of induction chemotherapy. To continue to refine and improve on the safety and results of chemotherapy we will continue to give chemotherapy before definitive treatments. By doing so we were able to introduce Cisplatin and 5-FU infusion as possible the best combination so far, and is widely used in patients with head and neck cancers and other malignant tumors.

Table 1. What was achieved with induction chemotherapy

1. High overall response rate (80 %-90 %).
2. High CR rate (up to 50 %).
3. High histological CR (up to 25 %).
4. Good response → good prognosis.
5. Higher CR with less nodal involvement.
6. Less distant metastasis.
7. Laryngeal preservation (with radiotherapy).

Concurrent chemo-radiotherapy

Since the late 1960s efforts are underway to combine chemotherapy, single and combination, with RT to improve on the results obtained with RT alone. Initially, single agents Methotrexate, Hydrea, 5-FU, or Bleomycin were administered during radiation treatment. These agents may produce mucositis of the oro-pharynx and the oral cavity, that lead to poor compliance and delay or termination of the chemotherapy or RT. Cisplatin is one of the best active single agent in patients with squamous cell carcinoma of the head and neck, does not produce mucositis, and is one of the better radio-potentiator and sensitizer. Presently, in patients with good renal function, Cisplatin alone or with other agent (especially 5-FU) are used commonly with radiotherapy.

Many randomized studies have been conducted utilizing single agent chemotherapy simultaneously with RT v.s. RT alone as total treatment in patients with inoperable or unresectable stage III and IV cancer. Common feature of most of these trials is the small number of patients entered and evaluated. The conclusions of these investigations, that chemo-radiotherapy produced higher clinical CR, improved disease free survival, and possible improved overall survival, as compared to RT alone. The incidence of systemic involvement was similar between the two groups, when single agent chemotherapy was used. Recently, Merlano et al reported the results of their important randomized study comparing Cisplatin, 5-FU, and RT v.s. RT alone. They confirmed the previously reported results of statistically better local control, disease free survival, and for the first time confirmed the survival advantage for the combined approach.

Other studies are underway for non-nasopharyngeal cancer, and patients with nasopharyngeal carcinoma to investigate further and improve on the role of chemotherapy as part of definitive RT.

Laryngeal preservation

It was observed that patients who responded to Cisplatin based chemotherapy, will respond to subsequent RT. While, among non-responder to chemotherapy, less than 10 % will respond to further RT. This was confirmed by prospective trial, and led to the pilots of laryngeal preservation. Randomized study was activated and completed by the V.A. Laryngeal Cancer Group, randomizing between standard S + RT v.s. chemotherapy of Cisplatin and 5-FU, good responders will receive RT. Poor responders to chemotherapy, had S followed by RT. About two thirds of the patients preserved their laryngeal function, while there were no difference in three year survival. Patients on the chemotherapy arm have higher loco-regional failure, especially those with N2-3, or T4 disease. While the incidence of distant metastasis was statistically less for the chemotherapy group. To improve further on these results, we gave two to three courses of Cisplatin and 5-FU infusion, followed by concurrent three courses of Cisplatin alone and RT. We do believe this is the most effective way for laryngeal or other head and neck site organ preservation and need to be confirmed in randomized trial.

Other timing of chemotherapy

Adjuvant chemotherapy of single agent Cisplatin, or Cisplatin combination have been investigated after definitive treatments in patients with resectable head and neck locally advanced cancers. Adjuvant chemotherapy resulted in significantly less distant metastasis, improved disease free survival, and possible improved survival. These results need to be confirmed by large randomized trials.

Post-operative Cisplatin concurrent with RT was initiated at our institution, and the feasibility and the effectiveness was confirmed by the Radiation Therapy Oncology Group (RTOG). One randomized trial comparing post-operative concurrent Cisplatin and RT v.s. RT alone, confirmed the statistically improved local control, disease free survival, and overall survival for the combined arm. No difference in the distant metastasis between the two groups were found.

Chemotherapy of Cisplatin and 5-FU infusion for three courses after surgery and followed by post-RT was conducted at our Center. After the feasibility of this CMT was confirmed by the RTOG, randomized and stratified trial was initiated. Patients with negative gross margins were randomized between standard RT or chemotherapy, followed by RT. Preliminary analysis of this trial is reported else where in this book, and showed statistically less distant involvement, and less nodal recurrence. This important study is too early for evaluation for disease free survival or overall survival.

Discussion and conclusions

Systemic chemotherapy were investigated as part of definitive treatments of S and/or RT in patients with locally advanced head and neck cancers, because of the poor results obtained with these traditional therapy. High overall response rate, and CR were achieved with Cisplatin based combination and especially, Cisplatin and 5-FU infusion. High CR response and improved disease free survival were also obtained with concurrent chemotherapy and RT especially with the administration of Cisplatin alone or with 5-FU. And recently, improved survival were documented with combination of chemoradiotherapy v.s. RT alone in resectable, and unresectable patients with head and neck cancers. With the utilization of Cisplatin and 5-FU infusion and RT we were able to achieve laryngeal preservation in two thirds of the patients. Further studies are underway, or need to be initiated to 1) document further of improved survival with chemo-RT in patients with unresectable cancers, 2) improve of the rate of laryngeal preservation and/or overall survival, 3) Document the efficacy of chemotherapy in patients with nasopharyngeal cancers, 4) Document the survival advantage in patients with resectable disease.

The future direction and investigation with chemotherapy are shown in Table 2.

Table 2. Future directions with chemotherapy

1.	Chemo-prevention trials.
2.	Identification of better and/or other active single agents.
3.	Identification of more effective and/or safer combination CT.
4.	Identification of better and more effective timing of CT.
5.	Identification of more effective and/or safer concurrent chemo-RT.

References

1. Merlans M, Vitale V, Rosso R et al (1992) Treatment of advanced squamous cell carcinoma of the hand and neck with alternating chemotherapy and radiotherapy. NEJM 327 : 1115-1121
2. Bachaud JR, David JM, Boussin G, Daly N (1991) Combined postoperative radiotherapy and weekly Cisplatin infusion for locally advanced squamous cell carci-

noma of the head and neck preliminary report of a randomized trial. I J Rad Biol Phys 20 : 243-246
3. Al-Sarraf M (1987) Adjuvant chemotherapy for advanced head and neck squamous cell carcinoma : Final report of the head and neck contract program. Cancer 60 : 301-311
4. Al-Sarraf M (1988) Head and neck cancer : chemotherapy concept. Sem Oncol 15 : 70-85
5. Schuller DE, Metch B, Stein DW et al (1988) Preoperative chemotherapy in advanced resectable head and neck cancer : final report of the SWOG. Laryngoscope 98 : 1205-1211
6. Al-Sarraf M, Kish JA, Ensley JF (1991) Head and neck cancer : The Wayne State University experience with adjuvant chemotherapy. Hem/Oncol Clin N Am 5 : 687-700
7. Ensley JF, Jacobs JR, Weaver A et al (1984) The correlation between response to Cisplatin combination chemotherapy and subsequent RT in previously untreated patients with advanced squamous cell cancers of the head and neck. Cancer 57 : 811-814
8. Jacobs C, Goffinet DR, Goffinet L et al (1987) Chemotherapy as a substitute for surgery in the treatment of advanced resectable head and neck cancer. Cancer 60 : 1178-1183.
9. Al-Sarraf M, Pajak T, Jacobs J et al (1990) Combined modality therapy in patients with head and neck cancer : timing of chemotherapy. RTOG Study. Adjuvant Therapy of Cancer, VI, Salmon S (ed) WB Saunders Company, pp. 60-70
10. Al-Sarraf M, Pajak T, Laramore G (1985) Timing of chemotherapy as part of definitive treatment for patients with advanced head and neck cancer. An RTOG study. Proc ASCO 4 : 141
11. Laramore GE, Scott CB, Al-Sarraf M et al (1991) Adjuvant chemotherapy for resectable squamous cell carcinomas of the head and neck : Report on Intergroup Study 034. Int J Radiat Oncol Biol Phys 21 (suppl 1) : 190
12. Al-Sarraf M (1991) Induction chemotherapy plus radiation compared with surgery plus radiation in patients with advanced laryngeal cancer. The Department of Veteran's Affairs Laryngeal Cancer Study Group. NEJM 325 : 1685-1690

Chemotherapy (CT) followed by radiotherapy (RT) vs. RT alone in patients with resected and negative margins squamous cell carcinoma of the head and neck : Phase III Intergroup Study

M Al-Sarraf, CB Scott, K Ahmad, JG Schwade, D Schuller, GE Laramore, J Jacobs

The traditional treatment of patients with resectable locally advanced (stages III & IV) squamous cell carcinoma of the head and neck has been surgery (S) followed by post-operative radiotherapy (RT). Usually those who receive post-operative radiotherapy are those with stage IV, nodal involvement, or patients with positive surgical margin(s). The overall results in these patients are poor, more than 60 % will recur loco-regionally in spite of the complete removal of all the disease by the surgeon and the adjuvant RT. Approximately twenty percent of the patients will develop distant metastasis, and 70 % are dead within five years. Not all the remaining living patients (30 %) at five year, are free of disease.

With the introduction of effective chemotherapy given before (Induction, Neo-Adjuvant) definitive treatments, many of the poor risk patients with resectable disease were included on these trials. In two randomized national trials in the USA, giving one or three courses of induction chemotherapy, followed by S and post-operative RT, failed to show survival advantage.

It is the believe of some investigators that timing of chemotherapy as part of combined modality treatment (CMT) is important factor that may influence the overall results. This is especially true in patients with resectable cancer, in which surgery is part of their planned therapy. Also, approximately 35 % of all patients received, and about 50 % of patients with good response to induction chemotherapy may refuse the best modality of treatment, surgery. The degree of S for the same stage disease may be different for those have or have not initial treatment of chemotherapy or RT, and the type of response achieved by these modality. This led to investigation of three courses of Cisplatin and 5-Fluorouracil (5-FU) post surgery, followed by radiotherapy in patients with stage IV head and neck cancer. With the feasibility of such study at local institution was accomplished, the same pilot was activated and the feasibility was confirmed in the Radiation Therapy Oncology Group (RTOG). In 1983 the RTOG activated a randomized trial in order to test this concept in a phase III study. In 1985, this study was adapted by the Head and Neck Cancer Intergroup in the USA, and activated by other cooperative national groups.

Wayne State University, Detroit, MI 48201, RTOG & ACR Statistical Unit, Philadelphia, PA, University of Miami, Miami, FL, Ohio State University, Columbus, OH, University of Washington, Seattle, WA, USA

Materials and methods

Patients with stages III or IV, MO resectable squamous cell carcinoma of the head and neck were entered into this study. Other eligibility criteria no previous history of invasive cancer, no previous radiotherapy or chemotherapy, and no prior surgery (except for diagnostic purposes) to the primary or nodal sites. In addition patients to have adequate bone marrow function with WBC $\geqslant$ 4,000/mm^3, and platelet count $\geqslant$ 100,000/mm^3, and creatinine clearance of at least 60 ml/minutes. All patients have to sign informed consent. Patients are evaluated by an otolaryngologist/head and neck surgeon, medical oncologist, and radiation oncologist prior to registration.

Patients after having surgery, and those with negative gross surgical margins, were stratified and then randomized to post-operative RT, or chemotherapy followed by same RT. The stratification criteria consist of Site, Stage, and Risks Factors (margins of less or more than 5 mm, presence or absence of carcinoma *in situ*, presence or absence of extra-nodal spread). The chemotherapy consist of three courses of Cisplatin 100 mg/m^2 intravenously with hydration and mannitol diuresis on day one. 5-FU 1 000 mg/m^2/24 hour infusion for five days. The chemotherapy were given every three weeks, and three weeks after end of chemotherapy, patients received the same RT as on the standard arm.

Radiation treatment was the same on each arm with a total of 50-54 Gy to be given to « low risk » volumes and 60 Gy given to « high risk » volume. The treatment being given in daily fractions of 1.8-2.0 Gy on a 5-day-a-week-basis.

Results

A total of 448 patients were randomized and evaluated for present analysis, 225 on the RT arm, and 223 were randomized to CT-RT arm. Table 1 shows the pretreatment patient characteristics by treatment arm. No statistical differences were found between the two groups in regards to be stratified or other prognostic factors. Toxicities of RT alone or CT + RT were as expected, and they were all acceptable and reversible. No fatal treatment induced side effects were reported on either arms.

Table 2 shows the pattern of first failures and subsequent failures by treatment group. There were 11 first failures in the regional nodes alone on the CT + RT arm compared to 22 first failures in the neck nodes alone on the RT arm (p = 0.03). Overall distant metastases were 15 % (33/222) on the CT + RT arm compared to 23 % (51/224) on the RT arrm (p = 0.03). With a minimal follow-up on all patients of about two years, no statistical differences were found in disease free survival and overall survival so far. At this analysis 119/224 (53 %) of patients have failed on the RT arm compared to 105/222 (47 %) of patients on the CT + RT arm. Calculated on an actuarial basis the 4-year disease were free survival is 38 % on the RT arm compared to 46 %

Table 1. Pretreatment patient characteristics by treatment arm

	RT (n = 225)	CT + RT (n = 223)
Primary site		
Oral Cavity	69 (31 %)	53 (24 %)
Oropharynx	51 (23 %)	62 (28 %)
Hypopharynx	34 (15 %)	42 (19 %)
Supraglottic	44 (19 %)	32 (14 %)
Glottic	26 (11 %)	30 (13 %)
Subglottic	1 (1 %)	4 (2 %)
T-Stage (Clinical)		
T1	6 (3 %)	4 (2%)
T2	55 (24 %)	52 (23 %)
T3	124 (55 %)	120 (54 %)
T4	40 (18 %)	47 (21 %)
N-Stage (Clinical)		
N0	71 (31 %)	81 (36 %)
N1	58 (26 %)	60 (27 %)
N2	63 28 %)	53 (24 %)
N3	32 (14 %)	29 (13 %)
NX	1 (1 %)	0
KPS		
60-80	92 (41 %)	90 (40 %)
90-100	132 (58 %)	133 (60 %)
Uknown	1 (1%)	0
Margins		
High risk	114 (51 %)	114 (51 %)
Low risk	111 (49 %)	109 (49 %)
Sex		
Male	188 (84 %)	186 (83 %)
Female	37 (15 %)	37 (17 %)
Age		
Mean	58.9	57.8
Range	33-80	20-79

on the CT + RT arm. Thus far 105/224 (47 %) of patients died on the RT arm compared to 98/222 (44 %) of patients on the CT + RT arm. Calculated on an actuarial basis the 4-year survival rate is 44 % on the RT arm compared to 46 % on the CT + RT arm with 35 patients being still « at risk ». Table 3 shows the four year actuarial rates for local/regional failure and survival as a function of risk factors. Patients with high risks factors have less loco-regional recurrences (p = 0.07), and improved survival (p = 0.06) on the CT-RT arm as compared to the RT group.

Table 2. Pattern of first failures and subsequent failures by treatment arm

First failure site / Subsequent failure site	RT	CT/RT
Primary	22	22
Nodes	2	2
Distant metastases	3	3
None	17	17
Nodes	22	11
Primary	2	3
Distant metastases	4	2
Primary and mets	4	0
None	12	6
Primary and nodes	3	5
Distant metastases	39	24
Primary	2	0
Nodes	2	1
Primary and nodes	1	0
None	34	23
Primary and mets	0	2
Nodes	0	2
None	0	2
Nodes and mets	1	0
Primary and nodes and mets	0	2

Table 3. Four year actuarial rates for local/regional failure and survival as a function of surgical margin status

	RT		CT/RT		
	%	at risk	%	at risk	
Local/regional failure					
Low risk	22 %	17	22 %	10	n.s.
High risk	34 %	15	28 %	25	p = 0.07
Survival					
Low risk	51 %	20	45 %	11	n.s.
High risk	39 %	15	50 %	26	p = 0.06

Discussion and summary

The overall results of « standard » treatment of patients with locally advanced and resectable head and neck cancer are poor. In spite of complete removal of all gross disease at surgery, and the adjuvant post-operative RT, about 60 % of these patients will have loco-regional recurrence. Many strategy have been investigated to improve on the disease free survival, and overall survival of these patients. Also, more than 20 % of the patients will develop distant metastases during the five years after planned therapy. For these reasons, systemic chemotherapy were investigated as part of the definitive treatments for these patients. The problems in administering chemotherapy before surgery, many of these patients will refuse the operation, especially the good responders to chemotherapy. Also, the type and extent of surgery performed after response to initial treatment may not be the same as compared to previously untreated patients. Since surgery will be performed, initial shrinking of the loco-regional cancer by chemotherapy may not change the results for these patients, except for the incidence of distant metastases.

The results of the present analysis should be considered preliminary. Since patients with positive gross surgical margins were excluded, it is necessary to have minimal follow-up of 5 year for final conclusions. So far, as predicted the incidence of systemic metastases are less for the CT group. Also, the incidence or first regional recurrence are in favor for the CT arm. The overall disease free survival, and survival is too small for statistical significance. The most important findings so far that may help us for future protocol design in resectable patients, that the addition of chemotherapy may help those with high risk disease, and not those with low risk factors.

Efforts need to be continued to reduce on the incidence of loco-regional recurrence, especially with concurrent chemoradiotherapy, and with the addition of CT to continue to reduce the incidence of systmic disease.

References

1. Kramer S, Gelber RD, Snow JB et al (1985) Pre-operative v.s. post-operative radiation therapy for patients with carcinoma of the head and neck. Progress report. Head and Neck Surgery 3 : 255
2. Al-Sarraf M (1987) Adjuvant chemotherapy for advanced head and neck squamous cell carcinoma : final report of the head and neck contract program. Cancer 60 : 301-311
3. Al-Sarraf M (1988) Head and neck cancer : chemotherapy concept. Sem Oncol 15 : 70-85
4. Schuller DE, Metch B, Stein DW et al (1988) Preoperative chemotherapy in advanced resectable head and neck cancer : final report of the SWOG. Laryngoscope 98 : 1205-1211
5. Al-Sarraf M, Kish JA, Ensley JF (1991) Head and neck cancer : The Wayne State University experience with adjuvant chemotherapy. Hem/Oncol Clin N Am 5 : 687-700
6. Al-Sarraf M, Kinzie J, Jacobs J et al (1982) A new way of giving chemotherapy as part of multi-disciplinary treatment for patients with head and neck cancers. Preliminary report. Prox AACR 23 : 134
7. Al-Sarraf M, Pajak T, Laramore G (1985) Timing of chemotherapy as part of definitive treatment for patients with advanced head and neck cancer. An RTOG study. Proc ASCO 4 : 141

Neo-adjuvant infusion Cisplatin, 5-FU and high-dose leucovorin for squamous cell carcinoma of the head and neck (SCCHN) : high rates of complete response (CR) and definitive radiotherapy as primary site management

J Clark, A Dreyfuss, P Busse, C Norris Jr, J Lucarini, R Rossi, J Andersen, D Casey, E Frei III

The role of Neo-Adjuvant chemotherapy for patients with advanced SCCHN remains controversial. While results from randomized trials of Neo-Adjuvant therapy have confirmed an association between response and treatment outcome, an improvement in survival has not been reported. Critical review of latter studies however, reveals flaws which limit the value of their findings [1]. An improvement in the survival of patients who receive Neo-Adjuvant therapy for SCCHN may not be confirmed until the rate of CR is consistently over 50 % and local-regional treatment is optimal [1].

The objective of this report is to update published results [2] of Neo-Adjuvant infusion Cisplatin, 5-FU and high-dose Leucovorin (PFL), a regimen which was evaluated at the Dana-Farber between 1987 and 1992. These results will be compared, to those of an institutional control group.

Materials and methods

Between 7/87 and 4/91, 90 patients with untreated advanced (84 % stage IV, all M_0) SCCHN received PFL (fig. 1) followed by surgery or RT. Criteria for eligibility, staging and response as well as the specifics of PFL administration and dose-reduction have been published [2].

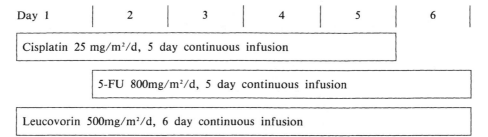

Fig. 1. Dana-Farber Protocol 87-005 : PFL

PFL was administered for a maximum of 3 cycles prior to surgery and/or RT. PFL was discontinued upon evidence of tumor progression or excessive toxicity, or after 2 cycles if response was less than partial.

Dana-Farber Cancer Inst., Harvard Medical School, Boston MA, 02115, USA

Treatment outcomes after PFL were compared to those from 202 age-matched patients (82 % Stage IV) with advanced SCCHN treated on three previous studies of Cisplatin-based Neo-Adjuvant chemotherapy at Dana-Farber (Table 1). Failure-free and overall survival were measured from treatment onset. Failure was defined as : *a)* tumor progression, the end of local-regional treatment or death, whichever came first, for patients not rendered free of disease ; *b)* relapse for patients rendered free of disease ; and *c)* death that was treatment associated.

Results

Two hundred and forty-six cycles of PFL were administered. A response to PFL was noted in 73/90 (81 %), including 51 (57 % ; 95 % C.I., 47 % to 67 %) CRs prior to local-regional treatment. Seventeen patients did not respond including 2 who expired during chemotherapy. The rate of CR to PFL is significantly higher ($p < .0001$) than that observed in 202 control patients (Table 1).

Table 1. PFL v.s. historical controls : response rates

Protocol	80-016	83-084	84-119	Total Controls	87-005
Chemotherapy §	PBM	PBM v.s. PF	PFM		PFL
Duration	2 m	2-4 m	2-3 m		2-3 m
Patients	92	89	21	202	90
Complete Response	25 %	28 %	38 %	28 %	57 %*
Total Response	78 %	67 %	86 %	74 %	81 %

§ P = Cisplatin, B = Bleomycin, M = Midcycle moderate-dose methotrexate with Leucovorin rescue, F = 5-FU
* PFL was independently associated with a CR in a multivariate analysis.

The primary site CR rate decreased with advancing T-stage for control patients ($p < 0.05$) but not for patients treated with PFL ($p = 0.094$) (Table 2). With PFL, CR rate remained high for all T-stages. Sixty-one of 86 (71 %) patients with evaluable primary site disease developed a CR at the primary. Of these, 50 (82 %) had pathologic evaluation of their primary site after PFL and 40 (80 %) had no residual disease at the time of rebiopsy prior to RT or surgical resection.

The principal toxicity of PFL is oral mucositis (> 90 % of patients). Diarrhea and rash occurred less frequently. These toxicities were controlled with dose reductions of F & L. Clinically important myelosuppression was unusual.

At the end of surgery and RT, 76 (84 %) patients treated with PFL were disease free in contrast to only 151 (75 %) of controls ($p = 0.07$, Table 3). With a median follow up of 34 months for PFL patients and > 5 years for controls, overall and failure-free survival, local control and sites of failure are presented in Tables 3 and 4.

Table 2. PFL v.s. controls : primary site responses

T-Stage	Controls			PFL patients		
	Pts	Clinical CR	Pts	Clinical CR	Pathology Evaluated	Pathologic CR
T0	4	NA	4	NA	NA	NA
T1	12	10 (83 %)	9	9 (100 %)	5	3 (60 %)
T2	31	21 (68 %)	18	13 (72 %)	11	8 (73 %)
T3	67	29 (43 %)	26	18 (69 %)	15	11 (73 %)
T4	88	26 (30 %)	33	21 (64 %)	19	18 (95 %)
Total	202	86 (83 %)	90	61 (71 %)	50	40 (80 %)

Table 3. PFL v.s. controls : outcomes after Neo-Adjuvant therapy

	Primary Surgery	NED after Treatment§	Actuarial estimates (3 years)		
			Overall Survival*	Failure Free Survival	Local Control
PFL	12 (14 %)	76 (84 %)	61 %	54 %	69 %
Controls	88 (45 %)	151 (75 %)	49 %	50 %	68 %

§ NED : no evidence of disease   * p = 0.057

Table 4. PFL v.s. controls : sites of failure in patients initially NED

		Sites of initial failure (P = primary ; N = neck ; D = distant)			
	Failed	P only	P and N only	N only	D ± P or N
PFL	24	12 (50 %)	1 (4 %)	5 (21 %)	6 (25 %)
Controls	56	18 (32 %)	6 (11 %)	11 (20 %)	21 (38 %)

Discussion

PFL is an active regimen that is associated with higher CR rates than observed with previous Cisplatin-based combinations. Remarkably however, PFL has had only a minor impact on the total response rate (CR + PR).

Neo-Adjuvant PFL was followed by a local treatment strategy that allowed for primary site preservation. By design, all primary site lesions were treated with definitive radiotherapy alone except those that achieved less than a CR after PFL and were operable and resectable. This approach resulted in a 3-fold decrease in primary site resections without a decrease in either the percent of patients disease free after treatment or in local control. An improvement in quality of life is apparent.

An analysis of sites of failure after Neo-Adjuvant PFL suggests that our policy of primary site preservation resulted in an increase in primary site failures relative to regional or distant failures. Given that local control is unchanged after PFL, the relative increase in primary site failure is in part due to an absolute decrease in regional and distant failure. The question remains whether PFL would have been associated with an increase in local control and failure free survival had all patients with resectable primary lesions undergone resection.

The increase in overall survival (p = 0.057), but not failure free survival after PFL is unusual and may relate in part to salvage surgical procedures which led to prolonged survival after failure in several patients treated with PFL.

These data support the contention that highly active regimens of Neo-Adjuvant therapy favorably impact on the natural history of this disease. The potential for chemotherapy to improve the survival of patients with SCCHN remains sound, but documentation of an improved survival awaits the creation of Neo-Adjuvant regimens that further increase the rate of CR. In addition, which patients can successfully avoid surgery after Neo-Adjuvant therapy must be further clarified.

References

1. Clark JR, Dreyfuss AI (1991) Cisplatin for squamous cell carcinoma of the head and neck. Semin Oncol 18 (suppl 3) : 34-48
2. Dreyfuss AI, Clark JR, Wright JE, et al (1990) Continuous infusion high-dose Leucovorin with 5-Fluorouracil and Cisplatin for untreated stage IV carcinoma of the head and neck. Ann Intern Med 112 (3) : 167-72

Abstract. Cisplatin (P) in combination with 5-FU (F) is a synergistic regimen that is active against SCCHN. Leucovorin (L) potentiates the cytotoxicity of F. In this study, Neo-Adjuvant PFL (P 25 mg/m²/d, d1-5 ; F 800 mg/m²/d, d2-6 and L 500 mg/m²/d, d1-6), was administered by continuous infusion every 28 days for 2-3 cycles prior to surgery or radiotherapy. As of 10/92, 90 patients (pts) with advanced (M_0) SCCHN (16 % Stage III, 84 % Stage IV) had received 246 cycles of PFL and been followed for a median of 34 months. Clinical responses after PFL were recorded in 81 % : CR 51(57 %), PR 22(24 %). Sixty-one (71 %) pts had a clinical CR at the primary site. Pathologic confirmation of a primary site CR was recorded in 40 of 50 (80 %) pts from whom tissue was available. Common toxicities included mucositis (93 % of cycles), diarrhea (53 %) and rash (26 %). Myelosuppression was generally mild. All patients have completed planned treatment and 76 (84 %) were disease-free after surgery or radiotherapy. Excluding two pts who died during PFL, primary site management consisted of radiotherapy alone in 76 (86 %) pts and surgery with radiation in 12 pts. Comparison with 202 similar pts treat-

ed with radiation in 12 pts. Comparison with 202 similar pts treated with previous P-based Neo-Adjuvant regimens reveals a significant increase in the rate of CR after PFL ($p < .001$). In addition, primary site management with surgery has decreased from 46 % to 14 % ($p < 0.01$) of cases. Despite this decrease in primary site resections, local control is unchanged. The 3 year actuarial estimates of failure free and overall survival after PFL are 54 % and 61 % respectively. PFL is a new and highly active regimen that warrants further study. A policy allowing primary site management with radiotherapy alone for the majority of pts has been successfully implemented.

Primary (Neo-Adjuvant) combined modality therapy in the management of locally advanced squamous cell carcinoma of the head and neck

G Mantovani*, E Proto**, L Contini*, S Littera*, L Curreli*, F Cossu***, P Puxeddu**, GS Del Giacco****

Recently, a combined modality therapy, usually chemotherapy (Neo-Adjuvant chemotherapy) followed by radiation therapy has been tested as an approach to sparing major surgery in patients with locally advanced head and neck cancer. Current choices for such patients include 1) a complete surgical resection with either preoperative or postoperative radiation therapy, 2) a Neo-Adjuvant chemotherapy followed by surgery and postoperative radiation therapy, or 3) a Neo-Adjuvant chemotherapy plus radiation therapy, and surgery if disease recurs [1].

Neo-Adjuvant chemotherapy has three main goals : *a)* to improve disease-free and overall survival, *b)* to render unresectable tumors resectable, and *c)* to eradicate local and distant (micro)metastases [1].

Although almost all of the clinical trials of Neo-Adjuvant chemotherapy have been uncontrolled, objective response rates (OR, i.e. complete response, CR, plus partial response, PR) are always greater than 50 % and sometimes above 90 % [2-8] and CR rates rise to 66 % [9]. Therefore, a CR proportion of 20 % to 30 % and a major response proportion of 60 % to 90 % can be reliably expected.

Aim of the study

Our phase II uncontrolled open study had two main goals, i.e. 1) to assess the results, in terms of OR rates, of the Neo-Adjuvant combined therapy with, for instance, Cisplatin based chemotherapy plus radiotherapy (with or without surgery) and 2) to substantially reduce the extent of surgery in the treatment of locally advanced squamous cell carcinomas (SCC) of the head and neck.

Patients and treatment plan

The patients (pts) were divided into two groups : the first included pts with SCC of the oral cavity, oropharynx and hypopharynx (HNC group) and the second included pts with laryngeal SCC (LC group). Pts were so divided mainly because of the well known different prognosis of the two cancer sites.

---

* Department of Medical Oncology, ** Department of Otolaryngology, *** Department of Radiation Therapy, **** Department of Internal Medicine, University of Cagliari Medical School, 09124 Cagliari, Italy

The primary chemotherapy (both for HNC and for LC) was the classical Al Sarraf's Regimen [10] : Cisplatin 100 mg/m^2 i.v. as a 60 min infusion on day 1 plus 5-FU 1,000 mg/m^2/day on days 1-5 as a continuous infusion by peripheral vein, repeated every 3 weeks.

The schedule for HNC was the following : a) Neo-Adjuvant treatment consisting of 1 chemotherapy cycle (days 1-5), followed by radiation therapy with a telecobalt unit, a total dose of 30 Gy at a daily dose of 2 Gy for five days weekly (on days 6-27), and further 2 cycles of chemotherapy (at this point responses were evaluated). Subsequently, the pts were submitted to radical surgery (in case of residual tumor) ; b) adjuvant treatment consisting of supplementary radiation therapy of up to 60-70 Gy (full dose) and further 3 cycles of chemotherapy. The schedule for LC was the following : 3 cycles of Al-Sarraf's Regimen, randomly followed by radiotherapy (60-70 Gy) or surgery. The clinical response was evaluated after at least 3 complete cycles of chemotherapy (including radiotherapy for HNC pts). The pts accrual was from February '90 to October '92.

The study included 35 pts (33 men and 2 women) with, 22 of whom (21 men and 1 woman ; mean age : 55.7 years, range 34-84 ; 1 pt stage II, 5 stage III, 16 stage IV, performance status ECOG 0-2) could be evaluated in December '92. The remaining 13 pts were not evaluable (5 too early, 4 early deaths, 3 refusing further therapy and 1 excluded for toxicity). The study also included 16 pts (15 men and 1 woman) with LC, 11 of whom (10 men and 1 woman ; mean age : 58.8 years, range 40-78 ; 1 pt stage II, 6 stage III, 4 stage IV, performance status 0-1) could be evaluated in December '92. Of the remaining 5 pts, 2 were too early, 1 died early, 1 was excluded for toxicity and 1 refused further therapy.

Evaluation of the results and toxicity

The clinical response was assessed by physical and conventional (often supplemented with CT) instrumental examination of the pts after the completion of the Neo-Adjuvant therapy. Furthermore, an updated evaluation was performed in December '92. The evaluation of the clinical response and the occurrence of systemic toxicity was evaluated according to the WHO criteria [11].

Results

The evaluation of the OR (CR + PR) after completion of the Neo-Adjuvant therapy is reported for the two groups of pts in Table 1.

In HNC pts an OR was achieved in 20/22 (91 %) : CR 11/22 (50 %), PR 9/22 (41 %) ; in LC pts an OR was achieved in 10/11 (91 %) : CR 7/11 (64 %), PR 3/11 (27 %). In HNC pts the mean time for response was 3.1 months (range 1-6.7) and in LC pts 2.6 months (range 2-5).

The mean follow-up time was 10.6 months (range 3.5-33) for HNC pts and 11.6 months (range 1.8-32) for LC pts. Preliminary data on overall survival

Table 1. Evaluation of tumor objective response (OR) after completion of Neo-Adjuvant chemotherapy. Analysis according to site and stage

Head and neck cancer

Site	Stage			Total
	II	III	IV	
Oral cavity	1/1 (1 CR)	1/1 (1 PR)	5/6 (2 CR, 3 PR)	7/8
Oropharynx		4/4 (3 CR, 1 PR)	5/6 (3 CR, 2 PR)	9/10
Hypopharynx			4/4 (2 CR, 2 PR)	4/4
Total	1/1 (1 CR) (100 %)	5/5 (3 CR, 2 PR) (100 %)	14/16 (7 CR, 7 PR) (87,5 %)	20/22 (11 CR, 9 PR) (91 %)

Laryngeal cancer

Site	Stage			Total
	II	III	IV	
Supraglottis		3/3 (2 CR, 1 PR)	2/2 (1 CR, 1 PR)	5/5
Glottis	1/1 (1 CR)	3/3 (2 CR, 1 PR)	1/2 (1 CR)	5/6
Total	1/1 (1 CR) (100 %)	6/6 (4 CR, 2 PR) (100 %)	3/4 (2 CR, 1 PR) (75 %)	10/11 (7 CR, 3 PR) (91 %)

Table 2. Mean overall survival for all patients and for responders ( ) : months.

Head and neck cancer

Site	Stage			Total
	II	III	IV	
Oral cavity	9 (9)	10.5 (10.5)	7.35 (6.62)	7.95 (7.51)
Oropharynx		12.25 (12.25)	18.58 (20.9)	16.05 (17.06)
Hypopharynx			6.03 (6.03)	6.03 (6.03)
Total	9 (9)	11.9 (11.9)	11.23 (11.55)	11.28 (11.51)

Laryngeal cancer

Site	Stage			Total
	II	III	IV	
Supraglottis		6.7 (6.7)	23 (23)	13.22 (13.22)
Glottis	5 (5)	5.33 (5.33)	21 (32)	10.5 (10.6)
Total	5 (5)	6.02 (6.02)	22 (26)	11.74 (11.91)

Table 3. Mean disease-free survival for all patients and for responders ( ) : months.

Head and neck cancer

Sites	Stage			Total
	II	III	IV	
Oral cavity	6.0 (6.0)	6.0 (6.0)	4.56 (3.67)	4.92 (4.34)
Oropharynx		10.5 (10.5)	12.17 (14.6)	11.5 (12.78)
Hypopharynx			1.55 (1.55)	1.55 (1.55)
Total	6.0 (6.0)	9.6 (9.6)	6.66 (6.97)	7.3 (7.58)

Laryngeal cancer

Site	Stage			Total
	II	III	IV	
Supraglottis		4.47 (4.47)	20 (20)	10.68 (10.68)
Glottis	3 (3)	3.13 (3.13)	17.5 (29)	7.9 (8.28)
Total	3 (3)	3.8 (3.8)	18.75 (23)	9.16 (9.48)

(OS) and disease-free survival (DFS) are reported for all pts and for responders in Tables 2 and 3. At the end of December '92 the following patients were alive and in OR : 14/22 (64 %) HNC pts (CR 9 and PR 5) and 10/11 (91 %) LC pts (CR 9 and PR 1). The causes for the death of the 8/22 HNC pts were disease progression (5), toxicity (1) and other causes (2). The death of the 1/11 LC pt was due to disease progression. Toxicity was on the whole acceptable : Grade IV (6 hematological with 1 death for toxicity and 6 gastrointestinal) and Grade III toxicity (2 hematological, 2 gastrointestinal, 1 neurologic and 1 cardiac) occurred.

As far as the second goal of our study is concerned, we can summarize our results by scoring the reduction of the extent of surgery made possible by Neo-Adjuvant chemotherapy versus the standard local therapy which would have been entailed to each pt.

Among the HNC pts we have obtained : 6/16 pts with score 3 (very highly reduced extent of surgery and/or function preservation), 5/16 pts with score 2 (highly reduced extent ...), 5/16 with score 0 (non reduced extent ...), and, among the 5 LC pts randomly submitted to surgery : 2 pts with score 3, 2 pts with score 2 and 1 pt with score 0.

Conclusions

Our results, in terms of OR, are certainly among the best obtained in the above reported studies, but it must be considered that :
1) The follow-up time was too short (approximately 1 year) to obtain very reliable data (a follow-up period at least 2 years should be adequate). For this

reason our data on OS and DFS are quite preliminary and can only be evaluated properly at the end of our study. 2) We have not yet been able to evaluate the results regarding surgery v.s. radiation therapy after Neo-Adjuvant chemo therapy in LC pts. As far as the second goal of our study is concerned, the results obtained may appear to be striking, but the number of pts included is too small to allow for statistical evaluations. The results of other randomized studies report that the survival in the total laringectomy-arm is identical to that of the larynx-sparing-arm [12]. It is however our opinion that we have given our pts an equal chance of cure and a better quality of life.

Nonetheless, the most important question as to whether Neo-Adjuvant chemotherapy improves overall survival when compared to standard local therapy still remains unanswered due to the inadequate number of pts enrolled in the randomized clinical trials [13]. For obvious reasons also our study cannot provide a substantial answer to this question. We believe that « through interdisciplinary study and integrated therapy, both survival and function end points should be addressed. Quality of life is as important as longevity, and patients deserve the best of both » [1].

Our study is still in progress with the aim of achieving more significant results in a larger number of patients over a longer follow-up period and we hope that the final results will lead to the design of a controlled phase III clinical trial.

Acknowledgments. This work was supported by CNR, Rome, AP « Clinical Applications of Oncological Research », Contract No. 92.02211.PF39.

References

1. Bosl GJ, Strong E, Harrison L, Pfister DG (1991) Chemotherapy and the management of the locally advanced squamous cell carcinoma of the head and neck : role in larynx preservation. In : DeVita VT Jr, Hellman S, Rosenberg SA (eds) Important Advances in Oncology. JB Lippincott Co, Philadelphia, pp 191-203
2. Al-Sarraf M, Pajak T, Jacobs J, Marcial V, Tupchung L, Banker FL, Cooper J (1990) Combined modality therapy in patients with head and neck cancer : timing of chemotherapy. Radiation Therapy Oncology Group (RTOG) study. 6th Int Conf on the Adjuvant Therapy of Cancer, Tucson, AZ, Mar 7-10, p 31
3. Frei E, Clark J, Dreyfus A, Miller D (1990) Advances in Neo-Adjuvant chemotherapy for head and neck cancer. 6th Int Conf on the Adjuvant Therapy of Cancer, Tucson, AZ, Mar 7-10, p 31
4. Martin M, Hazan A, Vergnes L, Peytral C, Mazeron JJ, Senechaut JP, Lelievre G, Peynegre R (1990) Randomized study of 5-Fluorouracil and Cisplatin as Neo-Adjuvant therapy in head and neck cancer : a preliminary report. Int J Radiat Oncol Biol Phys 19 : 973-975
5. Panis X, Coninx P, Nguyen TD, Legros M (1990) Relation between responses to induction chemotherapy and subsequent radiotherapy in advanced or multicentric squamous cell carcinomas of the head and neck. Int J Radiat Oncol Biol Phys 18 : 1315-1318
6. Vokes EE, Panje WR, Mick R, Kozloff MF, Moran WJ, Sutton HG, Gold-

man MD, Tybor AG, Weichselbaum RR (1990) A randomized study comparing two regimens of Neo-Adjuvant and adjuvant chemotherapy in multimodal therapy for locally advanced head and neck cancer. Cancer 66 : 206-213
7. Verweij J, de Jong PC, de Mulder PHM, et al (1989) Induction chemotherapy with Cisplatin and continuous infusion 5-Fluorouracil in locally far-advanced head and neck cancer. Am J Clin Oncol 12 : 420-424
8. Tannock IF, Broman G (1986) Lack of evidence for a role of chemotherapy in the routine management of locally advanced head and neck cancer. J Clin Oncol 4 : 1121-1126
9. Dreyfus AI, Clark JR, Wright JE et al (1990) Continuous infusion high-dose Leucovorin with 5-Fluorouracil and Cisplatin for untreated stage IV carcinoma of the head and neck. Ann Intern Med 112 : 167-172
10. Rooney M, Kish J, Jacobs J, Kinzie J, Weaver A, Crissman J, Al-Sarraf M (1985) Improved complete response rate and survival in advanced head and neck cancer after three-course induction therapy with 120-hour 5-FU infusion and Cisplatin. Cancer 55 : 1123-1128
11. Miller AB, Hodgstraten B, Staquet M, Winkler A (1981) Reporting results of cancer treatment. Cancer 47 : 207-214
12. Poplin J, Hong WK, Dorman B et al (1985) Voice preservation with sequential chemotherapy and radiation therapy without laryngectomy in patients with operable stage III, IV squamous cell carcinoma of the larynx and hypopharynx. Proc Am Soc Clin Oncol 4 : 149
13. Final Report of the Head and Neck Contracts Program (1987) Adjuvant chemotherapy for advanced head and neck squamous carcinoma. Cancer 60 : 301-311

A Phase II trial of induction Cisplatin, 5-FU, Leucovorin, and Interferon α-2B (PFL-α) followed by concurrent Hydroxyurea, 5-FU and radiation for Stage IV squamous cell cancers of the head and neck (HNC)

MS Kies, DJ Haraf, B Mittal, I Athanasiadis, M Kozloff, J McEvilly, R Mick, W Moran, W Panje, H Pelzer, TD Sheehan, R Weichselbaum, B Wenig, EE Vokes

Background

The combination of Cisplatin and Infusional fluorouracil has been widely used for the treatment of locally advanced squamous head and neck cancer, at diagnosis and recurrence [1-4]. When applied in the Neo-Adjuvant setting, it has resulted in high response rates and probably a reduced incidence of distant metastases. Overall survival, however, has not been proven to be increased and therefore use of this drug combination remains investigational in primary management [5, 6].

At Northwestern University and the University of Chicago we have attempted to increase the activity of Neo-Adjuvant chemotherapy through chemical modulation of the Cisplatin and 5-FU regimen and thereby increase the complete response rate in order to eventually effect prolongation of survival. Laboratory studies have suggested that interferons (IFN) enhance the activity of both Cisplatin and 5-FU [7-15]. Additionally, IFN-α may have moderate single agent activity [16, 17]. Our initial effort focused on the addition of Leucovorin to Cisplatin and 5-FU and in a phase I study in patients with recurrent or metastatic head and neck cancer, we identified recommended doses for 5-FU (800 mg/m^2/d × 5) and Leucovorin (100 mg orally q 4 hours) with mucositis dose-limiting toxicity [18]. Subsequently, this combination was given to previously untreated patients followed by local therapy with concurrent radiation and hydrea-5-FU. The CR rate after the Neo-Adjuvant treatment was 31 % and median survival has not yet been reached at a median follow up time of 3 years [19, 20].

To increase the activity of Cisplatin, 5-FU and Leucovorin through further biochemical modulation, we studied the pharmacologic interaction of 5-FU and IFN-α-2B [21]. Escalating doses of interferon from 0.5 to 4.0 × 10^{6}U/m^2/d were added to Cisplatin 100 mg/m^2, continuous infusion 5-FU 800 or 640 mg/m^2/d × 5 and leucovorin 100 mg orally q 4 hours. Twenty-one patients were treated during the phase I study with mucositis again dose-limiting toxicity. After decreasing the 5-FU dose to 640 mg/m^2/d, the maximally tolerated dose (MTD) of IFN was 2.0 × 10^{6}U/m^2/d. Mucositis and myelosuppression were dose limiting. Of 34 patients treated at this MTD, 56 % had a com-

---

Northwestern University and the University of Chicago, Chicago, IL, USA

plete clinical and radiographic remission. There was no clear correlation between 5-FU clearance and interferon dose, but analyses at the MTD showed that older age, female sex, and higher 5-FU area under the time v.s. concentration curve were associated with greater myelo-toxicity and increased mucositis. Diabetes appears to be a risk factor for enhanced toxicity as well as lower 5-FU clearance compared with non diabetics. Conclusions [21] from this project were that recommended doses for the PFL-α INF regimen are 640 mg/m^2/d for 5-FU and 2.0×10^6 U/m^2/d for IFN.

Based on this work a phase II project was developed with the Neo-Adjuvant PFL-α drug combination preceeding concurrent hydrea-5-FU/radiation.

Plan

Patients who enter this trial will have biopsy proven, previously untreated, stage IV M0 squamous carcinoma of the oral cavity, oropharynx, larynx or paranasal sinuses. For entry a joint medical and surgical evaluation is required as well as performance status 0-2 by ECOG criteria. Normal blood counts, renal and liver function studies, and an adequate staging evaluation including triple endoscopy with appropriate CT or MRI scanning are also to be obtained. Informed consent procedures will be required according to usual institutional guidelines.

The treatment plan as shown :

TREATMENT PLAN
PFL-α $\times$ 3 $\rightarrow$ HU/5-FU - RT

Details of the PFL-α Neo-Adjuvant schedule are given :

PFL-α REGIMEN

CDDP — 100 mg/m^2 on day 1

5-FU — 640 mg/m^2/d, continuous infusion $\times$ 5 days

L — LV 300 mg/m^2/d continuous IV over 5.5 days

IFN — 2×10^6 U/m^2 sc/d $\times$ 6 days
(Cycles repeat q 21 days $\times$ 3)

After induction chemotherapy patients are to proceed to concurrent chemotherapy and radiation (Patients achieving only partial response to PFL-α are considered for surgical resection before radiation) :

CONCURRENT CHEMOTHERAPY AND RT

Hydroxyurea, 1,000 mg po q 12° × 11 doses

5-FU, 800 mg/m^2/d continuous i.v. infusion × 5 days

and

RT, 200 cGy/d × 5 (to total 7,000 cGy)

(14 day cycles × 7)

The entire program is an intensive combined treatment schedule which will be highly toxic and require much supportive care. Virtually all patients are expected to have mucositis and myelosuppression. Much attention to symptom control with mouth rinses, analgesics, ancillary nutritional and fluid support, electrolyte replacement, and antibiotics will be necessary. Diabetes, again, may be a risk factor for extraordinary problems and these patients will be closely observed.

If anticipated high response rates obtain, the combined program may become suitable for randomized study against a more standard local treatment.

References

1. Rooney M, Kish J, Jacobs J et al (1985) Improved complete response rate and survival in advanced head and neck cancer after three-course induction therapy with 120-hour 5-FU infusion and Cisplatin. Cancer 55 : 1123-1128
2. Vokes EE, Mick R, Lester EP et al (1991) Cisplatin and 5-fluorouracil does not yield long-term benefit in locally advanced head and neck cancer : Result from a single institution. J Clin Oncol 9 : 1376-1384
3. Jacobs C, Lyman G, Velez-Garcia E et al (1992) A randomized phase III study comparing Cisplatin and Fluorouracil as single agents in combination for advanced squamous cell carcinoma of the head and neck. J Clin Oncol 10 : 257-263
4. Kies MS, Gordon LI, Hauck WW et al (1985) Analysis of complete responders after initial treatment with chemotherapy in head and neck cancer. Laryngol Head Neck Surg 93 : 199-205
5. The department of veterans affairs laryngeal cancer study group (1991) Induction chemotherapy plus radiation compared with surgery plus radiation in patients with advanced laryngeal cancer. N Engl J Med 324 : 1685-1690
6. Laramore GE, Scott CB, Al-Sarraf M et al (1991) Adjuvant chemotherapy for resectable squamous cell carcinomas of the head and neck : Report on intergroup study 0034. Am Soc Therapeut Radiat Oncol (abstr)
7. Wadler S, Schwarz EL (1990) Antineoplastic activity of the combination of interferon and cytotoxic agents against experimental and human malignancies : A review. Cancer Res 50 : 3473-3486
8. Wadler S, Wersto R, Weinberg V et al (1990) Interaction of Fluorouracil and interferon in human colon cancer cell lines : Cytotoxic and cytokinetic effects. Cancer Res 50 : 5735-5739

9. Chu E, Zinn S, Boarman D, Allegra CJ (1990) Interaction of α-Interferon and 5-Fluorouracil in the H630 human colon carcinoma cell line. Cancer Res 50 : 5834-5840
10. Houghton JA, Adkins DA, Rahman A et al (1991) Interaction between 5-Fluorouracil, Leucovorin and recombinant human Interferon-α-2a in cultured colon adenocarcinoma cells. Cancer Commun 3 : 225-231
11. Allegra CJ (1991) Biochemical modulation : A modality that has come of therapeutic age. J Clin Oncol 9 : 1723-1726
12. Von Hoff DD (1991) In vitro data supporting Interferon plus cytotoxic agent combinations. Sem Oncol 18 : 58-61 (suppl 7)
13. Sato M, Yoshida H, Urata M et al (1984) Effects of 5-Fluorouracil and the combination of 5-Fluorouracil and human leukocyte Interferon on human salivary gland adenocarcinoma cell in culture. Int J Oral Surg 13 : 35-44
14. Elias L, Sandoval JM (1989) Interferon effects upon Fluorouracil metabolism by HL-60 cells. Biochem Biophys Res Commun 163 : 867-874
15. Neefe JR, John W (1991) Mechanisms of interaction of Interferon and 5-Fluorouracil in solid tumors. Sem Oncol 18 : 77-82 (suppl 7)
16. Padovan I, Brodaree J, Ikic D et al (1981) Effect of Interferon in therapy of skin and head and neck tumors. J Cancer Res Clin Oncol 100 : 295-310
17. Vlock DR (1991) Immunobiologic aspects of head and neck cancer. Clinical and laboratory correlates. Hematol Oncol Clin North Am 5 : 797-820
18. Vokes EE, Choi KE, Schilsky RL et al (1988) Cisplatin, Fluorouracil, and high-dose Leucovorin for recurrent or metastatic head and neck cancer. J Clin Oncol 6 : 618-626
19. Vokes EE, Schilsky RL, Weichselbaum RR et al (1990) Induction chemotherapy with Cisplatin, Fluorouracil and high-dose Leurovorin for locally advanced head and neck cancer : A clinical and pharmacologic analysis. J Clin Oncol 8 : 241-247
20. Vokes EE, Weichselbaum RR, Mick R et al (1992) Favorable long-term survival following induction chemotherapy with PFL and concomitant chemoradiotherapy for locally advanced head and neck cancer. J Natl Cancer Inst 84 : 877-882
21. Vokes EE, Ratain MJ, Mick R et al (1993) Cisplatin, Fluorouracil and Leucovorin augmented by Interferon-α-2b in head and neck : A clinical and pharmacologic analysis. J Clin Oncol (in press)

Induction chemotherapy with Cisplatin (P), 5-Fluorouracil (FU) and Folinic Acid (FA) in locally advanced head and neck cancer

E Fonseca, JJ Cruz, J Garcia, A Panadero, P Sanchez, A Gomez, G Martin, MJ Garcia, JC Vallejo

It has been observed that a synergism exists between Cisplatin (P) and 5-Fluorouracil (FU) when these agents are jointly administered in continuous perfusion.

Additionally, the cytotoxicity of 5-FU can be potentiated by modulation with Folinic Acid (FA), which increases the inhibition of nimydalate synthetase, one of the enzymes necessary for DNA synthesis [1].

In the light of these data, we have designed a new scheme, adding FA to a previous protocol with Cisplatin and 5-Fluorouracil, both in continuous perfusion [2,3].

Materials and methods

Between June 1990 and June 1992, 73 patients with locally advanced carcinoma of the head and neck were treated with a induction chemotherapy protocol employing P, FU and FA (PFFA) followed by locoregional therapy.

This group consisted of 68 men and 5 women; the median age was 55 years. Histologically, 64 of the cases were epidermoid carcinomas and 9 were undifferentiated carcinomas. The initial location of the lesions was as follows: larynx 24; oral cavity 13; nasopharynx 12; oropharynx 11; hypopharynx 10; and paranasal sinuses 3. Patients were staged according to the classification of the AJC. 13 of them had stage III disease and 60 stage IV disease.

Treatment consisted of the administration of FA at a dose of 250 mg/m^2 infused over 2 h. followed by 25 mg/m^2 of P and FU at a dose of 1 000 mg/m^2 both in continuous perfusion over 24 h, repeated during 4 days. Courses were administered every 21 days, for a total of 4. Changes were no considered neither in the dosis of FA nor FU.

Patients were assessed for their response and toxicity after each course and at the end of locoregional treatment, following the WHO criteria.

Results

70 patients were evaluable for response. Three of them abandoned the protocol by own decision.

Service of Medical Oncology, University Hospital of Salamanca, Spain

After chemotherapy, 38 CR (54 %) were achieved, and 26 PR (37 %). The number of objective responses was 64 (91 %).

Responses according to location, stage and TNM are shown in Table 1. Of 35 patients with T3-4 N2-3 disease, 20 (57 %) achieved a complete response. Biopsy specimens of the primary tumor or specimens of definitive resection inmediately after PFFA therapy were available in 25 patients with CR. In 11 (44 %) patients, no residual tumor was found in the specimen.

Table 1. Response by characteristics of patients

Characteristics	N°	CR %	CR + PR %
Primary site			
Larynx	24	46	88
Nasopharynx	12	67	100
Oropharynx	11	64	91
Oral cavity	11	55	91
Hypopharynx	10	44	88
Paranasal	2	67	100
Stage			
III	12	50	92
IV	58	55	91
T Class			
T1	3	67	100
T2	4	50	75
T3	27	52	93
T4	36	56	92
N Class			
N0	18	55	94
N1	9	44	88
N2	23	61	96
N3	20	50	85

271 courses were administered. 63 patients received four cycles. The remaining ones didn't complete the protocol because of the toxicity. The commonest toxicity was mucositis (44 %). Three patients required to go to the hospital because of mucositis. Grade 2-3 stomatitis were noticed in 23 % of the courses. Diarrhea was seen in 11 % of the courses it tended to be mild and to resolve spontaneously. Three patients had grade 4 leukopenia, two of them died owing to sepsis after respiratory infection. Three patients had grade 3 thrombopenia but no one bled. The dose of Cisplatin was modified in three patients because of impaired renal function. One of the patients showed peripheral neuropathy.

Conclusion

Combined administration of Cisplatin, 5-Fluorouracil and Folinic Acid in locally advanced head and neck cancer proved to be very efficient, with an objective response of 91 %, with 54 % CR (confirmed histologically in 11 of the 25 patients in which it was possible to perform the histological study (44 %). Owing to the low number of patients, it is not possible to draw any conclusions about the role of the size of the tumor, nodes or the location of the disease in the response.

The toxicity was important. We observed moderate and severe stomatitis in nearly all the patients, and two patients died beacause of sepsis.

In conclusion, the protocol has proven to be very efficient in patients with locally advanced head and neck cancer, with a high percentage of CR and a severe degree of toxicity. This result should be confirmed in a larger serie and observations should be made of the impact of this result on the survival of this kind of patient.

References

1. Trave F, Zakrzewski S, Petrelli N (1987) Biochemical and pharmacologic basis for potentiation of 5-fluoracil action by leucovorin. NCI Monogr 5 : 165-170
2. Cruz JJ, Fonseca E, Gomez A et al (1991) Neoadjuvant chemotherapy in locally and advanced head and neck cancer with cisplatinum (P) and 5-Fluoracil (FU) both in continuous infusion. Proc Third International Congress on Neoadjuvant Chemotherapy, Paris
3. Bernal AG, Cruz JJ, Sanchez P et al (1989) Four-day continuous infusion of Cisplatinum and 5-Fluoracil in head and neck cancer. Cancer 63 : 1927-1930

A randomized study of CDDP and 5-FU as Neo-Adjuvant chemotherapy in head and neck cancer : an interim analysis

M Martin*, L Vergnes*, Lelièvre**, P Michel-Langlet*, C Peytral**,
JJ Mazeron*, E Malaurie*, R Peynegre**

A prospective randomized study of Cisplatin and 5-Fluorouracil (5-FU) preceeding loco regional treatment (LRT) as compared with LRT alone in squamous cell carcinoma (SCC) in head and neck cancer was conducted from September 1986 to October 1989. This study was designed to test the response rate of induction chemotherapy, the impact upon local regional control and survival.

156 patients were stratified by site (oral cavity 33, oropharynx 43, hypopharinx 37, larynx 43) and by stage (stage II-51, stage III-64, stage IV-41) and randomized to receive LRT (surgery and post-operative radiation or radiation alone) or induction chemotherapy followed by LRT. Chemotherapy consisted of 3 cycles of 120 hr 5-FU infusion 1 g/m^2/day plus Cisplatin 100 mg/m^2 on day 1 on each cycle. The overall objective response rate to chemotherapy was 75 % with 47 % complete response. The median follow-up is 60 months (min : 40, max : 74). After LRT, the complete response is 89 % in the chemotherapy group and 84 % in the control group. Actuarial overall survival at 5 years is 42 % in the chemotherapy group and 38 % in the control group (p = 0,2).

This interim analysis shows that in spite of initial tumor response, Neo-Adjuvant chemotherapy does not improve long-term control and survival.

Squamous cell carcinoma (SCC) of the head an neck represents 15 % of the malignant tumor seen in France. Despite favorable control rates for patients with Stages I and II, the ultimate control rate remains poor for patients with advanced disease such as Stages III and IV. The local regional control rates using combinations of radiation therapy and surgery are well below 40 %-50 %, and the frequency of distant metastasis is 15 %-20 %. Recent chemotherapy regimens incorporating Cisplatin with Belomycine or Fluorouracil (5FU) have show response rates of 60 % to 80 %, with complete response occuring in 10 to 50 % of patients [2, 4, 10]. Although effective drug regimens may achieve high rates of response, the impact of Neo-Adjuvant chemotherapy consisting of Cisplatin and 5-FU upon local/regional control and survival remains to be demonstrated.

Patients and methods

A randomized prospective trial of induction chemotherapy before standard irradiation or surgery and irradiation was conducted from September 1986 to

---

Dept. of oncology and otolaryngology, Créteil, Montfermeil, France

October 1989 in the Department of Oncology and Oto-laryngology of 2 institutions (Créteil-Montfermeil). The patients with Stages I, II, III, IV cancers of the oral cavity, oropharynx and hypopharynx, and Stage II, III, IV cancers of the larynx were included in this study. The age limit was 70 years. The criteria for patient exclusion were : distant metastasis, recent additional malignancy, estimated life expectancy for less than 12 weeks, pre-treatment with blood cell count < 3,500/μl, absolute granulocyte count < 2,000/μl, or platelet count < 100,000/μl, serum creatinine > 1.5 mg dl. The study was designed to test induction chemotherapy prior to planned surgery and irradiation. The chemotherapy regimen consisted of Cisplatinum 100 mg/m^2 diluted in normal saline and infused over 2.5 hr on day 1 after hydration. This was followed by 120 hr 5-FU infusion 1 g/m^2/day. The regimen was repeated every 3 weeks for three courses in patients with tumor regression. Then, they received definitive local treatment (DLT). Non responding patients were switched to DLT after 1 or 2 cycles of chemotherapy. The modalities of the DLT were definitively decided by the multidisciplinary team prior to randomization. The standard treatment for operable patients with or without chemotherapy consisted of radical surgical treatment of the primary and cervical nodes (based on the original tumor extent in the chemotherapy group, even if clinical complete response) followed by regional radiation therapy : 55 Gy fractions, 5 times each week, over a 6 weeks period ; post-operative residuel disease, if present, was boosted to 70 Gy.

For inoperable patients, primary radiation alone was delivered and consisted of 70 Gy over 8 weeks at 1.8 Gy per fraction. In some instances, primary irradiation alone was delivered for favorable tumor sites.

One hundred fifty six patients were entered into the study and were randomized and received chemotherapy, prior to standard treatment or standard treatment only. 150 patients were evaluable, 76 in the chemotherapy group and 74 in the control group.

Patients were stratified by site and stage with excellent balance (Table 1). The tumor response to chemotherapy and radiation was assessed by all members of the treatment team. The survival curves were estimated by the Kaplan Meier technique [7]. Survival was measured in months from the date of diagnosis.

Table 1. Distribution by stage and site

Site and stage	Chemotherapy group 76 patients	Control group 74 patients
Oral cavity	15	14
Oropharynx	23	20
Hypophraynx	18	18
Larynx	20	22
Stage II	24	26
Stage III	32	30
Stage IV	20	18

Results

Seventy six patients were randomized to the chemotherapy group and seventy four to the control group. The two groups were compared according to age, sex, site, stage and loco-regional treatment modalities ; there were no statistically significant differences.

Seventy two patients were evaluable for response to chemotherapy. The overall objective response rate was 75 % (54 patients) with 47 % complete response (34 patients).

Chemotherapy was delayed for 21 patients (28 %), dose was reduced for 28 patients (37 %) and discontinued for 23 patients (29 %). 76 patients were evaluable for toxicity : the most common side effects related to chemotherapy are reported in Table 2. They were 3 deaths related to drug toxicity.

Local regional relapse rate, second primaries, metastasis were similar in the two groups. Eight patientys in the chemotherapy group had persisted loco-regional disease at the completion of treatment and 12 in the control group (Table 3).

Table 2. Toxicity to chemotherapy 76 pts

	GR III	GR IV	Total (%)
Anemia	4	1	7 %
Neutropenia	10	6	21 %
Trombocytopenia	1	8	12 %
Renal	—	—	—
Gastrointestinal	10	2	15 %
3 toxic deaths : 2 septicemia			
1 cardiac			

Table 3. Pattern of failure

	CH + (76)	CH − (74)
Alived ned	30	28
L/R persistance	8	12
L/R relapse	16	14
Metastasis	4	4
2 nd Localisation	8	12
Dead ID	4	6

Division by tumor site, stage or nodal status revealed no significant difference in survival. The actuarial survival at five years is 42 % in the chemotherapy group and 38 % in the control group. Actuarial disease free survival showed no significant differences. At 5 years disease free survival in the chemotherapy group is 39 % and in the control group 35 %.

Discussion

The efficacity of systemic chemotherapy in cancer of the upper aerodigestive tract has been established with confirmed response rates exceeding 50-70 % in several trials [1, 5, 9]. To date, Neo-Adjuvant chemotherapy has not had a proven impact upon local regional disease control or survival. At our institution, a regimen with Cisplastinum and 5-FU was tested in a randomized, stratified, prospective study as Neo-Adjuvant therapy.The results revealed no significant difference in survival and loco-regional control in the two arms. The results of several randomized studies with induction chemotherapy using Cisplatinum combined with 5-FU or Bleomycine and for Methotrexate [4, 8, 9, 14] show no difference and in one trial, results were worse in the chemotherapy group. Thus, the hope that more effective chemotherapy may change these results has not yet been demonstrated. The initial good responses to induction Cis platinum and 5-FU may foster the problem of patient withdrawal prior to the completion of planned multimodality treatment.

Neo-Adjuvant chemotherapy seems only indicated for patients where a mutilating surgery is planned, as we have suggested it in a randomized prospective trial with Carboplatine-5-FU [10].

References

1. Carter SK (1977) The chemotherapy of head and neck cancer. Sem Oncol 4 : 413-424
2. Decker DA, Drelichman A, Jacobs J, Hoschner J, Kinsie J, Loh JJK, Weaver A, Al-Sarraf M (1983) Adjuvant chemotherapy with CDDP and 120 hours infusion 5-FU in stage III and IV squamous cell carcinoma of the head and neck. Cancer J1 : 1353-1355
3. Forestière A, Metch B, Schuller D, Ensley J et al (1992) Randomized comparison of Cisplatin plus Fluorouracil and Carboplatin plus Fluorouracil versus Methotrexate in advanced squamous cell carcinoma of the head and neck : a southwest oncology group study. J Clin Oncol 10 : 1245-1251
4. Hass C, Anderson T, Byhard R, Cox J, Duncavage J, Grossman T, Hass J, Libnoch J, Malin T, Ritch P, Toohill R (1986) Randomized Neo-Adjuvant study of 5-FU and CDDP for patients with advanced resectable head and neck cancer. Proc Am Assoc Cancer Res 27 : 185
5. Holoye PY, Byers RM, Gard DA, Goepfert H, Guillamondegui OM, Jesse RH (1978) Combination chemotherapy of head and neck. Cancer 42 : 1661-1669
6. Hong WK, Bromer (1983) Current concepts, chemotherapy in head and neck cancer. N Engl J Med 308 : 75-76
7. Kaplan E, Meier P (1958) Non parametric estimation from incomplete observation. J Am Stat Assoc 58 : 475-481
8. Martin M, Mazeron JJ, Glaubiger D, Brun B, Langlois A, Feuillade F, Lelièvre G, Strunsky W, Vergnes L, Denarnaud J, Peynègre R, Pierquin B (1986) Neo-Adjuvant polychemotherapy of head and neck cancer. Preliminary results of a randomized study. Proc Am Soc Clin Oncol J 141
9. Martin M, Schuller DE, Wilson H, Hodgson S, Mattox D (1984) Pre-operative reductive chemotherapy for stage III or IV operable epidermoid carcinoma of the oral cavity and oropharynx, hypopharynx or larynx phase III, a southwest oncolo-

gy group study. In : Vidockler HR (ed) Proceedings of international conference on head and neck cancer. Lancaster Press, Baltimore, p. 48

10. Martin M, Lelièvre G, Gehanno P, Depondt J, Guerrier B, Peytral C, Dubreuil P, Margotton A, Pellae Cosset B (1992) Induction Carboplatin and 5-FU treatment versus no chemotherapy before loco regional treatment for oro and pharyngo laryngeal cancers : preliminary results of a randomized study. Proc 11 Assoc : 769

11. Taylor SG (1987) Integration of chemotherapy into the combined modality therapy of head and neck squamous cancer. Int J Radiat Oncol Biol Phys 13 : 779-783

12. Vokes E, Schilsky R, Weichselbaum M, Kosloff M, Panje W (1990) Induction chemotherapy with Cisplatin, Fluorouracil, and high dose Leucovorin for locally advanced head and neck cancer : a clinical and pharmacologic analysis. J Clin Oncol 8 : 241-247

13. Wittes R, Heller K, Randolph V, Shah J, Sairo R, Strong E (1979) CDDP based chemotherapy as initial treatment of advanced head and neck cancer. Cancer Treat Rep 63 : 1533-1538

14. Wolf GT, Jacob C, Makuch RW, Vikram B (1984) CDDP and Bleomycine adjuvant chemotherapy in head and neck cancer : resultas of the head and neck contacts program. In : Vidockler HR, (ed.) Proceeding of the internationale conference on head and neck cancer. Lancaster Press, Baltimore, p. 43

Concomitant chemoradiotherapy in locally advanced head and neck cancers : a prospective study of 68 patients

S Walter*, C Hennequin*, MD Brette**, P Leblanc**,
PY Cheriff-Cheikh**, M Espie***, JP Monteil**,
M Marty***, C Maylin*

Rationale

For locally advanced, unresectable head and neck cancers, radiotherapy (RT) is the standard treatment but has poor results (25 % five year survival). Randomized trials showing improved survival in patients treated by concomitant chemoradiotherapy have been published for 5-FU, 5-FU-CDDP and Bleomycin [1, 2]. CDDP with 5-FU is a synergistic regimen against recurent and disseminated squamous cell carcinomas of the head and neck [3, 4]. To emphasize these results, we have attempted to increase the efficacy of RT with a concomitant and simultaneous Cisplatin (CDDP) and 5-Fluorouracil (5-FU) chemotherapy (protocol PURE).

The aim of this combination was to increase both local and systemic control by potentiation of cell killing based on an inhibition of the recovery of radiation induced damage (spatial cooperation), treatment of distant micrometastasis.

Patients

From february 1988 to July 1992, 68 patients with following elligible criteria were entered the study : histologically confirmed carcinoma, unresectable disease, age less than 70 years, performance status > 30, no impairment of liver, kidney, bone marrow or heart funtion. Characteristics of 68 patients treated are outlined in Table 1.

Twenty-five patients had previously been treated : 12 had recurrent tumors after surgery with or without radiotherapy, 18 had received a neoadjuvant chemotherapy.

Treatment

Combined radiochemotherapy consisted of courses of 21 days. CT was started on day 1 and delivered 5-FU 1,000 mg/m² in continuous infusion from day 1 to day 3, CDDP 45 mg/m² on day 1 and 2, CDDP 15 mg/m² on day 8. RT by supervoltage equipment with ^{60}Co was started on day 1 and delivered 45 or 70 Gy according to response :

---

* Service de Cancérologie-Radiothérapie, ** Service de Chirurgie ORL et Maxillofaciale, *** Service d'Oncologie Médicale, Hôpital Saint-Louis, 1, avenue Claude-Vellefaux, Paris, France

Table 1. Characteristics of the patients and tumors

Characteristic	Number	%
Sex		
Male	66	97
Female	2	3
Age (yr)		
≤ 60	47	69
> 60	21	31
Karnofsky Index		
≤ 60	13	19
> 60	55	81
Disease Stage*		
II	2	3
III	13	19
IV	52	77
Site of disease		
Oropharynx	26	38
Oral Cavity	21	31
Hypopharynx	15	22
Larynx	5	7
Paranasal sinuses	1	1
Two sites	21	31
Three sites	3	4
Histological Type		
Squamous	66	98
Carcinosarcoma	1	1
Cylindroma	1	1
Histological Grade		
Grade 1	34	50
Grade 2	2	3
Grade 3	2	3
Unknown	30	44

* Disease stage was determined according to the AJC Classification

- before 1991 (PURE I) : 15 Gy were delivered in 8 fractions over 11 days (1,8 Gy from day 1 to 4 and from day 8 to 11), 48 patients were treated ;
- after 1991 (PURE II) : 20 Gy were delivered in 10 fractions over 12 days (2 Gy from day 1 to 5 and from day 8 to 12), 20 patients were entered. There was a week rest and then the next cycle started on day 21.

When the total dose of 70 Gy was delivered, the duration of treatment was 105 days in PURE I and 63 days in PURE II.

Supportive care included enteral or parenteral nutrition with a caloric intake superior to 2 000 calories a day.

After 45 Gy, each patient was reconsidered for surgery. For good responders remaining unresectable, chemoradiotherapy was carried on until the total dose of 70 Gy. For non responders, RT was carried on alone. Response assessment was established two months after the end of the treatment.

Results

All patients were evaluable for toxicity and survival. Six patients were not evaluable for response because of early toxic death, there was no early patient lost to follow up.

Toxicity

The grade of toxicity was determined according to the scale of the World Health Organization (Table 2). Toxicity was moderate and acceptable with the same distribution according to the two groups : grade 3-4 leucopenia in 18 %, grade 3-4 mucositis in 22 %. There were 6 toxic death. Cause of death was : infection (septic shock, pyocyanic pneumopathy during aplasia), intracerebral hemorrhage induced by thrombocytopenia. The cause of death remained unknown for the last 3 patients.

Table 2. Toxic reactions

Reaction	Grade I-II	(%)	Grade III-IV	(%)
Leucopenia	2	(31)	18	(26)
Anemia	5	(7)	1	(1)
Thrombocytopenia	3	(4)	1	(1)
Mucositis	38	(55)	11	(16)
Infection	1	(1)	4	(6)
Nephrotoxicity	11	(16)	0	(0)
Neurotoxicity	1	(1)	0	(0)
Myocardial ischemia	0		1	(1)
Toxic death 8 %				

Response to treatment

Sixty two patients (91 %) completed their treatment and were included in the analysis of response. After 45 Gy, only six patients underwent surgery. Mean tumor dose was 70 Gy in PURE I, 69 Gy in PURE II, mean duration of treatment was 86 days (PURE I : 110 days, PURE II : 67 days). Dose intensity was upper than 80 % percent for 5-FU and in 81 percent for CDDP.

Mean tumor response was : 85 % (PURE I : 78 %, PURE II : 93 %), mean nodal response was : 76 % (PURE I : 76 %, PURE II : 97 %). Mean duration of treatment was 86 days (PURE I : 90 days, PURE II : 67 days).

At the end of the treatment, an objective response (> 50 %) was noted in 92 % (PURE I : 87 %, PURE II : 80 %). Complexe response was achieved in 61 % (PURE I : 56 %, PURE II : 75 %) (Table 3).

Table 3. Response to treatment according to regimens

Event	Total response n = 68	(%)	Pure I n = 48	(%)	Pure II n = 20	(%)
Complete response	42	(61)	27	(56)	15	(75)
Partial response	16	(24)	15	(31)	1	(5)
Overall response	58	(85)	42	(87)	16	(80)
Stable disease	1	(1)	1	(2)	0	(0)
Disease progression	3	(4)	3	(6)	0	(0)
Early death	6	(9)	2	(4)	4	(20)

Overall survival

Median survival is 18 months (PURE I : 14 months, PURE II : not reached). Two and three year overall survival are respectively 48 and 30 % (Fig. 1 et 2).

At the time of the present analysis, 30 patients are alive (PURE I : 16/48 ; PURE II : 14/20), 6 patients from regimen PURE I are lost to follow up and 32 are dead (PURE I : 26/48 ; PURE II : 6/20). Thirteen patients are long survival (19 %). Cause of death was locoregional involvment (59 %), infection (13 %) distant metastasis (9 %), other (18 %).

While we are waiting for longer follow-up before conducting a final analysis of this trial, there is a trend for the shorter treatment (PURE II) without statistically log rank difference between the two groups probably due to the lack of total strength.

Discussion and conclusion

In patients with advanced unresectable squamous cell carcinoma of the head and neck, a randomized trial was designed by Merlano et al [1] and determined that alternative radiochemotherapy with 5-FU and CDDP improved the survival of such patients comparing with radiotherapy alone : the median survival was 16.5 months in the combined-therapy group and 11.7 months in the RT group ; the three-year survival was 41 percent and 23 percent respectively ($P < 0.05$).

Our two treatment groups did not differ signicantly in their rate of objective response but they differed in their rates of complete and partial response (Table 3). This concomitant and simultaneous radiochemotherapy provides a complete response rate of 61 %, higher than alternative radiochemotherapy reported in litterature and similar median survival above 17 months, two and three year survival.

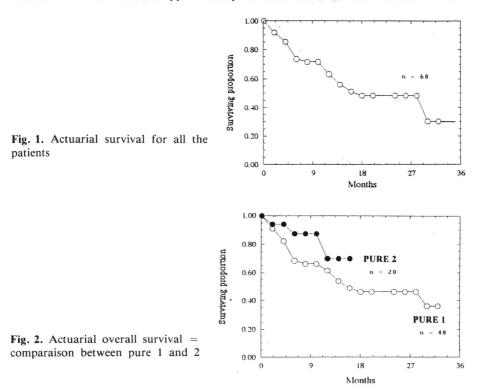

Fig. 1. Actuarial survival for all the patients

Fig. 2. Actuarial overall survival = comparaison between pure 1 and 2

To our knowledge, no trial has compared different schedules of fractionation and duration of treatment. Our results suggest there is an influence of total duration of treatment on complete response and overall survival. We are designing a randomized trial to determine the role of duration of treatment and analyze alterations of fractionation.

References

1. Merlano M, Vitale V, Rooso R et al (1992) Treatment of advanced squamous cell carcinoma of the head and neck with alternating chemotherapy and radiotherapy. N Engl J Med 327, 16 : 1115-1121
2. Vokes EE, Weichselbaum RR (1988) Concomitant chemoradiotherapy : rationale and clinical experience in patients with solid tumors. J Clin Oncol 8 : 911-934
3. Kish JA, Weaver A, Jacobs J et al (1824) Cisplatine and 5-Fluorouracil in patients with recurrent and disseminated epidermoid cancer of the head and neck. Cancer 53 : 1819-1824
4. Merlano M, Grimaldi A, Brunetti I et al (1987) Simultaneous Cisplatine and 5-Fluorouracile as second-line treatment of head and neck cancer. Cancer Treat Rep 71 : 485-488

Abstract. From January 1988 to July 1992, 68 patients with locally advanced and unresectable carcinomas of the head and neck were given 3 to 5 courses of chemotherapy (5-Fluorouracil 1,000 mg/m^2 day 1 to 3, Cisplatin 45 mg/m^2 day 1 and 2, 15 mg/m^2 day 8) combined with simultaneous radiotherapy (until the dose of 45/70 Gy according to response). Two regimens of radiotherapy were performed : the first delivered 70 Gy in 105 days and the second the same dose in only 63 days. The toxicity of this protocol was moderate and acceptable. Sixty-two patients completed their treatment : an objective response was obtained in 85 % (61 % complete response and 24 % partial response) with a higher complete response (80 %) with the shorter treatment. For all the patients, the median survival is 18 months. At 2 and 3 years, the overall survival is respectively 48 and 30 %. These results suggest an influence of total duration of treatment on complete response and overall survival.

Epidermal growth factor receptor in upper aerodigestive tract cancer

JL Formento, M Francoual, O Dassonville, J Santini, A Ramaioli, G Milano, M Schneider, F Demard

The epidermal growth factor receptor (EGFR) is a 170 Kd transmembrane glycoprotein with an intracellular component which is very similar to the v-erb-B oncogene of the avian erythroblastosis virus [1]. The presence of EGFR has been reported in different cancer types [2-9], and it was suggested that the overexpression of EGFR in tumors might be of poor prognosis in breast [10], bladder [5], oesophageal [11], cervical [12], ovarian [13], lung [14] and head and neck cancers [14].

Head and neck squamous cell carcinomas are characterized by local tumoral aggressiveness [15], multifocal lesions in 1 % to 20 % of cases [16], and early recurrences [15]. For head and neck cancer patients, the overall survival remains low and thus, in this cancer type, the identification of reliable tumor markers reflecting tumor aggressiveness could be useful tools for undertaking more or less aggressive treatment.

Material and methods

Patients and sample collection

Tumor biopsies were obtained from 109 consecutive patients with head and neck cancer (100 men and 9 women). Control biopsies were obtained from 94 patients in a symetrical non tumoral area of the same anatomic site. All biopsies were obtained at the time of patient examination for diagnosis when systematic biopsies were performed for histological examination by the pathologist. Tumor localizations were as follows : oral cavity (33), oropharynx (38), larynx (19), hypopharynx (16), nasopharynx (3). Biopsy specimens weighed between 5 and 70 mg. The median age of the study population was 60 years (range 30-85). Histolopathologic grading and tumor staging of the primary tumor were performed according to the specifications of the TNM classification of malignant tumors. For evaluation of results, differentiated tumors were classified as well differentiated, moderately differentiated and poorly differentiated tumors. Seventy-three patients, most of them with advanced tumors (49 stage IV, 13 stage III, 8 stage II, 2 stage I, 1 not determined), were treated by first-line chemotherapy consisting of the following : day 0, 6 hours hydration with 5 % dextrose (2 L), NaCl (6 g L^{-1}), and KCl (3g L^{-1}), followed by cisplatin (CDDP, 100 mg m^{-2}) 1 mg min^{-1} i.v. in normal saline (0.5 L) with 1.6 % mannitol (0.25 L) and then 5 % dextrose (1 L), NaCl (6 g L^{-1}), and KCl (3 g L^{-1}) ; days 1-5, 5-fluorouracil (5-FU) 1,000 mg m^{-2} 24 h^{-1} by continuous i.v. infusion with a controlled flow pump. The protocol called for 3 courses per patients every 3 weeks. Sixty patients were evaluable for response to chemotherapy. Response was evaluated by the same physician 2 weeks after completion of the last chemotherapy course. Clinical response was defined using the product of 2 perpendicular lesion diameters. Complete response (CR) corresponded to disappearance of all clinically visible or palpable lesions ; partial response (PR) was defined as tumor regression of more than 50 % ; no response (NR) corresponded to tumor regression of 50 % or less, stable disease, or progressive disease. The treatment for the 36 patients not treated by first line chemotherapy was surgery (n = 29), radiotherapy (n = 6), no treatment (n = 1). One hundred and three patients were involved in the follow-up. The median duration of follow-up was 18 months (range 3-35).

EGFR determination

Human recombinant ^{125}I-EGF [specific activity 900-1 300 Ci/mmole (ref IM 196)] and unlabeled human recombinant EGF (ref ARM 5 100) were from AMERSHAM (Les Ulis, France). Specific details for EGFR determination were previously published [17].

The single dose assay [18] was used because of the limited amount of biological material provided by most biopsies (5-30 mg). Briefly, 100 μl of each membrane preparation (0.2 − 0.8 mg/ml of membrane protein) were incubated 1.5 hours at room temperature with 100 μl ^{125}I-EGF (1 nM final) in a final volume of 250 μl in the absence (total binding) or in the presence of an excess of unlabeled EGF (160 nM final, non specific binding).

Results

Table I describes the overall distribution of EGFR values in the study population. The presence of detectable EGFR levels was found in all explored tumors with highly marked differences between patients (median 71, range 2-2302 fmol/mg protein). EGFR levels were measurable in only 75 % of cases for healthy control tissue. In 93/94 cases EGFR levels were higher in tumor samples as compared to healthy control zones (Wilcoxon signed rank test, p < 0.0001). There was no significant difference in EGFR expression according to the various anatomic sites explored (Kruskall-Wallis test). There was no significant link between EGFR expression and tumoral differentiation status (Kruskall-Wallis test). There was a significant difference of distribution for EGFR levels between stages I and II tumors (median = 46) and stages III and IV tumors (median = 87) (Mann and Whitney test, p = 0.03). The tumor EGFR levels were not linked to the response to first line chemotherapy by CDDP-5-FU (Mann and Whitney test).

Survival was evaluable for 103 patients for overall survival and for 81 patients for recurrence. The best EGFR cut-off value for overall survival was found located at 120 fmol/mg protein in tumors. Based on this threshold value, EGFR overexpression was associated with shorter relapse-free (p = 0.0125, log rank test) and overall survival (p = 0.028, log rank test) as com-

Table 1. Distribution of EGFR Levels (fmole/mg prot) in head and neck cancer patients

	N° patients	Mean	SD	Median	Range
Anatomic sites					
• *Control*					
All cases	94	12.2	17.8	6.0	0-98
- Oral cavity	32	9.7	14.4	5.0	0-60
- Oropharynx	31	10.9	16.9	3.0	0-63
- Hypopharynx	12	10.3	15.8	5.5	0-57
- Larynx	16	17.4	23.9	10.5	0-98
- Others	3	33.7	20.6	43.0	10-48
• *Tumors*					
All cases	109	165.6	311.6	71.0	2-2302
- Oral cavity	33	90.5	73.0	71.0	3-300
- Oropharynx	38	174.3	240.9	92.5	4-1042
- Hypopharynx	16	133.7	317.2	33.3	2-1307
- Larynx	19	192.4	321.7	64.0	13-1168
- Others	3	878.4	1236.4	259.0	74-2302
Tumor staging					
S I	9	26.1	22.4	24.0	5-74
S II	20	110.1	153.8	73.0	8-722
S III	21	166.7	257.7	61.0	16-2302
S IV	57	168.4	264.0	90.0	3-1168
Tumor differentiation status					
Poor	39	123.1	178.0	58.0	2-963
Moderate	13	436.0	674.1	134.0	19-2302
Well	31	161.2	260.9	88.0	3-1307
Response to chemotherapy					
CR	24	178.0	266.8	107.0	7-1168
NR + PR	36	145.8	246.7	65.0	2-1307

Keys: The chemotherapy protocol was a first line treatment including CDDP and 5-FU (see material and methods section). The statistical significance of the data is presented in the results section.

pared to patients exhibiting lower EGFR levels (Fig. 1). Table 1 compares the prognostic values between EGFR and the tumor staging. Analysing the overall survival by univariate mode revealed that both EGFR and tumor staging were significant variables, with tumor staging achieving the highest significance (p = 0.007) (Table 2). For relapse-free survival EGFR was the only significant parameter (p = 0.047). Confirmation of the respective prognostic values of EGFR and tumor staging comes from multivariate analysis where the only significant variable was EGFR for relapse-free survival and tumor staging for overall survival. The association of EGFR to tumor staging markedly improves the significance for overall survival predictability (p = 0.002). We checked there was no bias in the survival patient analysis introduced by the treatment ad-

Table 2. Prognostic value of tumor EGFR determination

	Relapse n = 81	
Univariate	Chi-2	p-value
Stage	1,58	0,208
EGFR	4,69	0,030
Mulitivariate		
EGFR	4,69	0,030
	Overall survival n = 103	
Univariate		
Stage	7,39	0,007
EGFR	3,94	0,047
Multivariate		
Stage	6,52	0,010
Stage + EGFR	12,58	0,002

ministered to patients [EGFR distribution in patients with chemotherapy versus other treatments (Mann and Whitney test)].

Figure 2 shows the overall survival according to response to first line chemotherapy for all patients treated by first line chemotherapy (CDDP-5-FU). Patients with a CR exhibited a longer survival ($p = 0.018$). The expression of EGFR in the primary tumor allowed CR and NR + PR patients to be discriminated for the overall survival. Thus the longest survival was achieved for patients showing a CR to chemotherapy and having the lowest EGFR levels. At the other end of the scale, the worst prognosis was found in patients with a PR or a NR to chemotherapy with high EGFR levels. Interestingly, there was no difference in the overall survival for patients exhibiting a CR with high EGFR levels and those with NR + PR with low EGFR levels ($p = 0.834$).

Discussion

We observed that EGFR levels were, in most cases (93/94), expressed at higher levels in the tumor as compared to the healthy control tissue of the same patient. One can wonder about the significance of detectable EGFR levels in an apparently healthy tissue of head and neck cancer patients. Scambia et al have shown that EGFR was expressed in the laryngeal mucosa of healthy subjects [19]. Interestingly, Berger et al [20] have reported higher EGFR levels in the mucosa of healthy subjects overexposed to alcohol and tobacco as compared to other controls with low or moderate consumption of alcohol and tobacco. It would be interesting to prospectively evaluate the relative propor-

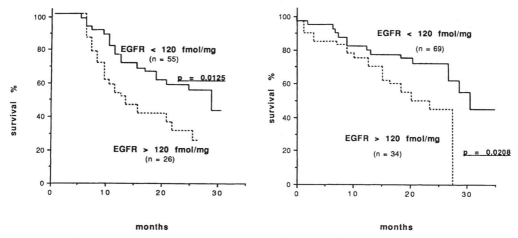

Fig. 1. Survival curves for study patients according to EGFR expression in the primary tumor. *Top :* relapse free survival ; *bottom :* overall survival

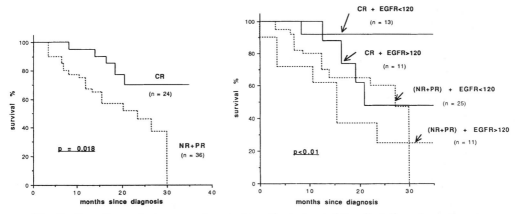

Fig. 2. Overall survival curves for study patients treated by first line chemotherapy including CDDP and 5-FU. *Top :* survival according to the response to treatment, *bottom :* survival according to the response to treatment and EGFR expression in the primary tumor

tion of cancers developed in high risk subjects showing different level of EGFR expression in the oral mucosa.

In the present study it was not possible to establish a relationship between the anatomic site of the tumoral lesion and the quality of EGFR sites. This is in line with the data reported by Ishitoya et al [21] who analyzed the presence of EGFR in head and neck cancers both by gene amplification and by its overexpression. As concerns the link between tumor differentiation and EGFR levels, the data are rather conflicting. Some investigators have shown that well differentiated tumors overexpressed EGFR [21], others reported high EGFR levels in undifferentiated tumors [14, 19, 22] and, finally, others found no relationship at all [23, 24]. We add to the confusion by noting that moderately differentiated tumors were those with the highest EGFR levels ; Ebrahim El-Zayat et al made a similar observation [25].

Previous studies on EGFR suggest its value as a prognostic marker for cancer [2-9]. Our preliminary work on EGFR in head and neck cancer strongly suggested its usefulness at a prognostic level as EGFR levels were linked to tumor size and disease staging [17]. The present data confirm the positive association between EGFR and tumor staging in head and neck cancer. The value of EGFR as an indicator of bad prognosis is established and EGFR is even more powerful than tumor stage for relapse-free survival ; this finding is not surprising by itself since the presence of EGFR is linked to the proliferative potential of the tumor cells. Santon et al [26] observed that the expansion rate of A 431 epidermal cells was associated to the expression levels of EGFR. Interestingly, EGFR expression was found to be complementary to the tumor staging for predicting overall survival. First line treatment of head and neck cancer by chemotherapy associating CDDP and 5-FU allows an interesting response rate to be obtained for advanced lesions [27, 28]. In a group of 406 head and neck cancer patients in our institute by this chemotherapy protocol, the response to treatment was shown to be linked to patient overall survival [29]. In our opinion, the most clinically relevant finding of the present study is the fact that EGFR expression in the primary tumor is able to stratify overall survival among the different groups of responders to chemotherapy ; thus, among CR patients, 90 % of those with the lowest EGFR levels were alive after 38 months of follow-up ; this percentage was close to 50 % for the CR patients whose primary tumor expressed high EGFR levels. Even more interestingly, there was no difference in survival between CR patients with high EGFR and NR + PR patients with low EGFR. Among the different groups of chemotherapy responders, the survival discrimination by tumor EGFR expression may be on the intrinsic tumor agressivity conferred by the presence of EGFR ; this can be true for NR + PR patients ; it is also possible that among CR there are patients with microscopic residual disease, the evolution of which differs according to the EGFR levels. For head and neck cancer patients, the benefit of first line chemotherapy by CDDP-5-FU is now discussed in terms of survival, as compared to other alternative treatments [30]. The possibility given by EGFR determination for early identification of those patients who will really benefit from a first line chemotherapy protocol is of potential clinical importance. Thus it is possible that for patients with high EGFR other treatment approaches could be considered. On the other hand, EGFR must not be taken solely as a prognostic marker but also as a tumor signal allowing specific treatment to be undertaken targeting EGFR. For instance, EGFR directed therapeutic tools are available and may include tyrosine kinase inhibitors [31] or monoclonal anti-EGFR antibodies [32].

In conclusion, EGFR determination should deserve particular attention in head and neck cancer since it carries a strong prognostic value by itself. It allows survival among first line chemotherapy responder categories to be discrininated and finally it may offer further treatment options based on specific EGFR tumor targeting.

References

1. Downward J, Yarden Y, Mayes E et al (1984) Close similarity of epidermal growth factor receptor and verb B oncogene protein sequences : Nature 307 : 521-527
2. Fitzpatrick SL, Brightwell J, Wittliff JL, Barrows GH, Schultz GS (1984) Epidermal growth factor binding by breast tumour biopsies and relationship to estrogen and progestin receptor levels. Cancer Res 44 : 3448-3453
3. Perez R, Pascual M, Macias A, Lage A (1984) Epidermal growth factor receptors in human breast cancer. Breast Cancer Res Treat 4 : 189-193
4. Veale D, Ashcroft T, Marsh C, Gibson GJ, Harris AL (1987) Epidermal growth factor receptors in non-small cell lung cancer. Br J Cancer 55 : 513-516
5. Neal DE, Marsh C, Bennett MK, Abel PD, Harris AL (1985) Epidermal growth factor receptors in human bladder cancer : comparisons of invasive and superficial tumors. Lancet i : 366-368
6. Liberman TA, Razon N, Bartal AD, Yarden Y, Schlessinger J, Soreq H (1984) Expression of epidermal growth factor receptors in human brain tumors. Cancer Res 44 : 753-760
7. Gullick WJ, Marsdeen JJ, Whittle N, Ward B, Bobrow L, Waterfield MD (1987) Expression of epidermal growth factor receptors on human cervical, ovarian and vulvar carcinomas. Cancer Res 46 : 285-292
8. Cowley G, Smith JA, Gusterson B, Hendler F, Ozanne B (1984) The amount of EGF receptor is elevated in squamous cell carcinomas. In : Levine AJ, Van de Wande GF, Toppe WC, Watson JD (eds) The cancer cell. Cold Spring Harbord Laboratory, New York, pp. 5-10
9. Ozanne B, Shum A, Richards CS et al (1985) Evidence for an increase in EGF receptors in epidermal malignancy. In : Ceramisco J, Ozanne B, Stiles (eds) Cancer cells growth factors and transformation. Vol 3. Cold Spring Harbor Laboratory, New York, pp. 41-49.
10. Sainsbury JRC, Farndon JR, Needham GK, Malcom AJ, Harris AL (1987) Epidermal growth factor receptor as predictor of early recurrence of and death from breast cancer. Lancet i : 1398-1402
11. Ozawa S, Ueda M, Ando N, Shimizu N, Abe O (1989) Prognostic significance of epidermal growth factor receptor in esophageal squamous cell carcinomas. Cancer 63 : 2169-2173
12. Pfeiffer D, Stellwag B, Pfeiffer A, Borlinghaus P, Meier W, Scheidel P (1989) Clinical implications of the epidermal growth factor receptor in the squamous cell carcinoma of the uterine cervix. Gynecol Oncol 33 : 146-150
13. Bauchnecht T, Kohler M, Janz I, Pfleider A (1989) The occurrence of epidermal growth factor receptors and the characterization of EGF-like factors in human ovarian, endometrial, cervical and breast cancer. J Cancer Res Clin Oncol 115 : 193-199
14. Hendler F, Shum Siu A, Nanu L, Ozanne B (1988) Overexpression of EGF receptors in squamous tumors is associated with poor survival. J Cell Biochem S 12A : 105
15. Slaughter DP, Southwick HM, Smejkal W (1953) « Field cancerization » in oral stratified squamous epithelium. Cancer 6 : 963-968
16. Hsairi M, Luce D, Point D, Rodriguez J, Brugere J, Leclerc A (1989) Risk factors for simultaneous carcinoma of the head and neck. Head and Neck 11 : 426-430
17. Santini J, Formento JL, Francoual M et al (1991) Characterization, quantification, and potential clinical value of the epidermal growth factor receptor in head and neck squamous cell carcinomas. Head and Neck 13 : 132-139
18. Formento JL, Francoual M, Formento P et al (1990) Epidermal growth factor recep-

tor assay : validation of a single point method and application to breast cancer. Breast Cancer Res Treat 17 : 211-219
19. Scambia G, Benedetti Panici P, Battaglia F et al (1991) Receptors for epidermal growth factor and steroid hormones in primary laryngeal tumors. Cancer 67 : 1347-1351
20. Bergler W, Bier H, Ganzer U (1989) The expression of epidermal growth factor receptors in the oral mucosa of patients with oral cancer. Arch Otorhinolaryngol, 246 : 121-125
21. Ishitoya J, Toriyama M, Oguchi N et al (1989) Gene amplification and overexpression of EGF receptor in squamous cell carcinomas of the head and neck. Br J Cancer 59 : 559-562
22. King I, Sartorelli AC (1987) Relationship between epidermal growth factor (EGF) receptor levels, its kinase activity, and the terminal differentiation of human squamous carcinoma cells. Proc AACR 28 : 61
23. Miyaguchi M, Olofsson J, Hellquist HB (1990) Expression of epidermal growth factor receptor in laryngeal dysplasia and carcinoma. Acta Otolaryngol (Stockh.) 110 : 309-313
24. Kamata N, Chida K, Rikimaru K, Horikoshi M, Enomoto S, Kuroki T (1986) Growth-inhibitory effects of epidermal growth factor and overexpression of its receptors on human squamous cell carcinomas in culture. Cancer Res 46 : 1648-1653
25. Ebrahim El-Zayat AA, Pingree TH, Mock PM, Clark GM, Otto RA, Von Hoff DD (1991) Epidermal growth factor receptor amplification in head and neck cancer. Cancer Journal 4 : 375-381
26. Santon JB, Cronin MT, Mac Leod CL, Mendelsohn J, Masui H, Gill GN (1986) Effects of epidermal growth factor receptor concentration on tumoregencity of A 431 cells in nude mice. Cancer Res 46 : 4701-4705
27. Amrein PC, Weitzman SA (1985) Treatment of squamous cell carcinoma of the head and neck with cisplatin and 5-fluorouracil. J Clin Oncol 3 : 1632-1639
28. Vokes EE, Schilsky RL, Weichselsaum RR, Kozloff MF, Panje NR (1990) Induction chemotherapy with cisplatin, fluororuacil and high-dose leucovorin for locally advanced head neck cancer : a clinical and pharmacologic analysis. J Clin Oncol 8 : 241-247
29. Thyss A, Schneider M, Santini J, Demard F (1986) Induction chemotherapy with cis-platinum and 5-Fluorouracil for squamous cell carcinoma of the head and neck. Br J Cancer 54 : 755-760
30. Vokes EE, Mikes R, Lester EP, Panje WR, Weichselbaum RR (1991) Cisplatin and fluorouracil chemotherapy does not yield longt-term benefit in locally advanced head and neck cancer : results from a single institution. J Clin Oncol 9 : 1376-1384
31. Schwartsmann G, Workman P (1992) Anticancer drug screening and discovery in the 19905 : a European perspective. Eur J Cancer 29 : 3-14
32. Fong CJ, Sherwood ER, Mendelsohn J, Lee C, Kozlowsky JM (1992) Epidermal growth factor receptor monoclonal antibody inhibits constitutive receptor phosphorylation, reduces autonomous growth and sensitizes androgen-independent prostatic carcinoma cells to tumor necrosis factor α. Cancer Res 52 : 5887-5892

Abstract. *EGFR was determined in tumor biopsies obtained from 109 consecutive patients with head and neck cancer (100 men and 9 women). Control biopsies were obtained from 94 patients in a symetrical non tumoral area of the same anatomic site. EGFR was measured by a binding assay using human recombinant ^{125}I-EGF.*

The presence of detectable EGFR levels was found in all explored tumors with highly marked differences between patients (median 71, range 2-2302 fmol/mg protein). In 93/94 cases EGFR levels were higher in tumor samples as compared to healthy control zones. There was a significant difference of distribution for EGFR levels between stages I and II tumors and stages III and IV tumors. The tumor EGFR levels were not linked to the response to first line chemotherapy by CDDP-5-FU.

The best EGFR cut-off value for overall survival was found located at 120 fmol/mg protein in tumors. EGFR overexpression was associated with shorter relapse-free ($p = 0.0125$) and overall survival ($p = 0.028$).

By multivariate analysis the only significant variable was EGFR for relapse-free survival and tumor staging for overall survival. The association of EGFR to tumor staging markedly improves the significance for overall survival predictability ($p = 0.002$).

The expression of EGFR in the primary tumor allowed CR and NR + PR patients to be discriminated for the overall survival. The longest survival was achieved for patients showing a CR to chemotherapy and having the lowest EGFR levels.

Concomitant α-Interferon and chemotherapy in advanced squamous cell carcinoma of the head and neck

M Benasso, M Merlano, F Blengio, M Cavallari, R Rosso, S Toma

Experimental and clinical data suggest a possible role of Biological Response Modifiers alone or in combination with chemotherapy in treatment of several human tumors [1, 3].

To date few clinical data have been published on head and neck cancer without definitive results [4, 8].

Therefore we started a phase II trial to test, in relapsed or persistent squamous cell carcinoma of head and neck, the feasibility and the activity of a combination of Cisplatin (CDDP), 5-Fluorouracil (5-FU) and recombinant Interferon alpha 2b (rIFN-α-2b).

From July 1990 and December 1991, 14 patients (pts) entered the study. Patients and tumor characteristics are shown in Table 1.

Table 1. Patients and tumor characteristics

N° PTS	14
Sex	
Male	12
Female	2
Age (yr)	
≤ 60	4
> 60	10
Performance status	
median	1
range	0-2
Site of primary	
Nasophraynx	2
Oropharynx	2
Oral cavity	4
Larynx	6
Site of involvement	
T	9
N	4
T + N	1
Pretreatment	
S + RT	8
RT	5
S + RT + CT	1

S = Surgery, RT = Radiotherapy, CT = Chemotherapy

Dept. of Medical Oncology I, Istituto Nazionale per la Ricerca sul Cancro, V. le Benedetto XV, 10, 16132 Genoa, Italy

In particular 3 pts had persistent and 11 relapsed disease after surgery and radiotherapy (9 pts) or radiotherapy alone (5 pts).

All patients but one had not been treated with prior chemotherapy.

Physical examination, chest X-ray, complete blood count and chemistry were performed as pretreatment evaluation.

All patients received a combination of CDDP (20 mg/m^2/day i.v.), 5-FU (200 mg/m^2/day i.v.) and rIFN-α-2b (3 MIU/day i.m.) for 5 consecutive days.

Recombinant IFNα-2b was also administered 3 times/week during cycles interval and, in responders, was continued at the same dosage from the end of treatment up to progression disease to maintain the response achieved.

Supportive therapies included Paracetamol (500 mg orally), 30' before rIFN-α-2b administration, to prevent « flu-like » symptoms. Paracetamol was repeated every 8 hours if necessary.

Toxicity was evaluated before each chemotherapy (CT) course and evaluation of response was performed after the second cycle and after every further cycle ; both toxicity and response were recorded according to WHO scale [6].

Time to progression was calculated from the beginning of treatment up to progression or last follow-up.

All the patients have been evaluated for toxicity (Table 2).

Table 2. Toxicity

Grade (WHO scale)	I	II	III	IV
Nausea-vomiting	4	3	1	—
Diarrhea	1	—	—	—
Mucositis	—	1	—	—
Leukopenia	1	6	2	—
Anemia	—	3	2	1
Thrombocytopenia	1	4	2	2
Anorexia		3		
Fatigue		7		
« Flu-like » symptoms (chill, fever, malaise, muscle pain)		6		

A grade III-IV haematological toxicity was observed in 43 % of pts (grade III-IV thrombocytopenia and anemia in 4 and 3 pts respectively and grade III leukopenia in 2 pts) ; grade III nausea and vomiting was recorded in 1 patient (pt).

« Flu-like » symptoms were observed in 43 % of pts. Fatigue and anorexia were experienced by most pts.

Only 5 pts underwent the treatment as planned due to toxicity : a CT delay was necessary in 9 pts and 5 pts needed a rIFN-α-2b discontinuation.

Because of severe thrombocytopenia (3 pts) and severe pancytopenia (1 pt), rIFN-α-2b administration was definitely stopped.

All the pts but one (lost to follow-up) were evaluable for response.

The overall response rate was 54 % (31 % CR, 23 % PR).

Four out of 5 pts who completed the treatment plan, achieved an objective response (2 CR and 2 PR).

Median time to progression for responders was 8 months (range 5-14).

Only 1 pt out of responders continue rIFN-α-2b at the end of treatment.

According to the « minimum 2 stage » design of Simon [7] 29 pts were foreseen for the study, but the accrual was early stopped due to toxicity.

In particular the haematological toxicity (50 % grade III-IV) has been higher than expected with CT alone with the same regimen [5] and entire compliance was generally lower.

The combination employed in our trial has an antitumoral activity similar, in terms of overall response rate, to that reported with the best CT regimen without rIFN-α-2b [2, 5].

However we observed 4/5 clinical response in pts who completed the treatment as planned.

Further investigation are mandatory.

References

1. Carmichael J, Fregusson RJ, Wolf CR et al (1986) Augmentation of cytotoxicity of chemotherapy by uman alpha-Interferons in human non small cell lung cancer xenografts. Cancer Res 46 : 4916-4920
2. Kish JA, Weaver A, Jacobs J et al (1984) Cisplatin and 5-Fluorouracil infusion in patients with recurrent and disseminated epidermoid cancer of the head and neck. Cancer 53 : 1819-1824
3. Mandelli F (1990) Maintenance treatment with recombinant Interferon-α-2b in patients with multiple myeloma responding to conventional induction chemotherapy. N Engl J Med 322 : 1430
4. Medenica R, Slack M (1985) Clinical results of leucocyte Interferon induced tumor regression in resistant human metastatic cancer resistant to chemotherapy and/or radiotherapy-pulse therapy schedule. Cancer Drug Deliv 2 : 53-76
5. Merlano M, Grimaldi A, Brunetti I et al (1987) Simultaneous Cisplatin and 5-Fluorouracil as second line treatment of head and neck cancer. Cancer Treat Rep 71 : 485-488
6. Miller AB, Hoogstraten B, Staquet M et al (1981) Reporting results of cancer treatment. Cancer 47 : 207-210
7. Simon R (1989) Optimal two-stage designs for phase II clinical trials. Controlled Clinical Trials 10 : 1-10
8. Vlock DR, Jonson J, Myers E et al (1991) Preliminary trial of nonrecombinant Interpheron-α in recurrent squamous cell carcinoma of the head and neck. Head and Neck 13 : 15-21

Thymidylate synthase activity and Folate levels in head and neck squamous cell carcinomas

O Parise Jr*, F Janot*, B Luboinski*, M Verjus**, A Gouyette**, GG Cabot**

Currently, the choice of the treatment strategy in head and neck squamous cell carcinoma (HNSCC) is based on the following clinical characteristics: tumor volume and site, loco-regional spread and/or metastatic dissemination of the primary. However, these clinical parameters may not take into account biological factors that could better predict the outcome of therapy.

The treatment of HNSCC is now based on the combination of surgery and radiotherapy. Although the role of chemotherapy in HNSCC remains controversial, a variety of drugs are being used as single agent, or in combination chemotherapy regimens.

The single most efficient agent in HNSCC is Cisplatin (CDDP) [1], usually administered in combination with 5-Fluorouracil (5-FU). Although CDDP/5-FU-containing neoadjuvant regimens yield high response rates (60-90 %), with 20-50 % of complete remissions [2], better survival rates are not yet achieved [3]. It is possible that the high response rates observed with current Neo Adjuvant regimens may reflect a patients selection with a good prognosis [4], rather than the chemotherapy efficacy.

Clinically, it is often observed that HNSCC which have similar histopathologic features exhibit various degrees of chemosensitivity. These differences in chemosensitivity may be partly due to drug-metabolizing enzyme systems involved in either activation and/or detoxication of drugs.

In an attempt to better understand the interpatient variability in terms of response to the major drugs employed in HNSCC treatment (i.e. 5-FU and CDDP), we have studied thymidylate synthase activity (TS) and folate levels in HNSCC and their corresponding normal adjacent mucosae from 24 untreated patients. The choice of TS is based on its involvement in chemoresistance to 5-FU [reviewed in 5], and its probable relation to CDDP resistance [6]. Folates are also involved in 5-FU sensitivity by stabilizing the ternary complex formed by the enzyme TS and 5-Fluoro-deoxyuridine monophosphate.

Patients and methods

Patients included in this prospective study had histologically proven head and neck squamous cell carcinoma, and were not previously treated with radiation or chemotherapy.

---

* Department of Head and Neck Surgery, ** Laboratory of Clinical Pharmacology, Institut Gustave-Roussy, rue Camille-Desmoulins, 94805 Villejuif Cedex, France

Tumor tissues were obtained from the surgical specimens, and normal mucosae from the disease-free margins of the same specimens, at least 1.5 cm from the tumor limits. All specimens underwent histopathological evaluation.

Tumors and normal mucosae were immediately frozen in liquid nitrogen after resection in the operating room, and tissues were stored in a freezer ($-80°$ C) until asssays for TS and folates.

For TS activity measurements, the tissue samples were homogenized in Tris-HCl buffer containing beta-Mercaptoethanol. Cytosols used for TS measurements were obtained by centrifugation (60 mn, 105 000 $\times$ g). TS activity was assayed by the method described by Houghton et al [7]. Briefly, the addition of ^{3}H-dUMP and the reduced folates promote the formation of the ternary complex ^{3}H-dUMP-TS-folates. Endogenous dUMP, as well as the free
^{3}H-dUMP (unbound to the ternary complex) were removed by filtering the samples through fiberglass filters. The radioactivity emitted from these samples is proportional to TS activity expressed in pmoles/mn/mg protein. To assess reproducibility, a duplicate internal standard control was included in each assay (liver of newborn mice). Cytosolic proteins were measured using the Bradford method [8] (Bio-Rad Protein Assay).

For folate measurement the tissue samples were homogenized in a solution containing Tris-HCl, mannitol and sucrose. Folate levels were assayed in the homogenates, using a commercially available kit for folates radiodetermination (Magic Lite Folated Ciba Corning kit). An internal standard control was included in each assay. Protein concentrations were determined by the bicinchoninic acid assay [9] using the Pierce BCA Protein Assay Reagent.

The Wilcoxon test was used for the statistical analysis of TS activity in tumors compared to mucosae, given that the standard deviations between the two tissue types were not comparable. The Student paired *t* test was used to compare folate levels in tumors and mucosae. Differences were considered significant when p value was below 0.05. Results are presented as mean $\pm$ SD.

Results

Patient characteristics

The patient population comprised 21 men and 3 women with ages ranging from 48 to 68 years (mean 59.9 years). The following primary sites included : oral cavity (2 patients), oropharynx (4), larynx (12) and hypopharynx (6). 21 patients had histologically proven well-differentiated HNSCC, and 3 patients had poorly-differentiated HNSCC. The clinical staging was as follows : 8 patients had clinical stage II, 4 patients had stage III, 11 patients had stage IV and 1 patient presented with a previous partial laryngectomy performed 6 years before the local recurrence.

Thymidylate synthase activity

TS activity was detected in all the 20 tumor specimens and in 17/22 specimens of normal mucosae assayed. The mean TS activity for tumor samples was 12.2 ± 39.4 pmol/mn/mg protein, and 0.6 ± 0.8 pmol/mn/mg protein (p = 0.0001) for mucosae. The interpatient variability was however high in tumors, with approximately a 180-fold difference between the lowest and the highest TS activity.

Folate levels

Folates concentrations were detectable in 15/18 tumor specimens and in 11/18 normal mucosa samples assayed. The mean concentration for tumor samples was 1.16 ± 1.05 pmol/mg protein and 0.82 ± 0.87 pmol/mg protein for mucosae (p = 0.1).

Discussion

Vokes and collaborators' clinical trial published in 1990 combining CDDP/5-FU/Leucovorin to treat 31 locally advanced HNSCC patients achieved 26 objective responses among 29 evaluable patients [10]. This result is noteworthy : the regimen was based on a rational drug combination which promoted the direct and indirect optimal inhibition of TS activity, and illustrates the therapeutic interest in the role of TS in sensitivity to these cytotoxic drugs in HNSCC.

In order to be active, 5-FU must be converted into Fluoro-deoxyuridine monophosphate (FdUMP). The main mechanism of action of 5-FU could result from the direct inhibition of TS by FdUMP which forms a stable ternary complex (FdUMP-TS-folates) in the presence of folates. TS is the enzyme that catalyzes the methylation of deoxyuridine monophosphate (dUMP) resulting in the formation of thymidine monophosphate, an essential precursor of deoxythymidine triphosphate (dTTP) one of the four deoxyribonucleotides required for DNA synthesis [reviewed in 5]. FdUMP cytotoxicity could also be due to its direct incorporation into RNA. Whether FdUMP is incorporated into DNA and as a consequence gives rise to cytotoxic activity remains unknown [11]. The synergistic relationship between 5-FU and CDDP is also related to TS activity [6].

Resistance to 5-FU may be related to TS in many ways : altered enzyme kinetics of TS, an increase in the level of dUMP or a decrease in FdUMP concentration, reduced stability of the ternary complex FdUMP-TS-folates, intracellular depletion of folates, increased TS synthesis or amplification of the gene coding for TS [11-17].

Since 5-FU cytotoxicity is linked to the inhibition of TS activity, and TS activity seems itself correlated to response to 5-FU in colorectal and breast cancers [11, 14, 18], it was of interest to investigate TS activity in HNSCC and their corresponding mucosae in a prospective study, in an attempt to find predictors of response in patients. We have found that tumor TS levels were significantly higher than their corresponding mucosae. These data are in accordance with other studies that have shown a 5-fold higher TS activity in lung and gastric squamous cell carcinomas [19, 20]. Also in accordance with other investigators studying TS activity in colorectal tumors [21], we also have found a high interpatient variability in our HNSCC population.

Since increased TS activity in HNSCC may be linked to an increased DNA synthesis rate, it seems worthwhile conducting further studies to determine whether a correlation exists between TS activity and DNA ploidy or doubling time.

Folates is a term used to define the different analogues of the pteroylglutamic acid, namely co-enzymes needed for a whole series of biosynthesis reactions [12]. The combination of 5-FU and folates (Leucovorin) in clinical practice has demonstrated its efficacy, particularly in the treatment of colorectal cancer [13-17].

Our data did not show a significant difference between tumors and mucosae in terms of folate concentrations. It is however difficult to interpret the significance of these data because of the variation in blood content of the samples may have biaised the assay. In spite of this possible technical drawback, the determination of folate levels in tissue samples will be an essential component of a prospective study of the relationship between TS activity and chemoresponsiveness to 5-FU and CDDP.

The clinical importance of interpatient variability in tumor TS activity still remains to be established in HNSCC, considering that in most cases the short clinical follow up does not yet allow the correlation of this activity with respect to prognosis.

In conclusion this study has focused on TS activity and folate levels in HNSCC which are both involved in cellular sensitivity to 5-FU and CDDP. Our results showed increased TS activity in tumors compared to mucosae, with an important degree of interpatient variability for tumor samples. The real significance of TS variability is now being explored in relation to chemosensitivity to 5-FU and CDDP, and also in relation to HNSCC behavior. Provided that correlations are found, it could then be possible to tailor HNSCC treatment to individual patients, and hopefully increase survival rate in this disease.

Acknowledgement. The authors are grateful to Ms Lorna Saint-Ange for revision of the manuscript.

References

1. Taylor SG (1987) Head and neck cancer. In : Pinedo HM, Chabner BA (eds) Cancer chemotherapy, vol. 7. Elsevier, Amsterdam, pp 287-301
2. Al-Sarraf M (1988) Head and neck cancer : Chemotherapy concepts. Sem Oncology 15 (1) : 70-85
3. Jacobs C (1989) Adjuvant chemotherapy for head and neck cancer, Editorial. J Clin Oncol 7 (7) : 823-826
4. Luboinski B, Richard JM, Wibault P, Sancho-Garnier H (1983) Pelvimandibulectomie après chimiothérapie première — A propos de 71 Cas. J Eur Radiother 4 (3) : 143-150
5. Grem JL (1990) Fluorinated Pyrimidines. In : BA Chabner, JM Collins (eds) Cancer Chemotherapy Principles and Practice. JB Lippincot Co, Philadelphia, pp 180-224

6. Scanlon KJ, Kashani-Sabet M, Miyachi H, Sowers LC, Rossi J (1989) Molecular Basis of Cisplatin Resistance in Carcinomas : Model Systems and Patients. Anticancer Research 9 : 1301-1312
7. Houghton JA, Radparvar S, Torrance PM, Williams LG, Houghton P (1987) Determination of Thymidylate Synthase Activity in Colon Tumor Tissues After Treatment with 5-Fluorouracil. Biochem Pharmacol 36 (8) : 1285-1289
8. Smith PK, Krohn RI, Hermanson GT et al (1985) Measurement of Protein Using Bicinchoninic Acid Anal Biochem 150 : 76-85
9. Bradford MM (1976) A Rapid and Sensitive Method for the Quantitation of Microgram Quantities of Protein Utilizing the Principle of Protein-dye Binding. Anal Biochem 72 : 248-254
10. Vokes EE, Schilsky RL, Weichselbaum RR, Kozloff MF, Panje WR (1990) Induction Chemotherapy with Cisplatin, Fluorouracil, and high-dose Leucovorin for locally advanced head and neck cancer : A Clinical and Pharmacological Analysis. J Clin Oncol 8 (2) : 241-247
11. Peters GJ, van Groeningen CJ (1991) Clinical Relevance of Biochemical Modulation of 5-Fluorouracil, Review. Ann Oncol 2 : 469-480
12. Devlin TM (1986) (Ed) Textbook of Biochemistry, 2nd Edition. John Wiley & Sons, New York
13. Spears CP, Gustavsson BG, Berne M, Frosing R, Brenstein L, Hay AA (1988) Mechanism of Innate Resistance to Thymidylate Synthase Inhibition after 5-Fluorouracyl. Cancer Res 48 : 5894-5900
14. Doroshow JH, Multhauf P, Leong L et al (1990) Propective Randomized Comparison of Fluorouracil Versus Fluorouracil and High-Dose Continuous Infusion Leucovorin Calcium for the Treatment of advanced measurable colorectal cancer in Patients Previously Unexposed to Chemotherapy. J Clin Oncol 8 : 491-501
15. Poon MA, O'Connell MJ, Moertel CG (1989) Biochemical Modulation of Fluorouracil : Evidence of Significant Improvement of Survival and Quality of Life in Patients with advanced colorectal carcinoma. J Clin Oncol 7 : 1407-1417
16. Erlichman C, Fine S, Wong A, Elhakin T (1988) A Randomized Trial of Florouracil and Folinic Acid in Patients with Metastatic Colorectal Carcinoma. J Clin Oncol 6 (3) : 469-475
17. Bleyer WA (1989) New Vistas for Leucovorin in cancer chemotherapy. Cancer 63 : 995-1007
18. Spears CP, Waugh W, Leichman L et al (1990) Salvage Therapy of breast cancer with Fluorouracil and high-dose of Leucovorin : Response Correlations with Tumor Pharmacodinamics. Proc Am Soc Clin Oncol (Abstract) 282, 9 : 73
19. Maehara Y, Kusumoto T, Kusumoto H et al 5-Fluorouracil and UFT-Sensitive Gastric Carcinoma has a High Level of Thymidylate Synthase. Cancer 63 : 1693-1696
20. Maehara Y, Moruguchi S, Emi Y et al (1990) Comparaison of Pyrimidine Nucleotide Syntheic Enzymes Involved in 5-Fluorouracil Metabolism Between Human Adenocarcinomas and squamous cell carcinomas. Cancer 66 : 156-161
21. Bardot V, Luccioni C, Lefrançois D, Muleris M, Dutrillaux B (1991) Activity of Thymidylate Synthase, Thymidylate Kinase and Galactokinase in Primary and xenografted human colorectal cancer in Relation to their Chromossomal Patterns. Int J Cancer 47 : 670-674

Abstract. Head and neck squamous cell carcinomas (HNSCC) present variable aggressivity and sensitivity to chemotherapy. Cisplatin (CDDP) and 5-Fluorouracil (5-FU) are the main drugs used for the treatment of HNSCC. The activity of thymidylate synthase (TS) is related to folate levels and is involved in 5-FU resistance. TS was also related to CDDP resistance.

We assayed the TS activity and the folate levels in HNSCC and their corresponding normal adjacent mucosae from 24 untreated patients.

Results showed a markedly higher activity of TS in tumors compared to mucosae : 12.2 versus 0.6 pmoles/mn/mg protein ($p = 0.0001$) with an important tumoral interpatient variability. The folate levels in tumors and mucosae were 1.16 and 0.82 pmoles/mg protein ($p = 0.1$), respectively.

These results may be useful to better understand the variability in the HNSCC behavior or interpatient differences in drug sensitivity.

Long term nephrotoxicity of Cisplatinum (CDDP) in man

Y Bahmed[*], M Déchaux[*], V Bassot, D Brasnu, C Kindermans[*], H Laccourreye, C Sachs[*]

The prognosis of solid malignant tumors has been largely improved by the use of Platinum compounds and specially of Cisplatin. This agent, both alone and in combination with other antineoplastic drugs has been shown to be effective in treating testicular, ovarian, and urinary bladder carcinomas and tumors of the head and neck. The therapeutic efficacity of this drug increases with increasing dose but in the same time, acute and may be long-term toxicity including nephrotoxicity is also dose-related. Nephrotoxicity has been dramatically reduced when systematic hydration has been given during or sometimes before and during administration of the drug. The different ways of hydration proposed in the literature include IV saline infusion, 2 to 3 liters a day, and less frequently osmotic diuresis with Mannitol or Furosemide (Hayes 1977, Vogl 198, Groth 1986).

In most papers, nephrotoxicity has been evaluated by creatinine clearance (Dentino 1978, Davila 1987, Reed 1991, Pinnaro 1986). As a matter of fact, creatinine could be a poor marker for GFR in these conditions (Meijer 1983, cancer, Hansen 1988, Daugaard 1988, Davila 1987, Reed 1991), and variation in true GFR not reflected by variations in creatinine clearances (Buahmah 1982, Meijer 1983, Markman 1991). When isotopic methods have been used (Fjelborg 1986, Groth 1986, Daugaard 1988), CDDP-induced fall in GFR has been estimated to be 15 to 30 % of pre-treatment values.

Our present study reports time-course of renal function following administration of high-doses of Cisplatin, CDDP being given as continuous IV continuous perfusions in ambulatory patients and prevention of nephrotoxicity performed with daily oral administration of 20 to 40 ml/kg/24 hours of tap water. Renal function has been measured by reference methods i.e. inulin and para amino hippurate (PAH) clearances for estimation of glomerular filtration rate (GFR) and renal plasma flow (RPF).

Material and methods

Patients included in this study protocol had malignant tumors in which Cisplatinum chemotheray was indicated. CDDP therapy was scheduled in out-patients and was given ambulatory via a pump permitting thus a sub-normal activity at home. A cycle of Cisplatin administration consisted in a continuous Cisplatinum infusion of 20 to 25 mg/m^2/24 h during 6 consecutive days. The next

---

[*] Department of Physiology and Head and Neck Surgery Department, Laennec Hospital, Paris, France

cycle was started after a 2 week stop period and when possible, doses were then increased to 25-30 mg/m²/24 h during 6 other consecutive days. Each patients received at least three cycles. When no surgery was proposed, a total of 6 cures was indicated. As a matter of fact, cumulative Cisplatin doses during this study ranged between 186 and 386 mg/m² body area. Chemotherapy protocol constantly associated 5-Fluorouracil at the dose of 1,000 mg/day during 6 days in parallel with CDDP. During the Cisplatin administration period, oral ingestion of 20 to 40 ml/kg/day of tap water was recommended ; as prevention of nauseas and vomiting, alizaprid, was constantly associated. All patients were informed of the aim of the study i.e. evaluation of CDDP nephrotoxicity, a free acceptance being obtained in each case. The protocol of follow-up of renal function included 4 determinations : the first one has been performed in all patients (n = 25) prior to Cisplatin administration and the 3 others scheduled 1 month (14 patients), 3 to 6 months (16 patients), and 12 months after the end of Cisplatin administration (15 patients). Thirteen patient has been investigated at least twice including basal time, 8 others at 3 times and 4 others at the 4 times. RBF and GFR were determined as PAH and inulin clearance : an I.V. priming dose of PAH (10 mg/kg b.w.) and of inulin (50mg/kg b.w.) was followed by infusion of a saline solution containing PAH and inulin, at a rate of 50 ml/hour during 3 hours. The first one-hour period was devoted to equilibration of PAH and inulin concentrations between the different hydric compartments. Thereafter, 4 urine collections were obtained from spontaneous voiding every 30 minutes. Oral water intake maintained an urine flow rate between 6 and 10 ml/minute in each case. Plasma samples for inulin and PAH determinations were obtained before infusion and as the mid-point of each urine collection time. Before the clearance period, total and ionized calcium, phosphate, magnesium, parathormone, Vitamin-D, 25 (OH) D_3 and 1.25 (OH) $_2D_3$, Osteocalcine were determined in the plasma, calcium, phosphate, and magnesium in the urine. inulin and PAH determinations were performed using a method adapted to Technicon auto-analyser. Intra and inter assay analytical reproducibilities for both methods were less than 3 %. Plasma calcium and phosphate were determined using colorimetric methods (RA 1000, Technicon), uonized calcium with a specific electrode (ICA II, Radiometer), plasma and urine magnesium, urine calcium with atomic absorption. PTH_{1-84} was measured using a commercial kit (Mallinkrot), 25 $(OH)D_3$ and 1.25 $(OH)_2D_3$ with competition methods, osteocalcin with a commercial kit (ORIS, France).

Results are expressed as mean ± SD. Paired « t » test was used for comparisons between values obtained in the same patients at different times of the study. Correlations between variables were made using method of least squares ; $p < 0.05$ was considered as significant.

Results

Renal function data are illustrated in fig. 1 : during the first month, RPF and GFR decreased significantly, $p < 0.001$, respectively, 420 ± 84 v.s. 510 ± 80 mL/min/1.73m² (− 18 %) and 77 ± 22 v.s. 105 ± 3 to mL/min/1.73

m² (− 26 %) and plasma creatinine increased, 111 ± 20 v.s. 90 ± 14 μmol/L, $p < 0.01$. No significative change in RPF, GFR and plasma creatinine values was observed between this period and the 3 to 6 month post-chemotherapy period. At the last examination, mean RPF and GFR increased significantly, $p < 0.01$, but did not reach pretreatment values : respectively a decrease of 25 % and of 19 % was noted (380 ± 69 and 85 ± 14 mL/min/1.73 m²). Plasma creatinine concentration was then 107 ± 14 μmol/L. No relationship was found between renal haemodynamic parameters and cumulative CDDP doses, whatever the time post chemotherapy studied.

No significant change was noted in plasma ionized calcium and plasma phosphate concentrations at the three post therapy determinations. In contrast, magnesemia decreased significantly, $p < 0.001$, 0.58 ± 0.15 v.s. 0.78 ± 0.09 mmol/L (pretreatment value) and reached 0.74 ± 0.07 mmol/L at the last determination without any supplementation. In parallel, plasma 1-84 PTH concentration was significantly increased, $p < 0.05$, 36 ± 13 v.s. 20 ± 6 ng/mL one month after the end of CDDP theray and returned to pretreatment values thereafter. Plasma 25-OH-D_3 concentration was low in most patients and no significant change was observed during the period of observation. No significant change has been noted in urine calcium and phosphate urine excretion at any time of the study.

Discussion

Administration of high doses of CDDP and consequently antimitotic CDDP efficiency are limited by the possible toxicity of the drug. In most studies, nephrotoxicity has been evaluated to occur in more than 50 % of the patients (Blachley). Acute nephrotoxicity includes proximal tubular necrosis, tubular atrophy of cortical nephrons and renal failure (Safirstein). The mechanisms of Cisplatin induced renal failure are still controversial : some authors incriminate renal hemodynamic disturbance and as a matter of fact reduced renal blood flow (RBF) and reduced glomerular filtration rate (GFR) are constantly observed. Alternatively, proximal or distal tubular dysfunction (Laurence) could be the primary defect (Safirstein 1986). The problem of long-term nephrotoxicity is not yet resolved : since the observation of irreversible renal insufficiency reported by Dentino 1978, the necessity of evaluation of this severe CDDP complication has been stressed out. The time-course of renal dysfunction after CDDP administration is still controversial (Fjelborg 1986, Pinnaro 1986, Hansen 1988). In our study, we observed a fall in GFR and RPF a month after CDDP, followed by a steady state status and an improvement, but not a total recovery, one year after the end of therapy. No correlation was found between renal parameters and cumulative dose of CDDP. Administration of Cysteamine, Penicillamin and N-Acetylcystein, inhibitors of Iangiotensin I-converting enzyme or calcium channel blocker Verapamil, have been proposed to prevent renal failure (Offerman 1985). Preliminary reports indicate that sodium thiosulfate could attenuate Cisplatin induced increase in serum creatinine and blood urea nitrogen. As these results are still controversial (Hirosawa 1988), massive hydration before and during Cisplatin infusion is yet considered as the only efficient therapeutic method. To our knowledge, no paper in the literature reports oral hydration as an efficient method for prevention of renal failure. Our paper demonstrates that renal function data observed, one month and furthermore, one year after the end of therapy, are not different from those obtained with IV hydration methods.

References

Hayes DM, Cvitovic E, Golbey RB, Scheiner E, Helson L, Krakoff I (1977) High-doses Cisplatinum-Diammiedichloride : amelioration of nephrotoxicity by mannitol diuresis. Cancer 39 : 1372-81

Vogl SE, Zaravinos T, Kaplan BH (1980) Toxicity of Cis-Diamminedichloroplatinum given in a two hour out-patient regimen of diuresis and hydration. Cancer 45 : 11-15

Groth S, Nielsen H, Sorensen JB, Christensen JB, Pedersen G, Rorth M (1986) Acute and long term nephrotoxicity of Cisplatinum in man. Cancer Chemother Pharmacol 17 : 191-6

Dentino M, Luft FC, Yum MN, Williams SD, Einhorm LH (1978) Long term effect of Cis-Diamminechloride platinum (CDDP) on renal function and structure in man. N° 41 : 1274-81

Davila E, Gardner LB (1987) Clinical value of the creatinine clearance before the administration of chemotherapy with Cisplatin. Cancer 60 : 161-4

Reed E, Jacob J, Brawley O (1991) Measures of renal function in patients with Cisplatin-related chronic renal disease. J Natl Med Assoc 83 : 522-6

Pinnaro P, Ruggeri EM, Carlini P, Giovanelli M, Cognetti F (1986) Cumulative or delayed nephrotoxicity after Cisplatin (DDP) treatment. Tumori 72 : 197-200

Meijer S, Sleijfer D, Mulder NH, Sluiter WJ, Marrink J, Koops HS, Brouwers TM, Oldhoff J, Van Der Hem GJ, Mandema E (1983) Some effects of combination chemotherapy with Cisplatinum on renal function in patients with nonseminomatous testicular carcinoma. Cancer 51 : 2035-40

Hansen S, Groth S, Daugaard G, Rossing N, Rorth M (1988) Long-term effects on renal function and blood pressure of treatment with Cisplatin, Vinblastin and Bleomycin in patients with germ cell cancer. J Clin Oncol 6 : 1728-31

Daugaard G, Rossing N, Rorth M (1988) Effects of Cisplatin on different measures of glomerular function in the human kidney with special emphasis on high-dose. Cancer Chemother Pharmacol 21 : 163-7

Buamah PK, Howell A, Whitby H, Harpur ES, Gesher A (1982) Assessment of renal function during high-dose Cisplatinum therapy in patients with ovarian carcinoma. Cancer Chemother Pharmacol 8 : 281-4

Markman M, Rothman R, Hakes T, Reichman B, Lewis JL, Rubin S, Jones W, Almadrones L, Hoskins W (1991) Late effects of Cisplatin based chemotherapy on renal function in patients with ovarian carcinoma. Gynecol Oncol 41 : 217-9

Fjelborg P, Sorensen J, Helkjer PE (1986) The long-term effect of Cisplatin on renal function. Cancer 58 : 2214-7

Blachley JD, Hill JB (1981) Renal and electrolyte disturbances associated with Cisplatin. Ann Intern Med 95 : 628-32

Safirstein R, Winston J, Goldstein M, Moel D, Dikman S, Guttenplan J (1986) Cisplatin Nephrotoxicity. Am J Kidney Dis 8 : 356-67

Offerman JJG, Meijer S, Sleijfer DT, Milder NH, Donker AJM, Schraffordt KH, Van der Hem (1985) The influence of Verapamil on renal function in patients treated with Cisplatinum. Clin Nephrol 24 : 249-53

Hirosawa A, Nijtani H, Kayashibara K, Tsiboi E (1988) Effects of sodium thiosulfate in combination therapy of Cisdichlori diammineplatinum and Vandesine. Invest New Drugs 6 : 135-42

Abstract. The aim of this study was to evaluate renal function in patients in whom CDDP administration is not an IV bolus but a continuous IV infusion, lasting 6 days a week, and in whom prevention of nephrotoxicity is based on oral hydration : 25 patients aged 41 to 66 years with aerodigestive squamous carcinoma have been studied. Each patient received a total dose of CDDP ranging between 186 and 386 mg/m². Renal plasma flow (RPF) and glomerular filtration rate (GFR) were measured as PAH and inulin clearances respectively. Creatinine clearance, phosphate, calcium and magnesium status were also evaluated. These determinations have been performed before treatment and 1 month, 3 to 6 months and 12 months after the end of therapy. A significant decrease in renal function has been observed one month after therapy. Later on, renal function improved progressively but did not reach pretreatment values. Magnesemia was decreased one month after the end of CDDP administration but returned into the normal range without any magnesium supplementation in all subjects.

In conclusion, continuous IV infusion does not induce more severe renal failure that the classic IV hydration compbined with repeated IV bolus of CDDP.

Prognostic factors in head and neck cancer patients included in a program of Neo-Adjuvant chemotherapy and radical radiotherapy

I Castillo, F Gomez, R Guerrero, P Sanchez, I Martin Lopez, J Cueto, JL Garcia Puche

Patients with advanced head and neck cancer (AHNC) generally haven't an optimal treatment. The 5 years survival is poor with Surgery and Radiotherapy (RT), combinated or separately (1). Neo-Adjuvant chemotherapy (NCT), initially hopeful specially with Al-Sarraf studies [2, 3], couldn't significatively increase the all patients survival compared with classical treatment [4, 5]. Just a little group of them can take advantage of a CT + RT programme, adding the agressivity of this treatment, it seems to be more and more necessary to select these patients.

In order to identify prognostic factors of patients who can really take advantage of NCT, we present the experience of our Service.

Material and methods

The evolution of 103 patients with head and neck squamous cell carcinoma have been analyzed. All of them had an advanced disease (40 stage III and 63 stage IV), 11 women and 92 men, and Karnofsky Index (KI) at least 60 %. The location of primary tumor was : Oropharynx 29, Oral Cavity 27, Larynx 21, Nasopharynx 17 and other locations 9. Average age of patient was 59 (34-83). The histological grade of differentiation was : well differentiated 18, moderately differentiated 41, undifferentiated 25 and unknown in the others 19.

All patients were included in a homogeneous therapeutic schedule : 2-3 courses of NCT (Cisplatinum and 5-FU), mean courses for patient 2.9 (minimum 2 and maximum 5) followed by external RT with 60-Co photons in primary area and bilateral neck and supraclavicular nodes (mean dose level 67 Gy).

The mean follow-up of the 103 patients (since the beginning of the NCT treatment) was 78 months (with a minimum of 12 and a maximum of 117).

Results

After NCT, 37 patients (36 %) were in complete remission (CR), 46 (45 %) were in partial remission (PR), then 83 patients (81 %) had a favourable response (FR), and the other 20 patients (19 %) were non-responders (NR) to NCT.

Servicio de Oncologia y Radioterapia, Hospital Clinico San Cecilio, Granada, Spain

At the end of the trial 29 patients (28 %) had no evidence of disease (NED), and the other 74 patients (72 %) were dead by tumor. The 5 years actuarial survival for all patients was 26 %. 74 patients had failure after treatment, 62 (84 %) had local recurrence only, 4 (5 %) had distal failure only, and the other 8 (11 %) had both patterns of failure.

The prognostic effect of different factors (tumoral, patient's, or therapeutical) over survival was analized with these results :

The more important factors in our study are :

— Clinical stage : probability of 5 years survival in stage III patients was 36 % versus 20 % in stage IV patients ($p = 0.04$).

— Response to NCT : probability of 5 years survival in FR patients was 33 % versus 0 % in NR ($p = 0.05$). The best survival in FR patients was found in CR patients, and in this group, the CR quickness (tumoral clearance velocity) has been decisive in survival : the 5 years actuarial survival of patients with CR obtained with only 1 course of NCT was 75 % versus 53 % in these with CR after the second course of NCT and only 20 % in these who need 3 courses or more to obtain CR. This observation should lead up us to explain some reasons of control tumor failure often observed after complete response. In our experience the quickness tumor clearance is the more important factor asociated to chemical treatment.

— Clinical disease in neck nodes : the actuarial 5 years survival was 36 % for N0 patients versus 21 % for N1-2-3 patients ($p = 0.05$).

— Tumoral site : the actuarial 5 years survival in oropharynx tumor was 43 % versus 0 % in oral cavity tumor ($p = 0.01$).

— RT dose : the actuarial 5 years survival for patients receiving more than 65 Gy was 36 %, versus 9 % for patients who received 65 Gy or less ($p = 0.03$). When for any reason is necessary to make a pause in RT treatment, the time of this pause influenced in survival : pause less of 14 days got an actuarial 5 years survival of 36 % versus 17 % if the pause was more than 14 days ($p = 0.06$). The dose rate in RT treatment (2 Gy/day or 1.7-1.9 Gy/day) had not influence in survival.

Factors without influence in survival, in our study, are :
— age of patients,
— sex,
— Karnofsky Index,
— histological grade of tumor,
— anatomo-clinical pattern (ulcerated, excrecent, infiltrating) of tumor.

After a multivariant analysis (Wilcoxon-Cox) with these 13 parameters, only 3 got an independent influence in patients survival : the tumoral clearance velocity to obtain CR to NCT, RT dose and site of primary tumor.

In conclusion, the NCT, seems to be effective in AHNC patients who obtained CR with only the first course of NCT always followed by high-dose of RT (more than 65 Gy). These conditions take advantage in oropharynx located tumors. The other patients should be treated with other schedules like : hyperfractionated RT, simultaneous CT-RT, etc.

References

1. Hong WK, Bromer R (1983) Current Concepts : Chemotherapy in head and neck cancer. N Engl J Med 308 : 75-78
2. Al-Sarraf M (1988) Head and neck cancer : Chemotherapy Concepts. Sem Oncology 15 (1) : 70-85
3. -Al-Sarraf M (1984) Chemotherapeutic strategies in squamous cell carcinoma of the head and neck. CRC Critical Rev Oncol/Hematol 1 : 323-325
4. Al-Kourainy K, Kish JA, Ensley JF, Tapazoglou E, Jacobs J, Weaver A, Crissman J, Cummings G, Al-Sarraf M (1987) Achievement of superior clinically complete responders to Cisplatinum combination in patients with locally advanced head and neck cancer. Cancer 59 : 233-238
5. TJ Ervin JR, Clark RR, Weichselbaum R (1987) An analysis of Induction and Adjuvant chemotherapy in the multidisciplinary treatment of squamous cell carcinoma of the head and neck. J Clin Oncol 5 : 10-20

Induction chemotherapy for larynx preservation in laryngeal and hypopharyngeal cancers

F Demard, M Schneider, O Dassonville, P Chauvel, A Thyss, J Santini

If controlled trials have failed to demonstrate a clear survival advantage with the addition of induction chemotherapy, another potential role of this treatment concerns reduction of tumor bulk in and around the larynx in order to reduce the need for partial or total laryngectomy with identical survival results and a better quality of life. In 1985, the department of Veterans Affairs Cooperative Studies Program initiated a prospective randomized clinical trial in patients with resectable stage III and IV laryngeal cancer. The results suggest than organ preservation can be achieved in over 60 % of patients randomized to chemotherapy plus radiotherapy [1].

Jacobs [2] Urba [3], Bosl [4], Karp [5] have reported non randomized pilot studies based on this treatment approach with induction chemotherapy used as a substitute for surgery in a selected group of patients in particular those who are complete responders. All demonstrate that combined chemotherapy and radiotherapy with the goal of larynx preservation, reserving surgery on primary site for non responders is feasible and effective. In light of there results and our previous study [6], this report describes a larger series of patients with cancer of the larynx and hypopharynx treated by a homogeneous induction chemotherapy protocol at the Centre Antoine-Lacassagne (Nice-France) in order to check the validity of this organ preservation concept.

Methods (Table 1)

Table 1.

DESIGN OF THE TRIAL

Centre Antoine-Lacassagne, Nice, France

Eligible patients included those with previously untreated, resectable squamous cell cancers, (stages II, III, IV) arising in larynx and hypopharynx. Before induction chemotherapy all patients had a complete history and physical examination, complete blood count, cervical ultra sonography and CTscan. Patients were further evaluated by direct endoscopy under general anesthesia with oesophagoscopy and bronchoscopy at the discretion of the examining head and neck surgeon. Patients were assigned a clinical TNM-UICC classification. Were excluded patients with stage I tumor, distant metastasis, previous treatment, Karnovsky performance status lower than 50 %, WBC count lower than 4,000/mm^3 and platelet count < 100,000/mm^3, creatinine clearance < 60 ml/mn or severe pulmonary disease.

Chemotherapy protocol: a central venous catheter was first inserted for all patients. The protocol consisted of administration of Cisplatinum: 100 mg/m^2 IV with hyperhydratation on day 1 and 5-FU 100 mg/m^2/day by continuous 120 hours infusion. Since 1988, at half cycle, the 5-FU dosage is adjusted according to the half cycle AUC. 3 cycles were administrated at 15 day intervals. Ten days after completion of the last chemotherapy course, response was assessed under the same conditions as for primary endoscopy. Multiple biopsies were obtained systematically. Response data were recorded separately for the primary tumor and regional nodes.

Definite treatment

If the patient achieved a complete clinical response (non visible or palpable disease with no microscopic residual disease on the biopsy specimen), the originally planned surgery on the primary tumor was eliminated, but if palpable disease remained in the neck, a neck dissection alone was performed. CR patients were treated by definite radiation therapy: 65 Gy to the tumor and 55 to 65 Gy to the nodes (5 fractions a week, 1.8 to 2 Gy per fraction). If patients were judged to have less than a CR (partial or non response, PR, NR) the initially programmed surgical indication was proposed to the patients. The extent of this surgical resection was determined by tumor size at initial evaluation and was not modified by the tumor response to induction chemotherapy. After surgical resection, patients received radiation therapy, 55 to 65 Gy. Patients were followed up every month the first year, every 2 months the second year, and every 3 months thereafter.

Results

Patients population

Between september 1983 and June 1991, 170 consecutive patients with laryngeal and hypopharyngeal tumors entered this trial. There were 160 men and 10 women. The primary tumor sites included: larynx 96 cases (glottic 35, supraglottic 61), hypopharynx 74 (piriform sinus 73, posterior pharyngeal wall 1). In the group of patients with laryngeal tumors, 35 had stade II disease,

26 had stage III and 35 stage IV. In the group of patients with hypopharyngeal tumors 5 had stage II, 21 had stage III and 48 stage IV. Thus in the entire group 130/170 (75.4 %) had advanced stage III-IV tumors (Tables 2, 3).

Table 2. TNM distribution larynx

	N0	N1	N2	N3	Total
T1	0	0	1	0	1 (1%)
T2	37	5	10	1	53 (55%)
T3	17	3	7	3	30 (31%)
T4	9	2	1	0	12 (13%)
	63 (66%)	10 (10%)	19 (20%)	4 (4%)	96

☐ Stage 1   ▨ Stage 2   ▓ Stage 3   ☐ Stage 4

Table 3. Distribution TNM hypopharynx

	N0	N1	N2	N3	Total
T1	0	0	0	1	1 (1%)
T2	5	6	5	1	17 (23%)
T3	9	6	15	6	36 (49%)
T4	1	4	10	5	20 (27%)
	15 (20%)	16 (22%)	30 (40%)	13 (18%)	74

☐ Stage 1   ▨ Stage 2   ▓ Stage 3   ☐ Stage 4

Toxicity

Most of the patients experienced nausea and vomiting. Toxicity, evaluable for more than 1,000 cycles, has been presented elsewhere [7]. 9 deaths during chemotheray were attribuable to the chemotherapy regimen but most of these patients had significant medical complications. No death occured after 1988 thanks to pharmacokinetic monitoring of the 5-FU AUC on day 3 which can predict and thus allows prevention of severe toxicity by reduction of drug dose [8].

Response

Response to chemotherapy was evaluated for 156/170 patients. 14 patients could not be evaluated (9 toxic death, 5 refusals). Response was considered complete for 43.8 % of the larynx tumors and 38.2 % of the hypopharynx tumors and partial (better than 50 % tumor regression or with persistent disease at multiple biopsies) for 42.7 % larynx and 42.6 % hypopharynx tumors. The objective response rate (CR + PR) was thus respectively 86.5 % and 80.8 % for the evaluable laryngeal and hypopharyngeal lesions. The response percentage for the primary tumor varied with tumor size (Tables 4, 5).

Table 4. Response to chemotherapy/T Stage (Larynx)

	RC	RP	NR	Total	NE	Total
T1	1	0	0	1	0	1
T2	30 (57%)	19	4	53	0	53
T3	7 (27%)	13	6	26	4	30
T4	1 (11%)	6	2	9	3	12
	39 (44%)	38 (43%)	12 (13%)	89	7	96

Table 5. Response to chemotherapy/T Stage (Hypopharynx)

	CR	PR	NR	Total	NE	Total
T1	1	0	0	1	0	1
T2	8 (47%)	9	0	17	0	17
T3	10 (31%)	14	8	32	4	36
T4	7 (39%)	6	5	18	2	20
	26 (38%)	29 (43%)	13 (19%)	68	6	74

Post-chemotherapy treatment

After chemotherapy, patients were treated according to the design of our trial, but in the group of patients with PR and NR, 13 patients still resectable refused the total laryngectomy required and they were referred for radiationtherapy and excluded from the study as were 4 others who refused all treatment and were rapidly lost to follow up. Pattern of failure and current status for the entire group of evaluable patients (median follow-up 28 months), causes of relapse and 5 year overall survival and disease free survival are outlined in Table 6.

Table 6. Pattern of failure/Current status

		Relapse				Five-year survival %	
		LF	NR	D	NR+D	Overall	Disease-free
LARYNX	T2	6	3	10	1	67%	51%
	T3	5	0	6	0	40%	44%
	T4	3	2	3	0	41%	33%
PHARYNX	T2	0	3	8	0	27%	28%
	T3	12	2	12	0	14%	15%
	T4	4	0	4	0	19%	18%

LF = local failure, NR = nodal recurrence, D = distant metastasis,
NR + D = nodal + distant. Survival calculated with Kaplan Meïer method

Table 7. Scheduled surgery/Larynx preservation

			LARYNX PRESERVATION			
			CR pts (65)		Population (170)	
SURGERY	TL	33	71%	76%	15%	22%
	TLP	55	78%	80%	25%	28%
	NTL	27	91%		37%	
	LP	36	81%	87%	47%	47%
	PPh	19	100%		47%	

Results were analyzed taking into consideration the initially scheduled extent of surgical laryngeal resection and patients were thus separated into 2 groups :

Candidate for conservative surgery on both larynx (partial laryngectomy PL, or partial pharyngectomy PPH) and patients who were considered for near total laryngectomy (NTL) or total laryngectomy ± partial pharyngectomy.

No difference in survival or DFS was seen between patients treated by the modified protocol and the patients treated by the non modified protocol. These data confirm that CR patients do not need to undergo surgery and can be treated by primary chemotherapy and radiotherapy without compromising survival (Table 7) : 71 % of CR patients previously scheduled for TL, 78 %

for TLP, 91 % for NTL retained their larynx, actually 80 % of the complete responders. For these patients initially scheduled to undergo conservative surgery (PL, PPH), 87 % of the complete responders preserved their larynx. Comparison of these figures with the entire population treated by induction chemotherapy reveals that the larynx preservation were respectively 28 and 47 %.

The results of our trial are encouraging and have shown the feasibility of such an approach which allows larynx conservation in a significant number of patients without compromising survival.

To attain better rates of organ preservation, new drugs regimens that can induce higher CR rates are a promising field of investigation, selection of patients including patients with other specific tumor sites requires study as do radiation treatment schedules with accelerated fractionation or concomitant chemoradiotherapy. Clinical and biological prognostic factors and methods of predicting radiosensitivity will also play an important role on the future, and may allow better selection of patients for organ preservation protocols.

References

1. Hong WK, Wolf GT, Fisher S et al (1989) Laryngeal preservation with induction chemotherapy and radiotherapy in the treatment for advanced laryngeal cancer. Proc Am Soc Clin Oncol 8 : 167
2. Jacobs C, Goffinet DR, Goffinet L et al (1987) Chemotherapy as a substitute for surgery in the treatment of advanced resectable head and neck cancer. Cancer 60 : 1178-1183
3. Urba S, Forastiere AA, Wolf GT et al (1989) Neo-Adjuvant chemotherapy with high-dose continuous infusion Cisplatin, 5-FU and Mitoguazone for head and neck cancer. Proc Am Soc Clin Oncol 8 : 172
4. Bosl JL, Strong E, Harrison L et al (1191) In : De Vita VI, Hellman S, Rosenberg SA (eds.) Important advances in Oncology — Larynx conservation. Lippincott, Philadelphia, pp 191-203
5. Karp DD, Vaughan CW, Carter R et al (1991) Voice preservation using induction chemotherapy plus radiation therapy as an alternative to laryngectomy in advanced head and neck cancer. Proc Am Soc Clin Oncol 11 : 152
6. Demard F, Chauvel P, Santini J et al (1990) Response to chemotherapy as justification for modification of the therapeutic strategy for pharyngolaryngeal carcinomas. Head and Neck 12 : 228-231
7. Schneider M, Demard F, Chauvel P et al (1991) Induction chemotherapy with Cisplatin and 5-FU for SCC of the head and neck 6 year experience at the Nice Cancer Center. In : Neo-Adjuvant chemotherapy. Springer-Verlag, Paris, pp 18-22
8. Milano G, Thyss A, Santini J et al (1989) Benefit of 5-FU pharmacokinetics for head and neck chemotherapy protocol associating Cisplatin and 5 days continuous 5-FU. Cancer Chem Pharm 23 : 2750-2710

A pilot study of vinorelbine on a weekly schedule in recurrent and/or metastatic squamous cell carcinoma of the head and neck

V Gebbia, A Testa, R Valenza, G Zerillo, S Restivo, F Ingria, G Cannata, N Borsellino, N Gebbia

Vinorelbine (VNR), 5'-nor-anhydrovinblastine, is a new semi-synthetic vinka alkaloid with selective affinity for mitotic microtubules, which has been shown to be active against several non small cell lung cancer lines *in vitro* [1]. VNR has been reported to yield a 34.7 % and 20 % overall response rate in patients with squamous cell lung carcinoma and bronchial adenocarcinoma respectively [2]. Moreover, VNR has been shown to be active in advanced breast carcinoma where it may induce a 30-50 % response rate depending on the extent of pretreatment [3]. We tested the activity and toxicity of single agent VNR given on a weekly schedule in a series of patients with recurrent and/or metastatic squamous cell carcinoma of the head and neck (SCHNC).

Patients and methods

All of the following criteria had to be fullfilled before entry : age < 75 years ; Karnofsky Index (KI) > 50 ; measurable disease ; expected survival > 2 months ; WBC > 4,000/mmc and PLT > 120,000/mmc ; BUN < 50 mg %, serum creatinine < 1.2 mg % ; serum bilirubin < 1.2 mg % ; no major cardiovascular, neurological, or metabolic disease ; no previous pretreatment with vinca alkaloids. Informed consent was required due to the investigative nature of the study.

Twenty-four patients with biopsy-proven recurrent and/or metastatic SCHNC were treated as follows : VNR 20 mg/m^2/wk i.v. diluted in 250 cc of NS over 20 min infusion was given to the first group of 3 patients, and then escalated by 5 mg/m^2/wk for subsequent groups of 3 patients until the maximally tolerated dose was reached. There were 22 males and 2 females with a mean age of 56 years (range 41-71), and mean Karnofsky Index of 75 (60-100). Patients included 10 laryngeal, 7 oropharyngeal, 3 hypopharyngeal, 3 rhinopharyngeal and 1 maxillary sinus SCHNC. Pretreatment included : surgery in 12 patients (50 %), radiotherapy in 8 patients (33 %), and chemotherapy in 6 (25 %). Two patients were previously untreated. Sites of disease included : locoregional disease (75 %), node (17 %), lung (12.5 %), liver (8 %), and soft tissue (8 %).

Standard WHO criteria were employed for definition of objective response and toxicity. Student's T test has been employed for survival anlysis, and ob-

---

Chair of Chemotherapy, and Division of Othorhinolaryngology, Policlinico, University of Palermo, Italy

jective responses have been reported as relative rates with 95 % confidence limits (CL).

Table 1. Dose escalation of weekly VNR and related side-effects

Dose level	Patients	Toxicity (WHO score)
20 mg/m²/wk	pt n.1	Leukopenia G 1
	pt n.2	Leukopenia G 1 — local pain G 1
	pt n.3	Leukopenia G 2 — constipation G 1 — Neurosensory G 1 (paraesthesias)
25 mg/m²/wk	pt n. 4	Leukopenia G 2 — PLT G 1 — constipation G1
	pt n.5	Leukopenia G 3 — nausea G 2
	pt n.6	Leukopenia G 2 — anemia G 1
30 mg/m²/wk	pt n.7	Leukopenia G 4 — PLT G 2 — nausea G 1
	pt n.8	Leukopenia G 3 — vomiting G 2 — Neurosensory G 1 (paraesthesias)
	pt n.9	Neuromotor G 2 (impaired speech) — Leukopenia G 3

Table 2. Type and duration of objective response

Type of response	N. of patients	(%)	Duration (months) mean	(range)	Survival (months) mean	(range)
Partial	5	(22 %)	5.8+	(3.4/8.3)	7.4+	(3.6/9.5)
No change	7	(30 %)	4.3+	(3.0+/5.8)	5.7+	(3.2+/6.8+)
Progression	11	(48 %)	-	-	4.6+	(2.5/5.8)

Results

Table 1 showes toxicity according to the dose escalation of VNR. While VNR 20 and 25 mg/m²/wk was quite well tolerated, however we were not able to increase VNR dosage above 30 mg/m²/wk because of grade 4 granulocytopenia and grade 2 neuromotor toxicity. Thus all further patients received VNR 25 mg/m²/wk.

A total of 286 weeks of VNR was given to patients (11.9 wks/pt). Seven patients (29 %) had grade 3 leukopenia, 2 patients (8 %) grade 4 leukopenia, and 8 patients (33 %) grade 1-2 thrombocytopenia. Nausea/vomiting was mild with grade 2 toxicity in 29 % of cases. Grade 1 stomatitis was seen in 2 cases (8 %), and a slight increase in serum bilirubin (< 2 times normal) in 2 additional cases. Four patients (17 %) had grade 1-2 constipation, 3 patients (12.5 %) had grade 1 paraesthesias, and 2 patients grade 1-2 impaired speech. Pain in the injection site was recorded in 4 cases (17 %). One patient experienced acute severe bone pain soon after VNR infusion, and an other patient complained of tumor pain after VNR. Pain was rapidly abolished by i.v. ketorolac-trimetamine in both cases.

Five patients (22 % ; 95 % CL 18 %-26 %) showed partial response (Table 2), 7 patients (30 %) had a stabilization of their disease, and 11 patients progressed. Among partial responders there were 2 previously untreated patients with locoregional disease at oropharynx, 2 patients pretreated with radiotherapy presenting soft tissue metastases of rhinopharyngeal carcinoma and locoregional recurrency of laryngeal tumor respectively, and 1 patient with nodal recurrency who had undergone surgery for laryngeal cancer. Survival analysis showed a slight, but not statistically significant, advantage for responders over non-responders.

Discussion

Present data, although preliminary, suggest that VNR is fairly active against SCHNC, being able to induce a 22 % partial response rate (95 % CL 18 %-26 %) in this series of 24 patients with recurrent and/or metastatic SCHNC. The mean duration of partial response was 6 months. VNR may be safely given on a weekly schedule at the dose of 25 mg/m^2/wk on an outpatients basis. We were not able to increase VNR weekly dose above 30 mg/m^2 due to the occurrence of severe leukopenia and mild neurotoxicity. Although the most frequent side-effect was hematological toxicity, it is noteworthy the acute bone or tumor pain experienced by 2 patients soon after VNR.

In conclusion it may be worthwhile to include VNR in further phase II trials in association with other drugs, such as 5-Fluorouracil and Cisplatin in order to increase response rates and duration of response.

References

1. Poitier P (1989) The synthesis of Navelbine prototype of a new series of Vinblastine derivatives. Sem Oncol 16 : 2-5
2. Cros S, Wright M, Morimoto C et al (1989) Experimental antitumor activity of Navelbine (5'-nor-Anydrovinblastine, Vinorelbine). Sem Oncol 16 : 15-20
3. Depierre A, Lemarie' E, Dabouis G et al (1989) Efficay of Navelbine (NVB) in non small cell lung cancer (NSCLC). Sem Oncol 16 : 26-29

Abstract. A series of 24 patients with recurrent and/or metastatic squamous cell head and neck cancer were treated with weekly vinorelbine achieving a 22 % partial response rate. Authors suggest to employ vinorelbine at 25 mg/m^2/wk in order to avoid severe leukopenia. Toxicity is also reported.

Concomitant radiotherapy and Cisplatin in head and neck cancer : a pilot study

P Olmi, C Fallai**, C Chiostrini*

Advanced tumors of the head and neck have a dismal prognosis. High-dose radiotherapy (rt) can achieve from 5 to 20 % survival at 5 years depending on site of origin, stage and histology.

In 1990 we began a preliminary study on advanced tumors of head and neck combining standard higt-dose rt with concomitant chemotherapy (ct).

We chose to administer Cisplatin (cddp) that, as a single agent, has activity itself against head and neck tumors and does not have mucositis as its dose limiting toxicity, what could be of great importance when combining treatments.

Cddp was delivered through continuous intravenous infusion (i.v. c.i.). As radiation enhancement may occur as result of cddp — dna adducts when cddp is delivered before irradiation or may result from postradiation inhibition of repair of sublethal damage and of potentially lethal damage [1], c.i. might benefit of both radiosensitizing actions.

Furthermore, c.i. seems to decrease the frequency of renal failure [2], and to cause minimal nausea vomiting and haematologic toxicity [3]. Our primary aim was to establish feasibility of such a combined treatment approach.

Materials

From August 1990 to August 1992 21 patients affected with advanced carcinoma of the head and neck were treated with radiotherapy and concomitant continuous infusion chemotherapy (rt-ct) at the radiotherapy department of Florence, Italy.

Age ranged from 35 to 67 years with a mean age of 55 years. There were 18 males and 3 females with a ratio of 6 to 1.

All cases were histologically proved epithelial carcinoma of squamous cell type except for 1 nasopharyngeal carcinoma of undifferentiated type, 3 adenocarcinomas and 1 adenoid cystic carcinoma (paranasal sinuses).

The distribution by site of origin was as follows : 2 nasopharynx (np), 8 oropharynx (op), 2 hypopharynx (hp), 3 oral cavity (oc), 5 paranasal sinuses (ps), 1 supraglottic larynx (la).

All previously untreated patients with stage III or IV (IICC 1987) head and neck cancer, with normal haematological, renal and liver values and not inclued in other trials were considered eligible for the present study. Patients older than 75 years and with a KPS less than 70 were excluded.

All recruited cases were, however, stage IV (UICC 1987) : there were 1 T2N2b, 3 T2N3, 1 T3N2c, 1 T3N3, 8 T4N0, 4 T4N1, 3 T4N2c.

Radioterapia — Universita'* e Ospedale** — Policlinico di Careggi Viale Morgagni 85, 50134 Firenze, Italy

Treatment

Eighteen patients were treated with rt-ct only, with surgery reserved for suitable cases at relapse : 1 patient was considered operable after 60 Gy and underwent surgery, 2 patients were administered rt-ct postoperatively due to questionable radicality.

All patients were irradiated with a cobalt 60 machine or a 6 MeV linear accelerator. The total dose ranged from 64 to 70 Gy with a mean dose of 68 Gy in 17 cases treated with rt-ct ; 1 patient was excluded due to its early death when only 42 Gy had been delivered. The patients treated preoperatively or postoperatively were administered 60 Gy. The fractionation of the dose was conventional (2 Gy a day × 5 days/wk).

Cddp was delivered by a computerized pump with an i.v. c.i. over 24 hours a day via a peripheral line, 5 days a week, concomitantly with the first three weeks of rt. The drug was diluted into 1,000 ml of saline (0,9 % NaCl) solution. In 2 patients, after implanting a subcutaneous port, the drug was delivered through a Hickman catheter.

Sixteen patients out of 21 completed the planned 3 weeks of treatment ; dose per square meter (sqm) ranged from 3.5 to 12 mg with a mean dose of 5.8 mg/sqm : their total dose ranged from 90 to 320 mg and the mean total dose was 147 mg.

The effective dose intensity was 26.3 mg/mq/wk in the group of patients completing the treatment.

Sequelae

Sequelae and results are analysed in 20 patients of 21. One patient, whose previous history was negative, died of a sudden massive haemorrhage due to perforated gastric ulcer ; he had been given 42 Gy and 105 mg of cddp. At autopsy he resulted free of disease in the oropharynx.

The main acute sequela due to radiotherapy is mucositis that causes a frequent prolongation of treatment. In the present series 8 patients completed their treatment in the scheduled time ; 7 had a prolongation of 7 to 13 days while 5 had a delay of 14 days or more. Chemotherapy was stopped in 4 patients because of the following causes (1 patient each) : intractable vomiting, episode of angina pectoris, hypertension crisis, laryngeal oedema due to rt.

Gastrointestinal, renal and haematologic toxicities were scored according to the recommendations of WHO grading system. Fifteen patients did not have any nausea or vomiting. Four patients had nausea (grade 1), well controlled with conventional therapy. In 1 case vomiting persisted in spite of antiemetic medications (grade 4) and the administration of cddp had to be interrupted.

Renal toxicity, always transient and completely revertible, as showed by increase of blood urea and/or creatinine, was graded 1 in 4 patients and graded 2 in 1 patient.

Haematologic toxicity was observed in 6 patients : 1 grade 1, 2 grade 2,

2 grade 3 ; nadir occured between 2 and 4 weeks after the end of chemotherapy (from the 5th to the 7th week of rt).

Results

Response was evaluated 3 months after the end of the treatment course. Evidence of response was obtained with standard diagnostic means ; special diagnostic means (computerized tomography, magnetic resonance imaging) were used for selected sites (e.g. np, ps) and in any other case, when considered necessary.

An objective response was observed in 14 patients out of 20 (70 %) : there were 9 complete response (cr) and 5 partial response (pr).

Current status of the present series includes 11 patients (55 %) alive without evidence of disease (ned). Two patients (1 oc lesion, relapsed at the primary site after cr ; 1 maxillary sinus, pr) underwent salvage surgery and are currently considered ned.

With a median follow-up of 14 months, mean survival is 10 months.

Conclusions

Combined rt-ct with ci of cddp (dose intensity of 26 mg/sqm/wk × 3 weeks) is feasible.

As far as acute mucositis and following treatment breaks are concerned, compliance to combined treatment has been the same as to radiotherapy only, according to our experience.

Acute gastroenteric, renal and haemathologic toxicities have turned out to be quite acceptable, transient and revertible.

No firm statements are possible considering that this is a small heterogeneous series with a short follow-up. However, 55 % of 20 patients are currently alive (ned) what would represent a fairly good result, considering that all patients were stage IV, if this datum will be confirmed after a longer follow-up and a larger recruitement.

References

1. Vokes E, Weichselbaum R (1990) Concomitant radiotherapy : rationale and clinical experience in patients with solid tumors. J Clin Oncol 8 : 911-934
2. Rotman M, Aziz H (1990) Concomitant continuous infusion chemotherapy and radiation. Cancer 65 : 823-835
3. Choi K, Aziz H, Stark R, Sohn C, Rosenthal J, Braverman A, Khil S, Isaacso S, Marti J, Rotmann M (1988) Concomitant radiation and infusion Cisplatinum in advanced cancers of the head and neck. Proc Ann Meet Am Soc Clin Oncol 7 : A607

Ifosfamide/Mesna plus Carboplatin as Neo-Adjuvant therapy for stage I-III head and neck cancer. Preliminary report

M Bruno

It is generally accepted that radiotherapy and surgery are both effective techniques in the management of head and neck cancer. But the possibility of diminishing the volume of the primary tumor with chemotherapy as first approach, appears to be the most significant achievement in recent years. It has been demonstrated that the use of preoperative adjuvant chemotherapy can increase disease-free survival in several kinds of tumors, such as osteogenic sarcoma [1], breast cancer [2], head and neck cancer [3]. Major advances in chemotherapy for head and neck cancer have been achieved recently. Several single agent regimens have induced significant tumor regression in 20 % to 40 % of patients with locally recurrent or metastatic head and neck cancer [4]. Cisplatin has been the basis for many new drug combinations, usually with the addition of Bleomycin and/or Methotrexate [5].

Response rates have varied from 25 % to 75 %. Carboplatin is a second generation platinum derivative currently been evaluated in clinical trials. In general, the antitumor activity of Carboplatin in pre-clinical studies is comparable with that of Cisplatin, although each agent shows some selectivity for certain tumors [6]. In general Carboplatin has proved to be well tolerated by patients with solid tumors in doses of 360 to 400 mg/m^2 every four weeks [7]. The dose limiting toxicity of Carboplatin is myelosuppression, including both leukopenia and thrombopenia and is less emetogenic than Cisplatin. In the last few years, ifosfamide has become a first line drug in some neoplasms such as ovarian cancer, testicular cancer, small cell lung cancer and sarcoma, and it appears to be very promising even in cancer of cervic [8], breast [9] and head and neck cancer [10]. There are only few reports showing some single agent activity of ifosfamide in head and neck cancer. According to various studies, results seemed to be dose dependent. Cervellino [10] reported 42.7 % objective response with high dose ifosfamide/mesna among 28 patients. Pai [11] observed 52 % objective response in recurrent or metastatic head and neck cancer. In order to test the activity of the combination Ifosfamide/Carboplatin as Neo-Adjuvant therapy, we conducted this study.

Material and methods

25 patients with stage I-III squamous cell head and neck cancer (scchn) were included. Other eligibility criteria included the presence of measurable lesions, no prior treatment, a performance status on the Karnofsky scale $\geq$ 60 ; age

---

Oncology service, Gas del Estado, Buenos Aires, Argentina

⩽ 75 years ; WBC ⩾ 4,000/ml ; platelet count ⩾ 100,000/ml ; creatinine and bilirubin serum levels ⩽ 1.5 mg %. Tumor localizations werre as follows : amygdala 7 ; gena 5 ; larynx 6 ; tongue 3 ; maxylar sinus, palate, lip and nasal fossa 1 each (Table 1). The treatment regimen consisted of Ifosfamide 2,500 mg/m^2, 3 hour i.v. infusion on days 1-3, and mesna 500 mg/m^2, i.v. bolus injection at 0.4 and 8 h, on days 1-3. Carboplatin 300 mg/m^2, 1 hour infusion on day 1. Cycles were repeated every 3 weeks for a total of 3 cycles (Table 2). This regimen was suitable for outpatient treatment. An adequate trial required administration of surgery or radiotherapy as complementary therapy. Complete response was defined as a complete disappearance of all clinical and/or detectable disease for at least 2 months. Partial response was defined as a greater than 50 % reduction in the sum of the diameters of all measurable lesions and the absence of any new lesion for at least 2 months. No change, a disease status or progression with no change of measurements for at least 2 months. Progression, more than 25 % increase in the sum of the diamenters of all measurable lesions and/or the appearance of new lesions. The trial sequence of procedures was as follows : 1) staging of tumor 2) Neo-Adjuvant chemotherapy and toxicity evaluation 3) evaluation of tumor response 4) conventional treatment (surgery or radiotherapy) 5) evaluation of response 6) follow-up and determination of sites of recurrences.

Table 1. Ifosfamide-Carboplatin/head and neck cancer

Characteristics of patients
Patients 25
Age : Median 55 years   Range : 42 - 69 years
Sex : M 16   F 9
Tumor localization
  Amygdala   7
  Larynx   6
  Gena   5
  Tongue   3
  Maxylar Sinus   1
  Palate   1
  Lip   1
  Nasal Fossa   1
Stage   I : 1   II : 14   III : 10

Table 2. Schedule of therapy

Ifosfamide 2,500 mg/m^2 i.v. days 1-3
Mesna 20 % of Ifo dose, i.v. hour 0, 4 and 8, days 1-3
Carboplatin 300 mg/m^2 i.v. day 1
Every 3 weeks - Three cycles

Results

25 evaluable patients were entered in the study. Mean age 55, with a range of 42-69 years, and a median performance status on the Karnofsky scale was 80. Nine patients were women. All patients received 3 courses of chemotherapy. Two patients achieved complete response and 15 achieved partial response for an overall response rate of 68 % (Table 3). Toxicity was reported for 75 cycles and ranged from mild to moderate (Table 4). No renal impairment and no CNS symptoms occurred. No death was registered from treatment. After giving conventional surgery or radiotherapy, objective response improved from 68 % to 80 % (CR 36 %, PR 44 %) (Table 3).

Table 3. Response

Tumor	Chemotherapy		OR/Pts	Radioth/Surg		OR/Pts
	CR	PR		CR	PR	
Amygdala	2	3	5/7	3	3	6/7
Larynx	0	3	3/6	1	3	4/6
Gena	0	4	4/5	3	2	5/5
Tongue	0	3	3/3	1	2	3/3
Maxylar Sinus	0	1	1/1	1	0	0/1
Palate	0	0	0/1	0	0	0/1
Lip	0	1	1/1	0	1	1/1
Nasal Fossa	0	0	0/1	0	0	0/1
Total	2	15	17/25	9	11	20/25
% obj resp	8	60	68	36	44	80

Table 4. Toxicity

	OMS	Grade		
	2	3	4	Total
Vomiting	1	3	1	5
Alopecia	12	4	0	16
Leukopenia	3	2	0	5
Anemia	1	0	0	1
Stomatitis	1	1	0	2

Conclusions

Squamous cell head and neck cancer is a Neo-Adjuvant chemosensitive tumor for Ifosfamide/Carboplatin combination. A remarkable increase in the number of CR from 8 % to 36 % were achieved after conventional surgery (5 pts) and radiotherapy (2 pts). Marked nausea and vomiting were trouble some side effects of Ifosfamide mainly, for 20 % of patients. The median survival time for responders was 11 + months with an overall survival of 10 + months (range 2-23 months). Six patients died (Table 5). Ifosfamide plus Carboplatin are very well tolerated and represent a reasonable alternative Neo-Adjuvant regimen for induction chemotherapy in patients with stage I-III head and neck cancer.

Table 5. Survival in months

Patients : 25	Median	Range
Overall	10+	2 – 23+
Responders	11+	3 – 23+

References

1. Rosen G, Caparros B, Huvos AG et al (1987) Preoperative chemotherapy for osteogenic sarcoma. Selection of post operative adjuvant chemotherapy based on the response of the primary tumor to preoperative chemotherapy. Cancer 49 : 1221-1230
2. Bonadonna G, Valagussa P, Tancini G et al (1986) Current status of Milan adjuvant chemotherapy trials for node positive and node negative breast cancer. NCI Monogr
3. Kish J, Drelichman A, Jacobs J et al (1982) Chemical trial of Cisplatin and 5-Fluorouracil infusion as initial treatment for advanced squamous cell carcinoma of the head and neck. Ca Treat Rep 66 : 471-474
4. Erwin T, Karp D, Weichselbaum R (1985) Multidisciplinary treatment of advanced squamous carcinoma of the head and neck. Sem Oncol 12 : 71-78
5. Schwert R, Jacobs J, Crissman J et al (1983) Improved survival in patients with advanced head and neck cancer achieving complete clinical response to induction chemotherapy. Proc Am Soc Clin Oncol 2 : 159
6. Boven E, Van der Vijgh W et al (1985) Comparative activity and distribution studies in five platinum analogues in nude male mice bearing human ovarian carcinoma xeno grafts. Cancer Res 45 : 86-90
7. Calvert A, Harland S, Newell D et al (1982) Early clinical studies with Cisdiammine-1,1-Cyclobutane dicarboxylate platinum II. Cancer Chemother Pharmacol 9 : 140-147
8. Coleman R, Clarke J, Slevin M et al (1988) Ifosfamide and Ifosfamide + Cisplatin chemotherapy for advanced cervical carcinoma. N° 58 : 273
9. Brade W, Herdrich K, Varini M (1985) Ifosfamide pharmacology, safety and therapeutical potential. Cancer Treat Rev 12 : 1-47
10. Cervellino J, Araujo C, Pirisi C et al (1991) Ifosfamide and Mesna for the treatment of advanced squamous cell head and neck cancer. Oncology 48 : 89-92
11. Pai V, Parikh D, Mazumdar A et al (1991) Phase II study of high dose Ifosfamide as single agent and in combination with Cisplatin in the treatment of advanced and/or recurrent squamous cell carcinoma of the head neck. ECCO 6, S/47 : 877

Role of Ifosfamide, Cisplatinum (IC) combination in the metastatic neck nodes

VR Pai*, DM Parikh**, AT Mazumdar*, RS Rao**

Many chemotherapeutic agent have been shown to have activity against head and neck cancer. Methotrexate, Bleomycin and Cisplatinum are considered the most active drugs. The search for new drug and effective drug combinations with acceptable toxicity is major task at present.

In head and neck cancer, Ifosfamide has not been studied extensively. So far, only three French studies have been reported, but the studies are incomplete. Legant [1] treated eighteen pretreated and twelve non-pretreated patients, reporting an ill-defined number of responses, but not giving any response criteria. In this study, Ifosfamide was also supposed to have activity in pretreated patients.

Freche [2] treated 20 patient with local recurrence after previous radiotherapy. They used three different dose regimen and obtained « objective improvement » in 75 % of the patients. However, besides a decrease in pain and dysphagia other response criteria were not given. Sennon [3] treated 16 similar patients, also claiming important clinical improvement without giving response criteria. For combination chemotherapy only one report is available. Focan et al [4] used Vincristine, Cisplatinum and Ifosfamide in seven patient achieving two complete and five partial remission. These patients were not pretreated but had stage IV disease without distant metastases.

Although these reports suggested activity of Ifosfamide in head and neck cancer, a definite proof for such activity was still lacking hence we initiated a Phase II trial using Ifosfamide as a single agent in advanced and/or recurrent squamous cell carcinoma of head and neck. After establishing role of Ifosfamide as a single agent in head and neck cancer we extended this study using combination chemotherapy with Cisplatinum and we observed, apart from the response in advance cases, this combination showed its effectiveness against lymph node metastases.

Material and methods

At Tata Memorial Hospital, Bombay 37 patients were entered into this study. All patients were uniformly treated with Ifosfamide, Cisplatinum combination chemotherapy.

---

* Division of Medical, ** Surgery Tata Memorial Hospital, Paral, Bombay, 400012, India

Eligibility criteria

1. Patient must have no prior exposure to chemotherapy.
2. Patient must have histologically confirmed metastatic carcinoma.
3. Patients must have a performance status 0 to 3 on the WHO scale. There is no age limit.
4. Patients must have a white blood count of 4,000/cmm or greater and platelet count of 100,000/cmm or greater.
5. Patient must have normal serum creatinine.
6. Patient must have normal liver function.
7. Patient must have no active gross infection.

Treatment design

Injection Ifosfamide	: 1.5 gm/m^2 IV infusion on day 1 to day 5.
Injection Mesna	: 400 mg IV push at 0 hr, 4 hr and 8 hr on day 1 to 5.
Injection Cisplatinum	: 10 mg/m^2 IV infusion on day 1 to day 5.

Daily schedule of Cisplatin therapy

Dextrose saline	: 500 ml.
Dextrose saline	: 500 ml – add required dose of Cisplatin in last 100 ml (1/2 hour drip).
Mannitol	: 350 ml intravenous.

IV fluid with Dextrose saline/Dextrose/Ringer's Lactate 2,500 ml. To this 1 gm/L Mgso4 was added and given over 6 hours. Urine output should be maintained at more than 2,000 ml/day. Diuretics were used when necessary. Blood urea and serum creatinine was normal before every course. Repeat cycle at an interval of every four week and such three cycles were administered.

After completion of three cycle of chemotherapy, patient was assessed for surgery/radiation.

The side effect from chemotherapy were generally well tolerated and reversible. All patients experienced some degree of anorexia and nausea which was controlled with metoclopramide hydrochloride. Alopecia and leucopenia were experienced by all. Care of oral hygiene was taken by povidone-iodine mouth wash.

Results

All the 37 patients entered into this study were evaluable for response and toxicity. The total group included 32 male and 5 female ranging in the age from 18 to 70 years (median age : 50 years). All patients had a significant measurable neck node with performance status (WHO) of 0-3. The general characteristic of the patient population were as follows (Table 1).

Table 1. Patient characteristics

No. entered	37
Sex M/F	32/5
Median age	50 years (18-70 years)
Performance status	0-3
Hystology	
Mets. squamous ca.	32
Mets. undiff. ca.	1
Mets. porly diff. ca.	4

Table 2. Nodal status of 37 patients

	Number of patients	
Node size	Unilateral	Bilateral
< 3 cm	6	2
3 – 6 cm	14	5
< 3 & 3 – 6 cm	—	3
3-6 & > 6 cm	—	1
> 6 cm	6	—

Discussion

There are approximately 4,300 new cases of head and neck cancer we see at our centre each year. The disease has a major impact on the quality of life.

In patients with locally advanced or inoperable HN carcinoma the main prerequisite to prolong overall survival is to obtain an initial local control of the disease, achieving clinical CR 5. This finding has been observed in nearly all trials employing RT, or induction chemotherapy, where CR predicted for longer survival 6.

In the past, chemotherapy consisted of the use of a single agent usually Methotrexate in HN cancer. However the past decade has yielded the development of new chemotherapeutic agents (Cisplatinum, Bleomycin, Fluorouracil) and multiple combination of chemotherapy.

In our experience with Ifosfamide as a single agent in advanced or recurrent squamous cell carcinoma of head and neck shows a total response of 53 % and in combination with Cisplatinun it is 67.5 % with a median duration of response of 2 and 4 months respectively which is comparable with other single agents mentioned above.

A notable feature of this combination is that it is effective against lymph node metastases. Most other chemotherapeutic regimens are very effective against the primary tumour but marginally effective against lymph node metastases. Uncontrolled cervical node metastases which are unresectable and not suitable for radiation because of sheer bulk, is a common problem. This combination help to reduce the bulk of the tumour permitting surgery of radiation therapy.

Table 3. Nodal regression in 37 patients

	Neck node size					
Nodal Regression	Unilateral nodes			Bilateral nodes		Total
	< 3 cm	3 – 6 cm	> 6 cm	<3 & 3 – 6 cm	3 – 6 cm*	>6 cm
100 %	2	7	1	—	—	10
> 70 %	—	6	1	1	1	9
> 50 %	4	3	—	—	—	7
25-50 %	1	1	2	—	—	4
Minimal	—	—	1	1	—	2
NC	—	2	1	1	—	4
PD	1	—	—	—	—	1

* and > 6 cm

Table 4. Treatment followed after 3 cycles of CT

Treatment	Number of patients
RT	10
Surgery	3
RT + CT	3
RT + Surgery	2
CT	3
No treatment/Progressive disease	10
Lost to follow up	6

Table 5. Results

No. entered	37
No. evaluated	37
Response : Complete	10 (27 %)
Partial	19 (51 %)
No change	2
Progression	6
Total response	29 (78 %)
Median duration of survival	6 months (1 to 36 months)

A notable feature of this regime was the effect of Ifosfamide, Cisplatinum combination on the metastatic nodes. There was a dramatic reduction in the size of lymph nodes (Figs. 1-3). Out of 37 patients with metastatic nodes CR was seen in 10 patients (27 %) and PR in 19 patients (51 %). In one case a block dissection was performed which showed no microscopic evidence of disease in the specimen.

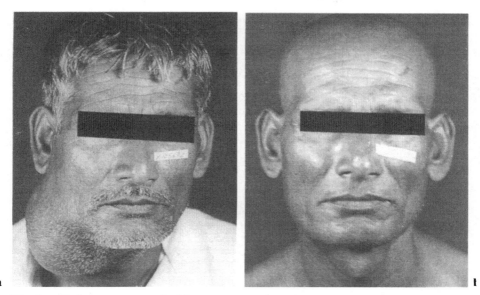

Fig. 1. a Before treatment, b After treatment

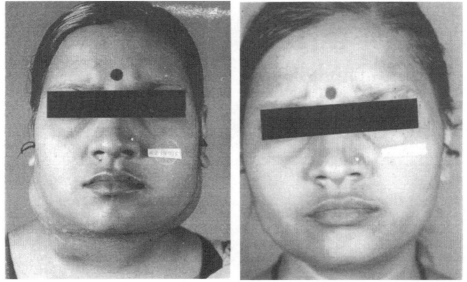

Fig. 2. a Before treatment, b After treatment

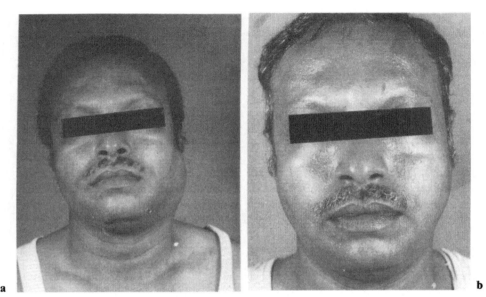

Fig. 3. a Before treatment, **b** After treatment

References

1. Legent F, Beanvillain C (1978) Experimentation clinique de l'Holoxan 1,000. Quest Med 6 : 377-380
2. Frenche Ch (1978) Essai de l'Holoxan 1,000 dans les cancers ORL. Gaz Med France 10 : 1081-1083
3. Sennon B (1978) Evaluation de l'Holoxan 1,000 dans les tumeurs ORL avancées. Extension aux cancers anaplasiques des bronches. RMSM. 2 : 137-138
4. Focan C, Salamon E, Le Hungs, Frere MM, Buyamb P, Claessens JJ. Efficacité d'une chimiothérapie séquentielle incluant la Vincristine, la Cisplatine et la Fosfamide dans le traitement des carcinomes de la tête et du cou stade IV et des mélanomes avec atteinte viscénale. Bull Cancer 71 : 105-107
5. Clark JR, Fallon BG, Dreyfuss AL, Norris CM, Anderson JW, Ervin TJ, Anderson RF, Claffy JT, Miller D, Frei III E (1988) Chemotherapeutic strategies in the multidisciplinary treatment of head and neck cancer. Sem Oncol 15 (suppl 3) : 35-44
6. Choksi AJ, Dimery IW, Hong WK (1988) Adjuvant chemotherapy of head and neck cancer : the past, the present and the future. Sem Oncol 15 (suppl 3) : pp 45-59

Abstract. *37 patients of advanced head and neck cancer with histologically proven metastatic squamous cell carcinoma were treated with Ifosfamide 1.5 gms/m^2 IV drip for half an hour in 125 ml of dextrose saline for 5 days and Mesna 20 % of the total Ifosfamide dose in 3 doses for 5 days in combination with Cisplatinum 10 mg/m^2 IV infusion for 5 days following Ifosfamide drip. The courses of treatment were repeated at the interval of every four weeks and total 3 cycles were given. Out of 37 patients with bulky nodes 10 patients showed total regression of nodes. 9 patients showed more than 75 % regression, 7 showed more than 50 % regression, 4 patients showed more than 25 % regression of nodes. There was no regression of nodes in 7 patients.*

This combination chemotherapy is very much effective against lymph node metastases.

Nausea, vomiting, alopecia and leucopenia was experienced by all patients.

Clinical pharmacokinetics of Pure 1 Folinic Acid and Fluorouracil during a phase I-II trial of Fluorouracil biomodulation in head and neck cancer patients. Preliminary data

MC Étienne*, G Milano*, M Schneider*, A Thyss*, O Dassonville*, M Bardon**, T Guillot**, F Demard*

5-Fluorouracil (5-FU) is increasingly used in the treatment of several types of malignancies, though not because of the efficacy of the drug itself. For example, even though 5-FU is widely used for the management of colorectal adenocarcinoma, it still has a disappointingly low efficacy when administered alone in this pathology [1, 2]. The renewed interest in 5-FU is linked to the results obtained when 5-FU is administered in combination with other drugs, in particular with Cisplatin (CDDP) for the treatment of head and neck cancer [3-5], and with Folinic Acid (FA) which significantly improves the response rate in colorectal carcinoma [6-9]. The improved efficacy obtained when 5-FU is administered in combination can be explained biochemically. Reduced folates enhance the inhibition of thymidylate synthase (TS) induced by the 5-FU anabolite, 5-fluoro-2'-deoxyuridine-5'-monophosphate [10, 11]. Although less work has been conducted on 5-FU potentiation by CDDP, the Cisplatin-induced increase in intracellular levels of reduced folates may be the main biochemical mechanism of 5-FU-CDDP synergism [12]. Administration of the triple association 5-FU-CDDP-FA was a logical consequence, which demonstrated objective responses in heavily pretreated patients with breast [13, 14], gastrointestinal [15, 16] and head and neck carcinoma [17]. However, severe toxicity has also occurred and caused a number of deaths [15]. Previous investigations from our group have shown that 5-FU-related toxicities can be predicted and controled by individual dose adjustment based on 5-FU pharmacokinetics [18].

Up to now, FA has usually been administered as the racemic mixture (dl-FA), whose biological activity is supported by natural 1 form (1-FA). Numerous pharmacokinetic studies have reported marked accumulation of d-FA in plasma relative to 1-FA during prolonged dl-FA administration [19, 20]. In addition, d-FA may compete with folyl polyglutamation [21] and folate membrane transport [22]. Thus there are objective reasons for using pure 1-FA instead of dl-FA. We present clinical and phamacokinetic preliminary data of a phase I-II trial, consisting in a 5-FU-CDDP-pure 1-FA combination administered as first line chemotherapy in head and neck cancer patients. Not only 5-FU plasma concentrations but also those of 1-FA and its active metabolite 5-methyltetrahydrofolate (5-MTHF) were analyzed.

---

* Centre Antoine-Lacassagne, 36 voie romaine, 06054 Nice Cedex ; ** Lederle Laboratories, 74, rue d'Arcueil, Silic 275, 94578 Rungis, France

Material and methods

Patients

This clinical trial was conducted on locally advanced (stage III-IV) head and neck cancer patients, all of whom not having been previously treated. The induction chemotherapy consisted in CDDP (100 mg/m^2, 1 mg/min IV) on day 1 followed by 5-FU (500 mg/m^2/d) plus pure 1-FA (200 mg/m^2/d) concomitantly administered by continuous venous infusion (day 2 to day 6). Three cycles were planned (day 1, day 22, day 43) and evaluation of response was done at day 53. This trial was initially planned to include 30 patients. So far, 21 patients have entered the study (20 men, 1 woman, median age 63, range 40-70). Primary site was oropharynx in 10 patients, oral cavity in 6 patients, hypopharynx in 3 patients, larynx in one patient and nasal fossa in one patient. Tumor size was T4 for the majority of patients (11/21 T4, 7/21 T3, 3/21 T2). Node involvement (N1, N2, N3) was observed in 16/21 patients.

Pharmacokinetic investigations

For each cycle, blood sampling was performed at H9, H24, H33, H48, H57, H81 and H105 after the start of the 5-FU-1-FA administration. 5-FU was analyzed in plasma using an HPLC assay initially described by Christophidis et al [23]. Pure 1-FA and 5-MTHF were analyzed in plasma using an HPLC assay previously developed in our laboratory. Area under the curve ($AUC_{0-105\,h}$) was calculated using the least square methodology and results were expressed as mean concentration over the cycle ($Cmean = AUC_{0-105\,h}/105$).

Statistics

5-FU, 1-FA and 5-MTHF concentrations did not fit a gaussian distribution, therefore non-parametric tests (Mann-Whitney, Speaman rank correlation) were used for studying the relationship between either toxicity or response to treatment and 5-FU or folate plasma concentrations. Statistical analysis was performed on Statgraphics solftware (Uniware, Paris, France).

Results

Up to now 13/21 patients have been assessable for response (1 death, 1 refusal, 6 on study) and 49 cycles have been analyzed for toxicity. Description of toxicity is presented in Table 1. The most frequent toxicity was mucositis, with grade 3-4 occurring in 45 % of cycles.

Overall objective responses (CR+PR) were observed in 77 % of patients (10/13). As concerns response on primary tumor, we observed 6 CR, 4 PR and 3 failures. Eleven patients assessable for response exhibited metastatic lymph nodes ; response on lymph nodes showed 5 CR, 2 PR and 4 failures.

At the present time, pharmacokinetic analysis has been performed for 47 cycles and results are reported in Table 2. 5-FU as well as 1-FA and

Table 1. Analysis of toxicity (49 cycles)

	OMS grade				grade
	1	2	3	4	3-4
Mucositis	3	10	17	5	45 %
Nausea-vomiting	5	3	3	—	6 %
Diarrhea	—	1	1	—	2 %
Alopecia	2	1	—	—	0 %
Rash	4	—	—	—	0 %
Neutropenia	8	11	6	1	14 %
Thrombopenia	4	—	1	—	2 %

Table 2. Pharmacokinetic analysis (Cmean, 47 cycles)

	5-FU (μM)	l-FA (μM)	5-MTHF (μM)
Mean	0.98	1.82	4.06
SD	0.34	1.06	1.38
Range	0.39-1.85	0.55-7.88	1.70-8.11

5-MTHF concentrations exhibited a great variability. Nevertheless, total active folate concentration (l-FA + 5-MTHF) was always above the micromolar level. Analysis of 5-FU-l-FA related toxicities (i.e. mucositis, hematological and digestive toxicities) as a function of pharmacokinetic data shows only a significant relationship between hematological toxicity and 5-FU concentrations (Mann-Whitney test, grade 0-1-2 *versus* grade 3-4, p = 0.01). Moreover, Fig. 1 illustrates the fact that the greater the hematological toxicity grade, the greater the 5-FU concentration (Spearman rank correlation, p = 0.009).

As concerns objective response to treatment, we were able to demonstrate a significant link between either 5-FU concentrations or total active folate concentrations and the response on primary tumor (Mann-Whitney test, CR + PR *versus* failure, p = 0.03 and 0.05 for 5-FU and folate concentrations respectively). Fig. 2 and 3 clearly show in fact that the 3 patients with treatment failure both exhibited low 5-FU and folate concentrations. No relationship was observed regarding response on lymph nodes.

Discussion

From these preliminary data it is certainly too early to draw any conclusions about the antitumor efficacy of this 5-FU-CDDP-l-FA combination. The 77 % response rate herein reported is very close to those recently published after induction chemotherapy with 5-FU-CDDP-dl-FA in head and neck carcinoma [24, 25]. Interestingly, a promising response rate on metastatic lymph nodes

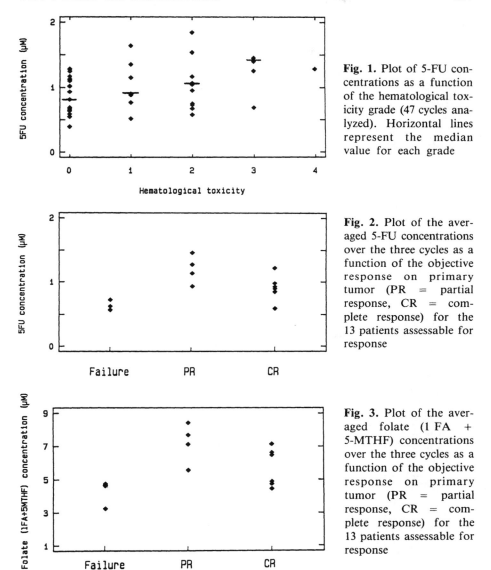

Fig. 1. Plot of 5-FU concentrations as a function of the hematological toxicity grade (47 cycles analyzed). Horizontal lines represent the median value for each grade

Fig. 2. Plot of the averaged 5-FU concentrations over the three cycles as a function of the objective response on primary tumor (PR = partial response, CR = complete response) for the 13 patients assessable for response

Fig. 3. Plot of the averaged folate (1 FA + 5-MTHF) concentrations over the three cycles as a function of the objective response on primary tumor (PR = partial response, CR = complete response) for the 13 patients assessable for response

was observed in the present study. Thus, the use of pure 1-FA in combination with 5-FU and CDDP leads to substantial tumor shrinkage in head and neck carcinoma. Whether or not the antitumor effects observed here with pure 1-FA are superior to those previously reported with dl-FA mixture should be prospectively tested in controled trials.

The present pharmacokinetic data on 5-FU and folate concentrations are instructive. The average active folate concentrations (1-FA + 5-MTHF) were above the micromolar level, which has been demonstrated to potentialize 5-FU toxicity on head and neck cancer cells *in vitro* [26]. The main limiting toxicity was mucositis, which would prevent the use of higher 5-FU doses. On average, 5-FU concentrations observed in the present study were around one half of that observed in patients treated with CDDP plus 5-FU alone (5 days CVI) [27]. Significantly higher 5-FU plasma concentrations were demonstrated in patients exhibiting severe hematological toxicities as compared to patients with no or moderate hematological toxicities. This is in line with previous data from our group which have shown a significant link between high 5-FU $AUC_{0-105 h}$ and 5-FU-related toxicity after 5-FU-CDDP chemotherapy in head and neck cancer patients [27]. More interesting is the fact that the three non-responsive patients exhibited both low 5-FU and active folate plasma concentrations. Taken together, these observations suggest the possibility of defining an optimal plasma concentration for 5-FU and folates allowing a maximal probability of efficacy and a limited risk of severe toxicities. A wider patient recruitment in the present trial will reveal whether this exciting hypothesis is to be confirmed or not.

References

1. Moertel CB (1978) Chemotherapy of gastrointestinal cancer. N Engl J Med 299 : 1049-1052
2. Cohen AM, Shank B, Friedman MA (1989) Colorectal cancer. In : De Vita VT, Hellman S, Rosenberg SA (eds) Cancer principles and practice of oncology. JB Lippincott Company, Philadelphia, p. 895
3. Kish J, Drelichman A, Jacobs J et al (1982) Clinical trial of Cisplatin and 5-FU infusion as initial treatment for advanced squamous cell carcinoma of the head and neck. Cancer Treat Rep 66 : 471-474
4. Amrein PC, Weitzman SA (1985) Treatment of squamous cell carcinoma of the head and neck with Cisplatin and 5-Fluorouracil. J Clin Oncol 3 : 1632-1635
5. Thyss A, Schneider M, Santini J et al (1986) Induction chemotherapy with Cisplatinum and 5-Fluorouracil for squamous cell carcinoma of the head and neck. Br J Cancer 54 : 755-760
6. Machover D, Goldschmidt E, Chollet P et al (1986) Treatment of advanced colorectal and gastric adenocarcinomas with 5-Fluorouracil and high-dose Folinic acid. J Clin Oncol 4 : 685-696
7. Rustum YM (1989) Toxicity and antitumor activity of 5-Fluorouracil in combination with Leucovorin. Role of dose schedule and route of administration of Leucovorin. N° 63 : 1013-1016
8. O'Connell MJ (1989) A phase III trial of 5-Fluorouracil and Leucovorin in the treatment of advanced colorectal cancer. A Mayo Clinic/North Central Cancer Treatment Group Study. Cancer 63 : 1026-1029
9. Arbuck SG (1989) Overview of clinical trials using 5-Fluorouracil and Leucovorin for the treatment of colorectal cancer. Cancer 63 : 1036-1039
10. Houghton JA, Schmidt C, Houghton PJ (1982) The effect of derivatives of Folic acid on the Fluorodeoxyuridylate-thymidylate synthetase covalent complex in human colon xenografts. Eur J Cancer Clin Oncol 18 : 347-350
11. Kerr DJ (1989) 5-Fluorouracil and Folinic acid, interesting biochemistry or effective treatment ? Br J Cancer 60 : 807-810
12. Scanlon KJ, Newman EM, Lu Y, Priest DG (1986) Biochemical basis for Cisplatin and 5-Fluorouracil synergism in human ovarian carcinoma cells. Proc Natl Acad Sci USA 83 : 8923-8926

13. Hart L, Chua C, Brophy L (1989) Salvage chemotherapy for metastatic breast carcinoma using Cisplatin, Fluorouracil and Leucovorin : a phase I-II study. Proc ASCO 8 : 43
14. Allegra CJ, Mayer A, Reed E et al (1989) Therapy of patients with metastatic breast cancer with 5-Fluorouracil, Leucovorin and Carboplatin. Proc ASCO 8 : 54
15. Leong L, Doroshow J, Ackman S et al (1989) Phase II trial of 5-FU and high dose Folinic acid with Cisplatin and Dipyridamole in advanced colorectal cancer. Proc ASCO 8 : 99
16. Fernandes JP, Oliveira J, Santos A et al (1989) Cisplatin, Fluorouracil and Folinic acid in advanced gastric cancer. Proc ASCO 8 : 115
17. Vokes EE, Schilsky RL, Weichselbaum RR et al (1989) Cisplatin, 5-Fluorouracil and high-dose oral Leucovorin for advanced head and neck cancer. Cancer 63 : 1048-1051
18. Santini J, Milano G, Thyss A et al (1989) 5-FU therapeutic monitoring with dose adjustement leads to improved therapeutic index in head and neck cancer. Br J Cancer 59 : 287-290
19. Schilsky RL, Ratain MJ (1990) Clinical pharmacokinetics of high-dose Leucovorin calcium after intravenous and oral administration. J Natl Cancer Inst 82 ; 1411-1415
20. Newman EM, Straw JA, Doroshow JH (1989) Pharmacokinetics of diastereoisomers of (6 R,S) — Folinic acid (Leucovorin) in humans during constant high-dose intravenous infusion. Cancer Res 49 : 5755-5760
21. Sato JK, Moran RG (1984) Interaction of Methotrexate and Citrovorum factor with folyl polyglutamate synthetase. Proc Am Assoc Cancer Res 1234 : 312
22. Bertrand R, Jolivet J (1988) The natural and unnatural diastereoisomers of Leucovorin : aspects of their cellular pharmacology. In : Rustum Y, McGuire JJ (eds) The expanding role of folates and fluoropyrimidines in cancer chemotherapy. Plenum Press, New York, pp. 13-22
23. Christophidis N, Mihaly G, Vadja F et al (1979) Comparison of liquid-and-gas liquid chromatographic assays of 5-Fluorouracil in plasma. Clin Chem 25 : 83-86
24. Vokes EE, Schilsky RL, Weichselbaum RR et al (1990) Induction chemotherapy with Cisplatin, Fluorouracil and high-dose Leucovorin for locally advanced head and neck cancer. J Clin Oncol 8 : 241-247
25. Dreyfuss AI, Clark JR, Wright JE et al (1990) Continuous infusion of high-dose Leucovorin with 5-Fluorouracil and Cisplatin for untreated stage IV carcinoma of the head and neck. Ann Int Med 112 : 167-172
26. Etienne MC, Bernard S, Fischel JL et al (1991) Dose reduction without loss of efficacy for 5-Fluorouracil and Cisplatin combined with Folinic acid. In vitro study on human head and neck carcinoma cells. Br J Cancer 63 : 372-377
27. Thyss A, Milano G, Renée N et al (1986) Clinical pharmacokinetic study of 5-FU in continuous 5-days infusions for head and neck cancer. Cancer Chemother Pharmacol 16 : 64-66

Long-term follow-up of the patients with recurrent or advanced head and neck cancer who received chemotherapy for palliation

Y Inuyama

Before Bleomycin (BLM) was developed, there were almost no reports on the 5-year survivals of the patients with recurrent or advanced head and neck cancer who was treated with chemotherapy alone. After the appearance of BLM, however, there are some reports on the long-term surviving patients cured with BLM, but only in early or small recurrent diseases. Since combination chemotherapy based on cell kinetics and Cisplatin (CDDP) appeared, we have observed the long-term survivals even in recurrent or advanced cancer [1]. The purpose of this paper is to present the long-term follow-up of the patients with recurrent or advanced head and neck cancer who received chemotherapy for palliation.

Material and methods

We have treated 250 patients with recurrent or advanced head and neck cancer with palliative chemotherapy for the purpose of prolonging life and improving quality of life for the past 17 years. Single agent chemotherapy or combined chemotherapy regimens used are as follows : Peplomycin (PEP), Cisplatin (CDDP), UFT (Uracil + Tegafur), new analogs of CDDP (Carboplatin, 254-S) for single agent chemotherapy, and BLM + Mitomycin C (MMC), Vincristine (VCR) + Methotrexate (MTX) + BLM, Price-Hill regimen, VCR + MTX + BLM + MMC, Vindesine (VDS) + MTX + PEP, CDDP + PEP [2], Adriamycin (ADM) or Pirarubicin (THP) + CDDP + PEP, VCR + CDDP + PEP, CDDP + 5-Fluorouracil (5-FU), CDDP + Etoposide (ETP). CDDP + ETP + MMC, etc. for combination chemotherapy.

Results

250 patients were treated with chemotherapy for palliation. The response rate of chemotherapy for recurrent or advanced head and neck cancer ranged from 32 to 71 % with no CR before we used CDDP. After we used CDDP, it looked almost similar, ranging from 35 to 68 %. But CR rate was much improved, ranging from 10 to 27 % (Table 1).

Out of the 250 patients, 150 patients with local-regional diseases and 50 patients with distant metastases were followed up and evaluated. For the rest of them, chemotherapy was discontinued and other treatment was performed. The long-term survival of the patients with local-regional diseases is

---

Department of Otolaryngology, Hokkaido University School of Medecine, Kita-15, Nishi-7, Kita-Ku, Sapporo, 060, Japan

Table 1. Response to chemotherapy in recurrent or advanced head and neck cancer

Chemotherapy	No. of patients	Response rate (%)	CR rate (%)
BLM, MMC	37	32	0
PEP	7	71	0
VCR, MTX, BLM	8	50	0
Price-Hill	8	50	0
VCR, MTX, BLM, MMC	22	68	0
CDDP	20	35	10
UFT	20	40	20
CDDP, PEP	72	67	26
ADM, CDDP, PEP	11	64	27

Table 2. Long-term survival of the patients with recurrent or advanced head and neck cancer who received chemotherapy for palliation

Chemotherapy	No. of patients	1	2	3	4	5	6	7	8	9	10	11	12	13
BLM, MMC	20		1	2										
PEP	4	1			1									
VCR, MTX, BLM	4	1												
Price-Hill	2													
VCR, MTX, BLM, MMC	18	2		1										
CDDP	7	1											1*	1*
UFT	24	8	3			1*								
CDDP, PEP	17	1	3	1										
VDS, MTX, PEP (VMP)	9	2												
ADM (THP), CDDP, PEP	10	1												
VCR, CDDP, PEP	20	5	1											
CDDP, 5-FU (CF)	1		1											
254-S	9	2												
VMP→CF	5	5												
Total	150	24	9	4	1	1							1	1

* surviving

shown on Table 2. 25 patients remained alive one to 2 years after chemotherapy, 10 patients 2 to 3 years, 4 patients 3 to 4 years, 1 patient 4 to 5 years, respectively. Meanwhile we have 3 patients who have been alive more than 5 years after chemotherapy. The survival years are 6, 12 and 13 years, respectively. So the survival curve steeply declined at 1 and 2 years, and then reached a plateau at 4 years. The 5 and 10-year survival rates were 2.6 % (3/114) and 2.1 % (2/96), respectively. These results suggested that combination chemotherapy did not always improve a prolongation of life, though it resulted in a higher complete response rate as compared with single agent chemotherapy.

In terms of the long-term survival of the patients with distant metastases, the median survival was 10 months, ranging from 2 to 53 months. So we have no patients who have survived more than 5 years.

Case reports

Two interesting cases are presented :

Case 1 : T S, 50-year-old male, cancer of the lower gingiva (well differentiated squamous cell carcinoma),T4N0M0. The tumor destroyed the mandible and invaded the skin of the upper neck. Therefore we administered combination chemotherapy consisting of VCR, MTX and BLM. At the completion of the 6th cycle, a near complete response was achieved. But 2 months later, regrowth of the tumor was observed, so we administered CDDP at the dose of 50 mg/m^2/cycle intravenously over 24 hours. After the completion of the second cycle, the tumor completely disappeared, but we added one more cycle. Thereafter the patients was given tegafur and Krestin® (a kind of biological response modifier) orally for 1 year and then Krestin alone. He had been disease free for 12 years. But now we lost his follow-up [3].

Case 2 : T K, 33-year-old male, maxillary sinus carcinoma (moderately differentiated squamous cell carcinoma), rT3N0M0. This patient was primarily treated with radiotherapy at the total dose of 50 Gy combined with intraarterial infusion of 5-FU, but the tumor recurred 4 months later. The patient, however, did not want to undergo an operation, so he was administered CDDP at the dose of 50 mg/m^2/cycle intraarterially. The tumor completely disappeared after the completion of the second cycle, but we added one more cycle. Then he was given 5-FU dry syrup and Krestin for 1 year. He has been disease free for 13 years.

Conclusion

The 5- and 10-year survival rates were 2.6 % and 2.1 %, respectively in patients with local-regional diseases who received chemotherapy for palliation. Higher complete response rates were achieved in combination chemotherapy as compared with single agent chemotherapy, but it did not always result in a prolongation of life. In the patients with distant metastases, the median survival was 10 months, ranging from 2 to 53 months.

References

1. Inuyama Y, Horiuchi M et al (1982) Clinical effect of Cisplatin (NK-801) on head neck cancer. Jpn J Clin Oncol 12 : 355-362
2. Inuyama Y, Fujii M et al (1986) Combination chemotherapy with Cisplatin and Peplomycin in squamous cell carcinoma of the head and neck. Auris Nasus Larynx 13 : 191-198
3. Inuyama Y, Fukuda S et al (1990) Prolongation of life and improvement of quality of life with use of chemotherapy for advanced or recurrent head and neck cancer. In : Sacristan T (ed) Otorhinolaryngology, Head & Neck Surgery. Kugler & Ghedini Publication, Amsterdam, p. 2651

Intensified concomitant chemoradiotherapy for poor prognosis head and neck cancer

EE Vokes, DJ Haraf, W Moran, B Wenig, D Brachman, S Rubin, JM McEvilly, P Luckett, WR Panje, RR Weichselbaum

Head and neck cancer presents most commonly as a locoregionally advanced malignant process [1]. Distant metastases are clinically rare, but may be present more frequently at the microscopic level. Patterns of failure following standard surgery and/or radiotherapy indicate the inability of that therapy to successfully eradicate locoregional disease in the majority of patients. Investigational therapy, therefore, must focus on increasing the efficacy of locoregional therapy as its primary goal. Eradication of systemic microscopic disease remains a secondary goal that may gain greater importance in patients whose locoregional disease can be controlled [2]. Finally, the prevention of second malignancies represents an important long-term goal that can help to maintain the cancer-free status in patients cured of their primary disease [3].

In pursuing more active locoregional therapy, the clinical Head and Neck Oncology Program at the University of Chicago has focused largely on the biochemical modulation of fluorouracil (5-FU) and the interaction of chemotherapy and radiation. The latter, in particular, has been shown to lead to improved disease-free survival and/or overall survival in randomized clinical trials [4-7].

In 1986, we initiated a phase I trial to investigate the interaction of 5-FU, hydroxyurea (HU) and radiotherapy (FHX) [8, 9]. Both chemotherapy agents have known systemic activity and can be postulated to contribute to systemic control of head and neck cancer and to locoregional tumor shrinkage. In addition, HU may modulate the activity of 5-FU. HU is a ribonucleotide reductase inhibitor that depletes cellular pools of deoxyuridine monophosphate (dUMP) and thus facilitates binding of the 5-FU metabolite 5-FdUMP to its target enzyme thymidylate synthase. Synergistic interaction of these two agents has been demonstrated in the laboratory [10]. Finally, both agents have been shown to act as radiation enhancers *in vitro* and *in vivo* [4, 5, 11]. Studies using two cell lines derived from patients with squamous cell cancer of the head and neck at our institution demonstrated additive activity for 5-FU and HU as single agents and in combination when administered with radiation. This effect was seen in a relatively radiation-resistant cell line, SQ-20B, with a D_0 of 239 cGy but not in SQ38, a more radiation responsive cell line with a D_0 146 cGy.

Our initial study was designed to identify the maximal tolerated doses of 5-FU and HU when administered with concomitant radiotherapy on a protract-

---

From the University of Chicago, Department of Medicine and Department of Radiation and Cellular Oncology; the University of Illinois at Chicago, Department of Otolaryngology-Head and Neck Surgery, and Rush-Presbyterian St. Luke's Medical Center, Department of Otolaryngology and Bronchoesophagology

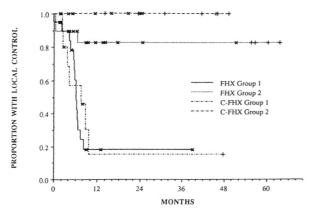

Fig. 1.

ed schedule. We identified as recommended dose of 5-FU 800 mg/m²/day administered as a 5 day continuous infusion. The maximal tolerated dose of HU was 1000 mg administered orally every 12 h for a total of 11 doses beginning prior to the 5-FU infusion and with one daily dose preceding radiotherapy by 2 hours. These doses resulted in moderate to severe mucositis and mild to moderate myelosuppression [8]. Radiotherapy was administered once daily at 180 to 200 cGy.

Patients treated with palliative intent were eligible for this study. There were no limitations on prior therapy, including prior radiotherapy. For the purpose of outcome analysis, we divided patients into two groups ; those having received prior local therapy (Group 1) and those not having received prior local therapy (Group 2). The latter group included patients with metastatic disease, those with poor renal or pulmonary function, and patients having received prior chemotherapy.

Response rates exceeded 90 % in both groups of patients. However, the majority of patients in Group 1 developed locoregionally recurrent disease and the median time to progression was 6 months. In Group 2, only 3 of 19 patients developed locoregional recurrence ; this included two patients who only received two cycles of chemoradiotherapy and then refused further therapy (Fig. 1).

These data suggested that this regimen had high locoregional activity and could be studied further in previously untreated patients in an attempt to improve locoregional control and thus contribute to improved survival. We have, therefore, since 1989 incorporated this FHX regimen into our overall treatment strategy for previously untreated patients with locoregionally advanced disease [12, 13]. Other authors have confirmed the high activity of this regimen [14, 15].

In parallel studies, we sought to further increase the activity of the FHX regimen by adding Cisplatin and/or Leucovorin to the combination (C-FHX) [2, 16, 17]. The choice of Cisplatin as third chemotherapy drug was based on its known single agent activity in head and neck cancer [1]. This activity might result in a further increase in the locoregional activity of this regimen while also increasing its systemic activity against micrometastatic disease. In addition, it has been shown to be synergistic with 5-FU and with HU. The mechanism of interaction between Cisplatin and 5-FU appears to be based on an increase of intracellular reduced folate pools following administration of Cisplatin ; therefore, it is similar to 5-FU modulation with Leucovorin [16]. HU on the other hand, depletes intracellular nucleotide pools and, thus, may decrease the cell's ability to repair Cisplatin DNA damage [16]. While the optimal schedule of Cisplatin administration has not been established, animal experiments have suggested, that its daily administration prior to a radiotherapy fraction may result in optimal radiation enhancement [5, 18]. Clinical studies have not identified a superior schedule of Cisplatin administration ; however, pharmacologic studies have suggested that administration as a continuous intravenous infusion might be superior since it may result in a higher area under the time versus concentration curve for non-protein bound platinum [19].

Based on this rationale, we conducted a broad phase I study that attempted to add continuous infusion Cisplatin to the previously described FHX regimen [16, 17]. At the initial dose of 10 mg/m^2/day for 5 days dose-limiting myelosuppression was observed. Therefore, we altered the regimen to administer Cisplatin only every other cycle (odd cycles) and utilize Leucovorin as a different (less myelosuppressive) 5-FU modulator on even cycles. The maximal tolerated dose of Cisplatin on this schedule was 20 mg/m^2/day of infusional Cisplatin with 600 mg/m^2/day of 5-FU on odd cycles and 400 mg/m^2/day of 5-FU with Leucovorin on even cycles. The dose of HU was decreased to 500 mg orally twice daily for eleven doses on all cycles. Using these doses, 33 % of patients developed grade 3 or 4 neutropenia during cycles 1 and 2 and 71 % at some time during their therapy. In patients receiving radiation to the head and neck a 69 % incidence of grade 3 or 4 mucositis was observed with this leucovorin containing regimen. This toxicity profile suggested that the addition of continuous infusion Cisplatin to the FHX combination came at the price of severe myelosuppression and that its alternation with leucovorin did not allow for further dose escalation of Cisplatin beyond 100 mg/m^2 every 4 weeks while increasing the incidence of severe mucositis. Response rates, local control and survival figures in this study were similar to that seen with FHX alone and again indicated excellent locoregional control in patients without previous surgery and/or radiation (Fig. 1).

We also tested the administration of Cisplatin as a daily short-term infusion at 20 mg/m^2/day on odd cycles and as a single 6 h infusion on day 2 of odd cycles. This change of cisplatin schedule did not result in a lower incidence of severe or life-threatening myelosuppression [unpublished data].

These data suggested that the clinical utility of this C-FHX regimen would be severely limited by its aggressive systemic toxicity profile. In an effort to ameliorate this severe toxicity, we have most recently added granulocyte-colony stimulating factor (G-CSF) to the combination. G-CSF is administered on days 6-12 of each cycle following 5 days of chemoradiotherapy with Cisplatin, 5-FU and HU. With G-CSF it has become feasible to administer this regimen with less myelosuppression. We have been able to escalate the dose of HU from 500 mg orally twice daily to 1 000 mg twice daily as originally given in this FHX combination without Cisplatin. In addition, the incidence of acute grade 3 or 4 mucositis appears reduced and intensification of the radiotherapy schedule to two daily fractions is currently being investigated. Should G-CSF allow for this intensified Cisplatin FHX regimen, we intent to test it in previously untreated patients with locoregionally advanced disease in the near future.

References

1. Vokes EE, Weichselbaum RR, Lippman S, Hong WK (1993) Head and Neck Cancer. N Engl J Med 328 : 184-194
2. Vokes EE, Weichselbaum RR, Mick R et al (1992) Favorable long-term survival following induction chemotherapy with PFL and concomitant chemoradiotherapy for locally advanced head and neck cancer. J Natl Cancer Inst 84 : 877-882
3. Hong WK, Lippman SM, Itri LM et al (1990) Prevention of second primary tumors with isotretinoin in squamous-cell carcinoma of the head and neck. N Engl J Med 3223 : 795-801
4. Vokes EE, Weichselbaum RR (1990) Concomitant chemoradiotherapy : Rationale and clinical experience in patients with solid tumors. J Clin Oncol 8 : 911-934
5. Vokes EE The interaction of chemotherapy and radiation. Sem Oncol (in press)
6. Merlano M, Vitale V, Rosso R et al (1992) Treatment of advanced squamous-cell carcinoma of the head and neck with alternating chemotherapy and radiotherapy. N Engl J Med 327 : 1115-1121
7. Bachaud JM, David JM, Boussin G, Daly N (1991) Combined postoperative radiotherapy and weekly cisplatin infusion for locally advanced squamous cell carcinoma of the head and neck : Preliminary report of a randomized trial. Int J Radiat Oncol Biol Phys 20 : 243-246
8. Vokes EE, Panje WR, Schilsky RL et al (1989) Hydroxyurea, 5-Fluorouracil and concomitant radiotherapy in poor prognosis head and neck cancer : A phase I-II study. J Clin Oncol 7 : 761-768
9. Haraf DJ, Vokes EE, Panje WR, Weichselbaum RR (1991) Survival and analysis of failure following hydroxyurea, 5-Fluorouracil and concomitant radiation therapy in poor prognosis head and neck cancer. Am J Clin Oncol 14 : 419-426
10. Moran RG, Danenberg PV, Heidelberger C (1982) Therapeutic response of leukemic mice treated with fluorinated pyrimidines and inhibitors of deoxyuridylate synthesis. Biochem Pharmacol 31 : 2929-2935
11. Vokes EE, Beckett MA, Karrison T, Weichselbaum RR (1992) The interaction of 5-Fluorouracil hydroxyurea and radiation in two human head and neck cancer cell lines. Oncology 49 : 454-460
12. Vokes EE, Haraf DJ, McEvilly JM et al (1992) Neo-Adjuvant PFL augmented by methotrexate and piritrexim followed by concomitant chemoradiotherapy for advanced head and neck cancer : a feasible and active approach. Ann Oncol 3 : 79-81
13. Vokes EE, Ratain MJ, Mick R et al (1993) Cisplatin, Fluorouracil and Leucovorin Augmented by Interferon α-2B in Head and Neck Cancer : A Clinical and Pharmacologic Analysis. J Clin Oncol (in press)
14. Guillot T, Wibault P, Cvitkovic et al (1990) Treatment of « favorable » recurrent head and neck squamous cell cancer with 5 days on/9 days off simultaneous chemoradiotherapy Vokes-Weichselbaum protocol. Proc Am Soc Clin Oncol 10 : 684 (Abstract)
15. Weppelmann B, Wheeler RA, Peters GE et al (1992) Treatment of recurrent head and neck cancer with 5-Fluorouracil, hydroxyurea and reirradiation. Int J Radiat Oncol Biol Phys 22 : 1051-1056
16. Vokes EE, Moormeier J, Ratain MJ et al (1992) 5-Fluorouracil, Leucovorin,

Hydroxyurea, and escalating doses of continuous infusion cisplatin with concomitant radiotherapy : a clinical and pharmacologic study. Cancer Chemother Pharmacol 29 : 178-184
17. Haraf DJ, Vokes EE, Weichselbaum RR, Panje WR (1992) Concomitant chemoradio-therapy with cisplatin, 5-Fluorouracil and Hydroxyurea in poor prognosis head and neck cancer. Laryngoscope 102 : 630-636
18. Kanazawa H, Rapacchietta D, Kallman RF (1988) Schedule-dependent therapeutic gain from the combination of fractionated irradiation and cis-diamminedichloroplatinum (II) in C3H/Km mouse model systems. Cancer Res 48 : 3158-3164
19. Vokes EE, Ackland SP, Vogelzang NJ (1990) Cisplatin, Carboplatin, and gallium nitrate. In : Lokich JJ (ed) Cancer Chemotherapy by infusion (2nd Edition). Precept Press, Chicago, p 176

Response to chemotherapy of ulcerative lymphoma of the midface

J Cabane*, Cl Grange*, G Lamas**, B Meyer***,
P Godeau****, JC Imbert*

It has recently been shown that the rare and ominous disease called « lethal midline granuloma » was in fact a true malignant lymphoma in most cases [1]. This disease represents a formidable challenge for the clinician : he has first to reach the diagnosis by the exclusion of dozens of other diseases capable of destroying the center of the face ; then he must select a curative treatment together with supportive measures including nutrition therapy in those cachectic patients ; and he must manage severe sepsis problems arising from the ulcerated face. We present here our 10-year experience of those ulcerative lymphomas of the midface (ULM).

Patients and methods

From 1986 on we conducted a nationwide protocol, headed by the French National Society of Internal Medicine (SNFMI) and with the help of the French ENT society, on the problem of diseases necrotizing the center of the face. The protocol gave to the clinician faced with such patients an exhaustive list of all diseases to search for and the diagnostic aids to ask ; then it gave loose treatment directions but asked for a precise report of the treatments given ; endly it proposed a biopsy protocol including light microscopy, cell surface immunotyping and molecular biology techniques on cryostored samples. We thus collected data about 40 cases. We will present here only the radio- and chemotherapy results observed among those patients who definitely had malignant lymphomas according to the microscopical and immunotyping criteria.

Results

Among the 27 ULM patients, 15 received radiation therapy (40 to 60 Gy to the face with the dose adjusted to the volume of the facial lesions according to the CT-scan). This treatment was given either alone (n = 7) or with chemo-

---

* Service de médecine interne, hôpital Saint-Antoine, 184, faubourg Saint-Antoine, 75571 Paris Cedex 12, France ; ** Service d'oto-rhino-laryngologie, hôpital de la Pitié, 87, boulevard de l'hôpital, 75013 Paris, France ; *** Service d'oto-rhino-laryngologie, hôpital Saint-Antoine, 184, faubourg Saint-Antoine, 75571 Paris Cedex 12, France ; **** Service de médecine interne, hôpital de la Pitié, 87, boulevard de l'hôpital, 75013 Paris, France

therapy (n = 8). One patient died from septic schock before treatment. One received different radiation treatments on three different facial sites (pharynx, frontal sinus and maxillary sinus) on successive relapses.

Chemotherapy was given alone to 9 patients with contra-indication of radiation therapy (mostly because of relapse following a previous treatment).

The response rate of the patients given radiation therapy alone was 6/7 (86 %) but only the half of these responders achieved a long-term remission. The others had relapses in the months following the end of the treatment (from 6 to 17 months) and were treated with chemotherapy or interferon.

The response rate for chemotherapy alone was 2/9 (22 %) ; of these two, one received then for a relapse radiation therapy and is a long-term survivor. The other relapsed after a year and eventually died from septic schock during a second chemotherapy trial. Unfortunately, there was a failure rate of 33 % (3/9 patients with extension of the facial necrosis despite chemotherapy) and a 45 % rate of severe septic complications including septic schock, facial cellulitis and pneumonia. These events obscured the evaluation of the response to chemotherapy, since many patients died after the first cycles of chemotherapy.

8 patients received combined radiation therapy and chemotherapy, yielding a response rate of 5/8 (62 %) but 3 relapsed ; hence only 2 patients remain as long-term survivors. Although the numbers are small, they do not markedly differ from those of the patients having received radiation therapy alone.

Comments

It has been known for 50 years since Stewart's first description [2] that midline granulomas are malignant diseases. Indeed, the only patient showing an improvement in the princeps paper by Stewart had received radiation therapy by means of radium needles inserted into his nose [2]. Although large comparative series are not available for this rare disease, some authors have tried radiation therapy and found it to be useful, at the expense of a risk of brainstem infarction [3]. On the other hand, chemotherapy has not met similar success : in some cases, patients have been given Cyclophosphamide-Prednisone combinations after Wegener's disease treatment protocols, with few or no responses ; the other cases published were given polychemotherapy after the malignant lymphomas protocols, mostly the ACVBP regimen (Adriamycin, Cyclophosphamide, Vincristine, Bleomycin, and Prednisone). The results in the literature parallel those in our patients : the few responses are outnumbered by numerous septic problems which often killed the patients in the first month of treatment.

Thus, other means of treatment are to be proposed for this disease. We think that a multidisciplinary approach is needed since ULM patients pose original problems :

— the lymphoid proliferation has a peculiar tendency to necrotize itself as it extends through the facial bones. Hence a new staging system should be used, with the help of the ENT specialist physician and the CT scan ;

— the infection control should be strenghened by systematic drainage and culture — oriented antibiotic therapy of every purulent retention in the facial cavities particularly the sinuses. The spontaneous and chemotherapy-induced neutropenia should be corrected with the help of growth factors ;

— radiation therapy remains the best first line of treatment : thus, it must be given to every patient to whom it can be. Careful dosimetry and delivery by an expert team should avoid radiation-induced problems (we observed no side-effects among our 17 radiation-treated patients) ;

— for those patients who cannot benefit from radiation therapy, a protocol with high-dose chemotherapy and growth factors is underway (we start an open pilot study with C2E2OP and GmCSF) ;

— the nutrition therapy of these cachectic and anorectic patients appears to be of prime importance. It can be delivered either by an intravenous line or preferably by the enteral route (either by a nasogastric tube or by gastrostomy).

We hope that such new directions of care will yield better results in those severely ill patients. Hopefully they will be included in ongoing protocols in order to give quickly the answers we need.

Conclusion

Ulcerative Lymphomas of the Midface (ULM) are peculiar lymphomas of difficult diagnosis and very poor response to conventional therapy. Owing to the mixture of different cells infiltrating the face around the necrotic areas, the diagnosis is always difficult, even with the help of good biopsies with immunotyping techniques. The patients are often in poor general status due to anorexia and local septic complications. Radiation therapy can cure the disease if it is possible to give it at high doses to the entire involved area. Chemotherapy has up to now given few good results ; however, innovative protocols with help of growth factors remain to be tried. Anyway, those patients should be managed in multidisciplinary teams with internist, maxillofacial, ENT, nutrition and oncology specialists working together.

References

1. Grange Cl, Cabane J, Dubois A, Raphael M, Chomette G, Lamas G, Godeau P, Meyer B, Imbert JC (1992) Centrofacial malignant granulomas. Clinicopathologic study of 40 cases and review of the literature. Medicine 71 : 179-196
2. Stewart JP (1933) Progressive lethal granulomatous ulceration of the nose. J Laryngol 48 : 657-701
3. Tsokos M, Fauci AS, Costa J (1982) Idiopathic midline destructive disease (IMDD). A subgroup of the patients with the « midline granuloma » syndrome. Am J Clin Pathol 77 : 162-168

A multicentric study of the GETTEC (Groupe d'Études des Tumeurs de la Tête et du Cou) about 408 clinically complete responders after Neo-Adjuvant chemotherapy for head and neck carcinomas

P Chauvel, JL Lefèbvre, B Luboinski, G Kantor, M Bolla, G Andry, J Brugère, JJ Pessey, F Demard

Material and methods

Clinically Complete Response (CCR) occuring after induction chemotherapy has often been considered as a good prognosis indicator. The routine use of CDDP-5-FU giving a relatively large amount of CCR, the GETTEC, a francophone study group, promoted in 1985 a multicentric study (ERCCACI : Enregistrement des Régressions Cliniques Complètes Après Chimiothérapie d'Induction) recording all these CCR in order to assess its value, the endpoints being survival, local and regional control, metastasis and second primaries. Retrospective inclusions were allowed and a total number of 408 cases were included by 8 institutions from april 1981 to may 1991 : almost a half of the patients has been included by the Centre Antoine-Lacassagne (215) in Nice, followed by the Centre Oscar-Lambret (55) in Lille, Institut Gustave-Roussy (36) in Villejuif, Fondation Bergonié (31) in Bordeaux, Hopital Michallon (23) in Grenoble, Institut Jules-Bordet (20) in Brussels, Institut Curie (18) in Paris, Hopital de Rangueil (10) in Toulouse.

The first patients were retrospectively included in the study by 4 centers performing induction chemotherapy for a long time (Bordeaux, Brussels, Nice and Lille) and the accrual was at its best on 1987, when some of us were convinced that chemotherapy could modify the prognosis of head and neck tumors.

Results

This series includes 358 men and 50 women, aged from 20 to 80 (mean 57.1). The repartition by sites is : oral cavity 74, oropharynx 158, larynx 79, hypopharynx 97. 88.2 % of the patients received a CDDP-5-FU combination ; 7.4 % have been lost for follow-up. UICC staging at presentation was : stage I : 2 %, stage II : 19 %, grouped in a first category of stages I-II, the stages III and IV represent a large majority of 79 % (321 patients). The repartition by stage varied widely from one institution to another (from 4.3 % to 33 % for stages I/II), but this does not represent a problem, the condition for inclusion being CCR. The proportion of patients without detectable nodes (No) at presentation, varied from one site to another : Oral Cavity and Larynx with

---

GETTEC c/o Centre A-Lacassagne, 36 voie Romaine, 06054 Nice, France

62 % and 60 % are opposed to oropharynx and hypopharynx with only 37 % and 30 %. The proportion of stages III-IV are respectively : 66 % and 68 % versus 82 % and 91 %. Crude actuarial survival at 1, 3, 5 and 7 years is : 88 %, 61 %, 48 % and 41 % respectively ; at the same intervals, the actuarial rates are :
— for tumor local relapse : 10 %, 26 %, 31 % and 35 % ;
— for nodal relapse : 5 %, 13 %, 15 % and 15 % ;
— for distant metastasis occurence : 6 %, 17 %, 22 % and 24 %. The 5 years actuarial survival for each tumor site is significantly different (p = 0.0004) : larynx 63 %, oropharynx 53.4 %, oral cavity 51 %, hypopharynx 24.4 %. The 5 years actuarial rates of tumor local relapse are 50 % for hypopharynx, 43 % for oral cavity, 25 % for oropharynx and 17 % for larynx (p = 0.0004). For nodal relapse, oropharynx, oral cavity, and larynx are grouped between 14 and 10 %, hypopharynx being at 32 %, but this difference is not statistically significant ;
— for distant metastasis, oropharynx, oral cavity and larynx are at 16 %, 17 % and 18 %, when hypopharynx is at 47 % (p = 0.0001) ;
— for second primary : the numbers are relatively close around 20 % (except for hypopharynx : 40 %) and the differences non significant.

The evolution is different from one site to another, local relapse seems to be the most frequent event in oral cavity (38.2 % versus 10, 12 and 22 % for nodal relapse, distant metastasis and second primary) ; for oropharynx the differences are quite smaller (25 v.s. 14, 12, 22 %). Larynx is affected by a very low incidence of relapses (13, 10, 17 %) and second primaries (12 %), these unfavourable events reaching their top for hypopharynx (37, 22, 40 % for the relapses, 12 % for the second primaries). From these results it is obvious that chemotherapy does not change anything to the well known poor prognosis of head and neck tumors.

The clinical stage at presentation (stages I-II versus stages III-IV) keeps its strong prognostic value for survival (74 v.s. 49 % at 5 years), local control (14 v.s. 32 %), nodal control (4 v.s. 18 %) and distant metastasis incidence (6 v.s. 23 %). It does not affect the incidence of second primaries (15 v.s. 19 %). This is true for the general population but we have to consider some differences regarding the tumor sites.

It seems that these assertions could be true for oropharynx (5 years survival 82 v.s. 57 %) and larynx (87 v.s. 53 %) excepted for the local control of laryngeal tumors which is always at a high level, whatever could be the initial UICC stage. But if we consider oral cavity and hypopharynx the differences between the stages disappear, whatever could the endpoint be. A trend only exists for hypopharynx when considering the local relapse incidence ; but the very small numbers for stages I-II do not allow to conclude. One possible explanation should be that the present treatment policies towards these tumor sites are really inadequate for curing the patient.

The next point to look for is the treatment policy following CCR. For a lot of patients, the surgical procedure initially planned was finally abandonned for the benefit of radiotherapy, in order to preserve a function as voice or chewing and an organ as larynx or mandible. Due to the different treatment policies between the institutions participating to the study, it was generally pos-

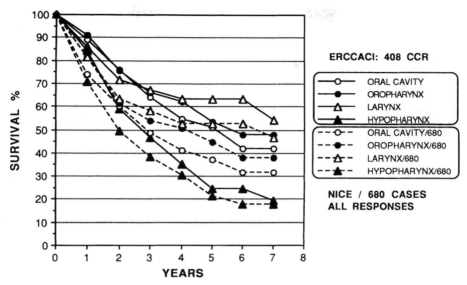

Fig. 1. Survival curves comparison between 408 CCR and 680 all responses from ERC-CACI and Nice

sible to have a sufficient number of patients treated by one or another procedure and to compare the patients outcome. No significant difference was found between surgery and radiotherapy, neither for survival nor for the different relapses. Oral cavity is the only one for which a doubt exists : it seems that a trend in favour of surgery could appear with a larger number of patients, 37 irradiated patients being compared to 9 operated. For oropharynx, no difference could be seen between the 124 irradiated and the 13 operated. For the larynx the comparison was impossible, due to the very small number of patient referred to or accepting a surgery after a CCR (2 patients over 60). Nevertheless the local relapse rate is very low and even if it could be 0 after surgery, the difference could not be considered as statistically significant. Again for hypopharyngeal tumors, no difference has been found between the 14 surgery and the 66 radiotherapy, validating the conservative policy relatively widely used in case of CCR.

This study lacking for a comparison with a general head and neck cancers population, we have superimposed (Fig. 1) the survival curves of the 408 CCR recorded in this study and these of the 680 cases treated in Nice by CDDP-5-FU, all responses included. At evidence, induction chemotherapy as presently used, does not modify the prognosis of head and neck tumors, even in the favourable situation of a clinically complete response.

Conclusion

Therefore, we are in the obligation to conclude that despite its apparent ability to remove some gross tumors, induction chemotherapy, as presently administered, does not affect the poor prognosis of head and neck tumors and, even worse, clinically Complete Response does not seem to be able to influence their usual outcome. The relative usefulness of these treatments could perhaps only be founded on an organ preservation policy. It seems reasonable to consider the problem of induction chemotherapy for head and neck cancer with a relative detachment and to keep in mind that a lot of work has to be done on the modalities of administration of chemotherapy in order to transform a tumor regression in a patient's cure.

Chemotherapy of undifferentiated thyroid cancer (UCT) and sarcoma of the thyroid gland (ST)

F Kober, A Heiss, B Neugebauer, R Roka

Anaplastic carcinoma and sarcoma of the thyroid gland are among the most lethal cancers in humans. Median life expectancy is usually less than 4 months after the initial diagnosis. Most tumors are unresectable when first seen, because of enormous size and infiltration of adjacent structures such as trachea and oesophagus. Between 1957-1989 a retrospective study on 169 patients with highly malignant thyroid tumors was carried out in the Kaiserin-Elisabeth-Hospital. The retrospective analysis clearly showed that if a radical resection of tumor (R0-R1) can be achieved the median survival time rises to 8 months in comparison with only two months after palliative surgery (R2). Conventional radiotherapy usually failed to induce any significant regression of the tumor. In 1985 on the basis of these results we decided to carry out a prospective study to evaluate the effect of highly malignant thyroid tumors by ChtX We selected the patients according to the following criteria.

Including criteria

Patients with undifferentiated carcinoma and sarcoma of thyroid gland.

Excluding criteria any of the following

1. Karnovsky index less than 50 %,
2. Tumor stage T2 N0 M0,
3. Chronic renal disease, thrombocytes < 100,000 and leucocytes < 3,000.

Between 1-1-1985 and 1-1-1991 32 patients with undifferentiated thyroid carcinoma or thyroid sarcoma were admitted to our clinic. According to these criteria 10 patients were excluded from ChtX and the others were treated among to the following protocol.

Attempt at a radical tumor resection (R0, R1).
Early postoperative commencement of chemotherapy :
— Day 3 postop. : Mitoxantrone 20 mg/m^2 BSA,
— Day 8 postop. : Cisplatin 100 mg/m^2 BSA,
— Chtx was repeated 6 times, 3 to 4 weeks apart.

On five patients we achieved an R0 and in another five an R1 resection, and in one further case the patient was operated in another hospital and we do not know the extent of the resection. In 11 patients only palliative resection of tumors was possible. The response of chemotherapy was defined as follows.

Department of Surgery, Kaiserin-Elisabeth-Hospital, Huglgasse 1-3, A-1150 Vienna, Austria

Complete remission

Total disappearance of the thyroid tumor and or the distant metastases. No local recurrence and no distant metastases up to 3 months after the end of ChtX, in case of R0 or R1 resection.

Response

More than 25 % reduction of the tumor mass or distant metastases. Local recurrence or distant metastases up to 3 months after start of ChtX, in case of R0 or R1 resection.

Progression

No effect on tumor or metastatic growth. Local recurrence or appearance of metastases up to 3 months after start of ChtX in case of Ro or R1 resection. Of the 22 patients who received ChtX 15 (7CR, 8PR) were responders and 7 were nonresponders.

Nonresponders

In the group of nonresponders the median and mean survival times were 3.7 and 4.8 months. All of the nonresponders died from the direct consequences of the tumor growth such as asphyxia or indirect consequences such as cachexia, during the first year.

Responders

Among the responders the mean survival time was 27 months and the median 17 months. 5 patients are still alive and tumor-free, between 20 and 78 months after the beginning of ChtX. Among the responders 2 of 9 patients died in neutropenic sepsis after ChtX. In the group of responders 7 patients had a complete remission (according to the above criteria). 3 of them underwent a second look operation at which local tumor control could be confirmed. 6 of 7 responders who died on consequences of the tumor showed local recurrences. It was remarkable that only one of the 15 responders developed metachronous metastases. All other patients remained either free of metastases. By contrast 5 of 7 patients among the group of nonresponders showed metachronous metastases.

Discussion

The results from our prospective unicenter study show a positive effect of ChtX in two third of patients suffering from a highly malignant thyroid tumor. Several factors probably contributed : ChtX was always the therapy of first choice and not a last, desperate attempt to influence advanced tumors resistant to other therapies. The dosage of ChtX was significantly higher than that used in most published studies and ChtX was started on the third postop. day. Patients with a low Karnovsky index were excluded from the study, because the retrospective study had showed that their general condition cannot be improved by aggressive therapy.

Studies evaluating the effect of ChtX on undifferentiated thyroid carcinoma based on a large number of patients are rare. In most studies the patients had already been treated by extensive radio therapy and/or high dose radio — Iodine — therapy, so that ChtX was the last resort.

Examples are the studies of Benker et al or Shimaoka [2, 5]. Benkers [2] study included 20 patients with undifferentiated thyroid carcinoma treated with Doxorubicin and Bleomycin. In 5 cases a partial remission was achieved, in another 5 no change. Shimaoka was able to show in a randomised comparative study of Doxorubicin versus Cisplatin and Doxorubicin that the combination therapy is superior to monotherapy particularly in the degree of response. He observed a complete remission in three of 18 patients and a partial remission in three patients who received Doxorubicin and Cisplatin (response rate was 33 %). In these clinical cases ChtX was used as second line therapy. It is worth mentioning in this context the therapeutic regimen of Auersperg [1] et al, who varied the ChtX according to the cytoflowmetric DNA analysis. Auersperg and Tallroth [7] et al, both observed a high local response rate to combined ChtX and hyperfractionated radio therapy.

In our prospective study we were able to show that early postoperative chemotherapy (Cisplatin 100 mg/m^2 BSA, Mitoxantrone 20 mg/m^2 BSA) is effective in patients with undifferentiated thyroid carcinoma and sarcoma of the thyroid gland. However 6 patients of the group of responders had some local recurrences after chemotherapy. Therefore we also recommend combination therapy with chemotherapy and hyperfractionated radiotherapy.

References

1. Auersperg M, Us-Krasovec M, Petric G, Pogacnik A, Besic N (1990) Results of combined modality treatment in poorly differentiated and anaplastic thyroid carcinoma. Wien Klin Wochenschr 102 : 267
2. Benker G, Reinwein D (1983) Ergebnisse der Chemotherapie des Schilddruesenkarzinoms. Dtsch Med Wochenschr 108 : 403
3. Holinsky Ch, Kober F, Hermann M, Loicht U, Keminger K (1990) Prognostische Faktoren bei hochmalignen Schilddruesentumoren. Wien Klin Wochenschr 102 : 249
4. Kim JH, Leeper RD (1983) Treatment of anaplastic giant and spindle cell carcinoma of the thyroid gland with combination adriamycin and ratiation therapy. Cancer 52 : 954
5. Shimaoka K, Schœnfeld DA, Dewys WD, Creech RH, De Conti R (1985) A randomized trial of doxorubicin versus doxorubicin plus cisplatin in patients with advanced thyroid carcinoma. Cancer 56 : 2155
6. Simpson WJ (1980) Anaplastic thyroid carcinoma, a new approach. Can J Surg 23 : 25
7. Tallroth E, Wallin G, Lundell G, Loewhagen T, Einhorn J (1987) Mulimodality treatment in anaplastic giant cell thyroid carcinoma. Cancer 60 : 1428

Retinoid chemoprevention of aerodigestive carcinogenesis

WK Hong, SM Lippman, SE Benner, JS Lee

Biology and retinoids

Epithelial cancers of the upper aerodigestive tract, lung and esophagus are a significant public health problem throughout the world. Despite improvement in local treatment and decreasing cigarette consumption in developing countries, the incidence of aerodigestive cancers unfortunately continues to increase worldwide. Clearly, new directions are needed.

Chemoprevention is a new approach which has the potential to reduce the morbidity and mortality of these devastating diseases. The term « chemoprevention » was coined by Michael Sporn, in 1976, and is defined as the use of specific natural or synthetic chemical agents to reverse, suppress, or prevent carcinogenic progression to invasive cancer [1]. Progress in our understanding of the carcinogenic process at the cellular and molecular level, combined with the availability of new chemopreventive agents, has buoyed up the entire field of chemoprevention research.

The primary biologic rationale for chemoprevention in aerodigestive carcinogenesis is provided by the concepts of both multi-step epithelial tumor development and field carcinogenesis. The multi-step process of epithelial cancer development is histologically characterized by the progression from premalignant lesions to the development of invasive carcinoma. Alterations in specific oncogenes such as *ras, myc,* and *erb-b* gene families, mutation of tumor suppressor genes such as retinoblastoma, p-53, and genetic changes involving chromosomes 3p, 7, and 17 have been reported in lung and head and neck cancer. Studies of non-neoplastic high risk tissue, such as premalignant lesions and/or tissue adjacent to invasive carcinoma, have identified genotypic and phenotypic changes which support the concept of multi-step carcinogenesis. Phenotypic alterations associated with epithelial carcinogenesis include altered cell differentiation markers and proliferation markers such as PCNA. Although the precise sequence of genotypic and phenotypic alterations in early and late-stage carcinogenesis is not clear, this multi-step process provides the opportunity to intervene pharmacologically to prevent the development of invasive carcinoma [2].

The second supporting concept for chemoprevention, « field carcinogenesis », describes the diffuse, field-wide carcinogenic effects of tobacco and alcohol on the aerodigestive tract epithelium, which predispose the entire region toward the development of multiple malignancies [3]. This hypothesis is supported by recent studies in humans which document the existence of clinical, histological, and biochemical premalignant abnormalities within the carcinogen-

---

Department of Thoracic/Head and Neck Medical Oncology, University of Texas, MD Anderson Cancer Center, 1515 Holcombe boulevard Box 80, Houston, Texas 77030, USA

exposed epithelium, as well as by the higher risk of synchronous and metachronous second primary tumors within the aerodigestive tract. In high risk patients, the various stages of multifocal premalignant foci can be found throughout the lung and other sites of the aerodigestive tract.

Retinoid data from *in vitro*, animal, and epidemiologic studies strongly support the role of retinoids and carotenoids in the prevention of epithelial carcinogenesis [4, 5]. The retinoids are well-established agents for epithelial cell growth and differentiation *in vivo* and *in vitro*. Retinoids can suppress carcinogenesis in a variety of epithelial tissues including the skin, trachea, lungs, and/or mucosa. Vitamin A deficiency leads to squamous metaplasia, which can be reversed by supplementation with Vitamin A or certain retinoids. Metaplasia, which also develops during Vitamin A deficiency, is similar to premalignant lesions caused by chemical carcinogens. Evaluation of Vitamin A or carotenoid status in patients with aerodigestive cancer has revealed reduced serum levels. Retinoids have also been found to be effective inhibitors of chemical carcinogenesis in several animal studies. The development of premalignant lesions and carcinoma was retarded in carcinogen DMBA-treated hamsters receiving retinoid or carotenoid. The precise mechanism of the anti-carcinogenic effect of retinoids is not fully understood; recent investigations suggest that retinoids modulate or inhibit carcinogenesis by directly regulating gene expression through mediation of nuclear retinoic acid receptors (RAR).

Clinical chemoprevention trials

Oral leukoplakia trials

Oral leukoplakia is a premalignant lesion of squamous carcinoma which consists of whitish patches in the oral cavity which cannot be scraped off or clinically classified as any other disorder. Oral leukoplakia is primarily tobacco-related, and is easy to monitor and biopsy. It is therefore the ideal human model for chemoprevention studies in aerodigestive tract carcinogenesis, and short-term chemoprevention studies in oral leukoplakia have been conducted for the past 20 years. Although early studies were not controlled, they made interesting observations regarding the activity of supplemental Vitamin A in reversing oral leukoplakia. Clinical work with synthetic retinoids now includes more than 10 trials, producing a response rate of over 50 %. In 1986, Hong et al conducted the first placebo-controlled Phase III chemoprevention study in oral leukoplakia [6]. This study opened new chemoprevention approaches worldwide by establishing the activity of high-dose 13-*cis*-retinoic acid (13-cRA) compared to placebo.

The trial was short-term, lasting only three months, but it revealed two major problems; first, the relapse rate exceeded 50 % within 2-3 months after stopping therapy, and second, the toxicity was unacceptably high for general chemoprevention use. Retinoid response must be maintained, but high-dose toxicity limits the duration of the therapy.

These problems led to our design of a randomized study comparing the abilities of low-dose 13-cRA and beta-carotene to maintain remission or nonprogression of oral carcinogenesis after high-dose 13-cRA induction [7]. This trial was conducted in two phases : The first was a three-month induction phase using high-dose 13-cRA in all patients, and the second was a nine-month maintenance phase in which patients were randomized to receive either low-dose 13-cRA or beta-carotene. Patients whose disease progressed at any time were taken off the study. The induction and maintenance phase of this study has been completed, with 70 patients enrolled. The high-dose 13-cRA induction produced a major response rate of 55 %. Beta-carotene was significantly less effective than low-dose 13-cRA ; after the maintenance phase, the progression rate in the low-dose 13-cRA group was 8 %, and in the beta-carotene group was 55 %. Furthermore, low-dose 13-cRA was well tolerated, and only 12 % of the subjects developed toxic effects of Grade III or higher severity, whereas 34 % of the total study population experienced such effects during the high-dose 13-cRA induction phase.

These two consecutive randomized trials established that high-dose and low-dose 13-cRA have significant activity in leukoplakia. The use of low-dose 13-cRA (30 mg/day) in the aerodigestive tract is currently being investigated through further chemoprevention studies, including adjuvant trials to prevent second primary tumors associated with head, neck and lung cancer.

Retinoids are unquestionably the most-studied chemopreventive agents in oral leukoplakia, with the second most-studied agent being beta-carotene. However, no Phase III data or controlled study data exist for beta-carotene, and the results of previously performed studies are quite conflicting.

High-dose 13-cRA adjuvant trial in head and neck cancer

A randomized adjuvant trial of high-dose 13-cRA has been conducted at Boston Veterans Affairs Medical Center and MD Anderson Cancer Center in cured head and neck cancer patients. Eligible patients included those with biopsy-proven disease (Stages I-IV) who were rendered disease-free after surgery and/or radiation treatment. Patients were stratified by tumor site and previous treatment to receive 13-cRA 50-100 mg/m^2/day or placebo for 12 months. The treatment was initiated no later than 10 weeks after surgery and/or 16 weeks after radiation treatment. The endpoint of this study was the recurrence of primary disease or the development of second primary tumors.

This study was initially reported in detail in 1990 [8], and at a median followup of 32 months, a significant reduction in second primary tumors was found in the high-dose 13-cRA group as compared to the placebo group. However, 13-cRA showed no impact on local, regional or distant recurrence of the original tumor. At 48 months median followup, the primary disease progression is now 33 % in both groups, but the rate of second primary tumor development is 8 % in the 13-cRA-treated group and 29 % in the placebo group (p = .07). In this adjuvant study, 16 of 19 patients developed a second primary of a squamous cell carcinoma type within the area of field cancerization — the lungs, upper two-thirds of the esophagus, or bladder. Survival was not prolonged in the 13-cRA group, probably because the rates of primary disease recurrence were identical. Treatment with 13-cRA is associated with significant toxicity, which kept many of the patients from completing the full 12 months of treatment.

Second primary tumors are the major cause of death in both early-stage head and neck and lung cancer patients. Second primary tumors develop out of pre-neoplastic lesions, either visible or invisible, which remain after local treatment. The adjuvant activity of high-dose 13-cRA against second primary tumors led to the development of two ongoing large randomized studies using low-dose 13-cRA to prevent second primary tumors in the early stages of head and neck cancer and non-small cell lung cancer. The choice of the 13-cRA dosage and administration schedules were based on the randomized maintenance trial in oral leukoplakia. The primary endpoint of these two large-scale trials will be second primary tumor development.

Bronchial metaplasia trial

Several studies have reported that invasive squamous cell carcinoma of the lung arises in association with areas of carcinoma *in situ* and progressive changes from metaplasia to carcinoma. These changes are very well accepted as the development path of squamous cell carcinogenesis. Saccomanno et al conducted a non-randomized trial on 26 subjects with documented atypia on sputum cytology, ranging from moderate atypical metaplasia to overt carcinoma. These subjects received 1-2.5 mg/kg/day of 13-cRA. There was no improvement in the degree of atypia after treatment with 13-cRA, but alteration in cellular morphology was noted [9]. The randomized trial of Arnold et al failed to demonstrate statistically significant reversal of sputum atypia with etretinate treatment. Using squamous metaplasia documented by histologic evaluation of bronchial biopsy as endpoint, Gouveia et al reported the retinoid etretinate was effective in reversing sputum atypia in heavy smokers. In an uncontrolled study by Gouveia et al, chronic smokers (more than 15 pack/years) were evaluated with fiberoptic bronchoscopy, during which biopsies were obtained from 6 standardized regions. Individuals with a metaplasia index of more than 15 % were treated with oral etretinate 25 mg/day for 6 months. The initial report showed that in 10 of the 11 patients who had completed the treatment, the metaplasia index had decreased. The follow up report showed a significant change in the metaplasia index, which decreased from 34.57 % prior to treatment to 26.96 % following etretinate therapy. However, the metaplasia indices of 4 patients who stopped smoking dropped to 0 % after treatment [10].

A prospective randomized study is underway at MD Anderson to evaluate the role of 13-cRA in the reversal of bronchial metaplasia. Volunteers with at least a 15 pack/year history of cigarette smoking underwent bronchoscopy, and biopsies were obtained from 6 standardized sites following the procedure previously reported by Gouveia et al. Individuals with dysplasia or a metaplasia index of at least 15 % were randomized to receive 13-cRA 1 mg/kg/day or placebo. Follow-up bronchoscopies were performed at 6 months, and patients who did not have any improvement of the metaplasia index were crossed over to the other arm. Accrual is now completed with 152 patients screened and 87 patients randomized, and the final data will be available later this year. The findings obtained from the multiple bronchoscopy biopsies will hopefully provide more reliable molecular and genetic biomarkers to serve as potential intermediate endpoints for lung cancer chemoprevention trials.

Conclusions

In summary, despite local and systemic therapy and smoking cessation programs, aerodigestive cancers remain the major cause of cancer-related death in the United States and worldwide. Chemoprevention is an exciting and promising investigational modality for the control of aerodigestive carcinogenesis. Aerodigestive carcinogenesis is an excellent model for chemoprevention approaches, and our studies have suggested that chemoprevention using retinoids has great potential for the suppression of oral premalignant lesions and the reduction of second primary tumors in head and neck cancer. The results of our ongoing studies in the prevention of second primary tumors with low-dose 13-cRA for head and neck and lung cancer patients will decide future multi-modality chemoprevention strategies in patients with aerodigestive cancer and individuals at high risk for cancer development. Further efforts to identify effective, non-toxic chemopreventive agents, combined with the identification of reliable biomarkers as intermediate endpoints, will ultimately lead to a major reduction in the morbidity and mortality of aerodigestive epithelial cancer.

References

1. Sporn MB (1976) Approaches to prevention of epithelial cancer during the preneoplastic period. Cancer Res 36 : 2699-2702
2. Wolf G, Lippman SM, Laramore G, Hong WK (in press) Head and neck cancer. In : Holland JF, Frei E, Bast RC Jr, Kufe DW, Morton DL, Weichselbaum RR (eds) Cancer medicine. Lea & Febiger, Philadelphia
3. Slaughter DP, Southwick HW, Smejkal W (1953) Field cancerization in oral stratified squamous epithelium : clinical implications of multicentric origin. Cancer 6 : 963-968
4. Lotan R (1980) Effects of Vitamin A and its analogs (retinoids) on normal and neoplastic cells. Biochem Biophys Acta 605 : 33-91
5. Peto R, Doll R, Buckley JD, Sporn MB (1981) Can dietary beta-carotene materially reduce human cancer rates ? Nature 290 : 201-208
6. Hong WK, Endicott J, Itri LM, Doos W, Batsakis JG, Bell R, Fofonoff SS, Byers R, Atkinson EN, Vaughan C, Toth BB, Kramer A, Dimery IW, Skipper P, Strong S (1986) 13-cis-retinoic acid in the treatment of oral leukoplakia. N Engl J Med 315 : 1501-1505
7. Lippman SM, Batsakis JG, Toth BB, Weber RS, Lee JJ, Martin JW, Hays GL, Goepfert H, Hong WK (1993) Comparison of low-dose Isotretinoin with beta-carotene to prevent oral carcinogenesis. N Engl J Med 328 : 15-20
8. Hong WK, Lippman SM, Itri LM, Karp DD, Lee JS, Byers RM, Schantz SP, Kramer AM, Lotan R, Peters LJ, Dimery IW, Brown BW, Goepfert H (1990) Prevention of second primary tumors with isotretinoin in squamous cell carcinoma of the head and neck. N Engl J Med 323 : 795-801
9. Saccomanno G, Moran PG, Schmidt R, Hartshorn DF, Brian DA, Dreher WH, Sowada BJ (1982) Effects of 13-cis-retinoids on premalignant and malignant cells of lung origin. Acta Cytol 26 : 68-85
10. Gouveia J, Hercend T, Lemaigre G, Mathe G, Gros F, Santelli G (1982) Degree of bronchial metaplasia in heavy smokers and its regression after treatment with a retinoid. Lancet 65 : 710-712

Definite radiation and concomitant Cisplatin administration in locally advanced head and neck cancer

G Fountzilas, D Skarlos, P Kosmidis, E Samantas, J Tzitzikas, P Makrantonakis, P Pantelakos, A Nicolaou, H Bacoyiannis, M Sinodinou, P Papaspyrou, C Banis, A Vritsios, J Daniilidis

The prognosis of patients with locally advanced head and neck cancer (HNC) is generally poor. Despite mutilating surgery and/or radical irradiation, 50-60 % of patients recur within 2 years and an additional 20-30 % develop distant metastases [1].

Induction chemotherapy followed by radiation therapy has been extensively investigated during the last decade. Unfortunately, it seems that there is no survival benefit from this combined modality approach with most of the patients developing locoregional recurrences [2]. Also another disadvantage from the use of induction chemotherapy is that there is a considerable number of patients who refuse local therapies after the completion of induction chemotherapy, and may be their survival is compromised. In an attempt to improve local control of the tumor, investigators administered several drugs, such as Cisplatin (DDP), Fluorouracil, Mitomycin, etc., which is known that they are radiation-potentiators concurrently with radiation. In this study we report our preliminary results in using DDP concurrently with radiation in patients with HNC.

Patients and methods

Only patients with locally advanced HNC were included in the present study. Eligibility criteria included measurable of evaluable disease, performance status (PS) > 40 % of Karnofsky's scale, normal renal and hepatic functions, WBC count > 4,000/ml, and platelet count > 100,000/ml, age < 75 years, no active ischemic heart disease and prior treatment. An informed consent according to our institutional policies was obtained from all patients. Initial examination included history, clinical examination, laryngoscopy, esophagography, complete blood count, sequential multiple analysis (SMA-12), electrocardiogram, chest x-ray, bone scan and computed tomography (CT scan) of the head and neck region. Audiogram was not routinely required. All patients were initially evaluated by an ENT surgeon, a medical oncologist and a radiotherapist and staged by AJC/UICC criteria [3]. From april 1991 until october 1992 47 patients were entered this study, conducted by the Hellenic Co-operative Oncology Group. There were 43 men and 4 women with a median age of

---

AHEPA Hospital, Thessaloniki, Macedonia, « Agii Anargiri » Cancer Hospital, Athens, « Evangelismos » Hospital, Athens, « Metaxa » Cancer Hospital, Piraeous, all in Greece

62 (range, 18-77) years and a median PS of 90 (range, 60-90) of Karnofsky's scale. Histology was squamous cell carcinoma in 41 and undifferentiated in 6 patients. Primary site was nasopharynx (8 patients), oropharynx (8), hypopharynx (5), oral cavity (5), larynx (18), salivary gland (1) and unkrown (2). The stage distribution is shown in Table 1. Thirty-four (72 %) of the patients presented with stage IV disease. All patients were irradiated with a ^{60}Co unit. According to the protocol they received 70 Gy to the tumor area and 45 Gy to the rest of the neck. DDP was infused in a 3-hour period at a dose of 100 mg/m^2 on days 2, 22 and 42.

Ten to twelve weeks after the completion of radiation therapy all patients were reevaluated with ENT examination, CT scan, chest x-ray and biochemistry. Tumor response was determined according to WHO criteria.

Results

Forty-six patients completed radiation as per protocol. One stopped treatment after he received all 3 courses of DDP while 3 patients were treated during the third course with reduced DDP dose because of toxicity. After the completion of the combined teratment 33 (70 %) patients achieved a complete response (CR) and 5 (11 %) a partial response. CRs were seen in all primary

Table 1. TNM staging

	No	N1	N2	N3
Tx				2
T1		2	1	1
T2	3	2	1	2
T3	6	2	5	2
T4	7	1	9	1

AJC/UICC criteria

Table 2. Relationship between primary site of the tumor and response to treatment (n = 43)

Site	Response			
	CR	PR	SD	PD
Nasopharynx	5	3		
Larynx	14	1	2	
Oropharynx	7			
Hypopharynx	3		1	
Oral cavity	2			2
Salivary gland	1			
Unknown	1	1		
Total	33	5	3	2

Table 3. Acute treatment toxicities (%)

	Grade*			
	1	2	3	4
Nausea/Vomiting	10	32	12	2
Stomatitis	56	29	2	2
Diarrhea	2		2	
Anemia	22	5		
Leukopenia	15	17	12	
Thrombocytopenia		2		2
Infection	2			
Alopecia	12	7		
Otitis	24	7	2	
Salivary gland	27	63		
Larynx	49	10	5	
Pharynx	51	22	2	2
Neurotoxicity	7			
Nephrotoxicity	7	12	5	
Weight loss	24	24	32	
Dermatitis	42	56		2

* WHO criteria
There were 2 treatment-related deaths.

sites (Table 2). Acute toxicities are shown in Table 3. Grade III toxicities included mainly vomiting, leukopenia and weight loss. Up to January 1, 1993 41 patients were alive. Five patients with CR relapsed after 6, 9, 10, 12 and 17 months respectively. Site of relapse was locoregional (3 patients), regional and liver (1) and bone, lung and liver (1).

Discussion

It has been shown in tissue cultures and in experimental animals that platinum analogs are acting radiation potentiators. The mechanism of potentition has been proposed to be the inhibition of the repair of potentially lethal damages induced by radiation [4-6].

The administration of DDP concurrently with radiation has been tested in locally advanced HNC by several investigators. The Radiation Therapy Oncology Group (RTOG) conducted a phase II study of concomitant radiation and DDP at a dose of 100 mg/m^2 every 3 weeks. The CR rate was 71 %, similar to that achieved in the present study. Moderate or severe acute toxicities are seen often with chemo-radiation. It is noteworthy that more than 1/2 of our patients suffered considerable weight loss. Also, two patients died at home a few days after the completion of treatment. Both were malnurished and dehydrated and thus three these deaths should be considered as treatment-related. This serious side effect can be partially prevented by hospitalizing the patient, especially during the last two weeks of treatment with proper administration of IV fluids.

In conclusion, concurrent radiation and DDP is a highly effective treatment and should be considered as standard therapy for patients with locally advanced HNC.

References

1. Merino OR, Lindberg RD, Fletcher GH (1977) An analysis of distant metastases from squamous cell carcinoma of the upper respiratory and digestive tracts. Cancer 40 : 145-151
2. Tannock IF, Browman G (1986) Lack of evidence for a role of chemotherapy in the routine management of locally advanced head and neck cancer. J Clin Oncol 4 : 1121-1126
3. American Joint Committee on Cancer (1988) Manual for staging on Cancer. 3rd edition. JB Lippincott, Philadelphia
4. Creagen ET, Fountain KS, Frytal S et al (1981) Concomitant radiation therapy and cis-diammine-dichloroplatinum in patients with advanced head and neck cancer. Med Pediatr Oncol 9 : 119-120
5. Leipzig B (1983) Cisplatin sensitization to radiotherapy of squamous cell carcinomas of the head and neck. Am J Surg 146 : 462-465
6. Coughlin CT, Richmond RC (1985) Platinum based combined modality approach for locally advanced head and neck carcinoma. Int J Radiat Oncol Biol Phys 11 : 915-919
7. Marcial VA, Pajak TF, Mohiuddin M et al (1990) Concomitant Cisplatin Chemotherapy and Radiotherapy in advanced mucosal squamous cell carcinoma of the head and neck. Long-term results of the Radiation Therapy Oncology Group Study 81-17. Cancer 66 : 1861-1868

Improved survival of patients with advanced squamous cell carcinoma of the head and neck with alternating chemotherapy and radiotherapy

M Benasso, R Corvó, M Cavallari, G Sanguineti, G Margarino, R Rosso, V Vitale, M Merlano and members of affiliated institutions

Radiotherapy is the standard approach to the treatment of advanced, unresectable squamous cell carcinoma of the head and neck. With radiotherapy alone the expected five-year survival is about 25 %, but it may be 1-2 % in the patients with very advanced disease (T4 and/or N3 disease). Experimental and clinical data suggest a possible advantage by integrating chemotherapy and radiotherapy in such a tumors even if the true impact of combined modalities over radiotherapy alone remain unclear. Therefore we designed a randomized trial to compare standard radiation (Arm B) to alternating chemotherapy and radiation (Arm A), in patients with advanced, inoperable and previously untreated SCC-HN.

Between February 1987 and December 1990, 157 patients (80 pts in Arm A and 77 pts in Arm B) entered the study.

Patients and tumors characteristics are shown in Table 1. In particular approximately 75 % of pts in both arms had stage IV disease including many with T4N2 or T4N3 disease. Patients elegibility was determined by a multidisciplinary team including a medical oncologist, a radiation oncologist and a head and neck surgeon. A physical examination, complete blood count, chemistry and chest films were obtained in all patients ; CT, endoscopy, liver sonogram and bone scan were performed when indicated. Patients randomized in Arm A received 4 courses of Cisplatin (CDDP) (20 mg/m^2/day) + 5-Fluorouracil (5-FU) (200 mg/m^2/day) for 5 consecutive days (wks 1, 4, 7, 10) alternated with 3 courses of radiotherapy (20 Gy each ; wks 2-3, 5-6, 8-9). The employed chemotherapy was a regimen, modified from the original Al Sarraf's scheduling (Kish, 1984), in which 5-FU is administered e.v. push to allow a full outpatients administration and to avoid possible toxic interaction on the mucosas between RT and continuous infusion of 5-FU.

Arm B consisted in RT alone, administered as single daily fraction of 2 Gy to a total dose of 65-75 Gy.

At the end of treatment each patient was revaluated. No further treatment was planned for pts with complete response ; pts with partial response underwent surgical evaluation and, when possible, resection of the tumor was performed.

Toxicity was evaluated before each chemotherapy course and recorded according to WHO scale (Miller, 1981).

Progression free survival (PFS) was computed from the time of randomi-

Dept. of Medical Oncology I, Istituto Nazionale per la Ricerca sul Cancro, v. le Benedetto XV, 10, 16132 Genoa, Italy

Table 1. Patients and tumor characteristics

	Arm A	(%)	Arm B	(%)
Randomized patients	80	(100)	77	(100)
Sex				
Male	66	(83)	65	(84)
Female	14	(17)	12	(16)
Age (yr)				
≤ 60	39	(49)	40	(52)
> 60	41	(51)	37	(48)
Performance status				
0	42	(52)	38	(49)
1	34	(43)	32	(42)
2	3	(4)	7	(9)
3	1	(1)	-	(-)
Site of primary				
Nasopharynx	6	(7)	7	(9)
Oropharynx	29	(37)	24	(31)
Oral cavity	24	(30)	22	(29)
Larynx	6	(7)	10	(13)
Hypopharynx	15	(19)	14	(18)
Stage				
II	1	(1)	-	(-)
III	20	(25)	18	(23)
IV	59	(74)	59	(77)

zation to that of disease progression and pts who died without disease progression were considered to have progression at the time of death.

Overall survival (OS) was computed from the time of randomization to that of the last follow-up observation or death.

All patients have been evaluated for toxicity (Table 2). Grade III-IV mucositis occured in 19 % and 18 % in Arm A and in Arm B respectively.

All patients were considered in the analysis of response (Table 3).

The analysis showed a significant difference in terms of complete response rate in favour to the experimental arm (43 % CR in Arm A v.s. 22 % CR in ArmB) (p 0.037). At the end of the treatment 12 partial responders (9 in Arm A, 3 in Arm B) underwent surgery. Therefore, including complete responses converted by surgery, the complete response rate was 53 % in the combined arm and 26 % in the control arm.

A statistically significant advantage in terms of PFS (p.002) and OS (p.048) in favour of combined treatment has been already odserved in a preliminary analysis (April 1992) (Merlano, 1992). On January 1993, at a median follow-up of 43 months, a mature analysis was performed. In comparison to the former analysis an increased difference either in terms of PFS (p.001) or OS (p.001) in favour of the experimental arm was observed. The medium survival is 16.6 month in Arm A and 11.4 month in Arm B (p.01) and the 4-years survival is 34 % v.s. 13 % in two arms respectively.

Table 2. Toxicity

Grade (WHO scale)	Arm A (%)				Arm B (%)			
	1	2	3	4	1	2	3	4
Nausea - Vomiting	38	34	4	1	1	-	1	-
Leukopenia	19	12	20	1	1	-	-	-
Thrombocytopenia	14	10	4	1	-	-	-	-
Anemia	90	3	5	1	-	-	-	-
Nephrotoxicity	4	1	-	-	-	-	-	-
Neurotoxicity	1	1	-	-	-	-	1	-
Mucositis	23	15	16	3	35	25	17	1
Xerostomia	18	7	1	-	23	9	3	-
Oedema	14	3	-	-	17	6	6	1
Dermatitis	1	-	3	-	6	1	-	-
Infections	3	1	-	-	1	1	-	-
Cardiotoxicity	-	-	-	-	-	-	-	-
Alopecia	-	-	-	-	-	-	-	-
Weight loss > 10 %		3				1		

WHO : World Health Organization

Table 3. Response to treatment

	Arm A		Arm B	
	N° pts	%	N° pts	%
CR*	34	42.5	17	22.1
PR	23	28.7	33	42.8
OR	57	71.2	50	64.9
SD	2	2.5	7	9.1
PD + ED	10	12.5	13	16.9
PV**	11	14.0	7	9.1
- refusal***	(7)	(8.8)	(6)	(7.7)
- toxicity	(2)	(2.5)	(-)	(-)
- inelegibility	(2)	(2.5)	(-)	(-)
- lost to follow-up	(-)	(-)	(1)	(1.3)
Total	80	100	77	100

* p = 0.037
** PV = protocol violations
*** Patients who refused to start treatment

Among in complete responders 36 pts in Arm A and 71 in Arm B had a loco-regional relapse. In the whole series of pts distant metastases were detected in 9 % and 8 % respectively while a majority of second primaries was recorded in Arm A (6 % v.s. 2 %).

In conclusion the updated analysis strongly confirms data reported in our previous paper (Merlano, 1992) : alternating chemo-radiotherapy is superior to standard radiotherapy and the improvement seems to be secondary to a better local control.

References

Kish JA, Weaver A, Jacobs J et al (1984) : Cisplatin and 5-Fluorouracil infusion in patients with recurrent and disseminated epidermoid cancer of the head and neck. Cancer 53 : 1819-1824
Merlano M, Vitale V, Rosso R et al (1992) : Treatment of advanced squamous cell carcinoma of the head and neck with alternating chemotherapy and radiotherapy. N Engl J Med 327 : 1115-1121

Treatment of patients with cancer of the head and neck or esophagus with carboplatin, 5-FU, Interferon-α and interleukin-2

O Schlappack, A Hainz, P Berghammer, M Grasl, M Kautzky, G Kment, W Dobrowsky, C Dittrich

We have treated 27 patients with cancer of the head and neck (18) or esophagus (9) according to the following protocol : day 1 carboplatin i.v. [dose in mg = 5 × (glomerular filtration rate + 25)] followed by 120 hrs of 5-FU at 750 mg/m^2/24 hrs. During the first week of treatment interferon alpha-2b (Intron A) was given 3 times s.c. at 5 Mio. I.U./m^2. In week 2 and 3 of each treatment course 2 Mio. I.U./m^2 (in locally advanced head and neck tumours) or 5 Mio. I.U./m^2 (in disseminated head and neck and esophagus cancers) of interleukin-2 (Proleukin) was administered s.c. 3 times per week. Cycles were repeated every 3 weeks. 5 women and 22 men were treated. Median age of the patients was 59 years (range : 41-78). Toxicities observed were mainly hematological with grade 3 & 4 in 12 % of cycles. The only other major toxicities were grade 3 mucosities in 2 cycles and grade 3 pulmonal toxicity, infection and constipation in 1 cycle each. Patients' quality of life during treatment was assessed weekly by visual analogue scales and showed no change over time. 20 patients received at least 3 cycles of treatment and were thus evaluable for response. 1 CR, 9 PR, 2 NC and 1 PD were found in head and neck and 5 PR and 2 NC in esophagus cancer patients. This is an effective treatment that caused significant toxicity but patients' quality of life was not compromised.

Standard treatment of recurrent squamous cell carcinoma of the head and neck and of advanced carcinoma of the esophagus consists of cisplatin and 5-FU. However, cisplatin is nephrotoxic and emetogen. Carboplatin is a second generation platinanalogue that is not nephrotoxic and less emetogen than cisplatin. The question is whether cisplatin can be replaced by carboplatin in the treatment of head and neck and esophagus cancer.

Reports by Forastiere, 1987, and Volling, 1989, suggest that in head and neck cancer equally good results can be achieved with the combination of carboplatin plus 5-FU as with cisplatin 5-FU. However, the carboplatin plasma clearance is linearly related to the glomerular filtration rate. Thus the area under the concentration versus time curve, AUC, for carboplatin is primarily dictated by the pretreatment glomerular filtration rate. If, therefore, the renal function is taken in account it is possible to minimize the variations in the AUC in different patients, Calvert, 1989.

Using a panel of 12 squamous cell carcinoma of the head and neck cell

---

University of Vienna, Alser Straße 4, A-1090 Vienna, Austria lines Sacchi, 1991, reported the sensitivity of these tumor cells to tumor necrosis factor-α, interferon-γ, and interferon alfa. Vlock, 1991, reported on a trial with IFN-α in 14 patients with head and neck tumors. They observed 1 complete remission, one patient had a mixed response, and 2 patients had stabilization of disease.

Interferon can potentiate the activity of cytotoxic agents against human tumors, Wadler, 1990 and Vokes, 1991, reported a 72 % clinical complete response rate in head and neck cancer patients treated with cisplatin, 5-FU, leucovorin and interferon alpha.

Interleukin-2 (IL-2) was used by Valone, 1991, to treat locally recurrent or metastatic head and neck cancer patients in combination with cisplatin and 5-FU. They achieved a response rate of 55 %. Heslop, 1991, reported that IL-2 may facilitate myeloid recovery when administered during the period of haemopoietic regeneration following ablative chemoradiotherapy.

In addition to immunomodulatory effects IL-2 was shown to directly inhibit the growth of human head and neck squamous cell carcinoma cell lines. This effect is mediated by IL-2 receptors on the surface of these tumor cell lines, Weidmann, 1992. Also, treatment of human head and neck cancer xenografts in nude mice with IL-2 resulted in inhibition of tumor growth, Sacchi, 1990. Cortesina, 1991, reported the treatment of patients with recurrent squamous cell carcinoma of the head and neck with low doses of IL-2 injected perilymphatically. Of 20 patients treated 65 % showed an objective response.

Thus, carboplatin plus 5-FU in combination with interferon alpha and IL-2 seemed an attractive approach to study in head and neck squamous cell carcinoma and esophagus cancer patients.

Patients and methods

18 head and neck cancer patients and 9 esophagus cancer patients were treated according to the following protocol :

Week 1

• Day 1 : carboplatin i.v.
The dose of carboplatin given was derived using the formula {dose in mg = 5 × (glomerular filtration rate + 25)} described by Calvert, 1989.
• Day 1-5 : 5-FU, 750 mg/m^2/day, given as continuous i.v. infusion plus alpha interferon 5 million IU/m^2 three times per week subcutaneously. Head and neck cancer patients with tumor in the head and/or neck received the s.c. injections in the neck.

Week 2 and 3

• Patients with tumor in the head and/or neck only : Recombinant interleukin-2 2 million IU/m^2 three times per week s.c. in the neck.
• Patients with disseminated head and neck or esophagus cancer : Recom-

binant interleukin-2 5 million IU/m² three times per week s.c. in the abdominal wall.

Week 4 = week 1 of next cycle

Toxicity according to WHO grading was assessed weekly.
Quality of life was assessed weekly by patient self report using linear analogue scales.
Tumor response was evaluated following termination of every third treatment cycle.

Table 1. Toxicity in head and neck cancer patients

WHO grade	1	2	3	4
Hematological	21 %	17 %	10 %	2.6 %
Gastrointestinal	25 %	6 %		
Renal	9 %			
Kardial				
Neurological	15 %			
Constipation	44 %	13 %		
Pain	39 %	15 %		
Pulmoral	11 %			
Skin	6 %	6 %		
Hairloss	6 %			
Infektion				
Fever	66 %	11 %		

Table 2. Toxicity of esophagus cancer patients

WHO grade	1	2	3	4
Hemotological	22 %	24 %	9 %	2 %
Gastrointestinal	12 %	3 %		
Renal	3 %			
Kardial	3 %			
Neurological	26 %			
Constipation	51 %	20 %		
Pain	43 %	11 %		
Pulmonal	6 %	14 %		
Skin	17 %	20 %		
Hairloss	14 %			
Infection	3 %			
Fever	63 %	11 %		

Results and discussion

Patient characteristics : 5 women and 20 men were treated. The median age was 59 years (range : 41-78). All head and neck cancer patients had a squamous carcinoma.

Quality of life showed no change over time during treatment : 1 CR, 9 PR, 2 NC and 1 PD were observed in head and neck and 5 PR and 2 NC in esophagus cancer patients. This is an effective toxic treatment that does not impair the patients' quality of life.

References

Calvert AH, Newell DR, Gumbrell LA, O'Reilly S, Burnell M, Boxall FE, Siddik ZH, Judson IR, Gore ME, Wiltshaw E (1989) Carboplatin dosage : prospective evaluation of a simple formula based on renal function. J Clin Oncol 7 : 1748-1756
Cortesina G, de Stefani A, Galeazzi E, Cavallo GP, Jemma C, Giovarelli M, Vai S, Forni G (1991) Interleukin-2 injected around tumor-draining lymph nodes in head and neck cancer. Head Neck 13 : 125-131
Forastiere AA, Natale RB, Takasugi BJ, Goren MP, Vogel WC, Kudla-Hatch V (1987) A phase I-II trial of carboplatin and 5-fluorouracil combination chemotherapy in advanced carcinoma of the head and neck. J Clin Oncol 5 : 190-196
Heslop HE, Duncombe AS, Reittie JE, Bello-Fernandez C, Gottlieb DJ, Prentice HG, Mehta AB, Hoffbrand AV, Brenner MK (1991) Interleukin 2 infusion induces haemopoietic growth factors and modifies marrow regeneration after chemotherapy or autologous marrow transplantation. Br J Haematology 77 : 237-244
Sacchi M, Snyderman CH, Heo DS, Johnson JT, d'Amico F, Herberman RB, Whiteside TL (1990) Local adoptive immunotherapy of human head and neck cancer xenografts in nude mice with lymphokine-activated killer cells and interleukin-2. Cancer Res 50 : 3113-3118
Sacchi M, Klapan I, Johnson JT, Whiteside TL (1991) Antiproliferative effects of cytokines on squamous cell carcinoma. Arch Otolaryngol Head Neck Surg 117 : 321-326
Valone FH, Gandara DR, Deisseroth AB, Perez EA, Rayner A, Aronson FR, Luce J, Paradise C (1991) Interleukin-2, cisplatin, and 5-fluorouracil for patients with non-small cell lung and head/neck carcinomas. J Immunotherapy 10 : 207-213
Vlock DR, Johnson J, Myers E, Day R, Gooding WE, Whiteside T, Pelch K, Sigler B, Wagner R, Colao D (1991) Preliminary trial of nonrecombinant interferon alpha in recurrent squamous cell carcinoma of the head and neck. Head Neck 13 : 15-21
Vokes EE, Wenig B, Haraf DJ, McEvilly JM, Ervin TJ, Ratain MJ, Barton K, Kozloff M, Kies M, Panje WR, Weichselbaum RR (1991) Interferon-alfa-2b (IFN) as modulator of PFL induction chemotherapy for stage IV head and neck cancer (HNC). Eur J Cancer 27 (Suppl. 2) : S199
Volling P, Schröder M, Rauschning W, Achterrath W, Stennert E (1989) Carboplatin, the better platinum in head and neck cancer ? Arch Otolaryngol Head Neck Surg 115 : 695-698
Wadler S, Schwartz EL (1990) Antineoplastic activity of the combination of interferon and cytotoxic agents against experimental and human malignancies : a review. Cancer Res 50 : 3473-3486
Weidmann E, Sacchi M, Plaisance S, Seog Heo D, Yasumura S, Lin W, Johnson JT, Herberman RB, Azzarone B, Whiteside TL (1992) Receptors for interleukin-2 on human squamous cell carcinoma cell lines and tumor *in situ*. Cancer Res 52 : 5963-5970

Surgical considerations in the treatment of well-differentiated thyroid cancer

I Roisman, V Barak, D Sapir, A Bitterman, N Livni,
J Honigman, Z Gimmon, J Manny, AL Durst

Well-differentiated thyroid cancer is the most common malignancy arising in the thyroid gland, but its optimal management remains controversial : surgical resection and its extent provokes discussion [1, 2], but most authors agree that some type of thyroidectomy is appropriate if possible as the initial management. Radioiodine is also frequently used, either as adjuvant therapy or primary treatment modality for patients with systemic disease [3].

Patients and methods

A review of records, including clinical presentation, management, and outcome, was conducted of 269 thyroid cancer patients treated at two major clinics in Israel between 1970 and 1989. Follow-up periods varied from months to more than 20 years, with an average of 10 years. There were 196 (73 %) females and 73 (27 %) males (a ratio of 2.68 : 1) between 15 to 85 years (mean = 50.4). The survey revealed 184 (68 %) patients with papillary carcinoma and 85 (32 %), follicular carcinoma. Codings for histological stages were taken from the American Joint Committee on Cancer [4].

Statistical methods

Survival was studied by standard life-table methods (Kaplan-Meier method), and survival tables were analyzed by the Lee-Desu statistical test, with prognostic scores based on stage, extent (local invasion, distant metastases), size of tumor, and patient age. Comparison between several parameters were made by the c^2 test.

Results

Our survey found that the highest rate of well-differentiated thyroid cancer in papillary carcinoma is in the fourth decade. Place of birth of patients included 31.6 % from Israel, 35.7 % Europe, and 32.7 % elsewhere or unknown. The c^2 test was used to correlate sex and ethnic origin ($p > 0.05$).

Physical findings

One-half of the patients surveyed had been referred because of a mass in the neck, and 8.2 % because of swelling in that region found by routine medical examination. Physical findings included : nodule in thyroid gland, 27 % ; diffuse goiter, 11.5 % ; growing goiter, 9.7 % ; multinodular goiter, 3.3 % ; hoarseness, 4.8 % ; transient paralysis of vocal cords, 2.6 % ; and, regional lymph nodes enlarged, 8.6 %.

Departments of Surgery and Oncology, Hadassah University Hospital, Jerusalem, Israel

	No Data	Israel	Asia	Africa	Europe	America	
Patients	35	85	16	34	96	3	= 269
%	13	31.6	5.9	12.6	35.7	1.2	= 100

The majority of the patients had good thyroid function tests (88.5 %), while only 3.7 % had hyperthyroidism. In 96.3 % there was no known familial anamnesis of thyroid cancer, and in 97.4 % no previous irradiation to head and neck region. Finally, 13.4 % had hypertension ; 8.2 % heart diseases ; 5.1 % diabetes mellitus ; and 67 % had no other diseases.

« Cold nodules » were found in 43.5 % of patients, 21 % of the patients had a normal thyroid scan, 2.4 % had a « hot » nodule, and no thyroid scan was performed in 31.1 %. Positive carcinoma cells were found in 40.1 % by FNA before surgery, none were found in 8.6 %, and no evidence of performance had been noted in the charts in 37.1 % of the cases.

Treatment

In our study, a total thyroidectomy was performed in 113 patients (42 %), subtotal thyroidectomy in 134 (50 %), and other surgical procedures in 22 (8 %). A post-operative scan showed if a total or subtotal thyroidectomy had been done.

Histology

Neoplasms were classified as papillary or the follicular variant of papillary carcinoma in 183 (68 %) patients, and as follicular carcinoma in 86 (32 %). Bilateral cancer in both lobes was found in 11 %.

Complications of surgery

Perioperative complications included tachycardia (0.4 %) and tachypnea (1.1 %) ; while post-operation problems included permanent paralysis of one vocal cord (3.0 %), transient paralysis which passed after 6 months (5.6 %), and hypocalcemia, which was mainly associated with total thyroidectomy (6.3 %). There were no postoperative complications in 74.7 % of the cases.

No local recurrence was found in 82.9 % of the cases. In 8.2 %, there was local recurrence within the first two years due to undetected residual carcinoma or invasion of the tumor to the capsule ; and a second primary tumor was found in 1-20 years after the first operation (2.2 %). Additional surgery was performed on 7.1 % of the patients for the following reasons : 1) a frozen section was not done in the first operation, and the final result indicated the operation had to be expanded ; 2) a frozen section was unable to determine a final result for the first operation ; 3) a total thyroidectomy had to be done after the final result due to invasion of the tumor into blood vessels.

Actuarial survival curves

Overall actuarial survival curves for well-differentiated thyroid cancer is shown on Table 1.

Table 1. Overall survival

	Overall Total	Post total Thyroidectomy	Post-subtotal Thyroidectomy
After 5 years	97 %	98 %	98 %
After 10 years	92 %	92 %	94 %
After 20 years	80 %	79 %	94 %

There is a significant recurrence 20 years after treatment, whatever the actual procedure used. Of these, the subtotal thyroidectomy offers the smallest incidence of recurrence ($p = 0.39$ for men ; $p = 0.64$ for women).

In Israel, no statistical difference is seen between Jewish women of Ashkenazi (European or western) and Sephardi (Arabic, African, or eastern) origin (86-95 % post operative survival rates ($p = 0.59$), respectively). Relatively few cases of thyroid cancer among the Christian population of Israel makes it difficult to establish comparative rates.

The survival curve is slightly better for younger than for older patients ($p = 0.29$) : $p = 0.09$ for subtotal thyroidectomy no statistical difference for total thyroidectomy.

Histology : there is a slightly better actuarial survival curve for papillary carcinoma as compared to follicular carcinoma, even if there is no statistically significant difference ($p = 0.90$).

The survival curve is better for stage I patients after 20 years (94 %) than for stage II patients (86 %), but the difference is not significant ($p = 0.87$). Stage III is not shown here because of the small number of patients in Israel.

There is an identical survival curve 20 years after surgery in stage I post subtotal thyroidectomy and total thyroidectomy (95 %) ($p = 0.65$). In stage II after 20 years there were 95 % in subtotal thyroidectomy and 82 % post total thyroidectomy ($p = 0.97$).

Survival rates according to histology and stage of disease show higher mortality rates for follicular carcinoma than for papillary carcinoma (stage I — 90 % to 95 % at 15 years post surgery, $p = 0.21$, ns ; and stage II — 60 % to 93 % after 20 years, $p = 0.83$, ns).

Discussion

Worldwide, the incidence rate of thyroid cancer ranges from 0.5 % to 10/100,000 persons. Israel has 2.5 patients per 100,000 persons [5], which is comparable to approximately 25 new cases per million in the UK [6]. In all countries, females are affected two to three times more often than males.

Prognosis. Several factors have been associated with a poor prognosis in differentiated thyroid cancer : tumor characteristics such as size (> 1.5 cm), capsular and vascular invasion, extent, type, and grade ; male sex ; and age (males > 40 years ; females > 50 years). Age at initial diagnosis is considered the single-most important indicator of eventual outcome [7]. No single ultrastructural or microscopic feature provides a reliable means of predicting a fatal outcome.

Thoresen *et al.* [8] state that age and stage are the only factors of prognostic importance obtained by the multivariate analysis. In the present study, patients' ages ranged from 15 to 85 (mean = 50.4 ; SD = 18.32). This compares with Shaw et al. [9], who reported a mean of 46 years. One explanation for the importance of age in prognosis is offered by Joensuu et al [10], who have shown an increasing aneuploidy of cellular DNA with age in both benign and malignant thyroid tumors.

Conclusion

Young patients with stage I well-differentiated thyroid cancer can be safely treated by subtotal thyroidectomy. Total thyroidectomy combined with radioactive ablation is indicated in patients with more advanced disease. Prognosis is related to age, stage of disease, and gender.

References

1. Clark OH (1982) Total thyroidectomy : The treatment of choice for patients with differentiated thyroid cancer. Ann Surg 196 : 361
2. Mazzaferri EL (1981) Papillary and follicular thyroid cancer : A selective approach to diagnosis and treatment. Ann Rev Med 32 : 73
3. Bellegie NJ, RH Baskin, GL Sims et al (1982) Experience with malignant tumors of the thyroid in a private surgical practice. Surg Gynecol Obstet 155 : 62
4. American Joint Committee on Cancer (1980) Staging of Cancer of Head and Neck Sites and Melanoma. DeVita VT, S Hallman, SA Rosenberg (eds) Cancer — Principles and Practice of Oncology, Third Edition. Lippincott, USA
5. Robinson E, Y Horn, A Hochmann (1966) Incidence of cancer in thyroid nodules. Surg Gynec Obstet 123 : 1024
6. Domizio P (1989) Thyroid cancer. Surgery (Israel edition) 62 : 1490
7. Cady B, CE Sedgwick, WA Meissner et al (1979) Risk factor analysis in differentiated thyroid cancer. Cancer 43 : 810
8. Thoresen SO, LA Akslen, E Glattre et al (1989) Survival and prognostic factors in differentiated thyroid cancer — A multivariate analysis of 1055 cases. Br J Cancer 59 : 231
9. Shaw JHF, P Dodds (1990) Carcinoma of the thyroid gland in Auckland, New Zealand. Surg Gynec Obstet 171 : 27
10. Joensuu H, P Klemi, E Eerola et al (1986) Influence of cellular DNA content on survival in differentiated thyroid cancer. Cancer 58 : 2462

Abstract. In the period 1970-1989, 269 patients, 15 to 85 years (mean age = 50.4), with well-differentiated thyroid cancer were treated by surgery with or without complementary treatment. Of 196 female and 73 male patients, 194 (68 %) had papillary carcinoma and 85 (32 %) had follicular carcinoma. A total thyroidectomy was performed on 113 patients (42 %), subtotal thyroidectomies on 134 (50 %), and 22 (8 %) had other surgical procedures.

The 20-year actuarial survival figures (p = 0.67) show : all patients, 80 % ; females, 89 % ; males, 37 % (p = 0.09) ; papillary carcinoma, 95 % ; follicular carcinoma, 90 % (p = 0.90) ; stage I, 94 % ; stage II, 86 % (p = 0.87) ; patients younger than 40 years, 100 % ; patients older than 40, 85 % (p = 0.29) ; patients treated by total thyroidectomy, 79 % ; patients treated by subtotal thyroidectomy, 94 % (p = 0.67)

It was concluded that young patients with stage I, well-differentiated thyroid cancer can be safely treated by subtotal thyroidectomy. Total thyroidectomy combined with radioactive ablation is indicated in more advanced systemic disease. All specimens were stained with thyroglobulin in accordance with immunohistochemical procedures : 66 % stained with CA19-9, and, surprisingly, 80 % stained with CA15-3.

Lung cancer

Intensive chemotherapy with recombinant-human granulocyte-macrophage colony stimulating factor (r-hu-gm-csf) for small cell lung cancer (sclc) : a pilot study

C Besana, E Bucci, A Borri, G Di Lucca, S Tognella, M Tresoldi, M Marcatti, C Corti, G Citterio, F Inversi, C Rugarli

Systemic chemotherapy is the treatment of choice for patients with small cell lung cancer (sclc), Myelosuppression is the limiting toxicity related to most combination regimens in sclc, inducing substantial morbidity, frequent dose reductions, and delay in administrating subsequent cycles. Vp-16, Ifosfamide and Carboplatin are all highly active as single agents against sclc, with a ramge of objective response between 60 % and 75 %, A combination of these 3 drugs (with concurrent chest radiotherapy) showed impressive activity) > 90 % objective response rate) in a previous report by another group (Smith, 1990), at the cost of a 100 % incidence of grade III-IV neutropenia, with 7 % therapy-related deaths and dose reductions required for 72 % of patients. The association of recombinant human granolocyte-macrophage colony stimulating factor (r-hu-gm-csf) to a chemotherapy regimen consisting of Carboplatin and Vp-16 could allow higher doses of cytotoxic drugs to be given, possibly resulting in much higher complete response rates, even in extended disease (Morstyn, 1989). Basing on these data, we designed a pilot study on the association of r-hu-gm-csf to intensive chemotherapy.

Patients and methods

The study included 10 patients (7 males, 3 females ; median age 58.5 ; range 49-68) with histologically proven sclc, not previously treated. Eight patients had extended disease. All patients had ecog performance status 0 or 1. The median number of metastatic sites was 2 (range 1-5). Lactic dehydrogenase was elevated in 6 patients. Invasion of bone marrow was documented in 2 cases. No patients had concurrent severe medical disease. Brain metastases were an exclusion criterion.

Treatment consisted of : vp-16 100 mg/sqm/day diluted in 250 ml normal saline i.v. over 60' day 1-2-3 ; Ifosfamide 1.500 mg/sqm/day diluted in 500 ml dextrose 5 % water i.v. over 120' day 1-2-3 with Mesna uroprotection (400 mg i.v. bolus every 4 hours × 3) ; Carboplatin 125 mg/sqm/day diluted in 250 ml dextrose 5 % water i.v. over 60' day 1-2-3. Antiemetic prophylaxis consisted of Metoclopramide, 0.5 mg/kg × 2 i.v. + lorazepam 1 mg × 2 p.o. Recombinant human gm-csf was administered subcutaneously, as a single daily injection, at the dose of 10 micrograms/kg/day from day 4 to day 14. Cycles

Divisione di medicina II, Instituto scientifico ospedale s. raffaele, via Olgettina 60, 20132 Milano, Italy

had to be repeated every 28 days. Chemotherapy had to be delivered for 4-6 cycles depending on response. Thereafter, patients with limited disease achieving cr or pr were scheduled to receive thoracic radiotherapy (46 Gy over 23 daily fractions). Prophylactic whole brain radiotherapy (30 Gy) was scheduled for all patients achieving CR. Dose reduction at 75 % of the dose administered in the previous cycle was scheduled for cytostatic drugs if grade IV neutropenia and/or thrombocytopenia occurred, regardless the incidence of infection or hemorrhage. Dose reduction at 50 % was planned for r-hu-gm-csf if any grade III-IV toxicity developed. In the case of severe of recurrent grade IV toxicity possibly related to r-hu-gm-csf patients had to be withdrawn from the study.

Results

Overall, 42 cycles of chemotherapy were given (median number per patient, 4 ; range 2-6). Only 2 courses were delayed due to prolonged neutropenia. However, full dose treatment was given only in 21/42 courses (50 %). Grade III-IV neutropenia was observed in 21/42 courses (50 %) ; median duration of neutrophil count < 1.000/mmc was 7 days (ranges 2-13). Granulocytopenic fever occurred in 5/42 courses (12 %) but infection was documented only in 3 cases and subsided after proper antibiotic therapy. Grade III-IV thrombocytopenia occurred in 11/42 courses (26 %) ; median duration of thrombocytopenia was 3 days (range 1-11). Only 1 patient was given platelet transfusions for platelet count < 20.000/mmc and bleeding was never observed. Except for hematologic toxicity, this chemotherapy was well tolerated. Vomiting > grade II, severe renal, hepatic, or mucosal toxicity were never reported. No treatment-related deaths occurred. Mean nadir of neutrophil count was significantly higher after the second cycle than after the first (1108 v.s. 428/mmc p = 0.001), reflecting the reduction of chemotherapy dose applied in most patients. No significant difference in neutrophil and in platelet count was observed in the subsequent cycles. Recombinant h-gm-csf at the dose of 10 micrograms/kg/day was associated to severe cardiovascular toxic side events in 2 patients. In the first case, severe hypotension with supraventricular tachycardia was observed starting on the third day of administration and r-hu-gm-csf had to be continued at 50 % of the dose. In the second case, the toxic event consisted of frequent ventricular ectopic beats which required antiarrhythmic therapy with amiodarone. Thereafter, r-hu-gm-csf dose was reduced to 5 micrograms/kg/day with no further report of cardiovascular toxicity. In 3 cases severe skin reactions were observed (generalized erythema or urticaria) ; 2 patients had to be excluded from protocol because of prolongation or recurrence of skin reactions. The drug was otherwise well tolerated, except for pain and erythemia at injection site. Concerning dose-intensity, the scheduled dose reductions caused a striking reduction of the actual dose-intensity from cycle 1 to cycle 2 (93.95 % v.s. 76.21 % p = 0.012), whereas no further reductions were needed in the subsequent cycles.

All patients were evaluated for respnse : 1 patient achieved complete response and 8 patients achieved partial response (pr) after chemotherapy. The only patient judged to have progressive disease had actually discordant response with reduction of pulmonary and nodal disease but progession of liver metastases. Two patients with limited disease, achieving a pr > 75 % were subsequently surgically treated with radical excision of residual lung disease ; 1 of them is currently alive without relapse at 14 + months. All other responses were short-lasting (median 4 months, range 2-7). At failure, patients were treated with various chemotherapy regimens, but only 1 partial response of brief duration was observed.

Median survival, estimated following Kaplan-Meier's method, is 500 days ; median time-to-treatment failure is 170 days.

Conclusions

Despite the introduction of new agents and new combination regimens, overall survival for sclc has not been significantly modified with respect to a decade ago. The combination of vp-16, Ifosfamide and Carboplatin seemed to be confirmed to have an extremely high level of activity in terms of objective response rate, even in this small study. However, median duration of response is disappointing. The contribution of hematopoietic growth factors to chemotherapy, both in terms of reduction of toxicity and enhancement of dose-intensity, is currently under evaluation in several studies. Recently, the addition of r-hu-g-csf to a chemotherapy regimen has been validated as a progress in supportive care of sclc patients in a randomized trial, obtaining a reduction of neutropenic events, infectious episodes, and days of hospitalization (Crawford, 1991). A reduction in myelotoxicity could be also suggested in our pilot study, with respect to the data reported by another group (Smith, 1990) with a similar regimen. However, a reduction at about 75 % of the planned dose-intensity was needed. The usefulness of hematopoietic growth factors to ameliorate results in cancer chemotherapy through an enhancement of dose-intensity remains questionable. Recombinant hu-gm-csf at the dose of 5 micrograms/hg/day by subcutaneous injection is well tolerated, whereas a two-fold increase of the dose seems to be related to some risk of cardiovascular toxic side effects.

References

1. Smith IE, Perren TJ, Ashley SA et al (1990) Carboplatin, Etoposide and Ifosfamide as intensive chemotherapy for small cell lung cancer. J Clin Oncol 8 : 899-905
2. Morstyn G, Bishop J, Stuart-Harris R et al (1989) Optimal dose and scheduling of GM-CSF for the abrogation of chemotherapy-induced neutropenia. Proceedings ECCO 5 ; Satellite Symposium on Intron-A and GM-CSF in clinical oncology : status and prospects (abstract)
3. Crawford J, Ozer H, Stoller R et al (1991) Reduction by granulocyte-colony stimulating factor of fever and neutropenia induced by chemotherapy in patients with small cell lung cancer. N Engl J Med 325 : 164-170

Sequential high-dose chemotherapy with r-metHu-G-CSF (Filgrastim) and infusion of peripheral blood progenitor cells (PBPC) in patients with small cell lung cancer (SCLC). A feasibility study

S Leyvraz, N Ketterer, JPh Grob, Ph Schneider, P Vuichard, V von Fliedner, F Lejeune

Despite the progress that has been made during the last decades in the treatment of small cell lung cancer, the emergence of drug resistant cells to chemotherapy remains a major problem. Dose-response relationship has been initially demonstrated in animal models [1]. Similarly, several clinical trials have confirmed that a dose-response exist for many chemotherapeutic agents [2, 3] and that intensive chemotherapy may achieve a high response rate in refractory tumors such as breast or small cell lung cancers [4, 5, 6]. To date however, the increase in complete response rate has not been translated into improvement in overall survival. But intensification has been limited to the administration of a single treatment under the protection of autologous bone marrow transplantation. The early delivery of multiple sequential, intensive treatments might improve these results.

Such an approach is limited by the hematological toxicity which may produce inacceptable morbidity and mortality. The avaibility of hematopoietic colony-stimulating factors (CSFs) has allowed safer administration of intensive regimens, by reducing the importance of neutropenia. CSFs have also been shown to expend the pool of peripheral blood progenitor cells (PBPC) that can be harvested by leucapheresis and used in conjonction with autologous bone marrow transplant or alone to reconstitute the marrow functions [7, 8, 9].

The aim of this trial was to test the possibility to mobilize by granulocyte colony-stimulating factor (r-metHuG-CSF, Filtrastim) alone and collect enough PBPC for multiple cycles of high-dose chemotherapy. We studied the feasibility of administering 4 sequential courses of chemotherapy considering the hematological and non hematological toxicities.

Patients and methods

Six patients with histological proven small cell lung cancer and 1 patient with stage IV breast cancer entered into the study to date. The patient characteristics are reported in Table 1. Four patients were not pretreated. One patient received radiotherapy before the first cycle because of a superior vena cava syndrome. One patient had received Adjuvant chemotherapy and radiotherapy for breast cancer 10 years previously. The patient with stage IV breast cancer

---

Centre Pluridisciplinaire d'Oncologie, Division d'hématologie, Centre de transfusion, Centre Hospitalier Universitaire Vaudois, Lausanne, Switzerland

was treated with Adjuvant chemotherapy 3 years previously and with mediastinal radiotherapy for recurrence 1 month before being included in the study.

Mobilization and collection of PBPC were performed before the first cycle of chemotherapy. Filgrastim was given subcutaneously at a daily dose of 12 µg/kg/day for 10 days. On the fifth day, leukaphereses were started for a maximum of 5 times. Mononuclear cells were obtained from leukapheresis collection and cryopreserved in 10 % DMSO. Bone marrow harvest was done in the first 4 patients for backup, but was never used.

Table 1. Patient characteristics

# patients		7
Age median (range)		50 (36-60)
Male/Female		2/7
Diagnosis :	— Small cell lung cancer	6
	— Breast cancer	1
Pretreatment :	— No	4
	— Yes	3
	Adjuvant chemotherapy	2
	Mediastinal radiotherapy	2
# cycles :	1	2
	2	2
	4	3

High-dose chemotherapy consisted in Cyclophosphamide 2.5 g/m² on days 1 and 2, Cisplatin 50 mg/m² on days 1 to 3 and Etoposide 300 mg/m² on days 1 to 3. The treatment was planed to be repeated every 21 days for a total of 4 cycles. One fourth of PBPC collection was reinfused 24 to 48 hours after the end of chemotherapy. Filgrastim was started the same day at the dose of 12 µg/kg/day subcutaneously for 14 days or less in case of early recovery. Ciprofloxacine ot Phenoxymethyl-penicillin were given during the periods of neutropenia, and broad-spectrum antibiotics were administered intravenously in case of febrile episode. Platelet transfusions were prescribed for thrombocytopenia lower than $10 \times 10^9/l$.

Results

Mobilization by Filgrastim alone given for a median of 8 days (range 7 to 10) produced an increase of leucocyte count to a median of $88.4 \times 10^9/l$ (range 50.7 to 153.0). After a median of 4 leukaphereses (range 3 to 5), the collection of mononuclear cells was a median of $5.46 \times 10^8/kg$ (range 3.61 to 19.87). The number of CD–34+ cells was a median of $5.25 \times 10^6/kg$ (range 0.68 to 26.48) and correlated with the obtained number of colony-forming unit for granulocyte-macrophage (CFU-GM) that reached $53.25 \times 10^4/kg$ (range 4.14 to 210.1).

Table 2. Hematological toxicity

		1st cycle median (range)	2nd cycle median (range)	3rd cycle median (range)	4th cycle median (range)
Days to Lc*	≥ 0.3	8 (8-11)	8 (7-10)	9 (8-10)	10 (9-11)
	≥ 0.5	10 (9-14)	10 (8-11)	11 (9-12)	10 (9-11)
	≥ 1.0	11 (9-15)	11 (8-11)	12 (9-12)	10 (10-12)
Days with Lc	≤ 0.3	7 (5-9)	6 (4-7)	7 (6-7)	7 (6-8)
	≤ 0.5	9 (6-12)	7 (6-9)	8 (7-9)	7 (6-9)
	≤ 1.0	9.5 (7-13)	8 (6-10)	9 (8-9)	10 (8-11)
Days to Plts*	≥10	9.5 (7-14)	9 (9-12)	10 (9-11)	12 (9-12)
	≥20	10 (9-15)	11 (9-12)	13 (10-14)	13 (9-14)
Days with Plts	≤10	6 (1-10)	2 (1-5)	4 (2-4)	7 (1-7)
	≤20	6.5 (1-11)	5 (3-8)	7 (6-9)	7 (2-9)

* Leucocyte and platelet unit : × 10^9/l.

Table 3. Clinical parameters

	1st cycle median (range)	2nd cycle median (range)	3rd cycle median (range)	4th cycle median (range)
Plts transfusion	3.5 (1-9)	2 (1-3)	3 (2-3)	
Hb transfusion	2 (1-4)	2 (1-2)	2 (1-3)	
Hospitalization (days)	19.5 (17-44)	19 (16-22)	18 (16-20)	
T° ≥38⁵ (# pat.)	6	1	2	(1-4)
Proven infection (# pat.)	3	1	1	(2-4)
Days with i.v. AB	11 (6-14)	8 (7-14)	8	(18-20)

Eighteen cycles of chemotherapy are evaluable, whereas the study is still ongoing. Three patients completed the 4 cycles, 2 patients received 2 cycles and 2 patients 1 cycle. The duration of leucopenia and thrombopenia was calculated from the day of PBPC reinfusion to recovery or as the number of days with a low leucocyte or thrombocyte count. The results are presented in Tables 2 and 3. The median time to leucocytes recovery $\geqslant 0.3 \times 10^9/l$ was 8 days (range 9 to 11). It was 10 days (range 9 to 14) and 11 days (range 9 to 15) to recovery $\geqslant 0.5$ and $\geqslant 1.0 \times 10^9/l$. The median time with a leucocyte count $\leqslant 0.3 \times 10^9/l$ was 7 days (range 5 to 9). It was respectively 9 days (range 6 to 12) and 9.5 days (range 7 to 13) with leucocyte count $\leqslant 0.5 \times 10^9/l$ and $\leqslant 1.0 \times 10^9/l$. The duration of leucopenia did not change with increased number of cycles, neither the number of days with intravenous antibiotics.

Thrombocytopenia was short-lasting and dit not cause any clinically significant bleeding. During the first cycle, the median time to platelet recovery $\geqslant 10$ and $\geqslant 20 \times 10^9/l$ was 9.5 days (range 7 to 14) and 10 days (range 9 to 15). The median time with platelets $\leqslant 10$ and $\leqslant 20 \times 10^9/l$ were respectively 6 days (range 1 to 10) and 6.5 days (range 1 to 11). The time to platelet recovery was not significantly longer in the fourth cycle compare to the first 1. The median number of platelet transfusions was 3.5 (range 1 to 9) for the first cycle, 1 (range 1 to 3) for the second cycle, 2 (range 1 to 3) for the third and 3 (range 1 to 4) for the fourth cycle. The median number of red blood cell transfusions did not change from cycle 1 to 4 and was a median of 2 (range 1 to 4) for each cycle.

The duration of hospitalisation was not longer between the first and the subsequent cycles. It reached a median of 19.5 days (range 17 to 44) in the first cycle. The longest period of hospitalisation was observed in the patient with the superior *vena cava* syndrom who experienced severe oesophagitis and bacteriaemia possibly enhanced by previous radiotherapy.

The limiting toxicity of this regimen appeared after the third and fourth cycle and consisted in neurotoxicity and ototoxicity. Indeed, the 3 patients receiving 4 cycles of treatment developed grade 2 ototoxicity and a median grade 2 (range 2 to 3) neurotoxicity.

Other toxicities consisted in moderate nausea and vomiting. All the patients complained of exhaustion and weight loss with a median of 3.5 kg for the patients who received 1 cycle and 8 kg (range 7 to 11) after the fourth cycle. Mucositis and diarrhea were mild except in 2 patients who developed grade 3 oesophagitis and in 1 patient, an episode of transient ileus and rectorragia.

Response evaluation was not the end point of this study. Among the 5 evaluable patients with small cell lung cancer, there were 3 complete and 2 partial responses.

Conclusion

Encouraging results have been observed with high-dose chemotherapy [10, 11, 12]. In small cell lung cancer, cure is infrequent even though the chemosensitivity is high. Current treatment generally fails to achieve permanent control of the tumor. However, intensification of chemotherapy may increase the response rate and the disease free survival in patients with limited disease [13]. Our study tested the possibility of increasing intensity of chemotherapy for the treatment of SCLC with the support of PBPC and Filgrastim.

We demonstrated that the dose of 12 µg/kg/day for 10 days mobilized enough PBPC for multiple sequential cycles of high-dose chemotherapy. PBPC could be collected safely by the mean of repeated leukaphereses. The amount of PBPC was large enough to allow complete recovery of marrow functions.

Reinfusion of PBPC after an intensive regimen simultaneously with the administration of Filgrastim alleviated the induced myelosuppression. We observed no obvious cumulative haematological toxicity in the patients who received 3 or 4 cycles of treatment.

An important finding was the disclosure of non hematological dose-limiting toxicity. All the patients receiving 4 cycles of therapy experienced severe ototoxicity and neurotoxicity. It prevented further administration of the fourth cycle in subsequent patients.

In conclusion, we demonstrated the feasibility of administering multiple, sequential, intensive chemotherapy with the support of PBPC and Filgrastim. The occurrence of severe dose limiting non hematological toxicity showed the limitation of such an approach. Chemotherapy regimen specific for intensification programs should be developed focusing in agents with strictly hematological toxicity pattern.

References

1. Schabel FJ, Griswold DP, Corbett TH et al (1984) Increasing the therapeutic response rates to anticancer drugs by applying the basic principles of pharmacology. Cancer 54 : 1160-1167 (suppl)
2. Frei E, Canellos GP (1980) Dose : A critical factor in cancer chemotherapy. Am J Med 69 : 585-594
3. Johnson DH, Wolff SN, Hainsworth JD et al (1985) Extensive-stage small cell bronchogenic carcinoma : intensive induction chemotherapy with high-dose Cyclophosphamide plus high-dose Etoposide. J Clin Oncol 3 : 170-175
4. Tannock IF, Boyd NF, De Boer G et al (1988) A randomized trial of two dose levels of CMF chemotherapy for patients with metastatic breast cancer. J Clin Oncol 6 : 1377-1387
5. Williams SF, Gilewski T, Mick R et al (1992) High-dose consolidation therapy with autologous stem-cell rescue in stage IV breast cancer : Follow-up report. J Clin Oncol 10 : 1743-1747
6. De Vita VT (1986) Dose-response is alive and well. J Clin Oncol 4 : 1157-1159
7. Neidhart JA, Mangalik A, Kohler W et al (1989) Granulocyte colony-stimulating factor stimulates recovery of granulocytes in patients receiving dose-intensive chemotherapy without bone marrow transplantation. J Clin Oncol 7 : 1685-1692
8. Vadhan-Raj S, Broxmeyer HE, Hittelman WN et al (1992) Abrogating chemotherapy induced myelosuppression by recombinant granulocyte-macrophage colony-stimulating factor in patients with sarcoma : Protection at the progenitor cell level. J Clin Oncol 10 : 1266-1277

9. Sheridan WP, Begley CG, Juttner CA et al (1992) Effect of peripheral-blood progenitor cells mobilized by Filgrastim (FILGRASTIM) on platelet recovery after high-dose chemotherapy. Lancet 339 : 640-664
10. Wheeler C, Antin JH, Churchill WH et al (1990) Cyclophosphamide, Carmustine and etoposide with autologous bone marrow transplantation in refractory Hodgkin's disease and non-Hodgkin's lymphoma : A dose-finding study. J Clin Oncol 8 : 648-656
11. Peters WP, Shpall EJ, Jones RB et al (1988) High-dose combination alkylating agents with bone marrow support as initial treatment for metastatic breast cancer. J Clin Oncol 6 : 1368-1376
12. Nichols CR, Tricot G, Williams SD et al (1989) Dose-intensive chemotherapy in refractory germ cell cancer. A phase I-II trial of high-dose Carboplatin and Etoposide with autologous bone marrow transplantation. J Clin Oncol 7 : 932-939
13. Humblet Y, Symann M, Bosly A et al (1987) Late intensification chemotherapy with autologous bone marrow transplantation in selected small cell carcinoma of the lung : a randomized study. J Clin Oncol 5 : 1864-1873

Cisplatinum and 5-Fluorouracil in small cell lung cancer

JF Morere*, A Duran*, F Tcherakian**, C Boaziz*, JP Battesti***, L Israel*, JL Breau*

Objective tumor regression can be obtained in the majority of small cell lung cancer patients using current chemotherapy. In spite of a high response rate, only a small fraction of patients can be cured because of treatment failure due to development of resistance to the drugs. Detecting new active combinations remains a goal in the management of such patients.

Cisplatin yields a response rate of less than 30 % when used alone [1]. But it is currently used in combination with VP16 achieving a 65 to 85 % response rate [2].

5-FU has not been adequatly tested as a single agent in small cell lung cancer. Brugarolas [3] did not observe any response in 5 patients treated by 5-FU used alone. Only one study by Havsteen [4] has found a low activity in a phase II study on 26 patients.

However the combination of Cisplatin and 5-FU is synergistic in animal systems. The biochemical basis for this synergy may be that Cisplatin increases the availility of the reduced folate necessary for 5-FU to be cytotoxic [5].

This advantage is confirmed in human in head and neck and in non-small cell lung cancer [6, 7]. On the basis of these observations, we have studied Cisplatin plus 5-FU as first line therapy in small cell lung cancer.

From November 1986 to February 1992, 110 patients with previously untreated small cell lung cancer were entered into this study at the oncology department of Avicenne hospital and pneumology department of Auxerre hospital. All patients were required to have measurable or evaluable pathologically confirmed small cell lung cancer. There were 57 males and 53 females, with a median performance status of 1.54 had localized and 56/110 had disseminated disease. One patient was not evaluable for response due to prior surgery. All were considered eligible for toxicity.

Patients received Cisplatin at a dose of 25 mg/m^2/day and 5-FU at a dose of 600 mg/m^2/day, day 1 through day 5, by continuous infusion for the first course and over 4 hours for the following out patient treatment. As first evaluation, the first 25 patients received only one course of Cisplatin plus 5-FU to avoid a too long delay before standard therapy.

For the other patients at least 2 courses were delivered. Cycles of chemotherapy were repeated every 3 weeks if toxicity permitted otherwise at 4 weeks with dose adjustment (20 % decrease in the dose). The median number of courses administered was 3.

---

* Service d'Oncologie Médicale, Hôpital Avicenne, 125 route de Stalingrad, 93000 Bobigny, France
** Service de Pneumologie, Centre Hospitalier d'Auxerre, 2 bis place St Germain, 89011 Auxerre, France
*** Service de Pneumologie, Hôpital Avicenne, 125 route de Stalingrad, 93000 Bobigny, France

After evaluation of the Cisplatin — 5-FU combination standard therapy Cyclophosphamide, Adriamycin, VP16 was given, followed in 59 patients by chest and or cerebral irradiation.

Follow-up

The primary end points of this study were response rate and toxicity. Chest radiographs were obtained at 3 weeks intervals. Patients in whom disease was documented by computed tomographic scan, magnetic resonance imaging, or bone scan had these tests repeated at regular intervals to assess their responses. A complete response was defined as disapearance of all measurable disease for 4 weeks. A partial response occurred when there was a reduction greater than 50 % in the sum of the products of the greatest perpendicular diameters of all measurable lesions for 4 weeks compared with the pretreatment measurements. For evaluable disease, a partial response was a definite decrease in tumor size assessed independently by 2 investigators.

Results

There were 85 objective responses in 109 evaluable patients corresponding to an overall response rate of 77 %. The 95 % confidence limits for this overall response rate were, 70-85 %. There were 23/109 complete responses and 62/109 partial responses. Stable disease was seen in 18/109 patients and progressive disease was documented in 6/109.

Responses occurred in all tumour sites : chest : 72, CNS : 21, liver : 21, pleura : 1, skin : 1, supraclavicular nodes : 3.

Toxicity

The acute toxicity of this regimen was mainly expressed on the thrombocytes. Thrombocytopenia was found in 10/110 of patients. In half cases thrombopenia occurred in cases of diffuse bone metastases. Grade 2-3 neutropenia was seen in only 4 patients. Three patients developped a grade 2 cardiac toxicity leading to stop 5-FU chemotherapy. No toxic death was attributed to this chemotherapy.

Conclusion

DDP-5-FU is active in small cell lung cancer. The overall response rate 77 % (CI : 70-85) can be favorably compared with that of currently used combinations. Toxicity (thrombopenia) was tolerable.

Association of this regimen with radiation therapy or leucovorin or VP16 seems interesting to be evaluated in further studies.

References

1. Cavalli F, Goldhirsch K, Siegaltthaler P et al (1980) Phase II study with cis-dichloro diammineplatinum in small cell anaplastic bronchogenic carcinoma. Eur J Cancer 16 : 617-621
2. Ihde DC (1992) Chemotherapy of lung cancer. N Engl J Med 327 : 1434-1441
3. Brugarolas A, Rivas A, Lacave AJ et al (1975) 5-Fluorouracil (NSC-19893) compared to Cyclophosphamide (NSC-26271) in bronchogenic carcinoma : results of a clinical study. Part J Cancer Chemother Rep 59 : 1025-1026
4. Havsteen N, Sorenson S, Rorth M et al (1981) 5-Fluorouracil in the treatment of small cell anaplastic carcinoma of the lung : a phase II trial. Cancer Treat Rep 65 : 123-125
5. Peters GJ, Van Groeningen CJ (1991) Clinical relevance of biochemical modulation of 5-Fluorouracil. Ann Oncol 2 : 469-480
6. Weiden PL, Einstein AB, Rudolph RH (1985) Cisplatin bolus and 5-FU infusion chemotherapy for non-small cell lung cancer. Cancer Treat Rep 69 : 1253-1255
7. Heim W, Wampler GL, Lokick JJ et al (1991) A study of infusional Cisplatin and infusion Fluorouracil for locally advanced or metastatic non-small cell lung cancer : a Mid-Atlantic Oncology Program Study. J Clin Oncol 9 : 2162-2166

Phase I-II study of oral Etoposide and modulation of drug resistance with ketoconazole in small cell lung cancer

D Dalley*, B Brigham**

Etoposide, an inhibitor of the enzyme Topoisomerase II has been used in the treatment of small cell lung cancer in various dose schedules including chronic daily oral administration [4]. Although considered one of the most active chemotherapeutic agents for this malignancy, invariably drug resistance occurs as with other agents singly or in combination. Both in the laboratory and in clinical studies attempts have been made to circumvent drug resistance.

Ketoconazole (KCZ), an antifungal agent, has been used in oncology patients as a manipulator of endocrine function, not only to treat hypercortisolaemia [1, 2, 3], but also to inhibit steroid synthesis and sex hormone production in prostate and breast cancers. This effect is by virtue of its inhibitory effect on the cytochrome P-450 system (CP_{450}) [5], and CP_{450} dependent enzymes. Auxiliary enzyme systems that involve NADPH and NADPH-CP_{450}-reductase (in endoplasmic reticulum) or NADPH-ferredoxin and a flavoprotein reductase (in mitochondria) are involved during all CP_{450} reactions [6]. Both CP_{450} and the glutathione related enzymes are involved in detoxification of cytotoxic and carcinogenic compounds [7, 8]. Their interrelationship is very complex, but both enzyme groups are present in virtually all tissues.

Because of an apparent synergism between the drugs KCZ and Etoposide in a patient reported earlier [3], we undertook a prospective phase I/II study in extensive small cell lung cancer patients.

Patients and methods

Eligibility criteria

For eligibility patients had to have histologically confirmed small cell undifferentiated lung cancer, and extensive disease on the basis of staging investigations. Patients were required to have adequate haematological parameters (leucocyte count of $\geq 4.0 \times 10^9/l$ and platelet count of $\geq 100 \times 10^9/l$), life expectancy of more than 1 month, no history of prior malignancy and either measurable or assessible disease not subject to prior radiotherapy. Patients were to have had no previous large field radiotherapy, no prior cytotoxic chemotherapy and had to be able to swallow tablets. They were only included on the study after giving informed consent in writing as dictated by the hospital ethics committees. Poor performance status was not an exclusion factor, but was recorded prior to entry and during treatment.

Medical Oncology Departments, * St Vincents Hospital, Darlinghurst NSW 2010, **Prince of Wales Hospital, Randwick NSW 2031, Australia

Pretreatment staging required for study entry included chest radiographs, liver/upper abdominal ultrasound or CT scan, CT head scans, radionucleide bone scan and bone marrow examination.

Treatment

Treatment for the first 15 patients consisted of oral Etoposide 200 mg/m^2/day for 3 days every 3 weeks, starting 3 days after commencement of Ketoconazole 200 mg qid with steroid replacement consisting of cortisone acetate 37.5 mg/day and Fludrocortisone 0.1 mg/day. The Ketoconazole and steroid replacement was given continuously before, during and after the treatment with Etoposide. Dose modification was according to tolerance.

After the first 15 patients, because of the toxicity seen, the treatment was changed such that the Ketoconazole was given for 3 days before, 3 days during and 3 days after the oral Etoposide. The initial dose of Etoposide was 150 mg/m^2/day for 3 days and was adjusted to 100 mg/m^2/day for ECOG performance 4 patients. If tolerance was satisfactory, then the dose of Etoposide was escalated to 200 mg/m^2/day. For response and toxicity the World Health Organisation criteria were used [9].

Results

Between April 1990 and November 1992, 21 patients were entered onto the study. There were 19 men and 2 women with an age range of 53 to 82 years (median age 66 years). Ten patients had ECOG performance status (PS) of 0.6 with PS 1 and 5 with PS 3. There have been no patients with PS 2 or 4 to date.

Four patients died early and are not evaluable for response. Two of these patients died toxic deaths. One died from a documented myocardial infarction prior to starting Etoposide, and 1 patient died from unknown causes.

All patients were evaluable for toxicity and the major toxicity was haematological (Table 1).

Table 1. Toxicities (WHO criteria)

	Grade 1	Grade 11	Grade 111	Grade 1V
Alopecia	5	10	—	—
Nausea/vomiting	0	1	1	1
Mucositis	5	3	1	—
Diarrhoea	2	2	0	—
Liver	0	0	0	0
Infection	0	2	0	2*
Adrenal suppression	0	0	0	1
Leucocytes	0	0	0	3*
Granulocytes	0	0	1	3*
Platelets	0	1	0	4*

* 2 deaths in patients with these toxicities

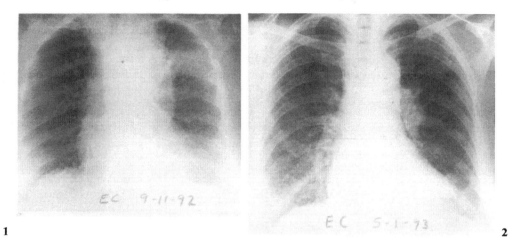

Fig. 1. Plain chest radiograph prior to treatment in patient EC
Fig. 2. Plain chest radiograph for EC following 2 cycles of Ketoconazole and Etoposide

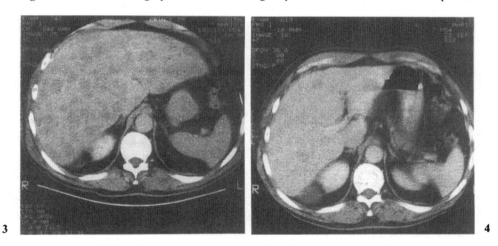

Fig. 3. CT scan of liver prior to treatment in ML
Fig. 4. CT scan of liver following treatment for ML

Of the 17 patients evaluable for response, there were 9 responders. Of these, 2 were complete responders and 7 were partial responders (Fig. 1-4). The median duration of response is 4+ months (range 1+ to 13 months). Seven patients had initial stable disease with a median duration of 2 months (range 1/2 to 3 months). Only 1 patient to date has had progressive disease.

Following the development of progressive disease after initial response or stable disease, in most cases patients were given alternative chemotherapy (various treatments), and this very likely had an influence on the overall survival. The median survival of the overall group (21 patients) was 155 days (range 2 to 439). For responders the median survival was 213 days, (range 61 to 439) and for stable disease patients median survival was 155 days (range 53 to 330).

Discussion

One of the most disappointing aspects of the treatment of small cell lung cancer is that although the disease is sensitive to therapy many patients do not have a tumour response in the first instance, or later have the development of resistance to anticancer therapy. So far attempts to modulate drug resistance have failed. Conventionally the use of combination chemotherapy attempts to reduce this likelihood but often leads to increased toxicity. Historically the response rates for single drug Etoposide have ranged from 20 to 75 % [10]. We assume therefore that for Etoposide alone the true response rate is probably about 45 %. Our patient numbers at present are too small to accurately estimate the true response rate; we hope to accrue 50-60 patients and should then have a better idea.

Recently the Vanderbilt University group have reported improved results with chronic low dose oral Etoposide [4]. It is not certain whether the improved results are due to a more prolonged exposure of the tumour to the drug (area under curve effect) or some other effect, at a cellular level.

Potentially of interest would be the use of a drug which interferes with the degradation of Etoposide, thereby altering its pharmacokinetics, or which more importantly, may interfere with tumour degradation of the drug. Of particular interest is the possibility that KCZ has an independent anti-tumour effect in this malignancy. Recent reports suggest that this may be the case for some human tumours [11, 12].

The problem encountered with excess haematological toxicity has been previously seen in a randomised study where KCZ was given prophylactically in an attempt to reduce the incidence of fungal infections in acute leukaemic patients [13]. The KCZ arm had more profound and prolonged neutropenia and subsequent incidence of bacteraemia compared to the placebo arm.

In our study, we believe that we have made appropriate changes to the dose scheduling to cope with the problem of excess haematological toxicity. Whether the use of Ketoconazole with Etoposide results in an improvement in the therapeutic index or not is yet to be answered. Although our study with larger patient numbers may demonstrate a high response rate, the question of whether this is the optimal scheduling is another important issue to be resolved in future studies.

Acknowledgements. Funding has been provided by Bristol-Myers Laboratories, Riverwood Rotary Club, and the friends/family of Mrs. Dulcie Keir, in whose memory this manuscript is dedicated. Thanks also to Dr.R.Golding for reviewing radiographs, and to Mrs J Thompson and Ms. M.Ng for help in preparation of the manuscript.

References

1. Shepherd FA, Hoffert B, Evans WK et al (1985) Ketoconazole : Use in the treatment of ectopic adrenocorticotrophic hormone production and Cushing's syndrome in small cell lung cancer. Arch Intern Med 145 : 863-864
2. Engelhardt D, Jacob K, Doerr HG (1989) Different therapeutic efficacy of ketoconazole in patients with Cushings syndrome. Klin Wochenschr 67 : 241-247
3. Hoffman DH, Brigham B (1991) The use of Ketoconazole in ectopic adrenocorticotrophic hormone syndrome. Cancer 67 : 1447-1449
4. Johnson DH, Greco FA, Strupp J et al (1990) Prolonged administration of oral Etoposide in patients with relapsed or refractory small cell lung cancer : a phase II trial. J Clin Oncol 8 : 1613-1617
5. Sonino MD (1987) The use of Ketoconazole as an exhibitor of steroid production. N Engl J Med 317 : 812-818
6. Guengerich FP (1988) Cytochromes P-450. Comp Bioch Physiol 89C (1) : 1-4
7. Guengerich FP (1988) Roles of cytochrome P-450 enzymes in chemical carcinogenesis and cancer chemotherapy. Cancer Res 48 (11) 2946-54
8. Chasseaud LF (1979) The role of glutathione and glutathione-S-transferases in the metabolism of chemical carcinogens and other electrophilic agents. Adv Cancer Res 29 : 175-274
9. Miller AB, Hoogstraten B, Staquet M et al (1981) Reporting results of cancer treatment. Cancer 47 : 207-214
10. Cohen MH, Perevodchikova NI (1979) Single agent chemotherapy of lung cancer. In : Muggia FM, Rozencweig M (eds) Progress in cancer research and therapy, vol 11, « Lung Cancer : progress in therapeutic research ». Raven Press, New York, pp. 343-374
11. Tzanakakis GN, Agarwal KC, Vezeridis MP (1990) Inhibition of hepatic metasatsis from a human pancreatic adenocarcinoma (RWP-2) in the nude mouse by prostcyclin, forskolin and Ketoconazole. Cancer 65 : 446-451
12. Naftalovich S, Yefenof E, Eilam Y (1991) Antitumour effects of Ketoconazole and trifluoperazine in murine T cell lymphomas. Cancer Chemother Pharmacol 28 : 384-90
13. Palmblad J, Lonngvist B, Carlsson G (1992) Oral Ketoconazole prophylaxis for candida infections during induction therapy for acute leukaemia in adults : more bacteraemias. J Intern Med 231 : 363-370

Abstract. Ketoconazole, an Imidazole derivative and potent inhibitor of steroid biosynthesis has been used in the palliation of Cushing's syndrome [1, 2, 3]. Following its use in 1 of our patients in combination with Etoposide [3], we were prompted to undertake a study in poor risk small cell lung cancer patients. Twenty-one patients have been treated to this point. Of the 17 evaluable for response there have been 9 responders, 7 with stable disease and 1 with progressive disease, with a median survival for the 21 patients being 5 months. Following 2 toxic deaths among the first 15 patients we have modified the treatment. Our results with poor risk patients are comparable to those treated with combination chemotherapy reported in the literature.

Angiogenesis : a novel target for Adjuvant chemotherapy in locally advanced non-small cell lung cancer

P Macchiarini*, G Fontanini**, E Dulmet**, V de Montpreville**, A Chapelier*, B Lenot*, J Cerrina*, F Le Roy Ladurie*, P Dartevelle*

Surgery remains the only curative treatment modality for non-small cell lung cancer (NSCLC). Long-term results are significantly influenced by the primary tumor (T) and lymph node (N) stages and the oncological radicality of operation. Early-staged (T1N0M0) tumors are highly curable by surgery alone and because of its cost-benefit ratio, adjuvant therapy is not recommended [1]. For more advanced disease (any T3-4, N1-2M0), operation still represents the only chance for cure but long-term results are largely influenced by the biological operability and dependent from the T and N subset categories [2].

Since more than 2/3 of patients with locally advanced disease undergoing resection ultimately die from systemic recurrence of their primary tumor [3], several efforts have been made to improve treatment outcome by administering adjuvant chemotherapy, radiationtherapy or both [4]. Unfortunately, all have failed and the advocated explanations have been the absence of independent predictors of tumor recurrence and efficacy of the chemotherapeutic regimens. In previous studies we demonstrated that the induction of new capillaries and venules (angiogenesis) significantly correlates with the development of metastasis in early-staged, node-negative (T1N0M0) NSCLC [1, 5]. In the present study, we have tested whether this hypothesis holds true for NSCLC invading the thoracic inlet, the most advanced node-negative subset of NSCLC.

Patients and methods

The surgical specimens of 28 consecutive patients treated between January 1980 and December 1991 were reviewed. There were 25 males and 3 females aged in median 56 years (range, 36-73 years). All patients presented with a NSCLC invading the thoracic inlet ; these tumors represent T4 lesions (stage IIIB) and have been usually considered an absolute surgical contraindication [2]. However, we designed a new surgical approach which enables these tumors to be completely resected at the expense of minimal morbidity and mortality and impressive long-term results [6]. Ten carcinomas were of a squamous type, 8 of an adenocarcinoma, 8 of a large cell type, and 2 were mixed cell neoplasms. Eighteen NSCLC were located in the left thoracic inlet. Fourteen tumors involved the lower trunk of the brachial plexus, 12 the subclavian vessels and 16 the first 2 ribs. The resection of the tumor-bearing inlet area was associated with 14 wedge pulmonary resections, 13 upper lobectomies and 1 pneumo-

---

Departments of * Thoracic and Vascular Surgery and Heart-Lung Transplantation and ** Surgical Pathology, Hôpital Marie-Lannelongue, Paris-Sud University, le Plessis-Robinson, France

nectomy. All but 1 patient had negative mediastinal lymph nodes. Twenty-five patients (89 %) received postoperative adjuvant radiotherapy (median, 60 Gy) with ($n = 14$) or without ($n = 11$) Cisplatin-based chemotherapy. Seventeen patients died from either local ($n = 2$) or systemic ($n = 15$) relapse ; 1 patient relapsed locally after 3 months from operation but is still alive while receiving local radiation therapy. One patient died from a sudden myocardial infarction after 15 months, without evidence of tumor disease. The remaining 9 patients are alive and disease-free.

Tumor immunohistochemical studies

All paraffin-embedded bouin-fixed blocks containing tumour tissue from each patient were analyzed for the presence of tumor emboli within blood or lymphatic vessels, p53 gene expression, proliferative activity and other histological variables according to previously described methods [1, 5, 7]. The presence of tumour emboli in endothelial-lined channels and their location in the specimen were assessed [1]. Analysis of p53 human protein was done with the ABC immunoperoxidase technique using the rabbit polyclonal antibody CM-1 recognizing the p53 nuclear protein (wild and mutant type). The areas of tumor containing the most intense angiogenesis were examined by light microscopy, screened by scanning the tumor sections at low power (40 × and 100 x) and by identifying them with the highest number of discrete microvessels, e.g. capillaries and small venules staining for factor VIII antigen [5]. The areas of high neovascularization were more frequent at the neoplasm margins and graded on a density scale of 0 to 4+. Microvessels in sclerotic areas within the tumor and adjacent areas of unaffected lung parenchyma were not considered in vessel count and served as internal controls for assessing the quality of staining for factor VIII. After the most vascularized area was identified, individual microvessels were counted on 200 x fields and each count was expressed as the highest number of microvessels identified within the area [5].

Cell kinetic studies were determined by estimating the expression of the proliferating cell nuclear antigen (PCNA) and mitotic count (MC) [1, 7]. Absolute counts of PCNA immunoreactivity were made by scoring a minimum of 5 HPFs and the percentage of proliferating tumors cells was determined (range, 0 to 100 %).

Statistical analysis

Survival was calculated from the date surgery until death or the date of the last follow-up (censored). The disease-free interval (DFI) was considered as the time elapsed form the date of surgery to the first documented evidence of recurrence (local or metastatic), while deaths related to causes other than NSCLC were censored. Survival and DFI were estimated by the product-limit method [8], and differences on their distribution were evaluated *via* the log rank test [9], for univariate analysis, and Cox's proportional hazards stepwise model [10], for multivariate analysis. Numbers were expressed either as median or as mean ± S.D. of *n* number of observations. The *a priori* level of significance was set at a $p < .05$. All tests were two-sided.

Results

Tumor characteristics are depicted in Table 1. 71 % of them ($n = 20$) presented areas of angiogenesis; the median density grade was 1 and the median number of neovessels 6.39 % lesions ($n = 11$) presented IBVI ($n = 5$), PBVI ($n = 4$) or both ($n = 2$) by tumor cells. With a median follow-up time of 3.5 years (range, 8 to 145+ months), the projected 2 and 5 year survivals for all patients were 46 % and 29 %, respectively; the median DFI was 23 months. By univariate analysis, BVI by tumor cells (+ vs −) and degree of angiogenesis were the most significant in predicting poor survival and DFI (Table 2). The density of angiogenesis ($<$ vs ≥ 1) and number of neovessels ($<$ vs ≥ 6) were the only independent and significant predictors of DFI (Table 3). Patients whose tumors had a density of angiogenesis ≥ 1 and a number of neovessel ≥ 6 (high-risk) had a significant worse DFI ($p = 0.0001$) (Fig. 1) and higher ($p = 0.0001$) RR (5.63 times [95 % CI, 1.56-20.2]) of developing systemic recurrence from their primary tumor than their low-risk counterparts. High-risk patients had tumors with a significantly higher ($p < 0.0001$) incidence of tumor emboli within their blood vessel than low-risk patients (66.1 % vs 7.6 %, respectively).

Table 1. Tumor characteristics of 28 non-small cell lung cancer involving the thoracic inlet

Characteristics	Values
Tumor size (cm) :	5.911 ± 4.02
	(5.5, [5.06-8.185])
Tumor grading (grade I vs II vs III) :	3 vs 10 vs 15
(1 to 3 scale) :	2.357 ± 0.731
p53 expression (absent vs present) :	17 vs 11
%	14.7 ± 14.9
	(10, [4.7-24.75])
Tumor proliferative activity* (%) :	42.268 ± 17.686
	(45, [35.4 − 49.12])
Mitotic count :	22.214 ± 14,004
	(18, [16.7 − 27.6])
Angiogenesis (present vs absent) :	20 vs 8
Angiogenesis-density (0 to 4 + scale) :	1.19 ± 1.157
	(1, [0.74-1.64])
Angiogenesis count (per 200 × field) :	7.64 ± 7.28
	(6, [4.81 − 10.46])
Blood vessel invasion (absent vs present) :	17 vs 11

Data are expressed as mean ± standard deviation (S.D.). Numbers in parenthesis indicate median and [95 % Confidence Intervals]. * Determined by PCNA staining

Angiogenesis

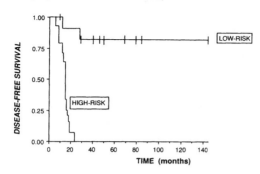

Fig. 1. Disease-free interval (DFI) stratified by risk-status. The relative risk of recurrence from the primary tumor was significantly highter in high-risk (angiogenesis density $\geq$ 1 and a microvessel count $\geq$ 6, $n = 15$), than low-risk patients (angiogenesis density < 1 and a microvessel count < 6, $n = 13$) ($p = 0.0001$). High-risk patients had a significantly ($p < 0.0001$) shorter disease-free interval than low-risk patients (projected 5-year rates of 0 and 82 %, respectively). Vertical bars indicate patients currently alive and disease-free.

Table 2. Univariate survival and disease-free interval (DFI) analysis

Features	Survival (P-*value*)	DFI (P-*value*)
Tumor size ($<$ vs $\geq$ median, 5.5 cm) :	NS	NS
Tumor grading ($<$ vs $\geq$ median, 2.5 cm) :	NS	NS
P53 Staining (present vs absent) :	NS	NS
PCNA° ($<$ vs $\geq$ median, 45 %)	NS	NS
Mitotic count ($<$ vs $\geq$ median, 18) :	NS	NS
Angiogenesis-density ($<$ vs $\geq$ median, 1) :	0.0005	0.0011
Angiogenesis count ($<$ vs $\geq$ median, 6) :	0.0005	0.0011
BVI* (absent vs present) :	0.036	0.046

NS : not statistically significant. No other discrete and continous variable met the 0.05 level of significance. *BVI : blood vessel invasion by tumour cells. °PCNA : Proliferating Cell Nuclear Antigen Reactivity

Table 3. Multivariate disease-free interval analysis

Features	β Coefficient	S.D.°	P-*value*
Microvessel-density grade : (<1 vs ≥ 1)	3.157	1.483	0.033
Microvessel count (*per* 200 × field) : ($<$ vs $\geq$ median, 6 cm)	1.062	0.402	0.008

° S.D. Standard deviation. No other variable met the 0.05 significance level

Discussion

Experimental evidence (32) indicates that after a new tumor has attained a size of few millimetre in diameter (10^6 tumor cells), further exponential expansion of the tumor-cell population requires the induction of new capillary blood vessels (angiogenesis) [11], process related to the release of tumour angiogenic factors [12] or deregulation of tumor differentiation [11]. These new capillaries arise from pre-existing capillaries or venules, never from arteries, arterioles, or veins, and represent the consequence of the ingrowth of columns of aligned endothelial cells. Adjacent columns contract to form loops which then develop a lumen, permitting blood flow to begin [11]. The new proliferating capillaries have fragmented basement membranes [13] and their leakness [14] facilitates their penetration by tumour cells as opposed to mature vessel [11]. Moreover, rapidly proliferating tumors may force the migration of tumour cells along lines of least resistance [15]. Thus, angiogenesis increases the opportunity for single or multiple tumor cells to enter into circulation [16, 17].

This study was performed to confirm our previous experiences with early-staged NSCLC [1, 5, 7]. In order to have locally-advanced but still node-negative tumors, we selected neoplasms invading the thoracic inlet because of their unique local aggressiveness and metastatic pathway. They were larger and less differentiated than T1N0M0 lesions and displayed a remarkable higher degree of angiogenesis, confirming the suggestion of Horak and associates [18] that degree of angiogenesis occurs as tumors enlarge or become more poorly differentiated. The degree of angiogenesis independently and significantly correlated with poor DFI, and this is in line with recent observations made in other solid tumors [19-20]. A plausible explanation of this phenomenon might be that above a threshold of neovascularization, metastasis is more likely to occur. This correlation is further demonstrated by the fact that high-risk patients had a significantly higher ($p < 0.0001$) incidence of tumor cells in their primary blood vessels than low-risk patients. Since this circumstance correlates with the development of tumor vascularization, results provide evidence that angiogeneis is an essential prerequisite for tumor growth and develpment of metastasis.

The univariate and multivariate DFI analysis data are particularly important from a clinical point of view, because we failed to find important predictors of relapse in our previous experiences examining only traditionally clinical parameters [6]. By identifying a low-risk group associated with a 5-year survival rate greater than 80 %, we clearly demonstrated that NSCLC involving the thoracic inlet are highly curable lesions. However, we were also able to select a group of high-risk patients associated with an extremely poor prognosis and the clinical implications of this finding is of paramount importance because newer treatment modalities might be used to treat or prevent angiogenesis. For instance, one might block the production of tumor angiogenic factors (fibroblast growth factors or transforming growth factors, heparanase) by the combination of Cortisone and Heparin [21]; this combination is a potent inhibitor of new vessel formation in tumour-bearing mice and is accompanied by the reduction in the size of the primary tumor mass and in the incidence of metastasis. An alternative to prevent angiogenesis would be to target the tumor vasculature by flavone acetic acid (an anticancer agent which induces procoagulant activity *in vitro* and inhibits tumor growth *in vivo* and has an established effect against tumor vasculature though not against developing vessels) [22], or α tumor necrosis factor or Vinblastine that act on solid tumors by a host cell-mediated mechanism which induces vascular damage by loss of blood flow within the tumor [23]. Unfortunately, most of these potentially fruitful therapeutic approaches are yet experimental and their clinical effectiveness remains to be demonstrated. However, they are likely to play in the near future an increasing and expanding role in preventing or treating the metastatic phenotype of angiogenic-dependent tumors [24].

In conclusion, presented results demonstrate that angiogenesis significantly correlates with late treatment failure and is acquired at a critical density and number of neovessels. Our findings provide also guidelines for targeting the risk of relapse and death in high-risk patients by administering antiangiogenic agents in the postoperative course.

References

1. Macchiarini P, Fontanini G, Hardin M, Pingitore R, Angeletti CA (1992) Most peripheral, node-negative non-small cell lung cancer have absence of intratumoral and peritumoral blood and lymphatic vessel invasion and low proliferative rates. J Thorac Cardiovasc Surg 104 : 892-899
2. Mountain CF (1988) Prognostic implications of the international staging system for lung cancer. Sem Oncol 15 : 236-245
3. Mountain CF (1985) The biological operability of stage III non-small cell lung cancer. Ann Thorac Surg 40 : 60-64
4. Holmes EC (1991) Surgical adjuvant therapy of non-small cell lung cancer. Lung Cancer 7 : 71-76
5. Macchiarini P, Fontanini G, Hardin M, Squartini F, Angeletti CA (1992) Relation of neovascularization to metastasis of non-small cell lung cancer. Lancet 340 : 145-146
6. Dartevelle P, Chapelier A, Macchiarini P et al (in press) Anterior transcervical-thoracical approach for radical resection of lung tumors invading the thoracic inlet. J Thorac Cardiovasc Surg
7. Macchiarini P, Fontanini G, Hardin M (in press) Blood vessel invasion by tumour cells predict recurrence in completely resected T1N0M0 non-small cell lung cancer. J Thorac Cardiovasc Surg
8. Kaplan EL, Meier P (1958) Nonparametric estimation from incomplete observations. J Am Stat Assoc 53 : 457-481
9. Peto R, Pike MC, Armitage P, Breslow NE, Cox DR, Howard SY (1977) Design and analysis of randomized clinical trials requiring prolonged observations of each patient : II. Analysis and examples. Br J Cancer 35 : 1-39
10. Cox DR (1972) Regression models in life tables. J R Stat Soc (B) 34 : 187-220
11. Hart IR, Saini A (1992) Biology of tumour metastasis. Lancet 339 : 1453-1457
12. Folkman J, Watson K, Ingberg D, Hanahan D (1989) Induction of angiogenesis during the transition form hyperplasia to neoplasia. Nature 339 : 58-61
13. Folkman J, Haudenschild C (1980) Angiogenesis in vitro. Nature 288 : 551-556
14. Nagy JA, Brown LF, Senger DR (1989) Pathogenesis of tumor stroma generation : a critical role for leaky blood vessels and fibrin deposition. Biochemic Biophys Acta 948 : 305-326
15. Eaves G (1972) The invasive growth of malignant tumors as a purely mechanical process. J Pathol 109 : 233-237
16. Liotta LA, Steeg PS, Stetler-Stevenson WG (1991) Cancer metastasis and angiogenesis : an imbalance of positive and negative regulation. Cell 64 : 327-336

17. Liotta L, Kleinerman J, Saidel G (1974) Quantitative relationships of intravascular tumour cells, tumour vessels, and pulmonary metastasis following tumor implantation. Cancer Res 34 : 997-1004
18. Horak ER, Leek R, Klenk N (1992) Angiogenesis, assessed by platelet/endothelial cell adhesion molecule antibodies, as indicator of node metastases and survival in breast cancer. Lancet 340 : 1120-1224
19. Frost P, Levin B (1992) Clinical implication of metastatic process. Lancet 336 : 1458-1461
20. Weidner N, Semple JP, Welch WR, Folkman J (1991) Tumor angiogenesis and metastasis-correlation in invasive breast carcinoma. N Engl J Med 324 : 1-8
21. Folkman J, Langer R, Linhart RJ, Haudenshild C, Taylor S (1983) Angiogenesis inhibition and tumor regression caused by heparin or a heparin fragment in the presence of cortisone. Science 221 : 719-725
22. Mahadevan V, Hart IR (1991) Divergent effects of flavone acetic acid on established versus developing tumor blood flow. Br J Cancer 63 : 889-892
23. Murray JC (1992) Vascular damage and tumor response. Eur J Cancer 28 : 1593-1594
24. Macchiarini P (1993) L'angiogènese, un nouveau marquer prognostique dans la maladie cancéreuse. Sang Thrombose Vaisseaux 5 : 1-4

A statistical model for investigating Adjuvant chemotherapy in T1N0M0 non-small cell lung cancer

JM Hardin*, P Macchiarini**, KP Singh*

The use of Adjuvant chemotherapy in NSCLC has been greatly debated in the literature [6]. Because of the favorable outcomes associated with the use of surgery alone and its high cost-effectiveness, as well as the lack of evidence that adjuvant therapy has a significant effect on survival or on recurrence, it has not been recommended for T1N0M0 NSCLC [11]. However, as noted in a previous paper [9], we share the view of [11], that the absence of positive adjuvant trials in NSCLC reflects the ineffectiveness of drug regimens and the inappropriateness of patients selected for the therapy.

In a recent investigation [9], we observed that patients with a prognosis similar to that of patients with mediastinal lymph node [12], were at a high risk for recurrence of NSCLC. Further we observed that patients with positive intratumoural and/or peritumoral blood vessel invasion (BVI^+) by tumour cells have a significant tendency to relapse systemically in the first 5-years. Thus, it was suggested that since there is some evidence that adjuvant therapy is beneficial for mediastinal lymph node [8], perhaps BVI^+ patients would be suitable for adjuvant systemic chemotherapy.

From our previous analysis, we observed that BVI was a highly significant prognostic factor for disease free time (DFI) using a Cox proportional hazards model. However, the relative risk of BVI over 5, 10, and 15 year periods calculated using the methods of [10], revealed a changing pattern over time, thereby suggesting that the constant relative risk assumption of the Cox model may be violated. Thus, to better model and understand this data, we consider in this paper the use of the generalized log-logistic regression model [14].

Statistical methods

In various types of cancers including breast and lung cancers [4, 5, 7] and others have provided sufficient evidences that non-monotone convergent hazard functions are associated with clinical covariates. In fact, Harris and Albert have provided several examples of survival data that clearly violate the assumption of constant relative risk of the Cox model, that is, hazard rate is constant over time.

Briefly, recall that [2] proposed a model in which no assumption is made

---

* Department of Biostatistics University of Alabama at Birmingham, Alabama 35294, USA
** Department of Thoracic and Vascular Surgery and Heart-Lung Transplantation, Hospital Marie-Lannelongue (Paris-Sud University), 92350 le Plessis-Robinson, Paris, France

about the mathematical form of the underlying hazard function, i.e., baseline hazard function, $h_0(t)$. The model for the ith individual is given by

$$h_i(t, Z) = h_0(t) \exp(\hat{\beta} Z_i) \quad (2.1)$$

This model is in fact partially parametric or semi-parametric since 1 needs to estimate the regression coefficient-vector β. The relative hazard function exp (βZ_i) is constant through time and the survival distributions for different Z_i are related as powers of each other, i.e., power law relation.

A family of non-proportional hazard models have been recently proposed by Singh et al [14]. These models are defined as follows. Let T be the survival time for an individual and let Log(t) be a generalized logistic random variable with shape parameters m_1 and m_2. Then T is a generalized log-logistic random variable with shape parameters m_1 and m_2 and the probability distribution function is given by

$$F(t) = \int_0^{F_0(t)} B(m_1, m_2)^{-1} W^{m_1 - 1} (1-W)^{m_2 - 1} dW \quad (2.2)$$

and the density function is given by

$$f(t) = \frac{\alpha B(m_1, m_2)^{-1} [F_0(t)]^{m_1} [1 - F_0(t)]^{m_2}}{t}, \quad m_1 > 0, m_2 > 0 \quad (2.3)$$

where $B(m_1, m_2)$ is the complete β function and $F_0(t)$ is the log-logistic function and given by

$$F_0(t) = \frac{1}{1 + \exp(-\alpha \log t - \beta_0 - \beta'Z)}, \quad \alpha > 0, t > 0 \quad (2.4)$$

We also call F(t) the β-logistic distribution, the generalized β of second type or the generalized F distribution (Prentice 1975, Ciampi et al 1986, Sibuya and Hirotsu 1984). For notational simplicity let T GLL (m_1, m_2).

When $m_1 = m_2 = 1$, GLL(m_1, m_2) becomes the log-logistic random variable and thus

$$\text{logit}[S_0(t)] = \hat{\beta}_0 + \alpha \log t + \hat{\beta} Z \quad (2.5)$$

Note that (2.5) gives a linear relation of the logarithm of odds ratio to the logarithm of survival time and to the covariate regression function βZ assumed independent of time.

The family of the generalized log-logistic models has limit distributions including generalized γ distributions, reciprocal γ distribution, Weibull distribution and log-normal distribution. Following Glaser [3], Singh [13] showed that this family provides models for many of the different shaped hazard rates, for example, strictly increasing (I), constant (C), strictly decreasing (D), bathtub shaped (ψ) and upside down bathtub shaped. Because of space limitation we refer the interested readers to Singh [13]. In applying the family to real data computational difficulties occur because of the flatness of the loglikelihood over m_1 and m_2. This suggests the considerations of submodels GLL (m,1) and GLL (1,m). Note that the shape parameter m still retains the property of measuring the structure of heavy tail. For the model GLL (m,1), m < 1 reflects the heavy tail. For GLL (1,m) also reflects such a tail.

Using these methods, we attempted to better model our T1N0M0 NSCLC data.

Application

The data for this study was obtained from a group of 95 consecutive T1N0M0 NSCLC patients treated with surgery alone. The study design and patient characteristics for this data has been previously described [9].

Table 1. Estimates and standard errors of log-logistic model

Covariates	GLL (1, 1) Estimates ± S.E. (p-value)	GLL (1, M) Estimates ± S.E. (p-value)
Log_e (T)	0.886 ± 0.179 (<0.001)	1.270 ± 0.038 (<0.001)
Intercept	−8.307 ± 0.659 (<0.001)	−8.538 ± 0.073 (<0.001)
Tumor Size	0.448 ± 0.350 (<0.001)	0.569 ± 0.078 (<0.001)
BVI	−0.960 ± 0.825 (<0.001)	−1.666 ± 0.044 (<0.001)
PCNA	2.172 ± 0.538 (<0.001)	2.753 ± 0.000 (<0.001)
MC	0.029 ± 0.021 (<0.001)	0.036 ± 0.020 (<0.001)
M2	--------	0.320 ± 0.058 (<0.001)
2 Log (X)	−162.542	161.601

Multicollinearity among the variables was examined using standard procedures and highly collinear variables were deleted. The resulting variables used to model disease free time (or time to recurrence) were surgery, side, local, tumor size, BVI, PCNA, MC. We then fit both GLL (1, 1) and GLL (1, M) generalized log-logistic models to the data. For both models only the variables tumor size, BVI, MC, PCNA were found to be significant. The regression coefficients and estimates of the standard errors are given in Table 1.

The GLL (1, M) model appears to give a slightly better fit to the data. Both models seem to fit the data better than the Cox model which had 2*log-likelihood of -213.543. Also note that the coefficient for log(t) is significantly greater than 0 reflecting the time dependence seen in the relative risks. Further, the estimate of m (M2 = .320) indicates the heavy tail of the hazard function. These results are similar to those observed in other cancer studies, e.g. [1].

Discussion

In this paper we have examined the use of the generalized log-logistic model for the modeling of recurrence time (DFI) in a group of patients with T1N0M0 NSLLC. Four variables were found to be significant covariates in the model. The generalized log-logistic models also were seen to provide a better fit to the data than previous Cox models. Interesting, BVI was a significant in all models. Presently, we are developing the software to allow the fitting of the more general GLL (m_1, m_2) model to this data. Once this task is complete, our intentions are to develop a patient profile model to select individuals with a high risk of NSCL recurrence, and hence candidates for Adjuvant chemotherapy. The current models, however, give evidence to support a recommendation of adjuvant therapy for individuals with BVI.

References

1. Bartolucci AA, Singh KP (1991) A two-step procedure for survival analysis. Presented at joint meeting of the Society for Clinical Trials and the International Society for Clinical Biostatistics, Brussels, Belgium, July 8-12
2. Cox DR (1972) Regression models and life table (with discussion). JRSS B34 : 187-220
3. Glaser RE (1980) Bathtub and related failure rate characteristics. JASA 75 : 667-672
4. Gore SM, Pocock SJ, Kerr GR (1984) Regression models and non-proportional hazards in the analysis of breast cancer survival. Appl Stat 33 : 176-195
5. Harris EK, Albert A (1991) Survivalship analysis for clinical studies. Marcel Dekker, Inc
6. Holmes EC, Bleehen NM, Le Chevalier T et al (1991) Postoperative adjuvant treatments for non-small cell lung cancers : A consensus report. Lung Cancer 7 : 1-13
7. Langlands AO, Pocock SJ, Jerr GR, Gore SM (1979) Long-term survival of patients with breast cancer : a study of the curability of the disease. Br Med J 2 : 1247-1251
8. Macchiarini P, Hardin JM, Angeletti CA (1991) Long-term evaluation of intrapleural Bacillus Calmette and Guerin with or without Adjuvant chemotherapy in completely resected stages II and III non-small cell lung cancer. Am J Clin Oncol 14 : 291-297
9. Macchiarini P, Fontanini G, Hardin JM, Chuanchieh H, Bigini D, Vignati S, Pingitore R, Angeletti A (1993) Blood vessel invasion by tumour cells predicts cancer recurrence in completely resected T1N0M0 non mall cell lung cancer. J Thorac Cardiovasc Surg (in press)

10. Sackett DL, Haynes RB, Tugwell P (1985) Clinical epidemiology : A basic Science for clinical medicine. Little Brown, Boston, MA, pp. 47-138
11. Shields TW (1989) Carcinoma of the lung. In : Shields TW (ed) General Thoracic Surgery, 3rd ed. Lea & Febiger, Philadelphia, pp. 890-934
12. Shields TW (1990) The significance of ipsilateral mediastinal lymph node metastasis (N2 disease) in non-small cell lung carcinoma of the lung. J Thorac Cardiovasc Surg 99 : 48-53
13. Singh KP (1989) A generalized log-logistic regression model for survival analysis : hazard rate characteristics. Biom Praxim 29 : 63-74
14. Singh KP, Lee C, George EO (1988) On generalized log-logistic model for censored survival data. Biom J 30 : 843-850

A combination chemotherapy with Ifosfamide (I), Cisplatin (P) and Etoposide (E) for advanced non-small cell lung cancer (NSCLC)

G Martin, MJ Garcia, JJ Cruz, A Gómez, A Panadero, E Fonseca, P Sánchez, P Soria, J Garcia, JC Vallejo

The role of combination chemotherapy in the treatment of NSCLC remains controversial. One of the most widely used conbinations is PE which yielded a 32 % response rate in 682 patients [1]. Efforts to improve the efficacy of this regimen by adding a third agent have not been particularly successful. Recently, however, interest has focused on the promise of I in this role [2].

We report here the results of our prospective phase II study of IPE in previously untreated patients with advanced NSCLC.

Patients and methods

Thirty-one previously untreated patients were eligible for study if they had cytologically or histologically proven NSCLC (Squamous 19, Adenocarcinoma 11, Undifferenciated 1), considered unresectable for cure. This included patients with Stage III-A (4/31), III-B (11/31) and IV (16/31) according to the 4th edition of the UICC. Inclusion criteria were : measurable or evaluable disease, age < 75, (ECOG) performance status < 2, normal baseline renal, hepatic and cardiac functions, and baseline neutrophils $2 \times 10/L$ or more and platelets $100 \times 10/L$ or more. Patients with brain metastases were excluded.

The protocol consisted of the administration of I 4 gr/m^2 intravenously (i.v.) with Mesna uroprotection (800 mg/m^2, 30 minutes before and 0.4 and 8 hours after 1 administration) day 1. P 100 mg/m^2 i.v. day 2, and E 80 mg/m^2 i.v. days 1 to 3. Courses were repeated every 28 days for a total of 3-4 cycles.

Results

Of 31 elegible patients, 29 were evaluables for response and toxicity (2 of them abandoned voluntarily the protocol). Objective responses (OR) to IPE chemotherapy were obtained in 15 patients. Among them a complete response (CR) was achieved in 3 patients (10 %) and a partial response (PR) in 12 patients (41 %). Non response (NR) was observed in 14 patients (48 %).

According to the stages responses were as follow : Stage III-A (4 patients) : none CR, 2 PR and 2 NR ; Stage III-B (9 patients) : 2 CR, 4 PR and 3 NR ; Stage IV (16 patients) : 1 CR, 6 PR and 9 NR. There were no significant differ-

Servicio de Oncologia, Hospital Clinico, Salamanca, Spain

ences between Stage III (OR 61 %) and Stage IV (OR 49 %) responses, or according to performance status : ECOG I, 56 % (9/16) and ECOG II, 46 % (6/13).

Responses according to histology were : squamous (18) : 2 CR, 11 PR and 5 NR (OR 72 %) ; adenocarcinoma (10) : 1 CR, 1 PR and 8 NR (OR 20 %) ; undifferenciated (1) : 1 NR. One patient underwent surgery showing histological complete response. This patient died because of sepsis after surgery.

Thoracic radiotherapy (60 cGy) was administered to 17 patients after chemotherapy. Two of them in CR, 9 in PR and 6 with NR. There was no change in responses after local therapy except in 1 patient who do not respond to chemotherapy, and then, he achieved CR.

Actuarial survival at 15 months is 70 % for responders and 33 % for non-responders (p = 0.284). There was no difference in survival between Stage III and IV or among different histology.

Toxicity was mild and manageable. A total of 103 cycles were administered. Neutropenia was showed in only 3 courses (2.9 %). One patient died because of sepsis after severe neutropenia and coma owing to encephalopaty due to I. Gastrointestinal toxicity was moderate (37 %). Doses of P were reduced in 3 patients because of renal toxicity (Creatinine level between 1.5 and 2 mg/dL (2.9 %). Alopecia was universal.

Discussion

We conclude that IPE protocol is an active treatment of advanced NSCLC with a 51 % of OR rate and 10 % of CR rate. These results are similar to those achieved by others authors [3, 4, 5]. Pujol et al [4] with this same protocol, obtained a rate of 70 % OR in Stage III patients. However, the hematopoietic toxicity was pronounced.

Table 1. Response to IPE

	N° Patients	CR (%)	PR (%)	NR (%)	OR (%)
Overall responses	29	3 (10)	12 (41)	14 (48)	15 (51)
Stage :					
III-A	4	—	2 (50)	2 (50)	2 (50)
III-B	9	2 (22)	4 (44)	3 (33)	6 (66)
IV	16	1 (6)	6 (37)	9 (56)	7 (43)
Histology :					
Squamous	18	2 (11)	11 (61)	5 (27)	13 (72)
Adenocarcinoma	10	1 (10)	1 (10)	8 (80)	2 (20)
Undifferenciated	1	—	—	1 (100)	
ECOG :					
I	16	2 (12)	7 (43)	7 (43)	9 (56)
II	13	1 (7)	5 (38)	7 (53)	6 (46)

Median survival was 8 months. There were no significant difference in any group (responders and non-responders, Stage III and IV and among different histology). It is necessary longer follow-up in order to get difference at the survival.

References

1. Klastersky J (1986) Therapy with Cisplatin and Etoposide for non-small cell lung cancer. Sem Oncol 13 : 104-114 (suppl 3)
2. Eberhardt W, Niederle N (1992) Ifosfamide in non-small cell lung cancer : a review. Sem Oncol 19 : 40-48 (suppl 1)
3. Shepherd FA, Evans WK, Goss PE et al (1992) Ifosfamide, Cisplatin and Etoposide (ICE) in the treatment of advanced non-small cell lung cancer. Sem Oncol 19 : 54-58 (suppl 1)
4. Pujol JL, Ross JF, Le Chevalier T et al (1990) Phase II pilot study of Ifosfamide-Cisplatin-Etoposide in locally advanced non-small cell lung cancer. Eur J Cancer Clin Oncol 26 : 798-801
5. Shirinian M, Lee JS, Dhingra HH et al (1992) Phase II study of Cisplatin, Ifosfamide with Mesna and Etoposide (PIE) chemotherapy for advanced non-small cell lung cancer. Sem Oncol 19 : 49-53 (suppl 1)

Mitomycin, Ifosfamide and Platin (MIP) in advanced and disseminated non-small cell lung cancer (NSCLC)

PJ Souquet, C Bohas, T Zenone, E Michaud, MT el Khoury, P Romestaing, JP Bernard

The usefulness of chemotherapy in advanced non small cell lung cancer is still controversial, but our recent meta-analysis [1] clearly shows that the polychemotherapy reduces the mortality during the first year.

Nevertheless the most effective regimen of chemotherapy is not yet established. There are only few drugs (Cisplatin - Ifosfamide - Mitomycine - Vinblastine - Vindesine or Vinorelbine) which when tested as single agents produce major responses in 15 % or more of cases [2, 3].

Between January/91 and July/92 we performed a phase II study of Mitomycine - Ifosfamide - Platin in inoperable NSCLC.

Patients and methods

Previously untreated (except surgery) ambulatory (WHO performance status 0,1 or 2) patients aged 70 years or less, with non resectable (stage IIIB or IV) and histologically confirmed NSCLC, were eligible for this phase II study. All patients had normal blood counts and normal renal function. Thoracic and cerebral tomodensitometry and abdominal ultrasound scan were done as a part of the staging procedure. Isotopic bone scan was performed when indicated.

Chemotherapy consisted of 90 mg/m^2 of Platin day 1 in 1 hour infusion, 6 mg/m^2 of Mitomycin day 1 intravenously and Ifosfamide 2 g/m^2 days 1 and 2 infused during 2 hours with Mesna 1 g given intravenously 30 minutes before Ifosfamide and Mesna 0.5 g 4 hours and 8 hours after.

Antiemetic treatment was either ondansetron or granisetron with Methylprednisolone.

The courses were repeated every 28 days.

Patients were fully reassessed after 3 courses of chemotherapy and after 6 courses (in stage IV) and 1 month after the end of thoracic radiotherapy (stage IIIB). Response was assessed clinically and with chest X-Ray, thoracic tomodensitometry, fiberoptic bronchoscopy and reassessment of all the involved sites, using the WHO criteria.

In stage IV, 3 other courses (Mitomycine only in courses, 1, 2, 4, and 6) were performed only in responders. In stage III-B a thoracic radiotherapy was performed (2 Gy by fraction, 5 fractions by week for 5 weeks), after the 3 cycles of chemotherapy.

Department of Pneumology and Thoracic Oncology, Centre Hospitalier Lyon Sud, 69310 Pierre Bénite, France

Results

Between January/91 and July/92, 27 patients entered this study. Patient characteristics is reported in Table 1.

Table 1. Patient characteristics (n = 27)

Age		
	Range	36-70 years
	Median	56 years
	Men-Women	26-1
WHO performance status		0 10
		1 16
		2 10
Stage		
	IIIB	12
	IV	15
Histology		
	Squamous cell carcinoma	18
	Adenocarcinoma	9

All patients were considered evaluable for response, toxicity and survival.

After 3 courses of chemotherapy, 8 patients achieved partial remission (29.5 %) (3 stage IIIB, 5 stage IV) but there was no complete remission.

In stage IIIB after thoracic radiotherapy there was only 3 partial remission.

In stage IV after the end of the 6 courses there were 1 complete remission and 1 partial remission.

The median overall survival was 9 months.

The toxicity was quite large and is detailed in Table 2.

Table 2. Toxicity observed in 82 courses (WHO grade)

	Grade 3	Grade 4
Alopecia (after 3 courses)		
(28 patients assessibles)	28	0
Leucopenia	4	2
Thrombopenia	1	2
Nausea vomiting	6	1
Raised serum creatinine	1	0
Neurotoxicity	1	0
N° cycles delayed 2		
N° cycles reduced 6		

One patient died 10 days after the first course of chemotherapy (aplasia and sepsis) 3 patients had only 2 courses of chemotherapy because of unacceptable toxicity (renal grade III, major nausea and vomiting, neurotoxicity with severe transient confusion). Nausea and vomiting were severe in 5 patients despite the use of 5 HT3 antagonists. Alopecia occured in all patients.

Myelosuppression was moderate.

Discussion

An objective response rate of 29.5 % (despite no complete response) suggest that the MIP regimen (with this dosage) has a quite good activity in non small cell lung cancer. Others studies of the M.I.P. regimen with various dosage had shown better results (34 to 69 % in a total of 205 patients [4].) M. Cullen [5] has reported 50 % of overall response rate (with 11 % of complete response) with Ifosfamide 3.0 g/m^2, Cisplatin 50 mg/m^2, Mitomycine 6 mg/m^2, day 1-22 but Kardamakis [6] with the same regimen had only 34 % of response.

Giron [7] and Anton-Torres [8] with increased dosage of Cisplatin (100 and 80 mg/m^2 respectively) reported 69 and 56 % of response.

In our study, the response rate of stage IIIB was disappointing with only 3 responders in 12 patients (worst than in stage IV). The effect of radiotherapy was also disappointing with no complete remission after the planned treatment of radiotherapy. In general patients with limited disease NSCLC respond better to combination chemotherapy than do those with extensive disease [9].

In our report, the myelosuppression was moderate with 1 treatment related death due to repsis. Non hematological toxicity was most important (renal toxicity, neurotoxicity with transient agitation and confusion and nausea and vomiting despite the use of 5 HTA antagonists).

The combination of Mitomycine, Ifosfamide and Platin produces objective response rate comparable with those obtained with other Cisplatin containing regimens (MVP) ; Nevertheless the optimal dosage and schedule of Cisplatin and Ifosfamide needs to be studied.

References

1. Souquet PJ, Boissel JP, Bernard JP (1991) Utility of the chemotherapy in advanced and disseminated non-small cell lung cancer : Results of a meta analysis. VI Congress of IASLC, Melbourne, Australia, 10-14 November
2. Bakowski MT, Creacj JC (1983) Chemotherapy of non-small cell lung cancer. A reappraisal and a look to the future. Cancer Treat Rev 10 : 159-165
3. Splinter TAW (1990) Chemotherapy in advanced non-small cell lung cancer. Eur J Cancer Clin Oncol 26 : 1093-1099
4. Eberhardt W, Niederle N (1992) Ifosfamide in non-small cell lung cancer : a review. Sem Oncol 19-1 (suppl 1) : 40-48
5. Cullen MH, Joshi R, Chetiyawardana AD et al (1988) Mitomycine, Ifosfamide and Cisplatin in non-small cell lung cancer. Treatment good enough to compare. Br J Cancer 58 : 359-361
6. Kardamakis D, Corcoran K, Trask CWL (1990) A multidrug chemotherapy regime (MIC) in inoperable non-small cell lung cancer. J Cancer Res Clin Oncol, 116-121 - (abstr) B1 : 137-147
7. Giron CG, Ordonez A, Jalon JL et al (1987) Combination chemotherapy with Ifosfamide, Mitomycine and Cisplatin in advanced non-small cell lung cancer. Cancer Treat Resp 71 : 851-853
8. Anton-Torres A, Aranda E, Barnetto IC et al (1990) Treatment of squamous lung cancer with Mitomycine, Ifosfamide, Cisplatin (MIC 2). Ann Oncol, 1-62 - (abstr) P7 : 46
9. Klatersky J, Sculier JP, Libert P et al (1989) Cisplatin versus Cisplatin Etoposide in the treatment of advanced non-small cell lung cancer J Clin Oncol 8 : 1087-1092

Phase III randomized study of Neo-Adjuvant chemotherapy surgery in non-small cell lung cancer (NSCLC) preliminary results

A Depierre, B Milleron, Cl Chastang, B Lebeau, P Terrioux,
E Quoix, D Moro, G Miech, N Paillot, JL Breton, H Danicot,
JN Lombard, J Clavier, E Lemarie, P Jacoulet

Adjuvant treatments of non-small cell lung cancer (radiotherapy and chemotherapy) before or after surgery, have been tested in numerous trials, more particularly as regards postoperative chemotherapy. For a long time the results were disappointing, and in randomized studies none of the therapeutic regimens prescribed could improve the patient's survival. New hopes of advances in this matter were raised by Goldie and Coldman [1] whose mathematical concept recommended a systemic treatment applied as early as possible in cases with localized tumour. The advent of Platinum [2], the results obtained in metastatic tumours by some associations with Platinum and those obtained in localized tumours by chemotherapy-radiotherapy [3] have been promising. Many phase II studies have shown that surgery was feasible after 2 or 3 cycles of chemotherapy [4, 8] even thought 1 of them [9] had observed a high rate of progression after chemotherapy which prevented surgery.

In order to determine the efficacy of Neo-Adjuvant chemotherapy on survival of resectable NSCLC, we initiated a randomized phase III study in June 1991. The aim of this trial is to compare 2 therapeutic strategies : 1 induced by 2 cycles of chemotherapy before surgery and the other induced by surgery without chemotherapy. The major points of analysis will be survival and disease-free survival. Others points will be the toxicity of the chemotherapy-surgery association, the efficacy of the chemotherapy and the prognostic significance of chemotherapy response.

The study is being conducted in untreated histologically proved NSCLC. These tumors have to be resectable before Neo-Adjuvant chemotherapy. The others eligibility criteria are : stages I (except T1N0), II and IIIa ; patients must be operable (no chronic heart or hepatic disease). They must have a performance status inferior to 3, they must be 75 years old or less and have signed an informed consent. A progression during the 2 cycles of chemotherapy before surgery must not make the tumor unresectable : if this event has been initially anticipated, the patient must be considered as ineligible before the randomisation. The trial is a two-arms study. In the first group, surgery is done first immediately after the randomization. If the surgical specimen is classified as T3 or N2, additional radiotherapy is carried out after surgery. If it is classified as T1-2 or N0-1, the patient is followed up until relapse. In the second randomized group, 2 cycles of chemotherapy are performed cycles are administered immediately after surgery. As in the first group, readiotherapy

---

Service de Pneumologie, CHU St-Jacques, 25000 Besançon, France is carried out if the tumor is classified as T3 or N2 on the surgical specimen. After treatment, the minimal duration of follow up will be five years, or until progression of the disease and the death of patient. The chemotherapy used is the M.I.P. association. The schedule is as follow : Mitomycine 6 mg/m²/day 1, Ifosfamide 1 200 mg/m²/day 1-3, completed by Mesna 800 mg/m&/day 1-3 and Cisplatinum 75 mg/m²/day 1. The treatment is repeated on day 22. After surgery, the schedule of M.I.P. is the same (2 cycles with a 3 weeks interval).

From june 91 to december 92, 96 patients were included from 26 French institutions, 48 in each group. 74 of them have completed their therapy program : 36 in the group of surgery alone and 28 in the chemotherapy-surgery group. We want to analyse the faisability of the chemotherapy-surgery association. In this group, 1 patient refused treatment association after the randomisation procedure and asked to have surgery alone. One patient died from multiple arterial embolisms of legs after the second cycle of chemotherapy and before surgery. All the other patients underwent thoracotomy although 1 of them had a tumoral progression after 2 cycles of chemotherapy. Surgery was potentially curative in all these cases. Mediastinal fibrosis did not alter resecability when it was present. The time period from randomization to surgery is represent in Table 1. According to the protocol, the surgery has to take place during the seventh week and before the nineth week in the chemotherapy-surgery group. For 80 % of the patients, this timing was respected. Only 3 patients were undergone the operation during the tenth week. Toxicity observed after surgery in the first 74 patients of the 2 groups is shown in Table 2. Four patients died of iatrogenic toxicity : 3 in the surgery group and 1 in the chemotherapy-surgery group. All of them died from infectious pulmonary disease. Four patients had infectious complication in pleural cavity (3 after pneumonectomy, 1 after lobectomy). Three of them were in the chemotherapy-surgery group, and 1 in the surgery group.

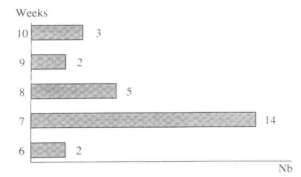

Table 1. Delay from randomization to surgery

At this point of the trial, surgery is feasible after 2 cycles of chemotherapy by M.I.P. Toxicity of surgery after M.I.P seems acceptable. The rate of tumoral progression after 2 cycles of M.I.P was low and did not prevent surgery. We feel that it is ethical to continue the study.

Table 2. Toxicity observed after surgery in the first 74 patients of the 2 groups.

Toxicity	Surgery Alone	Chemotherapy plus sugery
Pythorax	1	2
Infectious Empyema	—	1
Pneumonia	3	2
• Fatal Pneumonia	3	1
Complete Arythmia	1	—
Intra-Thoracic Hermorrage	1	1

References

1. Goldie DH, Coldmann AJ (1979) A mathematic model for relating the lung sensibility of tumors to their spontaneous mutation rate. Cancer Treat Rep 63 : 1727-1733
2. Albain K, Growley Y, Leblanc M et al (1990) Does cisplatin-based therapy improved survival in extensive non-small cell lung cancer ? Southwest oncology Group (SWOG) Studies. Proceedings ASCO, A 887
3. Dillman R, Seagren S, Propert K et al (1988) Protochemotherapy improves survival in regional non-small cell lung cancer (NSCLC). Proceedings ASCO, A 753
4. Burkes R, Ginsberg R, Shphred S et al (1988) Phase II pilot program of Neo-Adjuvant chemotherapy for stade III (T1-3, N2, M0) unresectable non-small cell lung cancer. Proc Lung Cancer 4 (abstr) n° 8.2.28
5. Gralla RJ, Kris MG, Martini M, Zaman M (1988) A Neo-Adjuvant in stage IIIA non-small cell lung cancer in patients with clinically apparent mediastinal node involvement with MVP chemotherapy (Mitomycine + Vinca Alkaloid + Cisplatin). Proc Lung Cancer 4 (abstr) n° 8.2.05
6. Curie D, Miles D, Drake J et al (1990) Mitomycine, Ifosfamide and Cisplatin in non-small cell lung cancer. Cancer Chemother Pharmacol 25 : 380-381
7. Artal A, Garrido P, Baron M et al (1990) Randomized trial comparing Ifosfamide, Cisplatin, Mitomycine v.s. Ifosfamide, Cisplatin-Vindesine in patients with advanced non-small cell lung cancer. Proceeding ASCO, A 979
8. Rosell R, Gomez-Codina J, Camps C et al (1992) Favorable outcome and anenploidy reversion following Neo-Adjuvant chemotherapy in stage IIIA non-small cell lung cancer (NSCLC). Proceeding ASCO, A 954
9. Dautzenberg B, Benichou J, Allard Ph, Lebeau B, Coetmeur D, Brechot JM, Postal M, Chastang Cl (1990) Failure of the perioperative PCV Neo-Adjuvant Polychemotherapy in resectable bronchogenic non-small cell carcinoma. Results from a randomized phase II trial. Cancer 65 : 2435-2441

Vinorelbine, 5-Fluorouracil, Folinic acid and Cisplatin in non-small cell lung cancer : Vindesine for Vinorelbine ?

H de Cremoux*, I Monnet*, N Azli**, S Voisin***, P Ruffié**, L Vergnes*, J Huet***, JC Saltiel***, JP Armand**, E Cvitkovic****, ATTIT*****

In order to extend our experience in the treatment of non-small cell lung cancer (NSCLC) [1], we undertook a phase II study maintaining Cisplatin (CDDP), continuous infusion of 5-Fluorouracil (5-FU) + Folinic acid (FA), but replacing Vindesine for Vinorelbine (VNB). Indeed the recent comparison of Vindesine (3 mg/m²/weekly) with VNB (30 mg/m²/weekly), both in association with the same dose of CDDP, has shown that VNB could be more active at least in term of response rate but could be more toxic than Vindesine [2]. The aim of the present study were to estimate the effects of this substitution (on activity and toxicity), by comparison with our previous results.

Patients and methods

Eligibility

The criteria for inclusions were : unresectable or metastatic NSCLC, age ⩽ 75 years, measurable (bi-dimentionally — CT scan) target(s), performance status ⩾ 70 %, normal bone marrow, renal and hepatic functions. A complete staging procedure was performed for each patients. For patients with limited disease, resection was not attempted before chemotherapy, if the tumor was assessed as T4, and/or if the mediastinal lymph node(s) were assessed as N 3 or N 2 (> 20 mm on CT scan, or biopsy proven).

Chemotherapy protocol

The first patients (series a) received every 3 weeks, 5-FU (600 mg/m²/day) by 24 hours continuous infusion day 1-4, Leucovorin (600 mg/m²/day) by 20 min infusion every 6 hours day 1-5, VNB (20 mg/m²/day) IV days 1 and 8 and CDDP (100 mg/m²) was given on day 1 over 30 min with hydration. For the following patients (series b), doses were decreased in view of toxicities. Dose reductions were 20 % for 5-FU (480 mg/m²/day), 33 % for Leucovorin (400 mg/m²/day) and 10 % for VNB (18 mg/m²/day).

Hematological toxicities were systematically monitored at days 10, 14 and

---

* CHI Créteil, 40 av de Verdun, 94000 France ; ** IGR La-Grange, 77175 Savigny Le Temple ; *** CH Corbeil, 59, bd Henri-Dunant, 91100 Corbeil Essonne, France ; **** Hôpital Paul Brousse, 14, av. P Vaillant Couturier, 94804 Villejuif ; ***** ATTIT, Association pour le Traitement des Tumeurs Intra-Thoracique

21. The doses were adapted on the basis of tolerance. CDDP was attenuated by 50 % if creatinine clearance was between 45 and 54 ml/mn. VNB and 5-FU were attenuated by 20 % if the neutrophil count presented grade 4 toxicity at day 10 or 14 and by 50 % in case of neutropenic fever in the previous cycle. VNB and CDDP were witheld in case of grade 2-4 neurological toxicity. Treatment was postponed for 1 week if at day 21 the white blood cells count < 4 000 leucocytes/mm^3 or < 150.000 platelets/mm^3, as in the case of unresolved mucositis.

Evaluation of response

Evaluation of response, according to Eagan's criteria, was performed either after the second cycle for stage III patients, when surgical option was reconsidered ; or after the third cycle for all other patients. In case of clinical suspicion of progressive disease or of premature discontinuation for toxicity reasons, evaluation was performed earlier.

Local therapy

After response evaluation, stage III patients underwent either exploratory surgery with radical resection intent or full dose radiotherapy.

Results

Study population

From November/90 to September/92, 92 previously untreated patients'were entered. Results are given separately for series a (n = 17) and b (n = 75). Patients characteristics are shown in Table 1.

Table 1. Characteristics of the 92 patients and chemotherapy protocol

Characteristics	Series a n = 17	Series b n = 75
Age mean (years)	56	55
range	28-70	38-68
Male (%)	94	88
Karnosky status > 70 %	100	100
Squamous (%)	59	53
Adenocarcinoma (%)	18	28
Large cell (%)	24	19
Limited (%)	59	56
VNB	20 mg/m^2 days 1 and 8	18 mg/m^2 days 1 and 8
5-FU	600 mg/m^2 day 1-4	480 mg/m^2 day 1-4
Leucovorin	600 mg/m^2 day 0-4	400 mg/m^2 day 0-4
CDDP	100 mg/m^2 day 1	idem

Table 2. ATTIT 003 and ATTIT 005 (series a and b) : main results

	ATTIT 003 (n = 53)	ATTIT 005 Series a (n = 17)	(a)	ATTIT 005 Series b (n = 75)	(b)
Activity : OR/NC/PD (%)					
Limited :	39/50/11	80/20/0	(ns)	50/40/10	(ns)
Metastatic :	25/58/17	43/42/14		30/39/30	
Mediane survival (months) :	11	11		To early	
Mediane response duration :	15	17		To early	
Mediane follow up :	31	23		12	
Toxicities*					
Neutropenia (grade III-IV) :	41	31	(ns)	24	(.05)
Stomatitis (grade III-IV) :	19	33	(.001)	10	(.01)
Neutropenic fever :	4	20	(.001)	1	(.01)
Doses Intensity**					
Vindesine :	0.92 (86)	—			
Vinorelbine :	—	10.6 (75)		10.7 (89)	
5-Fluorouracil :	703 (88)	617 (77)		576 (90)	
Cisplatin :	29.5 (89)	29.8 (89.6)		31.3 (94)	

* : Mean the percentage of complicated courses. ** : Mean the actual received doses (mg/m^2/week and % of the planned doses), taking in account the doses reductions and the delays for toxicities. a and b : mean respectively the statistical differences between series a and b, ATTIT 003 and series b

Toxicities

Toxicities, were mainly neutropenia and stomatitis, usually observed concurrently. In series a, toxicities after the first cycle were alarming (neutropenia grade 4 : 7/17 cycles - 41 %, stomatitis grade 4 : 7/17 cycles - 41 %), leading to dose reduction and delays during the treatment period (Table 2). Global toxicities for the 51 cycles of series a are shown in Table 2. Parenteral support for toxicities was indicated in 12 instances (10 patients) with 3 toxic deaths. In series b, toxicities after the first cycle were mild (neutropenia grade 4 : 9/75 cycles − 12 %, stomatitis grade 4 : 0/75 cycles − 0 %), and dose intensities were preserved. Global toxicities for the 244 cycles of series b are shown in Table 2. Only 1 neutropenic fever and no toxic death were observed in series b.

Response rate, local therapy and survival

In series a, 11/17 patients achieved objective response (OR) (65 % - 95 % CI 37 % - 89 % - complete response, n = 2), among them, 8/10 patients with limited disease achieved OR (80 %). In series b, 31/75 patients achieved OR (41 % - 95 % CI 28 % - 52 % - complete response, n = 3), among them, 21/42 patients with limited disease achieved OR (50 %). No differences for response rate were observed according to histology : squamous cell carcinoma, 10/29 (34 %) ; adenocarcinoma : 4/12 (33 %) and large cell carcinoma, 3/11 (27 %).

After restaging workup, 15 patients could have an effective resection : 9 among the 12 patients in stage IIIa (75 %), and 7 among the 28 in stage b (25 %). At time of analysis median survival time has not been reached.

Discussion

The comparison of our 2 previous pilot studies (ATTIT 002 v.s. ATTIT 003 protocol), suggested that the introduction of Leucovorin induces an increase of stomatitis (in spite of dose reduction for 5-FU) but in the other hand could improve the response duration and to confer a survival advantage mainly in patients with metastatic disease [1]. In the present study (ATTIT 005 protocol), we attempted to increase the therapeutic index of this combination, by substituting Vindesine for VNB. Although our 2 trials were consecutive phase II studies, it is licit to compare the main data of these studies. Indeed our group has done these trials over 2 years, with the same investigators, referal pattern and standards of evaluation.

This study demonstrate that, in absence of doses adjustment for 5-FU and Folinic acid, the introduction of VNB (20 mg/m^2/days 1 and 8, i.e. 40 mg/m^2/cycle) instead of Vindesine (0.8 mg/m^2/day by 24 hours by continuous infusion day 1-4, i.e. 3.2 mg/m^2/cycle) was associated with an unacceptable increase in toxicities mainly mucositis or neutropenia.

After dose reductions (for VNB, 5-FU, AF) the early results in the series b, compare favourably in toxicity (in term of neutropenia and stomatitis) and activity, with our previous data obtained with Vindesine (ATTIT 003 protocol). Those data suggest that VNB and subtle doses adjustment for 5-FU - Folinic acid have improved the therapeutic index of this regimen (Table 2). Moreover it is noteworthy that we have compared 2 drugs but also 2 schedules of administration : continuous infusion for Vindesine and bolus for VNB. Continuous infusion could confere an improvement in therapeutic index of Vindesine [3] and the best schedule for VNB has to be determined. The evaluation of the general activity of this regimen needs a longer follow up period to evaluate the response duration and the survival.

References

1. de Cremoux H, Azli N, Voisin S, Monnet I, Ruffié P, Riggi M, Vergnes L, Huet J, Saltiel JC, Cvitcovic E (1991) Cisplatin, 5-Fluorouracil + Leucovorin and Vindesine in non-small cell lung cancer : a phase II study. Proc 3rd International Congress on Neo-Adjuvant Chemotherapy, pp. 447-447
2. Le Chevalier T, Pujol JL, Douillard JY, Alberola V, Monnier A, Rivière A, Lianes P, Chomy P, Cigolari S, Berthaud P, Gottfried M, Panizo AG, Besenval M, Brisband D (1992) A European multicentre randomized study comparing Navelbine alone v.s. Navelbine-Cisplatin v.s. Vindesine-Cisplatine in 612 patients with advanced non-small cell lung cancer. Proc ASCO 11 : 963 (abstr)
3. Yap HY, Blumenschein GR, Bodev GP, Hortobagy GN et al (1981) Vindesine in the treatment of refractory breast cancer : improvement in therapeutic index with continous 5-day infusion. Cancer Treat Rep 65 : 775-779

Preoperative chemotherapy in non-small cell lung cancer (NSCLC) — A pilot study

JR Fischer, C Manegold, D Branscheid, I Vogt-Moykopf, P Drings

At the time of diagnosis, 30 % of patients with non-small cell lung cancer have a localized tumor. In these patients in tumor stage I or II, surgical resection is the treatment of choice and may result in definite cure. Locally advanced or disseminated non-small cell lung cancer in most cases is not curable at the present time. 70 % of patients are inoperable at the time of diagnosis. Patients in stage IIIA are considered operable in selected cases, stage IIIB in most cases is considered inoperable. Thus, in the majority of cases surgical treatment is not possible due to the local extend of tumor spread. Survival of patients in advanced stage without treatment is in the range of 4 to 6 months. Surgery of selected patients or radiation therapy in these cases results in a median survival of 10 to 18 months. Because 30 to 50 % of patients with non-small cell lung cancer respond to chemotherapy, however, we tested whether in patients with primarily inoperable, locally advanced tumor chemotherapy would induce sufficient tumor regression to allow for subsequent surgery with curative intent.

Patients and treatment

Patients

All patients had histologically confirmed NSCLC. Performance status of all patients was good (ECOG performance status 0-II). All patients had a tumor stage IIIA or IIIB. Median age was 54 years.

Chemotherapy

At least 2 cycles of CT have been given consisting of Cisplatinum (100 mg/m^2) and Vindesine (3 mg/m^2), Ifosfamide (10 g/m^2) and VP-16 (360 mg/m^2), or a combination of Cisplatinum (75 mg/m^2), Ifosfamide (6 g/m^2), VP-16 (360 mg/m^2). Chemotherapy was repeated every 4 weeks. In part of the pts treated with cisplatinum, ifosfamide and VP-16, chemotherapy was repeated every 3 weeks by including an acceleration of neutrophil recovery with the use of hematopoetic growth factors.

Thoraxklinik der LVA Baden, Amalienstraße 5, 6900 Heidelberg-Rohrbach, Germany

Surgery

In patients considered operable after chemotherapy the tumor was resected within 4-6 weeks after the last cycle of cytotoxic treatment.

Results

So far 52 patients (histologically confirmed NSCLC, tumor stage III, ECOG performance status 0-II and median age 54 years) have been included (Table 1). At least 2 cycles of CT have been given consisting of Cisplatinum (100 mg/m^2) and Vindesine (3 mg/m^2), Ifosfamide (10 g/m^2) and VP-16 (360 g/m^2), or a combination of Cisplatinum (75 mg/m^2), Ifosfamide (6 g/m^2), VP-16 (360 mg/m^2) (Table 2). At present 48 patients are evaluable for CT. Twenty-five patients responded to CT (16 PR, 9 MR), 23 patients did not respond (11 NC, 12 PD) (Table 3). In 28 patients tumor was resected within 4-6 weeks after CT (14 in PR, 8 in MR, 6 in NC) (Table 4). In 16 patients complete resection could be achieved. Twenty patients are evaluable for 2 years survival. Of these 20 patients 9 responded to CT (4 PR, 5 MR). In 12 patients tumor was resected. The 9 patients with response to CT and consecutive resection are alive 45+, 44+, 39, 27+, 17, 15, 15, 8, 4 months after diagnosis. The 11 pts without response to CT, including 3 pts with resection are alive 24, *24*, 23+, 13, 9, 7, 7, 6, 4, *4*, 4 months after diagnosis (Table 5). Our results indicate improved survival after response to chemotherapy followed by tumor resection. Furthermore, preliminary data indicate, that accelerated chemotherapy with hematopoetic growth factors may increase response rates (not shown).

Discussion

A variety of phase II studies have investigated the effect of preoperative chemotherapy in locally advanced NSCLC. In several investigations, preoperative chemotherapy was combined to preoperative radiotherapy. Most investigators concentrated on stages IIIA and IIIB. Occasionally, stage I and II patients were also included in these trials. Several cooperative groups now try to initiate phase III trials. In these projects, again, the main focus is on stage III patients. A French study seems to look mainly on preoperative chemotherapy in patients in stage II. The whole variety of these studies reflects the complex problems and questions with regard to the search for the best treatment of these patients. Should we really include stages, that may be operated initially with curative intent ? In our institution, so far only patients regarded inoperable were included in this feasibility study. What is the best form of chemotherapy ? Some reports demonstrate an objective response rate of over 70 % with a high rate of complete remissions [1]. On the other hand, a meta-analysis of results of chemotherapy in NSCLC over the last 15 years reported an objective response rate of 30 to 40 % [2]. Do chances exist, to improve

Table 1. Characteristics of patients

NSCLC histologically confirmed
Stage III A/B
ECOG 0-II
median age 54

Table 2. Chemotherapy : at least 2 cycles

Cisplatinum 100 mg/m^2
Vindesine 3 mg/m^2

Ifosfamide 10 g/m^2
Etoposide 360mg/m^2

Cisplatinum 75 mg/m^2
Ifosfamide 6 g/m^2
Etoposide 360 mg/m^2

Accelerated chemotherapy including G-CSF

Table 3. 48 patients evaluable for chemotherapy

25 responders : 16 PR, 9 MR
23 non responders : 11 NC, 12 PD

Table 4. Tumor resection 4-6 weeks after CT

28 pts	14 in PR
	8 in MR
	6 in NC

Table 5. 20 patients are evaluable for 2 years survival

9 responders : 4 PR, 5 MR	
12 resections : 4 in PR, 5 in MR, 3 in NC	
9 responders to CT with OP alive	45+, 44+, 39, 27+, 17, 15, 15, 8, 4 mts after diagnosis
1 non responders alive	24, *24*, 23+, 13, 9, 7, 7, 6, 4, 4, 4 mts after diagnosis
(including 3 underlined pts undergoing OP after CT)	

these response rates ? Preliminary results from our investigation indicate, that by accelerated chemotherapy including hematopoetic growth factors the rate of partial responses may be increased. Furthermore, local response rates may be increased by the addition of preoperative radiotherapy. Taken together, our preliminary results indicate, that a combined treatment modality including preoperative chemotherapy, surgery and postoperative radiation may improve survival in patients with locally advanced NSCLC. For further evaluation of combined treatment, there is now an urgent need to overcome the obstacles of a multidisciplinary as well as multicenter cooperation and to carry out well conducted randomized trials.

References

1. Strauss G, Langer M, Elias A, Skarin A, Sugarbaker D (1992) Multimodality treatment of Stage IIIA non-small cell lung carcinoma : A cricical Review of the Literature and Strategies for Future Research. J Clin Oncol 10 : 829-838
2. Donnadieu N, Paesmans M, Sculier J.P (1991) Chemotherapy of non-small cell lung cancer according to desease extent : a meta-analysis of the literature. Lung Cancer 7 : 243-252

Neo-Adjuvant Cisplatin and Etoposide for stage IIIA (clinical N2) non-small cell lung cancer

S Darwish, V Minotti, R Rossetti, G Ciccarese, L Crinò,
P Fiaschini, U Mercati, E Maranzano, P Latini, M Tonato

Prognosis for regionally advanced non-small cell lung cancer (NSCLC) patients is poor. Treatment with either surgery or radiation has been unsatisfactory and 5 years survival rates of less than 10 % are reported for these patients [1]. In an attempt to increase the complete resection and survival rates in stage IIIA disease, several pilot studies have explored multiple therapeutic modalities including Neo-Adjuvant chemotherapy or concomitant chemotherapy and radiotherapy [2, 3, 4].

In 1988 we began a phase II trial with DDP/VP-16 in patients with clinically apparent mediastinal node involvement (clinical N2) to assess the feasibility and efficacy of Neo-Adjuvant chemotherapy.

Patients and methods

From June 1988 to July 1991, 46 untreated patients with stage IIIA NSCLC with clinical evidence of mediastinal node involvement (N2) at chest X-rays or at computed tomography (ipsilateral lymph nodes $\geqslant$ 2 cm) or with evidence of widened carina or main bronchus compression by the node were included in the study. Inclusion criteria were : age $\leqslant$ 70, a performance status of 0-2 (ECOG), normal cardiac, renal and pulmonary functions. All patients received 2 or 3 cycles of chemotherapy consisting of Cisplatin 120 mg/m^2 on day 1 and Etoposide 100 mg/m^2 on days 1-3. The cycle was repeated every 21 days.

Toxicity was assessed by the WHO scale. Response to treatment was evaluated by standard criteria. Only patients achieving major response (CR or PR) were surgically explored in an attempt to resect all measurable disease and perform mediastinal lymph node dissection.

Results

Patient characteristics are shown in Table 1. Forty-five patients were evaluable for response : 1 patient died from an undetermined cause after the first cycle. As shown in Table 2, the overall major response rate to Neo-Adjuvant chemotherapy was 82 %. Three patients (7 %) achieved complete response and 34 (75 %) had a partial response. Toxic effects were primarily hemotologic.

Thirty-five patients (2/3 CR, 31/34 PR and 2/5 SD) underwent surgical exploration ; 8 were considered non-surgical candidates : 3 had progressive dis-

Divisions of Medical Oncology, Surgery, Radiotherapy, Perugia Hospital, 06122 Perugia, Italy

Table 1. Patient characteristics

No. of patients	46
Males/Females	39/7
Median age (range)	58 (45-70)
HISTOLOGY	
epidermoid ca	34
adenocarcinoma	10
large cell	1
large cell/squamous	1
STAGE	
T1	12
T2	20
T3	14
N2 Involvement by :	
chest X-ray	30
bronchoscopy	11
lymph node $\geq$ 2 cm on CT scan	40

Table 2. Treatment results

	Chemotherapy response				
	Complete response	Partial response	Stable	Prog.	Total
Completed therapy	3	34	5	3	45
Surgically explored	2	31	2	0	35
Complete resection	2	25	1	0	28
Partial resection	0	4	1	0	5
Unresectable	0	2	0	0	2
No tumor in resected spec.	2	2	0	0	4

Table 3. Side effects (WHO classification)

Toxicity		No.	(%)
Anemia	(1-2)	26	(57)
	(3-4)	5	(11)
Leucopenia	(1-2)	20	(43)
	(4)	5	(11)
Anaphylaxis		1	(2)
Nausea/vomiting	(1-2)	13	(28)
Blood creatinine	(1)	7	(15)
Ototoxicity		4	(9)

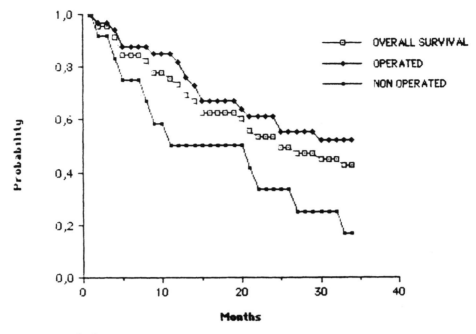

Fig. 1. Survival curves

ease, 2 had pulmonary complications following Neo-Adjuvant chemotherapy, and 3 had stable disease.

Of the 35 patients who underwent surgical exploration a resection was possible in 33 patients (73 % of evaluable patients) without technical difficulties. A complete resection was achieved in 28 patients (62 % of all evaluable patients and 80 % of surgically explored patients). In 4 patients (2 CR, 2 PR) no tumor was found in the biopsy specimen.

The median survival for all 46 patients was 24.5 months with a 2 years survival rate of 53 % (Fig. 1). Nine of the 28 patients who underwent complete resection relapsed with a median time to recurrence of 12 months (range 8-28). There were 5 loco-regional relapses and 4 distant metastases (1 brain, 2 liver, 1 heart). To date 26 patients have died. Three deaths were considered surgery-related (1 ventricular fibrillation, 1 bronchus-pleural fistula, 1 enteric hemorrhage).

Discussion

This pilot trial with Neo-Adjuvant chemotherapy in a selected and homogeneous group of patients with regionally advanced NSCLC shows that the DDP/VP-16 regimen is very active with an overall objective response of 82 % including a 7 % CR rate. This high activity may be partially explained by the better performance status and lower tumor burden compared to patients with metastatic NSCLC.

Toxicity consisted primarily of moderate myelosuppression and did not result in severe morbidity. 62 % of patients were ultimately rendered completely disease-free. It is note-worthy that 4 patients had pathologically negative biopsy specimens. The median survival of 24.5 months for all 46 patients was better than that usually reported for patients with regionally advanced NSCLC. The apparently improved survival may be partially explained by patient selection. None of our patients underwent mediastinoscopy. It is possible, therefore, that some of our patients had mediastinal reactive nodes.

Despite some differences, our results are consistent with those reported by Gralla et al [4]. These authors treated 73 patients with clinically staged N2 with 2-3 cycles of MVP induction chemotherapy. Of these patients, 58 went to thoractomy and 44 were completely resected. After a 5 years follow-up, the authors reported a 24 % survival in completely resected patients.

Although further follow-up is required, the resection and survival rates observed in this study justify randomized trials to assess the role of Neo-Adjuvant chemotherapy.

References

1. Burt ME, Pomerantz AH, Bains MS et al (1987) Results of surgical treatment of stage III lung cancer invading the mediastinum. Clin Chest Med 67 : 987-1000
2. Vokes EE, Bitran JD, Hoffman PC et al (1989) Neo-Adjuvant Vindesina, Etoposide and Csplatin for locally advanced non-small cell lung cancer. Chest 96 : 110-113
3. Pujol Jl, Ross JF, Le Chevalier T et al (1990) Phase II pilot study of Neo-Adjuvant ifosfamide, Cisplatin and Etoposide in locally advanced non-small cell lung cancer. Eur J Cancer 26 : 798-801
4. Gralla RJ, Kris MG, Martini N et al (1991) Neoadjuvant chemotherapy in NSCLC : Long term follow-up in a 73 patients trial with IIIA staging and clinically apparent mediastinal node involvement. Lung Cancer 7 (abstr) : 134

Concomitant chemoradiotherapy with Cisplatin dose escalation as palliative therapy for advanced malignancies of the chest

C Lee Drinkard, J Daniel Haraf, C Philip Hoffman, M Harvey Golomb, K Mark Ferguson, J Nicholas Vogelzang, E Everett Vokes

The concept of concomitant chemoradiotherapy

The simultaneous or concomitant administration of a chemotherapeutic agent with radiation therapy has been employed as a unique treatment modality in a number of locally advanced malignancies including head and neck cancer, limited stage small cell lung cancer, and squamous cell carcinoma of the anus, as well as in esophageal carcinoma. Concomitant chemoradiotherapy is aimed at improving local control by overcoming radioresistance, and at eradicating distant micrometastasis to decrease systemic failure rates [1].

Most patients with non-small cell lung cancer present with loco-regionally advanced disease and presumed microscopic dissemination or clinically overt metastases [2]. Treatment of non-small cell lung cancer as well as other intrathoracic malignancies centers around local and systemic tumor control. Local tumor control is obtained by either surgery or radiotherapy. Systemic tumor control with traditional chemotherapy is frequently not achieved using current regimens.

However, 2 trials of Neo-Adjuvant chemotherapy prior to radiation therapy in locally non-small cell lung cancer have shown a survival benefit when compared with radiotherapy alone. In addition, response rates to chemotherapy in this setting were higher than what is usually seen in chemotherapy for metastatic disease [3, 4, 5].

In addition, Schaake-Konig et al randomized patients with locally advanced non-small lung cancer to receive either radiotherapy or radiotherapy combined with 3 different dose schedules of Cisplatin [6]. While local tumor control was improved in this study, distant failure rates were the same regardless of treatment. A definite survival benefit was seen on the treatment arm that received concomitant chemoradiotherapy with daily Cisplatin.

Chemotherapy may enhance the effect of radiation in the treatment of locally advanced non-small cell lung cancer and thereby improve local tumor control. The most affective regimen of concomitant chemoradiotherapy that provides for both radiation enhancement to improve local control and is systemically effective has not been identified.

University of Chicago, IL Chicago, USA

Concomitant chemoradiotherapy at the University of Chicago

At the University of Chicago, concomitant chemoradiotherapy has been investigated in esophageal, head and neck, and non-small cell lung cancers. The underlying themes in all of these regimens are the principles of radiation enhancement, spatial cooperation, and nonoverlapping toxicity as outlined in section 1.3.1. In this section we will describe the rationale and development of two concomitant chemoradiotherapy regimens and their incorporation into a proposed multimodality program for esophageal cancer.

Interferon and Cistaplin

Interferon has been demonstrated to be a radiosensitizer when studying several cell lines including mouse 3T3 cells [7], bronchogenic carcinoma cells [8], and cervical carcinoma cells (HeLa cells) [9]. The exact mechanism by which radiosensitization occurs is unknown. One possible mechanism is blockage of the cell cycle at the G2-M phase [10].

Phase I trials of Interferon with radiotherapy by Torrisi [11] established a maximum tolerated dose range of 2-5 Mu/m^2 administered 3 or 5 times a week. Toxicities included enhancement of radiation dermatitis, esophagitis, and « flu-like » symptoms.

Holsti et al [12] treated 12 patients with limited stage small cell carcinoma of the lung with 2 schedules of Interferon and radiotherapy. Response rate overall was 100 %, with a complete response rate of 50 % suggesting radiation enhancement by the Interferon.

Cisplatin is a chemotherapeutic agent with a very broad spectrum of antitumor activity. It has also been found *in vitro* and in animal models to be a radiation sensitizer. The precise mechanisms of radiation enhancement are unknown but possible mechanisms include the inhibition of radiation induced sublethal DNA damage as well as killing of radioresistant hypoxic cells by Cisplatin [13].

In a phase I study, at the University of Chicago we evaluated the combination of Interferon-α-2A and Cisplatin given with concomitant twice daily (hyperfractionated) radiation therapy. The recommended dose of Interferon was 5 million U/m^2 daily for 5 days. The recommended dose of Cisplatin was 50 mg/m^2 on day 1. Significant activity was found in non-small cell lung cancer both inside and outside of the radiated field [14].

Cisplatin, 5-FU, Hydroxyurea and radiotherapy

5-Fluorouracil is a fluorinated Pyrimidine which *in vivo* is ultimately converted to Fluorodeoxyuridine monophosphate (FdUMP). FdUMP is a potent inhibitor of thymidylate synthase and by this mechanism inhibits DNA synthesis. The precise cellular mechanism by which 5-FU and radiotherapy interact is unknown. One theory includes inhibition of DNA repair of radiation-induced DNA damage, but experimental evidence is lacking [15].

Hydroxyurea is a potent inhibitor of ribonucleotide reductase, and thereby depletes pools of deoxyribonucleotides, thus modulating the action of purine and pyrimidine antimetabolites. Hydroxyurea also inhibits DNA repair and enhances the DNA damaging effects of radiotherapy [21]. Studies in mouse L1210 leukemia show a synergistic effect of 5-FU and Hydroxyurea [16].

At the University of Chicago, pilot studies of 5-FU, Cisplatin, Hydroxyurea and radiotherapy in head and neck cancer have shown high overall response rates in previously untreated as well as pretreated patients (92 % and 60 % respectively) [17].

We have also explored the use of 5FU, Hydroxyurea, Leucovorin and radiotherapy in locally advanced non-small cell lung cancer. Significant responses were seen in non-small cell lung cancer. In 23 patients entered there was a 57 % partial response rate and a 4 % complete response rate [18]. Median survival was 12 months with median time to tumor progression 6 months. There was a 52 % systemic failure pattern, a 13 % failure rate inside of the radiated field, while 4 % of patients failed in both locations. Dose limiting toxicities were mucositis, dermatitis, and hand-foot syndrome.

Concomitant chemoradiotherapy for chest malignancies

We are currently completing a phase I dose escalating study that combines both concomitant chemoradiotherapy regimens together in the treatment of chest malignancies [19]. The design employs a split course of radiotherapy given over 6 weeks with a 1 week break in the fourth week of treatment. During the first week of treatment radiotherapy is administered concomitantly with Interferon (5×10^6 Units/m²/day for 5 days) and escalating doses of Cisplatin. During the second week radiotherapy is administered concomitantly with 5-FU (800 mg/m²/d for 5 days continuous infusion), Hydroxyurea (1.000 mg/day for 5 days), and escalating doses of Cisplatin. All radiotherapy is administered in once daily fractions of 200cGy. During the third week radiotherapy is given alone. The above regimen is repeated during the fifth, sixth, and seventh weeks of treatment.

Toxicities observed have been primarily mucositis, with esophagitis and dysphagia, as well as myelosuppression. G-CSF was added between weeks of treatment and during the first and fifth week of treatment to counteract the myelosuppression seen with high-doses of Cisplatin. Interferon dosage was reduced to 2.5×10^6 U/m²/d x 5 days during weeks 1 and 5 in order to ameliorate renal toxicity. With the addition of G-CSF, we have been able to escalate the dose of Cisplatin to 100 mg/m² during both weeks of treatment. This dose is currently the maximum tolerated dose of Cisplatin.

In an attempt to reduce the incidence of severe esophagitis and to shorten treatment duration, we incorporated hyperfractionated radiotherapy (150 cGy Bid) with a slightly reduced dose of 5-FU (600 mg/m²/day × 5 days) into a final dose level. Our experience in 4 patients treated to date is that esophagitis is less severe during therapy but becomes severe in the weeks following completion of the regimen. Thrombocytopenia has become the dose limiting toxicity of this regimen.

References

1. Vokes EE, Weichselbaum RR (1990) Concomitant chemoradiotherapy : rationale and clinical experience in patients with solid tumors. J Clin Oncol 8 : 5 911-34
2. Haraf DJ, Devine S, Ihde DC, and Vokes EE (1992) The evolving role of systemic therapy in carcinoma of the lung. Sem Oncol 19 (suppl 11) : 72-87
3. Dillman RO, Seagren SL, Propert K et al (1990) A randomized trial of induction chemotherapy plus high-dose radiation versus radiation alone in stage III non-small cell lung cancer. N Engl J Med 323 : 940-945
4. Le Chevalier T, Arriagada R, Quoix E et al (1991) Radiotherapy alone versus combined chemotherapy and radiotherapy in nonresectable non-small cell lung cancer : First analysis of a randomized trial in 353 patients. J Natl Cancer Inst 83 : 417-423
5. Le Chevalier T, Arriagada R, Tarayre M et al. (1992) Significant effect of Adjuvant chemotherapy on survival in locally advanced non-small cell lung carcinoma. J Natl Cancer Inst 84 : 58
6. Schaake-Konig C, van den Bogaert W, Dalesio O et al (1992) Effects of concomitant Cisplatin and radiotherapy on inoperable non-small-cell lung cancer. N Engl J Med 326 : 524-530
7. Dritschillo A, Mossman K et al (1982) Potentiation of radiation injury by Interferon. Am J Clin Oncol 5 : 79-82
8. Gould MN, Kakria RC, Olson S, Bordon EC (1984) Radiosensitization of human bronchogenic carcinoma cells by Interferon-β. J Interferon Res 4 : 123-128
9. Namba M, Yamamoto S et al (1984) In vitro and in vivo studies on potentiation of cytotoxic effects of anticancer drugs or cobalt 60 γ-ray by Interferon on human neoplastic cells. Cancer 54 : 2262-2267
10. Chang AYC, Keng PC (1987) Potentiation of radiation cytotoxicty by recombinant Interferons, or phenomenon associated with increased blockage at the G2-M phase of the cell cycle. Cancer Res 47 : 4338-4341
11. Torristi J, Berg C et al (1986) The combined use of interferon and radiotherapy in cancer management. Sem Oncol 13 (suppl 2) : 78-83
12. Holsti LR, Mattson K et al (1987) Enhancement of radiation effects by α-Interferon in the treatment of small cell carcinoma of the lung. Int J Radiat Oncol Biol Phys 13 : 1161-1166
13. Schilsky RL Biochemical pharmacology of chemotherapeutic drugs used as radiation enhancers. Sem Oncol 19, 4 (suppl 11) : 2-7
14. Vokes EE, Haraf DJ, Hoffman PC (1993) Escalating doses of Interferon-α-2A with Cisplatin and concomitant radiotherapy : a phase I study. Lung Cancer (in press)
15. Byfield JE, Calbro-Jones P, Klisak I et al (1982) Pharmacologic requirements for obtaining sensitization of human tumor cells in vitro to combined 5-Fuorouracil 2 or 2 ftorafur and x-rays. Int J Radiat Oncol Biol Phys 8 : 1923-1933
16. Moran RG, Danberg PV, and Heidelberger C (1982) Therapeutic response of leukemic mice treated with Fluorouracil pyrimidines and inhibitors of Deoxyuridylate synthesis. Biochem Pharmacol 31 : 2929-2935
17. Vokes EE, Haraf DJ, Weichselbaum RR et al (1992) Prospectives on combination chemotherapy with concomitant radiotherapy for poor prognosis head and neck cancer. Sem Oncol 19, 4 (suppl 11) : 47-56

18. Vokes EE, Vijayakumar S, Hoffman PC et al (1990) 5-Fluorouracil with oral Leucovorin and Hydroxyurea and concomitant radiotherapy for stage III non-small cell lung cancer. Cancer 66 : 437-442
19. Hoffman P, Drinkard L, Haraf H et al (1993) Concomitant chemoradiotherapy with Cisplatin dose escalation in advanced chest malignancies : A phase I study. Proc Am Soc Clin Oncol (abstract, in press)

Concomitant chemoradiotherapy for inoperable non-small cell carcinoma of the lung : results of continuous infusion Cisplatin in 85 patients

F Reboul, P Vincent, B Chauvet, Y Brewer, C Felix Faure, M Taulelle

Despite the fact that radiation therapy is widely accepted as the standard treatment of locally advanced and/or inoperable non-small cell carcinoma of the lung, long term results are disappointing. Two-year survival after radiation therapy alone remains around 15 % due to early distant metastasis and poor local control. Previous experimental and clinical data support the concept of radiosensitization by Cisplatin while continuous infusion provides better tolerance and possibly enhanced interactions. On the other hand, Cisplatin is the most effective drug and is an essential component of chemotherapy regimens in non-small cell carcinoma of the lung. It may have an impact on subclinical dissemination at a dose level of 60-100 mg/sqm. Based on these data, we initiated a pilot study in which concomitant radiation therapy and high-dose continuous infusion Cisplatin were evaluated in terms of tolerance, local control and survival.

Material and methods

From July 1989 to july 1991, 110 consecutive randomly selected, previously untreated patients with inoperable biopsy-proven non-small cell carcinoma of the lung were entered into this pilot study. There were 18 ineligible patients because of metastasis at initial work-up (10), unknown histology (4) or initial surgery (4). Seven patients were excluded from study because early death prior to chemotherapy (5) or protocol violation (2). Thus, 85 patients werer fully evaluable for response, toxicity and survival. Median age was 66 years (35-81) and sex ratio (M/F) 78/7. Performance status according to the WHO classification was 0 (18.8 %), 1 (76,5 %), and 2 (4.7 %).
Histologic type was squamous cell carcinoma in 77.7 %, adenocarcinoma in 12.9 % and undifferentiated large cell carcinoma in 9.4 %. Histologic grade was well differentiated in 24.7 %, moderately differentiated in 16.5 %, poorly differentiated in 38.8 % and unknown in 20 %. Predominant anatomic sites of the tumor were upper lobe in 61.2 % and lower lobe in 21.2 %. Clinical staging analysis showed a predominance of T2 (33.0 %) and T3 (60.0 %), N1 (12.9 %) and N2 (57.7 %) with 14.1 % stage I/II, 75.3 % stage IIIA and 10.6 % stage IIIB. Thoracic irradiation was delivered to the entire mediastinum at a dose of 40 grays in 20 fractions over 4 weeks by A-P fields with

---

Lung Cancer Treatment Unit, Clinique Sainte-Catherine, 84082 Avignon, France

individualized cerrobend blocks. After a 2 weeks rest period, an additional boost of 30 grays in 15 fractions over 3 weeks was delivered to the original tumor volume with oblique fields sparing the spinal cord with CT scan computerized dosimetry. Continuous infusion Cisplatin was delivered at a constant rate of 20 mg/sqm/24 hours for 5 days (120 hours) during the second week of each radiation cycle for a total dose of 200 mg/sqm per patient. No prophylactic cranial irradiation or maintenance chemotherapy was added after this treatment. Radical surgery became feasible after the first cycle of treatment in 11 patients (13 %).

Results

Compliance was acceptable with 90.6 % of patients receiving the first cycle at full dose of radiation and Cisplatin. Rest period varied between 2 weeks (62.5 %) and 3 weeks (23.6 %). During the second cycle of treatment, radiation was delivered at full dose in 84.7 % and Cisplatin in 65.3 %. Acute toxicity was mainly hematologic (39.8 %) and gastro-intestinal (nausea and vomiting 20.5 %, esophagitis 8.4 %) but there were only 3.6 % grade 3-4 complications. Late pulmonary fibrosis (grade 3-4) occurred in 5.2 % of patients. Two treatment-related deaths occured (hemoptysis, fibrosis). Response was evaluated with CT-scan and fiberoptic bronchoscopy with biopsy at the initial tumor site in all patients 6 weeks following completion of treatment.

Complete response (CR) was observed in 65.9 % with an additional 15.8 % major response. At the time of analysis, local relapse had occured in 15.3 %, distant metastasis in 28.2 % or both in 7.1 %. With a median follow-up of 27 months (16-39), actuarial survival at 1, 2 and 3 years are 48.2 %, 27.5 % and 25 % respectively with a median survival of 11.4 months. No local relapse or distant metastasis were recorded after 3 years. Age, gender, histologic type and grade, and clinical stage were not significant prognostic factors. 2 factors significantly influenced survival at two years : complete response (42.1 % p = .0001) and surgery (75.8 % p = .0013).

Conclusions

High-dose radiation therapy with concomitant continuous infusion Cisplatin is well tolerated with a low incidence of acute and late toxicity. This regimen provides a high complete response rate (65.9 %) and good local control with substantial improvement of 2 years survival (27.5 %) as compared to standard radiation alone. This improvement is particularly encouraging in the CR group (42.1 %) and for patients that become operable after the first course of treatment (75.8 %). These results are comparable to other studies with radiation and concomitant Cisplatin given on different schedules. However, if local control appears substantially improved by this approach, the incidence of distant relapses remains significant during the first 2 years. Further studies with concomitant chemoradiotherapy should focus on incorporating a second drug with activity against subclinical disseminated disease.

Late results of Neo-Adjuvant chemoradiotherapy for primary inoperable non-small cell lung cancer

JL Rebischung, JM Vannetzel, P Dartevelle

Locally advanced non-small cell lung cancer keep always a very poor prognosis, because the high risk of metastatic progression despite chemotherapy, and the difficulty to obtain a local control without surgery. Recently, the interaction between 5-FU, Cisplatin and thoracic irradiation led to an increase of clinical response rates. Therefore we conduct a Phase II study of Neo-Adjuvant cyclic concomitant chemoradiotherapy (CCCR) which final results are here reported.

Patients and methods

From 1988 to 1990, 73 consecutive patients, median age 58 years, with histological proof of NSCLC, have been included after initial evaluation detailed in Table 1. Thirty-six Stage A and 37 Stage IIIB were treated with Vindesine 3 mg/m^2 d1, 5-FU 600 mg/m^2 d1-4 by continuous infusion, Cisplatin 20 mg/m^2 d1-4 immediately after irradiation delivering 2.5 Gy on the tumor mass, mediastinal lymph nodes, supra-clavicular area, each 3 three weeks (d1 = d21).

Table 1. Inclusion cirterias

Respiratory insuffisency	22
Mediastinal T4	13
N3 involvement	9
Pancoast-Tobias	2
Pleural effusion	2
Tracheal extension	3
Vena cava syndrom	4
Recurrent paresia	3
Left pulm. artery obs.	2
Histological N2	13

Evaluation was performed after 4 cycles according to OMS criteria (40 Gy). Responders were assigned to surgery within 1 month after CCCR, if functionnal parameters allowed it, followed-up after radical resection, or treated with 2 post-operative cycles of CCCR after palliative surgery.

Definitively inoperable patients received two other cycles of chemoradiotherapy (60 Gy).

Response rates, survival, pattern of failures, toxicities and histological results have been analysed.

J Sauvaget and the GEARC

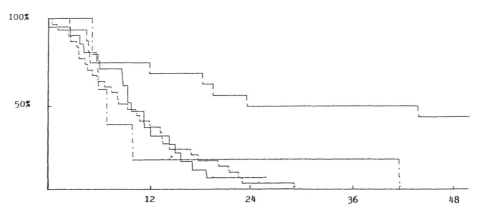

Fig. 1. Actuartial survival

Results

Because 4 early deaths (1 IIIA, 3 IIIB) by fatal hemoptysis, acute migration, infarction under 5-FU, tumor necrosis, 69 patients are evaluable with 54 objective reponses (78 %), 11 stabilisations and 4 progressions.

Twenty-four patients have been evaluated surgically, 1 by mediastinoscopy only, 2 by thoracotomies and 21 resected with 10 lobectomies, 1 bilobectomy, 10 pneumonectomies.

One initial T1, 6 T3 and 1 T4 were sterilized ; among 13 histological N2 at presentation, 9 were negative ; finally 7 patients (33 %) were pT0N0.

Forty-eight non resected patients received 6 cycles of CCCR.

With a median follow-up of 2.5 years, 63 patients died ; 18 of non tumoral causes within 11 of the non resected group.

Forty-five relapses have been registred ; 20 local, 3 local and metastatic and 13 metastatic in the non-resected group (48 p.) versus 2 local and 7 metastatic in the resected group (21 p.).

Median survival of non-resected patients is 9.5 months with 43 % alive at 1 year, 18 % at 18 months, versus 20 months for the resected group with 62 % at 1 year, 57 % at 18 months.

Toxicities

We noted 6 toxic deaths, 1 infarction under 5-FU, 1 acute tumor necrosis after 1 cycle, 1 sepsis after 4 cycles without aplasy and 3 postoperative deaths (2 ADRS, 1 rythmic disorder).

Other toxicities were acceptable ; only 1 cycle was delayed ; **90 % for Stage IIIA and 77 % for Stage IIIB** of the planified doses of chemotherapy were delivered.

Conclusion

CCCR is a feasible Neo-Adjuvant approach of locally advanced NSCLC.

Survival of definitively inoperable patients is similar to these obtained with conventional treatment.

Surgery after CCCR, specially for Stage IIIA, confirmed a complete tumor control in 33 % of the resected patients, and led to a significant increase of survival by reduction of local recurrences and delay to metastatic progression.

Gastro-intestinal tumors

Conservative treatment of esophagus cancer concomitant chemoradiotherapy treatment. First results of a 143 patients serial[1]

JH Jacob, A Roussel, JM Ollivier, JPh Izard, JC Vernhes

Since the first publication in 1981 from the Wayne State University by Steiger and Franklin [1], the concomitant radio-chemotherapy has been used by many teams in the world for the treatment of œsophageal cancer.

Recently, 2 randomized North American trials have demonstrated the advantages of the combined modality in comparison with radiotherapy alone [2]. But the benefice is obtained with an increased toxicity.

To decrease this toxicity, « split-course » radiotherapy with concomitant chemotherapy was adopted in our institution since 1987.

Characteristics of patients

- patients : 137 men, 6 women, mean age 63
- histology :
    epidermoïd : 124
    undifferentiated : 12
    adenocarcinoma : 4
    anaplastic : 1
    unprecised : 2
- location :
    middle third : 56 %
    lower third : 28 %
    upper third : 16 %
- TNM staging (UICC 1978)
    stade I : 24 %
    stade II : 36 %
    stade III : 30 %
    stade IV : 9 %

[1] From January 1987 to December 1991, 143 patients with cancer of esophagus have been treated by concomitant chemoradiotherapy in our institution.

Centre François-Baclesse, 14021 Caen Cedex, France

Characteristics of the treatment

Radiotherapy

Megavoltage radiation therapy was used with the modality of the « split-course » in 2 courses of 5 daily fractional dose of 3,70 Gy. Two weeks without treatment separate the 2 courses.

The radiation field extented at least 5 cm above and below the tumor. The supra-clavicular fossa and coeliac region was required for respectively upper third and lower third of the esophagus.

Multi field techniques were used to limit the total dose to normal structures. All the fields were treated daily.

Chemotherapy

It was delivered at the same time as radiotherapy. Fluorouracil (1.000 mg/m^2/jour) was administred as a continous intra-veinous infusion for the day 2, 3, 4 of each radiotherapy course.

Cisplatin 100 mg/m^2 was given on the first day of each courses or delivered on the first 4 days (25 mg/m^2/j) in patients with hypertension, cirrhosis or with heart failure treatment.

For 25 patients with too high level of creatinenia or with a deafness, Mitomycine was used instead of Cisplatine with the dose of 10 mg/m^2 during the first course of radiotherapy.

Results

Toxicity

The toxicity has been gastro-intestinal, hematologic, renal and neurologic. The gastro-intestinal toxicity, the most frequent, included stomatitis, oesophagitis, diarrhea, emesis. It has been always mild or moderate, and never led to discontinue the course of treatment.

The severe toxicities grade III or IV have been hematologic (10 cases) and renal (1 case). They led to discontinue the treatment for 10 patients.

One case of lethal toxicity has been observed under administration of 5-FU and Cisplatinum preceded by a coma without neurologic localisation symptoms.

Local response

It has been evaluated 1 month after the later course of chemoradiotherapy on improvement of swallow, barium œsophagography and endoscopy.

If normalisation of the œsophageal mucosa at endoscopy was obtained, the response was estimated as complete.

The total response local rate was estimated at 68 % with 55 % of complete response.

Survival

The global survival course with the Kaplan and Meier method estimates the survival rate at 1 year and 2 years respectively at 60 % and 30 % ; the median survival at 15 months.

Three major pronostic factors influence the survival with a significant statistical difference :
- the staging TNM
- the weight loss
- the local response

Conclusions

- The modality of split course in this combined chemoradiotherapy schedule does not lead to a loss of efficiency in local response rate and in survival.
- With concomitant chemotherapy, the « split-course » radiotherapy can obtain a benefit in confort treatment with a shorter time of hospital stay and less severe mucosal toxicity than a classical modality.
- But only a randomized trial with a comparison between radiotherapy split course and classical radiotherapy will be able to give a response at the question of optimal schedule.
- The results with the limited lesions classified stade I, suggest that concomitant chemoradiotherapy is, may be, equal to surgical excision alone.

References

1. Steiger Z, Franklin R, Wilson RF et al (1981) Eradication and palliation of squamous cell carcinoma of the esophagus with chemotherapy, radiotherapy and surgical therapy. J Thorac Cardio Vasc Surg 82 : 713-719
2. Herskovic A, Martz K, Al-Sarraf M, Leichman L, Brindle J, Vaitkevicius V, Cooper J, Byhardt R, Davis L a,d Emani B (1992) Combined chemotherapy and radiotherapy compared with radiotherapy alone in patients with cancer of the esophagus. N Engl J Med 24 : 1593-1598

Induction chemotherapy, surgery and concomitant chemoradiotherapy for carcinoma of the esophagus

PC Hoffmann, MK Ferguson, DJ Haraf, LC Drinkard, HM Golomb, EE Vokes

In an effort to combine the 3 major cancer treatment modalities against esophageal cancer, we designed a study building on our institution's interest in 5-Fluorouracil modulation and concomitant chemoradiotherapy. From 1989 through 1992, we entered 41 patients with carcinoma of the esophagus into a study using induction chemotherapy, surgical resection, and concomitant chemoradiotherapy. Patients had to have no known distant metastases, a calculated creatinine clearance of $\geq$ 50 ml/hr, and a good performance status (Cancer and Leukemia Group B 0,1, or 2). Patients with adenocarcinoma and squamous cell carcinoma were eligible. Written informed consent was required.

Induction chemotherapy consisted of 2 21-day courses of Cisplatin, 100 mg/m^2 IV day 1 ; 5-Fluorouracil 800 mg/m^2 IV daily for 5 days by continuous infusion ; and Leucovorin 100 mg/m^2 orally every 4 hours for 5 days. After a re-evaluation with esophagoscopy, thoracic CT scan, and barium esophagram, surgical resection was performed if the patient was a suitable candidate both medically and surgically. Four to 6 weeks following surgery, chemoradiotherapy was begun. Surgery prior to Cisplatin-Fluorouracil-Leucovorin chemotherapy was allowed in 4 cases, either due to bleeding from the tumor or patient insistence. Radiotherapy was delivered to the mediastinum and upper addomen, in 200 cGy fractions daily, 5 days per week, every other week for 5-6 treatment weeks (total dose 5.000-6.000 cGy). Radiotherapy was given concomitantly with 5-Fluorouracil 800 mg/m^2 continuous IV infusion daily for 5 days, and Hydroxyurea 1.0 Gm twice daily for 5 days.

Of the 41 patients entered, 18 had squamous cell carcinoma, 22 had adenocarcinoma, and one had poorly differentiated carcinoma. Toxicities of induction chemotherapy were significant but manageable : moderate to severe mucositis, moderate myelosuppression, and mild renal toxicity. Diarrhea and nausea and vomiting were generally mild to moderate. There was 1 toxic death from sepsis. Responses to induction chemotherapy are summarized in Table 1.

Surgical resection was performed in 31 patients. Ten were not resected : 3 were not resectable due to extensive disease, 4 were medically poor surgical candidates, 1 refused surgery, 1 had a toxic death during induction, and 1 was lost to follow-up after first cycle of induction therapy. Three patients had no residual tumor on pathological examination of the surgical specimen (all had squamous cell histology). There were 2 deaths from surgical complications - 1 from respiratory failure at 37 days after surgery in a patient who also had rapidly progressive disease ; and 1 from a pulmonary embolism at 8 days after surgery.

Twenty-nine patients underwent concomitant chemoradiotherapy, of whom Twenty-four had undergone surgical resection. Twelve patients did not under-

Table 1. Response to induction chemotherapy

n = 37 evaluable for response
(4 pts not evaluable because they were resected first)

Cell Type	Complete Resp. (CR)	Partial Resp. (PR)	CR + PR	95 % C.I.
Adenocarcinoma (n = 18)	0	5 (28 %)	5 (28 %)[#]	(7-49 %)
Squamous (n = 18)	3 (17 %)*	8 (44 %)	11 (61 %)[#]	(38-84 %)
Total (n = 37[+])	3 (8 %)	13 (35 %)	16 (43 %)	(27-59 %)

* Pathological complete responses
+ Includes 1 poorly differentiated carcinoma, lost-to-follow-up
# Chi square test, P = .05

Table 2. Survival data

	Adenocarcinoma	Squamous	All
n	21	18	39*
Median Survival	11.0 month[+]	Undefined[+]	12.5 months
Survival at 1 year	33 ± 13 %	70 ± 11 %	52 ± 9 %
Survival at 2 years	Only 1 pt alive ≥ 24 months	63 ± 12 %	49 ± 9 %

* Two pts lost to follow-up
+ Log rank test p = .08

go the concomitant therapy for the following reasons : 1 toxic death during induction therapy, 2 postoperative deaths, 2 lost to follow-up after induction, 1 left the area after induction, 2 had metastatic disease to abdominal nodes found at surgery, 2 had prolonged poor performance status after surgery with early progressive disease, and 2 refused (1 received radiotherapy alone). Toxicities were well-tolerated : mild to moderate mucositis/esophagitis, mild dermatitis, mild to moderate leukopenia, and occasional mild thrombocytopenia.

Eighteen patients have died - 14 from progressive tumor, 2 from surgical complications (1 with progressive tumor), 1 from drug toxicity, and 1 from therapy-related toxic pneumonitis. Twenty-one patients are alive (median follow-up time 13 months), 1 with active tumor. Two are lost to follow-up. Table 2 details survival data.

We conclude

1. This induction chemotherapy regimen of Cisplatin, 5-Fluorouracil and Leucovorin is tolerable, and active in patients with both adenocarcinoma and squamous cell carcinoma of the esophagus.
2. Concomitant chemoradiotherapy is well-tolerated, and in conjunction with surgery produces good local control of tumor in this study.
3. Response rates are significantly higher in patients with squamous cell carcinoma than in those with adenocarcinoma.
4. Median survival, and 1 and 2 years survival rates in patients with squamous cell carcinoma appear to be superior to those in patients with adenocarcinoma.

Superiority of combined chemoradiotherapy to radiotherapy alone in patients with esophageal cancers. An intergroup study

M Al-Sarraf, K Martz, A Herskovic, L Leichman, JS Brindle, VK Vaitkevicius, J Cooper, R Byhardt, L Davis, B Emami

Superiority of combined chemoradiotherapy to radiotherapy alone in patients with esophageal cancers. An intergroup study.

The traditional treatment of patients with localized cancer of the esophagus are surgery and/or radiotherapy. The type of therapy will depend on the location and the histopathology of the primary tumor, tumor stage, the resectability of the lesion and operability of these patients. Unfortunately the overall results of the standard treatments are very poor. The median survival is about 9 months, 2 year survival is 10 %, and the 5 year survival is less than 5 %. Better results were reported from some institutions for selected patients, especially those patients with T1 or T2N0M0 disease. In part, one of the reasons for this poor results, is the high postoperative mortality rate, especially those who have resection and anastomosis performed. The mean mortality rate reported is about 10 %, and may go as high as 25 %. Added morbidity problem are re-stenosis and possible leakage. It has been stated but has not been proven, that surgical resection v.s. non-surgical options may improve the patients quality of life by relieving their dysphagia.

These poor results led to the investigation of effective systemic chemotherapy especially Cisplatin based combination as part of combined modality therapy. These agents given before surgery, or radiotherapy, and concurrent with radiotherapy. The concomitant chemoradiotherapy given as total treatment, preoperative or occasionally postoperatively. The best results obtained with chemotherapy alone or in combination with radiotherapy was with the use of Cisplatin and 5-FU infusion. This resulted in improvement of the overall results in patients eligible for these cooperative groups or single institutions phase II trials. The median survival for the combined modality treatment was about 13 months, and the 2 year survival was about 25 %.

Two of these pilots were carried out in the Radiation Therapy Oncology Group (RTOG), and the Southwest Oncology Group (SWOG). The trial consist of 2 courses of Cisplatin day 1 and 5-FU 96 hours infusion every 3 weeks concurrently with 3.000 cGy radiotherapy were given before surgery. Three weeks postchemotherapy, the patients were operated for possible complete resection. It was learned from these trials, that surgery may not influence the patients survival or overall outcome. Of course, these studies was not design to answer the important question of the role of surgery in these patients. Also, it

---

Wayne State University, Detroit, MI ; RTOG Heardquarters, Philadelphia, PA ; Oakwood Hospital, Dearborn, MI ; University of Southern California, Los Angeles, CA ; University of North Dakota, Bismarck, ND ; New York University, New York, NY ; Medical College of Wisconsin, Milwaukee, WI ; Emory University, Atlanta, Georgia ; Washington, University, St-Louis, MO

was learned that the incidence of systemic recurrences continued to be high, and these patients may need more chemotherapy. These encouraging results, led to the activation in the RTOG of phase III randomized and stratified trial to compare chemoradiotherapy to radiation treatment alone. After the activation of this trial in the RTOG, SWOG and the North Central Cancer Treatment Group joined the study.

Material and methods

Patients with T1-3, N0-1, and M0, with either squamous cell carcinoma or adenocarcinoma of the esophagus were entered in the study. These patients did not have tracheo-esophageal fistula, history of previous invasive cancer, or prior radiotherapy or chemotherapy. All patients have adequate renal and bone marrow functions. Patients were stratified according to type of histopathology, size of primary tumor, and amount of weight loss and randomized to treatment arms.

On the standard arm, patients to receive 6.400 cGy of total radiotherapy. On the investigational arm the radiotherapy dose was 5.000 cGy. Chemotherapy started on the same day of radiation treatment. Cisplatin 75 mg/m^2 i.v. given with hydration and mannitol diuresis on day 1. 5-FU 1.000 mg/m^2/day, 96 hours infusion day 1-4. Two courses of chemotherapy given during radiotherapy with 4 weeks apart. Additional 2 courses of the same chemotherapy were given 3 weeks apart after the end of radiotherapy.

Results and discussion

Between 1st February 1986 and 30th April 1990, 129 patients were entered for randomization. One hundred and twenty-three patients were evaluable. Sixty-two were randomized to receive RT alone, and 61 for chemoradiotherapy. The other 6 patients were either excluded or not evaluable. During the preliminary analysis, it was found that 1 arm was statistically superior, this led to the early closure of this important trial.

The stratification prognostic factors were the same between the 2 groups. No significant differences were found in evaluating other factors between the 2 arms. These include age, sex, race, symptoms, performance status, and T and N stages. The local toxicities were similar between the treatment methods. While, as expected, more patients had systemic side effects on the chemotherapy arm. No treatment related death occurred on either therapy.

The incidence of persistent disease, loco-regional failure, distant metastasis at 12 months, were significantly less for patients treated on the chemoradiotherapy (Table 1). The median survival was 12.5 months for patients treated with combined chemoradiotherapy, v.s. 8.9 months (p = 0.0013) for had radiation treatment only. The overall survival at 12 and 24 months between CT + RT and RT alone were 50 % v.s. 33 %, and 37 % v.s. 10 % (p = 0.0009) respectively. At the most recent update, 3/62 (5 %) are alive on the RT arm, and

20/61 (33 %) (p = 0.0004) are alive on the CT-RT arm. None of the survival on the RT treatment is beyond 3 years, while, 15 patients are alive more than 3 years, 14 of them continued without evidence of disease on CT-RT.

Table 1. Intergroup esophageal study

	Overall results		
	RT ± CT	RT	P-Value
Median survival (Mo)			
Overall	12.5	8.9	0.0013
Completed Treatment	14.9	9.9	0.0036
(43 pts on each arm)			
Survival : at 12 Mo	50 %	33 %	
at 24 Mo	38 %	10 %	0.0009
Loco- Regional Failure	45 %	65 %	0.02
Persistant Disease	25 %	33 %	
Failed Post-Treatment	20 %	32 %	
Distant Metastasis	22 %	38 %	0.005
(At 12 Mo)			

Table 2. Madian survival and overall 2 years survival according to treatment

	Surgery and/or radiotherapy	Chemotherapy radiotherapy ± surgery pilots	Present study
Medain Survival (Months)	9	13	13
2-years Survival	10 %	25 %	37 %

The important results reported here had confirmed without doubt the previous reported observations from the phase II pilots incorporating chemotherapy as part of surgery and/or radiotherapy in patients with esophageal cancers (Table 2). The median survival, and overall survival at 2 and 3 years, are similar what have been reported and known for many decades. In spite of less dose of RT on the combined arm, the incidence of treatment failure, and incidence of recurrence in the radiation field (loco-regional) is statistically less with chemoradiotherapy v.s. higher dose of RT alone. Further, the addition of systemic chemotherapy, reduced significantly the incidence of distant metastasis. These important effects, resulted in improvement of overall survival of more than 6 times with CT + RT over RT alone.

We concluded that concurrent Cisplatin, 5-FU infusion and RT followed by maintenance CT is superior to RT alone in patients with localized cancer of the esophagus. Further studies are needed to continue to improve on these results.

References

1. Earlam R, Cuhna-Melo JR (1980) Oesophageal squamous cell carcinoma. I. A critical review of surgery. Br J Surg 67 : 381-390
2. Harlam R, Cuhna-Melo JR (1980) Oesophageal squamous cell carcinoma. II. A critical review of radiotherapy. Br J Surg 67 : 457-461
3. Leichman L, Steiger Z, Seydel HG, Vaitkevicius VK (1984) Combined preoperative chemotherapy and radiation therapy for cancer of the esophagus : the Wayne State University, Southwest Oncology Group and Radiation Therapy Oncology Group experience. Sem Oncology 11 : 178-185
4. Kelsen DP, Bains M, Hilaris B et al (1982) Combination chemotherapy of esophageal carcinoma using Cisplatin, Vindesine, and Bleomycin. Cancer 49 : 1174-1177
5. Leichman L, Berry BT (1991) Experience with Cisplatin in treatment regimens for esophageal cancer. Sem Oncology 18 (suppl 3) : 64-72
6. Forastier AA (1992) Treatment of loco-regional esophageal cancer. Sem Oncology 19 (suppl 11) : 57-63
7. Al-Sarraf M (1990) The Current Status of Combined Modality Treatment Containing Chemotherapy in Patients with Esophageal Cancer. Guests Editorial. Inter J Radiat Oncol Biol Phys 19 : 813-815
8. Herskovic A, Martz K, Al-Sarraf M, Leichman L, Brindle J, Vaitkevicius V, Cooper J, Byhardt R, Davis L, Emami B (1992) Combined Chemotherapy and Radiotherapy Compared with Radiotherapy Alone in Patients with Cancer of the Esophagus. New Engl J Med 326 : 1593-1598

Neo-Adjuvant chemotherapy for advanced gastric cancer : a pilot study with angiotensin II induced drug delivery system

K Sugiyama, H Sato, M Hoshi, M Urushiyama, K Ishizuka, R Kanamaru

Tumor microcirculation is one of the important factors in cancer chemotherapy. Tumor blood flow is known to be very poor and in-homogeneous, so it is supposed that conventional systemic administration of anticancer drug(s) would not deliver sufficient dose of drug(s) into whole tumor tissue.

It is reported that angiostensin II (A-II) infusion brings remarkable increase in tumor blood flow, while normal tissue blood flow remains stable [1]. According to this phenomenon, we attempt to administer anticancer drug(s) with A-II infusion in order to enhance selective drug delivery to tumor tissue. We call this method « A-II induced hypertension chemotherapy (IHC) », and have applied it to many cancer patients since 1978 [2].

Recently, we reported a randomized controlled study of a combination chemotherapy using DXR, 5-FU and MMC with versus without A-II for advanced gastric cancer [3], and showed clinical advantage of A-II combined chemotherapy (Table 1).

Table 1. Result of randomized controlled study for advanced gastic cancer : combination chemotherapy of DXR, 5-FU, MMC with v.s. without A-II

	Registered	Eligible	Completed	CR	PR	NC	PD	Response rate*
With A-II	36	34	32	4	6	10	12	31.3 %
Without A-II	39	36	30	0	2	14	14	6.7 %

* $p < 0.05$ (χ^2 test)

In present report, we show our experience of usage of this method as Neo-Adjuvant chemotherapy for advanced gastric cancer.

From 1980 to 1990, 14 advanced gastric cancers received a few courses of preoperative chemotherapy with a 3-drugs combination of DXR, 5-FU and MMC under A-II induced hypertensive state (Fig. 1). Postoperative chemotherapy was done differently in each case, with or without A-II.

We estimated staging based on pretreatment clinical examination (clinical stage : CS), based on surgical macroscopic findings (surgical stage ; SS) and based on histopathological findings in resected material (pathological stage ; PS) in each case (Table 2). SS revealed some false positive estimation of lymphnodes, so we defined « down staging (DS) » when improvement of PS compared with CS was observed. According to this definition, 7 cases (50 %) achieved DS.

Dept. of Clin. Cancer Chemother., Res Inst for Tbc and Cancer, Tohoku Univ., 4-1 Seiryomachi, Aobaku, Sendai, Japan 980

Fig. 1. Schedule of Neo-Adjuvant chemotherapy : A-II is infused to keep mean blood pressure at 150 mmHg during injection of anticancer drugs

Regimen A (1978-1983)

Day	1	2	3	4	5	6	14	15	16	17	18	19
DXR 33 mg/m²						X						
5-FU 330 mg/m²	X	X	X	X	X		X	X	X	X	X	
MMC 5 mg/m²												X
A-II	X	X	X	X	X	X	X	X	X	X	X	X

q 4-5 weeks

Regimen B (1984-1990)

Day	1	2	3	8	9	10
DXR 33 mg/m²			X			
5-FU 330 mg/m²	X	X	X	X	X	X
MMC 5 mg/m²				X		
A-II	X	X	X	X	X	X

q 4 weeks

Table 2. Characteristics, staging, and survival of 14 gastric cancers

No.	Age	Sex	Clinical TNM	CS	Surgical TNM	SS	Pathological TNM	PS	DS	Survival (days)
1	73	M	420	IV	310	IIIA	000	0	+	>1514
2	63	M	301	IV	210	II	100	IA	+	>1251
3	62	F	400	IIIA	310	IIIA	220	IIIA	−	> 881
4	56	M	420	IV	321	IV	310	IIIA	+	> 795
5	69	M	420	IV	310	IIIA	000	0	+	> 781
6	50	M	421	IV	321	IV	300	II	+	699
7	71	M	42X	IV	410	IIIB	400	IIIA	+	481
8	70	M	420	IV	320	IIIB	320	IIIB	+	> 446
9	60	M	3XX	II	421	IV	321	IV	−	286
10	49	M	401	IV	321	IV	321	IV	−	258
11	69	M	421	IV	421	IV	321	IV	−	246
12	34	M	421	IV	421	IV	321	IV	−	220
13	41	M	400	IIIA	411	IV	411	IV	−	164
14	41	M	421	IV	321	IV	321	IV	−	162

CS : clinical stage, SS : surgical stage, PS : pathological stage. DS : down staging

Then, histopathologic grade, dose intensity of each anticancer drug and response rate were compared between DS group and non-DS group. The well and moderately differentiated histology showed higher rate of achievement of DS. The dose intensities of DXR and 5-FU of DS group were lower than those

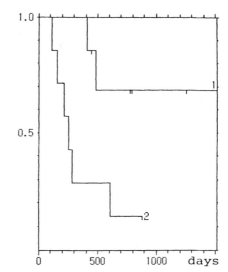

1 : Down staging group (n = 7)
2 : Non down staging group (n = 7)

1 vs 2 : p < 0.01 (generalized Wilcoxon test)

Fig. 2. Cumulative survival rate (Kaplan-Meier) of gastric cancer patients received Neo-Adjuvant chemotherapy with angiotensin II

of non-DS group. No other factor showed statistically significant differences between the 2 groups (not shown).

The mean survival time of DS group was 1 206.2 days, while that of non-DS group was 316.8 days (Kaplan-Meier method). DS group survived significantly longer than non-DS group ($p < 0.01$, generalized Wilcoxon test) (Fig. 2).

We conclude that Neo-Adjuvant chemotherapy contributes to survival when « down staging » is achieved, and A-II combined chemotherapy (IHC) seems to be a favorable method for neoadjuvant chemotherapy in terms of drug delivery.

References

1. Suzuki M, Hori K, Abe I, Saito S, Sato H (1981) A new approach to cancer chemotherapy : Selective enhancement of tumor blood flow with angiotensin II. JNCI 67 : 663-669
2. Sato H, Sato K, Sato Y, Asamura M, Kanamaru R, Sugiyama Z et al (1981) Induced hypertension chemotherapy of cancer patients by selective enhancement of drug delivery to tumor tissue with angiotensin II. Sci Rep Res Inst Tohoku Univ -C 28 : 32-44
3. Sato H, Wakui A, Hoshi M, Kurihara M, Yokoyama M et al (1991) Randomized controlled trial of induced hypertension chemotherapy (IHC) using angiotensin II human (TY-10721) in advanced gastric carcinoma. Jpn J Cancer Chemother 18 : 451-460

Combination of 5-FU, Leucovorin and Cisplatin (CDDP) : an efficient low-toxic chemotherapy in advanced gastric adenocarcinoma

M Ychou, Y Fedkovic, A Christopoulou, B Saint-Aubert, Ph Rouanet, C Astre, H Pujol

Metastatic gastric cancer remains a frequent disease with spontaneous median survival of about 6 months [1]. FAM regimen (5-FU, Doxorubicin and Mitomycin) was until the nineteens, considered as standard treatment of advanced gastric cancer. Recent publication of EORTC data showed significant improvement of survival in patients treated with FAMTX (5-FU, Methotrexate, Doxorubicin) in comparison to FAM [11].

In the last 3 years, other polychemotherapy associations showed similar results in term of objective responses (about 50 %) and median survival (9 to 11 months) [4, 7, 9, 10]. Actually 3 of these regimens are tested in a randomized study conducted by EORTC gastrointestinal group (ELF v.s. 5-FU Cisplatin v.s. FAMTX). One of this regimen is a combination of 5-FU in continuous infusion (day 1 to 5) with Cisplatin at day 1 or 2 [5,8].

The rational of our phase II study is the modulation of 5-FU by Leucovorin [6], demonstrated in metastatic colorectal cancer and the association with Cisplatin, 1 of the major drug in gastric cancer.

Patients and methods

Patients : Eligibility criteria included advanced of metastatic gastric carcinoma pathologically confirmed by laparotomy or biopsy having measurable or evaluable disease and performant status grade O to 2 according to World Health Organization (WHO).

Method : Patients were treated every 28 days with : Leucovorin : 200 mg/m^2/day, day 1 to 5 in fifteen minutes infusion ; 5-FU : 400 mg/m^2/day, day 1 to 5 in 1 hour infusion ; Cisplatin : 100 mg/m^2/day, day 2 in 1 hour infusion. Clinical, biological and radiological evaluation were performed before treatment and after 2 or 3 courses. WHO-criteria were used for the definition of tumor response and toxicity.

Results

Among 30 patients included in this study, 5 patients have less than 3 courses and have not been yet evaluated. Characteristics of the evaluated 25 patients

---

CRLC Val d'Aurelle, 34094 Montpellier, France

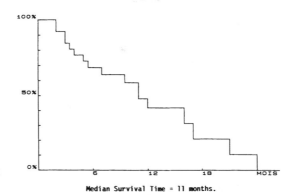

Fig. 1. Results on survival (Kaplan-Meier)

Median Survival Time = 11 months.

are summarized in Table 1. A total of 124 courses of chemotherapy were administered with a median of 5 per patients (range 2 to 9). Four complete responses were assessed (16 %), 2 were confirmed by laparotomy and 1 by endoscopic biopsy (local recurrence). We observed 9 partial responses (36 %) resulting in an overall response rate of 52 %.

Table 1. Characteristics of evaluable patients

No of patients	25
Median age (range)	65 (35-78)
Male/Female	1/4
Performance status (WHO)	
0	11
1	7
2	7
Cardia/Non cardia	9/16
Extent of disease	
Primary plus metastases	14
Only metastases	11
No Metastatic sites	
1	16
2	8
3	1
Location of metastases	
Liver	16
Peritoneum	9
Lymph nodes	5
Bone	1
Local recurrence	4

Nine patients are still alive with actually follow up of 4 to 16 months.

Median survival of the 25 evaluable patients is 11 months with a 1-year survival of 42 % (Kaplan-Meier).

Toxicity of this chemotherapy was very moderate with only 3 digestive toxicities grade 3-4 according to the WHO-criteria. There was no toxic related death.

Conclusion

With 52 % response rate and a median survival of 11 months, the FLP regimen has very similar results than the other actives chemotherapy in gastric carcinoma (EAP, FAMTX, FP, ELF) [4, 7, 8, 10]. Netherless it is necessary to confirm these encouraging results in a larger trial including at least 40 patients. If these results are confirmed in term of response rate and low toxicity, it will be interesting to compare the FLP regimen to others standard chemotherapy in a randomized phase III study.

References

1. Allum WH, Powell DJ, McConkey CC, Fielding JW (1989) Gastric cancer : a 25 years review. Br J Surg 76 : 535-540
2. Cullinan SA, Moertel CG, Fleming TR et al (1985) A comparison of three chemotherapeutic regimens in the treatment of advanced pancreatic and gastric carcinoma. Fluorouracil v.s. Fluorouracil and Doxorubicin v.s. Fluorouracil, Doxorubicin and Mitomycin. JAMA 253 : 2061-2067
3. De Lisi V, Cocconi G, Tonato M et al (1986) Randomized comparison of 5-FU alone or combined with Carmustine, Doxorubicin and Mitomycin (BAFMi) in the treatment of advanced gastric cancer. A phase III trial of the Italian Clinical Research Oncology Group (GOIRC). Cancer Treatm Rep 70 : 481-485
4. Kelsen D, Atiq OT, Niedzwiecki D, Ginn D, Chapman D, Heelan R, Lightdale C, Vinciguerra V, Brennan M (1992) FAMTX versus Etoposide, Doxorubicin and Cisplatin : a random assignment trial in gastric cancer. J Clin Oncol 10, 4 : 541-548
5. Lacave AJ, Buesa JM, Gracia JM et al (1989) Cisplatin and 5-Fluorouracil in the treatment of advanced gastric cancer. Abstr. EORTC Symp Adv in Gastrointest Tract Cancer Res and Treatm 44
6. Machover D, Golfschmidt E, Chollet P, Metzger G, Zittoun J, Marquet J, Vandenbulcke JM, Misset JL, Schwarzenberg, Fourtillan JB, Gaget H, Mathe G (1986) Treatment of advanced colorectal and gastric adenocarcinomas with 5-Fluorouracil and high-dose folinic acid. J Clin Oncol 4, 5 : 685-696
7. Preusser P, Wilke H, Achterrath W et al (1989) Phase II study with the combination Etoposide, Doxorubicin and Cisplatin in advanced measurable gastric cancer. J Clin Oncol 7 : 1310-1317
8. Rougier Ph, Mahjoubi M, Oliveira J et al (1989) Treatment of advanced gastric adenocarcinoma (AGC) with 5-FU/platinum combination. Abstr. EORTC Symp Adv in Gastrointest Tract Research and Treatm 45
9. Wilke H, Preusser P, Fink U, Achterrath W, Lenaz L, Stahl M, Schober C, Link H, Meyer HJ, Lucke B, Schmoll HJ (1990) High-dose folinic Acid/Etoposide/5-Fluorouracil in advanced gastric cancer — a phase II study in elderly patients or patients with cardiac risk. Investigational New Drugs 8 : 65-70
10. Wilke H, Preusser P, Fink U, Stahl M, Meyer HJ, Achterrath W, Köhne-Wömpner CH, Schöber Ch, Harstrick A, Lenaz L, Meyer J, Schmoll HJ (1991) Pilot study with Folnic Acid, Etoposide, 5-Fluorouracil, and Cisplatin in advanced gastric and esophageal cancer. Tumordiag. u. Ther 12 : 21-24
11. Wils JA, Klein HO, Wagener DJ et al (1991) Sequential high-dose Methotrexate and Fluorouracil combined with Doxorubicin - a step ahead in the treatment of advanced gastric cancer : a trial of European Organization for Research and Treatment of Cancer Gastrointestinal Tract Cooperative Group. J Clin Oncol 9 : 827-831

Adjuvant chemotherapy and radiotherapy in liver transplantation for primary hepatocellular carcinoma: a feasibility study

JY Pierga*, P Piedbois*, D Cherqui**, C Duvoux***,
A Ramouni****, JM Métreau***, D Mathieu****, M Julien**,
D Dhumeaux***, PL Fagniez**, JP Le Bourgeois*

Despite considerable advances in knowledge of tumor biology and diagnosis, the overall prognosis of hepatocellular carcinoma remains poor. When possible, hepatic resection is the treatment of choice, but less than 30 % of HCCs can be considered for resection (Dusheiko 1992, Haug 1992, Ringe 1988). The experience with liver transplantation for hepatic malignancies is still limited, and the results are far to be impressive. Tumor recurrences are usual (43 to 60 %), liver and the lung being the 2 most commonly involved sites of relapse (Calne 1982, Iwatsuki 1991). In an attempt to reduce the high risk of relapse rate in patients with liver transplantation for HCC, we underwent a pilot study of a adjuvant treatment combining preoperative chemoembolization, preoperative radiotherapy and postoperative chemotherapy.

Material and methods

From November 1989 to March 1992, 10 consecutive patients with primary hepatocellular carcinoma were included in this study. Patient characteristics are listed in Table 1. Most of them had post-hepatitis B or alcoholic cirrhosis. Informed consent was obtained from all patients.

Chemoembolization consisted of repeated Adriamycin 50 mg bolus infusions, associated with ethiodized oil (Lipiodol) and gelatin sponge. The treatment started several weeks before surgery if the portal circulation was correct. Contraindications to CE were portal venous thrombosis at or below the hilar convergence, reverse portal flow, stage C cirrhosis and significant bilirubin level.

Radiotherapy was administered immediately before transplantation at the total dose of 5 Gy in one fraction by a cobalt unit with antero-posterior and postero-anterior portals.

Hepatectomy and liver replacement were performed by conventional methods. One patient with terminal chronic renal insufficiency had in the same time a kidney transplantation.

Chemotherapy was started within the 24-hour following liver transplantation, and consisted of Mitoxantrone 5 mg/m^2 intravenous bolus injection weekly for 12 weeks.

Postoperative immunosuppression consisted of a combination of Ciclospo-

---

* Department of Oncology, ** Department of Surgery, *** Department of Hepatogastroenterology, **** Department of Radiology, Henri Mondor Hospital, Créteil 94000, France

Table 1. Patients' characteristics

Patient	Date of transplantation	Sex	Age (year)	Cause of cirrhosis	α foeto-protein	Number of tumors	Size of tumor	Intrahepatic portal involvement	Diaphragmatic involvement
1	11.07.89	m	48	B Hepatitis	< 15	9	4 cm	yes	no
2	01.16.90	m	40	B Hepatitis	1.500	3	6 cm	no	no
3	09.30.90	m	48	Hemochromatosis	700	diffuse	8 cm	yes	yes
4	10.18.90	f	51	PBC	60	diffuse	2 cm	yes	yes
5	04.12.91	m	56	Alcohol	71.5	4	7 cm	yes	no
6	04.28.91	m	50	Alcohol	< 15	2	3 cm	no	no
7	05.16.91	m	27	B Hepatitis	17.200	4	4 cm	no	no
8	08.22.92	m	53	B Hepatitis	701	1	5 cm	no	no
9	03.25.92	m	52	Alcohol	262	5	3.5 cm	no	no
10	not done	m	42	Alcohol	<15	1	2 cm	unknown	unknown

rine, Azathioprine and Prednisone. Toxicity of the chemotherapy was assessed clinically and biologically, according to the World Health Organization grading (WHO).

Results

Eight patients received 1 to 4 chemoembolizations (CE) (mean 2). One patient (patient 5) with a hepatofugal portal flow and another (patient 3) with a complete portal thrombosis did not receive CE. One patient died 10 days after the first CE course of an acute hepatic failure. Retrospectively, he was considered with a Child C cirrhosis. Tumor response to CE was assessable in 7 patients by histological tumor examination (Table 2).

Two transplanted patients were not irradiated : 1 who received both an hepatic and renal transplantation, and 1 who had severe reactions after CE. There was no radiotherapy related complication or late toxicity.

Standard orthotopic liver transplantation was performed in 9 patients. One patient (patient 8) died 4 days after surgery from an heart failure.

Eight patients received 4 to 12 courses (mean 9) of chemotherapy consisting of Mitoxantrone. The main toxicity of chemotherapy was leucopenia (Table 3) : 18 Grade I, 16 Grade II, 4 Grade III and 3 Grade IV leucopenia were observed out of a total of 62 courses (WHO grading). Early thrombopenia was observed in 6 patients during the first week after surgery, probably related to the cumulative hematotoxicity of Azathioprine and Mitoxantrone. There were no hemorragic complication. Five patients presented septic complications associated to leucopenia which led to stop definitively the chemotherapy : Pneumocystis pneumonia after 11 courses in patient 1, pyelonephritis after 4 courses in patient 2, abdominal wall abscess after 8 courses in pateint 5, zona after 5 courses in patient 7, and biliary complications after 8 courses in patient 9. The outcome was favorable in all cases.

Six out of 9 transplanted patients are alive without evidence of disease 10, 20, 21, 21, 36 and 38 months after liver transplantation. Two patients with initial diaphragmatic tumor extension relapsed : one at 4 months (brain and pulmonary metastasis) and one at 9 months (liver recurrence).

Discussion

Up to now, very few attemps have been made to reduce the risk of relapse after LT for HCC (Karlberg, 1992), which is considered a chemoresistant tumor (Stone 1989). Various cytostatic agents have been tested in patients with advanced disease, as 5-FU, Streptozotocin, Methyl-CCNU or Cisplatin (Falkson 1988), with response rates between 0 and 25 %. Doxorubicin has been reported to be the most active drug, with response rates of 20 to 25 % (Stone 1989).

Mitoxantrone is considered less toxic than Doxorubicin for nausea, vomiting, alopecia, cardiotoxicity and stomatis (Stuart-Harris 1986). Mitoxantrone

Table 2. Transplanted patients outcome

Patient	Chemoembolization	Tumor necrosis	Radiotherapy	Number of chemotherapy courses	Relapse	Status	Duration of survival in months
1	1 at d-27	no	yes	11	no	alive NED	38+
2	1 at d-29	complete	yes	4	no	alive NED	36+
3	no (portal thrombus)	no	yes	4	lung	dead	7
4	2 at d-57 and d-8	> 50 %	yes	11	liver	dead	11
5	no (reverse portal flow)	no	yes	8	no	alive NED	21+
6	1 at d-45	about 50 %	no	12	no	alive NED	21+
7	4 at-10 to-6 months	< 50 %	no	5	no	alive NED	20+
8	2 at d-120 and d-75	about 50 %	yes	0	no	dead at d + 4	0
9	3 at d-240, d-150 and d-14	< 50 %	yes	8	no	alive NED	10+

can be administered on a weekly schedule, which permit to adapt the dose according to the observed toxicity.

Chemoembolization (CE) is considered a relatively safe treatment for HCC. Because CE does not preclude subsequent resection, it is now often used in patients with resectable cancer, in an attempt to reduce the tumor size (Bismuth 1992). In our series, we have obtained a high rate of tumor necrosis (Table 2).

Conclusion

The present study demonstrates that the combinaison of preoperative CE and radiotherapy and postoperative systemic chemotherapy is feasible for patients receiving a LT for HCC.

The result suggest that outcome of patients was improved by the adjuvant treatment, since 6 out of 10 patients are alive without evidence of disease at 10, 20, 21, 21, 36 and 38 months.

This promising results should be confirmed in a randomized trial comparing combined adjuvant treatment and control.

References

1. Bismuth H, Morino M, Sherlock D, Castaing D, Miglietta C, Cauquil P, Roche A (1992) Primary treatment of hepatocellular carcinoma by arterial chemoembolization. Am J Surg 163 : 387-394
2. Calne RY (1982) Liver transplantation for liver cancer. World J Surg 6 : 76-80
3. Dusheiko GM, Hobbs Kef Dick R, Burroughs AK (1992) Treatment of small hepatocellular carcinomas. Lancet 340 : 285-288
4. Falkson G, Cnaan A, Schutt AJ, Ryan LM, Falkson HC (1988) Prognostic factors for survival in hepatocellular carcinoma. Cancer Res 48 : 7314-7318
5. Haug CE, Jenkins RL, Rohrer RJ, Auchincloss H, Delmonico FL, Freeman RB, Lewis WD, Cosimi AB (1992) Liver transplantation for primary hepatic cancer. Transplantation 53 : 376-382
6. Iwatsuki S, Starzl TE, Sheahan DG, Yokoyama I, Demetris AJ, Todo S, Tzakis AG, Vanthiel DH, Carr B, Selby R, Madariaga J (1991) Hepatic resection versus transplantation for hepatocellular carcinoma. Ann Surg 214 : 221-229
7. Karlberg I (1992) Liver transplantation in primary liver malignancy. Transplant Proc 24 : 382
8. Stillwagon GB, Order SE, Guse C, Klein JL, Leichner PK, Leibel SA, Fishman EK (1989) One hundred ninety-four hepatocellular cancers treated by radiation and chemotherapy combinations. Int J Radiation Oncology Biol Phys 17 : 1223-1229
9. Stone MJ, Klintmalm G, Potter D, Husberg B, Egorin MJ (1989) Neo-Adjuvant chemotherapy and orthotopic liver transplantation for hepatocellular carcinoma. Transplantation 48 : 344-347
10. Stuart-Harris R, Coates AS, Raghavan D, Sullivan A, Kefford R, Tattersall MHN (1986) Patient acceptatibility of chemotherapy in advanced breast cancer : a radomized cross-over study of Mitoxantrone versus Doxorubicin. Proc AACR 27 : 701

Abstract. This paper presents a feasibility study of an adjuvant treatment in patients receiving an orthotopic liver transplantation for hepatocellular carcinoma. This treatment consisted of preoperative chemoembolization and radiotherapy, and postoperative chemotherapy with Mitoxantrone for 12 weeks. Ten patients entered this study. Tumor sizes ranged from 2 to 8 cm. CE was well tolerated in patients with child A or B cirrhosis. There was no radiotherapy related toxicity. The main toxicity of CT was leucopenia : 18 grade I, 16 grade II, 4 grade III and 3 grade IV leucopenia according to the WHO grading were observed in 62 chemotherapy courses. In five cases, leucopenia was associated with a septic complication, which led to stop the chemotherapy. One patient died 4 days after surgery from an heart failure. Six patients are alive without evidence of disease between 7 and 35 months after liver transplantation.

Intensive weekly chemotherapy for advanced gastric cancer using 5-Fluorouracil, Cisplatin, Epirubicin, 6S-Leucovorin and Granulocyte-colony stimulating factor

S Cascinu, A Fedeli, S Luzi Fedeli, G Catalano

Although declining in frequency gastric cancer remains one of the leading cause of death in western countries [1].

Cure for patients with gastric carcinoma is currently available only in those in whom a complete surgical resection can be performed. Unfortunately it is possible in only 30 % to 35 % of patients and, however, also in these patient relapse is common. Consequently advances in the treatment of gastric cancer (both in the adjuvant and advanced disease) will require the development of effective systemic therapy. At the present time 4 drugs (5-Fluorouracil [5-FU] ; Doxorubicin [ADR] ; Cisplatin [CDDP] and Mitomycine-C [Mit-C]) have been identified as having reproducible modest to moderate single-agent activity in patient with advanced gastric cancer [2]. Clinical trials combining these cytotoxic agent have reported response rate of 30 % to 40 % but, unfortunately, complete responses have been uncommon, the duration of response has been short, and the impact on survival uncertain [3].

Recently 2 clinical trials with more agressive regimens, than those of earlier combination chemotherapy, have reported response rates exceeding 50 % with high complete responses. A 64 % response rate (21 % complete responses) was observed in patients treated with combination of Etoposide, Doxorubicin and Cisplatin (EAP). The median response duration was 7 months while the median survival time was 9 months [4].

In the other clinical trial, designed to modulate 5-FU biochemically with sequential methotrexate (FAMTX), a 59 % response rate was reported with 12 % of the patients achieving complete response ; the median survival time was 9 months [5].

The initial successes of these regimens were not confirmed, however, in recent trial in which patients with metastatic gastric carcinoma were randomly treated with EAP (21 % response rate) or FAMTX (31 % response rate). Few complete responses were documented for both regimens, with consistent toxicity, above all for EAP combination [6].

On the basis of these discouraging results and in order to identify a more effective and less toxic regimen we tried to determine new combination with low individual doses but weekly treatment of 5-FU, Epidoxorubicin (epiADR), CDDP, 6S-Leucovorin (6-LV) with the support of Granulocyte-Colony Stimulating factor (G-CSF). The choice of these drugs and schedule depend on :

5-FU, ADR and CDDP remain the most active single agents in gastric cancer (we substituted ADR by EpiADR because of the same activity but lower toxicity) [7].

Servizio di Oncologia, Ospedali Riuniti. P. le Cinelli 4, 61100 Pesaro, Italy

Leucovorin can enhance 5-FU activity [8].

the weekly administration, allowing more drug to be administered per unit time and minimizing side-effects, can increase dose intensity (DI) of these drugs, that is probably an important factor in determining activity of 5-FU, ADR, CDDP a reported in several tumors (i.e. ovary ; breast ; colon) [9].

G-CSF could contribute to this weekly administration reducing the incidence of leukopenia.

Patients and methods

Thirty-four patients with advanced gastric carcinoma entered this clinical trial.

Eligibility criteria included unresectable locally advanced or metastatic gastric carcinoma pathologically confirmed by laparotomy or biopsy ; measurable disease ; performance status ECOG grade 0 to 2 and normal liver, renal, cardiac and bone marrow functions. Patients were excluded from the study if they had received any prior chemo or radiotherapy, if their age was greater than 70 years, or for the presence of CNS metastases.

Measurable disease was defined as presence of at least one lesion clearly bidimensionally measured by computed tomography scan. In patients with locally advanced disease the primary tumor was evaluated by CT scan or endoscopy.

Patients received 5-Fluorouracil 500 mg/sqm intravenously (i.v.) weekly ; 6 S-Leucovorin 250 mg/sqm i.v. in 4 hours infusion weekly ; Cisplatin 40 mg/sqm i.v. weekly ; Epidoxorubicin 35 mg/sqm i.v., weekly. Cisplatin was administered a 2 hours infusion in 1.5 L 0.9% sodium chloride and posthydration was performed with total of 1.5 L of 0.9% sodium chloride. From the day after to the day before each chemotherapy administration Granulocyte-Colony Stimulating Factor wa administered at the dose of 5 microgram/Kg. We chose this way of administration to avoid the theoretical risk of sensitizing hematopoietic precursor cells to chemotherapy-induced damage. G-CSF therapy in fact should not be begun until sufficient time has elapsed to permit clearing of all active chemotherapy metabolites and should be stopped at least 1 day before chemotherapy. One cycle of therapy consisted of 9 weekly treatment.

Full doses of anticancer drugs was given if the leukocyte count was >4.000/mm^3 ; if the platelets count >130.000/mm^3.

When less we delayed week. Protocol followed 2 stage design. Initially we intended to include 17 patients. In the presence of or more responses other 17 patients would be included. If the trial continued to 34 patients and at least 10 responses were seen it would be considered promising.

Evaluation of response was performed after 9 weeks while toxicity wa evaluated weekly according to standard WHO criteria [10]. All patients provided informed consent.

Results

Thirty-four patients were included in this clinical trial.
Demographic characteristics for the entire patients cohort are summarized in Table 1. All patients were evaluable for response and toxicity.

Table 1. Patients' characteristics

Age (years)	
median	58
range	44-74
Sex	
M/F	25/9
Performance Status (ECOG)	
0	12
1	13
2	9
Symptoms	
Weight loss >10 %	10
Abdominal pain	10
Dyspnoea	1
Dysphagia	5
Prior surgery	
None	10
Curative	19
Palliative	5
Sites of primary tumors	
Gastroesophageal junction	4
Proximal stomach	6
Body	13
Distal stomach	10
Unknown	1
Histology type	
Well differentiated	12
Moderately differentiated	13
Poorly differentiated	8
Anaplastic	1
Sites of metastases	
Liver	16
Abdomen/peritoneum	12
Lymph nodes	12
Lung	5
Bone	2

Results are shown in Table 2. Five patient (14 %) achieved a complete response and 20 partial response, resulting in an overall response rate of 72 % (95 % confidence interval, 59 % to 88 %). Median remission duration was 8 months for complete responses and 7 for partial responses. Median survival time was 12 months for all the patients, and it was 13 months for responding patients. After chemotherapy, 2 patients with partial responses had resectable disease by CT scan and endoscopy criteria. One underwent curative gastrectomy, and the other underwent palliative resection.

Toxicities are delineated in Table 3. Side-effects principally in the form of leukopenia, anemia and thrombocytopenia determined reduction of the planned dose-intensity of about 10 %.

Table 2. Results

Evaluable patients No 34			
Complete response	5	(14 %)	72 %
Partial response	20	(58 %)	
Stable disease	5		
Progressive disease	4		
Median duration response (months)			
complete response	8		
partial response	7		
Median duration survival (months)			
responders	13		
overall	12		

Table 3. Toxicity

| Toxic effects | | No of patients | | |
	WHO grade 1	2	3	4
Leukopenia	1	5	3	—
Anemia	2	3	4	—
Trombocytopenia	1	3	1	—
Nausea/vomiting	2	3	—	—
Diarrhea	1	3	—	—
Stomatitis	2	2	—	—
Neurotoxicity	2	4	1	—

Discussion

The identification of active systemic therapy in advanced gastric cancer is a very high priority, since resulting 5 years survival statistics range from 5 % to 15 % of all patients. Up to day the efforts of finding an active chemotherapeutic combination failed. Even EAP and FAMTX regimens, claimed as innovative treatment in gastric cancer, cannot be considered resolutive. EAP show in fact a moderate activity with an alarming rate of life-threatening toxicity [11, 12]. FAMTX was found by Kelsen et al less toxic but no significantly more effective than EAP [6]. Moreover the method of Methotrexate administration is expensive and demanding, requiring patients' hospitalization.

Retrospective analyses have shown correlations between outcome and DI of chemotherapy for a variety of drugs against variety of diseases. DI was particularly demonstrated an important factor in determining activity of 5-FU, CDDP, ADR, that represent the most active single agents in gastric carcinoma [2].

In order to test the hypothesis that larger doses of antineoplastic drugs are more effective also in gastric cancer 5-FU, CDDP, EpiADR combination was constructed to maximize DI and minimize associated toxicity. We thought in fact that with low individual doses but weekly treatments and with the support of G-CSF to limit the problem of leukopenia, the DI of these drugs could be increased without severe toxicity. Data from our study seem to confirm this hypothesis. The objective response rate of 72 % with a 14 % of complete responses is in fact noticeably even if these results are based on a limited sample and must therefore be viewed as preliminary.

Another point of interest arising from this work can be the efficacy and safety of the support by G-CSF to a weekly administration of cytotoxic drugs. We are not aware of trials using this schedule. We hypothesized this G-CSF administration on the basis of preclinical and clinical studies. It was demonstrated in fact that the absolute neutrophil count rise on days 4-5 after the first administration of G-CSF [13]. Furthermore it is possible that therapy with G-CSF before chemotherapy may increase the efficacy of G-CSF given following chemotherapy [14]. In phase III study the duration of neutropenia following chemotherapy in the patients randomized to receive G-CSF was shorter during cycles 2 through to 6 than in cycle 1, suggesting that prior G-CSF treatment may prime the marrow to augmented response to subsequent G-CSF [14].

Finally, we would like to point out that we registered very few episodes of gastrointestinal toxicity, even using weekly administration of 5-FU and LV, at the same dosage as Buffalo regimen, that cause diarrhea and stomatitis [15]. A possible explanation of this low incidence of gastrointestinal toxicity is that G-CSF may reduce the incidence of mucositis by increasing the number of neutrophilis as well as their functional ability to guard mucosal barriers more efficiently [14].

In conclusion, although the small number of patients suggesting caution in the interpretation of results we think that this regimen seems to be promising and suitable for further studies in gastric cancer.

References

1. Silverberg E (1989) Cancer Statistic 38 : 3-20
2. Moertel CG, Lavin PT (1979) Phase II-III chemotherapy studie in advanced gastric cancer. Cancer Treat Rep 63 : 1863-1869
3. Wilke H, Preusser P, Finkk U et al (1990) New development in the treatment of gastric carcinoma. Sem Oncology 17 (suppl) : 61-70
4. Preusser P, Wilke H, Achterrath W et al (1989) A phase II study with the combination Etoposide, Doxorubicin, and Cisplatin in advanced measurable gastric cancer. J Clin Oncol 7 : 1310-1317

5. Wils J, Bleiberg H, Blijhan G et al (1986) An EORTC gastrointestinal group evaluation of the combination of sequential methotrexate (MTX) and 5-Fluorouracil (F), combined with Adriamycin (A) (FAMTX) in advanced measurable gastric cancer. J Clin Oncol 4 : 1799-1803
6. Kelsen D, Atiq OT, Saltz L et al (1992) FAMTX versus Etoposide, Doxorubicin and Cisplatin random assignment trial in gastric cancer. J Clin Oncol 10 : 541-548
7. Roth A, Zupanc D, Luetic J, and Kolaric K (1990) Open phase II with 5-Fluoruracil, 4-Epi-Doxorubicin and Mitmycin C (FEM) in advanced gastric cancer. Tumori 76 : 51-53
8. Arbuck SG, Douglas HO, Trave F, et al (1987) A phase II trial of 5-Fluorouracil and high-dose intravenous leucovorin in gastric carcinoma. J Clin Oncol 5 : 1150-1156
9. Hryniuk WM (1987) Average relative dose intensity and the impact on design of clinical trials. Sem Oncology 14 : 65-74
10. Miller AB, Hoodgstraten B, Staquet M, and Winkler A (1981) Reporting results of cancer treatment. Cancer 47 : 207-214
11. Lerner A, Gonin R, Steel G and Mayer RJ (1992) Etoposide, Doxorubicin and Cisplatin chemotherapy for advanced gastric adenocarcinoma results of phase II trial. J Clin Oncol 10 : 536-540
12. Sparano JA, Wiernik PH (1991) Toxicity of Etoposide, Doxorubicn and Cisplatin in gastric cancer. J Clin Oncol 5 : 938-939
13. 13. Gabrilove JL, Jakubowsky A, Scher H et al (1988) Effectof granulocyte colony-stimulating factor on neutropenia and associated morbidity due to chemotherapy for transitional-cell carcinoma of the urothelium. N Engl J Med 318 : 1414-1422
14. Glaspy JA, Golde DW (1992) Granulocyte Colony-Stimulating Factor preclinical and clinical studies. Sem Oncology 19 : 386-394
15. Petrelli N, Douglas HO, Herrer L, Russel et al (1989) The modulation of Fluorouracil with Leucovorin in metastatic colorectal carcinoma : a prospective randomized phase III trial. J Clin Oncol 7 : 1419-1426

Neo-Adjuvant chemotherapy for inoperable gastric cancer via local and general delivery routes (FLEP Therapy)

T Nakajima, S Ishihara, H Motohashi, Y Kitamura, Y Nakajima, M Fujii, A Tokunaga, K Matai, H Anzai, M Nishi

Though some improvement has been observed in the treatment result of gastric cancer in Japan over the recent 40 years, inoperable gastric cancer still has a poor prognosis. To improve the treatment result of advanced cancer, a novel Neo-Adjuvant chemotherapy was conducted by a multi-institutional clinical trial group since 1989. This paper deals with a local effect of Neo-Adjuvant chemotherapy, and survival benefit in patients treated with and without surgery.

Patients and methods

Thirty-nine patients with inoperable gastric cancer entered the study. The reasons of unresectability were extended lymph node metastasis along the abdominal aorta in 64 %, peritoneal dissemination in 38.5 %, local extension to the adjacent organs or retroperitoneal spaces, and liver metastasis in 31 %. Some patients had more than 2 reasons of unresectability simultaneously.

Chemotherapy: on days 1 to 5, 370 mg/m^2 of 5-Fluorouracil and 30 mg/body of Leucovorin were given intravenously by 1 shot injection. On days 7 and 21, CDDP, 70 mg/m^2 and Etoposide, 70 mg/m^2 were given intraarterially via a catheter placed in the aorta (the level of nineth thoracic vertebra), or in the celiac artery over 60 minutes by infusion pump. The regimen was repeated 2 times every 4 or 5 weeks. Response was evaluated according to the WHO criteria. Patients who responded to chemotherapy were subjected to surgery with an intent of resection. Survival rate and median survival time were computed by Kaplan-Meier method.

Results

Out of 39 cases entered the study, 24 cases (61.5 %) completed the 2 or more than two courses of chemotherapy. Remaining cases did not complete the 2 course regimen due to the side effect, or disease progression.

Toxicity of grade 3 (WHO criteria) was observed in 48.7 % of all cases. Main limiting factors were the bone marrow suppression and gastrointestinal disturbances. Leukopenia was observed in 23.7 %, thrombocytopenia in 10.5 %, and anemia in 28.9 %. Nausea and vomiting were observed in 15 % of cases,

---

Neo-Adjuvant chemotherapy study group and cancer institute hospital, Tokyo

which were controlled by granisetron. Stomatitis was also a common toxicity, and 5 % of patients were impossible to take meal because of severe stomatitis. Depletion of creatinine clearance was observed in 11.8 %, and 1 patient died of acute renal failure and bone marrow suppression. Local effect of chemotherapy was evaluated in 35 of 39 cases which had measurable lesions (Table 1). All-over response rate was 51.4 % (18/35). Response rate according to the site of lesions was 32.3 % for primary lesions, 53.8 % for liver metastasis, and 75.0 % for lymph node metastasis, which included complete disappearance of supraclavicular node swelling.

Table 1. Response rates according to sites of tumor

Target	CR	PR	NC	PD	RR (%)
Primary		10	17	4	32.2
Liver		7	3	3	53.8
Lymph node	2	16	31	1	75.0
		All-over response rate			51.4

Sixteen patients who responded to chemotherapy and 4 patients who had no measurable tumors were subjected to surgery. Resectability rate was 52.6 % for all cases. Curative surgery was carried out in 4 of 12 cases with complete chemotherapy, and 1 of 8 cases with incomplete chemotherapy. All 20 cases had total gastrectomy, and some associated with combined resection of adjacent organs, and with extensive lymphadenectomy along the both sides of the aorta. Hepatectomy was not carried out for the patients with liver metastasis, but intraoperative biopsy revealed no cancer cells microscopically in the obtained specimen of some patients.

Observation time ranged 3 to 36 months, and 12 of 39 cases are still alive. The longest survivor is alive without recurrence for 36 months. One patient died of toxicity, 2 died of postoperative complication, and remaining 24 cases developed recurrent diseases. Median survival time (MST) was 245+ days for non-responders, and 164 + days for non-responders, 401+ days for curative surgery, and 243+ days for non-curative surgery.

Discussion

Neo-Adjuvant chemotherapy with recent regimens utilizing biochemical modulation, or new drugs seems to have an impact on the life-span of the advanced gastric cancer. EAP therapy [1] had a high response rate and long survivors among the unresected cancers, but it causes, at the same time, severe side effects. In order to reduce the systemic toxicity, high drug concentration at the tumor site and low in the systemic circulation might be desirable. Clinical benefit of regional chemotherapy in the liver tumors are reported previously. Stephans [2] and Aigner [3] have reported the advantage of celiac axis infusion chemotherapy for advanced gastric cancer. If the tumor extends only to the adjacent organs, celiac delivery is preferable to systemic delivery. However, our patients had wider tumor extension to the paraaortic nodes or peritoneal dissemination. We employed semiselective intraaortic delivery of CDDP and Etoposide, plus systemic delivery of 5-FU and Leucovorin to cover the wider distribution of tumor.

The overall response rate of FLEP regimen was 51.4 %, which is fairly good compared with those of recent studies [4, 6], ranging from 30 % to 50 %. This regimen has high response rate in the liver metastasis (53.8 %), and in the distant hymph node mestastasis (75.0 %). A high response of lymph node and liver metastasis to chemotherapy are reported by the previous literatures and could be explained by the sensitivity of cancer cells to the drugs. FLEP therapy succeded in the down-staging in half of the primarily unresectable cancer, rendering enough to resection. Median survial time (MST) was 245 + days for all patients, 330 days for responders, and 401 + days for cases with curative resection. Comparing with MST of non-resected cases (95 days) in Cancer Institute Hospital, Tokyo, MST of patients treated with FLEP therapy (and with surgery) are much longer than the natural history. While 1/4 of the patients are still alive, longer observation in needed to confirm the clinical significance of this therapy.

References

1. Preusser P, Wilke H, Achterrath W et al (1989) Phase II study with the combination Etoposide, Doxorubicin, and Cisplatin in advanced measurable gastric cancer. J Clin Oncol 7 : 1310-1317
2. Stephans FO, Adams BG, Crea P (1986) Intra-arterial chemotherapy given preoperatively in the management of carcinoma of the stomach. Surg Gyn Obstet 162 : 370-374
3. Aigner KR, Benthin F, Mueller H (1991) Celiac axis infusion (CAI) chemotherapy for advanced gastric cancer. In : Sugarbaker PH (ed) Management of gastric cancer. Kluwer Academic Publishers, Boston, 357-362
4. Machover D, Goldschmidt E, Chollet P et al (1986) Treatment of advanced colorectal and gastric adenocarcinomas with 5-Fluorouracil and high-dose Folnic acid. J Clin Oncol 4 : 685-696
5. Kremer B, Henne-Bruns D, Weh HJ et al (1989) Advanced gastric cancer. A new combined surgical and oncological approach. Hepatogastroenterol 36 : 23-26
6. Anderson H, Scarffe JH, Ranson M et al (1991) MMAF for advanced gastric cancer. Eur J Cancer 27 : 1234-1238

Gastric cancer — a place for preoperative induction regional chemotherapy

BY DW Storey, PJ Gallagher, RC Waugh, FO Stephens

Gastric cancer is still amongst the 10 most common causes of cancer death in both sexes even though its incidence in Europe, North America and Australia has been decreasing in recent years [1]. Until recently gastrectomy has been the only treatment offering any real prospect of cure for patients with gastric cancer but when they present and have a diagnosis established in only little more than half of the patients is the tumour localised sufficiently for there to be any prospect of cure by gastrectomy. Five years survival results of patients treated by gastric resection with apparent total removal of the tumour have in the past rarely been reported as better than 25 % [2, 3, 4, 5].

In Japan and Korea where gastric cancer is the most common cancer affecting adult males the situation is quite different. Mass screening campaigns and more intense routine diagnostic techniques have resulted in earlier detection and treatment of the disease with consequent improved 5-years survival statistics after gastrectomy [6, 7]. The remarkable improvements seen in the Japanese studies appear not to have been matched in similar studies in the United States [8].

Whilst the main thrust in preventing death from gastric cancer has been in attempts at cancer prevention especially by better food preservation and dietary practices as well as early detection of disease at a more operable stage, other attemps at improvement have included more radical surgical procedures [2, 9], and radiotherapy in combination with operative surgery [10]. Chemotherapy given post-operatively as adjuvant treatment has also been used in attemps to improve life-expectancy after gastrectomy but proven benefit from this approach has yet to be established [11, 12]. An interesting integrated management approach using early postoperative intraperitoneal Adrimaycin as an adjuvant treatment is presently under study in Washington by Paul Sugarbaker [13].

Induction (Neo-Adjuvant) chemotherapy given prior to operative surgery, especially when given by intra-arterial infusion on a regional basis, in treating advanced localised cancers in other situations has yielded encouraging results [14]. By using a similar approach with delivery of chemotherapy by constant infusion into the coeliac axis for a period of approximately 5 weeks prior to subsequent gastrectomy we have, in our group, improved our 5-years survival for patients with gastric cancer from about of 25 % to about 50 %. The program of chemotherapy used has been a once only dose of BCNU followed by continuous infusion of Adriamycin, Mitomycin-C, and 5-FU on daily rotation [5].

Although encouraged by considerably improved results the former program

---

The Royal Prince Alfred Hospital and the Department of Surgery, The University of Sydney, Sydney, Australia

of preoperative treatment has been expensive in terms of a minimum of 5 weeks preoperation hospitalisation requiring close supervision and continuous monitoring of patients having continuous intra-arterial infusion chemotherapy.

The present paper reports an attempt at making a program of preoperative chemotherapy more economically feasible and hopefully more effective with less demand upon hospital bed usage by the introduction of an intermittent regimen of intra-arterial chemotherapy at 3-week intervals.

Materials and methods

A pilot study of an intermittent chemotherapy regimen was introduced on July 4th 1991. Ten patients (4 males and 6 females) with invasive gastric cancer have been studied to date. No patient with minimal or mucosal disease was included. Pre-operative investigations included gastroscopy with biopsy, CT of chest and abdomen, and laparoscopy. Patients found to have carcinoma in liver, nodes beyond the N2 gastric node drainage or peritoneal seedings were not included in the study.

Radiological catheterisation of the coeliac axis was established via the femoral artery. A guide wire was inserted through the lumen of the catheter further into the coeliac axis or 1 of its branches to hold the catheter in place and avoid its falling out into the aorta. Catheters with multiple side holes in the end 2 cm were used.

After catheterisation gastroscopy was performed and blue dye (Patent Blue or Disulphine Blue) was injected into the catheter during gastroscopy in order to confirm that the flow of agent through the catheter infused the gastric cancer and surrounding gastric tissues.

The regimen of agents used was Mitomycine-C 8 mg/m^2 over 2 hours, then Cisplatinum 80 mg/m^2 over 2 hours, then Adriamycin 40 mg/m^2 over 6 hours followed by 5-FU 500 mg/m^2 daily for 3 days.

Full blood counts were then carried out weekly. Three weeks after commencement of the first treatment a second treatment was given including gastroscopic assessment of the tumour response. A third treatment was carried out approximately 3 weeks after commencing the second treatment giving a total of 3 treatments in all at 3-week intervals.

Three to 4 weeks after the final treatment (provided blood count had returned to within normal limits) total or subtotal radical gastrectomy was carried out at the R2 node clearance level.

Results

Tumour-response

In 1 patient the tumour had apparently completely disappeared after one treatment only. For this reason the total number of cannulations used was 28 rather than the anticipated 30 in this series.

Of the 10 patients 3 showed apparent complete response; in 6 there was partial response and in 1 patient no tumour regression was detected. In no patients was there evidence of tumour progression.

Side-effects

All patients suffered temporary alopecia which in most cases was near complete. All patients experienced nausea for 1-5 days. Bone marrow depression necessitated deferment of treatment on 2 occasions.

Catheter complications

In 28 catherisations the catheters remained in place on 26 occasions. There was need to replace the catheters on 2 occasions. One patient suffered dissection and occlusion of the iliac artery requiring treatment with an internal stent.

Operation complications

Gastrectomy was uneventful in all patients with normal wound healing. There was no evidence of anastomotic leak, however 1 patient developed an intra-abdominal abscess which was drained by aspiration under radiological control and 1 patient suffered a moderate wound infection.

Survival

The period of study is quite short but to date there have been 2 treatment failures. The 1 patient without evidence of tumour response suffered tumour recurrence postoperatively and subsequently died of the disease. One other patient, initially diagnosed as having a *linitis plastica* but with partial response to chemotherapy, subsequently developed recurrent and progressive pelvic disease and died. All of the remaining 8 patients are alive and well to date (3-18 months post-treatment).

Discussion

Although the incidence of gastric cancer has been progressively declining over the past 3 or 4 decades, particularly in Westernised Societies but also in Japan, there is still clearly a need for improved management for those patients who have invasive gastric cancer at the time of initial diagnosis.

The concept of tumour reduction by initial use of regional chemotherapy prior to surgical resection has been shown to be feasible and has been shown to offer potential for significantly improved results [5]. However the management program initially used by our group is time consuming and expensive particularly in the need for continuous hospitalization for 5-6 weeks prior to gastrectomy.

The modified regimen of intermittent induction chemotherapy management was conceived in order to reduce the expense and extensive hospitalisation required and hopefully to increase the tumour response. Although the number of patients studied to date has been small and the period of study has been too short for overall conclusions to be made, the results to date do confirm that the treatment program is practicable and feasible and can be carried out with a low incidence of morbidity. This small series also suggests that the rumour response may be greater than the tumour response achieved by the former and more time consuming and expensive treatment protocol.

These encouraging results achieved to date suggest that such a study is worthy of more intensive investigation in multicentre trials.

Summary and conclusions

In Western Societies gastric cancer still has a poor prognosis. When diagnosed only about half of the patients have a potentially resectable cancer and of those resected only about 25 % of patients have a long-term (5 years) tumour free survival. In Japan and Korea, where the disease is more prevalent, detection at an earlier stage allows a better patient prognosis but in Western Societies the disease is almost invariably infiltrating and comparatively advanced before patients present and the diagnosis is established. Prognosis has been improved in Japan and Korea mainly due to operative treatement at an earlier stage often as a result of mass screening and early investigations of people at special risk. In Western Societies attempts at improving results by the addition of chemotherapy after surgical resection have largely failed. However, attempts at improving prognosis with the use of preoperative induction chemotherapy have been more hopeful [15].

Intra-arterial induction chemotherapy as used in our unit over 16 years has indicated considerable potential for improved prognosis but the use a continuous intra-arterial regimen requiring hospitalization for a period of 5 to 6 weeks is expensive and time-consuming. Since 1991 a new regimen using intermittent intra-arterial infusion of 5-FU, Mitomycine-C and Adriamycin has been used in treating 10 patients with locally advanced, but apparently localised, gastric cancer. Patients have been hospitalized for 4 days only on 3 occasions at 3-week intervals for this treatment. All patients except 1 showed endoscopic regression of the cancer. In 3 patients regression appeared to be complete and in 6 patients there was more than 50 % tumour regression. Morbidity has been low and to date only the patient without response and 1 patient with *linitis plastica*, who had a partial response, developed recurrence after the staged resection. Multi-centre randomised trial studies are warranted.

References

1. Silverger E (1985) Cancer statistics. Cancer 35 : 19-35
2. Scott HW Jr, Adkins RB Jr, Sawyer JL (1985) Results of an aggressive surgical approach to gastric carcinoma during a 23-years period. Surg 97 : 55-59

3. Baddie AW, McBride CM, Balch CM (1989) Gastric cancer. Am J Surg 157 : 595-606
4. De Calan L, Portier G, Ozoux JP et al (1988) Carcinoma of the cardiac and proximal third of the stomach. Results of surgical treatment in Ninety-one consecutive patients. Am J Surg 155 : 481-485
5. Stephens FO (1988). Management of gastric cancer with regional chemotherapy preceding gastrectomy — 5-years survival results. Regional Ca Treat 1 : 80-82
6. Okamura T, Tsujitani S, Korenage D et al (1988) Lymphadenectomy for cure in patients with early gastric cancer and lymph node metastases. Am J Surg 155 : 476-480
7. Yamazaki H, Oshima A, Murakami R et al (1989) A long-term follow-up study of patients with gastric cancer detected by mass screening. Cancer 63 : 613-617
8. Leanert T, Sternberg S, Sprossmann M, De Cosse JJ (1989) Early gastric cancer. Am J Surg 157 : 202-207
9. Salo JA, Saario I, Kibilaakso EO et al (1988) Near total gastrectomy for gastric cancer. Am J Surg 486-489
10. Moertel CG, Childs JS, O'Fallon JR et al (1984) Combined 5-FU and radiation therapy as a surgical adjuvant for poor prognosis gastric carcinoma. J Clin Oncol 2 : 1249-1254
11. Clark PI, Slevin ML (1987) Chemotherapy for stomach cancer. Br Med J 295 : 870-871
12. Fielding JW (1988). The value of multidisciplinary approach in management of gastric cancer. Rec Res Cancer Research 110 : 57-64
13. Sugarbaker PH (1991) Management of gastric cancer. Kluwer Academic Publishiers, Boston
14. Stephens FO, Marsden FW, Storey DW, Thompson JF et al (1991) Developments in surgical oncology — past, present and future trends. Med J Aust 155 : 803-807
15. Stephens FO (1991) Induction chemotherapy using intra-arterial infusion. In : Sugarbakar P (ed) Management of Gastric Cancer. Kluwer Academic Publishers, Boston, pp. 161-170

α-2b-Interferon (IFN) plus chemotherapy in inoperable biliary-tract carcinoma, preliminary data

G Frasci*, M Monaco**, L Cremone***, U Sapio****,
F Faiella****, G Persico*

Biliary tract cancers are relatively uncommon tumors in western countries. However, they represent a significant health problem because of their high lethality [1]. In fact, most of the patients present invasive, inoperable cancer at diagnosis. Generally, the median survival, from diagnosis, of these patients is 6 months. Five-years survival does not exceed 3 % in the largest series.

Chemotherapeutic management of biliary tract cancer has rarely been studied sistematically because of inadequate numbers of patients at individual institutions. Generally, a 30-40 % response rate has been achieved by mono or polychemotherapy, with a median duration of response of 8.5 months. Fluorouracil and Adriamycin seem to be the most effective drugs [2].

Interferons have shown *in vitro* and *in vivo*, a clear antitumor activity. Unfortunately, they did not show significant results when used alone in patients suffering from solid tumors. However, they seem able to potentiate antitumor activity of some cytotoxic drugs, including 5-FU Epirubicin etc. [3, 4].

On the basis of these considerations we started a phase II clinical trial employing an α-2b-Interferon-chemotherapy combination, in patients with locally advanced or metastatic gallbladder or bile duct cancer.

Patients and methods

Twenty-three patients (pts) with histologically confirmed diagnosis of locally advanced or metastatic biliary-tract carcinoma, median age 67 (49-77), received a combined immuno-chemotherapy starting in September 1987. Thirteen had gallbladder and 10 extrahepatic bile-duct cancer. Four out of 23 pts had distant metastases (3 lung and 1 bone). Median ECOG performance status was 1 (0-2).

Fifteen out of 23 pts had obstructive jaundice at diagnosis. Ten out of 15 underwent laparotomy. In 7/10 biliary-intestinal anastomoses were performed. In the remaining only trans-stenotic catheter was positioned. In the 5 other pts showing jaundice, trans-hepatic internal biliary drainage was performed. Treatment consisted of α-2b-IFN subcutaneous administration (3 Mil. IU/m^2 3 times a week) plus weekly intravenous administration of 5-FU (10 mg/kg) and Epydoxorubicin (30 mg/m^2). The treatment was continued until the achieve-

*VII Division of General Surgery, II Faculty of Medicine Naples, Divisions of General Surgery USL 48*** and 50** (SA), Division of Internal Medicine USL 50* (SA), Italy

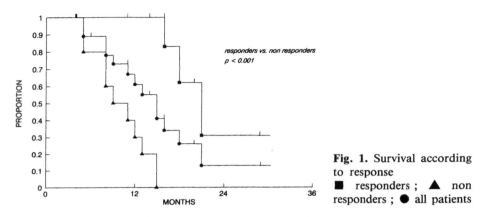

Fig. 1. Survival according to response
■ responders ; ▲ non responders ; ● all patients

ment of complete response or progression of the disease. CT was discontinued after a maximum of 15 courses in the patients showing partial regression of the tumor. Full doses of chemotherapics were administered if WBC > 3.000, platelets > 100.000, Bilirubine < 2 mg, and the hepatic enzymes did not exceed twice the normal values. A 50 % dose reduction was performed if WBC ranged between 2.000 and 3.000, platelets 75,000 and 100,000 and Bilirubin levels 2.5 and 5 mg.

Statistical analysis : survival curves were calculated by using the Kaplan Meier method, and the Mantel Haenszel test have been employed to compare survival of responders and not-responders.

Results

Overall 157 courses have been administered up to now. One patient had to discontinue IFN since grade 3 WHO fatigue. Two pts showed grade 4 leukopenia, but none had to be hospitalized because of the occurrence of sepsis. To date, 20 pts are evaluable for response to treatment. Two complete (1 pt had gallbladder and 1 bile-duct cancer), 5 partial and 2 minor responses for a 45 % overall response-rate (95 % C.I. : 25-65) were observed. Additional 3 pts showed stable disease and 6 progression. Median duration of response was 11 (2+ - 29+)months. Median survival was 14 months, with a 2 year survival rate of 13 % (95 % C.I. : 2-24). Responders showed significantly better outcome than non responders (median 19 v.s. 9 months, chi-square = 16.337, $p < 0.0001$), with a 2 year survival rate of 31 % (95 % C.I. : 7-55) (Fig.1).

Discussion

The role of medical treatments in improving prognosis of advanced biliary tract cancer is still unclear, since the lack of clinical trials in which a large number of patients have been treated. The main purpose of this study was to demonstrate whether the combination of IFN and chemotherapy might achieve a high objective response rate, and significantly lengthen the duration of survival in these patients. We cannot yet draw definite conclusions in this regard, because the number of patients is too small and the follow-up too short. However, we succeeded in achieving near to 50 % clinical objective responses. Moreover, despite the short-term follow-up it is of interest to point out that survival was significantly longer in the responders.

References

1. Nagorney DM, McPherson GAD (1988) Carcinoma of the gallbladder and extrahepatic bile ducts. Sem Oncol 15 : 106-115
2. Falkson G, MacIntyre JM, Moertel CG (1984) Eastern Cooperative Oncology Group experience with chemotherapy for inoperable gallbladder and bile duct cancer. Cancer 54 : 965-969
3. Langyel P (1982) Biochemistry of Interferons and their actions. Ann Rev Biochem 51 : 251-282
4. Wadler S, Schwartz EL (1990) Antineoplastic activity of the combination of Interferon and cytotoxic agents against experimental and human malignancies. A review. Cancer Res 50 : 3473-3486

Abstract. Twenty-three patients with locally advanced or metastatic biliary-tract carcinoma received a IFN-chemotherapy combined treatment starting in September 1987. Thirteen had gallbladder and 10 extrahepatic bile-duct cancer. Treatment consisted of α-2b-IFN (3 Mil. IU/m^2 s.c. 3 times a week) plus weekly i.v. 5-FU (10 mg/kg) and Epydoxorubicin (30 mg/m^2). Overall 157 courses have been administered up to now. One patient had to discontinue IFN since grade 3 WHO fatigue. Two pts showed grade 4 leukopenia, but none had to be hospitalized since the occurrence of sepsis. To date, 20 pts are evaluable for response to treatment. Two complete (1 pt had gallbladder and 1 bile-duct cancer), 5 partial and 2 minor responses for a 45 % overall response-rate (95 % C.I. : 25-65) were observed. Median duration of response was 11 (2+ - 29+)months. Median survival was 14 months, with a 2-years survival rate of 13 % (95 % C.I. : 2-24). Responders showed significantly better outcome than non responders (median 19 v.s. 9 months, chi-square = 16.337, $p < 0.0001$), with a 2-years survival rate of 31 % (95 % C.I. : 7-55).

A phase II study of weekly 48 hours infusion with high-dose Fluorouracil (FU) in colorectal cancer

E Aranda, E Díaz-Rubio, C Camps, C Fernández-Marto, A Carrato, A Antón, A Cervantes, JJ Cruz-Hernández, A Tres, J Belón, J Sánchez, M Garciá-Paredes

Colorectal cancer has been traditionally considered a tumoral type resistant to chemotherapy. During the last decades, 5-Fluorouracil (FU) has been the standard single agent treatment of colon and rectum cancer with a low response rate (not higher than 20 %) and without significant effect on survival [1, 2]. Combination chemotherapy has not yet shown significant benefit over FU alone [3]. However, the utilization of daily [4] or weekly 48-hours infusion FU [5, 6] allows to increase the maximal tolerated dose (MTD). We recently pointed out [7] that weekly high-dose 48-hours continous infusion FU can be given at a dose of 3.5 mg/m^2. The limiting toxicities were diarrhea and mucositis. The response rate of previously untreated patients was 43 %. On this basis the TTD Group (Spanish Cooperative Group for the treatment of Gastro-Intestinal Tumors) decided to start on June 90 a phase II study with weekly high-dose 48-hours infusion FU (3.5 gr/m^2).

Patients and methods

All patients entered in this study had histollogically proven colorectal carcinoma, were previously untreated and had at least 1 bidimensionally measurable lesion confirmed by Rx, TAC or ultrasonography (ECHO). Karnofsky index > 70 %, age < 75 years, expectancy of life at least of 2 months, leukocytes > 4.000/mm^3, platelets > 150.000/mm^3, bilirrubin < 1.5 mg/dl and Creatinine < 1.2 mg/dl were other inclusion criteria.

After giving their informed consent, 89 patients have been entered in the study (Table 1) and received a weekly 3.5 mg/m^2 of FU in 48-hours infusion by portable pumps or central catheter. Treatment was continued until progression or unacceptable toxicity.

Toxicity was assessed weekly and a minimum of 6 weeks on treatment was required for the evaluation of response.

Toxicity and response were defined according to WHO grade criteria [8]. At entry, all patients were required to have complete history and physical examination, tumoral measure (Rx, TAC, ECHO), complete blood count, ionogram, liver and renal function tests and CEA levels assessment.

E Aranda, Medical Oncology Service, University Hospital « Reina Sofía », Avenida Menendez Pidal s/n, 14001 Córdoba, Spain

Table 1. Patient characteristics

Parameter	N° patients
Entered	89
Evaluable for response	83
Evaluable for toxicity	86
Median age (range years)	60 (34-75)
Primary tumor	
Colon	47
Rectum	42
Previous treatment	
Radical/palliative surgery	77/4
Radiotherapy	6
Histologycal grade G2-G3	28
ECOG 0	42
1	32
2	14
DFI = 0	41

Results

Of 89 patients included in this study 83 were evaluable for response and 86 for toxicity, the median age was 60 (34-75). At entry, 74 patients had an acceptable performance status (ECOG 0-1). The median number of cycles administered per patient was 12 (1-60). Fifty-three patients had liver metastases, 18 lung metastases, 25 local relapse and 16 a primary tumor. Objective responses were obtained in 38.5 % (32/83) of the patients with a confidence limit at 95 % equal to 28-50 %. 8 % achieved complete response and 24 % partial response and no change was observed in 45 % of the patients. Referring responses by site of disease (Table 2) : liver metastases 17 of 53 patients with objective response (32 %), local relapse 7 of 25 responses (28 %) and lung metastases 4 of 18 (22 %).

Table 2. Localization and response

Localization	Responses
Liver	17/53 (32 %)
Local relapse	7/25 (28 %)
Lung	4/18 (22 %)
Peritoneal	0/8 (0 %)
Bone	0/7 (0 %)
Lymp node	2/6 (33 %)
Abdominal	2/4 (50 %)
Subcutaneous	1/2 (50 %)

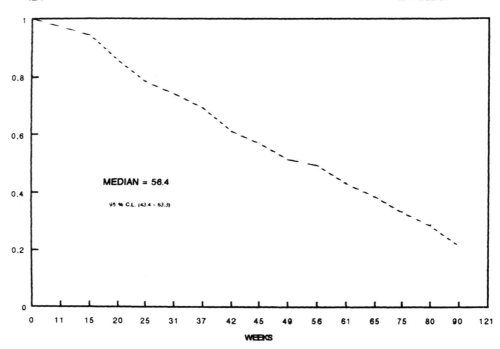

Fig. 1. Time to progression

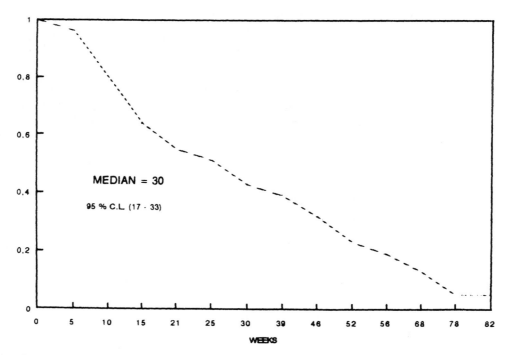

Fig. 2. Overall survival

The median time of follow-up was 50 weeks. The median time to progression was 30 weeks (Fig. 1) and the median survival was 56.5 weeks (Fig. 2) with 17 % of patients alive at 2 years follow-up.

The limiting toxicity, as reported (Table 3), was diarrhea with 10 % G-3 and 2 % G-4, and G-3/G-4 mucositis in 11 % of the cases. Two cases developed G3-G4 leukopenia and 5 patients presented hand-foot symdrome (5.5 %).

Table 3. Toxicity

Parameter	G3 (%)	G4 (%)
Nausea	2	1
Emesis	3	0
Diarrhea	10	2
Fever	1	1
Mucositis	11	0
Phlebitis	4,5	0
Hand-foot syndrome	2	3
Infection	0	2
Leukopenia	1	1
Anemia	3	1
Trombopenia	0	1

Discussion

The optimal FU schedule in advanced colorectal cancer, needs to be still defined, in spite of the numerous studies performed with FU alone. It has been accepted an average of response rate of 20 % [1] and myelosupression is the dose-limiting toxicity [8, 9].

The introduction of continuous infusion in the treatment of colorectal cancer is recent. Prospective and randomized trials have demonstrated higher response rates and activity in the continuous infusion FU than bolus FU regimens [5, 7], but the impact on survival is poor [10].

The utilization of continuous infusion FU (300 mg/day) [4] has been shown superior to the bolus FU 500 mg/m^2/day × 5 days every 5 weeks regimen with a response rate of 30 % and 7 % respectively.

Apparently, weekly 48-hours infusion FU seems to be superior to other FU regimens with lower toxicity [2, 3, 4, 5]. In the same way, it has also been reported that high-dose continuous infusion FU (60 mg/m^2) was well tolerated [5, 6].

The concept of biochemical modulation has been introduced in the treatment of colorectal cancer and represents a promising field to be explored. Four of 7 randomized studies with FU and Leucovorin (LV) versus FU alone, have shown higher response rate with the combination. In 2 studies survival was increased [12, 13, 14, 15, 16, 17, 18]. LV provides a source of reduced folates to the cell, promoting the binding of FdUMP to thymidylate synthetase.

Last year, a meta-analysis of all randomized studies that had been performed with FU alone versus FU + LV confirmed the superiority of the combination regimen regarding to response rate, but impact on survival was not significant, probably due to a low overall survival and to the fact that at progression 20 % of the patients treated with FU alone were rescued with FU + LV [19].

In our study an overall response rate of 38.5 % was obtained with a confidence limits at 95 % equal to 28-50 %, achieving a median dose intensity of 3 gr/m^2/week, the limiting toxicities were diarrhea (G3 10 %, G4 2 %) and mucositis (11 %). The response rate with the combination regimen is higher than the standard FU alone. It seems that the activity of weekly high-dose 48 hours infusion FU is similar to the FU + LV regimen, the levels of FdUMP achieved with high-doses FU could be similar to both regimens.

There is a lot of controversy about the utilization of continuous infusion FU or biomodulated regimens. The most important questions raised are : 1- Optimal duration of infusion and its relationship to dose intensity. 2- The relative cost of the infusion FU in comparison with bolus FU (which is usually combined with LV and Interferon).

The obvious benefit of the utilization of continuous infusion FU instead of standard treatment with FU alone is the quadrupling the overall response rates and amelioration of toxicity even if the response rates achieved were similar to modulated FU.

At the same time, it has been demonstrated that the duration of treatment is associated with dose intensity which is related to response rate [20].

Further prospective, randomized studies comparing continuous infusion FU regimens with different duration of treatments are needed to define the best continuous schedule. It is also important to know which are the possibilities of modulating the weekly high-dose 48-hours continuous infusion FU with LV. Trying to answer these questions TTD. Group has started other study in colorectal cancer.

References

1. Carte SK (1976) Large bowel cancer. The current status of treatment. J Natl Cancer Inst 56 : 3-10
2. Cohen AM, Shank B, Friedman M (1989) Colorectal cancer. In : de Vita VT, Hellman SY, Rosenberg SA (eds) Cancer : Principles and Practice of Oncology. Lippincott Co., 3rd Edition, Philadelphia, pp. 895-952
3. Diaz-Rubio E (1990) Avances en el tratamiento del cáncer colorectal avanzado. Rev Clin Esp 186 : 68-76
4. Lokich JL, Alhgren JD, Gullo JJ et al (1989) A prospective randomized comparison of continuous infusion Fluorouracil with a conventional bolus schedule in metastatic colorectal carcinoma : a mid-Atlantic Oncology Program Study. J Clin Oncol 7 : 425-432
5. Shah A, MacDonald W, Goldie J et al (1985) 5-FU infusion advanced colorectal : a comparison of three dose schedules. Cancer Treat Rep 69 : 739-742
6. Blijham GH, Bleiberg H, Duez N et al (1989) EORTC experience with very high-dose Fluorouracil. Pre EORTC symposiums on Advanced in Gastrointestinal Tract Cancer Research and Treatment, Frankfurt

7. Diaz-Rubio E, Aranda E, Martín M et al (1990) Weekly high-dose infusion of 5-Fluorouracil in advanced colorectal cancer. Eur J Cancer 26 : 727-729
8. Miller AB, Hoogstraten B, Staquet M, Winkler A (1981) Reporting results of cancer treatment. Cancer 47 : 207-214
9. Moertel CG (1975) Clinical management of advanced gastrointestinal cancer. Cancer 36 : 675-682
10. Ansfiled F, Klots J, Nealon T et al (1977) A phase III study comparing the clinical utility of four regimens of 5-Fluorouracil. Cancer 39 : 34-40
11. Lokin JJ, Colon and rectal cancer (1990) In : Lokich JJ (ed) Cancer chemotherapy by infusion. Precept Press, 2nd Ed., Chicago, pp. 323-339
12. Poon MA, Onconell MJ, Moertel CG et al (1989) Biochemical modulation of Fluorouracil : evidence of significant improvement of survival and quality of life in patients with advanced colorectal carcinoma. J Clin Oncol 7 : 1407-1417
13. Petrerrera L, Rustum Y et al (1987) N H Prospective randomized trial of 5-Fluorouracil v.s. 5-Fluorouracil and high-dose Leucovorin v.s. 5-Fluorouracil and Methotrexate in previously untreated patients with advanced colorectal carcinoma. J Clin Oncol 5 : 1559-1565
14. Erlichman C, Fine S, Wong A, Elhakim T (1988) A randomized trial of 5-Fluorouracil and Folnic acid in patients with metastatic colorectal carcinoma. J Clin Oncol 6 : 469-475
15. Nobile MT, Vidilli MG, Sobrero A et al (1988) 5-Fluorouracil alone or combined with high-dose Folnic acid in advanced colorectal cancer patients : A randomized trial. Proc Am Soc Clin Oncol 7 : 97
16. Doroshow JH, Bertrand P, Multhauf P et al (1987) Prospective randomized trial comparing 5-FU versus high-dose Folnic acid for treatment of advanced colorectal cancer. Proc Am Soc Clin Oncol 6 : 96
17. Valone FH, Friedman NA, Wittlinger PS et al (1989) Treatment of patients with advanced colorectal carcinoma with Fluorouracil alone, high-dose Leucovorin plus Fluorouracil or sequential Methotrexate, Fluorouracil and Leucovorin : A randomized trial of the Northern California Oncology Group. J Clin Oncol 7 : 1427-1436
18. Petrelli N, Douglass HO, Herrera M et al (1989) The modulation of Fluorouracil with Leucovorin in metastatic colorectal carcinoma. A prospective randomized phase III trial. J Clin Oncol 7 : 1419-1426
19. Piedbois P, Buyse M, Rustum Y et al (1992) Modulation of Fluorouracil by Leucovorin in patients with advanced colorectal cancer : Evidence in terms of response rate. J Clin Oncol 10 : 896-903
20. Anderson N, Lokich J (1992) Controversial issues in 5-Fluorouracil infusion use. Dose intensity treatment duration and cost comparisons. Cancer 70, 4 : 998-1002 (suppl)

Phase II trial of Fluorouracil, Leucovorin and Interferon-α

RM Bukowski, V Gibson, S Murthy, D McLain, T Olencki, GT Budd

Recent reports of randomized clinical trials have demonstrated the combination of Folinic acid (LV) and Fluorouracil (5-FU) may have superior therapeutic value compared to 5-FU alone [1, 2]. The biochemical basis is the enhanced inhibition of DNA synthesis by the binding of 5-Fluoro-Deoxyuridine monophosphate to thymidilate synthetase in the presence of 5, 10 Methylene Tetrahydrofolate [3].

It has also been reported there is synergistic cytotoxic activity when 5-FU and Interferon are combined *in vitro* and tested against a variety of murine and human cell lines [4, 5]. The exact biochemical mechanism for this therapeutic enhancement has not been clearly defined. Several possibilities include the enhanced inhibition of Thymidine kinase activity and Thymidine's incorporation into DNA [6], inhibition of Thymidilate synthetase [7] and the abrogation of tumor resistance to natural killer cell cytotoxicity by 5-FU [8]. Studies with this combination reported response rates of 26 to 76 % in patients with metastatic colorectal cancer [9-12]. The interactions of all 3 agents *in vitro* have also been examined in several human colon cancer cell lines [13]. Further potentiation of cytotoxicity was noted, and interactions at the level of Thymidilate synthetase a DNA were proposed as mechanisms.

In view of this data, and the *in vitro* pre-clinical data a phase I clinical trial of 5-FU, IFNα and Leucovorin (LV) was performed at The Cleveland Clinic Foundation [14]. The Maximum Tolerated Dose, defined as the dose level below which 3 of 6 patients developed grade 3 or 4 toxicity during cycle 1, was determined and a phase II trial to assess the response rate was initiated in 1989.

Patients and methods

Study design

Therapy consisted of 5 consecutive days of administration of bolus intravenous 5-FU and Leucovorin (LV), with Interferon-α given subcutaneously. The rHuIFNα-2b utilized in this trial was obtained from Schering-Plough, Kenilworth, NJ, the 5-FU was commercially obtained from Hoffman LaRoche, Nutley, NJ, and the LV from Lederle Laboratories, Pearle River, NY. The treatment schema consisted of fixed doses of rHuIFN-2b/4 × 10^6/u/m², 5-FU 430 mg/m², and LV 200/mg/m² administered in an out patient setting. Week-

---

Experimental Therapeutics Program, Cleveland Clinic Cancer Center, Cleveland, Ohio 44195 ly evaluations of toxicity and complete blood counts with differential smears were performed with each cycle (28 days). Additional cycles of therapy were given when the white blood cell count (WBC) was ≥ 4.000/ul, platelets > 100.000/ul, the absolute granulocytes > 1.500/ul, and all gastrointestinal side-effects related to the previous cycle of therapy had resolved. Dose escalation of the study drugs was not permitted. Dose reductions of 5-FU and IFN-α were made in subsequent cycles as follows : 25 % for ≥ Grade II gastrointestinal toxicity or 50 % for ≥ Grade 3/4 hematologic toxicity.

Patient selection criteria

Patients (≥ 18 years) with metastatic adenocarcinoma of the colon or rectum, with histologic proof of malignancy and measurable disease were eligible. No chemotherapy for metastatic disease was allowed, but patients with prior radiation were eligible. A performance status (PS) of ≤ 2 (Eastern Cooperation Group), and a life expectancy of at least 6 months were required. Adequate organ function was required and was defined as a WBC ≥ 4.000/ul, ANC ≥ 2.000/ul, a platelet count ≥ 100.000 /ul, serum creatinine ≤ 1.5 mg/dl, and a serum Bilirubin ≤ 1.5 mg/dl. Exclusion criteria included a history of brain metastases, a second malignancy (with the exception of carcinoma *in situ* of the cervix, basal or squamous cell carcinoma of the skin, and transitional cell of the bladder) within 5 years of study entry, severe cardiac disease (New York Heart Association Class III or IV) or serious cardiac arrhythmia, and/or, pregnancy. Informed consent was obtained as required by Institutional and National Cancer Instituted guidelines.

All pre-treatment parameters were repeated every 28 days, with the exception of CT scans which were repeated every 56 days.

Response criteria

A complete response was defined as disappearance of all clinically detectable tumor for a minimum of 4 weeks. A partial response of malignant hepatomegaly consisted of a 30 % decrease in the sum of liver measurements below the costal margin(s) in the midclavicular lines and xiphoid process or a 50 % decrease of the sums of the products of the perpendicular diameters of all measured lesions for at least 4 weeks. Progressive disease included appearance of new lesions or greater than 25 % increase in the sum of the products of individual measured lesions. The duration of response was measured from the time of response to progression.

Results

Twenty-nine patients were entered into the study between November 1989 and December 1992, and 28 are evaluable at present. The median age of the patients was 61 years (range 35 to 82 years), 17 being male and 11 being females. The performance status of the group was as follows : 0 : 15 (54 %), 1 : 10 (36 %) and 2 : 3 (10 %). The median number of cycles administered was 5, with a range of 1 to 17. All patients completed at least 1 course of therapy and 27 are evaluable for response (1 too early) and 28 for toxicity. There were 9 (32 %, 95 % C.I., 16 - 52 %) partial responders to therapy (Table 1). The median time to response was 12 weeks and median response duration was 32 weeks. Responding sites included lung 5, liver 4, and pelvic mass 1. The median survival for all patients is 49 weeks.

Table 1. 5FU/Leucovorin/IFN-α. Responding patients

Patient No.	Site of response	Time to response (wks)	Duration of response (wks)	Site of progression
35	Lung	8	25	Lung
57	Liver	12	9	Liver
58	Lung	16	24	Lung
61	Rectum	16	49	Rectum
65	Liver Lung	16 8	37 44	Liver
66	Liver	8	32	Liver
67	Lung	18	42+	----
70	Lung	5	38	Lung Subcutaneous (scalp)
71	Liver	8	37+	----

The toxicity of 5-FU, LV and IFN-α therapy has been moderate in nature. The majority of the 28 patients experienced mild fatigue (39 %), skin reaction (35 %), anorexia (39 %) and fever with chills (75 %). The most frequent toxicities were hematologic, gastrointestinal, and hepatic. Gastrointestinal toxicity in the form of Grade 1-2 diarrhea occurred in 19 (68 %) of the patients. Nausea and vomiting was seen 13 (46 %) patients. Mucositis was the most common toxicity seen and occurred in 23 (82 %) patients. Hepatic toxicity in the form of increased serum alkaline phosphate was seen 15 (54 %) patients. This was moderate to severe in 5 instance, but was unrelated to therapy and secondary to disease progression. Hematologic toxicity appeared as anemia (89 %), leukopenia (60 %), neutropenia (68 %) and thrombocytopenia (25 %). A normochromic, normocytic anemia was seen in 24 patients which was mild to moderate and did not require transfusions. Grade 3 and 4 neutropenia was seen in 9 patients, requiring a 50 % dose adjustment of the 5-FU and IFN-α dose. Thrombocytopenia was mild to moderate and occurred in 7 patients.

Overall most toxicities abated with the cessation of the treatment and the majority were moderate. Dose reductions of 5-FU and IFN-α were required in 82 % of patients. No treatment related deaths were seen.

Discussion

The combination of Fluorouracil, Leucovorin and Interferon-α as administered in this study was well tolerated. Dose reductions for mucositis or neutropenia were required in most patients, and generally this occurred after the initial cycle of treatment. The majority of these were for mucositis, and no treatment related deaths or life threatening toxicity was seen.

The results seen in this study suggest the regimen is active, and response rates resemble those reported for the combinations of 5-FU and Leucovorin or 5-FU and Interferon. The most relevant comparison however is with the five day regimen of 5-FU and Leucovorin which utilized similar dose levels of 5-FU and Leucovorin [15]. Response rates in our trial and that of Erhlichman et al [15] are similar (32 v.s. 33 %). Survivals are likewise comparable (12.6 months v.s. 49 weeks). Direct comparisons will require randomized trials, and in view of the clinical *in vitro* data these appear reasonable.

References

1. Poon MA, O'Connell MJ, Moertel CG et al (1989) Biochemical modulation of Fluorouracil evidence of significant improvement of survival and quality of life in patients with advanced colorectal carcinoma. J Clin Oncol 7 : 1407-1418
2. Erlichman C, Fine S, Wong A et al (1988) A randomized trial of Fluorouracil and Folnic acid in patients with metastatic colorectal carcinoma. J Clin Oncol 6 : 469-475
3. Danenberg PV, Danenberg KD (1978) Effect of 5,10 Methylene-Tetrahydrofolate on the disassociation of 5-Fluor-2-Deoxyuridylate from Thymidylate synthetase : Evidence for an ordered mechanism. Biochemistry 17 : 4018-4024
4. Stolfi RL, Martin DS (1985) Modulation of chemotherapeutic drug activity with Polyribonucleotide or with Interferon. J Biol Response Modif 4 : 634-639
5. Namba M, Muyoshi T, Kanamosi T, Nobuhara M, Kimoto T, Ogawa S (1982) Combined effects of 5-Fluorouracil and Interferon on proliferation of human neoplastic cells in culture. Dann 73 : 819-824
6. Dewert DR, Shah S, Clemens MJ (1981) Inhibition of cell division by Interferons : changes in the transport and intracellular metabolism of the Thymidine in human lymphoblastoid (Daudi) cell. Eur J Biochem 116 : 487-492
7. Elias L, Crussman HA (1988) Interferon effects upon the Adenocarcinoma 38 and HL-60 cell lines : Antiproliferature responses and synergistic interactions with halogenated Pyrimidine antimetabolites. Cancer Res 48 : 4868-4873
8. Neefe J, Glass J (1991) Abrogation of Interferon-induced resistance to Interferon activated major histo-compatibility complex unrestricted killers by treatment of a melanoma cell line with 5-Fluorouracil. Cancer Res 51 : 3159-3163
9. Ajani JA, Rios AA, Ende K, Abbruzzese JL, Edwards C, Faintuch JS, Shah S, Gutterman J, Levin BJ (1989) Phase I and Phase II studies of the combination

of recombinant human Interferon-γ and 5-Fluorouracil in patients with advanced colorectal carcinoma. J Biol Response Modif 8 : 140-146
10. Wadler SW, Schwartz EL, Goldman M (1989) Fluorouracil and recombinant Interferon-α-2A : an active regimen against advanced colorectal carcinoma. J Clin Oncol 7 : 1769-1775
11. Pazdur R, Ajani JA, Patt YZ, Winn R, Jackson D, Shepard B, DuBrow R, Campos L, Quaraiski M, Faintuch J, Abbruzzese JL, Gutterman J, Levin B (1990) Phase II study of Fluorouracil and recombinant Interferon-α-2A in previously untreated advanced colorectal carcinoma. J Clin Oncol 12 : 2027-2031
12. Kenny N, Younes A, Sertar K, Kelsen D, Sammarco P, Adams L, Derby S, Murray P, Houston C (1990) Interferon-α-2A and 5-Fluorouracil for advanced colorectal carcinoma : assessment of activity and toxicity. Cancer 66 : 2470-2475
13. Houghton JA, Adkins DA et al (1991) Interaction between 5-Fluorouracil [6RS] Leucovorin and recombinant human Interferon-α-2A in cultured colon adenocarcinoma cells. Cancer Comm 3 : 225-231
14. Bukowski RM, Inoshita G, Yalavarthi P, Murthy S, Gibson V, Budd GT, Sergi J, Bauer L, Prestifilippo J (1992) A Phase I trial of 5-Fluorouracil Folnic acid and α-2A-Interferon in patients with metastatic colorectal carcinoma. Cancer 69 (4) : 889-892
15. Erlichman C, Fine S, Wang A, Elkakin T (1988) A randomized trial of Fluorouracil and Folnic acid in patients with metastatic colorectal carcinoma. J Clin Oncol 6 : 469-475

Continuous simultaneous intra-arterial and intravenous therapy of liver metastases of colorectal carcinoma. Results of a prospective randomized study

F Safi, KH Link, HG Beger

In about 25 % of patients with colorectal cancer liver metastases are already apparent when the carcinoma is established; in a further 30 % to 40 % of patients, metachronic metastases of a primary tumor settle in the liver, leading to the conclusion that liver metastases should be regarded as a significant factor in the prognostication of colorectal carcinoma [1]. When compared with systemic therapy, hepatic arterial chemotherapy significantly increases the response rate of hepatic metastases arising from colorectal carcinoma and appears to be a more effective treatment [5].

In the last years, the literature shows that response rates of liver metastases to regional intra-arterial perfusion of FUDR can vary between 43 % and 80 %. On the basis of these rates, median survival time is said to range between 17 and 26 months [6, 9]. The literature reports different incidence rates, ranging from 42 % to 75 %, concerning the occurrence of extrahepatic metastases after beginning the regional chemotherapy. It is the formation of metastases that causes the death of most patients, even those responding to regional chemotherapy [7, 8].

The role of continuous hepatic-artery infusion of the liver and, in addition, systemic therapy in the adjuvant setting is a related area of investigation. This study addresses both issues in a randomized prospective fashion in an attempt to establish the efficacy of both regional and systemic therapy using FUDR in the treatment of isolated hepatic metastases from colorectal cancer. The aim of additionally applied adjuvant systemic therapy is to delay or prevent occurrence of extrahepatic metastases during the course of regional chemotherapy.

Patients and methods of treatment

All patients with histologically confirmed adenocarcinoma of the colon and rectum who had measurable hepatic metastases were eligible for the study. Entry requirements included a Karnofsky performance status of 60 % or more and no evidence of extrahepatic disease. The localisation of colorectal cancer, postoperative tumor stage and volume of metastases are shown in Table 1. The 71 patients were stratified by primary tumor stage (TNM classification) and the percent of liver involvement (< 50 % compared with > 50 %) and were then randomly assigned before surgery to receive either intrahepatic or intrahepatic and systemic therapy. The i.a. group (n = 34) were treated only intra-

---

Department of General Surgery, University of Ulm Steinhövelstr. 9, 7900 Ulm, Germany arterially. In the i.a./i.v. group (n = 37), i.a./i.v. dual catheter Infusaid pumps were implanted. The characteristics of the patients are shown in Table 1. The patients in the 2 randomized groups were comparable with respect to the stage of primary tumor, metastatic spread in the liver, age and sex. Preoperative evaluation of the patients, surgical technique of i.a. and dual i.a./i.v. pump-implantation and monitoring of the therapy have been described before [2, 3, 4, 6].

Table 1. Patient characteristics

	Total n = 71	Randomized study	
		IA n = 34	IA/IV n = 37
Age (years)*			
Min-Max	36-77	46-72	40-73
Average	57	58	57
Sex* male	24	n = 13	n = 11
Female	47	n = 21	n = 26
Localisation of primary tumor*			
rectum	35	17	18
Sigma	19	12	7
colon	17	5	12
Primary tumor stage*			
$T_{1-3} N_0$	33	15	18
$T_{1-3} N_1$	30	15	15
$T_{1-3} N_2$	8	4	4
Volume of metastases*			
<50 % of liver volume	56	27	29
>50 % of liver volume	15	7	8

Dept. of General Surgery, University of Ulm, Germany   * = NS

No patient had previously been treated with cytostatic drugs. The FUDR therapy was initiated on the 8th to the 14th day after pump implantation. FUDR was the basic chemotherapeutic agent (0.2 mg/kg/day) administered in 2-week cycles alternating with double distilled water. This was the dose administered to all patients who had ia pumps. Patients with i.a./i.v. pumps were given FUDR at a dose of 0.3 mg/kg/day, during the course of which 0.21 mg/kg was infused intraarterially (regionally) and 0.09 mg/kg intravenously (systemically). Thus, the regional dose was the same in both the i.a. and i.a./i.v. group. We refer to « chemical hepatitis » when a 2-fold increase of 2 liver parameters above the normal values (GOT, GPT, APH, γ-GT) is present. Biliary sclerosis indicates bilirubinemia and strictures of the biliary truct ; intrahepatic tumor progression and metastases in the liver hilum must be excluded. Patients follow-up was supervised regularly in the outpatient department and sometimes by the patients general practitioner.

Statistics : Patient survival time from the time of pump implantation was calculated in accordance with Kaplan-Meier [10]. The test of Mantel and Haenzel was used for comparison of survival rates [11]. For categorical variables, the chi-squared test and Fisher exact test were used [12].

Results

FUDR Toxicity (Table 2). In 23 % of the patients, gastroduodenitis or duodenal ulcers occurred. In 52 % of the patients, a 2-fold elevation above the standard values of liver parameters was observed. The elevation was due to a chemical hepatitis resulting from the FUDR medication. This risk increases proportionally according to duration and dosage of FUDR. In an additional 17 patients (24 %), a sclerosing cholangitis could be detected by means of ERCP or PTC after elevation of serum Bilirubin. Eight patients (2 in the i.a. group, 6 in the i.a./i.v. group) complained of diarrhea that was severe enough for them to be hospitalized for hydration. Stomatitis, which was cured after reduction of FUDR dosage, was seen in 4 patients (1 in the i.a. and 3 in the i.a./i.v. group). Myelosuppression, alopecia and emesis did not occur with either treatment (i.a. and i.a./i.v.). Gastrointestinal tract and liver toxicities were not significantly different between the i.a. and i.a./i.v. treated patients.

Table 2. FUDR-Toxicity

	Total		Randomized study*			
	n = 71	%	IA n = 34	%	IA/IV n = 37	%
Stomatitis	4	6	1	3	3	8
Diarrhea	8	11	2	6	6	16
Ulcer/Gasrtritis	16	23	7	20	9	24
Chemical hepatitis	37	52	18	53	19	51
Sclerosing cholang	17	24	8	24	9	24

Dept. of General Surgery, University of Ulm, Germany   * = NS, p>0.1

With regard to the development of intrahepatic metastases, the control angio-CT scans showed a complete response in 14 patients. Another 27 patients showed a reduction in metastatic volume by more than 25 %. In 17 other cases no change in metastatic size was seen via a CT-scan. Progression of metastases in spite of FUDR therapy was also observed in 13 patients (Table 3). In accordance with the identical intra-arterial dose, the metastases in both groups (i.a., i.a./i.v.) responded equally to regional chemotherapy. During treatment 79 % (n = 27) of the i.a. and 51 % (n = 19) of the i.a./i.v. group developed extrahepatic metastases whose localisations are given in Table 4. This spreading of the carcinoma was found in a median observation period of 24 months. The difference between the 2 randomized groups is significant at that point in time (p < 0.01). The difference in extrahepatic diseasefree survival was significant between the two randomized groups (Fig. 1).

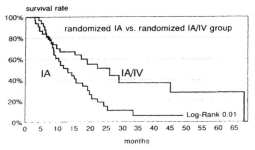

Fig. 1. Extrahepatic disease free survival

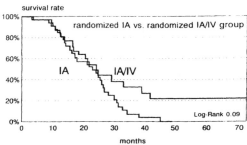

Fig. 2. Survival IA vs. IA/IV

Table 3. Response CT-Scan

	Total		Randomized study*			
			IA		IA/IV	
	n = 71	%	n = 34	%	n = 37	%
Complete Remission	14	6	1	3	3	8
Partial Remission	27	38	14	41	13	35
Stable Disease	17	24	8	23	9	24
Progression	13	18	6	18	7	19

Duration of response of liver metastases

Median (Min-Max) Month	Compl. remission 15 (6-39)	Part. remission 14 (6-27)	Stable disease 15 (6-24)

Dept. of General Surgery, University of Ulm, Germany   * = NS, p>0.1

Table 4. Extrahepatic spread of metastases

Randomized study*

	Total n = 71	IA n = 34	IA/IV n = 37
Extrahepatic metastases	46 (65 %)	27 (79 %)	19 (51 %)
Location of metastases			
Lung	24	11	13
Bone	2	—	2
Peritoneum	14	10	4
Pelvis	5	5	—
Cerebrum	1	1	—
Follow-up period (month)			
Median (Min-Max)	24 (2-72)	24 (3-49)	24 (2-72)

Dept. of General Surgery, University of Ulm, Germany   * = p<0.01

No significant difference in survival rate was found between the i.a. and i.a./i.v. treated patients (Fig. 2). The one year survival rate was 80 %, 2 years survival rate 55 % in each group and 5 years survival rate was 21 % in the i.a./i.v. and 0 % in the i.a. group.

Discussion

The efficacy of hepatic-artery infusion of FUDR, using a implantable pump, for the treatment of hepatic metastases from primary colorectal carcinoma, has yet to be proven in a prospective, randomized study. Several preliminary reports have observed varied response rates and survival times with this treatment. The advantage of this type of therapy has been controversial up to now. The main reason is the development of extrahepatic metastases which are responsible for the patient's death [7, 14]. Patients in the randomized study were stratified by the percent of liver involvement and primary colorectal cancer stage. The i.a. and i.a./i.v. arms were well matched by these important prognostic factors, as well as by other prognostic values, such as initial liver function tests and CEA serum levels.

Surgical implantation of the pump and insertion of the catheter do not cause mortality or any major morbidity. The pumps were accepted by the majority of patients, who were able to continue their usual work and daily activities. Skin necrosis in the region of the pump sideports was treated successfully in 3 patients by transposition and subfascial placing of the pump in another abdominal region.

Side effects due to regional chemotherapy did occur during treatment. Gastritis or duodenal ulcers and, in some patients induced cellular atypias, all of which followed the chemotherapy, are probably due to the antimitotic effect of FUDR [15, 16]. The time of occurrence of epigastric pain was, according to our observations, independent of duration and dosage of FUDR therapy [13]. Incidence of gastritis, as quoted in the literature, is variable between 15 % and 56 % [6, 7, 17]; in our patient population it was 23 %. The reported difference in the incidence is linked to the question of whether a regular gastroscopy was carried out or whether this was performed only when symptoms appeared. Chemical cholecystitis, whose incidence was 25 % [18], can be avoided by routine cholecystectomy during implantation of the pump. According to the literature, chemical hepatitis occurs in 13 % to 83 % of the patients [6, 18]; in our group it was 52 %. It subsides when the FUDR dose is reduced or the therapy discontinued. The difference in the reported frequency stems from the fact that no uniform definition for chemical hepatitis yet exists. Bilirubinemia must be excluded since it is caused only by progression of the intrahepatic metastases, by malignant occlusion of the bile duct or by sclerosing cholangitis.

As a result of FUDR infusion, biliary strictures (sclerosing cholangitis) of the intra- and extrahepatic bile ducts developed. This occurred independent of duration and dosage of the FUDR therapy. In the literature, the incidence rate varies between 17 % and 25 % [19]. In our patients it was 24 %. The pathogenesis of this complication is not yet known. The best marker for early detection of sclerosing cholangitis is a short-term determination of Bilirubin in serum. This assumption relates to the fact that the other liver parameters were elevated in more than 50 % of the patients who did not have any signs of sclerosing cholangitis.

The additional intravenous administration of FUDR in a dose of 0.09 mg/kg/day in the i.a./i.v. group did not cause further significant systemic side effects when compared to the i.a. group. The FUDR toxicity, both regional and systemic, was the same in both groups.

Evaluation of the response of hepatic metastases of this type of therapy was carried out by estimating several parameters : patients survival time, arterial angio-CT and follow-up of CEA. The i.a. and i.a./i.v. groups responded similarly to chemotherapy (59 % v.s. 57 % CT criteria, respectively). This observation is not surprising since, prior to the therapy onset, the metastatic spread in the 2 groups had been identical and the FUDR intra-arterial dose amounted to 0.2 mg/kg/day in the i.a. resp. i.a./i.v. treated patients. The literature documents different response rates : Balch et al report 80 % [6], Niederhuber et al 83 % [7] and Cohen et al 51 % [9]. This discrepancy is the result of response criteria that are not yet uniform.

The i.v. therapy in the adjuvant setting appeared to prevent extrahepatic spread of metastases which occur during regional therapy. In 79 % in the randomized i.a. group and in only 51 % in the randomized i.a./i.v. group, extrahepatic tumor progression occurred. This difference is statistically significant ($p < 0.01$). The literature shows high-rates concerning the frequency of extrahepatic metastases after the onset of regional chemotherapy. Balch et al report an incidence of 42 % [6], Niederhuber et al 73 % [7], Rothmund et al 77 % [20] and Kemeny et al 56 % [5]. Ultimately, most patient deaths, even among those who responded to regional chemotherapy, result from extrahepatic metastases. Owing to the high incidence of patients with extrahepatic carcinoma spread (42 % to 77 %) regional as well as systemic chemotherapy is indicated. The success of this additional therapeutic principle can be expected particularly in patients responding to regional chemotherapy.

Using the pump catheter system and treatment with FUDR, Balch and Urist [6] achieved a median survival time of 26 months, and Ensminger et al reported 21 months [21]. The response rate in their studies was above 80 %. In all of our patients (n = 71) the response rate was 57 % CT criteria. Median survival time of these patients is 24 months since the beginning of the therapy. We could not find an improvement of short term survival in the 2 randomized groups during the 36-months period. Later (long term survival), however, only 6 % of the patients in the i.a. group survived beyond this period. In the i.a./i.v. group 21 % of the patients survived beyond 36 months.

References

1. Kemeny N, Golbey R (1980) A chemotherapeutic approach to colorectal carcinoma. In : Stearns MR Jr (ed) Neoplasma of the colon, rectum and anus. John Wiley and Sons, New York, pp. 155-165

2. Safi F, Roscher R, Bittner R, Schumacher KA, Gaus W, Beger HG (1989) Regionale Chemotherapie von Lebermetastasen kolorektaler Karzinome. Dtsch Med Wschr 114 : 1478-1483
3. Safi F, Bittner R, Roscher R, Schumacher K, Gaus W, Beger HG (1989) Regional chemotherapy for hepatic metastases of colorectal carcinoma (Continuous intra-arterial versus continuous intra-arterial/intravenous therapy) — Results of a controlled clinical trial. Cancer 64 : 379-387
4. Safi F, Schumacher K, Roscher R, Bittner R, Beger HG (1990) Regional chemotherapy on liver metastases of colorectal carcinoma : Monitoring with arterial computed tomography. Cancer Invest 8 : 123-134
5. Kemeny N, Daly J, Reichmann B, Geller N, Botet J, Oderman P (1987) Intrahepatic or systemic infusion of Fluorodeoxuridine in patients with liver metastases from colorectal carcinoma. Ann Int Med 107 : 459-465
6. Balch CM, Unist MM (1984) Intra-arterielle Chemotherapie mit einer implantierbaren Infusionspumpe bei Lebermetastasen kolorektaler Tumoren und Hepatomen. Chirurg 55 : 485-493
7. Niederhuber JE, Ensminger W, Gyves J, Thrall J, Walker S, Cozzi E (1984) Regional chemotherapy of colorectal cancer metastatic to the liver. Cancer 53 : 1336-1343
8. Reed ML, Vaitkevicius VK, Al-Sarraf M, Vaughn CB, Singhakowinta A, Sexon-Porte M, Izbicki R, Baker L, Straatsma GW (1981) The practicality of metastatic hepatic malignancies : Ten-year results of 124 patients in a prospective protocol. Cancer 47 : 402-409
9. Cohen AM, Greenfield A, Wood WC, Waltman A, Novelline R, Athanasoulis Ch, Schaeffer NJ (1983) Treatment of hepatic metastases by transaxillary hepatic artery chemotherapy using an implanted drug pump. Cancer 51 : 2013-2019
10. Kaplan E, Meier P (1958) Nonparametric estimation from incomplete observations. J Am Stat Assoc 53 : 457-481
11. Mantel N (1966) Evaluation of survival data and two new rank order statistics arising in its consideration. Cancer Chem Rep 50 : 163-170
12. Conover WJ (1980) Practical nonparametric statistics. John Wiley and Sons, 2nd ed., New York, pp. 143-212
13. Safi F, Roscher R, Heymer B, Bittner R, Beger HG (1987) Erosive Gastroduodenitis mit schweren Epitheldysplasien als Komplikation der loco-regionalen intra-arteriellen Chemotherapie bei Lebermetastasen. Akt Chir 23 : 69-73
14. Ensminger WD, Rosowsky V, Raso DC, Glode M, Come S, Steele G, Frey E (1978) A clinical-pharmacological evaluation of hepatic arterial infusions of 5-Fluoro-2-Deoxyuridine and 5-Fluorouracil. Cancer 38 : 3784
15. Chuang VP, Wallace S, Stroehlein J, Xap HG, Patt YZ (1981) Hepatic artery infusion chemotherapy : Gastroduodenal complications. Am J Radiol 137 : 347
16. Hall DA, Clouse ME, Gramm HF (1981) Gastroduodenal ulceration after hepatic arterial infusion chemotherapy. Am J Radiol 136 : 1216
17. Kemeny MM, Goldberg DA, Browning S, Metter GE, Miner PA, Terz JJ (1985) Experience with continuous regional chemotherapy and hepatic resection as treatment of hepatic metastases. Cancer 55 : 1265
18. Kemeny N, Daly J, Oderman P, Shike M, Chun H, Petroni G, Geller N (1984) Hepatic artery pump infusion : Toxicity and results in patients with metastatic colorectal carcinoma. J Clin Oncol 2 : 595
19. Kemeny MM, Battifora H, Douglas W, Blayney GC, David AG, Lucille AL, Kim AM, Jose JT (1985) Sclerosing cholangitis after continuous hepatic artery infusion of FUDR. Ann Surg 202 : 176
20. Rothmund M, Brückner R, Keller E, Quint B, Knuth A, Schicketanz KH (1986)

Regionale Chemotherapie bei Lebermetastasen kolorektaler Karzinome mit implantierbaren Druckpumpen. Dtsch Med Wschr 17 : 652-658
21. Ensminger W, Niederhuber J, Dakhil S, Thrall J, Wheeler R (1981) Totally implanted drug delivery system for hepatic arterial chemotherapy. Cancer 65 : 393

Abstract. Seventy-one patients with biopsy-proven colorectal cancer metastatic to the liver were treated regionally. These patients were entered on a randomized prospective protocol to evaluate the effectiveness of continuous hepatic artery and intravenous infusion versus hepatic artery infusion alone via implanted pumps. Thirty-four patients (i.a. group) received only intraarterial FUDR perfusion. The another 37 patients (i.a./i.v. group) obtained simultaneous intra-arterial and intravenous infusion of FUDR. Intervention : continuous 14 days infusion of FUDR each month (0.2 mg/kg/day in all i.a. treated patients and 0.3 mg/kg/day in the i.a./i.v. treated patients). The complete and partial response rate in all of our patients (n = 71) was 58 % (59 % v.s. 57 % in the i.a. and i.a./i.v. randomized groups, respectively). No difference in the toxicity of FUDR between the 2 randomized groups was found. 79 % (n = 27) of the i.a. group and 51 % (n = 19) of the i.a./i.v. group developed in a median follow-up time of 24 months extrahepatic spread of cancer in the course of therapy. No significant difference in survival was found between the i.a. and i.a./i.v. groups. Intra-arterial FUDR infusion provided control of hepatic metastases. The combination of intra-arterial and intravenous therapy seemed to prevent extrahepatic tumor spread during therapy in most of the patients.

D-Verapamil and Adriamycin in the treatment of advanced colorectal cancer

W Scheithauer, G Kornek, S Globitz, M Raderer, T Schenk, CH Müller, CH Tetzner

One of the reasons for the primary resistance of colorectal cancer to a wide variety of cytotoxic drugs may be the high frequency of multidrug resistance (MDR) encountered in this disease [1]. Several classes of agents have been demonstrated to overcome MDR phenotype in experimental tumor systems. Verapamil (VPM) is the prototype of these drugs, but in early clinical studies it had to be recognized that VPM because of its potent effects on the cardiovascular system, could not be administered in the optimal concentration required for reversal of MDR *in vitro*. An attractive alternative to the use of the marketed drug Verapamil (a racemic DL mixture) is the D-isomer of VPM, which has equal resistance-reverting potential but a least 3-fold less cardiovascular potency [2]. Based on the potentially favourable therapeutic index of this second generation modulator, and histological studies indicating that colon cancer expresses high levels of p-glycoprotein that might be related to its inherent refractoriness to conventional anticancer agents, the present phase II study of DVPM plus Doxorubicin has been initiated.

Patients and methods

Sixteen patients with measurable metastatic colorectal cancer were entered onto this study, all of whom had failed or relapsed after prior palliative 5-Fluorouracil/Leucovorin-based chemotherapy. Patients had to have, WHO performance status < 2, wbc count of $> 4.000/\mu L$, platelet count $> 100.000/\mu L$, serum Bilirubin of < 1.5 mg/dL, and serumcreatinine of < 1.5 mg/dL. All patients had normal ECGs, resting systolic BP > 110 mmHg, and a normal pretreatment echocardiogram and all gave written informed consent. Treatment consisted of oral D-Verapamil (DVPM ; Knoll AG, Ludwigshafen, Germany) given at a starting dose of 300 mg every 6h for 3 consecutive days, and Doxorubicin (75 mg/m^2) administered by i.v. bolus injection on day 2.

Treatment was repeated every 3-4 weeks. If no cardiovascular symptoms occurred during the first treatment cycle, the dose of DVPM was to be increased to 4×350 mg/day. In case of chemotherapy-related WHO grade 3/4 systemic toxicity or minor DVPM-related cardiovascular side effects, the DVPM starting dose was maintained and the Doxorubicin dose was lowered to 60 mg/m^2. Tumor response, remission duration and non cardiovascular side effects were classified according to WHO standard criteria.

Departments of Internal Medicine I and IV, Vienna University Medical School, Waehringer Guertel 18-20, A-1090 Vienna, Austria, and Knoll AG, Ludwigshafen, Germany

Results

Sixteen patients were enrolled in this clinical trial and received a total of 47 courses of treatment. There were 10 men and 6 women, the median age was 59 years (range, 46 to 66), and the WHO performance status was 0 in 12 and 1 in 4 patients. Metastatic involvement included the liver in 13, lung in 8, abdominopelvic mass in 7, and peripheral lymph nodes and bone in 1 patient each. One patient was considered inevaluable for response, since after discontinuation for Doxorubicin-related acute cardiotoxicity during the first course, he refused further follow-up examinations. All other patients were assessable for response and toxicity. Side effects observed during this study are summarized in Table 1.

Table 1. Non cardiovascular side effects on DVPM plus Doxorubicin

Toxicity (WHO Grade)	0	1	2	3	4
Leukopenia	2	3	2	3	6
Granulocytopenia	2	1	1	2	10
Anemia	3	7	3	3	0
Trombocytopenia	9	2	2	3	1
Nausea/vomiting	9	6	0	1	0
Stomatitis	8	1	1	6	0
Constipation	13	3	0	0	0
Diarrhea	15	1	0	0	0
Infection/fever	8	4	2	2	0
Alopecia	0	0	9	7	0

Adverse reactions consisted mainly of myelosuppression and cardiovascular side effects. Granulocytopenia with neutrophil counts below $500/\mu L$ was encountered in 10 patients (62 %).

Transient hypotension, defined as systolic BP < 90 mmHg for at least 1 measurement, occurred in all 16 patients (36/47 treatment courses) though it was rarely symptomatic. A systolic BP of < 70 mmHg was seen in 4/16 cases only. Sinus bradycardia (< 60 beats per minute) occurred in 8 patients (50 %). First-degree heart block occurred in 5 (31 %), Wenckebach block, auriculoventricular rhythm and a trial ectopy were observed in 1 patient each. All dysrhythmias resolved with in 2-3 hours following temporary discontinuation of oral DVPM. Seven patients required modification of the dose of Doxorubicin at some point during their treatment course, primarily for hematologic toxicity and/or stomatitis. The dose of DVPM was increased to 4 × 350 mg/day according to the study protocol in 10 patients. In 4 patients the DVPM starting dose of 4 × 300 mg/day was maintained (n = 3) or reduced to 4 × 250 mg/day (n = 1) because of dysrhythmia, hypotension and/or occurrence of chemotherapy-related grade 3/4 systemic toxicity. One out of 15 evaluable patients (7 %), who had a pelvic recurrence of rectal cancer, had a partial response, documented on CT-scan. Another 7 patients (47 %) had stable disease for 3 to 7 months. The median duration of survival of all patients entered on protocol is + 4 months (range 1 to + 8 months).

Discussion

In this phase II study, we treated 16 patients with metastatic colorectal cancer, all of whom had failed or relapsed after prior 5-FU/LV combination chemotherapy.

Although we observed 1 partial response in a pretreated patient, it is evident that we were unsuccessful in circumventing the clinical resistance of colorectal cancer to chemotherapy. There are several explanations for the disappointing therapeutic outcome : 1) Overexpression of p-glycoprotein may be heterogenous within a given population of tumor cells. 2) There are other mechanisms by which resistance to agents such as anthracyclines might develop or preexist such as topoisomerase II mutations. 3) The bolus administration of Doxorubicin might have been inadequate for optimal MDR modulation. 4) The concentration of DVPM at the molecular site of action, particularly in patients with a large tumor volume, might have been inadequate. 5) Finally, we can not exclude that our selection of pretreated patients for study might have adversely influenced the treatment outcome. Cardiovascular side effects associated with the present regimen were frequent though generally did not require active medical intervention. There was evidence from this trial that DVPM may potentiate some of the noncardiac toxicity of Doxorubicin : Severe mucositis was observed in almost half of our patients and WHO grade 4 granulocytopenia, frequently associated with infections, occurred in 62 %. The increased toxicity of Doxorubicin might be related to inhibition of drug efflux from normal cells or enhanced distribution of the anthracycline/altered disposition as suggested in a previous pilot pharmacokinetic study [3]. Without realization of certain refinements of the concept of MDR modulation it would seem from our study results that colorectal cancer — despite histological demonstration of high levels of p-glycoprotein — would not be an appropriate target for future studies with MDR modulators. As it concerns the primary toxicity data observed in this study, whether related to inhibition of drug efflux from normal cells or to a pharmacokinetic interaction between DVPM and Doxorubicin, we would suggest that careful consideration should be given to the anthracycline dose in other clinical studies using resistance modulators such as DVPM.

References

1. Goldstein LJ, Galski H, Fojo A et al (1983) Expression of multidrug resistance gene in human tumors. J Natl Cancer Inst 81 : 116-124
2. Plumb JA, Milroy R, Kaye SB (1990) The activity of Verapamil as a resistance modifier in vitro in drug-resistant human tumour cell lines is not stereospecific. Biochem Pharmacol 39 :787-792
3. Scheithauer W, Schenk T, Czejka M (1992) Pharmacokinetic interaction between Epirubicin and the multidrug resistance reverting agent D-Verapamil. Br J Cancer (submitted)

Perioperative multimodal treatment of locally advanced rectal cancer. Results of a pilot study

P Schöffski, HR Raab, I Wildfang, CH Köhne-Wömpner, JH Karstens, R Pichlmayr, HJ Schmoll

Despite the advances in surgical techniques, local and systemic failure still remain common but serious complications in the clinical course of patients with resectable rectal cancer. Following potentially « curative » surgery, the incidence of local failure in TNM stages $T_{1-2} N_0 M_0$ is almost negligible; however, it increases to 15 % to 35 % in stages $T_3 N_0 M_0$ and $T_1 N_1 M_0$ and up to 45 % to 65 % in stages $T_{3-4} N_{1-2} M_0$ [1, 4]. Since rectal cancer is a very common condition, and the outcome of relapsed disease is fatal in the majority of cases, there is an urgent need for more efficient and widely practicable first line therapies, leading to a significant reduction in rectal cancer mortality.

Non-randomized trials of postoperative pelvic radiation therapy (RT) reveal an improvement in local control and survival compared with historical controls of surgery alone [5, 6]. Randomized postoperative trials have demonstrated a significant survival advantage of RT + chemotherapy versus surgery alone, RT + chemotherapy versus RT, and chemotherapy versus surgery alone [7, 10]. Postoperative radiochemotherapy is now the recommended standard approach for patients with resected locally advanced rectal cancer.

There are a number of potential advantages of preoperative compared with postoperative RT in the treatment of patients with rectal cancer. These include (1) increasing the resectability rate in case of irresectable disease, (2) decreasing RT-associated morbidity, (3) increasing the chance of performing a sphincter-sparing procedure and (4) downstaging in the primary tumor and pelvic lymph nodes. Given the advantage of chemotherapy reported in the postoperative adjuvant radiation rectal cancer trials [7, 10], the benefit of Folinic acid (FA) plus 5-Fluorouracil (FU) compared with FU alone in patients with metastatic disease [11] and the *in vitro* and *in vivo* evidence of FU sensitization of RT [12], it appears reasonable to combine FA/FU with RT in the preoperative setting [13].

Since postoperative chemotherapy alone is improving the relapse rate, disease-free and overall survival in patients with resected locally advanced colon cancer [14, 15], the potential benefit of Adjuvant chemotherapy in rectal cancer needs to be reevaluated. Various FA/FU combinations have been tested in both metastatic colon and rectal cancer [26]. The doses and schedules vary widely. The response rates are usually higher for the combination than those reported with FU alone. Although some trials report an advantage of FA/FU, it is not yet clear whether the increased response rate of FA/FU translates into an increase in survival compared with FU alone [16, 17].

Hannover University Medical School, Konstanty-Gutschow Str. 8, D-3000 Hannover 61, FRG
Department of Hematology/Oncology, Department of Abdominal and Transplant Surgery, Department of Radiation Therapy and Special Oncology

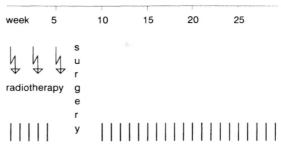

Fig. 1. Treatment schedule

Based on these considerations, we designed a single-center non-randomized pilot trial of combined preoperative RT (50 Gy in 25 fractions) and chemotherapy (weekly FA 300 mg/m² and FU 700 mg/m²), followed by surgery and Adjuvant chemotherapy (weekly FA 300 mg/m² and FU 700 mg/m²) for the treatment of non-pretreated patients with locally advanced rectal cancer, here being defined as biopsy-proven primary adenocarcinoma stage uT_{3-4} $uN_{+/-}$ M_X (u = rectal ultrasound). The main goal of this pilot trial was to determine the feasibility of a multimodal therapeutic approach for patients with poor risk resectable rectal cancer (Fig. 1).

Patients and methods

Patient population : The patients enrolled in this trial between February 1990 and September 1992 were mainly sent by private practitioners to the Department of Abdominal and Transplant Surgery at our institution for confirmation of clinical diagnosis of rectal cancer, and conventional surgery. The pretreatment evaluation here included a complete history and physical examination, proctoscopy and/or colonoscopy with biopsy, chest X-ray, abdominal and pelvic computed tomography (CT), rectal ultrasound, complete blood cell and platelet counts, sequential multiple serum analysis and tumor marker assays (CEA, TPA and CA 19.9). Twenty-one patients with locally advanced primary rectal cancer stage uT_{3-4} $uN_{+/-}$ M_X were enrolled in the trial after informed consent. Among these were 9 nodal positive, 12 nodal negative, 16 male and 5 female patients with a median age of 58 (38-72) years. We excluded patients who were pretreated with RT or chemotherapy, who had concurrent malignancies or multiple synchronous colorectal primary tumors.

Preoperative radiotherapy : RT (multiple-field technique) was administered once per day, 5 days per week at 200 cGy/day for 5 weeks, resulting in a cumulative dose of 50 Gy in 25 fractions. Procedures to minimize the small bowel toxicity of pelvic RT were used as previously described [18] whenever possible.

Preoperative chemotherapy : Concurrent chemotherapy was administered once per week for 5 weeks. Metoclopramide was used for prevention of nausea and vomiting at a standard i.v. dose of 20 mg. FA was given as a short i.v. infusion at a dose of 300 mg/m², directly followed by a 2 hours i.v. infusion of FU at a fixed dose of 700 mg/m², resulting in a cumulative preoperative dose of FA of 1.5 g/m² and FU 3.5 g/m², respectively.

Surgery : The patients underwent curative surgery 5 weeks after completion of external-beam RT and chemotherapy. The preoperative staging again included history and physical examination, proctoscopy, chest X-ray, abdominal and pelvic CT scans, blood counts, serum analysis and tumor marker assays. Rectal ultrasound was performed whenever possible.

Postoperative chemotherapy : Adjuvant chemotherapy was scheduled once per week for 20 weeks starting week 5 after surgery. Again, i.v. Metoclopramide was used for prevention of nausea and vomiting at a standard dose of 20 mg. FA was applied as a short i.v. infusion at a dose of 300 mg/m², directly followed by a 2 hours i.v. infusion of FU at a fixed dose of 700 mg/m², resulting in a cumulative postoperative dose of FA of 6.0 /m² and FU 14.0 g/m², respectively.

Toxicity assessment : For standardized evaluation of therapy-associated toxicity, the WHO toxicity criteria were used to determine the severity, clinical course and outcome of unwanted side effects.

Clinical follow-up : After completion of postoperative chemotherapy the patients underwent restaging including history and physical examination, chest X-ray, abdominal and pelvic CT scans, blood counts, serum analysis and tumor marker assays. Proctoscopy is being performed every 6 months. The patients are currently seen 4 times a year and followed for at least 5 years after surgery.

Results

Feasibility : 20 out of 21 patients received the full 5-week course of preoperative radiochemotherapy without dose reductions or significant delays. One patient died during the first week of RT due to preexisting cardiovascular disease ; this death was not related to cancer treatment. All other patients underwent curative pelvic surgery and could be evaluated for feasibility, toxicity and response. In our hands, preoperative radiochemotherapy did not compromise operability and was not associated with an increase in postoperative complications. However, we observed 2 cases of bowel obstruction, 1 of these requiring further surgery. Fourteen out of 20 patients consented to postoperative chemotherapy and received the full 20 weeks course of FA/FU as scheduled. In all patients enrolled in this trial, RT and chemotherapy could be administered on an outpatient basis.

Toxicity : RT and chemotherapy were tolerated well by the majority of patients. Only minor non-hematological side effects were observed. Common toxicities were mucositis °I, diarrhea °I, nausea/vomiting °I and skin rash °I according to WHO criteria. Some of the diarrhea was preexisting and potentially related to the rectal primary. All side effects observed in this trial were short in duration and fully reversible. Severe organ toxicity or toxic deaths did not occur.

Resectability : All patients underwent curative surgery, here defined as complete resection of the rectal tumor and regional lymph nodes with negative mar-

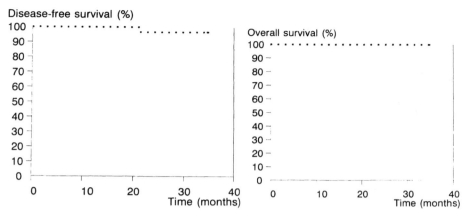

Fig. 2. Overall survival after a median follow-up of 24 (8-35) months

Fig. 3. Disease-free survival after a median follow-up of 24 (8-35) months

gins. Due to the small number of patients and the lack of randomized controls in this pilot trial, the objective impact of preoperative therapy on the resectability of the rectal tumor cannot be assessed. According to the well experienced surgeons involved in the management of our patients, the number of nerve-sparing resections was unexpectedly high as compared with historical controls.

Response evaluation : Prior to definite surgery, a proctoscopy was repeated in all patients enrolled in this trial, commonly revealing a significant reduction in tumor size after preoperative radiochemotherapy, being confirmed by the macroscopic appearance of the tumors during surgery. Microscopically, changes consistent with tumor regression, such as ulceration, necrosis, scarification, fibrosis and chronic inflammation were present in all surgical specimen after preoperative therapy. In one case, initially a uT_3 uN_1 M_X rectal adenocarcinoma, a complete response to radiochemotherapy could be confirmed by the pathologists. When comparing rectal ultrasound tumor stage prior to study entry, and pathological staging at time of definite surgery (uTNM versus ypTNM stage), a downstaging of the T-stage was observed in 8 out of 20 patients (40 %). A downstaging of the N-stage occurred in 7 out of 9 initially nodal positive patients (78 %). In 12 out of 20 patients who underwent surgery, either the T- and/or the N-stage improved, resulting in a response rate of 60 %. We did not observe any tumor progression during the preoperative phase. During follow-up, only 1 local relapse in case of a ypT_3 ypN_0 M_0 tumor occurred after a disease-free interval of 22 months. This patient initially underwent salvage laparotomy, and is currently being treated with second line chemotherapy for an irresectable pelvic tumor. None of our poor risk patients developed systemic metastasis after multimodal therapy up to now. All patients are alive after a median follow-up of 24 (8-35) months (Fig. 2). Nineteen out of 20 patients are without any evidence of disease (Fig. 3). Due to the lack of randomized controls and the small patient number in this pilot study, the objective response to multimodal therapy cannot be assessed.

Discussion

The rate of radiation-induced downstaging or rectal cancer is a function of the fraction size, total dose and time interval between the completion of RT and surgery. The highest rate of downstaging is reported from series in which patients received full-dose pelvic radiation ($\geqslant$ 45 Gy in conventional fractionation) and underwent surgery 4 to 5 weeks after the completion of RT [19, 25]. This approach is associated with maximum tumor shrinkage, and was therefore combined with pre- and postoperative chemotherapy in this trial.

In our hands, multimodal perioperative therapy for locally advanced rectal cancer was clearly feasible and was accepted by both patients and physicians involved. The toxicity of both pre- and postoperative therapy was almost negligible. Our data suggests, that FA and FU can be given concomitantly to RT at the dose and schedule chosen in this trial without a significant increase in toxicity. The ideal chemotherapy agents, doses and schedules in this setting still need to be determined. Furthermore, the effect of FA on the radiosensitizing capacity of FU should be tested *in vitro*.

The complete response rate of 5 % after preoperative multimodal therapy in our small series is comparable to data from published RT trials. The number of patients without tumor in their surgical specimen is commonly ranging between 10 to 15 % [13, 19, 23]. The true impact of a complete pathological response on survival in rectal cancer remains to be determined in future phase III trials.

The incidence of positive pelvic nodes seen at time of surgery was lower in our series (10 %) compared with all data from other institutions, where it usually ranges between 16 and 48 % [13]. It is unclear, whether this difference indicates a potential advantage of combined preoperative radio and chemotherapy as compared with RT alone, or may be due to concurrent factors such as patient selection and other clinicopathologic variables as well. Again, the ultimate impact of decreasing the incidence of pelvic nodes by preoperative therapy on disease-free and overall survival demands further reevaluation in clinical trials.

In our hands, preoperative therapy did not compromise the operability of locally advanced rectal cancer when compared with historical controls. All patients underwent curative resection, the number of sphincter-sparing procedures was unexpectedly high and postoperative complications were rare.

We cannot evaluate the potential advantage associated with postoperative chemotherapy, which was offered to all patients enrolled in this trial. Confirming the experience of other groups, patients' compliance with postoperative chemotherapy was somewhat lower than with preoperative therapy [15].

After a median follow-up of 2 years, the relapse rate, disease-free and overall survival of our patient group appears promising when compared with published historical data on the clinical course of the disease after « curative surgery » only. However, we cannot exclude a patient selection bias in this small series.

Taking into account that this pre- and postoperative treatment was associated with only minor toxicity and downstaging of the primary tumor and its loco-regional nodal metastasis was clearly evident, we feel encouraged by multimodal therapy strategies in poor risk rectal cancer.

References

1. Gunderson LL, Sosin H (1974) Areas of failure found at reoperation (second or symptomatik look) following « curative surgery » for adenocarcinoma of the rectum. Clinicopathologic correlation and implications for adjuvant therapy. Cancer 34 : 1278-1291
2. Mendenhall WM, Million RR, Pfaff WW (1983) Pattern of recurrences in adenocarcinoma of the rectum and rectosigmoid treated with surgery alone : implications in treatment planning with adjuvant radiation therapy. Int J Radiat Oncol Biol Phys 9 : 977-985
3. Minsky BD, Mies C, Recht A (1988) Resectable adenocarcinoma of the rectosigmoid and rectum. (1) Patterns of failure and survival. Cancer 61 : 1408-1416
4. Rich T, Gunderson LL, Lew R (1983) Patterns of recurrence of rectal carcinoma after potentially curative surgery. Cancer 52 : 1317-1329
5. Tepper JE, Cohen AM, Wood WC (1987) Postoperative radiation therapy of rectal cancer. Int J Radiat Oncol Biol Phys 13 : 5-10
6. Vigliotti A, Rich TA, Romsdahl MM (1987) Postoperative adjuvant radiation therapy for adenocarcinoma of the rectum and rectosigmoid. Int J Radiat Oncol Biol Phys 13 : 999-1006
7. Gastrointestinal Tumor Study Group (1985) Prolongation of the disease-free interval in surgically treated rectal carcinoma. N Engl J Med 312 : 1465-72
8. Gastrointestinal Tumor Study Group (1986) Survival after postoperative combination treatment of rectal carcinoma. N Eng J Med 315 : 1294-1295
9. Krook J, Moertel C, Gunderson LL (1991) Effective surgical adjuvant therapy for high-risk rectal carcinoma. N Engl J Med 324 : 709-715
10. Fisher B, Wolmark N, Rockette C (1988) Postoperative Adjuvant chemotherapy or radiation therapy for rectal cancer : Result from NSABP protocol R-01. J Natl Cancer Inst 80 : 21-29
11. Erlichman C, Fine S, Wong A (1988) A randomized trial of Fluorouracil and Folnic acid in patients with metastatic colorectal carcinoma. J Clin Oncol 6 : 469-475
12. Rotman M, Aziz H (1990) Concomitant continuous infusion chemotherapy and radiation. Cancer 65 : 823-835
13. Minsky BD, Cohen AM, Kemeny N (1992) Enhancement of radiation-induced downstaging of rectal cancer by Fluorouracil and high-dose Leucovorin chemotherapy. J Clin Oncol 10 (1) : 79-84
14. Laurie JA, Moertel CG, Fleming TR (1989) Surgical adjuvant therapy of large-bowel carcinoma : an evaluation of levamisole and the combination of levamisole and fluorouracil. J Clin Oncol 7 : 1447-56
15. Moertel CG, Flemming TR, Macdonald JS (1991) Levamisole and Fluorouracil for adjuvant therapy of resected colon carcinoma. N Engl J Med 322 :352-358
16. Buyse M, Zeleniuch-Jacquotte A, Chalmers TC (1988) Adjuvant therapy of colorectal cancer. Why we still don't know ? JAMA 259(24) : 3571-3578
17. Piedbois P, Buyse M, Rustum Y (1992) Modulation of 5-Fluorouracil by Leucovorin in patients with advanced colorectal cancer : a meta-analysis. Proc Am Soc Clin Oncol 11 : 167
18. Minsky BD, Cohen AM (1988) Minimizing the toxicity of pelvic radiation therapy. Oncology 2 : 21-25

19. Mohiuddin M, Marks J (1991) High-dose preoperative irradiation for cancer of the rectum, 1976-1988. Int J Radiat Oncol Biol Phys 20 : 37-43
20. Kodner IJ, Shamesh EI, Fry RD (1988) Preoperative irradiation for rectal cancer. Improved local control and long term survival. Ann Surg 209 : 194-199
21. Mendenhall WM, Bland KI, Pfaff WW (1987) Initially unresectable rectal adenocarcinoma treated with preoperative irradiation and surgery. Ann Surg 205 : 41-44
22. Doseretz DE, Gunderson LL, Hedberg S (1983) Preoperative irradiation for unresectable rectal and rectosigmoid carcinoma. Cancer 52 : 814-818
23. Mendenhall WM, Bland KI, Rout R (1988) Clinically resectable adenocarcinoma of the rectum treated with preoperative irradiation and surgery. Dis Colon Rectum 31 : 287-290
24. Fortier GA, Constable WC, Meyers H (1986) Preoperative radiation therapy for rectal cancer. An effective therapy in need of a clinical trial. Arch Surg 121 : 1380-1385
25. Haghbin M, Sischy B, Hinson J (1988) Combined modality therapy in poor prognostic rectal adenocarcinoma. Radiother Oncol 13 : 75-81
26. Köhne-Wömpner CH, Schmoll HJ, Harstrick A (1992) Chemotherapeutic strategies in metastatic colorectal cancer : an overview of current clinical trials. Sem Oncol 19 (suppl 3) : 105-125

Abstract. To determine the feasibility of a multimodal perioperative treatment approach for patients with poor risk rectal cancer, 21 non-pretreated individuals with biopsy-proven, locally advanced rectal adenocarcinoma TNM stage uT_{3-4} $uN_{+/-}$ M_X (u = rectal ultrasound) underwent preoperative radiochemotherapy, pelvic surgery and postoperative chemotherapy. The 5 week preoperative regimen consisted of weekly Folnic acid (FA) 300 mg/m² i.v. short infusion, followed directly by 5-Fluorouracil (FU) 700 mg/m² 2 hours i.v. infusion, combined with external-beam radiation to the pelvis with a cumulative dose of 50 Gy in 25 fractions. Curative surgery was scheduled for week 5 after preoperative therapy, 5 weeks later followed by postoperative weekly chemotherapy again involving FA at a dose of 300 mg/m² and FU 700 mg/m² over a period of 20 weeks.

Radio and chemotherapy were tolerated well. Only minor non-hematological side effects were observed, including nausea/vomiting, diarrhea, mucositis and skin rash. No treatment related deaths, but 1 early death due to cardiovascular disease occurred. The preoperative therapy did not compromise operability of the rectal primary ; the number of nerve-sparing resections was higher than expected. Comparing rectal ultrasound stages prior study entry with pathological staging at time of definite surgery, a downstaging of the T-stage was observed in 8/20 patients (40 %). Seven of 9 initially nodal positive patients were nodal negative after preoperative radiochemotherapy (78 %). In 12 out of 20 patients either the T- and/or N-stage improved, resulting in an 60 % response rate. One pathologically confirmed complete response was seen. After a median follow-up of 24 (8-35) months, all patients are alive, 19 of these are without any evidence of disease (95 %). Only one local relapse, but no systemic metastasis occurred so far.

Perioperative radiochemotherapy in locally advanced rectal cancer appears both feasible and effective, being associated with only minor toxicity and not compromising operability. This promising approach needs further reevaluation in randomized trials, comparing it with the current therapeutic standard of adjuvant radiochemotherapy.

Gynecologic cancer

Neo-Adjuvant chemotherapy for advanced ovarian cancer

Y Shimizu, S Umezawa, N Takeshima, T Kato, K Hasumi

Standard treatment modality for advanced (FIGO stage III/IV) ovarian cancer has been the initial debulking surgery followed by CDDP-based combination chemotherapy. If this modality is a best treatment method, patients not amenable to such a modality must have a poor prognosis. However, there is a considerable number of patients having a long-term survival who underwent an exploratory laparotomy at initial surgical effort because the disease were deemed « inoperable », but afterward received an unexpected optimal debulking (OD :residuum < 2 cm) subsequent to passive Neo-Adjuvant (NA) chemotherapy. Moreover, such a successful case has been noted even in patients who did not undergo initial debulking because of extremely poor performance status (PS). Thus, we conducted a retrospective study to reappraise the therapeutic power of the standard modality and also to assess the efficacy of NA chemotherapy for advanced ovarian cancer.

Patients and methods

1. Patients

The patient population consists of 138 patients with stage III ovarian cancer and 27 with stage IV treated at department of Gynecology, Cancer Institute Hospital in Tokyo between 1970 to 1991. The treatment policy of our department has been almost same as the widely accepted standard modality, namely initial debulking with a basic procedure followed by CDDP-based chemotherapy.

Only 6 cases were unexplored because of extremely poor performance status (PS) during the observation period. Seventy-seven patients considered to be optimal received primary debulking followed by a postoperative chemotherapy (PO). Eighty-two patients felt to be unsuitable for a curative surgery underwent an exploratory laparotomy, among whom 74 received NA chemotherapy and the remaining 8 did not have a planned chemotherapy because of poor PS. Therefore, NA group had more aggressive disease and had poorer PS than PO. Fourteen patients, including 6 without laparotomy due to extremely poor PS and 8 with incomplete NA chemotherapy following exploratory laparotomy, were defined as an untreated (U) group. The profiles of patients were shown in Table 1.

Department of Gynecology, Cancer Institute Hospital, 1-37-1, Kami-ikebukuro, Toshima-ku, Tokyo 170, Japan

Table 1. Profiles of patients with stage III and IV ovarian cancer

Variables	Postoperative (n = 77)	Neo-adjuvant (n = 74)	Untreated (n = 14)
Age			
Mean (range)	53 (21-80)	55 (32-83)	54 (20-77)
< 50	40	24	5
≥ 50	37	50	9
PS			
0-1	19	11	1
2	40	23	3
3-4	18	40	10
FIGO stage			
III	68	63	7
IV	9	11	7
Histologic subtype			
Serous	51	54	3
Mucinous	14	10	1
Endometrioid	1	2	0
Clear	8	2	0
Undifferentiated	1	1	0
MMT/sarcoma	0	1	1
Germ cell	2	1	1
Granulosa	0	1	0
Unknown	0	2	6
Regimen			
CAP/CP	50	53	4
FAMT	21	21	6
Others	5	0	1
None	1	0	3
Response			
CRIPR	13/15	12/38	0/0
NCIPD	20/18	14/10	0/0
NE	11	0	14
Primary debulking			
HBSO. 0m ± PLA ~PALA	74	31	0
More extensive	3	12	0
Biopsy	0	31	8
None	0	0	6
Total dose of CDDP	603 (0-1550)	626 (300-1260)	110 (0-180)
Mean (range)	(n = 56)	(n = 53)	(n = 5)

2. Debulking procedure

The basic surgical procedure of debulking performed at initial surgical attempt for PO group or carried out at secondary laparotomy subsequent to NA chemotherapy for NA group was semi-radical hysterectomy, bilateral adenectomy, omentectomy, appendectomy, and pelvic lymphadenectomy. In occasional cases, more extensive surgery including bowel resection, peritoneal stripping, paraaortic lymphadenectomy, and removal of other organs was performed.

3. Chemotherapy

The following chemotherapeutic regimens were applied to patients 7 days after the operation.

a) FAMT : 5-FU 250 mg/body, day 1-5
Cyclophosphamide (CPM) 350 mg/m^2, day 1
Mitomycin-C (MMC) 7 mg/m^2, day 1
Toyomycin (Chlomomycin A$_3$) 0.5 mg/body, day 1-5

b) CAP : CPM 500 mg/m^2, day 1
Doxorubicin (ADM) 35 mg/m^2, day 1
CDDP 50 mg/m^2, day 1

c) CP : CPM 500 mg/m^2, day 1
CDDP 10 mg/m^2, day 1-7

FAMT was used from 1970 to 1979, CAP from 1980 to 1987, and CP from 1988 to 1991.

Results

1. Debulking surgery performed at initial laparotomy

One hundred and fifty-nine patients received initial laparotomy. Initial debulking by basic procedure of 77 patients considered to be resectable at initial surgical attempt resulted in 35 optimal debulking (OD :residual < 2 cm) and 42 suboptimal debulking (subOD : residuum ≥ 2 cm). This means that the percentage of patients with stage III/IV disease optimally cytoreduced was 35/165 (21.2 %) when all the patients received basic surgery at initial surgical attempt. Eighty-two patients deemed unresectable at initial laparotomy had exploratory laparotomy. The remaining 6 did not receive a laparotomy because of extremely poor PS.

Table 2. Response of stage III/IV ovarian cancer patients by a timing of chemotherapy

Regimen	Postoperative (n = 77)						Neo-adjuvant (n = 74)					
	CR	PR	NC	PD	NE	CR + PR/evaluable	CR	PR	NC	PD	NE	CR + PR/evaluable
CAP	7	12	8	9	5	19/36 (53 %)	6	20	4	3	0	26/33 (79 %)
CP	3	1	1	2	2	4/7 (57 %)	4	13	1	2	0	17/20 (85 %)
FAMT	2	1	10	6	2	3/19 (16 %)	2	5	9	5	0	7/21 (33 %)
Others	1	1	1	1	2	2/4 (50 %)	0	0	0	0	0	0/0 (0 %)
Total	13	15	20	18	11	28/66 (42 %)	12	38	14	10	0	50/74 (68 %)

2. Response to chemotherapy

As shown in Table 2, the response rate to chemotherapy of NA group was significantly higher than that of PO group (p = 0.0001). There was no significant difference in the response rate between CAP and CP, regardless of a timing of chemotherapy.

3. Debulking subsequent to NA chemotherapy

Secondary laparotomy was carried out on 43 patients out of 74 having NA chemotherapy, and 34 (45.9 %) received OD. Among 31 patients not undergoing second laparotomy, 18 were chemo-responders.

4. Survival time by a timing of chemotherapy (PO v.s. NA)

There was no significant difference in the survival time between PO and NA group (Fig. 1). NA group showed a trend of longer survival (5 year :34 %, median : 31 mo) than PO (19 %, 21 mo) though not significant, despite a selection bias was set at initial laparotomy.

Next, we compared the survival of subgroup by radicality of debulking, which was carried out at initial laparotomy on PO group and at second laparotomy on NA group. For comparison, survival of patients with stage I and II disease registered during the same observation period were also shown in Figure 2.

Survival (5 year, median) for each subgroup was 42 %, 38 mo for OD → PO (35 cases), 6 %, 18 mo for subOD → PO (42 cases), 66 %, 82 mo for NA → OD (34 cases), and 7 %, 18 mo for NA → subOD (40 cases). Survival time for NA → OD was significantly longer than that for OD → PO and was almost equal to that for stage II (54 %, 72 mo).

5. Comparison of survival for chemo-responsive patients

The comparison of survival for OD → PO with that for NA → OD in Figure 2 was imbalanced because the former included chemo-resistants while the latters were all chemo-responders. Thus, we next made a comparison of survival of only chemo-responders of both groups (Fig. 3).

Patients with P_2-E (OD followed by an effective chemotherapy) in Figure 3, the most ideal group receiving standard modality, survived longest, but this group occupied only 17 % (13/77) of patients receiving debulking at initial laparotomy. Moreover, the survival of this group was not significantly longer than that of patients with N_2-E (NA followed by OD) which occupied 43 % (32/74) of patients receiving initial exploratory laparotomy followed by NA chemotherapy. However, this comparison was hard to assess the efficacy of NA chemotherapy because the tumor diameter of the NA group before the start of chemotherapy was significantly larger than that of PO. Then, we compared the survival of N_2-E with that of Px-E (subOD followed by an effec-

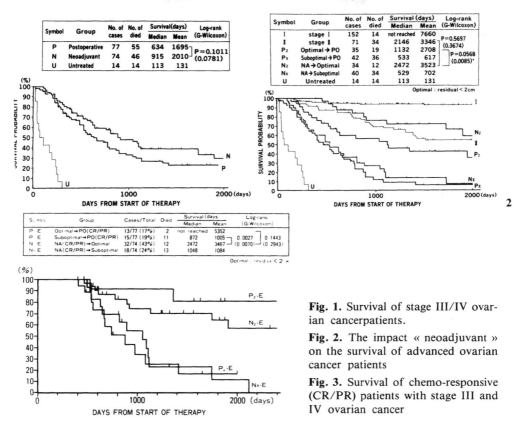

Fig. 1. Survival of stage III/IV ovarian cancer patients.

Fig. 2. The impact « neoadjuvant » on the survival of advanced ovarian cancer patients

Fig. 3. Survival of chemo-responsive (CR/PR) patients with stage III and IV ovarian cancer

tive chemotherapy). Even under this condition, it remains a hard comparison for NA group, because the tumor size is still significantly larger in NA group. As shown in Figure 3, patients with N_2-E survived significantly longer than those with Px-E. These results clearly showed a predominance of NA chemotherapy followed by a debulking over the standard treatment modality in the context of survival as well as response rate.

6. Comparison of survival for chemo-resistant patients

When NA chemotherapy was ineffective, OD was impossible as a matter of course. Such a worst group (Nx-R) was not different in survival as compared with patients with Px-E (subOD followed by an ineffective chemotherapy).

Discussion

When patients with stage III/IV ovarian cancer are subjected to a standard modality (maximal debulking at initial surgical attempt followed by PO chemotherapy), prognosis depends on the residual tumor size [1]. Indeed, patients with OD survived longer than those with subOD [2]. We have a question for this standard modality, since the primary debulking carried out at initial laparotomy produced only 21 % of patients with OD having good prognosis, with leaving 79 % of patients with subOD having poor prognosis. The rate of OD at initial laparotomy was reported to vary from 17 % to 87 %[3]. This rate depends partly on the eligibility criteria for admission of patients. Our hospital accepts all the patients who desire to receive a treatment, regardless of PS. The OD rate also varies by the definition of « optimal » which is defined in general as residuum < 2 cm.

It is apparent that even in the best surgical centers, OD can only be achieved in about one third of patients [3]. Thus, if the debulking is applied to all the patients at initial laparotomy, it will produce about two third of patients with poor prognosis, which cannot be converted by any treatment modality performed afterwards. Now, gynecological oncologists must reappraise the therapeutic power of current standard modality for advanced ovarian cancer.

There has been no randomized study to assess the efficacy of NA chemotherapy to date. Recent studies have reported that NA chemotherapy can increase the rate of OD in advanced ovarian cancer patients [4, 5]. However, the impact of NA chemotherapy followed by a debulking on survival has been controversial [6, 7]. The present retrospective study with selection bias set at the initial laparotomy clearly indicates that NA chemotherapy followed by debulking is a recommended modality to improve the prognosis of advanced ovarian cancer patients. The favorable results unexpectedly obtained in the present study are possibly due to the following two factors:

1) Response to chemotherapy is higher in NA group than in PO.

2) As a result of effective NA chemotherapy, OD was successfully performed in 46 % of patients deemed « unresectable » at initial laparotomy. In addition, radicality of debulking carried out on each patient may also be improved in NA group.

The present data warrants the worth of prospective study of NA chemotherapy followed by a debulking surgery for advanced ovarian cancer patients.

Conclusion

The present retrospective study concerning the mode of treatment for advanced ovarian cancer patients with selection bias set at the initial laparotomy clearly shows that NA chemotherapy followed by debulking surgery is a promising treatment modality for advanced ovarian cancer patients and warrants the worth of prospective study.

References

1. Griffiths GT (1975) Surgical resection of tumor bulk in the primary treatment of ovarian carcinoma. Natl Cancer Inst Monograph 42 : 101-104

2. Hoskins WJ (1989) The influence of cytoreductive surgery on progression-free interval and survival in epithelial ovarian cancer. Bailliere's Clin Obst Gynecol 3 : 59-71
3. Ozols RF, Rubin SC, Dembo AJ, Robboy S (1992) Epithelial ovarian cancer. In : Hoskins WJ, Perez CA, Young RC (eds) Principles and practice of Gynecologic Oncology. JB Lippincott Company, pp. 731-781
4. Lawton FG, Redman CWE, Luesley DM, Chan KK, Blackledge G (1989) Neo-Adjuvant (cytoreductive) chemotherapy combined with intervention debulking surgery in advanced, unresected epithelial ovarian cancer. Obst Gynecol 73 : 61-65
5. Chambers JT, Chambers SK, Voynick IM, Schwartz PE (1990) Neo-Adjuvant chemotherapy in stage X ovarian carcinoma. Gynecol Oncol 37 : 327-331
6. Neijt JP, Ten Bokkel Huinink WW, Van der Burg MEL, Van Oosterom AT, Willemse PHB, Heintz APM, Van Lent M, Trimbos JB, Bouma J, Vermorken JB, Van Houwelingen JC (1987) Randomized trial comparing two combination chemotherapy regimens (CHAP-5 v CP) in advanced ovarian carcinoma. J Clin Oncol 5 : 1157-1168
7. Jacob JH, Gershenson DM, Morris M, Copeland LJ, Burke TW, Wharton JT (1991) Neo-Adjuvant chemotherapy and interval debulking for advanced epithelial ovarian cancer. Gynecol Oncol 42 : 146-150

Hyperfractionation using weekly Cisplatin, Cyclophosphamide and Adriamycin (CAP) in advanced epithelial tumors of the ovary

K Tonkin, L Levin

Cisplatin (Cis) is an essential component in chemotherapy regimens for ovarian carcinoma. There are many multiagent regimens which suggests none has marked superiority (Young 1984, Pasmantier 1985).

Dose intensity

Dose intensity (DI) is a powerful approach in treatment. Average DI, of Cis, is a determinant of clinical response and survival (Levin 1987). Current analysis (Levin, personal communication) shows Cyclophosphamide (C) and Adriamycin (A) may enhance Cis response.

Weekly chemotherapy should increase the fractional cell kills (Skipper 1964). Minimizing intervals should restrict emergence of resistant clones. Its effect on toxicity is unknown.

Clinical data

Previously published data (Columbo 1991, O'Connell 1987) has shown the feasibility of weekly Cis but problems with toxicity when A was used as well.

The DI's of CAP used relative to standard Greco CHAP are 0.92, 1.05 and 1.14 respectively.

This equates to C 125 mg/week at all dose levels, A 10 mg/m^2/week increasing to 15 mg/m^2/week for levels 2 and 3, and Cisplatin 30 mg/m^2/week for levels 1 and 2, increasing to 35 mg/m^2 at level 3. All CAP was given weekly × 18.

Trial objectives

These are (a) determine the toxicity of hyperfractionated CAP ; (b) to evaluate the quality of life.

London Regional Cancer Centre, London, Canada

Study population

Criteria of eligibility, design and response criteria. A diagnosis of epithelial ovarian carcinoma must have been made histologically. No prior radiotherapy or chemotherapy should have been administered. Performance status should be ECOG 0-3. All other eligibility criteria were as per local requirements.

This is a pilot study with a total of 9 patients reported thus far.

Response was measured using standard WHO criteria as published previously.

Toxicity and dose reductions for myelosuppression. This is a major endpoint of the study, and is documented using ECOG toxicity criteria.

If the treatment day neutrophil count is less than $1.2 \times 10^9/L$ and/or the platelet count is less than $100 \times 10^9/L$, treatment should be delayed by 1 week.

Once recovery occurs, the same dose is given, but a further delay in treatment requires modifications. If a second 1 week delay occurs, C is omitted from further cycles. Further treatment delays leads to a decrease in A dose level or discontinuation.

Results

Renal, neurotoxicity and gastrointestinal toxicity was not seen in any patient.

Table 1: Patients Nos 1 and 2 received 100 % of their projected DI in 20 or 21 weeks. No 3 refused the 18th treatment.

Results of Level 2 are shown in Table 2. Nos 4 and 6 completed treatment in 24 or 23 weeks respectively. No 4 had asymptomatic neutropenia, and C was omitted after 7 doses, and the dose of A was reduced from 15 mg/m² to 10 mg/m² from the 10th dose. In patient 5, 15 treatments were given over a 16 week period, but the patient had fatigue and anorexia, and after gastrostomy tube, went into septic shock and died. Laparotomy done prior to death revealed minimal residual disease.

Results of Level 3 are illustrated in Table 3. No 7 was able to complete 14 weeks of the treatment over 19 weeks. She received 1 course of C 500 mg/m² and Cis 75 mg/m². She remains disease-free 4 months after. No 8 received 9 cycles over 14 weeks and then had treatment as for patient 7, but received 3 further cycles. She is disease-free 3 months after competion. No 9 received 3 weekly treatments then developed febrile neutropenia, was found to have cholecystitis and had cholecystectomy.

Discussion

The patients tolerated the first 2 dose levels, but at Level 3 the treatment could not be completed as scheduled.

Table 1. Level 1

	Doses given mg/m²/wk			% of projected dose			Time to complete (weeks)
	C	A	P	C	A	P	
01	125	10	30	100	100	100	20
02	125	10	30	100	100	100	21
03	118	9.4	28.3	94.4	94.4	94.4	21

Table 2. Level 2

	Doses given mg/m²/wk			% of projected dose			Time to complete (weeks)
	C	A	P	C	A	P	
04	69.4	8.3	27.5	55.5	55.5	91.6	24
05	125	15	30	100	100	100	16*
06	41.6	15	30	33	100	100	23

* Patient deceased - calculations for 15 weeks of treatment

Table 3. Level 3

	Doses given mg/m²/wk			% of projected dose			Time to complete (weeks)
	C	A	P	C	A	P	
07	59.2	11	25.8	50	77.8	77.8	19 (14)
08	80.4	9.6	22.5	50	50	50	14 (9)
09	125	15	35	100	100	100	3*

( ) Refers to number of weekly treatments received
* Patient deceased - only had 3 weeks of treatment

Further patients are being accrued on a 2 weekly regimen. This is C 500 mg/m², A 30 mg/m² and Cis 60 mg/m², all 2 weekly × 9. The DI is 1.24.

We will accrue 10-14 patients then prospectively evaluate it against 3 weekly DI inpatient CAP.

Conclusions

We found weekly outpatient CAP was feasible, but psychologically difficult to tolerate. We are pursuing DI treatment using 2 weekly outpatient treatment.

References

1. Columbo N, Pitelli MR, Marzola M et al (1991) Randomized study of two different Cisplatin (P) dose-intensity regimens in patients (pts) with advanced epithelial ovarian cancer (EOC). VIth Int Symposium on Platinum and Other Metal Coordination Compounds in Cancer Chemotherapy 173 : 139
2. Levin L, Hryniuk W (1987) Dose intensity analysis of chemotherapy regimens in ovarian carcinoma. J Clin Oncol 5 : 756-767
3. O'Connell G, Shelley W, Carmichael J et al (1987) High-dose intensity regimen of weekly Doxorubicin and Cisplatin in the treatment of patients with stage III and IV epithelial ovarian carcinoma. Cancer Treat Rep 71 (5) : 455-458
4. Pasmantier MW, Coleman M, Silver RT et al (1985) Treatment of advanced endometrial carcinoma with Doxorubicin and Cisplatin : Effects on both untreated and previously treated patients. Cancer Treat Rep 69 : 539-542
5. Skipper HE, Schabel FM Jr, Wilcox WS (1964) Experimental evaluation of potential anti-cancer agents. XII On the criteria and kinetics associated with « Curability » of experimental leukemia. Cancer Chemotherapy Reports 35 : 1-111
6. Young RC (1984) Ovarian cancer treatment : progress or paralysis. Sem Oncol 11 : 327-329

Adjuvant treatment of ovarian carcinoma[1]

IB Vergote, CG Tropé, LN De Vos, J Kærn, VM Abeler, M Winderen, EO Pettersen

Postoperative adjuvant treatment with alkylating chemotherapeutic agents or irradiation, either as intraperitoneal isotope (radioactive gold [^{198}Au] or phosphorus [^{32}P] colloid) instillation or as total abdominal irradiation, has been evaluated in various prospective randomized trials, but the value of postoperative adjuvant treatment is still controversial [1-7]. The key questions regarding adjuvant therapy [8] of ovarian carcinoma are : (1) What therapeutic options are reasonable and justifiable ? (2) Which patients possess a prognosis poor enough to justify subsequent adjuvant therapy ? (3) Do any of the existing adjuvant therapies benefit patients ?

What therapeutic options for adjuvant treatment are reasonable and justifiable ?

We compared adjuvant intraperitoneal ^{32}P therapy with 6 cycles of Cisplatin, the most active chemotherapeutic agent in ovarian carcinoma in a group of 347 patients without residual tumor following primary laparotomy. No difference in actuarial crude or disease-free survival between the 2 treatment groups was observed [9]. However, late bowel obstruction occurred more often in the group treated with ^{32}P compared with the Cisplatin group. In a second study we analyzed the treatment complications in 313 patients treated with intraperitoneal ^{32}P therapy. It was concluded that the morbidity was substantial since 2 patients died of complications which at least partly could be attributed to the ^{32}P therapy, and since 22 (7 %) patients suffered from small bowel complications treated surgically or medically, 2 from a colon fistula and 1 from an ileo-vaginal fistula. No significant relation existed between the incidence of small bowel complications and the ^{32}P dose, the ^{32}P distribution scintigram, treatment with ^{32}P after primary surgery or at second-look laparotomy, the type of surgery at instillation, the number of prior laparotomies, or whether ^{32}P was given on the same day as surgery or the next day.

Because of the well-established risk of leukemia after adjuvant treatment with alkylating agents, Young et al [6] recommended ^{32}P as the standard treatment for subsequent studies. In the absence of a therapeutic difference in our study between the ^{32}P and Cisplatin group, in addition to a low frequency of irreversible toxicity following Cisplatin therapy and a higher occurrence of bowel complications after ^{32}P therapy, we suggest that Cisplatin (or eventually other platin analogues) should be the standard treatment.

The Norwegian Radium Hospital, 0310 Oslo, Norway.
[1] Supported by The Norwegian Cancer Society Grants 88/222, 88/234 and 88/290.

Which patients possess a prognosis poor enough to justify subsequent adjuvant therapy?

It is widely recognized that the presence of residual tumor following primary surgery is one of the most important prognostic factors in ovarian cancer. Although the survival in patients with disease localized to the pelvis is better than in patients with more advanced disease, the relapse risk is high enough in some subgroups of patients to warrant postoperative treatment. FIGO Stage II disease is one of these subgroups since the 5-year actuarial survival is approximately 57 % only [10].

FIGO Stage I disease should be divided in different subgroups. Earlier large reports identified degree of differentiation, histological type, dense adhesions, large volume ascites, and patient age as independent prognostic characteristics [6, 11, 12]. In the current study we analyzed the traditional clinicopathological characteristics and DNA content in a series of 290 patients with FIGO Stage I epithelial invasive ovarian carcinoma. In graded tumors (i.e. not containing clear cell elements) a multivariate analysis identified degree of differentiation as the most powerful predictor of disease-free survival, followed by DNA ploidy and, finally, FIGO (1986) substage. When the effects of degree of differentiation, DNA ploidy and FIGO substage were accounted for, then none of the following were prognostic : dense adhesion, ascites, age, extracapsular growth, rupture during surgery, FIGO (1973) substage, size of the tumor, and type of adjuvant treatment. These findings confirm earlier studies suggesting that the degree of differentiation is an important independent prognostic indicator in FIGO Stage I ovarian cancer. In addition, this study identifies DNA ploidy and FIGO (1986) substage as new independent prognostic factors in FIGO Stage I disease. Results of studies evaluating the association between DNA ploidy and grade have been inconsistent. In our 219 tumors that were graded and had an interpretable DNA histogram, DNA ploidy was significantly associated with grade. However, despite this correlation 32 % of the well differentiated tumors were DNA non-diploid suggesting that the DNA content may not be predicted by the degree of differentiation.

Table 1. Relapse in stage I epithelial ovarian carcinoma according to prognostic groups

	Degree of differentiation			
	Well	Moderate	Poor	Not Graded (Clear Cell)*
Diploid	0/77 (0)§	HIGH	35/142 (25)	
Non diploid		RISK		
Stage Ia				1/15 (7)
Stage Ib-c				25/46 (54)

Numbers between parentheses denote percentages
* Including mixed epithelial tumors with clear cell elements

As in previous reports clear cell tumors had a worse prognosis than the other histological types in the present study. When considering DNA ploidy and FIGO (1986) substage in clear cell tumors and mixed epithelial tumors with clear cell elements, FIGO (1986) substage was an important prognostic variable while DNA ploidy was not significant.

Based on these analyses the patients were divided in prognostic groups (Table 1). None of the 77 patients with well differentiated DNA diploid tumors relapsed. This low-risk group had a significant better survival than well differentiated DNA non-diploid tumors or moderately differentiated DNA diploid tumors. The high-risk group was constituted of all moderately and poorly differentiated tumors, and highly differentiated DNA non-diploid tumors. No significant differences were observed between any of the « neighboring » subgroups in this high-risk group. When adding tumors with clear cell elements in FIGO (1986) Stage Ib and Ic to this high-risk group, 60 (32 %) of 188 patients relapsed. This rate should be high enough that most investigators feel a trial of adjuvant therapy is warranted.

Do any of the existing adjuvant therapies benefit patients ?

Comparison of survival results between non-randomized studies using different types of adjuvant treatment or no adjuvant treatment at all, is difficult. Most randomized trials compared 2 or 3 different adjuvant treatment modalities. However, without an untreated observation group the efficacy of adjuvant treatment can not be established. Only 2 randomized studies included a control arm. In a first study of the Gynecologic Oncology Group only 86 patients were randomized between pelvic irradiation, melphalan therapy or no treatment [4]. A second trial is reported of the Ovarian Cancer Study Group and the Gynecologic Oncology Group [6]. In this study only 81 patients with well or moderately differentiated FIGO (1973) Stage Ia_i or Ib_i were randomized between adjuvant melphalan therapy or no treatment. However, 1 patient in 3 was later declared on central pathological review to have a tumor of borderline malignancy. The estimated 5-year overall survival rates for untreated patients and patients treated with melphalan were 94 % and 98 %, respectively. This difference was not significant or even suggestive. This might have been expected since approximately 1000 patients are required, when a difference in survival of 5 % is to be detected at a significance level of 5 % and a power of 90 % in patients with a survival of 90 % [13]. Hence, only a large prospective trial of poor prognosis early ovarian cancer patients with an untreated control arm will be able to resolve the question whether any adjuvant therapy confers survival advantage.

In an effort to answer this question we started a Scandinavian randomized trial in May 1992 in high-risk FIGO (1986) Stage I ovarian carcinoma comparing carboplatin with a no treatment arm (Fig. 1). Carboplatin is used instead of Cisplatin because it has been shown that carboplatin is equally effective in ovarian cancer but possesses lower ototoxic, nephrotoxic, and neurotoxic properties than cisplatin. The carboplatin dose was related to the glomerular filtration rate (GFR) since Calvert et al [14] demonstrated that the toxicity and therapeutic efficacy of the drug are dictated primarily by the pretreatment GFR, and recommended 7 (GFR + 25) mg as dosage of choice for single-agent carboplatin therapy.

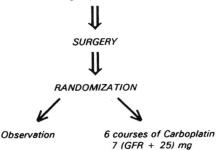

Fig. 1. Study design of the Scandinavian randomized adjuvant trial on stage I ovarian carcinoma. GFR : Glomerular Filtration Rate

References

1. Smith JP, Rutledge FN, Delclos L (1975) Postoperative treatment of early cancer of the ovary : a random trial between postoperative irradiation and chemotherapy. J Natl Cancer Inst 42 : 149-153
2. Kolstad P, Davy M, Hoeg K (1977) Individualized treatment of ovarian cancer. Am J Obstet Gynecol 128 : 617-625
3. Dembo AJ, Bush RS, Beale FA, Bean HA, Pringle JF, Sturgeon J, Reid JG (1979) Ovarian carcinoma : Improved survival following abdominopelvic irradiation in patients with a completed pelvic operation. Am J Obstet Gynecol 134 : 793-800
4. Hreshchyshyn MM, Park RC, Blessing JA, Norris HJ, Levy D, Lagasse LD, Creasman WT (1980) The role of adjuvant therapy in stage I ovarian cancer. Am J Obstet Gynecol 138 : 139-145
5. Klaassen D, Shelley W, Starreveld A, Kirk M, Boyes D, Gerulath A, Levitt M, Fraser R, Carmichael J, Methot Y (1988) Early stage ovarian cancer : a randomized clinical trial comparing whole abdominal radiotherapy, melphalan, and intraperitoneal chromic phosphate. A National Cancer Institute of Canada Clinical Trials Group report. J Clin Oncol 6 : 1254-1263
6. Young RC, Walton LA, Ellenberg SS, Homesley HD, Wilbanks GD, Decker DG, Miller A, Park R, Major FJ (1990) Adjuvant therapy in stage I and stage II epithelial ovarian cancer. Results of two prospective randomized trials. N Engl J Med 322 : 1021-1027
7. Sell A, Bertelsen K, Andersen JE, Stryer I, Panduro J (1990) Randomized study of whole-abdomen irradiation versus pelvic irradiation plus Cyclophosphamide in treatment of early ovarian cancer. Gynecol Oncol 37 : 367-373

8. Young RC (1991) Editorial. Gynecol Oncol 43 : 193-194
9. Vergote I, Vergote-De Vos L, Abeler V, Aas M, Lindegaard M, Kjorstad K, Trope C (1992) Randomized trial comparing Cisplatin with radioactive phosphorus or whole abdomen irradiation as adjuvant treatment in ovarian cancer. Cancer 69 : 741-749
10. Pettersson F (1991) Annual report on the results of treatment in gynecological cancer. Twenty-first volume. Statements of the results obtained in patients 1982 to 1986, inclusive 3- and 5-year survival up to 1990. Int J Gynecol Obstet (suppl) : 238-255
11. Dembo AJ, Davy M, Stenwig AE, Berle EJ, Bush RS, Kjorstad K (1990) Prognostic factors in patients with stage I epithelial ovarian cancer. Obstet Gynecol 75 : 263-273
12. Finn CB, Luesley DM, Buxton EJ, Blackledge GR, Kelly K, Dunn JA, Wilson S (1992) Is Stage I epithelial ovarian cancer overtreated both surgically and systemically ? Results of a five-year cancer registry review. Br J Obstet Gynecol 99 : 54-58
13. Freedman LS (1982) Tables of the number of patients required in clinical trials using the logranktest. Stat Med 1 : 121-129
14. Calvert AH, Newell DR, Gumbrell LA et al (1989) Carboplatin dosage : Prospective evaluation of a simple formula based on renal function. J Clin Oncol 7 : 1748-1756

Abstract. Between October 1982 and July 1988, 347 patients with ovarian cancer without residual tumor after primary laparotomy were randomized between intraperitoneal ^{32}P therapy and 6 courses of Cisplatin (50 mg/m²). Disease-free and crude survival were similar in both groups, but adjuvant ^{32}P therapy was associated with more bowel complications. No significant relation existed between the incidence of bowel complications and ^{32}P dose, ^{32}P distribution scintigram, type of surgery at ^{32}P instillation and number of prior laparotomies. The traditional clinical and pathological prognostic variables and DNA ploidy were analyzed in 290 patients with FIGO Stage I invasive epithelial ovarian carcinoma. A multivariate analysis identified degree of differentiation as the most powerful prognostic indicator, followed by DNA ploidy and, finally, FIGO substage. A high-risk group with graded tumors in FIGO Stage I was identified and consisted of all moderately and poorly differentiated tumors, and well differentiated DNA non-diploid tumors. The relapse rate in this group was 25 %. None of the patients with well differentiated DNA diploid tumors relapsed. Clear cell tumors were not graded and a relapse rate of 43 % was observed in this group with FIGO Stage I disease. Based on these results a Scandinavian randomized trial in high-risk FIGO Stage I ovarian carcinoma was initiated comparing adjuvant carboplatin therapy with a no treatment arm.

Cyclophosphamide (CTX) and high-dose 4-Epidoxorubicin (EPI) in advanced ovarian cancer (OC) treatment

G Cartei, M Signor, E Vigevani, M Giovannoni, A Sibau,
G Clocchiatti, M Mansutti

Cancer of the ovary is the fifth cause of cancer death in women, and the majority of patients have advanced stage disease at the time of presentation [1]. Clinical responses can be achieve with current regimens in over half of patients but only a minority enjoy prolonged disease free survival [2]. Consequently there is a need for innovative strategies to improve the prognosis in advanced stage patients. We have treated 52 consecutive patients, since september '87, with advanced ovarian cancer, utilizing a combination regimen based on the association between CTX and high-dose EPI-ADM in delayed administration.

This therapeutic option was purposed on the basis of following suggestions:
— remission rate % given by CTX and EPI-ADM, single and in association [2];
— lower cardiotoxicity of EPI-ADM with delayed administration;
— better chemoresponsivity utilizing high-dose of EPI-AD [3];
— lower efficacy of these agents in 2nd line approach and instead better therapeutic choice of CDDP in refractory patients [4];
— no neurologic and renal toxicity in women that often are compromized by natural history of cancer disease;
— choice of better management of therapeutic arms in pharmacological treatment;
— advanced disease stage with low possibilities of definitive cure even utilizing CDDP in first line [5];
— in office treatment or day hospital regimen.

Aim of the study was to estimate effectiveness and tolerability of CTX and high dose EPI-ADM combination chemotherapy in patients with advanced ovarian cancer. End points were: response rate — response duration — toxicity and tolerance — overall survival — correlation between prognosis factors and response plus survival.

Patients and methods

The study has enrolled 52 patients.
Criteria for entry were: *a)* histologic or cytologic diagnosis of epithelial ovarian carcinoma; *b)* International Federation of Gynecologies and Obstretics stage III or IV [6]; *c)* age younger than 75 years; *d)* Karnofsky Performande Status > = 60; *e)* no previous chemotherapy or radiotherapy; *f)* in-

Med Oncology Dep, Gen Hospital Udine, Italy

formed consense ; g) no medical controindications to combination chemotherapy, h) no cardiac risk factors.

Where possible, the extent of disease was determinated by surgical exploration ; as much of the tumor as possible was removed by total hysterectomy, bilateral salpingo-oophorectomy and omentectomy or, however, an optimal surgical debulking was performed. In other conditions, a clinical and radiologic stage assessment was achieved.

Treatment plan

Patients received 4-Epidoxorubicin 30 mg/m^2 and 300 mg/m^2 CTX h 08.00 a.m. and h 02.00 p.m. day 1,2 every 3 weeks. Combination of Lorazepam 2.5 x os, Methylprednisolone 125 mg x i.v. bolus (h. 0-6) and Metoclopramide 1.5 mg/Kg x i.v. (h. 0-6) was the suggested administered antiemetic regimen. Courses were repeated at 21 days intervals (provided that the WBC count was greater than 4,000, the PLT count was greater than 100,000).

Dose of all drugs were not modified but chemotherapy administration was delayed of 7 days until correct hematologic parameters were obtained. Patients were treated for 4-6 cycles or until progression ; clinically disease free women were submitted, whenever possible, to second look laparatomy. Then, patients in pathologic Complete Remission (pCR) or with microscopic residual disease received 3 courses of CDDP based combination chemotherapy regimen.

In the same manner, patients with macroscopic residual disease or in progressing during or relapsing after induction therapy received CDDP based polichemotherapy. Patients were considered evaluable after 2 or 3 cycles by the same diagnostic methods utilized for measurable lesions. Response duration was determined from the time of first clinical radiologic restaging to the moment of progression. Overall survival was assessed from first course to time of death. WHO criteria were utilized for defining toxicity and principal side effects.

Results

Since September '87 we enrolled 52 pts ; analysis at September '92 is available in the first 30 patients.

Patients'characteristics were : median age = 56 with range 38-72 ; median PS = 85 with range 60-100.

Histologic type : papillary serous = 21 (70 %), endometrioid = 4 (13.3 %), mucinous = 2 (6.6), undifferentiated = 2 (6.6 %), mesonephoid = 1 (3.3 %).

Histologic grade : I = 7 (23.3 %), II = 9 (30 %), III = 14 (46.6 %). Stage : IIIA = 6 (20 %), IIIB = 5 (16.6 %), IIIC = 15 (50 %), IV = 4 (13.3 %).

Prior surgery was : radical = 8 (26.6 %), cytoriductive = 1 (3.3 %), partial = 16 (53.3 %), explorative = 5 (17.6 %).

141 courses were administered with average of 4.7.

We obtained 8 (26,6 %) pathological complete remission (pCR), 6 [20 %] clinical complete remission (cCR) and 9 [30 %] partial remission (PR) with an overall response (OR) of 76,6 %.

Average duration of response, in months, was:
pCR = 334/8 = 43
cCR = 193/6 = 32.1
PR = 88/9 = 9.7

Second look laparotomy was performed in 18 (60 %) patients. Between the potential prognostic factors, only histologic grade had apparent importance in our study.

Toxicity was predictable mild to severe and included (grade and pts).

Nausea and vomiting: I = 3 (10 %), II = 14, (46.6 %), III = 10 (33.3 %). IV = 3 (10 %)

Hematological: I = 4 (13.3 %), II = 9 (30 %), III = 14 (46.6 %) IV = 3 (10 %).

Alopecia: I = 0, II = 16 (53,3 %), III = 14 (46,6 %)

Cardiac: I = 0, II = 4 (13,3 %), III = 1 (3,3 %)

There were no toxic deaths.

We observed that nausea and vomiting of moderate to severe intensity was experienced by the majority of the patients but we want to make you remember you that, with new antiemetic regimen based on ondansetron, chemotherapy is well tolerated. Furthermore the use of hematopoietic growth factors may permit further dose intensification and increase of dose intensity of EPI ADN and CTX containing regimens.

Discussion

Since September 87, we have treated 30 women with stage III-IV disease, median age: 56, PS ⩾ 60. We have obtained 14 CR and 8 PR for an overall response rate of 76.6 %.

We have administered 141 cycles.

There were no toxic deaths and we observed mild to severe toxicity particularly for nausea, vomiting and myelosuppression but no severe cardiac compromission. Aim of the study was to assess a scheme with characteristics of good response rate and accetable toxicity. Obviously we aren't sure to achieve the goal, however we have demonstered that on optimal treatment regimen has not been established particularly if we want to utilize pharmacological agents during history of ovarian malignancies to give our patients a significant improvement on the prognosis.

The results of our experience, in terms of overall response and toxicity, are good and more over they are positively comparable with studies utilizing CDDP based schemes although our number of patients is not large. We considered important that high-dose of EPI ADM gives us a good therapeutic option and in such way we can have another choice for optimal second line chemotherapy with CDDP based regimens those may be able to give high response rate. In other words might be that high dose EPI ADM combination chemotherapy followed by CDDP based second line can improve the poor prognosis of patients with advanced ovarian cancer and, perhaps, for this reason, it is necessary to assess randomized studies.

References

1. Young RC, Fuks Z, Hoskins WJ (1989) Cancer of the ovary. In : De Vita VT, Hellman S, Rosenberg SA (eds) Cancer : Principles and practice of oncology. Lippincott, Philadelphia, pp. 1162-1196
2. Thigpen JT, Blessing JA, Vance RB et al (1989) Chemotherapy in ovarian carcinoma : present role and future prospectives. Sem Oncol 16 : 58-65
3. Wheeler R, Ensminger WD, Thrall JH et al (1982) High-dose Doxorubicin : an exploration of the dose response curve in human neoplasia. Cancer Treat Rep 66 : 493-498
4. Omura G, Blessing JA, Ehrich CE (1986) A randomized trial of Cyclophosphamide and Doxorubicin with or without Cisplatin in advanced ovarian carcinoma. Cancer 57 : 1725-1730
5. Hainsworth HD, Grosh WW, Burnett LS et al (1988) Advanced ovarian cancer : long terms results of treatment with intensive Cisplatin based chemotherapy of brief duration. Ann Inter Med 108 : 115-170
6. International federation of gynecology and obstetrics (1987) Changes in definitions of clinical staging for carcinoma of the cervix and ovary. Am J Obstet Gyn 154 : 236-237

High-dose chemotherapy (HDC) and autologous bone marrow transplant (ABMT) in 39 advanced ovarian cancers : long-term results

A Legros*, H Curé*, J Fleury*, F Suzanne**, J Dauplat*, Ph Chollet*, R Plagne*

Commun epithelial ovarian carcinoma, in particular stage III and IV (FIGO) have a poor prognosis with a survival rate < 20 % at 5 years. Paradoxically ovarian cancer is very responsive to chemotherapy with high overall response rates demonstrated consistently using Cisplatin based combination regimens. It is this contrast of high response rates with major reductions in tumor burden, yet low numbers of durable complete remissions, that let us to use a high-dose chemotherapy and ABMT in poor risk patients.

Patients and methods

Patients

Out of the 39 patients, the initial FIGO stade was III in 31 patients, IV in 7 patients and II in 1 patient on relapse. All patients had initial surgery with 7 complete initial excision, 19 optimal surgery (residual tumor < 2 cm), 10 suboptimal surgery (residual tumor > 2 cm) and for 3 patients debulking surgery was impossible.

All patients received 4 to 8 courses of Cisplatinum based chemotherapy.

The patients had further a second-look operation (SLO) to evaluate results of chemotherapy : 10 of them have a negative SLO and 29 a positive SLO (5 microscopic, 24 macroscopic). At the initiation of HDC and ABMT, 16 patients had no tumor, 20 minimal excised residual disease, 6 had a tumor > 2 cm.

Methods

39 patients received 42 ABMT (3 double transplantation).

21 patients received high-dose Melphalan (140 mg/sq.m.) given as an IV bolus throught a central venous live.

21 patients received a combination of Carboplatine (1 to 1.5 g/sq.m.) and Cyclophosphamide (6 g/sq.m.) total dose fractionnated in 4 days.

All patients were well hydrated with coutinuous IV fluids started 24 hours before and continued 24 hours after HDC. Bone marrow was reinfused

From : * Centre Jean Perrin, BP 392, 63011 Clermont-Ferrand Cedex, ** Maternité, Hôtel-Dieu, 63000 Clermont-Ferrand, France

48 hours after chemotherapy by intravenous infusion ; patients received 2 x 10^8 autologous marrow cells/kg (range 0.3-4.5).

Patients were managed in single rooms with reverse isolation.

Complications

All patients experienced profound aplasia after HDC with a neutrophil count < $0.1 \times 10^9/l$ and platelet count < $20 \times 10^9/l$.

Prompt haematological recovery was observed in most patients, most patients experienced febrile episode and we observed 3 cytomegalovirus meningitis and 1 enterococcus septicemia.

Two patients had a completly reversible cardiac toxicity. No death due to treatment was observed.

Results

Overall 24 of the 39 patients are alive, 14 with non progressive disease at a median follow-up of 64 months after HDC (96-6 months) (Fig. 1). At present the projected disease-free survival is 23 % at 5 years and overall survival is 40 % at 5 years.

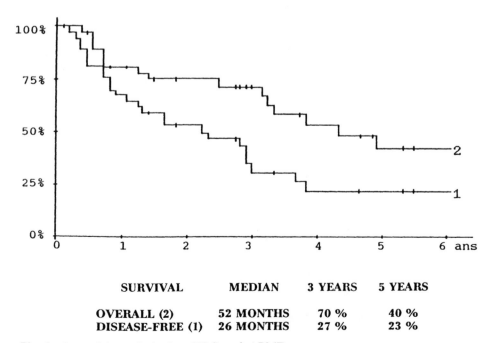

SURVIVAL	MEDIAN	3 YEARS	5 YEARS
OVERALL (2)	52 MONTHS	70 %	40 %
DISEASE-FREE (1)	26 MONTHS	27 %	23 %

Fig. 1. Actuarial survival after HDC and ABMT

Discussion

This study retrospectively evaluated results obtained with HDC and ABMT in a single institution. The results confirmed in this population the feasibility of such a therapy with a good long-term results. HDC + ABMT is a safe procedure and one third a long-term survivor can be expected in selected patients with poor risk prognosis factors. Survival is of good quality with non long-term toxicity and no more treatment. For patients who relapsed we observed a very good tolerance and efficacity of the conventionnal chemotherapy.

Concomitant chemotherapy and radiotherapy in the treatment of advanced cervix carcinomas

M Resbeut, M Noirclerc, G Gravis, Cl d'Ercole, P Pechikoff, G Houvenaeghel, JR Delpero, JL Blache, P Viens

Although early stages of cervix carcinomas can be controled successfully by radiotherapy (RT) alone or by surgery and RT, with high 5-years survival rates : about 90 % in stages (st.) IB patients (pts) and 80 % in st. IIA pts [13], the influence of the tumor volume is well documented and advanced lesions carry a bad prognosis.

Failures of the treatment become more frequent in st. IIB pts. In these st., 5-y survival rates are 60 % up to 70 [13] but less than 50 % in case of bulky disease (> 5 cm). In st. IIIB pts, these rates range from 25 % to 50 % [3] with markedly worse results in case of tumor fixation to both pelvic side walls [1]. Long term survivors are less than 20 % in st. IV pts [17]. Lymph node involvment implies a poor pronosis specially, in some series [7] if there are 3 or more positive nodes.

In case of bulky tumors, local control decreases in each st. [13] and pelvic appears to be the first site of failure in two/third of the cases [16].

Attempting to improve this local control we analyze in this paper a pilot study of concurrent chemo-radiation (CCR).

Methods and patients

Between February 1988 and July 1992, 33 pts (group A) with epidermoïd carcinomas underwent this CCR as their first treatment (st. IB> 5 cm : 4, st. IIB with distal parametrial involvment : 14, st. IV : 15). In group B, 7 pts with more than 3 metastatic nodes and/or capsular invasion on a previous lymphadenectomy received CCR after surgery. Median age was 47 years (29-70 years) and median Karnofsky index was 70 (50-100). Staging was checked under anaesthetic examination with an intracavitary ultra-sonography [6].

CCR was a RT on the whole pelvis delivering 45 Gy/25F/33d. (2 fractions a day in the last 14 pts) and a chemotherapy (CT) on days 1 and 21 which delivered CDDP 60 mg/m^2 followed by 5-FU IV continuous infusion for 96 hours. (respectively 40 and 400 mg in the last 16 pts). In groups A pts., CCR was followed by a brachytherapy (15 Gy) and a parametrial boost (55-60 Gy) if indicated, then by a surgery in 29 pts. In group B pts, a 9 Gy boost was delivered on positive areas.

---

* Institut Paoli-Calmettes, 232 Boulevard de Sainte Marguerite, 13009 Marseille, France

Results

Tolerance is evaluable in the 40 pts. A WHO grade 3 or 4 diarrhea was observed in 16 pts and led to a RT break in 7 cases (4 to 15 days). All the pts but 1 were given 2 cycles of chemotherapy (CT), with a second cycle delay in 3 cases (1-2 weeks). A pt died after the CCR with a septic episod without leucopenia. 5 postoperative intestinal or bladder complications required a second surgical procedure. Among these pts, 1 died with a small bowed fistula and 2 developed intestinal late complications. None postoperative or late complication was observed in pts treated with bi-fractionated RT.

Sites of failure were : pelvic : 4 ; metastase : 5 ; both : 3. With a median follow-up of 36 months (6-58), pelvic rate control was 82.5 %. Two years survival and DFS rates were 71.4 % and 61 % in the whole serie. In the group A pts. these rates were respectively 60 % and 61 % in st.IB-IIB pts and 78 % and 58 % in st. IV pts but these differences are not statistically significant ($p = 0.33$ and $p = 0.08$).

Discussion

Cure rates in pts with advanced solid tumors remain low as well in pts with advanced cervix carcinomas. Neo-Adjuvant CT was disappointing in randomized trials [2, 15]. In the same way the use of radiosensitizers [9], hyperbaric oxygen therapy and neutron therapy [11] have met with limited or no success. On the other hand, 13 Cis-Retinoïc Acid plus Interferon-α-2A seems to be a highly active therapy [10]. This is an important consideration since we observed metastatic and pelvic failures in a simular proportion. In this study we tried to improve the local control by using CT drugs as radio-potentiators. Cervix tumors can be sensitive to 5-FU and CDDP [14] and this fact could increase interaction between CT and RT [18]. Toxicity independence against the small bowel is not achieved in this CCR but a bi-fractionated RT is better tolerated and furthermore, the potentiator effect of CDDP and 5-FU could be enhanced with this kind of RT [8, 12]. Even after a major surgery such as anterior pelvectomy, none pt experencied serious complication with CCR including a bi-fractionated RT. Others autors [4, 16] used a fractionated RT at least in part of their treatment and our results are comparable to those reported by Thomas [16]. Post-RT surgery appears to be an important step in order to obtain a local control if we consider our st. IV treatment results, and such important surgical procedures seem to be possible in this protocol. When the RT is fractionated we think with Thomas [16] that results of CCR in the treatment of advanced cervix carcinomas are encouraging but these studies remain few and prospectives studies are needed. Systemic therapies as the Lippman's one [10] must be considered because the incidence of metastases increases with the bulk of the local tumors.

References

1. Benstead K, Cowies UJ, Blair V, Hunter RD (1986) Stage III carcinoma of the cervix. The importance of increasing age and extent to parametrial infiltration. Radiother Oncol 5 : 271-276

2. Chauvergne J, Rohart J, Heron JF, Ayme Y, Berlie J, Fargeot P, George M, Lebrun-Jezekova D, Pigneux J et al (1990) Essai randomisé de chimiothérapie initiale dans 151 carcinomes du col utérin étendus (T2b-N1, T3b, M0). Bull Cancer 77 : 1007-24
3. Hanks GE, Herring DF, Kramer S (1983) Patterns of care outcome studies. Results of the national practice in cancer of the cervix. Cancer 51 : 959-967
4. Heaton D, Yordan E, Reddy S, Bonomi P, Lee MS, Lincoln S, Graham J, Dolan T, Miller A, Phillips A, Kirschner C, Bergen S, Wilbanks G (1990) Treatment of 29 patients with bulky squamous cell carcinoma of the cervix with simultaneous Cisplatin, 5-Fluorouracil, and split-course hyperfractionated radiation therapy. Gynecol Oncol 38 : 323-327
5. Hill BT (1991) Interaction between antitumour agents and radiation and the expression of resistance. Cancer Treat Rev 18 : 149-190
6. Houvenaeghel G, Rosello R, Delpero JR, Resbeut M, Jacquemier J, Guerinel G (1991) Extension loco-régionale des cancers avancés du col utérin : évaluation prospective des résultats de l'examen clinique, des échographies endocavitaires, de la TDM, de l'IRM et de l'histologie. Bull Cancer 78 : 969-978
7. Inone T, Morita K (1990) The pronostic significance of number of positive nodes in cervical carcinoma. Cancer 65 : 1923-1927
8. Korbelik M, Skov KA (1989) Inactivation of hypoxic cells by Cisplatin and radiation at clinically relevant doses. Radiat Res 119 : 145-156
9. Leibel S, Bauer M, Wasserman T et al (1987) Radiotherapy with or without misonidazole for patients with stage IIIB or stage IVA squamous cell carcinoma of the uterine cervix : preliminary report of a Radiation Therapy Oncology Group randomized trial. Int J Radiat Oncol Biol Phys 13 : 541-549
10. Lippman SM, Kavanagh J, Paredes-Espinoza M, Delgadillo-Madrueno F, Paredes-Casillas P, Hong WK, Holdener E, Krakoff IH (1992) 13-Cis-Retinoïc acid plus Interferon-α-2A : highly active systemic therapy for squamous cell carcinoma of the cervix. J Natl Cancer Inst 84 : 241-245
11. Maor MH, Gillespie BW, Peters LJ et al (1988) Neutron therapy in cervical cancer : results of a phase III RTOG study. Int J Radiat Oncol Biol Phys 14 : 885-891
12. Myers CE, Diasio R, Eliot HM et al (1976) Pharmacokinetics of the fluoropyrimidines : implications for their use. Cancer Treat Rev 3 : 175-183
13. Perez C, Grigsby P, Nene S, Camel H, Galakatos A, Kao M, Lockett M (1992) Effect of tumor size on the prognosis of carcinoma of the uterine cervix treated with irradiation alone. Cancer 69 : 2796-2806
14. Rotmensch J, Senekjian KE, Ghodratollah J, Herbst A (1988) Evaluation of bolus Cisplatinum and continuous 5-Fluorouracil infusion for metastatic and recurrent squamous cell carcinoma of the cervix. Gynecol Oncol 29 : 76-81
15. Souhami L, Gil R, Allan S, Canary PC, Araujo CM, Pinto LH, Silveira TR (1991) A randomized trial of chemotherapy followed by pelvic radiation therapy in stage IIIB carcinoma of the cervix. J Clin Oncol vol 9 : 970-977
16. Thomas G, Dembo A, Fyles A, Gadalla T, Beale F, Bean H, Pringle J, Rawlings G, Bush R, Black B (1990) Concurrent chemoradiation in advanced cervical cancer. Gynecol Oncol 38 : 446-451
17. Upadhyay SK, Symonds RP, Haeferman M, Watson ER (1988) The treatment of stage IV carcinoma of cervix by radical dose radiotherapy. Radiother Oncol 11 : 15-19
18. Vokes E, Weichselbaum R (1990) Concomitant chemoradiotherapy : rationale and clinical experience in patients with solid tumors. J Clin Oncol 8 : 911-934

Adjuvant chemotherapies for small cell carcinoma of the uterine cervix

TC Chang, HC Chang, CH Lai, S Hsueh*, SF Huang**,
HK Chang***, YK Soong

Small cell undifferentiated carcinoma of the uterine cervix is a rare and very aggressive tumor with a tendency toward early recurrence and a high incidence of distant metastasis to parenchymal organs such as lung, bone, liver, and brain [1-4]. Patients with small cell carcinoma of the uterine cervix usually die within 1 year, with a median survival of 11 to 12.5 months [5, 6]. Some chemotherapeutic regimens have been used in this disease after local treatment, but their efficacy is still under evaluation. This is a preliminary report of our experiences in the therapy of small cell carcinoma of cervix with focus on the impact of chemotherapies to patients' survival.

Materials and methods

There were 28 patients with small cell undifferentiated carcinoma of the uterine cervix (SCCUC) primarily treated at Chang Gung Memorial Hospital between 1983 through 1991. The diagnosis of SCCUC was based on light microscopic findings as described by Warner and Albores-Saavedra [7, 8].

Patient was staged according to the International Federation of Gynecology and Obstetrics (FIGO) criteria for cervical cancer. The observation interval extended from diagnosis to death or until November 31 st, 1992.

Before September 1988, most patients with stage Ib, IIa (less than 2 cm of upper vaginal involvement from the cervico-vaginal junction), and some with stage IIb of primary cervical cancers, without medical contraindications, and age less than 70, were treated with radical hysterectomy and pelvic lymphadenectomy. Adjuvant radiation therapy or chemotherapy with Cisplatinum (60 mg/m^2), Vinblastine (1.4 mg/m^2), and Bleomycin ($15 \text{ mg/m}^2\text{/day} \times 3$ days) (PVB) every 3 weeks for 4-8 courses were given if the histopathology study showed full-thickness of cervical depth invasion, or parametrial invasion, or lymph node metastasis or marked lymphatic permeation of the cervix [9]. Patients with localized disease who did not undergo radical operation underwent pelvic radiation (4400 rads for the whole pelvis, 5800 rads to bilateral parametra and brachytherapy with intracavity radium insertion, 720 rads to point A, for 3 times) with or without chemotherapy with PVB. Staging operation for the definitive diagnosis of pelvic and para-aortic lymph node status was performed on some patients with local advanced disease, mostly stage III, and chemother-

---

From the Division of Gynecologic Oncology, Department of Obstetrics and Gynecology ; the * Department of Pathology ; and the *** Division of Hematology and Oncology, Department of Internal Medicine, Chang Gung Memorial Hospital and Chang Gung Medical College ; and the ** Department of Pathology, National Taiwan University Medical College ; Taipei, Taiwan

apy was administrated to those with histologically diagnosed positive lymph node(s) in addition to radiation therapy.

Since September 1988, small cell carcinoma was treated differently from other cervical cancers. Stage Ib and IIa (less than 2 cm of upper vaginal involvement) disease was treated by radical hysterectomy and bilateral pelvic lymphadenectomy followed by combination chemotherapy, mostly with Cyclophosphamide (1,000 mg/m^2/day × 1 day), Adriamycin (40 mg/m^2/day × 1 day), and Vincristine (1.4 mg/m^2/day × 1 day, up to 2.0 mg) (CAV), alternating with Cisplatinum (25 mg/m^2/day × 3 days) and Etoposide (100 mg/m^2/day × 3 days) (PE) every 3 weeks for 6 courses (CAV courses 1, 3, and 5 ; PE courses 2, 4, and 6). Informed consent was obtained from all patients who received adjuvant chemotherapy. Patients with IIb or more advanced diseases were treated primarily with the same chemotherapy (CAV/PE), and concurrent or consecutive radiation therapy.

Results

Nine of 12 stage I patients, 3/4 stage II patients, and 4/4 stage III patients died of disease. The median survivals (diagnosis to death) were 11 months, 4.3 months, and 13 months in stage I, II, and III respectively. Five patients who did not receive definitive surgery (radical hysterectomy) had persistent primary tumor after therapy (radiation or chemotherapy), and all died of disease. Intrapelvic recurrence or distant metastasis were observed in 11 of the 15 patients who underwent radical operation with disease free intervals ranged from 1.3 to 19.6 months, and all of these 11 patients died. The median survival was 9.6 months. Among these 11 patients, one had local recurrence only, 4 patients had local recurrence and distant metastasis, 6 had distant metastasis without evidence of pelvic recurrence. The most frequent site of distant metastasis are lung, bone and liver.

Among the 8 patients treated by new protocol, there were 6 of 7 stage I patients treated by radical hysterectomy and adjuvant CAV/PE still survive with a median follow up of 17.7 months. The other patient died of disease at 17.4 months. One stage III patient, treated by staging operation and CAV/PE survived for 6.9 months and died of uremia and infection.

Discussion

SCCUC is an aggressive malignancy and tumor recurrence with distant metastasis occurs frequently even in early stage patients. It may have been a systemic disease process even at the time of initial treatment. In this study, all the still surviving patients had received combination chemotherapy, and all patients who had not received adjuvant chemotherapy developed recurrent disease, except for one patient with small primary tumor.

PVB and CAV/PE are the 2 main chemotherapies used in this study. Although patients who received CAV/PE usually have longer survivals than patients who received PVB by historical comparison. There are 2 patients that received adjuvant PVB after radical hysterectomy, one with stage Ib, and one with stage IIb disease, both had multiple pelvic lymph node metastasis, experienced long term survival over 6 years and still survive. PVB may have a substantial effect on these patients.

Before a better protocol is established, the regimen for small cell carcinoma of lung should be the standard adjuvant therapy for this disease.

References

1. Huang SF, Shueh S, Chang TC (1988) Small cell carcinoma of the uterine cervix : pathologic analysis of 9 cases. J Formosan Med Assoc 87 : 297-303
2. Swan DS, Roddick JW (1973) A clinical-pathological correlation of cell type classification of cervical cancer. Am J Obstet Gynecol 116 : 666-670
3. Van Nagell JRJ, Rayburn W, Donaldson ES, Hanson M, Gay EC, Yoneda J, Marayuma Y, Powell DF (1979) Therapeutic implications of patterns of recurrence in cancer of the uterine cervix. Cancer 44 : 2354-2361
4. Van Nagell JR, Powell DE, Gallion HH, Elliot DG, Donaldson ES, Carpenter AE, Higgins RV, Kryscio R, Pavlik EJ (1988) Small cell carcinoma of the uterine cervix. Cancer 62 : 1586-93
5. Walker AN, Mills SE, Taylor PT (1988) Cervical neuroendocrine carcinoma : a clinical and light microscopic study of 14 cases. Int J Gynecol Path 7 : 64-74
6. Gersell DJ, Mazoujian G, Mutch DG, Rudloff MA (1988) Small-cell undifferentiated carcinoma of the cervix. A clincopathologic, ultrastructural and immunocytochemical study of 15 cases. Am J Surg Pathol 12 : 684-698
7. Warner TFCS (1978) Carcinoid tumor of the uterine cervix. J Clin Pathol 31 : 990-995
8. Albores-Saavedra J, Larraza O, Poucell S, Rodriguez-Martinez HA (1976) Carcinoid of the uterine cervix, additional observations on a new tumor entity. Cancer 38 : 2328-2342
9. Lai CH, Lin TS, Soong YK, Chen HF (1989) Adjuvant chemotherapy after radical hysterectomy for cervical carcinoma. Gynecol Oncol 35 : 193-198

Neo-Adjuvant M-VAC (Methotrexate, Vinblastine, Doxorubicin, Cisplatin) chemotherapy for locally advanced or metastatic cervical and vaginal cancer

GR Garton*, TO Wilson**, LC Hartmann***, HJ Long***, KC Podratz**

Based on previous reports of an approximate 70 % response rate to M-VAC chemotherapy in patients with metastatic gynecological malignancies (Long, 1990 and 1991), we administered Neo-Adjuvant M-VAC chemotherapy to patients with locally advanced or metastatic cervical and vaginal cancer.

Materials and methods

Since 1989, 23 women with gynecological cancer received Neo-Adjuvant M-VAC (Methotrexate, Vinblastine, Doxorubicin, Cisplatin) chemotherapy. The primary site was cervix in 21 pts and vagina in 2 pts. The stage distribution in pts with cervical cancer was stage IIB- 7 pts ; stage IIIA- 1 pts ; stage IIIB- 8 pts ; stage IVA- 2 pts, and stage IVB- 3 pts. Both pts with vaginal cancer had stage IVA.

The median number of cycles of M-VAC was 4. Treatment schedule consisted of Methotrexate (30 mg/m² IV), days 1, 15, and 22 ; Vinblastine (3 mg/m² IV), days 2, 15, and 22 ; Doxorubicin (30 mg/m² IV) ; and Cisplatin (70 mg/m² IV), day 2. Each cycle was repeated every 28 days. Following M-VAC chemotherapy, 12 pts underwent radical surgery and postoperative irradiation, 5 pts received radiation therapy alone ; 2 pts had surgery only ; and 4 patients received no further treatment. The median follow-up for the entire group of patients was 8 months (range, 4 to 34.5).

Results

Clinical response to M-VAC was observed in 20 of 23 pts (87 %), and was considered partial in 16 (70 %), and complete in 4 (16 %). Of the 3 remaining patients, 2 pts progressed after a partial response and 1 did not have a response. Of the 14 patients undergoing surgery, 9 pts had minimal gross residual disease in the hysterectomy specimen, 4 pts had only microscopic disease, and 1 pts had no tumor found in the resected specimen. At the completion of surgery, only 1 pt had a positive surgical margin. With a median follow-up of 8 months, 7 of the 23 patients (30 %) presented tumor recurrence or

From the *Division of Radiation Oncology, **Section of Gynecological Surgery, and ***Division of Medical Oncology, Mayo Clinic and Mayo Foundation, Rochester, MN 55905, USA

progression. Of the 23 pts, 14 (61 %) are alive without evidence of disease (median, 8 months ; range, 5 to 30), 6 pts (26 %) have died of disease, (median, 10.5 months ; range, 4-34.5), 2 pts (9 %) are alive with disease at 6 and 7 months and 1 pts (4 %) died of a pulmonary embolism 2 weeks following surgery. Of 23 pts, 12 (52 %) experienced 18 instances of grade 3 or higher treatment-related toxicity (vomiting, alopecia, leukopenia, anemia, stomatitis, thrombocytopenia and pulmonary embolism).

Discussion

The treatment for locally advanced (stage IIB to IVA) cervical or vaginal cancer has traditionally been external beam irradiation plus brachytherapy. Reported survival rates range from 28 % to 66 % in cervical cancer patients according to stage (Hanks, 1983, Montana, 1985 ; Montana, 1986), and from 19 % to 45 % in vaginal cancer patients (Kucera, 1985), also depending on the stage of their disease. In an attempt to improve tumor control and survival an aggressive program of Neo-Adjuvant M-VAC followed by surgery and radiation therapy was initiated at our institution. The clinical response rate to M-VAC chemotherapy was very high (87 %), allowing 14 of 23 pts (61 %) to proceed with potentially « curative » surgery. At the time of last follow-up, 14 pts (61 %) are alive without evidence of disease (median, 8 months ;). The toxicity associated with this aggressive multimodality treatment was moderate to severe. Of 23 pts, 12 (52 %) experienced 18 instances of grade 3 or higher treatment-related toxicity.

Conclusion

Neo-Adjuvant M-VAC chemotherapy in patients with advanced cervical of vaginal cancer resulted in very high clinical response and resectability rate. The resulting treatment related toxicity was considerable. Longer follow-up and a larger number of patients is needed before we can compare these results to standard radiation therapy.

References

1. Long HJ, Cross WG, Wieand HS (1990) M-VAC : A highly active combination chemotherapy regimen in advanced-recurrent cancer of the uterine cervix and vagina. Proc ASCO 9 : 158
2. Long HJ, Langdon RM, Wieand HS (1991) Phase II trial of Methothrexate, Vinblastine, Doxorubicin and Cisplatin (M-VAC) in women with advanced cancer of the uterine cervix and vagina. Proc ASCR 32 : 188
3. Hanks GE, Herring DF, Kramer S (1983) Patterns of care outcome studies. Results of the national practice in cancer of the cervix. Cancer 51 : 959-967

4. Montana GS, Fowler WC, Varia MA, Walton LA, Mack Y (1985) Analysis of results of radiation therapy for stage II carcinoma of the cervix. Cancer 55 : 956-962
5. Montana GS, Fowler WC, Varia MA, Walton LA, Mack Y, Shemanski L (1986) Carcinoma of the cervix, stage III. Results of radiation therapy. Cancer 57 : 148-154
6. Kucera H, Langer M, Smekal G, Weghaupt K (1985) Radiotherapy of primary carcinoma of the vagina : management and results of different therapy schemes. Gynecol Oncol 21 : 87-93

A phase II trial of Neo-Adjuvant chemotherapy (CT) with Ifosfamide (I), Mesna and Cisplatinum (C) in stage IIA-IIIB cervical cancer

A Erazo, L Torrecillas, G Cervantes, B Ortega

The most frequent malignant tumor in Mexico is cervical carcinoma and more than a half of the cases are first diagnosed as inoperable disease.

Prognosis of patients (pts) with advanced cervical carcinoma (ACC) treated with radiotherapy (RT) is poor.

Chemotherapy (CT) in patients with ACC can reduce bulky tumors, increase subsequent RT efficacy, and decrease the out side irradiation field recurrences.

Currently, Cisplatin (C) based regimens are widely used for palliative and Neo-Adjuvant treatment of cervical cancer [1]. Ifosfamide (I) also has a clearcut activity in the treatment of cervical tumors with response rates of 20 % to 50 % in previously untreated pts [2]. Also, I displays synergism with C *in vivo* models. We evaluate an I-C combination in a Neo-Adjuvant setting, to attempt improve local and distant long-term control of patients with ACC.

Patients and methods

Untreated pts with inoperable ACC stages IIA-I IIIB, entered the study. Eligibility criteria were : histological confirmation of squamous-cell cervical cancer, age < 65 years, ECOG performance status (PS) < 2, Leucocyte count > 3,500/ml, platelet count > 150,000/ml, hemoglobin > 12 g/L, creatinine clearance > 50 ml/min. The size of the neoplasm was obtained before treatment onset, prior each cycle and 4 weeks after the last cycle. Previous listed laboratory parameters were monitored before the start of each new cycle and 4 weeks after the last. WHO criteria were used to evaluate tumor responses and toxicity and modified to include minimal partial response (mPR) for tumor regression of 50 %-80 %, and major partial response (MPR) for response > 80 % but < 100 %. Survival (S) was measured from the first day of therapy until the last clinical evaluation ; disease free interval (DFI) was determined from the end of the treatment until tumor recurrence.

Treatment

Treatment schedule repeated every 28 days : Ifosfamide 1.5 g/m^2/day on day 1-4 as a 120 minutes infusion, Mesna as bolus injection (20 % of daily Ifos-

---

Servicio de Oncologia Hospital 20 de Noviembre ISSSTE, Felix Cuevas 540 Colonia del Valle 31000, Mexico City

famide dose given at 0.4 and 8 hours) and Cisplatinum 50 mg/m^2 on day 1 as an i.v. infusion over 30 minutes. Anti-emetic regimen : high-dose Methoclopramide, Dexamethasone, Diphenhidramine and Diazepam. Treatment was delayed a maximum of 2 weeks if myeloid or renal toxicity developed. Patients received 4 cycles before radical conventional RT : whole pelvis 50 Gy/5 weeks and intracavitary therapy 50 Gy to point A. Quality of life was assessed with standardize questionnaires.

Results

Between May '90 and July '91, 19 pts were treated. Pts' characteristics were : median age 49 years ; PS 0-1 ; 1 stage IIA, 13 stage IIB and 5 IIIB stage. CT response was evaluable in 17 pts (2 pts had a delay > of 2 weeks no treatment related). Responses were : 3 CR (18 %), 7 MPR (41 %), 4 mPR (23 %), and 3 SD (18 %). Fourteen pts were evaluable for RT response after CT (2 pts refuse irradiation despite MPR and SD after CT ; the patient with stage IIA was surgical treated with mPR after CT). Responses were : 12 CR (86 %), 1 PR (7 %), and 1 PD (7 %).

Toxicity

Toxicity for the 67 CT delivered cycles was : neutropenia grade 3-4 in 1.5 %, renal grade 1-2 in 13 %, macroscopic hematuria in 3 %, nausea and vomit grade 2-3 in 88 %, alopecia grade 2 in 90 %. Neo-Adjuvant CT did not enhanced the acute toxic effects of pelvic irradiation.

Current state and quality of life

Current state of the 17 pts treated with CT is : alive tumor-free 7 pts with S of 20 to 25 months and DFI of 14 to 22 months ; alive with tumor 1 patient with S of 24 months and DFI of 15 months ; lost of follow-up tumor free 3 pts with S of 5 to 15 months ; lost of follow-up with tumor 6 pts with S of 3 to 20 months. CT treatment modified the pts routine life due to : intense fatigue, persistent nausea, depression or anxiety and personal feeling of unpleasant appearance. Family relationships were not affected and they could carry out daily housework and physical activities.

Discussion

Based on the results of the major study by the Gynecologic Oncology Group (GOG) [3], we routinely prescribed 50 mg/m^2 in combination regimens for palliative or Neo-Adjuvant treatment. Our pts had a favorable OR (14 of 17 objective responses, 82 %) with 18 % of CR and 41 % of MPR. The OR rates were higher than those reported by Lara et al [1] with a total Cisplatin dose of 100 mg/m^2 and Ifosfamide 7.5 g/m^2. We must consider, the small number of pts in both trials and the clinical stage of the disease ; Lara et al included only pts with III B stage. Our results according to the clinical stage, are similar with these authors ; thus, 10/11 stage II B pts had tumor regression while 3/5 pts stage III B responded.

Although, the objective responses were not satisfactory in advanced stages, no tumor progression was observed during the CT induction phase ; in other words, CT does not delay the final radical RT treatment.

Neo-Adjuvant CT is not a curative and routinely recommended treatment, so we have to procure a minimal aggression to the patients' quality of life. CT treatment temporarily impaired social and work activities with complete recovery after the treatment withdrawal. The CT did not enhance the radiation morbidity ; hematologic and gastrointestinal toxic effects were treatable in all patients.

We conclude, that Neo-Adjuvant treatment based on Ifosfamide-Cisplatin combination is feasible and could be valuable in the management of cervical advanced tumors. However, bulky disease did not showed an over tumor reduction as smaller neoplasms.

References

1. Lara PC, Garcia-Puche JL, Pedraza V (1990) Cisplatin-Ifosfamide as Neo-Adjuvant chemotherapy in stage III B cervical uterine squamous carcinoma. Cancer Chemother Pharmacol 26 : S36-S38
2. Meanwell CA, Mould JJ, Blackledge G et al (1986) Phase II study of Ifosfamide in cervical cancer. Cancer Treat Rep 70 : 727-730
3. Bonomi P, Bruckner H, Cohen C, Marshall R, Blessing J, Slayton R (1982) A randomized trial of three cisplatin regimens in squamous cell carcinoma of the cervix. Proc Am Soc Clin Oncol 18 : 110 (abstr)

Abstract. We assessed the efficacy of I-C combination as Neo-Adjuvant induction chemotherapy (CT) before radical radiotherapy (RT) in advanced cervical carcinoma stages IIA-IIIB. Nineteen patients were treated with 6 g/m^2 i.v. Ifosfamide and 50 mg/m^2 Cisplatin. CT evaluable patients (17/19) achieved 3 (18 %) complete responses (CR) and 11 (64 %) partial responses (PR). Responses for 14 evaluable RT patients were 12 CR (86 %), 1 PR (7 %) and 1 progressive disease. I-C regimen is well tolerated with a high rate of remissions (82 %) and no enhanced radiation morbidity.

Bleomycin, Ifosfamide and Carboplatin in advanced uterine cervix carcinoma : preliminary results

C Louvet, S Moreau, A de Gramont, C Varette, B Demuynck, K Beerblock, L Marpeau, D Zylberait, A Pigné, D Soubrane, M Krulik

Several cytotoxic drugs are active in advanced squamous cell cancer of the cervix. Cisplatin results in a 20 to 38 % response rate with a short duration of response [1]. More recently, Ifosfamide was reported active in second-line therapy (11.1 % partial response) after Cisplatin-based regimen [2] and in first line with 50 % response rate using high-doses [3]. Analogues of Cisplatin are also active ; among them, Carboplatin is the best tolerated without significant renal and neurological toxicities [4, 5]. Other active single agents are Bleomycin, Vincristine and Methotrexate [1]. Combined regimens improve response rate : regimens such Cisplatin — Ifosfamide, Carboplatin — Ifosfamide, Bleomycin — Ifosfamide — Cisplatin or Bleomycin — Ifosfamide — Carboplatin were reported active with over 50 % response rate in advanced patients [6, 7, 8, 9, 10]. We report preliminary results of a phase II study with a combination of Bleomycin, Ifosfamide and Carboplatin (BIC) in advanced squamous cell carcinoma of the cervix.

Patients and methods

Seventeen patients (mean age : 45.9 years, range 26 to 67) were included. Eligibility criteria were pathologically-proven squamous cell carcinoma of the cervix, age < 70 years, performance status (WHO) 0 to 2, no previous chemotherapy, FIGO stage IIA to IV, measurable disease, normal liver and renal functions.

BIC regimen consisted in Bleomycin 20 mg/m^2 IV day 1 and 5 mg/m^2 IM twice a day from day 2 to 5, Ifosfamide 1 g/m^2 in 1 liter D5 % in 2 hours day 1 to 5 and Carboplatin 300 mg/m^2 in 250 ml D5 % day 1. Bleomycin was given only for the 2 first courses (total administered dose : 120 mg/m^2). This combination was repeated every 28 days.

Three courses were performed for locally advanced cancer patients before surgery and external pelvic radiotherapy. In metastatic patients, evaluation was made after 3 courses. Three additionnal courses were administered in case of response.

Median follow-up time in January 1993 was 26 months. Response duration was calculated from start of treatment to evidence of progression. Survival was calculated using the Kaplan-Meier method.

GERCOD (Groupe d'Etude et de Recherche sur les Cancers de l'Ovaire et Digestifs), Hôpital Saint-Antoine, service du Pr Krulik, 184, rue du Faubourg Saint-Antoine, 75012 Paris, France

Results

Six patients received BIC for locally advanced diseas : 2 stage IIA, 2 IIB and 2 IIIB. Three complete and 3 partial responses were observed. Two patients relapsed after 8 and 13 months respectively, the 4 others remaining disease-free.

Eleven patients received BIC for metastatic disease : 3 metastatic at diagnosis (stage IV), 1 relapse after surgery alone, and 7 relapses after surgery and radiotherapy. Two complete and 5 partial responses were observed (response rate : 63.6 %). Complete responses in metastatic patients lasted 9 and 11 months, while partial responses lasted 6, 8+, 12, 13 and 13 months.

Characteristics of patients, response and survival are summarized in Table 1.

Seventy-one courses were administered, including 11 with concomitant radiotherapy. Toxicity of the 60 remaining courses is summarized in Table 2. Main toxicity was hematological with 23.5 % and 23.5 % WHO grade 3 and 4 neutropenia respectively. However, only 2 febrile neutropenia episodes occured (3.3 % of courses). Nausea-vomiting (grade 2 : 29.5 %, grade 3 : 23.5 %) and alopecia (grade 2 : 35.3 %, grade 3 : 64.7 %) were also recorded. No neurological nor renal toxicity over grade 1 was observed.

Table 1. Characteristics of patients, response and survival (n = 17 patients)

Locally advanced patients

Pt	Age	FIGO satge	PS	Response to BIC	Status after surgery + RT	Survival (months)
1	67	IIB	0	CR	CR	48+
2	26	IIB	0	CR	CR	36+
3	61	IIIB	1	CR	CR	3+
4	38	IIIB	1	PR	CR	13
5	30	IIA	0	PR	CR	13+
6	37	IIA	1	PR	CR	15

Metastatic patients

Pt	Age	Metastatic site	PS	Response	Response duration (months)	Survival (months)
6	53	lung + lymph nodes	0	CR	9	22+
7	40	lymph nodes	0	CR	11	26+
1	42	lymph nodes	0	PR	13	22
2	42	bone + soft tissue	0	PR	12	18+
3	31	lymph nodes	0	PR	6	9
8	50	lymph nodes	2	PR	13	14
9	48	liver + lymph nodes	1	PR	8+	8+
5	63	lymph nodes	1	SD	—	6+
10	60	lymph nodes	1	SD	—	17
4	41	lung	0	PD	—	4+
11	52	lymph nodes	1	PD	—	5

PS : performance status ; RT : radiotherapy ; CR : complete response ; PR : partial response ; SD : stable disease ; PD : progressive disease

Table 2. Toxicity (n = 17 patients, 60 courses)

	Grade 0-1	Grade 2	Grade 3	Grade 4
Hematological	4 (23.5 %)	5 (29.5 %)	4 (23.5 %)	4 (23.5 %)
Nausea-vomiting	8 (47 %)	5 (29.5 %)	4 (23.5 %)	—
Alopecia	—	6 (35.3 %)	11 (64.7 %)	—
Renal	17 (100 %)	—	—	—
Neurologic	17 (100 %)	—	—	—

Conclusion

With 76.4 % response rate including 63.3 % in metastatic patients and a manageable hematological toxicity, this combination is active in advanced squamous cell carcinoma of the cervix. Results are in the same range than the best reported combinations. The BIC regimen needs further evaluation.

References

1. Perez CA, Disaia PJ, Knapp RC, Young RC (1987) Carcinoma of the uterine cervix. In : de Vita VT, Hellman S, Rosenberg SA (eds) Cancer : Principes and Practice of Oncology. JB Lippincott, Philadelphia, pp. 1013-1081
2. Sutton GP, Blessing JA, Adcock L et al (1989) Phase II study of Ifosfamide and Mesna in patients with previously-treated carcinoma of the cervix. Invest New Drugs 7 : 341-343
3. Cervellino JC, Aranjo CE, Pirisi C et al (1990) Ifosfamide and Mesna at high-doses for the treatment of cancer of the cervix. A GETLAC study. Cancer Chemother Pharmacol 26 (suppl) : S1-S3
4. Lira-Puerto V, Silva A, Groshen S et al (1989) Carboplatin (CBDCA) or CHIP : final report of the third phase II NCI-PAHO study in advanced cervical cancer. Proc Am Soc Clin Oncol 8 : 160
5. Mc Guire JC, Arsenau J, Blessing FT et al (1989) A randomized comparative trial of Carboplatin and Iproplatin in advanced squamous carcinoma of the uterine cervix : a Gynecologic Oncology Group study. J Clin Oncol 7 : 1462-1468
6. Kumar L, Bhargava VL (1991) Chemotherapy with Bleomycin, Ifosfamide and Cisplatin in recurrent and advanced cervical cancer. Gynecologic Oncology 40 : 107-111
7. Blackledge G, Buxton EJ, Mould JJ et al (1990) Phase II studies of Ifosfamide alone and in combination in cancer of the cervix. Cancer Chemother Pharmacol 26 (suppl) : S12-S16

8. Lara PC, Garcia-Puche JL, Pedraza V (1990) Cisplatin, Ifosfamide as Neo-Adjuvant chemotherapy in stage IIIB cervical uterine squamous-cell carcinoma. Cancer Chemother Pharmacol 26 (suppl) : S36-S38
9. Kühnle H, Meerpohl HG, Eiermann W et al (1990) Phase II study of Carboplatin/Ifosfamide in untreated advanced cervical cancer. Cancer Chemother Pharmacol 26 (suppl) : S33-S35
10. Murad AM, Santiago FF, Triginelli SA (1992) A phase II trial of BIC (Bleomycin, Ifosfamide and Carboplatin) in advanced cervical cancer. Proc Am Soc Clin Oncol 11 : 228

Urological and germinal tumors

Surveillance in stage I non-seminomatous germ cell tumors of the testis (NSGCTT). Experience at the Instituto Nacional de Cancerología of México

JW Zinser, R Gaona, A Mendoza, O Ocampo, H Domínguez, L Vicencio

Most patients with metastatic NSGCTT have an excellent prognosis due to the effectiveness of Cisplatin based chemotherapy. This has permitted to hold treatment in stage I patients to only those who relapse. Orchiectomy alone will cure 60-80 % of the patients, avoiding unnecessary morbidity in more than half of the patients. Surveillance results published in the english literature come from centers in industrialized countries were follow-up of patients is easier and better [1, 3]. In Mexico there is some reluctance against the surveillance policy, arguing that follow-up is very poor and that it would represent a high risk to the patient. Compliance is certainly a problem in our country, but a RPLND should not be considered a substitute for a potential poor follow-up. Another option for stage I NSGCTT has been Adjuvant chemotherapy for high risk patients such as those with vascular invasion [4]. This alternative overtreats some patients, adding unnecessary toxicity. And at our institution due to financial reasons we limit the administration of chemotherapy in patients with NSGCTT only to those with metastatic disease. In July 1985 we decided to submit to surveillance all patients with stage I NSGCTT and give additional treatment only at relapse.

Patients and methods

Since July 1985 all stage I patients with NSGCTT were submitted to surveillance. Other patients were included ; they had orchiectomy during the prior year and had not received any other treatment.

After orchiectomy patients had : Physical examination (PE) negative for metastatic disease, normal α-Fetoprotein (AFP), normal β-human-chorionic-gonadotropin (BHCG) and a chest X-ray and CT scan of the abdomen and pelvis negative for metastatic disease. Lymphangiogram was only done in selected cases. Follow-up included monthly PE, markers and chest X-ray during the first year. Every 2 months the second year, every 3 months the third year, every 4 months the fourth year, every 6 months the fifth year, and yearly thereafter. CT scan was done as follows : If preoperative markers were negative or unknown, every 4 months during the first year, every 6 months during the second year and yearly thereafter. If markers were positive preoperatively, every 6 months during the first year and yearly thereafter. Data of all patients

Instituto Nacional de Cancerología San Fernando 22, Tlalpan México, D.F. 14000 México

will be analyzed, however not all patients are included in the follow-up analysis as some patients elected not to be followed at the Institute.

Results

Between 1984 and 1990, 70 patients with stage I NSGCTT were seen at the Instituto Nacional de Cancerología of México. Sixty-one patients were followed. All patients had normal post orchiectomy AFP and BHCG, and chest X-ray, CT scan of the abdomen and pelvis and PE negative for metastasis. Seven patients had lymphangiogram : 6 were negative and 1 suggestive of metastasis. Five of the 6 patients in whom it was negative remain NED, the other relapsed at 8 months. The patient with the study suspicious of metastases was not treated and 33 months later remained NED.

Median age of all patients is 26 years (17-43). Sixty-two had surgery before their referral to the Institute, 16 of them, transcrotal. Five patients had cryptorchidism, in one case contralateral to the primary. Histology : 12 patients had pure histologic subtypes and 58 were mixed. There were 7 cases of choriocarcinoma in the later group.

Relapses

Fifteen patients have relapsed at a median of 5 months (2-96), 13 patients within 10 months and the other 2 at 33 and 96 months. One patient developed a contralateral stage I seminoma 5 years after surgery.

Sites of relapse : Retroperitoneum 2 patients, retro + supraclavicular 1 patient, retro + supraclav + markers 1 patient, retro + markers 3 patients, lung plus markers 1 patient, inguinal ipsilateral 2 patients, inguinal contralateral 1 patient and markers 4 patients. Three patients had transcrotal orchiectomy, none of whom relapsed in the inguinal region. Seven patients had mixed histologies harboring choriocarcinoma. Two cases relapsed at 4 months. Late relapses : In the patient who relapsed at 33 months the orchiectomy specimen revealed only teratoma. At relapsed he had a retroperitoneal mass and a BHCG of 5.403 mU/ml with gynecomastia. The patient who relapsed at 96 months had an embryonal carcinoma plus seminoma and recurred with a BHCG of 23 in retroperitoneum and supraclavicular area.

Treatment and outcome of patients at relapse

All patients were treated with Cisplatin based chemotherapy and 10 patients also had surgery. Fourteen patients achieved CR. One of them with an initial pulmonary nodule, relapsed again in the lung 8 months later ; had surgical excision and 2 courses of chemotherapy and remains in CR 30 months after completion of the last course. One patient who relapsed 3 months after orchiectomy with an AFP of 304 ng/ml, refused further follow-up and chemotherapy after one course. His status is unknown. Follow-up of the other 14 patients after completion of chemotherapy is 29 months (5-59).

Overall follow-up

Forty-eight patients (79 %) were in follow-up either continuously or at the time of relapse at a median of 51 months (3-104). Thirteen patients (21 %) were lost to follow-up without evidence of disease at a median of 16 months (3-47). Four patients within 5 months which was the median time to relapse and 6 patients within 10 months which is the length of time that 87 % of the relapses occurred. All but one had orchiectomy before been seen at the Institute. Regarding their histology, 3 had choriocarcinoma and were lost to follow-up at 3, 6 and 30 months respectively.

Prognostic factors

We were not able to evaluate spermatic cord and vascular invasion as there were only few slides per patient. The same was true for pre-orchiectomy serum markers since most patients operated before their referral to the institution did not have them. Regarding the surgical excision, 3/11 patients relapsed among those that were followed and had a transcrotal orchiectomy. Of the 7 patients with choriocarcinoma there are 2 relapses at 4 months each one, 2 patients are continuously free of disease at 70 and 89 months and 3 patients are lost to follow-up at 3, 6 and 30 months.

Conclusions

86 % of the stage I patients with NSGCTT seen at the Instituto had orchiectomy prior to their referral. Lymphangiogram should be done only in selected patients such as those with pre-orchiectomy negative markers, teratoma as the major histologic component and the goal that if retroperitoneal metastasis are diagnosed, probably a RPLND would be the best initial approach.

There is a 25 % relapse rate at a median of 5 months with only 13 % (2/15) of the relapses after 10 months. Since 1 patient relapsed after 8 years, we should be aware of possible recurrences even after a long time. Therapy at relapse is very effective, the only patient whose outcome after relapse is unknown had minimal tumor burden and refused further treatment after one course of chemotherapy.

References

1. Gelderman WAH, Koops HS, Sleijfer DTH et al (1987) Orchiectomy alone in stage I nonseminomatous testicular germ cell tumors. Cancer 59 : 578-580
2. Sturgeon JFG, Jewett MAS, Alison RE et al (1992) Surveillance after orchiectomy for patients with clinical stage I nonseminomatous testis tumors. J Clin Oncol 10 : 564-568
3. Read GP, Stenning SP, Cullen MH et al (1992) Medical research council prospective study of surveillance for stage I testicular teratoma. J Clin Oncol 10 : 1762-1768
4. Pont J, Höltl W, Kosak D et al (1990) Risk-adapted treatment choice in stage I nonseminomatous testicular germ cell cancer by regarding vascular invasion in the primary tumor : A prospective trial. J Clin Oncol 8 : 16-20

Combination chemotherapy with Etoposide, Cisplatin, Bleomycin, and Cyclophosphamide for advanced metastatic non-seminomatous germ cell tumors

A Gerl*, C Clemm*, M Hentrich**, R Hartenstein**, P Kohl*, W Wilmanns*

Cisplatin-based chemotherapy dramatically improved the outlook for patients with metastasized germ cell tumors. However, patients with a large tumor burden or specific sites of metastatic spread still are at a high risk of treatment failure [1]. As the PVB protocol including Cisplatin, Vinblastine, and Bleomycin in conventional doses led to long-term survival in only 44 % of patients with poor-prognosis metastatic disease [2], in 1983 we began to treat high risk patients with a dose-intensified chemotherapy schedule. This report summarizes our 10-years experience with ECBC chemotherapy for poor-risk nonseminomatous germ cell tumors (NSGCT).

Patients and methods

Sixty-four patients (median age 26, range 16-65 years) were treated with ECBC (Etoposide 120 mg/m^2, Cisplatin 30 mg/m^2, Bleomycin 12 mg/m^2, and Cyclophosfamide 300 mg/m^2 for 4 days, and 15 mg Bleomycin bolus injection on day 1). Bleomycin was given as continuous 24-hours infusion and was withdrawn, if pulmonary function deteriorated or if the total dose exceeded 400 mg. The patients received Mesna 0.4 and 8 hours after administration of Cyclophosfamide. Chemotherapy cycles were repeated at 3-week intervals if feasible.

All patients were not pretreated with other Cisplatin-based chemotherapy regimens. Fifty-two patients (81 %) presented with tumors of testicular, 12 (19 %) of extragonadal origin. Fourty-six patients (72 %) had « advanced disease » according to Indiana classification, 15 (23 %) patients had unresectable retroperitoneal disease (without haematogenous spread). The retroperitoneum and the lung were involved in 51 (80 %) and 37 (58 %) patients, respectively. Nineteen patients (30 %) presented with a mediastinal mass. Ten patients (16 %) had hepatic and 4 (6 %) cerebral metastases.

Pretreatment investigation consisted of physical examination, laboratory testing including serum tumor markers Human chorionic gonadotropin (HCG) and α-Fetoprotein (AFP), chest X-ray and thoracic and abdominal computed tomography (CT) scan. Serum tumor markers were measured frequently, at least prior to each chemotherapy course. After normalization of tumor markers usually 2 further cycles were given for consolidation. Patients with marker-negative

---

* Medizinische Klinik III, Klinikum Großhardern der Universität München, Marchioninistraße 15, W-8000 München 70 and **IV. Medizinische Klinik, Städtisches Krankenhaus Harlaching, Sanatoriumsplatz 2, W-8000 München 90, Bundesrepublik Deutschland

residual disease after chemotherapy underwent surgical resection of all masses if feasible. If there were viable tumor cells in the surgically removed tissue, 2 (or 3) further chemotherapy cycles were administered on an individual basis. Exceptionally, resection of residual masses was performed in patients who experienced no complete normalization of tumor markers (3 cases). Follow-up examinations were performed as described elsewhere [3].

Results

Presently, 62 patients (97 %) are evaluable for response. Fifty-one patients (80 %) received 4 to 6 cycles of ECBC. Two patients were given 7 and 9 cycles, respectively. Forty patients (65 %) achieved a no evidence of disease (NED) status. The NED rate was 60 % if considering patients with advanced disease according to Indiana classification. Thirty patients (75 %) who attained NED status underwent post-chemotherapy surgery. Seven patients (11 %) achieved a marker-negative partial remission. Considering both patients with NED status and marker-negative partial remission, the favorable response rate was 76 %.

3 patients with NED status relapsed after 6, 9, and 21 months, respectively, all of whom died of disease progression. Four patients with marker-negative residual lesions developed disease progression. Two of these patients died and 1 is alive with a large growing teratoma. One patient achieved a second remission after irradiation for cerebral metastases.

There were 5 early deaths (within 90 days after the start of chemotherapy), 2 of these patients died from treatment-related septic shock. Fifteen further patients died due to disease progression, 8 after they had undergone salvage chemotherapy on an individual basis. Forty-two evaluable patients (68 %) are currently alive. The relapse-free survival rate is 57 % for patients with « advanced disease » and 88 % for patients with « moderate disease » according to Indiana staging system. Minimal and median follow-up are 16 and 51 months, respectively.

The haematologic toxicity of the ECBC schedule was considerable. 79 % of 52 evaluable patients experienced a leucocyte nadir $< 1.0 \times 10^9/l$, 46 % a platelet count nadir $< 20 \times 10^9/l$ at least after one treatment course. 33 patients (52 %) required erythrocyte and 20 patients (32 %) platelet transfusions. 45 % of patients had dose reductions due to haematologic toxicity (30 % during the first 3 chemotherapy cycles). 32 patients (51 %) experienced at least one febrile episode which required hospitalization and antibiotic treatment. 7 patients (11 %) experienced bleeding complications due to thrombocytopenia.

Discussion

Presently, the PEB regimen including Cisplatin, Etoposide, and Bleomycin is regarded as standard treatment for metastasized NSGCT [1]. As a considerable proportion of patients with advanced metastatic disease is not cured by standard therapy, various attempts have been undertaken to improve treatment results. These approaches included dose escalation of Cisplatin [4, 5, 6] and Etoposide [6], the most active single agents against testicular cancer. Other investigators tried to improve treatment results by the inclusion of additional drugs such as Cyclophosphamide, Ifosfamide, Vincristine, Methotrexate and Actinomycin D [7, 8]. Alternating chemotherapy cycles are a further treatment option [7, 8]. Recently, early administration of high-dose chemotherapy with autologous bone marrow rescue was described [9].

Although some authors described a dose-response relationship for chemotherapy of germ cell tumors [7, 10], there is presently no proof that dose-intensified chemotherapy regimens are superior to standard treatment. Our treatment results for patients with « advanced disease » according to Indiana classification do not significantly differ from the best results with standard treatment [1]. However, a comparison is limited by the fact that the authors of the aforementioned report included patients with seminomas. In our own experience, seminomas had a better prognosis than NSGCT [11] and were therefore not included in this poor-risk trial. In general, as no conclusion has been reached about eligibility criteria for poor-risk studies, it is very difficult to compare treatment results of different investigators.

The ECBC regimen had a considerably higher haematologic toxicity than standard treatment with PEB [1]. But this higher toxicity seemed manageable and did not lead to more treatment-related deaths compared to standard treatment [1].

In conclusion, uniform eligibility criteria are necessary for patients who enter poor-risk trials. The superiority of dose escalation regimens can only be proven by randomized studies. Probably, the inclusion of new active drugs will be necessary to improve treatment results markedly.

References

1. Williams SD, Birch R, Einhorn LH et al (1987) Treatment of disseminated germ-cell tumors with Cisplatin, Bleomycin and either Vinblastine or Etoposide. N Engl J Med 316 : 1435-1440
2. Gerl A, Clemm C, Lamerz R, Mann K, Wilmanns W (1993) Prognostic implications of tumour marker analysis in nonseminomatous germ cell tumours with poor-prognosis metastatic disease. Eur J Cancer (in press)
3. Clemm C, Berdel WE, Hartenstein R et al (1986) Münchener Nachsorge-Schema bei fortgeschrittenen nicht-seminomatösen Hodentumoren — Nutzen und Kosten. Dtsch Med Wschr 111 : 1181-1185
4. Ozols RF, Ihde DC, Linehan M et al (1988) A randomized trial of standard chemotherapy v a high-dose chemotherapy regimen in the treatment of poor prognosis nonseminomatous germ-cell tumors. J Clin Oncol 6 : 1031-1040
5. Nichols CR, Williams SD, Loehrer PJ et al (1991) Randomized study of Cisplatin dose intensity in poor-risk germ cell tumors : A Southeastern Cancer Study Group and Southwest Oncology Group protocol. J Clin Oncol 9 : 1163-1172
6. Daugaard G, Rorth M (1992) Treatment of poor-risk germ-cell tumors with high-dose Cisplatin and Etoposide combined with Bleomycin. Ann Oncol 3 : 277-282
7. Crawford SM, Newlands ES, Begent RHJ, Rustin GJS, Bagshawe KD (1989) The

effect of intensity of administering treatment on the outcome of germ cell tumours treated with POMB/ACE chemotherapy. Br J Cancer 59 : 243-246
8. Bosl GJ, Geller NL, Vogelzang NJ et al (1987) Alternating cycles of etoposide plus cisplatin and VAB-6 in the treatment of poor-risk patients with germ cell tumors. J Clin Oncol 5 : 436-440
9. Droz JP, Pico JL, Biron P et al (1992) High-dose chemotherapy with ABMT in the first line treatment of poor risk non-seminomatous germ cell tumors. Bone Marrow Transplant 10 (suppl 2) : 27
10. Samson MK, Rustin SE, Jones SE et al (1984) Dose response and dose survival advantage for high versus low dose Cisplatin combined with Vinblastine and Bleomycin in disseminated testicular cancer. Cancer 53 : 1029-1035
11. Clemm C, Hartenstein R, Willich N, Boeninig L, Wilmanns W (1986) Vinblastine-Ifosfamide-Cisplatin treatment of bulky seminoma. Cancer 58 : 2203-2207

Extented resection after primary chemotherapy for residual malignant non-seminomatous germ-cell tumors of the mediastinum : is it worthwhile ?

P Macchiarini*, E Dulmet**, V de Montpreville**, A Chapelier*, B Lenot*, J Cerrina*, P Dartevelle*

Primary malignant non-seminomatous germ cell tumours are rare neoplasms accounting for only 1 to 3.5 % of all mediastinal malignancies and 1 to 2 % of all germ cell tumours in male patients [1]. Although they share many histological and serological features [2], their clinical and biological behaviour is different from their testicular counterparts [3, 4]. Most of them present as bulky anterior mediastinal masses that frequently involve surrounding structures or organs, lack of radiosensitivity, are rarely cured by surgical resection alone and have a poor prognosis [5].

However, treatment outcome is improving with modern therapy. Integration of induction cisplatin-based chemotherapy with surgical excision of all vestiges of residual disease, if present, followed by aggressive post-operative chemotherapy has become the standard treatment modality and associated with 5-year survival rates of approximately 50 % [1]. In this report, we addressed whether extended operations are worthwhile in patients presenting with residual masses and/or normalization of serum tumour markers after induction chemotherapy. Moreover, we have evaluated the biological characteristics of the tumour specimens with regard to the expression of the p53 suppressor gene, angiogenesis, proliferative activity and other early and late parameters of the process of metastatis.

Patients and methods

Between 1988 and 1992, 7 consecutive, previously untreated male patients affected by primary malignant non-seminomatous germ cell tumours of the mediastinum were observed. Eligibility included histologically proven non-seminomatous germ cell tumours of the mediastinum and or mediastinal mass with elevated serum tumour markers (STM), i.e. α-fetoprotein (α-FP), β-fraction of human chorionic gonadotropin (β-HCG), normal bone, liver, renal and cardio-pulmonary function, ECOG performance status of 0-3 and measurable disease. Patients with major intrathoracic structures or organs involvement were eligible if in the surgeon's judgement all known disease was completely resectable. Initial evaluation included history and physical examination,

---

Departments of *Thoracic and Vascular Surgery and Heart-Lung Transplantation and **Surgical Pathology, Hopital Marie-Lannelongue (Paris-Sud University) Le Plessis-Robinson, France

biochemical profile including STM, chest X-ray, bronchoscopy, computed tomography (CT) of the chest, abdominal ultrasound and bone scans. Other investigations were made to delineate the extent and operability of the noeplasms, as necessary. Our preferred policy was to determine the histological type of tumour by either surgical of non-surgical biopsy.

Patients received 2 to 4 courses of cisplatin, vinblastine and bleomycin (PVB) regimen [6, 7]. Those obtaining a complete response after induction chemotherapy were followed without further therapy. Those patients with normalization or a reduction > 90 % of STM and residual radiologic abnormalities underwent operation. At the time of surgery, resection attempted to remove the entire tumour area present at the time of initial staging and was defined as complete if all known disease was completely resected and the proximal resection margins were microscopically free of tumour. Incomplete resection was defined as such if gross (R2) or microscopically (R1) identifiable tumour was left in place. All margins were checked by frozen section.

All surgical specimens were classified histopathologically according to the WHO classification [8]. Paraffin-embedded bouin-fixed blocks containing tumour tissue from each patient were analyzed for the presence of tumour emboli within blood or lymphatic vessels, p53 gene expression, proliferative activity and other histological variables according to our previously described methods [9-11]. The presence of tumour emboli in endothelial-lined channels and their location in the specimen were assessed. Analysis of p53 human protein was done with the ABC immunoperoxidase technique using the rabbit polyclonal antibody CM-1 recognizing the p53 nuclear protein (wild and mutant type). The areas of tumour containing the most intense angiogenesis were examined by light microscopy, screened by scanning the tumour sections at low power (40x and 100x) and by identifying them with the highest number of discrete microvessels, e.g. capillaries and small venules staining for factor VIII antigen. The areas of high neovascularization were more frequent at the neoplasm margins and graded on a density scale of 0 to 4+. Microvessels in sclerotic areas within the tumour and adjacent areas of unaffected lung parenchyma were not considered in vessel count and served as internal controls for assessing the quality of staining for factor VIII. After the most vascularized area was identified, individual microvessels were counted on 200x fields and each count was expressed as the highest number of microvessels identified within the area. Cell kinetic studies were determined by estimating the expression of the proliferating cell nuclear antigen (PCNA) and mitotic count (MC). Absolute counts of PCNA immunoreactivity were made by scoring a minimum of 5 HPFs and the percentage of proliferating tumours cells was determined (range, 0-100 %). After operation, patients whose tumours displayed persistent germ cell malignancy underwent additional 2 courses of chemotherapy.

Statistical Analysis

Survival was calculated from the date of surgery until death or the date of last follow-up (censored), estimated the product-limit method [12], and differences on its distribution were evaluated *via* the log rank test [13]. Numbers

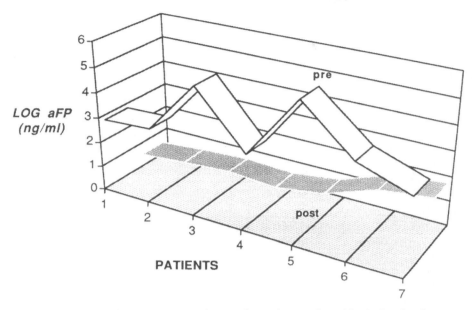

Fig. 1. Comparison between pre- and post-chemotherapy logarithmic levels of serum α-fetoprotein (α-FP) ($p < 0.01$). 5 patients had their initially elevated α-FP serum levels normalized and 2 reduced of $>$ than 90 %

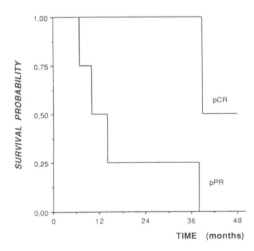

Fig. 2. Survival comparison between patients whose tumours were completely sterilized at pathological examination ($n = 3$, pCR) and those whose tumours showed viable tumour cells ($n = 4$, pPR). The difference was highly significant ($p < 0.01$).

are expressed either as median or as mean ± S.D. of n number of observations. Significancy was set at a $p > .05$; all tests were two-sided.

Results

There were 8 male patients aged in median 34 years (range, 21-45 years). All presented an anterior mediastinal mass associated with elevated α-FP levels. Pre-treatement histological diagnosis was obtained in 5 patients and included 3 mixed and 2 pure yolk sac tumours. After a median of 3 PVB courses (range, 2-5) partial responses were observed. 5 patients had their initially elevated STM normalized and 2 reduced more than 90 % (Figure 1).

All patients underwent a complete surgical excision of their tumour. 6 patients had multiple sites of involvement. Resection of the primary tumour was extended to the anterior pericardium in 6 patients, phrenic nerve in 6, right upper lobe in 3 and superior vena cava in 3. In these last three patients the superior vena cava was reconstructed with PTFE grafts. There was no operative mortality or major early and late post-operative complications. Analysis of the surgical specimens revealed 3 pure 4 mixed yolk sac tumours ; the mixed component included choriocarcinomas in 3 patients and teratocarcinoma in 1. A complete sterilization of the tumour was observed in 3 patients (43 %). The remaining 4 patients had viable tumour cells in their postchemotherapy residual lesions and their biological characteristics are depicted in Table 1. Only tumour displaying carcinomatous elements had expression of the p53 gene, proliferating cells and angiogenic dependent neoplasms ; the majority of tumours had abnormal expression of the p53 suppressor gene, high rate of tumour cells in the proliferating phases of the cell cycle (G_1, S, G_2), high degree of angiogenesis and no intratumour blood vessel tumour emboli.

With a median follow-up time of 37.5 months, overall 2 and 4 year survivals were 57 and 19 %, respectively. 5 patients died ; 3 from systemic progression of their tumour and two from the development of systemic mastocytosis after 38 and 39 months. The systemic mast cell disease was diagnosed on bone marrow and liver biopsies ; both patients had tumour containing yolk sac ele-

Table 1. Tumour characteristics of the 4 patients whose neoplasms displayed viable tumour cells within the surgical specimens.

Characteristics	Values
p53 expression (absent *vs* present) :	1 *vs* 3
count :	35 ± 11.9 (0-50)
Tumor proliferative activity* (%) :	52.5 ± 5 (50-60)
Mitotic count :	1.5 ± 0.5 (1-3)
Angiogenesis (present *vs* absent) :	4 *vs* 0
Angiogenesis-density (0 to 4 + scale) :	1.75 ± 0.25 (1-2)
Angiogenesis count (*per* 200x field) :	11.7 ± 5.4 (4-16)
Blood Vessel Invasion (absent *vs* present) :	4 *vs* 0

Data are expressed as mean ± standard deviation (S.D.). Numbers in parenthesis indicate median values. *Determined by PCNA staining.

ments and were without evidence of primary disease. The only factor able to influence survival significantly was whether or not a complete sterilization of the tumour was observed on the surgical specimens (Figure 2).

Discussion

Management of patients with mediastinal non-seminomatous germ cell tumours who have normalized the elevated serum tumour markers after induction chemotherapy but still have a residual disease is a common clinical scenario. Only 50 % of patients who achieve disease-free status do so with chemotherapy alone suggesting that surgical resection of all residual vestiges remains an important step in the overall management of these tumours [5]. Unfortunately, they have a very aggressive local behaviour and often present with multiple involvement of vital structures or organs [14]. Since there is no role for debulking surgery, surgeons are reluctant to perform extended resections because of the high cost-benefit ratio. Presented provide evidence that extended resections of residual mediastinal non-seminomatous germ cell tumours after induction chemotherapy in patients with normal serum a-FP levels or reduced > 90 % after induction chemotherapy are feasible and might be obtained at the expense of low morbidity, no mortality and encouraging long-term survival. Data clearly demontrate that multiple structure/organ involvements should not preclude the eligibility of a sinlge patient for this multimodality treatment, provided a complete resection of all tumour vestiges present at the time of initial evaluation might be anticipated. It should be noted that there bas been an increasing number of new surgical techniques developed in the last few years, and their application in the field of solid malignancies is likely to increase [15].

Surgical resection does allow the tumour not only to be resected but gives precise information about tumour biology. So far, patients with residual viable germ cells received additionally 2 courses of PVB chemotherapy while those with teratomas or necrosis were simply observed closely [5]. In this study, 46 % of the patients who had a clinical partial remission of their initial measurable disease had a complete sterilization of their tumour ; further supporting that surgical excision of the residual mass is the only way to know about the effectivness of a given chemoterapuetic regimen and the biological status of the residual neoplams. According to the afornementioned guidelines, they didn't receive any further treatment. On the other hand, the analysis of the surgical specimens of those tumours displaying viable tumour cells demonstrated that those germ cell tumours with carcinomatous components (e.g. teratocarcinoma choriocatcinoma) display a particular aggresive phenotype. They had aberrations of the p53 gene, a nuclear phosphoprotein involved in cell regulation and apoptosis which can function as a supressor of transformation and tumorigenesis. Different mutations of the p 53 gene may have diverse early and/or late effects on tumuor development [16] and the fact that we found p53 aberrations in 3 out of 4 lesions suggests that p53 alterations may be involved in the initiating steps of tumour progression and that this confers the particular aggressive phenotype of germ cell tumours.

Tumours consist of three populations of cells, i.e., proliferating cells that are involved in the growth and division (S, G_2, M, G_1), nonproliferating cells (G0) that may be triggered to reenter the cell cycle, and dying cells that have permanently loss the capacity to divide. It is well known that the rate of growth of any tumour reflects its subsequent behaviour pattern, and that increased proliferative rates are peculiar findings of aggressive tumours [17]. We were unable to find nonproliferating cells in the surgical specimens and the percentage of proliferating cells was remarkably high, suggesting that tumour cells might have acquired a degree of autonomy from normal regulatory controls on cellular proliferation and may facilitate emergence of new clones with propensity to invade locally and metastasise [18]. Experimental evidence [19] indicates that after a new tumour has attained a siz of few milimetre in diameter (10^6 tumour cells), further exponential expansion of the tumour-cell population requires the induction of new capillaries blood vessels (angiogenesis) [20]. All tumours were angiogenic-dependent and their degree of angiogenesis was remarkable. Since highly proliferating tumours are more sensitive to chemotherapy, on might postulate that the tumours displaying a high proliferative rate may be treated with more intensive chemotherapeutic regimens. Hence, anti-angiogenic factors might be associated in the preoperative setting to reduce or minimize the risk of tumour cells to enter into the circulation.

References

1. Wright CD, Kesler KA, Nichols CR et al (1990) Primary mediastinal non-seminomatous germ cell tumours. J Thorac Cardiovasc Surg 99 : 210-217
2. Patcher MR, Lattes R (1964) Germinal tumours of the meidastinum : A clinicopathological study of adult teratomas, teratocarcinomas, choriocarcinomas and seminomas. Dis Chest 45 : 301-310
3. Nichols CR, Hoffman R, Einhorn LH et al (1985) Hematological malignancies associated with primary mediastinal germ cell tumours. Ann Intern Med 102 : 603-609
4. Nichols CR, Saxman S, Williams SD et al (1990) Primary mediastinal non-seminomatous germ cell tumours. A modern single Institution experience. Cancer 65 : 1641-1646.
5. Nichols CR (1992) Medisatinal germ cell tumours. In : Mediastinal tumours. Sem Thorac Cardiovasc Surg 4 : 45-50.
6. Hainsworth JD, Einhorn LH, Williams SD, Stewart M, Greco FA (1982) Advanced extragonadal germ-cell tumours. Successful treatment with combination chemotherapy. Ann Intern Med 33 : 333-339.
7. Vogelzang N, Raghan D, Anderson R, Rosai J, Levitt S, Kennedy B (1982) Mediastinal non-seminomatous germ cell tumours : The role of combined modality therapy. Ann Thorac Surg 33 : 333-339
8. Mostofi FK, Sobin LH (1977) Histopathological typing of testicular tumours. In : International histological classification of tumours. N. 16. Geneva. World Heatlh Organization 27-31
9. Maccharini P, Fontanini G, Hardin M, Pingitore R, Angeletti CA (1992) Most peripheral, node-negative non-small cell lung cancer have absence of intratumoral

and peritumoral blood and lymphatic vessel invasion and low proliferative rates. J Thorac Cardiovasc Surg 104 : 892-899.
10. Macchiarini P, Fontanini G, Hardin M, Squartini F, Angeletti CA. (1992) Relation of neovascularization to metastasis of non-small cell lung cancer. Lancet 340 : 145-146.
11. Macchiarini P, Fontanini G, Hardin M et al. (in press) Blood vessel invasion by tumour cells predicts recurrence in completely resected T1N0M0 no-small cell lung cancer. J Thorac Cardiovasc Surg.
12. Kaplan EL, Meier P (1985) Nonparametric estimation from incomplete observations. J Am Stat Assoc 1958 ; 53 : 457-481.
13. Peto R, Pike MC, Armitage P, Breslow NE, Cox DR, Howard SY (1977) Design and analysis of randomized clinical trials requiring prolonged observations of each patient : II. Analysis and examples. Br J Cancer 1977 ; 35 : 1-39.
14. Ginsberg R (1992) Mediastinal germ cell tumours : The role of surgery. In : Mediastinal tumours. Sem Thorac Cardiovasc Surg 4 : 51-54
15. Dartevelle P, Chapelier A, Pastorino U, et al. (1991) Long-term follow-up after prosthetic replacement of the superior vena cava combined with resection of mediastinal-pulmonary malignant tumours. J Thorac Cardiovasc Surg 102 : 259-265
16. Levine AJ, Momand J, Finlay C (1991) The p53 tumour suppressopr gene. Nature (Lond.) 351 : 453-456.
17. Quinn CM, Wright NA. The clinical assessment of proliferation and growth in human tumours : evaluation of methods and applications as prognostic variables. J Path 1990 ; 160 : 93-102.
18. Volm M, Hahn EW, Mettern J, Muller T, Vogt-Moykopf I, Weber E. Five-year follow-up study of independent clinical and flow cytometric prognostic factors for the survival of patients with non-small cell lung carcinoma. Cancer Res 1988 ; 48 : 2923-2928
19. Folkman J. What is the evidence that tumours are angiogenesis dependent ? J Natl Cancer Inst 1990 ; 82 : 4-6
20. Hart IR, Saini A. Biology of tumour metastasis. Lancet 1992 ; 339 : 1453-1457
21. Austen KH. Systemic mastocytosis. New Engl J Med 1992 ; 326 : 639-640.
22. Ladany M, Samaniego F, Reuter VE et al. Cytogenetic and immunohistochemical evidence for the germ cell origin of a subset of acute leukemias associated with mediastinal germ cell tumours. JNCI 1991 ; 82 : 221-227

The prediction of treatment outcomes in non-seminomatous extragonadal germ cell tumors (NSEGCT) by using different criteria of « poor » and « good » risk

F Gutierrez Delgado, A Garin, S Tjulandin, M Ramirez Mendoza, A Khlebnov

Multivariate analysis allowed to identify prognostic factors on the treatment outcome and led to perform the current « good risk » and « poor risk » criteria for patients with germ cell tumors (GCT). In spite of common histology, an inferior CR rate in the treatment of NSEGCT patients, in comparison with those reached in testicular cancer have been reported by the most of authors and led to include them in « poor risk » group [1]. Thus all patients with extragonadal primary are automatically include in the « poor risk » definition of the Memorial Sloan Kettering Cancer Center (MSKCC)[2] and the National Cancer Institute criteria [3]. In this study we applied the objective criteria of « good » and « poor » risk performed for testicular tumors to assign NSEGCT patients in risk groups and to predict their treatment outcome.

Patients and methods

From 1979 to 1991, 40 patients with NSEGCT were treated in our institution with Cisplatin based chemotherapy (PVB, VAB-6 and BEP). Patients characteristics and treatment results of the NSEGCT patients included in this study have been detailed elsewhere [4]. Twelve patients achieved a CR with chemotherapy alone and 3 more after chemotherapy and cytoreductive surgery. Overall CR rate was 37 %. All other patients were considered as incomplete response (IR). At a median follow-up of 26 (3-116) months 14 [35 %] patients are alive with no evidence of disease, and 26 died from disease progression.

The MSKCC [2], NCO [3], Indiana University [5], Institute Gusto Rouse [6], and the European Organization for Research on Treatment of Cancer (EORTC)/Medical Research Council [7] have been compared to assignment to a « good risk » or « poor risk » groups utilizing a similar method described by Bajorin [2]. The probability of achieving a CR was calculated according to mathematical formulas performed at MSKCC [8] and IGR [6], which included patients in « poor risk » group with value less than 0.5 and 0.7 respectively. Specificity, sensitivity, and correct overall prediction of all criteria also have been calculated. Specificity was defined as the number of correct prediction of IRs divided by the number of IRs. Sensitivity was defined as the number of correct prediction of CRs divided by the number of CRs. Correct overall prediction was defined as the number of correct prediction of IRs + CRs divid-

---

Cancer Research Center [CRC], 24 Kashirskoe sh, Moscow, Russia ed by the total number of patients. Survival curves for « good risk » and « poor risk » groups designed by each criteria were constructed separately and compared by log rank test. All univariate comparisons of proportions were made using a chi-square test.

Results

The median and range of probability to achieve a CR calculated by mathematical formulas were : MSKCC 0.60 (0.15-0.90), and for IGR 0.89 (0.51-1). A significantly statistical difference was found in the number of patients designated « poor risk » by the different criteria (p = 0.001).The lowest proportion of « poor risk » patients was assignated by IGR (23 %) with progressively higher proportion of patients designated « poor risk » by MSKCC (40 %), EORTC (60 %), NCO (70 %) and IU (83 %). The proportion of patients considered « good risk » varied from 17 % (IU) to 77 % (IGR) CR rate between two prognostic groups reached a statistical significant difference if patients had been assigned by MSKCC and EORTC criteria (Table 1). Results of specificity, sensitivity and overall correct prediction by each criteria are showed in Table 1. The EORTC, IU, and NCI criteria had a high specificity to identify the patients with IR after chemotherapy. On the other hand IGR and MSKCC with better accuracy could predict a achievement of CR. However none of the criteria had a sensitivity and specificity more than 0.5 simultaneously. Only survival curves for « good » and « poor » risk patients constructed according to the IU criteria showed a significant difference (p = 0.03).

Table 1. Percentage of NSEGCT patients allocated to « good risk » (GR) and « poor risk » groups. CR rate and prediction rules for risk group

Criteria	Percentage of pts allocated to		CR rate		Specifity	Sensitivity	Correct overall prediction
	GR	PR	GR	PR			
EORTC	40	60	75	28	0.92	0.40	0.72
			p = 0.008				
IGR	77	23	39	33	0.28	0.86	0.50
			p = 0.54				
IU	17	83	71	30	0.92	0.33	0.70
			p = 0.005				
MSKCC	60	40	50	19	0.48	0.80	0.60
			p = 0.004				
NCI	30	70	33	29	0.92	0.06	0.60
			p = 0.68				

Discussion

Although NSEGCT are considered « poor risk » tumors, the most interesting observation of our study was that, from 17 % to 77 % of patients with NSEGCT has been assigned to « good risk » group. The proportion of « poor risk » group also varied significantly : from 23 % to 83 %. A statistical difference in CR rate between « good risk » and « poor risk » groups defined by the EORTC and MSKCC has been also registered, however, only the IU criteria showed significative difference when compared survival between « good » and « poor » risk groups.

In conclusion, results obtained in our study suggest that clinical parameters considered prognostic factors in primary testicular are insufficient to define NSEGCT patients as « poor risk » group, and to predict their treatment outcome. Due to rarity of this neoplasm, a international cooperation is required to include a large number of patients to identify and assessment new prognostic factors.

References

1. Hainsworth JD, Greco FA (1992) Extragonadal germ cell tumors and unrecognized germ cell tumors. Sem Oncol 19 : 119-127
2. Bajorin D, Katz A, Chan E et al (1988) Comparison of criteria for assigning germ cell tumors patients to « good risk » and « poor risk » studies. N° 6 : 786-792
3. Ozols RF, Ihde DC, Lineham WM et al (1988) A randomized trial of standard chemotherapy versus a high-dose chemotherapy regimen in the treatment of poor prognosis nonseminomatous germ cell tumors. J Clin Oncol 6 : 103-114
4. Gutierrez Delgado F, Tjulandin SA, Garin AM (1993) Eur J Cancer (in press)
5. Loehrer PJ, Williams SD, Einhorn LH (1988) Testicular cancer : the quest continues. JNCI 80 : 1373-1382
6. Droz JP, Kramar A, Ghosn M et al (1988) Prognostic factors in advanced non-seminomatous testicular cancer. A multivariate logistic regression analysis. Cancer 62 : 564-568
7. Horwich A, Stenning S, Mead et al (1990) Prognostic factors for survival in advanced non-seminomatous germ cell tumors. A study by the Medical Research Council (MRC). Testicular Tumour Subgroup. Proc Amer Soc Clin Oncol 9 : 132 (abstr C-513)
8. Bosl GJ, Geller NL, Cirrincione C et al (1983) Multivariate analysis of prognostic variables in patients with metastatic testicular cancer. Cancer Res 43 : 3403-3407

Advanced seminoma treated with chemotherapy (CT)

JW Zinser, R Gaona, A Mendoza, O Ocampo,
H Domínguez-Malagón, E Gómez, L Vicencio

Seminoma is highly radio-sensitive. Patients with low-volume disease have an excellent prognosis. But as tumor volume increases, the relapse rate can be as high as 80 %. CT in advanced disease is effective [1, 2] and there are even regimens with low myelosuppression or neurotoxicity [1, 3].

Patients and methods

Since September 1985 patients with metastatic testicular seminoma or primary extragonadal seminoma with tumor masses > 5 cm have been treated similarly as reported by the M.D. Anderson group with the following regimen : Cisplatin 100 mg/m^2 i.v. over 4 hours on days 1, 8, 15, 43 and 50 and Cyclophosphamide 1.000 mg/m^2 i.v. over 30 minutes prior to Cisplatin on days 1 and 43. All patients had CAT scan to evaluate measurable disease and all patients without an obvious testicular primary had ultrasound of both testis. All patients were required to have a normal AFP and a BHCG either negative or moderately elevated, as judged according to the tumor volume. After 5 courses of Cisplatin if there was residual disease > 5 cm they received radiotherapy, otherwise they were followed without treatment unless they develop progressive disease.

Results

Between September 85 and December 90 fifty-four patients with advanced seminoma were seen : 40 testicular and 14 mediastinal. Mean age : Testis 34.7 years (19-56) and mediastinal 27.7 years (19-38), (p = 0.007). Tumor size : Testis : < 5 cm : 3 (7 %), 5-10 cm : 24 (60 %) and >10 cm : 13 (33 %). Mediastinum : 5-10 cm 4 (29 %) and > 10 cm 10 (71 %). Among patients with tumors < 5 cm, one patient had prior radiotherapy, another multiple lymph node metastatic sites below the diaphragm and the third a large retroperitoneal mass partially resected. Five testicular patients (13 %) had disease above the diaphragm. All patients had negative AFP and 63 % elevated BHCG, median 40 mIU/ml (10-890). Only 3 patients > 100 mIU/ml, two testis patients (155 and 156) and one mediastinal (890). Elevation of BHCG according to the primary was : mediastinum 11/14 (79 %) and testis 23/40 (58 %), (p = 0.27). Three patients had hypercalcemia which resolved after the first course. Prior treatment : Three patients had radiotherapy and 1 patient non Cisplatin CT

Instituto Nacional de Cancerología, San Fernando 22, Tlalpan Mexico, D.F. 14000 Mexico

plus radiotherapy. Eighty five percent received 5 courses (2 had Doxorubicin, one due to a BHCG of 890 mIU/ml and the other one during the first course due to an initial diagnosis of thyroid carcinoma). One patient 6 courses, and the other 7 patients 3-4 courses. Two patients with elevated creatinine were started with Cyclophosphamide at 700 mg /m^2 i.v. on day 1 and Etoposide 400 mg i.v. in two days. Cisplatin was added within the following 2 weeks when renal function normalized and treatment continued as planned. One 56-years old patient with Creatinine in the upper limit received a total dose of Cisplatin of 270 mg/m^2. Relapsed and salvaged.

Response : Complete 37 %, partial 57 % and not evaluable 6 %. Of the later 3 patients 1 refused further follow-up and CT after 3 courses and was known to be asymptomatic after 12 months. One lost to follow-up after 3 courses and the third lost to follow-up after 5 courses. BHCG normalized at a median of 1 course [1-3]. Three testicular patients with residual disease received radiotherapy.

Relapses : All mediastinal patients remain progression-free and five testicular patients have relapsed (p = 0.31) at a median of 13 months [4-19]. Three patients did not have residual disease after initial CT. The other 2 patients had residual masses (1 and 8 cm). The later patient did not receive radiotherapy after CT. BHCG values prior to CT in these 5 patients were 94, 16, 25, 0 and 15 mIU/ml. One patient relapsed at 13 months in the retroperitoneum and liver with negative markers, was considered to have a non seminomatous component but refused further treatment and died. The other 4 patients were treated with 2-3 courses of Cisplatin, Cyclophosphamide and Doxorubicin (50-80 mg/m^2). Three patients also had radiotherapy and remain progression free at 11, 41, 43 and 68 months. The 4th patient had been treated with radiotherapy when first diagnosed.

Relapses according to tumor size prior to CT were : 1/13 when >10 cm, 2/24 when 5-10 cm, and 2/3 when < 5 cm. There are no relapses among patients with mediastinal primary in spite that 71 % had tumor masses > 10 cm, and 50 % residual masses the largest of 5.8 cm and no one received radiotherapy. Overall follow-up : Forty-two patients remain in continuous follow-up at a median of 41 months (17-82). Twelve patients are lost to follow-up. Among those 12 patients, 4 did not complete 5 courses and were lost at 1, 1, 1 and 12 months, the other 8 patients were lost to follow-up at a median of 2 months (0-20).

Toxicity : Nausea and vomit : 80 % of patients, with 25 % > grade 1. Myelosuppression : Among the 50 patients who received only Cisplatin and Cyclophosphamide, the median nadir of blood counts was as follows : Hemoglobin 12.0 g/dl (8.5-14.9), two patients required transfusion of packed red blood cells. Leukocytes 2,300/mcl (800-6,100), only one patient had less than 1,000 WBC and no one developed fever. Platelets 180,000/mcl (74,000-389,000). The two patients who initially received Etoposide instead of Cisplatin due to renal failure had a nadir of Hg, WBC and platelets of : 7, 200, 175,000 and 9.8, 300 and 174,000 respectively. History of radiotherapy did not affect the blood counts significantly. Neurotoxicity : 24 % symptomatic peripheral neuropathy and 17 % clinically disturbing hearing loss. Audiometric studies not done.

Nephrotoxicity : No patient had abnormal creatinine at completion of treatment.

Discussion

Among 54 patients with advanced seminoma there were 26 % of mediastinal origin and no retroperitoneal primaries. Over 90 % were untreated and with tumor masses > 5 cm. BHCG elevated in 63 %. Some differences were noted among patients with either testicular or mediastinal primaries ; the most relevant, although not statistically significant was that the relapses have been only among patients with a testicular primary even though most of the patients with mediastinal origin had a high tumor volume and half of them residual disease. Patients with mediastinal primaries were 7 years younger ($p = 0.007$). Although BHCG was elevated in 63 % of the patients and in spite that 43 % had tumor masses > 10 cm, in only 3/34 it was > 100 mIU/ml. We believe that in any patient with a BHCG > 200 mIU/ml the presence of non seminomatous elements should always be considered.

Cisplatin and Cyclophosphamide are an effective therapeutic regimen. All patients responded and 9 % relapsed at a median of 13 months (4-19). Except for the patient with a probable non seminomatous component all were salvaged and Doxorubicin seems to play an important role. Relapses after 19 months are unlikely as follow-up extends to a median of 41 months (17-82) and there have been no additional recurrences. One relapse was not unexpected as the patient had an 8 cm residual tumor and did not receive radiotherapy. However three of the other relapses occurred in patients without residual disease, and without having a pretreatment tumor larger > 6 cm and only a moderately elevated BHCG. Therefore, patients should be closely followed with CAT scan mainly during the first year and a half. We do not think it would be appropriate to add radiation therapy to all patients at completion of CT, as in most patients it would represent overtreatment. In patients with normal renal function this is a well tolerated regimen, neurotoxicity should be considered the major side effect, with no significant myelosuppression, although in occasional patients blood counts may drop to dangerous levels. Nausea and vomiting were present in 80 %, but can be ameliorated with the use of serotonin-blocking agents.

References

1. Logothetis CJ, Samuels ML, Ogden SL et al (1987) Cyclophosphamide and sequential Cisplatin for advanced seminoma : Long-term follow-up in 52 patients. J Urol 138 : 789-794
2. Loehrer PJ, Birch R, Williams SD et al (1987) CT of metastatic seminoma : The southeastern cancer study group experience. J Clin Oncol 5 : 1212-1220
3. Horwich A, Dearnaley DP, Duchesne GM et al (1989) Simple nontoxic treatment of advanced seminoma with carboplatin. J Clin Oncol 7 : 1150-1156

Concomitant 5-FU-CDDP and bifractionated split course radiation therapy for invasive bladder cancer

C Maulard*, M Housset*, Y Chrétien**, S Delanian*, F Colardelle*, JP Hallez**, B Dufour**, F Baillet*

Till now, radical cystectomy is considered the most effective treatment for local control of invasive bladder cancer but failed to cure more than 50 % of patients because the subsequent frequency of metastatic disease. Recent encouraging results, using exclusive chemo-radiotherapy without surgery, have been reported and such a conservative treatment could appear as a tangible reality for selected patients [1-3].

In 1988, we began a prospective study of Neo-Adjuvant chemo-radiotherapy, using a 5-FU Cisplatin combination and a concomitant bifractionated split course radiation therapy followed by cystectomy or additional chemo-radiotherapy in patients with muscle-invasive bladder cancer. This is a report of the results in a series of 54 patients with 18 months minimum follow-up.

Patients

From Febrary 1988 through June 1991, 54 patients were referred to Necker Hospital (Paris) for an operable untreated bladder cancer. There were 45 males and 9 females. The age ranged between 37 and 82 years (median : 66). All patients had a biopsy proven invasive transitionnal cell carcinoma confined to the pelvis. All patients were staged according to the TNM classification (1987). There were 14 T2 and 40 T3-T4 (25 T3a and 15 T3b-T4). Four patients presented a radiological N1 pelvic nodal involvment (1 T2 and 3 T3). The histological grading was III-IV in all patients.

Methods

Treatment

Trans-urethral resection : All patients initially underwent a trans-urethral resection (TUR). Complete macroscopic removal of the tumor by TUR was achieved in 25 cases (9 of 14 T2, 12 of 25 T3 and 4 of 15 T3b) and failed in 27 patients. Result of the resection was unknown in 2 cases.

Neo-Adjuvant chemo-radiotherapy combination :
- Radiotherapy : All patients were treated on a 4.5 MV linear accelerator

---

* Service d'Oncologie, Radiothérapie, Hôpital Necker ; ** Service d'Urologie, Hôpital Necker 149, rue de Sèvres, 75015 Paris, France

to the whole pelvis by four fields box technique. The Neo-Adjuvant irradiation dose was 24 Gy delivered in 8 fractions over 17 days, according to a modified bifractionated split course schedule. All portals were treated twice on day D1, D3, D15 and D17. Each fraction delivered 3 Gy. The interval of time between both daily fractions was at least 4 hours.

• *Chemotherapy* : The patients received concomitant intraveinous 5-FU — Cisplatin combination with radiation therapy. Cisplatin (15 mg/m^2/d) and 5-FU (400 mg/m^2/d) were administered as a short infusion over 2 hours on day D1, D2, D3 and D15, D16, D17. On day D1, D3, D15 and D17, chemotherapy infusion began 2 hours before irradiation.

Evaluation of Neo-Adjuvant chemo-radiotherapy combination and additionnal treatment planning : A control cystoscopy with deep biopsies was systematically performed on week 6. Patients with persistent tumor immediately underwent a radical cystectomy with pelvic nodes dissection. For patients achieving a complete histologic response, two different therapeutic approaches were used : immediate radical cystectomy or Adjuvant chemo-radiotherapy combination. For these responders, the additional treatment was not randomly planned. It depended on age, performance status, bladder capacity, the risks of operative morbidity and on patient preference. Additional radiation therapy consisted in a 20 Gy boost to the bladder. All portals were treated twice on day D64, D66, D78 and D80. Each fraction delivered 2.5 Gy, with a 4 hours interval between both daily fractions. Finally, the total bladder irradiation dose was 44 Gy in 16 fractions over 80 days. As for Neo-Adjuvant treatement, the same 5-FU Cisplatin combination schedule was used for additional therapy.

Statistical methods

Data were evaluated in an univariate study using contingency table analysis and the chi-square test (with Yates adjustment or with Fisher's exact test if necessary). Survival curves were calcultated by Kaplan-Meïer method and compared by log-rank testing.

Results

Objective response to Neo-Adjuvant chemo-radiotherapy combinaison

All patients were evaluated for immediate response on control cystoscopy. An histologic complete remission was obtained in 40 of the 54 patients (74 % ; responder group) ; persistent tumor was found in 14 patients (26 % ; non responder group) with a pT1 G1 residual tumor staging in 4 cases. Ten of 14 T2 patients (71 %) and 33 of 40 T3 (75 %) achieved a complete remission. Complete response was seen in 21 of the 25 patients (84 %) with complete debulking by TUR and in 17 of the 27 patients (62 %) with incomplete resection (p = 0.08). No progression tumor was seen. Among the 14 non responder patients, twelve underwent the planned radical cystectomy. For all these

12 patients, pathological examination of the bladder pointed out an evolutive tumor (3 pT1, 1 pT2, 8 pT3). Both remaining non responders refused surgery and received the additional chemo-radiotherapy treatment. Among the 40 responder patients, 22 were treated by conservative chemo-radiotherapy combination (group A) and 18 underwent a radical cystectomy (group B). Groups A and B were comparable for age, sex, TNM, histological grading and quality of resection by TUR. In all group B patients, the bladder was found free of tumor on pathological examination (18 pT0), confirming the cystoscopy findings ; all these 18 patients were free of nodal involvment too.

Pelvic recurrences

With a follow-up of 27 ± 12 months, 4 patients locally relapsed. Local relapse occurred at 6, 9, 11 and 46 months. Concerning the responders, there were one invasive and two superficial bladder relapses (1 pTa and 1 pT1) in group A and one pelvic relapse in group B.

Systemic disease

A systemic disease (para-aortic involvment and/or metastatic spread) occurred in 16 patients (30 %) with a mean time of 12 ± 8 months. Systemic disease occurence was significantly correlated with the previous response to Neo-Adjuvant treatment : 6 of the 40 responder patients (15 %) presented a systemic spread versus 10 of the 14 non responders (71 % ; $p < 0.001$). Systemic disease appeared in a mean time of 13 ± 8 months for the responders and 7 ± 4 months for the non responders. There were 3 systemic diseases in group A and 3 in group B.

Survival

The 3 year overall survival and the 3 year disease free survival were 59 % and 62 % respectively. The 3 year disease free survival was 66 % for T2 patients and 53 % for T3. The 3 year survival was significantly better for the responders (77 %) than for the non responders (23 % ; $p = 0.0001$). There was no significant difference in survival between group A (81 %) and group B (77 %).

Tolerance

Mild to moderate acute side effects of radiotherapy frequently occurred but did not required hospitalization. Chronic sequelae as contracted bladder or small bowel obstruction caused by radiation therapy, have not been observed until now. Chemotherapy was well tolerated even in elderly patients. Surgical morbidity was tolerable. Post-operatively, two patients presented a spontaneously resolutive digestive fistula. Four bladder replacements were performed without additional morbidity.

Discussion and conclusions

Treatment of invasive carcinoma of the bladder remains a double challenge : first the eradication of local disease and second the therapy of potential occult metastases. For that, we developed a prospective study based on a chemoradiotherapy association. Rationale for this combination was the potential synergy between 5-FU, Cisplatin and X-rays as well as the potential effect of chemotherapy on micrometastases. A 74 % complete response rate was achieved with such a therapeutic approach. Our results were quite comparable to other published series using a similar pre-operative schedule with a pelvic irradiation dose up to 40-45 Gy [4, 5, 6]. The achievement of a complete response by Neo-Adjuvant chemo-radiotherapy combination must be considered as the most important prognostic factor. In our series, the 3 year survival was significantly higher for the responder group than for the non responders, probably because a lesser metastatic spread incidence. Finally this Neo-Adjuvant chemo-radiotherapy combination with a concomitant bifractionnated split course radiation therapy is easily achievable and does not require systematic hospitalization. It can be proposed in most patients, even in elderly because an acceptable tolerance and a high complete response rate. A next prospective randomized study, comparing radical cystectomy and additional chemo-radiation therapy is needed to specify the exact place of a conservative treatment for the responder patients. Moreover, this chemo-radiation therapy as exclusive treatment may be a promising and worthwhile regimen for inoperable patients.

References

1. Coppin C, Brown E, the GU Tumor group (1986) Concurrent Cisplatin with radiation for locally advanced bladder cancer : a pilot study suggesting improved survival. Proceedings of ASCO, A 382
2. Shipley W, Einstein A, Coombs L et al (1987) Cisplatin and full dose irradiation for patients with invasive bladder carcinoma : a multi institutional group experience. Proceedings of the American Radium Society, A 1
3. Jakse G, Frommhold H, Dieter zur Nedden (1985) Combined radiation and chemotherapy for locally advanced transitional cell carcinoma of the urinary bladder. Cancer 55 : 1659-1664
4. Russel KJ, Boileau MA, Higano C, Collins C, Russel AH, Koh W, Cole SB, Chapman WH, Griffin TW (1990) Combined 5-Fluoro-uracile and irradiation for transitional cell carcinoma of the urinary bladder. Int J Radiat Oncol Biol Phys 19 : 693-699
5. Tester W, Porter A, Asbell S, Coughlin C, Heaney J, Martz K, Venner P, Hamond E (1989) Combined modality program with possible organ preservation for invasive bladder carcinoma : preliminary results of RTOG protocol. Proceedings of ASCO, A 548
6. Eapen L, Stewart D, Danjoux C, Genest P, Futter N, Moors D, Irvine A, Crook J, Aitken S, Petterson R, Rasuli P (1989) Intra-arterial Cisplatin and concurrent radiation for locally advanced bladder cancer. J Clin Oncol 7 : 230-235

Neo-Adjuvant treatment for locally advanced bladder cancer : a randomized prospective clinical trial

A Pellegrini, E Cortesi, N Gioacchini, E Ballatori, RA Virdis

The role of Neo-Adjuvant chemotherapy in locally advanced bladder urothelial tumors is not yet established : a number of prospective studies are evaluating the role of chemotherapy in DFS, OS and bladder preservation in selected patients.

In January 1989 GISTV[1] (Italian Bladder Tumor Study Group) started a cooperative randomized phase III study to compare, in locally advanced urothelial bladder tumors (T2-4, N0, M0), cystectomy alone versus Neo-Adjuvant chemotherapy + cystectomy.

End points of the study are : a) evaluation of DFS and OS ; b) comparison of the accuracy of clinical versus pathological staging ; c) identification of prognostic factors for possible bladder preservation ; d) evaluation of clinical activity of the M-VEC schedule (MTX 30 mg/sq days 1, 15, 22, VBL 3 mg/sq days 2, 15, 22, CDDP 70 mg/sq and 4-EPI 40 mg/sq d. 2) and tolerability of the combined treatment.

From January 1989 to June 1992 were enrolled 171 patients, stratified (T stage and grading) and randomized in two arms :

A : M-VEC x 3 cycles + cystectomy,
B : cystectomy alone.

Clinical characteristics of patients (age, previous local treatments, PS and associated diseases) are well balanced in both arms. At this time 134 patients are evaluable.

Arm A results (68 pts)

Overall responses are 49 % (33/68) with CR 31 % (21/68) and pCR 24 % (16/68), no clinical complete response in T4 stage ; Partial responses were 18 % (12/68) all confirmed at pathological staging (Fig. 1).

Myelotoxicity was the most important chemotherapy side effect : the related schedule modifications lead to the omissions of days 15 and/or 22, in 20 % (d 15) and 9 % (d 22) of pts at the first cycle, 36 % (d 15) and 15 % (d 22) at second cycle, 40 % (d 15) and 23 % (d 22) at third cycle. Renal toxicity and micositis occurred in mild grade and in a small number of patients.

Members of the GISTV Coordinating Center and Writing Committee ; Clinician from the following hospital are co-authors of the paper
[1] GISTV* (Italian Bladder Study Group)

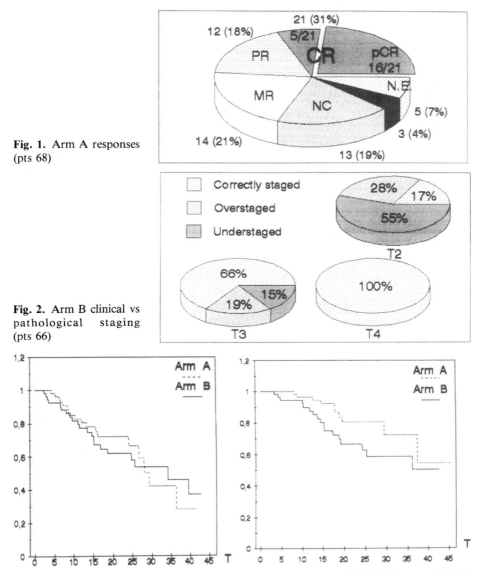

Fig. 1. Arm A responses (pts 68)

Fig. 2. Arm B clinical vs pathological staging (pts 66)

Fig. 3. Disease free survival (surgery > progression) Log-Rank 0.8202 Wilcoxon 0.4703

Fig. 4. Overal survival (random > deaths) Long-Rank 0.0777 Wilcoxon 0.0287

Arm B results (66 pts)

Pathological outcome reported a 46 % of patients correctly staged versus 32 % understaged and 22 % overstaged (Fig. 2). Pathological nodal involvement was showed in 18 % of pts in arm A and 26 % of pts in arm B.

Odds events (relapses or tumor related deaths) are still balanced in both arms, althought at 24 months of median follow-up there seem to be a little advantage in arm A. Relapses were 18 in arm A with 10 tumor related deaths versus 19 and 17, respectively, in arm B. The study is closed for recruitment and a longer follow-up is needed to show conclusive results on any possible difference in DFS (Fig. 3) and OS (Fig. 4).

We thank L Miano (Urology Dept. Civil Hosp., Teramo), T Lotti (Urology Dept. University II, Naples), N Cerulli (Urology Dept. University « La Sapienza », Rome), R Zolfanelli (Urology Dept. S. Croce Hosp., Cuneo), M Ventura (Urology Dept. S. Andrea Hosp., Vercelli), A Zincone (Urology Dept. Cardarelli Hosp., Naples), G Calderini (Urology Dept. Civil Hosp. Cassino-Frosinone), A Pinna (Urology Dept. S. Francesco, Nuoro) and G Francini (Oncology Dept. University of Siena), for including their patients in the study.

References

1. Scher HI (1990) Chemotherapy for invasive bladder cancer : Neo-Adjuvant versus Adjuvant. Sem Oncol 17 : 555-565
2. Soloway MS (1990) Invasive bladder cancer : selection of primary treatment. Sem Oncol 17 : 551-554
3. Sternberg CN, Yagoda A, Scher HI et al (1985) Preliminary results of Methotrexate, Vinblastine Adriamycin and Cysplatin (M-VAC) in advanced urothelial tumors. J Urol 133 : 403-407
4. Fair WR (1991) Neo-Adiuvant therapy in invasive bladder cancer : problems and pitfalls. Urol Clin North Am 18 : 539-542
5. Raghavan D, Pearson B et al (1991) Cytotoxic chemotherapy for advanced bladder cancer : Cysplatin containing regimens. Sem Oncol 18, 1 (suppl 3) : 55-63

Ultrastructural and clinical study of the urothelium after Interferon α-2b treatment

P Stravoravdi*, J Belivanis**, Th Dimopoulos**, J Hatzigiannis**, M Polyzonis***

Superficial bladder tumors will recur after initial treatment in 40 % to 85 % of pts usually within 6 to 12 months [1, 2]. Thus the management of the tumor should be directed both towards its treatment and the prevention of its recurrence. To this end a number of agents have been tried. Among them Interferons give promising relults. However there is a complete lack of information concerning the effect of Interferons on the ultra-structural morphology of the non-involved urothelium of SBC bearing pts. This study was, therefore, planned to evaluate the efficacy of Interferon to restore the ultrastructural morphology of the non-involved, but probably already initiated, urothelium of tumor bearing pts.

Materials and methods

Nine male pts with macroscopic hematuria but without any other urinary bladder symptoms were screened for this study. On cystoscopic examination they all had a new solitary SBC stage pTA, but the surrounding urothelium was normal. The tumor was completely resected by TUR with cold cup biopsy, and a second specimen for Electron Microscopy (EM) was taken from the posterior wall of the bladder from the non-involved urothelium away from the tumor. Histological examination showed that the tumor was totally resected and was either grade I or II. The specimens of the non-involved urothelium did not present signs of pathology. Six to 9 days after resection adjuvant therapy with Interferon was started. All instillations were administered intravesically with 50 MU of Interferon dissolved in 60 ml of saline. Each pt received a total of 22 instillations in 12 months : once a week for 8 weeks, followed by the same dosage bimonthly for the next 4 months, and finally 1 instillation per month for a further 6 months. At the end of therapy, when all pts were clinically free of recurrence, specimens for EM were taken again from the non-involved urothelium.

Results

Before treatment the free surface of the urothelia appeared flat and the AUM was missing. The superficial cytoplasm, lying between the luminal surface of

---

* Theagenion Cancer Hospital, Thessaloniki ; ** Panagia General Hospital, Urology Clinic Thessaloniki ; *** University of Thessaloniki Medical School (Technicians : K Lazopoulos, P Oustambasidis)

the cell and its nucleus appeared deserted, with very few mitochondria, sparce vesicles and few lysosomes. The Golgi apparatus was small. After therapy the pretreatment missing AUM reappeared, but although its laminar structure was apparent, its distribution was in isolated islands. The apical cytoplasm was gradually repopulated by increasing numbers of vesicles, mitochondria and lysosomes. The Golgi apparatus increased in size and complexity. NB's were also found in the nuclei with increasing frequency. Although centrioles were never found in the pretreatment specimens, they were quite frequent afterwards. Rarely found were intracytoplasmic inclusions of interwoven microtubules, known as tubuloreticular inclusions (TRI's) which were continuous with the SER system and the Golgi apparatus. Of the 9 cases studied 3 pts are tumor free after 2 years of follow-up. Three others had a recurrence after 14 months, and the last 3 are tumor free so far, after 16 months of follow-up.

Discussion

The prognosis of human SBC depends not only on the make-up of the initial tumor but also on the status of the surrounding urothelium [3]. According to Hicks « preneoplastic » changes may be present in disparate sites of the urothelium of pts with SBC [4]. Jacob et al [5] support that the urothelium from non-involved areas of tumor-bearing pts reflects some aspects of the underlying epithelial disease and Soloway [6] has shown that the tumor recurrence may be the result of a « restless » urothelium. Therefore Koss's suggestion [7] that an ultrastructural investigation of the urothelium peripheral and/or away to visible tumors (non-involved urothelium) may contribute to promote our knowledge and may prove of prognostic value in the management of the human SBC, is of importance. The non-involved urothelium of our cases, before Interferon treatment showed several deviations from the normal. After therapy, we observed a gradual enlargement of the Golgi apparatus, which is considered a specialized structure marking the cellular differentiation and functional maturity of the cell [8]. In the superficial cells of the urothelium the Golgi apparatus is in addition the site of synthesis and a kind of « packaging station » of the AUM [7, 9], which is the ultimate manifestation of differenciation [7]. Thus the AUM is considered a marker of functional end stage of epithelial differentiation [7] and a marker of urothelial normality [10]. After treatment, although it was difficult to determine whether the AUM covered the entire urothelial surface, there was structural evidence indicating its existence at least in some samples. NB's are a common complement of the cell nuclei in both normal and pathological tissues [8]. They are a normal feature in human urothelium too [9]. A review of the literature indicates that cells stimulated by a variety of means, among others drug action and immunological stimulation, show an increase in numbers, size and complexity of the NB's [8]. More difficult to interpret was the appearance of centrioles and cilia after treatment. Several drugs have been implicated in centriologenesis and ciliogenesis, as well some special conditions i.e. cell dehydration [11] and alteration of the cell metabolism [12]. Thus, we may also assume that the presence of cilia and centrioles is the result of the alteration of the surface cells metabolism due to the effect of Interferon. Further examination demonstrated that Interferon induced the formation of TRI's in the superficial cells. These inclusions have not been previously reported. TRI's are well documented in cases of lupus, in human immunodeficiency infections and in T-cell leukemia [13]. Our pts had none of the coincidental pathological conditions associated with the occurrence of TRI's. TRI's are considered a useful ultrastructural marker for Interferon response evaluation although their biological significance remains obscure. Our cases are too few and the time of observation only 24 months, to draw any conclusions about the efficacy of Interferon to restore the ultrastructural morphology of the non-involved but initiated urothelium of tumor bearing pts to the normal stage. However we cannot but take notice of the documented facts presented and suppose with some degree of certainty that the pretreated urothelium does show deviations from the normal mainly described by Jost [9] and that Interferon treatment did to some degree reestablish some of its normal features.

References

1. Torti MF, Lum LB (1987) Superficial bladder cancer. Risk of recurrence and potential role for Interferon therapy. Cancer 59 : 613-616
2. Williams RD (1988) Intravesical Interferon-α in the treatement of superficial bladder cancer. Sem Oncol 15 (suppl 5) : 10-13
3. Koss LC (1975) Tumors of the urinary bladder In : Atlas of tumor pathology. Armed Forces Institute of Pathology, Washington, 2nd series, p. 11
4. Hicks RM (1977) Discussion of morphological markers of early neoplastic change in the urinary bladder. Cancer Res 37 : 2822-2823
5. Jacob J, Ludgate CM, Forde J, Selby Tulloch W (1978) Recent observations on the ultrastructure of human urothelium. I. Normal bladder of elderly subjects. Cell Tissue Res 193 : 543-560
6. Soloway MS (1970) Intravesical and systemic chemotherapy of murine bladder cancer. Cancer Res 30 : 1309-1313
7. Koss LG (1977) Some ultrastructural aspects of experimental and human carcinoma of the bladder. Cancer Res 37 : 2824-2835
8. Ghadially FN (1988) Ultrastructural pathology of the cell and matrix, 3rd ed. Butterworths, London Boston Singapore Sydney Toronto Wellington
9. Jost PS, Gosling AJ, Dixon JS (1989) The morphology of normal human bladder urothelium. J Anat 167 : 103-115
10. Hicks RM (1975) The mammalian urinary bladder : an accomodating organ. Biol Reviews 50 : 215-246
11. Hubert FJ, Flament-Durand, Dustin P (1974) Centrioles and cilia multiplication in the pituitary of the rat after furosemid and colchicine treatment. Cell Tiss Res 149 : 349-361
12. Stubblefield E, Brinkley BR (1967) Architecture and function of the mammalian centriole. In : Warren BK (ed) Formation and fate of cell organelles. Academic Press, New York, pp. 175-218
13. Szakacs GE, Kasnik G, Walling AK (1992) Soft tissue sarcoma with complex membranous and microtubular inclusions. Annals Clin Lab Sci 21 : 430-440

Abstract. The ultrastructural effect of Interferon α-2b (Intron-A) treatment of the non-involved urothelium of 9 male patients (pts) with new solitary superficial bladder cancer (SBC) grade I or II was investigated along with the clinical course. Adjuvant topical treatment with Interferon was started 6-9 days after total resection. At the end of 1 year of follow-up, when this ultrastructural study was performed, none had recurrence. We noted a partial restoration of the urothelium to its normal morphology as compared to our controls. It concerned the Golgi apparatus, a partial restoration of the Asymmetric Unit Membrane, (AUM) appearance of nuclear bodies (NB's), and the presence of Tubuloreticular Inclusions (TRI's) which are considered markers of Interferon treatment. These structures in the cytoplasm of urothelial cells by the action of exogenous Interferon, have not been previously reported. Of the 9 pts studied, 3 were tumor free after 2 years of follow-up. Three others presented a recurrence after 14 months and the last 3 are tumor free after 16 months of follow-up. The significance of the appearance of Interferon markers and the beneficial outcome of therapy is discussed. The prevention of tumor recurrence by restoring the ultrastructural morphology of the urothelium by Interferon is a subject worth of further investigation.

Chemo-radiotherapy in locally advanced bladder cancer : Neo-Adjuvant and definitive treatment

L Canobbio*, F Boccardo*, A Curotto**, M Pace*, D Guarneri*,
A Rubagotti*, M Venturini*, M Orsatti*, V Vitale*, M Schenone**,
M Cussoto**, C Pegoraro***, GB Traverso****, G Salvia*****,
G Martorana**, L Giuliani**

Actually the standard treatment for patients with invasive bladder cancer remains radical cystectomy [1]. Radical radiotherapy is usually only recommended by urologic surgeons for use in patients unsuitable for cystectomy [2]. However, despite of improved surgical and radiotherapeutic techniques, the 5-years survival rates, following radical surgery, radical radiotherapy or combinations of both, remain at about 50 % or less, and regardless of local control the majority of patients develop distant metastases [3, 4]. In view of this relatively low cure rate from conventional treatment of invasive bladder cancer, attempts have been made to develop innovative approaches to this problems. Based upon the high response rates with the use of systemic chemotherapy for metastatic disease, several trials have been initiated to assess the efficacy of chemotherapy as Neo-Adjuvant or definitive treatment in concurrent administration with radiotherapy [5, 6].

Several such treatment programs have been assessed in nonrandomized and randomized studies. From the available data preemptive and concurrent chemotherapy appears to be safe and yelds objective local response rates of approximately 50 to 70 % with an high rate of complete responses sustained beyond 1 to 2 years [7, 9]. Moreover, promising preliminary results have been obtained from the investigation of bladder-sparing approaches as the primary treatment of localized bladder carcinoma employing various chemo-radiotherapy combinations [10, 14]. In order to define more clearly the potential benefits of this approach, a randomized controlled trial has been initiated comparing radical cystectomy alone and cystectomy plus a Neo-Adjuvant treatment. Contemporary patients who were not elegible for cystectomy or that refused surgery were treated with an alternated chemo-radiotherapy with bladder sparing.

Patients and methods

Randomized study

From 1988 patients with infiltrating bladder cancer, stage T2-T4N0M0 were prospectively randomized to receive radical cystectomy alone or cystectomy and

---

* National Institute for Cancer Research, Genoa ; ** Dept of Urology, University of Genoa ; *** Dept of Urology, Mantova ; **** Dept of Urology, Genoa Sanpierdarena ; ***** Dept of Urology, Catania-Italy

a previous Neo-Adjuvant alternated chemo-radiotherapy. Chemotherapy consisted of 2 cycles of Cisplatin 20 mg/sqm and Fluorouracil 200 mg/sqm days 1-5 every 3 weeks. Radiotherapy at a daily dosage of 200 cGy for a total dose of 2,000 cGy was administered between the 2 cycles of chemotherapy. Radical cystectomy was performed within 3 weeks from the end of treatment. The major end-point of the study was death due to whatever cause. Times to death were measured from the date of randomization. Overall survival and progression free survival curves were drawn using the method of Kaplan and Meïer and compared by the log-rank test [15]. All « p » values were derived from a 2-sided test for significance [16]. During a 3 years of accrual 104 patients were recruited, 53 in the surgery alone arm (A) and 51 in the combined arm (B). The major features of patients are shown in Table 1.

Table 1. Patients characteristics

	Surgery (n = 53)	CT-RT/Surgery (n = 51)
Median age	62 (44-72)	64 (42-74)
PS = 0	79.3 %	80.3 %
Clinical T		
T2	47.2 %	51.0 %
T3a	30.2 %	25.5 %
T3b	18.9 %	15.7 %
T4	3.7 %	3.9 %
Unknown	—	3.9
Clinical N		
N0	86.8 %	88.2 %
N1	3.8 %	5.9 %
N2	7.5 %	—
Unknown	1.9 %	5.9 %
Grading		
G1	—	2.0 %
G2	20.8 %	23.5 %
G3	77.4 %	70.6 %
Gx	1.8 %	3.9 %
Neoplasia		
Single	75.5 %	68.6 %
Multiple	22.6 %	27.5 %
Unknown	1.9 %	3.9 %
Siez		
<3 cm	45.3 %	43.1 %
>3 cm	52.8 %	51.0 %
Unknown	1.9 %	5.9 %
TUR		
Complete	43.4 %	39.2 %
Incomplete	43.4 %	47.1 %
Not carried out	9.4 %	5.9 %
Unknown	3.8 %	7.8 %

Phase II study

Patients who refused cystectomy or that were not considered elegible for radical surgery, stage T1 (G3)-T4N0M0, were treated with an alternated chemo-radiotherapy definitive treatment. The first 18 patients received 4 cycles of the same regimen of chemotherapy described above during the weeks 1, 4, 7 and 10 alternated with radiotherapy. Fourty Gy were administered in 20 fractions during the weeks 2, 3, 8 and 9. A second group of 33 patients received 3 cycles of the 5 days regimen of chemotherapy with Cisplatin and Fluorouracil during the weeks 1, 4 and 7 and 50 Gy of radiotherapy administered in 20 fractions during the weeks 2, 3, 5, 6. The last 11 patients received the same treatment of the second group except the replacement of Fluorouracil with Methotrexate at the dose of 40 mg/sqm days 1 and 8. The major characteristics of these 62 patients are presented in Table 2.

Table 2. Characteristics of patients

N° of pts	62
M/F	57/5
Median age (range) yrs.	63 (44-76)
Median ECOG PS	0 (0-1)
T1	7 (11 %)
T2	29 (47 %)
T3	20 (32 %)
T4	6 (10 %)
N0	57 (92 %)
N1	5 (8 %)
G2	24 (39 %)
G3	38 (61 %)

Patients selection

Both studies included patients with histological evidence of localized bladder infiltrating cancer, ECOG performance status ⩽ 2, no previous chemo-and/or radiotherapy, no evidence of cardiopathies, jeopardized renal and hepatic functions and insufficient marrow reserve. The initial assessment included the patient's history, objective examination, complete blood count, serum creatinine, liver functions tests, electrolytes, urography, chest X-rays, abdominopelvic CT scan, staging bioptic TUR and bone scintigraphy. Patients receiving full chemotherapy-radiotherapy undergo repeat cystoscopy, tumor-site biopsy and urinary cytology, pelvic and abdominal CT scans every 3 months. Clinical and radiological examination for patients undergoing radical cystectomy were also every 3 months. Moreover at interval follow-up clinical evaluation, complete blood count, serum creatinine, liver function tests, electrolytes, chest X-ray and performance status were recorded.

Response criteria

Clinical urological evaluation of the response of the primary bladder tumor is categorized with the following criteria: complete response requires the absence of any endoscopically visible tumor, the absence of any tumor in the tumor-site biopsy specimen and a negative urine cytology specimen, while partial response requires a clinical tumor down staging. Patients with stable or progressive disease are considered non responders.

Results

Randomized study

The pathologic assessment after radical surgery showed a significant biologic activity of our chemo-radiotherapy Neo-Adjuvant treatment. The complete pathologic response is 27.5 % and 0 % of patients in the arm B and A respectively (Table 3).

Table 3. Results in 61 evaluable patients

	cCR (%)	cPR (%)	cNR (%)
T1	7/7 (100)	—	—
T2	28/29 (97)	1/29 (30)	—
T3	16/19 (84)	2/19 (11)	1/19 (5)
T4	4/6 (66.6)	—	2/6 (33.3)
Total	55/61 (90)	3/61 (5)	3/61 (5)

After a median follow-up of 24 months, in the surgery only arm 21/53 (39 %) patients are alive and disease free, 8/53 (15 %) had a local recurrence (6 alive and 2 dead), 18/53 (34 %) had a distant relapse (3 alive and 15 dead) and 1 (2 %) patient dead for unrelated causes. Five patients were lost to follow-up. The median survival of the surgery only group was 25.5 months and the median disease free survival was 16 months.

In the combined arm 28/51 (55 %) patients are alive and disease free, 5/51 (10 %) had a local recurrence (1 alive and 4 dead), 10/51 (20 %) had a distant relapse (1 alive and 9 dead) and 7/53 patients dead for unrelated causes. One patient was lost to follow-up. The median survival of the combined treatment group was 25.6 months and the median disease free survival was 16 months.

The 4 years overall survival is 44 % and 41 % (p = 0.5) and the disease free survival is 29 % and 28 % (p = 0.4) in the group B and A of patients respectively (Fig. 1 and 2).

If patients dead of unrelated causes without evidence of relapsing bladder cancer were censored, the cancer specific survival is 55 % and 43 % (p = 0.08) and the cancer specific disease free survival is 43 % and 30 % (p = 0.06)

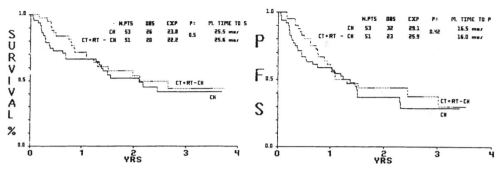

Fig. 1. Actuarial overall survival

Fig. 2. Actuarial progression free survival

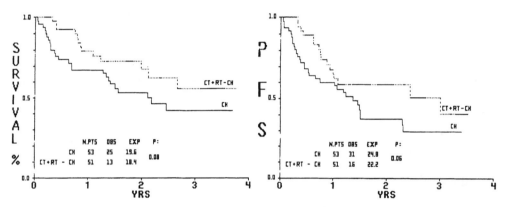

Fig. 3. Actuarial cancer specific survival

Fig. 4. Actuarial cancer specific progression free survival

in the combined treatment group and in the cystectomy only group respectively (Fig. 3 and 4).

The toxicity reported with the Neo-Adjuvant treatment was mild: nausea/vomiting G2-3 in 29 %, of patients, leukopenia G1-2 in 32 %, diarrhea G2 in 6.5 %, cystitis and proctitis in about 10 %.

Major intra-operative complication were present only in 5.6 % of patients randomized in the cystectomy alone arm, major postoperative complications were present in 17 % and 15.7 % of patients in arm A and B respectively.

Definitive chemo-radiotherapy

Sixty-one out of 62 entered patients were fully evaluable. One patient refused the treatment after the first week of chemotherapy. Of the 61 evaluable patients with a median follow-up of 25 months (range 8 to 65 months) 77 % are alive, 75 % have an intact bladder, 77 % have not had distant metastases, 69 % have a bladder remaining that has been continously free of tumor and 79 % have maintained the bladder either without a tumor or with a superficial recurrence. The 4 years overall survival and the disease free survival of all 62 patients by actuarial analysis was 76 % and 54 % respectively.

The local response of the primary bladder tumor by endoscopic re-evaluation, tumor-site biopsy and urinary cytology was evaluated at the end of the chemo-radiotherapy treatment. A cCR was observed in 55/61 patients (90 %), cPR in 3/61 patients (5 %) and a cNR in 3/61 (5 %). A cCR was achieved in 100 % of patients with T1 primary tumor, 97 % of patients with T2, 84 % with T3 and 66 % with T4.

Systemic side effects were mild : G1-G2 nausea and vomiting occurred in 57 % of patients, G1-G2 anemia in 35 %, G2-G3 leukopenia in 49 %, G3-G4 thrombocytopenia in 21 % and G3 stomatitis in 7 %. A moderate or severe local toxicity was reported in half of the patients. A severe cystitis, proctitis and diarrhea was observed in 21 %, 21 % and 7 % of patients respectively.

All the patients received the full radiotherapy planned dosage while 6 had a dose reduction of chemotherapy for haematological toxicity.

Discussion

Although conclusive results cannot be drawn from our randomized study for the low accrual of patients, some important aspects must be emphasized.

Although in our study a low accuracy of clinical stage has been observed, in fact only 30 % of patients were correctly evaluated while about 50 % of patients were understaged.

In spite of 43.4 % of TUR were considered complete by the surgeons, none patients were found stage P0 after radical cystectomy in the surgery only arm. This observation must suggest extreme caution in considering TUR the only efficient local therapy for infiltrating bladder cancer.

Our chemo-radiotherapy Neo-Adjuvant treatment has shown an high biological activity, 16/40 (40 %) patients has shown a pathological down staging and 11/40 (27.5 %) a pathological complete response. Our data are in the range of the results reported with Neo-Adjuvant treatments. Despite differences in case selection and treatment schedules the pCR range from 20 % to 40 % [17]. These data show that for the majority of patients the treatments employed are still inadequate to control disease within the bladder. These results give also an estimate of the proportion of patients for whom bladder preservation can be considered.

The high percentage of tumor regression reported and the better cancer specific survival warrants a further evaluation of Neo-Adjuvant treatments.

In our phase II study the chemo-radiotherapy definitive treatment employed has been quite well tolerated by most of this older and ill patients. The achievement of a local complete response and its maintenance is necessary in the treatment of patients treated with a bladder sparing approach. The role of transurethral resection in the bladder sparing approach must not be underestimated. Infact, though it could induce only few complete eradication of tumor, the minimal burden of tumor achieved could significantly help the local tumor control by the following cytotoxic treatment. In fact, the performance of a

TUR considered « complete » by the surgeons achieved a 2 years 71 % disease free survival while only 25 % of patients who had a TUR considered « incomplete » were disease free after 2 years. The results achieved in our group of patients treated with a definitive chemo-radiotherapy are well comparable with the results reported with other bladder-sparing approaches. Infact the results reported in the largest series treated with a sequential chemo-radiotherapy seems slightly worst than that observed in our group. Infact Prout et al observed a 3 year overall survival of 64 % and a 74 % cCR [18].

In conclusion our experience in the treatment of infiltrating bladder cancer shows that : 1) alternated chemo-radiotherapy is a safe treatment for infiltrating bladder cancer ; 2) Neo-Adjuvant treatment seems to improve the results achieved by cystectomy alone ; 3) although this comparison is not correct, our group of patients submitted to definitive treatment allowed bladder sparing and a better quality of life achieving also a better disease free survival and overall survival compared to patients treated with surgery in randomized study.

References

1. Raghavan D, Shipley WV, Garnick MB et al (1990) Biology and management of bladder cancer. N Engl J Med 332 : 1129-1138
2. Gospodarowich MK, Hawkins NV, Rawlings GA et al (1989) Radical radiotherapy for muscle invasive transitional cell carcinoma of the bladder. J Urol 142 : 1448-1450
3. Batata M, Whitmore WF, Chu C (1980) Patterns of recurrence in bladder cancer treated by irradiation and/or cystectomy. Int J Radiat Oncol Biol Phys 6 : 155-159
4. Skinner DG, Leiskovsky G (1984) Contemporary cystectomy with pelvic node dissection compared to preoperative radiation therapy plus cystectomy in management of invasive bladder cancer. J Urol 131 : 1069-1072
5. Sternberg CN, Yagoda A, Scher HI et al (1988) M-VAC (Methotrexate, Vinblastine, Doxorubicin and Cisplatin) for advanced transitional cell carcinoma of the urothelium. J Urol 139 : 461-469
6. Harker WG, Meyers FJ, Freiha FS et al (1985) Cisplatin, Methotrexate and Vinblastine (CMV) : an effective chemotherapy regimens for metastatic transitional cell carcinoma of the urinary tract : a Northern California Oncology Group study. J Clin Oncol 3 : 1463-1468
7. Raghavan D (1988) Preemptive (Neo-Adjuvant) intravenous chemotherapy for invasive bladder cancer. Br J Urol 61 : 1-4
8. Zincke H, Sen SE, Hahn RG et al (1988) : Neo-Adjuvant chemotherapy for locally advanced transitional cell carcinoma of the bladder : do local findings suggest a potential for salvage of the bladder ? Mayo Clin Proc 63 : 16-20
9. Scher HI, Yagoda A, Herr HW et al (1988) Neo-Adjuvant M-VAC (Methotrexate, Vinblastine, Doxorubicin and Cisplatin) effect on the primary bladder lesion. J Urol 139 : 470-474
10. Sauer R, Dunts J, Altendorf-Hofmann A et al (1990) Radiotherapy with and without Cisplatin in bladder cancer. Int J Radiat Oncol Biol Phys 19 : 687-691
11. Jakse G, Frommhold H, Nedden DZ (1985) Combined radiation and chemotherapy for locally advanced transitional cell carcinoma of the urinary bladder. Cancer 55 : 1659-1664
12. Rotman M, Macchia R, Silverstein M et al (1987) Treatment of advanced bladder carcinoma with irradiation and concomitant 5-Fluorouracil. Cancer 59 : 710-714

13. Waxman J, Barton C, Biruls R et al (1992) Bladder cancer : Inter-relationships between chemotherapy and radiotherapy. Br J Urol 69 : 151-155
14. Shipley WU, Kaufman SD, Prout GR (1988) The role of radiation therapy and chemotherapy in the treatment of invasive carcinoma of the urinary bladder. Sem Oncol 15 : 390-394
15. Kaplan EL, Meier P (1958) Non-parametric estimation from incomplete observations. J Am Stat Assoc 53 : 457-481
16. Mantel N (1966) Evaluation of survival data and two new rank order statistics arising in its consideration. Cancer Chem Rep 50 : 163-170
17. Scher HI (1990) Chemotherapy for invasive bladder cancer : Neo-Adjuvant versus adjuvant. Sem Oncol 17 : 555-565
18. Prout GR, Shipley WU, Kaufman DS et al (1990) Preliminary results in invasive bladder cancer with transurethral resection, Neo-Adjuvant chemotherapy and combined pelvic irradiation plus Cisplatin chemotherapy. J Urol 144 : 1128-1136

Interferon-α (IFN-α) combined with 5-Fluorouracil (5-FU) is an active regimen in metastatic renal cell cancer

A Sella, L Finn, R Amato, C Logothetis

Recurrent or metastatic renal cell cancer has a poor prognosis, with 96 % mortality at 3 years [1]. This poor outcome reflect the low response rate to systemic therapy [1, 2]. The theoretical basis for combining interferon-α (IFN-α) and chemotherapy for metastatic renal cell cancer is the *in vitro* synergism of IFN-α with a wide variety of cytotoxic agents [3]. In a pilot clinical trial, a 30 % response rate was noted in selected patients who failed initial IFN-α therapy with combination chemotherapy consisting of 5-Fluorouracil (5-FU), Doxorubicin, Mitomycin-C (MMC) and Cisplatin (FAMP) [4]. A phase III randomized study of INF-α administered sequentially with FAMP chemotherapy achieved only 12 % response rate in both groups [5]. We report here the results of a prospective trial of combined administration of IFN-α and 5-FU-based chemotherapy.

Materials and methods

Study design

The study population was divided into 2 groups : 1) patients with a prior nephrectomy and 2) patients who underwent angioinfarction of the primary tumor prior to therapy.

Treatment

Therapy was designed for the simultaneous delivery of IFN-α and the chemotherapy, with the intention of continuously exposing the patient to IFN-α and intermittent chemotherapy (Table 1). Therapy was adjusted for any grade 3-4 toxicity (WHO).

Table 1. Dose regimens for interferon-α-2α and chemotherapy

Agent				Dose level			
			Day	0	−1	−2	−3
Interferon-α*	(1×10^6 units/m²)	Daily		5	4	3	2	1
5-Fluorouracil	(mg/m²)		1-5	750	600	450	300
Mitomycine	(mg/m²)		1,2	5	4	3	2	2

* Interferon-α preceded chemotherapy by 5 days.
Chematherapy was given every 28 days.

Eligibility criteria

Only patients with histologically proven metastatic renal cell cancer were included in the study. Patients with sarcomatoid renal cell cancer were excluded [6]. Patients with brain metastases were eligible if the metastatic disease stabilized following radiation therapy or surgery and if the patient had not received steroids.

Response criteria

Response was classified according to WHO criteria. Duration of response was measured from the time of maximum response, until progression or surgical resection of residual tumor.

Patients

Between December 1988 and June 1990, 49 patients received IFN-α combined with 5-FU and MMC, while 20 patients were subsequently treated with INF-α and 5-FU only. The clinical characteristics of sex, age, and performance status were similar for both group of patients (Table 2).

Table 2. Comparison of patient characteristics

	IFN-α + 5-FU + MMC	IFN-α + 5-FU
Males	34 (69 %)	16 (80 %)
Females	15 (31 %)	4 (20 %)
Age (years)	57 (32-72)	54 (36-68)
Performance status	0-16 (33 %)	0-7 (35 %)
	1-27 (55 %)	1-10 (50 %)
	2-6 (12 %)	2-3 (15 %)
Metastatic sites		
Lung	39 (80 %)	14 (70 %)
Mediastinum	10 (20 %)	5 (25 %)
Lymph nodes	13 (27 %)	4 (20 %)
Soft tissue	18 (38 %)	5 (25 %)
Liver	11 (29 %)	2 (10 %)
Bone	11 (22 %)	4 (20 %)
Brain	4 (8 %)	1 (5 %)

Results

Response

Twenty-five patients (36 %, 95 % confidence interval, 24-48 %) demonstrated objective response, 4 of them (6 %) had complete response. A comparison of response rates for the 2 treatment groups revealed the same objective response rate (Table 3). Distribution of response according to metastatic sites is outlined in table 4. The outcome of the 29 patients who were treated following angioinfarction of the primary tumor (41 % objective response) was similar to the outcome of the 40 patients who had a relapse following nephrectomy (33 % objective response).

Within the INF-α, 5-FU and MMC group, the median response duration was 4.7 months (range, 2.0-12.0) and 3 patients (17 %) are still responding. The median response duration with IFN-α and 5-FU was 8.0 months (range, 1.1-13.7) with 1 patient (15 %) still maintaining his response. The median survival of all the patients was 13.0 months (range, 0.9-35.1), 12 patients are alive. The median survival duration of the patients treated with IFN-α 5-FU was 24.7 months (range, 2.7-35.1) v.s. 11.4 months (range, 0.9-28.5) for the patients treated with additional MMC (p = 0.001).

Nine patients underwent surgical resection of residual disease which rendered them in complete radiographic response. Their median survival was 28.5 months (range, 8.6-35.1). Five of them are alive, and 3 patients remain free of disease.

Table 3. Comparison of response rate

	IFN-α/5-FU/MMC	IFN-α/5-FU
Complete response	0	4 (20 %)
Partial response	19 (39 %)	3 (15 %)
Complete or partial response	19 (39 %)	7 (35 %)
Total number of patients	49	20

Table 4. Response rate by organ sites

Organs	IFN-α + 5-FU + MMC		IFN-α + 5-FU	
	Total number of patients	Complete or partial response	Total number of patients	Complete or partial response
Lung	39	20 (51 %)	14	5 (36 %)
Lymph nodes	13	6 (46 %)	4	2 (50 %)
Mediastinum	10	3 (30 %)	5	0
Liver	11	2 (18 %)	2	0
Bone	11	0	4	2 (50 %)
Soft tissue	18	0	5	0

Toxicity

With the IFN-α and 5-FU combined treatment there was significant less grade 3-4 trombocytopenia and neutropenia than with IFN-α, 5-FU and MMC (neutropenia, 83 % v.s. 25 % ; and thrombocytopenia, 49 % v.s. 0 % respectively). Non-hematologic toxicity was similar for both treatment groups and

Table 5. Grade 3-4 non-hematological toxicity

Toxicity	IFN-α/5-FU/MMC	IFN-α/5-FU
Stomatitis	18 %	31 %
Diarrhea	8 %	0
Liver	15 %	2 %
CNS	18 %	15 %

occurred significantly with the first treatments (Table 5). Three patients treated with IFN-α, 5-FU and MMC developed hemolytic uremic syndrome.

Discussion

Results of this trial suggest that renal cell cancer is responsive to IFN-α combined with 5-FU-based chemotherapy. This 36 % objective response rate is promising, as it was achieved in a population who reflect the natural history of untreated metastatic renal cell cancer [7]. In addition, responses were observed in sites such as the liver and lymph nodes, where IFN-α as a single agent has limited activity [1]. We suggest that the increased response rate compared with that from our previous trial [6] was due to the simultaneous delivery of the IFN-α and the chemotherapy, as was implied from the *in vitro* data [3].

Adjunctive nephrectomy or angioinfarction of the primary tumor does not prolong survival, nor does either procedure induce significant responses in patients with renal cell cancer [8]. The increased response rate achieved by various biological agents such as Interleukin-2, and IFN-α among patients who underwent prior nephrectomy raises the possibility that the primary tumor has a negative impact on the response to therapy [1, 2]. Thus, control of the primary tumor was accomplished in our patients without nephrectomy. Our study showed that debulking of the primary tumor was accomplished in our patients without nephrectomy. Our study showed that debulking of the primary tumor was not required to achieve response in the metastatic sites. However, because the study was not designed to evaluate the impact of angioinfarction on response to the therapy, its role requires further studies.

Nine patients underwent complete resection of the residual disease, suggesting that this modality can be integrated into the management of metastatic renal cell cancer. The potential benefit of combined treatment modalities in metastatic renal cell cancer is not defined, and requires prospective evaluation.

The toxicity spectrum of our treatment suggests that IFN-α and 5-FU are the most important components of the therapy, whereas MMC added toxicity without enhancing the activity of IFN-α and 5-FU. In an attempt to expand the efficacy of this combination, a trial of adding Interleukin-2 to this therapy is being conducted now.

References

1. Muss HB (1987) Interferon therapy for renal cell carcinoma. Sem Oncol 14 : 36-42
2. Fisher RI, Coltman CA Jr, Doroshow JH et al (1988) Metastatic renal cell cancer treated with Interleukin-2 and lymphokine-activated killer cells. A Phase II clinical trial. Ann Intern Med 108 : 518-23
3. Welander C, Morgan T, Homesley H et al (1985) Combined recombinant human Interferon-α-2 and cytotoxic agents studied in a clonogenic essay. Int J Cancer 35 : 721-9
4. Dexeus F, Logothetis C, Quesada J et al (1986) Potential increase in efficacy of chemotherapy after treatment of patients (PTS) with metastatic renal cell carcinoma (RCC) with Interferon (IFN). Proceedings ASCO 6 : 100
5. Dexeus F, Logothetis C, Sella A, Finn L (1989) Interferon alternating with chemotherapy for patients with metastatic renal cell carcinoma. Am J Clin Oncol 12 : 350-4
6. Sella A, Logothetis C, Ro J et al (1987) Sarcomatoid renal cell carcinoma. Cancer 60 : 1313-18
7. Dekernion J, Ramming K, Smith R (1978) The natural history of metastatic renal cell carcinoma : a computer analysis. J Urol 120 : 148-52
8. Montie J, Stewart B, Straffon R et al (1977) The role of adjunctive nephrectomy in patients with renal cell carcinoma. J Urol 117 : 272-5

Comparative efficacy of hormonal therapy used alone or in combination for treatment of prostatic carcinoma

W Mulloy

The current study was undertaken to evaluate the comparative efficacy of hormonal therapy used alone or in combination with an antiandrogen in palliative treatment of prostatic carcinoma. A lutenizing hormone releasing hormone (LHRH) agonist was injected into one group, while the other arm received this agent in combination with the antiandrogen, Flutamide. Progress was measured by comparison of tumor markers and serial studies of tumor size and metastatic lesions.

Many studies affirm the value of prostatic specific antigen (PSA) as a serologic marker for this entity, and strongly suggest its reliability for : 1) first line population screening, 2) prognostic indicator of tumor aggressiveness, and 3) detecting residual or recurrent disease following hormonal therapy. It is this third for which it was used in the current study, combined with other aucillary tests. These were : prostatic acid phosphatase (PAP) which has been shown to be useful in evaluating persistent disease ; neuron specific enolase (NSE), a marker present in many adenocarcinomas, including small cell lung cancer ; and human milk fat globulin (HMFG), found in this carcinoma as well as others in the body. It is therefore necessary to rule out other malignancies in the body to use them effectively.

Since PSA has emerged as the most valuable tool for this study, it is important to choose one assay format throughout the study. The PSA-EIA Hybrid-Tech Tandem-R method was used here, and has Food and Drug Administration (FDA) approval for this purpose. It is also noted that a frozen specimen is required for its determination, as well as for PAP, used concurrently with PAS.

The current study included patients with Stage D2 Carcinoma by the Whitmore system. This involved spread to pelvic lymph nodes and distant bone metastases. Those with a lesser classification or a concomitant malignancy from another source were excluded from the clinical trial. The TNM Class was : T4, tumor invaded adjacent structures ; N3, spread to lymph nodes more than 5 centimeters ; M2, distant metastases.

Pre-trial studies included : biopsy of primary tumor, pelvic CT scan, and bone scan to document metastases. Additionally, complete blood counts, lever function tests, and baseline serum level of tumor markers were determined. These were repeated at frequent intervals during the study : monthly for pelvic CT scans, every 3 months for bone scans, and at 2 or 3 month intervals for tumor markers. After careful screening and Karnofsky rating, subjects were randomized to 1 of 2 arms of the study. One group of 23 subjects received

---

Department of Medicine, Graduate Hospital, Philadelphia, PA, USA

a monthly injection of depot LHRH agonist alone, and no other medication except analgesics as required. The other 20 patients were given this medication in combination with the antiandrogen, Flutamide, in the amount of 750 milligrams daily in divided doses by mouth.

Results of these ongoing studies showed moderate regression of the primary tumor and surrounding lymph nodes. A computerized graph of these composite findings is presented here, showing some shrinkage of the lesions by the 2 treatment methods. There is no statistically significant difference noted in this graph of the results. Similarly, Technicium 99m phosphate bone scans demonstrated only moderate decrease in metastatic lesions, but again the 2 arms of the study were only slightly different in results.

There was more progress achieved in diminution of tumor markers, shown here for the LHRH agonist group. A mean level of 89 mg/ml was decreased by 7.8 % during the one year of this study. A slightly more significant reduction was effected in PAP, from 5 mg/ml maximum by a 16.2 % margin. The graph shows that the other 2 tumor markers, NSE and HMFG decreased somewhat more, but these are considered less important findings. The other arm of the study showed little variation from the one here presented. On the basis of these results it is concluded that subjects with Stage D2 carcinoma of the prostate can be treated with some effectiveness using monthly injections of LHRH agonist. The addition of the antiandrogen, Flutamide, does not measurably improve results of this single medication.

Etoposide in treatment of hormone refractory advanced carcinoma of the prostate

MD Firouz Daneshgari, E David Crawford, BA Susan A Majeski

Prostate cancer is the leading cause of cancer in US males, accounting for 22 % of all new cancers diagnosed. It is projected that 132,000 new cases will be diagnosed in the US during 1992. While localized prostate cancer can be cured with radical prostatectomy or radiation therapy, up to 2/3 of patients with this disease present in an advanced stage (Stage C or D) [1]. Since the pioneering work of Huggins and Hodges in 1940's [2], androgen deprivation remains the mainstay of management of advanced prostate carcinoma, orchiectomy, Diethylstilbestrol (DES), and analogues of Luteinizing Hormone Releasing Hormone (LHRH) have all been used to remove androgens of gonadal origin. The resultant modification of the biologic behaviour of this neoplasm has provided some of the most spectacular palliative treatment known for metastatic cancer. While newer methods of endocrine manipulations have been introduced to the therapeutic armamentarium, none of these methods have significantly changed the median progression free survival of 12-18 months and a median survival of 24-30 months.

Evidence of tumor progression mostly unaffected by subsequent hormonal manipulations develops in an almost predictable fashion following first-line treatment. The development of endocrine resistance in this disease is a much more definitive and irreversible phenomenon than in other endocrine dependent cancers, i.e ; breast. Development of hormone resistance tumor cells may be explained either by multi clones theory in which expansion of pre-existing androgen independent cells predominated the growth of the tumor or by mutation of previously sensitive tumor cell clones or, most likely, both [3, 4, 5, 6, 7]. These observations strongly support the need for continuing to focus vigorous efforts on the development of non-endocrine approaches.

Evaluation of response

In most solid tumors, response to chemotherapy is easily quantitated by measuring changes in tumor diameter clinically or radiographically. Using the conventional criteria in assessing response to treatment in prostate cancer, however is a difficult task to perform [8]. Because measurable disease in the lung, lymph nodes, and soft tissue is uncommon and bone remains the most common clinically apparent site of metastasis with osteoblastic bone lesions or mixed blastic and lytic lesions. The accurate measurement of these lesions are very difficult. Therefore this creates variability in defining criteria for patient eligibility and response criteria for clinical trials.

Division of Urology University of Colorado Health Sciences Center Denver, Colorado, USA

Quantitation of the primary prostatic tumor nodule, pain index, serum acid phosphatase, serum alkaline phosphatase and more recently measurement of serum prostatic specific (PSA) habe been suggested as objective parameters for assessment of response in patients with hormone refractory carcinoma of the prostate.

Use of single agents

Formation of the National Prostatic Cancer Project (NPCP) as a part of the Organ Site Program for Prostate Cancer, in 1973, marked the beginning of a new era of clinical trials for chemotherapy of the prostate cancer. Table 1 lists alphabetically the drugs that have been evaluated thus far [9].

Table 1. Single agents studied in prostatic cancer

AMSA	Esorubicin	MGBG	Nitrogen Mustard
AZQ	Estracyt	ME-CCNU	Prednimustine
BCNU	Etoposide	Melphalan	Procarbazine
Bisantrene	5-FU	Methotrexate	Spirogermanium
CCNU	GANO$_3$	Mitomycin-C	Streptozotocin
Cyclophosphamide	HMM	Mitoxantrone	Vinblastine
Cisplatin	Hydrea	Neocarcinostatin	Vincristine
Doxorubicin	Ifosfamide		Vindesine

Modified from Eisenberger M et al A (1985) re-evaluation of non-hormonal cytotoxic chemotherapy in the treatment of prostatic carcinoma. J Clin Oncol 3 : 827

Abbreviations : AMSA : Amsacrine ; AZQ : Aziridinyl Benzoquinone ; BCNU : Carmustine ; CCNU : Lomustine ; 5-FU : 5-fluorouracil ; GANO$_3$: Gallium Nitrate ; HMM : Hexamethylmelamine ; MGBG : Mitoguazone

However, a wide divergence in response rates reported with use of these drugs confirms the assessment problems alluded earlier.

Adjuvant chemotherapy and chemo-hormonal therapy

Tumor cell heterogenicity data [1, 6] has attracted attention to define the role of combination of hormonal ablation and chemotherapy in the treatment of prostatic carcinoma. Early data suggests that early combined therapy may be superior to treatment with either modality alone [10]. However the difference in antitumor activity of chemotherapeutic agents between human and prostate cancer and Dunning tumor model should be undertaken cautiously [11].

Following is the list of trials for combined chemo-hormonal therapy :

Coordinator	*Regimen*
NPCP	Diethylstibestrol (DES) or orchiectomy v.s.
	DES plus Cyclophosphamide versus
	Cyclophosphadice plus Estramustine Phosphate

NPCP   DES v.s. DES + Cyclophosphamide
or DES + Estramustine Phosphate

No response or survival differences were observed in either study [12, 13].
Southeastern Cancer DES v.s. DES + Cyclophosphamide.
Study Group.
No advantage for the combination arm was reported with this study [14].
Southwest Oncology Group Orchiectomy v.s. Orchiectomy + Cyclophosphamide + Doxorubicin.
Results of this study is not published yet.

Use of Etoposide in treatment of hormone refractory advanced prostate cancer

Etoposide is semisynthetic podophyllotoxin and has antineoplastic properties in man and in animals. In mammals, the primary mechanism of action is inhibition of DNA synthesis and DNA strand breakage. Etoposide has been shown effective in many human malignancies. Initially given as bolus intravenous dose, greater effectiveness has been achieved with a 5 days course of administration. It has also been shown effective in stopping growth od prostatic cancer in rats and in tissue culture. However, trials of intravenous Etoposide in humans have shown disappointing results. This may be due to long doubling time associated with adenocarcinoma of the prostate.

Recently, an oral form of Etoposide has become available. Orally administered Etoposide is similar in efficacy and toxicity to intravenous dosing [15]. There are no major differences in serum half-life, clearance, or volume of distribution between oral or intravenous routes. The fraction of orally administered drug absorbed is 52. The oral form allows for continuous dosing. Etoposide was administered at 25 mg/m^2/d and was well tolerated in a Phase I study. At higher doses, myelosuppppression was the dose limiting toxicity. Nadir counts were noted from days 21-28. At the University of Colorado Health Sciences Center, we have designed a study to evaluate the effectiveness of Etoposide on hormone refractory prostate cancer (Stage D3).

The objectives of the study are :
1. To determine the response rate and remission duration of hormone refractory adenocarcinoma of the prostate when treated with oral Etoposide.
2. To define the qualitative and quantitative toxicities of oral Etoposide administered in a Phase II study.

Patients eligibility criteria were as follows :
a. Previous treatement with hormonal ablation, i.e. ; orchiectomy, estrogens with evidence of castrate testosterone levels of LHRH agonist treatment.
b. Areas of measurable or evaluable disease.
c. Evidence of progession according to NPCP criteria after initiation of hormonal therapy.
d. Performance status of 2 or better by SWOG protocol.
e. Elevated PSA.

Restricted to the above criteria 18 patients were recruited to the study to receive 50 mg capsule Etoposide for 20 days every 28 days. The parameter for evaluation of response were :
1. Measurable/Evaluable metastasis (bone scan, CT scan).
2. Performance status.
3. Pain index.
4. PSA level.
5. Acid phosphatase.
6. Alkaline phosphatase.

The following table summarizes the most recent results of this study (also see Tables 2 and 3) :
Entered : 20.
Evaluated (received > 3 cycles) : 10.
Non-Evaluated (received < 3 cycles) : 10.
Maximum course today : 13.
On study : 2.

As of the day of this report, the following conclusions can be made :
I. We are too early in the study to conclude the advantages or disadvantages of use of Etoposide in the treatment of hormonal refractory carcinoma of the prostate.
II. With regard to evaluation parameters, the findings are :
a. Performance status : worsen in 5, no changes in 4, better in 1.
b. PSA : increased in 4, decreased in 6.
c. Pain index : worsen in 3, unchanged in 5, improved in 2.
d. Acid phasphatase : increase in 4, decreased in 3, unchanged in 3.
e. Alk Phosphatase : decreased in 6, increased in 3, unchanged in 1.

Table 2. Oral Etoposide in TX of hormone refractory CaP non-evaluable patients (< 3 cycles)

Name/age	Cycles	Reason off	Best response
CG/65	1	Spinal Com	Progression
WM/69	2	Thrombocytopenia	Progression
PB/75	2	↓ PS	Progression
SW/65	2	↓ PS, GI Tox.	Expired
TD/68	2	Changed M.D.	—
JA/63	2	↓ PS, RTx	Progression
WD/61	2	Ref. Neutropenia	Progression
LH/66	1	↑ Pain, Hip RTx	Progression
RB/55	2	Pain, ↓ PS	Progression
RaB/68	1	Ref. G.I. Tox	Expired

Table 3. Oral Etoposide in TX of hormone refractory CaP non-evaluable patients (> 3 cycles)

Name/age	Cycles	Reason off	Best response
GW/81	3	Bone Mets	Progression
JC/68	5	Rectal erosion	Expired
DR/78	3	Sepsis	Expired
AL/72	3	Bone Mets	Progression
CW/70	4	Ureteral Obs.	Stable
DL/75	6	PS,RTx	Stable
HH/78	10	↓ PS, ↑ Pain	Stable
RC/67	13	On study	Stable
JD/71	3	↑ Pain, ↓ PS	Progression
GG/67	10	On study	Stable

References

1. Sogani PC, Whitmore WF Jr (1987) Update in staging systems. In : Bruce AW, Trachtenberg J (eds). Springer-Verlag, New York, pp 107-115
2. Huggins C, Hodges CV (1941) Studies on prostatic cancer. I. The effect of Castration, of Estrogen and of Androgen injection on serum phosphatases in metastatic carcinoma of the prostate. Cancer Res 1 : 293-7
3. Isaacs JT et al (1982) Genetic instability coupled to clonal selection as a mechanism for tumor progression in the Dunning R-3327 rat prostatic adenocarcinoma system. Cancer Research 42 : 2353
4. Issacs JT et al (1979) Models for development of non-receptor methods for distinguishing androgen-sensitive and insensitive prostatic tumors. Cancer Research 39 : 2657
5. Isaacs JU, Coffey DS (1981) Adaptation versus selection on the mechanism responsible for the relapse of prostatic cancer to androgen ablation therapy studied in the Dunning R-3327-H adenocarcinoma. Cancer Research 41 : 5070
6. Isaacs JT et al (1986) Establishment and characterization of seven dunning rat prostatic cancer cell lines and their use in developing methods for predicting metastatic abilities of prostatic cancer. Prostate 9 : 261
7. Cunha GR et al (1987) The endocrinology and developmental biology of the prostate. Endocrine News 8 : 338
8. Yagoda A (1984) Response in prostate cancer : An enigma Semin Urol 1 : 311
9. Eisenberger MA (1990) Chemotherapy in prostate cancer. In : Crawford Ed, Das S (eds) Current genitourinary cancer surgery, p 509
10. Isaacs JT (1984) The timing of androgen ablation therapy and/or chemotherapy in the treatment of prostatic cancer. Prostate 5 : 1
11. Block NL, Canuzzi F, Denefrio J (1977) Chemotherapy of the transplantable adenocarcinoma (R-3327) of the Copenhagen rat. Oncology 34 : 110
12. Murphy GP, Beckley S, Brady DF et al (1983) and NPCP investigators. Treatment of newly diagnosed prostate cancer patients with chemotherapy agents in-combination with hormones versus hormones alone. Cancer 51 : 1264
13. Gibbons RP et al (1983) The addition of chemotherapy to hormonal therapy for treatment of patients with metastatic carcinoma of the prostate. J Surg Oncol 23 : 133

14. Moore M (1982) Chemohormonal therapy for stage D prostatic cancer. Preliminary results of a randomized trial. Proc ASCO, Abstract C-461
15. Hainsworth JD, Johnson DH, Frazier SR, Greco FA (1989) Chronic daily administration of oral Etoposide-A phase I trial. J Clin Oncol 7 : 396-401

Abstract. Hormone ablation remains the mainstay of management for advanced carcinoma of the prostate. Recurrent disease however, is invariably refractory to further hormone therapy. Thus, development of nonhormonal treatment for treatment of refractory disease is exceedingly needed. Interpretation of outcome results of newer treatments however, presents a challenge in assessing the effects of chemotherapeutic agents on refractory disease. In this article, we presented the interim findings on use of oral Etoposide in the treatment of hormone-refractory advanced carcinoma of the prostate. Twenty patient with hormone-refractory disease have entered into the study. Despite changes in PSA value, performance status and pain index, we concluded that it is too early in the study to interpret the advantages or disadvantages of this treatment modality. We will continue to recruit more patients for the study.

Sequential therapy with recombinant Interleukin-2 (rIL-2) and α-interferon (IFN) for advanced renal cell cancer (rcc) : a preliminary report

C Besana, E Bucci, A Borri, A Schoenheit, G Citterio, P Matteucci, S Tognella, C Baiocchi*, G Landonio*, E Ghislandi*, C Rugarli

Recombinant Interleukin-2 (rIL-2) and α-interferon (IFN) are both active as single agents in advanced renal cell cancer (rcc), with objective response rates around 15-20 % (Quesada, 1988 and Buzaid, 1989). The rationale for the combination, suggested by *in vitro* studies, is that α-IFN, enhancing the expression of tumour-associated antigens, could make tumour cells more susceptible to rIL-2 activated mononuclear cells. The combination of rIL-2 and α-IFN is currently being administered in various regimens, most of them based on the concurrent administration of both drugs (Rosenberg, 1989). We performed a phase II trial to test the clinical activity of sequential, rather than concurrent administration of rIL-2 and α-IFN, with the aim to reduce the risk of additional toxicity and to enhance the expression of mhc class I antigens on tumour cell surface and augmentation of specific recognition and lysis by rIL-2-activated effector cells.

Patients and methods

The original treatment schedule consisted of rIL-2 at a dose of 18×10^6 IU/m²/day be continuous intravenous infusion days 1-5 (120 hours), and α-IFN, at a flat dose of 9×10^6 U by subcutaneous or intramuscular injection thrice in a week, from day 8 to day 28 of each treatment cycle. Recombinant IL-2 was resumed on day 29. Treatment was planned for at least 3 cycles before performing evaluation of response, and was stated to be continued for 6-8 cycles depending on clinical response. Twelve patients, affected by histologically confirmed unresectable progressive or metastatic rcc, previously untreated with rIL-2, were initially treated. As severe toxicity, mainly cardiovascular, was experienced in this set of patients, subsequently 10 further patients were treated with half-dose rIL-2 (i.e. 9×10^6 IU/m²/day). During rIL-2 infusion, patients were hospitalized in a general medicine ward and were carefully monitored with regard to vital signs. Hypotension was managed by 20 % human albumin i.v. infusion and, when severe, with discontinuation of rIL-2 and institution of dopamine. α-INF was self-administered in a home-setting by the patients themselves.

Divisione di medicina II, Istituto scientifico ospedale S. Raffaele and *Divisione di oncologia medica « falck », Ospedale Niguarda, Ca'granda, Milano, Italy

Results

Of 22 enrolled patients (males : 16, females : 6 ; median age : 58, range 35-69), 16 (73 %) completed at least 1 cycle of treatment and were evaluated for response. Among excluded pts, 2 (9 %) experienced cardiac toxicity (ischaemia, SVPT) during rIL-2 infusion ; 1 patient (4 %) did not complete the first cycle for PT elongation > 3" over baseline and did not start the second cycle for early progression ; another patient (4 %) experienced severe thrombocytopenia (< 10,000/ml) after rIL-2 infusion : 2 pts (9 %) were not evaluable because of major protocol violation. We observed 6 major responses (1 complete response [cr] and 5 partial responses [pr]), for an objective response rate of 37 % (95 % CL 18-61 %). Five additional patients remained stable : 1 of them reached cr after surgical extirpation of a lung mass. Sites of response included lung, nodes, and bone. Duration of response is 11 + months for cr ; 17, 13 +, 11 +, 10 and 8 + months for prs. Stabilisation of disease lasted 20 +, 8, 6 and 4 months (surgically converted cr patient is not included). The complete responder patient, affected by lung metastates (tumor area : 4 sqcm), is still alive and disease-free. Of the 5 pr patients, 2 presented with bone metastases. In 1 case, the ischiopubic branch was involved requiring opioid therapy. After 3 courses of treatment, pain decreased until complete recovery and we observed partial recalcification on X-ray examination. In the other case, vertebral metastases with spinal chord compression were present. After 3 cycles we observed a partial regression of vertebral involvement with no evidence of spinal canal invasion. These 2 patients are still in pr and symptom-free. Two of the pts classified as sd achieved a reduction of tumour masse of about 30 %. One of them, affected by lung involvement (tumour area 5 sqcm) underwent surgical eradication after 10 months from the start of treatment. All the 5 non responder patients were affected by extensive disease at the start of treatment. Median follow-up is 14 Months. Estimated survival at 20 months is 51 %. Response was not significantly different between full-dose and half-dose rIL-2 regimen. Considering stable diseases as responses, there was a trend for a higher chance of response for patients with smaller tumour burden ($p = 0.065$, corrected chi-square).

Toxicity of rIL-2 treatment, mainly cardiovascular, was substantial : in 10 pts (45 %) treatment was interrupted due to severe toxic effects related to rIL-2. Five of the first 12 pts treated with full-dose rIL-2 went off protocol for cardiovascular toxicity (EKG signs of ischaemia, major arrhythmias, hypotension requiring pressors), and 2 other pts went off protocol for hematological toxicity (PTT elongation > 3" over baseline and severe thrombocytopenia). In view of such relevant toxicities, subsequent pts were treated with half-dose rIL-2 (9×10^6 IU/sqm/day). Again, 2/10 pts treated with this last regimen, went off protocol due to cardiac toxicity (EKG signs of ischaemia), and a third patient went off protocol due to severe exfoliative dermatitis requiring corticosteroids, that did not resolved after rIL-2 withdrawal. Another patient treated with half-dose rIL-2 experienced a CK elevation 1 month after first rIL-2 infusion. The patient was asymptomatic and there were no EKG signs ; however a myocardial radionuclide scan demonstrated a cardiac damage. Treatment was interrupted and we could not determine wether toxicity was specifically attributable to rIL-2 or α-rIFN. Complete resolution of the toxicity occurred in 7/10 pts, while in 2 pts cardiac abnormalities persisted after rIL-2 infusion withdrawal, even if asymptomatic.

Otherwise, treatment was well tolerated ; rIL-2 related toxicities promptly recovered after rIL-2 discontinuation and no treatment related deaths were reported. The half-dose rIL-2 regimen resulted significantly less toxic as far as concerned hypotension, fever, and oliguria ($p < 0.05$ Fisher's exact test, 2-sided). α-IFN was not related to major toxicities. Immunological studies showed a higher percentage of peripheral CD4+ bearing CD25 and CD29 cells during rebound lymphocytosis with the full-dose regimen, which was related even with a more relevant increase of CD56+ cells during infusion. With respect to an historical group of renal cell cancer patients treated with continuous infusion rIL-2 alone, the CD25+ cell subset seemed to have a more relevant increase.

Conclusions

The sequential administration of rIL-2 by continuous intravenous infusion and α-IFN by intramuscular or subcutaneous injection following this treatment schedule is feasible and active in renal cell cancer. In our series, response to treatment has seemed to be related to total amount of rIL-2 received. The analysis of the results obtained with the 2 rIL-2 dosages shows that the high-dose regimen is slightly more effective (4/12 major responses and 7/12 drops out for toxicity), while the half-dose regimen is less toxic (2/10 and 4/10 respectively). However, cardiovascular toxicity remains a major problem ; particularly, arrhythmias and ischaemic events are poorly predictable and preventable. Considering that toxic side effects frequently occur after 72 hours of rIL-2 infusion, our current trial is investigating feasibility and activity of a schedule in which rIL-2 infusion is shortened to 3 days.

References

1. Buzaid AC, Todd MB (1989) Therapeutic options in renal cell carcinoma. Sem Oncol 16 (suppl 1) : 12-19
2. Quesada JR (1988) Biologic response modifiers in the therapy of metastatic renal cell cancer. Sem Oncol 15 : 396-407
3. Rosenberg SA, Lotze MT, Yang JC et al (1989) Combination therapy with Interleukin-2 and α-Interferon for the treatment of patients with advanced cancer. J Clin Oncol 7 : 1863-1874

No advantage for the use of an early high-dose chemotherapy with autologous bone marrow transplantation in first-line treatment of poor risk non-seminomatous germ cell tumors

H Curé*, JP Droz**, JL Pico**, P Biron***, P Kerbrat****,
C Chevreau*****, JF Héron******, B Chevallier*******,
P Fargeot********, J Bouzy**, A Kramar**
and the Urologic Group of the French Cancer Centers Federation

The results of the treatment of non-seminomatous germ cell tumors (NSGCT) have been dramatically improved by Cisplatin-based chemotherapy regimens and selective indication of surgery. Approximately 80 % of all patients will enter in complete remission (CR) and 70 % will be cured [1].

Nevertheless about 10 % of patients in CR relapse and 30-40 % of patients with poor risk disease fail to respond to first-line treatment. Patients with NSGCT must be assigned to prognostic groups according to prognostic factors the most important of which are : the site of primary and metastatic disease, the tumor burden and the seric tumor marker levels. The 2 first classifications for the assignment of patients to the poor risk group were published by the Memorial Sloan Kettering Cancer [2] and by the Indiana University [3]. A prognostic model was developed at the Institut Gustave Roussy which was based on the seric human Chorionic Gonadotrophines (hCG) and α Fœto Protein (AFP) levels [4]. Patients with a probability to enter in CR less than 70 % were considered as poor prognosis patients.

In this poor risk patient group the major data from randomized trials on the result of treatment was provided by the Indiana University and the National Cancer Institute (NCI). At Indiana University, the combination of Bleomycin, Etoposide and Cisplatin (BEP regimen) was superior to a combination of Bleomycin, Vinblastine, Cisplatin (PVB regimen) [5]. On the other hand investigators at the NCI showed a higher cure rate with a regimen containing Etoposide and a double-dose Cisplatin (PVeBV) than a standard PVB regimen of chemotherapy [6]. Moreover, at the Institut Gustave-Roussy (IGR) high-dose chemotherapy (HDC) with autologous bone marrow transplantation (ABMT) was also tested and allowed to obtain long term non evolutive disease patients in the salvage setting [7] and the first-line treatment [8].

It was decided to conduct a randomized trial which compared the NCI regimen (PVeBV) to the original regimen developed at IGR with high-dose chemotherapy. This study was designed to recognize a 20 % improvement in the response rate.

* Centre Jean-Perrin, F 63011 Clermont-Ferrand Cedex 1 ; ** Institut Gustave-Roussy, F 94805 Villejuif Cedex ; *** Centre Léon-Bérard, F 69373 Lyon Cedex ; **** Centre Eugène-Marquis, F 35011 Rennes Cedex ; ***** Centre Claudius-Regaud, F 31052 Toulouse Cedex ; ****** Centre François-Baclesse, F 14021 Caen Cedex ; ******* Centre Georges-François Leclerc, F 21034 Dijon Cedex

Methods

Adult male patients with poor risk metastatic NSGCT were eligible randomization in a trial to study the role of early HDC + ABMT in first-line treatment. Twelve French cancer centers entered patients in this trial. The data management and the statistical analysis were performed in the Department of Biostatistics of the IGR. This trial was approved by an Ethics Committee ; the patients had to give oral informed consent.

The inclusion criteria were :
- untreated NSGCT of either testicular or extragonadal origin,
- at least 1 metastatic site,
- and poor prognosis according to the model developed at the IGR.

Patients were randomized to either Arm A, the standard treatment, or Arm B, the experimental treatment. Arm A (PVeBV) consisted of 3 or 4 cycles, repeated every 3 weeks, with Cisplatin : 40 mg/m^2/day (day 1 to day 5) + Vinblastine : 0.2 mg/kg (day 1) + Bleomycin : 30 mg i.v. bolus weekly + Etoposide : 100 mg/m^2/day (day 1 to day 5). Arm B consisted of 2 cycles of a slightly modified PVeBV regimen (Bleomycin in continuous infusion for 5 days and 4 week-interval between the 2 cycles) followed by the intensified chemotherapy whatever the response to the 2 first conventional cycles of chemotherapy was. High-dose regimen was a combination of Cisplatin : 40 mg/m^2/day (day 1 to day 5) + Etoposide : 350 mg/m^2/day (day 1 to day 5) + Cyclophosphamide : 1,600 mg/m^2/day (day 2 to day 5) with Mesna ($\approx$ PEC regimen). Bone marrow was reinfused at day 8.

In both Arms patients with residual disease and normal tumor markers at the end of the chemotherapy protocol were submitted to the surgical exeresis of the residual disease.

Results

Between January 1988 and June 1991, 115 patients (pts) were entered in this trial. Except 1 ineligible patient (because of good prognostic characteristics) all are evaluable for toxicity and efficacy (114 pts). There were 81 testicular, 18 mediastinal and 15 retroperitoneal primaries. The metastatic sites were : intrathoracic in 81 pts, lomboaortic nodes in 84 pts, liver in 17 pts, brain in 9 pts.

Seven pts in Arm A and 16 pts in Arm B failed to complete the planned treatment : 6 early deaths due to pulmonary failure related to bulky pulmonary involvement in Arm B and 3 toxic deaths, 5 treatment refusals, 4 progressive diseases, 5 contra-indications to treatment continuation in Arms A and B.

Efficacy

Thirty-three CR (58 %) in Arm A and 24 CR (42 %) in Arm B were observed.

There were 7 and 6 pts with PR and normal tumor marker in Arms A and B respectively. In Arm A there were 30 % failures and 47 % in Arm B. The difference is not statistically significant.

Relapses occurred in 4 pts in Arm A and 2 pts in Arm B. Fourty pts treated in Arm A and 33 pts in Arm B are continuously free of disease with a median follow-up of 30 months. The 2-years overall survival rate is 80 % and 60 % for Arms A and B respectively (not statistically significant in the log rank test, p = 0.08).

Toxicity

There was no major difference in the rate of Grade 4 leucopenia (77 % of the cycles), Grade 3-4 mucositis (20 % of the cycles) and in the occurrence of infections (40 % of the cycles) and renal dysfunction (creatinine > 150 μmole/l in 7 % of the cycles) between Arm A and the conventional chemotherapy of Arm B. Interestingly the rate of grade 1 or more neurotoxicity was 40 % in both arms. There were 5 toxic deaths (3 pts in Arm B and 2 in Arm B).

The toxicity of the intensive PEC regimen was : mean duration of aplasia of 16 days, fever 100 %, Grade 3-4 mucositis 55 %, renal dysfunction 7 %. There was no toxic death.

Conclusion

The results of this trial are consistant with the published results of the NCI (PVeBV regimen) on the one hand [6], and with the results of the former phase II trial at the IGR on the other hand [7, 8].

However this trial shows that early intensified chemotherapy fails to induce a higher complete remission rate and a higher 2-year overall survival rate than chemotherapy without early intensification.

We conclude that HDC + ABMT protocol is not indicated in the first-line treatment of poor risk nonseminomatous germ cell tumors.

References

1. Einhorn LH (1990) Testicular cancer : a new and improved model. J Clin Oncol 8 : 1777-1781
2. Bosl GJ, Geller NL, Cirrincione C et al (1983) Multivariate analysis of prognostic variables in patients with metastatic testicular cancer. Cancer Res 43 : 3403-3407
3. Birch R, Williams S, Cone A et al (1986) Prognostic factors for favorable outcome in disseminated germ cell tumors. J Clin Oncol 4 : 400-407
4. Droz JP, Kramar A, Ghosn M et al (1988) Prognostic factors in advanced non-seminomatous testicular cancer. A multivariate logistic regression analysis. Cancer 62 : 564-568

5. Williams SD, Birch R, Einhorn LH et al (1987) Treatment of disseminated germ-cell tumors with Cisplatin, Bleomycin and either Vinblastine or Etoposide. N Engl J Med 316 : 1435-1440
6. Ozols RF, Ihde DC, Linehan WM et al (1988) A randomized trial of standard chemotherapy v a high-dose chemotherapy regimen in the treatment of poor prognosis non-seminomatous germ cell tumors. J Clin Oncol 6 : 1031-1040
7. Droz JP, Pico JL, Ghosn M et al (1991) Long-term survivors after salvage high-dose chemotherapy with bone marrow rescue in refractory germ cell cancer. Eur J Cancer 27 : 831-835
8. Droz JP, Pico JL, Ghosn M et al (1992) A phase II trial of early intensive chemotherapy with autologous bone marrow transplantation in the treatment of poor prognosis non-seminomatous germ cell tumors. Bull Cancer 79 : 497-507

Bone and soft tissue sarcomas

Initial experience with autologous transplantation of 7 days non-cryopreserved peripheral blood stem cells, mobilized with G-CSF, in rhabdomyosarcoma

P Sobrevilla-Calvo, E Reynoso-Gomez, J de la Garza-Salazar

Advanced soft tissue sarcomas in adults are considered as non curable tumours with standard dose chemotherapy. Response to alkylating agents is at least partially dependent on the dose level. To reach the best dose intensity, myelosuppression must be minimized. This can be done by autotransplantation of bone marrow or peripheral blood stem cells (PBSC) with or without colony stimulating factors (CSF) [1]. Most transplants centers cryopreserve the stem cells [1]. Cryopreservation entails the use of an expensive equipment, not widely available and a mild, but significant toxicity due to the DMSO used to cryoprotect the cells. There has been a few reports of autotransplantation with non-cryopreserved bone marrow, stored for 1 or 2 days [2, 3]. We report our initial experience with a simple method of hematopoietic support with PBSC stored at 4° C for 7 days.

Method

PBSC were mobilized with G-CSF (Filgrastim, Hoffman La Roche Laboratories) 5 µg/kg/day subcutaneous on days −11 to −6, the PBSC were harvested in a Fenwall 3,000 machine on days −7, −6 and −5. We processed 7 litres of blood at a flow rate of 50 ml/min. The PBSC collected, without further manipulation, were stored at 4° C in a blood bank refrigerator. Chemotherapy was given on days −4, −3 and −2. On day 0, 1 unit and on day 1, 2 units of PBSC were reinfused rapidly. G-CSF was given again at the same dose from day 0 and until the absolute neutrophil count was $> 1,000/\mu l$. We counted the number of mononuclear cells/kg, the number of CD34+ cells/kg and determined the cell viability with the trypan blue method. This variables were measured just after the apheresis and at the time of reinfusion, 7 days after the PBSC collection.

Case report

A 28 years old female presented with a large pelvic mass in March 1992. An alveolar rhabdomyosarcoma was diagnosed with an open biopsy. After and incomplete surgical resection, she received 3 cycles of standard dose Doxorubicin, Dacarbazine and Ifosfamide, because of the known poor prognosis in this disease, we decided to consolidate the treatment with 3 cycles of high-dose chemo-

---

Instituto Nacional de Cancerologia de Mexico, Ave. San Fernando 22, Tlalpan, Mexico, D.F. Mexico 14000

therapy; on June 1st, 1992 she received 14 g/m² of Ifosfamide and on June 29, 16 g/m² of Ifosfamide + Doxorubicin 70 mg/m². A new CT scan showed a complete response, that was surgically confirmed. This good response was consolidated with a third course of Ifosfamide 14 g/m² on September and on December 92, with 50 Gy to the pelvis. There is no evidence of disease up to the present time.

Results

Table 1 summarizes the number of mononuclear and CD34+ cells harvested just after each apheresis and after 7 days of 4° C storage. Table 2, the total number of mononuclear and CD34+ cells infused after each cycle of chemotherapy.

The number of days with an absolute neutrophil count was 0 on cycle 1, 4 on cycle 2 and 2 on cycle 3. A platelet count of 14,000/μl was observed after cycle 2, but without bleeding signs and no platelet transfusion was given. The number of days on G-CSF was 10 for the first and second cycles and 7 for the third. The patient had, on the 3 cycles, nausea and vomiting grade II (WHO) despite the use of ondansetron. We observed mucositis grade I after the first cycle and grade III on the second.

Table 1. Mean cells collected per apheresis

Day	Mononuclear cells ×10⁸/kg immediate	7 days	CD34+ cells ×10⁶/kg immediate	7 days	V* %
1	1.3	1.2	9.4	7.5	66.6
2	1.4	1.0	8.9	22.6	74.3
3	0.9	0.9	12.3	9.3	68.6

* Cell viability at 7 days.

Table 2. Cells infused per cycle of high dose chemotherapy

Cycle No	Mononuclear cells ×10⁸/kg Immediate	7 days	CD34+ ×106/kg Immediate	7 days
1	4.1	3.0	30.2	45.2
2	3.1	2.4	26.7	23.7
3	4.0	4.2	34.8	49.4

Discussion

It is accepted that, if high-dose chemotherapy is followed by the infusion of cryopreserved PBSC, there is a complete reconstitution of the bone marrow [4], but if there is no stimulation of the hematopoiesis with G or GM CSF, the neutropenic period lasts for 20 to 30 days [5]. The collection of PBSC without any previous stimulation requires several apheresis procedures [4]. Our method uses the ability of the G-CSF to mobilize the stem cells [3, 5], this allowed us to harvest enough stem cells in just 3 apheresis procedures, resulting in a higher number of mononuclear cells collected than the usually reported with direct bone marrow aspiration (2.4×10^8/kg) [4]. In developping countries facilities for cryopreservation are scarce and this has been a limitation for the wider use of high-dose chemotherapy. There have been reports of autotransplantation with noncryopreserved marrow for periods of 1 or 2 days, in this report after 7 days, the number of cells, the number of CD34+ cells and the cell viability is practically the same as in the immediate sample and compares favourably with the number of cryopreserved PBSC reported by others [5]. Also with this method the neutropenic period is short and compares favorably with the achieved with cryopreserved bone marrow. These observations suggest that the combination of non-cryopreserved PBSC and G-CSF is an effective method to attenuate the myelotoxicity that follows high-dose chemotherapy. It might be possible that these results could have been obtained with the support of only G-CSF, but other reports mention that if CSF's are used by themselves the neutropenic period is still too long and the mortality is high [8], since the most important factor in predicting a toxic death is the number of days with severe neutropenia. Since this report was submitted, we have put into practice the method described in other 3 cases, with the following diagnosis : Hodgkin's disease, soft tissue sarcoma and lymphoma. The chemotherapy regimen used in each cycle was : Ifosfamide 6-10 g/m^2, Etoposide 1.8-2.2 g/m^2 and Carboplatin 1.2-1.5 g/m^2, the neutropenic period lasted between 9 and 12 days. Although these satisfactory results should be seen as preliminary, it has encouraged us to continue accruing patients in a pilot study.

References

1. Goldstone AH (1990) Autologous bone marrow transplantation in solid tumours. Curr Opin Oncol 2 : 269-276
2. Carella AM, Santini G, Giordano D et al (1984) High-dose chemotherapy and non-frozen autologous bone marrow transplantation in relapsed advanced lymphoma or those resistant to conventional chemotherapy. Cancer 54 : 2836-2839
3. Carey PJ, Proctor SJ, Taylor P et al (1991) Autologous bone marrow transplantation for high grade-lymphoid malignancy using melphalan/irradiation conditioning without marrow purging or cryopreservation. Blood 77 : 1593-1598
4. Kessinger A, Armitage JO, Landmark JD, Smith DM, Weisenburger DD (1988) Autologous Peripheral hematopoietic stem cell transplantation restores hematopoietic function following marrow ablative therapy. Blood 71 : 723-727
5. Taylor KM, Jagannath S, Spitzer G et al (1989) Recombinant human granulocyte colony-stimulating factor hastens granulocyte recovery after high-dose chemotherapy and autologous bone marrow transplantation in Hodgkin's disease. J Clin Oncol 7 : 179-199
6. Gianni AM, Bregni M, Stern AK et al (1989) Granulocyte-macrophage colony-stimulating factor to harvest circulating hematopoietic stem cells for autotransplantation. Lancet ii : 580-584

7. Molineux G, Pojda Z, Hampson IN, Lord BI, Dexter TM (1990) Transplantation potential of peripheral blood stem cells induced by granulocyte colony-stimulating factor. Blood 76 : 2153-2158
8. Shea TC, Mason JR, Storniolo AM, Newton B, Breslin M et al (1992) Sequential cycles of high-dose Carboplatin administered with recombinant human granulocyte-macrophage colony — stimulating factor and repeated infusions of autologous peripheral blood progenitors cells : A novel and effective method for delivering multiple courses of dose-intensive therapy. J Clin Oncol 10 : 464-473

High-dose chemotherapy with granulocyte colony-stimulating factor in advanced and/or metastatic soft tissue sarcomas

S Toma*,**, R Palumbo*, U Folco***, G Canavese*, E Aitini****, E Cantoni*****, M Vincenti*, R Rosso*

It is well known that the treatment of patients with locally advanced and/or metastatic soft tissue sarcomas is in most cases merely palliative, remaining overall survival very poor [1]. As in other advanced tumors, several clinical-biologic parameters have been tested as possible prognostic factors in the outcome of disease [2, 3, 4, 5]. At today, it is not yet known if the type of clinical response to chemotherapy could modify prognosis in these patients, but is general opinion that the achievement of an objective response (expecially complete response) may be, also in advanced and/or metastatic stage, an important factor for survival. With regard to soft tissue sarcomas, a dose-response relationship is suggested for Doxorubicin [6, 7] or his analogue Epidoxorubicin [8, 9], although with an increased cardiotoxicity. Similarly, in a review performed on the efficacy of Ifosfamide (a new effective drug more recently introduced in the management of sarcoma patients) combined with anthracyclines, the highest percentage of responses were reported in studies using the higher doses of Doxorubicin or Epidoxorubicin [10]. On the other hand, an increase of the administered dose of chemotherapy has been demonstrated effective in enhance the response in different tumours, also in advanced or metastatic stage [11]. However, in all reported experiences, the major limiting factor for dose escalation is the increasing in overall toxicity, both cardiac and haematologic. About this, the use of Epidoxorubicin consents the administration of higher doses, having shown a cytotoxic potential similar to Doxorubicin while producing significantly less cardiac and myelosuppressive effects [12] ; cardiotoxicity is also clearly reduced when Doxorubicin is administered by continuous infusion [13]. If it is true, as appears to be the case, that dose and dose-intensity of administered drug may increase the probability of successful therapy, the knowledge of possible prognostic factors predicting the response to chemotherapy, could allow a better selection of patients who can benefit from the treatment and, eventually, to have a longer survival. Based on this consideration, we began a phase II study, performed on patients with locally advanced and/or metastatic soft tissue sarcomas, all treated with the same chemotherapeutic scheduling : Ifosfamide (at fixed dose of 6 g/m^2/cycle) plus Epidoxorubicin at escalating doses, starting from 50 mg/m^2/cycle ; cycles were repeated every 3 weeks. The aims of the analysis which we are reporting were, first of all, to verify if the dose and dose-intensity of delivered chemotherapy may enhance

---

* Istituto Nazionale per la Ricerca sul Cancro-IST, Genova, Italia : ** Istituto di Oncologia Clinica e Sperimentale, Università di Genova, Italia ; *** Osp. S. Corona, Pietra Ligure, (SV), Italia ; **** Divisione di Oncologia Medica, Ospedale di Mantova, Italia ; ***** Divisione di Chirurgia Maxillo-Facciale — Università di Modena, Italia

the probability of objective response. Next, we attempt to improve the effectiveness of the treatment, using granulocyte colony-stimulating factor, which was demonstrated to permit the safer administration of higher or more frequent doses of chemotherapy, through an enhanced myeloprotection [14].

Finally, we wished to identify possible prognostic factors predicting the response to chemotherapy and affecting survival. A multivariate analysis, performed on the first 45 consecutive patients [15], showed that high-dose-intensity of Epidoxorubicin was positively correlated with the probability of response : objective responses were 16.7 % (2/12) in patients treated with doses of 50-65 mg/m^2, 35.3 % (6/17) for doses of 70-80 mg/m^2 and 56.2 % (9/16) for doses of 85-100 mg/m^2 (p = 0.04). The overall response rate was 38 % (17/45), reaching 44 % (17/39) in previously untreated patients. The overall survival time was found positively correlated with the achievement of objective response : 10 months for all evaluable patients versus 21 months in complete or partial responders (p < 0.01). In non responder patients the median survival was of 9 months. Treatment resulted effective and generally well tolerated. On the base of these results, we treated the following patients at doses progressively increasing of Epidoxorubicin, from 100 to 120 mg/m^2/cycle ; we added G-CSF (200 mg/Kg/day, subcutaneously, from day 8 to day 13) and a cardioprotector in the treatment scheduling (we used ICRF-187, at dose of 1,000 mg/m^2/cycle, e.v. infusion, 30 minutes before the Epidoxorubicin administration). For uroprophylaxis, we continued in using Mesna, which even in our previous experience has been proven effective in prevening or reducing the haemorragic cystitis induced by Ifosfamide [8]. In terms of effectiveness, the results of present study confirm our previous data [15] ; overall response rate was 37 % (24/53), with 7 complete (11 %) and 17 (26 %) partial responses ; specifically, we found that the higher percentage of objective responses was achieved in patients treated with the higher dose of Epidoxorubicin (objective response rate of 53.3 % for median dose-intensity of 34.5 mg/m^2/week). The treatment resulted feasible and toxicity generally acceptable ; especially, no case of evident carditoxicity occurred, neither in patients treated at the higher doses of Epidoxorubicin. The use of growth factors has been demonstrated effective in enhancing myeloprotection and permitting dose-intensification of chemotherapy in patients affected with sarcomas [16, 17]. In our experience, the use of granulocyte colony-stimulating factor was found effective in reducing the duration rather than the intensity of leucocyte-nadir, taking into account the cumulative thrombocytopenia, especially occurring with the higher doses of anthracycline. However, haematological toxicity was reversible in all cases. In conclusion, we think that a combined regimen with Ifosfamide plus Epidoxorubicin at doses ranging from 100 to 120 mg/m^2/cycle is feasible and effective in patients with advanced and/or metastatic soft tissue sarcomas. At present time, we are attempting to increase the Ifosfamide dosage, using different administration modalities, such as continuous infusion and new more effective uroprotectants. In addition, a multivariate analysis is ongoing, to verify and confirm the importance of dose-intensity of Epidoxorubicin for predicting clinical response to chemotherapy and outcome in these patients.

References

1. Elias AD, Antman KH (1989) Treatment of advanced sarcomas. Adv Oncol 5 (4) : 11-18
2. Fielding LP, Fenoglio-Preiser CM, Freedman S (1992) The future of prognostic factors in outcome prediction for patients with cancer. Cancer 70 : 2367-2377
3. Leyrez S, Costa J (1989) Issues in the pathology of sarcomas of the soft tissue and bone. Sem Oncol 16 : 263-280
4. Ueda J, Aozasa K, Tsujimoto M, Ohsawa M, Uchida A, Aoki Y, Ono K, Matsumoto K (1989) Prognostic significance of Ki-67 reactivity in Soft Tissue Sarcomas. Cancer 63 : 1607-1611
5. Alvergard AT, Berg NO, Baldetorp B, Ferni M, Killander D, Ranstam J, Rydholm A, Akerman M (1990) Cellular DNA content and prognosis of high-grade soft tissue sarcoma : The Scandinavian Sarcoma Group experience. J Clin Oncol 8 : 538-547
6. Schoenfeld D, Rosenbaum C, Horton J, Wolter JM, Falkson G, De Conti RC (1982) A comparison of Adriamycin versus Vincristine and Adriamycin, and Cyclophosphamide versus Vincristine, Actinomycin-D and Cyclophosphamide for advanced sarcoma. Cancer 50 : 2757-2762
7. Pinedo HM, Bramwell VH, Mouridsen HT, Somers R, Vendrik CP, Santoro A, Buesa J, Wagener T, Oosterom AT van, Unnik JA van (1984) CYVADIC in advanced soft tissue sarcoma : a randomized study comparing two schedules. A study of the EORTC Soft Tissue Sarcoma Group. Cancer 53 : 1825-1832
8. Toma S, Coialbu T, Biassoni L, Folco U, Gatti C, Canavese G, Giacchero A, Rosso R (1990) Epidoxorubicin plus Ifosfamide in advanced and/or metastatic soft tissue sarcomas. Cancer Chemother Pharmacol 26 : 453-456
9. Elli A, Hernandez Moran JC, Pasccon G, Negro A, Litowska S, Mendez A, Barg S, Santos R, Koliren L, Morgenfeld E, Goldfarb A, Rivarola E, Marantz A, Gercovich F (1991) Ifosfamide (Ifo), 4-Epidoxorubicin (4 Epi) chemotherapy (CT) for advanced soft tissue sarcomas (STS). Proc Ann Meet Am Soc Clin Oncol 10 : A1246
10. Toma S, Palumbo R, Sogno G, Venturino A, Santi L (1992) Doxorubicin (or Epidoxorubicin) combined with Ifosfamide in the treatment of adult soft tissue sarcomas. Ann Oncol 3 (suppl 2) : S119-S123
11. Bronchud MH, Hoxell A, Crowther D, Hopwood P, Souza L, Dexter TM (1989) The use of granulocyte colony-stimulating factor to increase the intensity of treatment with Doxorubicin in patients with advanced breast and ovarian cancer. Br J Cancer 60 : 121-125
12. Mouridsen HT, Bastholt L, Somers R, Santoro A, Bramwell V, Mulder JH, Oosterom AT van, Buesa J, Pinedo HM, Thomas D (1987) Adryamicin versus Epirubicin in advanced soft tissue sarcomas. A randomized phase II/phase III study of the EORTC Soft Tissue and Bone Sarcoma Group. Eur J Cancer Clin Oncol 23 : 1477-1483
13. Allen A (1992) The cardiotoxicity of chemotherapeutic drugs. Sem Oncol 19 : 529-542
14. Antman KA, Griffin JD, Elias A, Socinski MA, Tyan L, Cannistra SA, Oette D, Whitlev M, Frei E, Schnipper LE (1988) Effect of recombinant human granulocyte-macrophage colony-stimulating factor on chemotherpy-induced myelosuppression. N Engl J Med 319 : 593-598
15. Toma S, Palumbo R, Canavese G, Albanese E, Cantoni E, Barisone A, Reggiardo G, Rosso R, Santi L (1993) Ifosfamide plus Epirubicin at escalating doses

in the treatment of locally advanced and/or metastatic sarcomas. Cancer Chemother Pharmacol, in press
16. Steward WP, Verweij J, Somers R, Blackledge G, Clavel M, Van Oosterom AT, Greifenberg B, Soedirman J, Thomas D, Van Glabbeke M (1991) Doxorubicin plus Ifosfamide with rhGM-CSF in the treatment of advanced adult soft-tissue sarcomas : preliminary results of a phase II study from the EORTC Soft-Tissue and Bone Sarcoma Group. J Cancer Res Clin Oncol 117 (suppl 4) : S193-197
17. Vadhan-Raj S, Broxmeyer HE, Hittelman Wl, Papadopoulos NE, Chawla SP, Fenoglio C, Cooper S, Buescher ES, Frenck RW, Holian A, Perkins RC, Scheule RK, Gutterman JU, Salem P, Benjamin S (1992) Abrogating chemotherapy-induced myelosuppression by recombinant granulocyte-macrophage colony-stimulating factor in patients with sarcoma : protection at the progenitor cell level. J Clin Oncol 10 : 1266-1277

Treatment of osteosarcoma with Cisplatin and Doxorubicin either as Adjuvant or Neo-Adjuvant chemotherapy

JW Zinser, N Castañeda, A Alfeirán, E Maafs, M Durán, G Flores, R Gaona, L Vicencio

Improved survival in osteosarcoma patients treated with Adjuvant chemotherapy was reported since the early 70s [1, 2]. However it was strongly disputed [3] and it was not until the 80s, after the results of randomized clinical trials [4, 5] that Adjuvant chemotherapy became widely accepted. As chemotherapy has improved the cure rate, further steps have been taken in the management of these patients, such as limb-salvage surgery with preoperative chemotherapy [6]. Up to 100 % necrosis can be found in the surgical specimen and for such patients, disease free survival is significantly longer than for those with an initial poor response to chemotherapy [7, 8]. Nevertheless, it has not been demonstrated that Neo-Adjuvant chemotherapy has a survival advantage over adjuvant treated patients. Various active agents have been utilized but there is not a standard regimen [1, 2, 4-8]. Among the combinations utilized, systemic Doxorubicin and intra-arterial Cisplatin have yielded a 76 % 3-year disease-free survival [8]. At our institution in 1988 we began utilizing i.v. adjuvant Doxorubicin and Cisplatin and in 1989 conservative surgery.

Patients and methods

Chemotherapy : Cisplatin 100-120 mg/m^2 i.v. on day 1 over 4 hours with forced mannitol diuresis and Doxorubicin 80-90 mg/m^2 i.v. by continuous infusion over 72 hours, starting on day 1. Courses every 3 weeks for a total of 6 courses. On Neo-Adjuvant patients, 3 courses before surgery, and for those patients whose prosthesis were not ready, chemotherapy was continued until the patient was operated. After surgery patients continued with the same drugs to complete 6 courses and 3 patients also received Methotrexate. All patients had CT scan of the chest if the chest X-ray was negative for metastasis. CT scan of the primary tumor was performed in all patients considered to be candidates for limb-salvage surgery. The grade of necrosis of the surgical specimen was reported as 90-100 %, 60-80 %, and < 60 %.

Instituto Nacional de Cancerología, San Fernando 22, Tlalpan México, D.F. 14000 México

Results

Between 01/88-08/91, 21 patients were treated, 13 males and 8 females. Median age : 18 years (13-32). Location of the primary : Femur 12, tibia 4, humerus 2, fibula 1, iliac 1 and phalanx 1. Radiographic findings : Blastic 12, lytic 3 and mixed 6 patients. Periosteal reaction 18 and 1 fracture. Histology : Osteoblastic 13, fibroblastic 2, condroblastic 2, telangiectatic 2 and periosteal 2 patients. Symptoms before diagnosis : Median duration of tumor 3 months (0-10), median duration of pain 3 months (0-7).

Treatment : Adjuvant chemotherapy 8 patients, Neo-Adjuvant chemotherapy 13 patients. Conservative surgery : 8 patients. Courses administered : A median of 6 (4-9). Dose intensity : Median dose of Cisplatin : 27 mg/m^2/week (18-40), median dose of Doxorubicin : 21 mg/m^2/week (13-28). For the 3 patients who also received Methotrexate the dose ranged from 239 mg/m^2/week to 866 mg/m^2/week.

Relapses : Adjuvant treatment : 4/8 have relapsed and died at 4, 27, 32 and 36 months. All 4 with pulmonary metastasis and one also with brain metastases. Neo-Adjuvant treatment : 6/13 have relapsed at a median of 14 months (4-21). 3 of those patients, whose relapses were at 4, 6 and 7 months relapsed in the lungs and died. The other three patients relapsed at 21 months, 2 with a solitary nodule in the lung, which was resected and remain NED without further treatment at 22 and 9 months after thoracotomy. The third patient had a local relapse and underwent amputation. He is NED 3 months after surgery.

Overall follow-up and survival : Median follow-up for all patients until death or last visit is 24 months (4-53). Median time to relapse is 21 months (4-36). Eleven patients (52 %) remain continuously disease-free at a median follow-up of 23 months (12-53). Fourteen patients (67 %) are alive and disease-free at a median follow-up of 27 months (12-53). Seven patients (33 %) died at a median of 14 months (4-36). Survival according to dose intensity : Doxorubicin : > 80 % : 7/11 alive, < 80 % : 7/10 alive. Cisplatin : > 80 % : 8/11 alive and < 80 % 6/10 alive.

Survival according to number of courses : < 6 courses 5/8 alive, 6 courses 8/10 alive and > 6 courses 3/3 alive. Survival according to grade of necrosis : When 90-100 % 5/5 alive, 60-80 % 1/2 alive and < 60 % 3/5 alive. In 1 patient who is alive necrosis was not evaluated. Survival according to type of surgery : Conservative : 7/8 alive. Amputation : 7/13 alive.

Toxicity : Myelosuppression was the most important side effect. Anemia : Eleven patients (52 %) had hemoglobin < 8.0 g/dl and 16 patients (76 %) were transfused a median of 2 units of PRBC (1-4). Leukopenia : Median nadir of leukocytes was 700 mcl (300-2.400). Sixteen patients (76 %) were admitted to the hospital with fever. Thrombocytopenia : Median nadir of platelets was 33.000 mcl (7.000-238.000). Seven patients (33 %) required platelet transfusion. Sixteen patients (76 %) were hospitalized due to myelotoxicity after 44/121 (36 %) courses of chemotherapy. All patients had nausea and vomiting with 57 % > grade I. Nephrotoxicity : Two patients had transient elevations of Creatinine but all patients had normal Creatinine at completion of treatment.

Conclusions

We treated 21 osteosarcoma patients with Cisplatin and Doxorubicin at similar doses as has been reported by the M.D. Anderson group. However, both drugs were given systemically rather than intra-arterial Cisplatin. Treatment was given either as an adjuvant modality or Neo-Adjuvant in 62 % of the patients with an attempt to perform conservative surgery which was possible in 8/13 (61 %) such patients. Median follow-up of all patients is 24 months (4-53). There have been 10 relapses (48 %) at a median of 21 months (4-36). All 4 patients who relapsed in the adjuvant group are dead, whereas 3/6 of the patients who relapsed in the Neo-Adjuvant group are alive and disease-free after surgical treatment of recurrence at 3, 9 and 22 months. Median survival for the 33 % of patients who died was 14 months (4-36). 52 % of patients remain continuously disease-free at 23 months (12-53) and 67 % of patients are alive and disease-free at 27 months (12-53) after completion of initial chemotherapy. We did not find a survival correlation with dose intensity, however there seems to be a benefit for those patients who received at least 6 courses of chemotherapy. In these group of patients, grade of necrosis has not been found to significantly correlate with survival in contrast to what has been reported [11-13]. Less tumor volume in the Neo-Adjuvant group may explain a better prognosis. At 2 years, survival is similar to some of the reported results [6, 7, 12, 13], however, this is a very myelotoxic regimen as 3/4 of the patients required red cell transfusions and were admitted to the hospital with fever and neutropenia and 1/3 received platelets. The potential addition of G-CSF is likely to improve tolerance.

References

1. Jaffe N, Frei E, Traggis D et al (1974) Adjuvant Methotrexate and citrovorum-factor treatment of osteogenic sarcoma. N Engl J Med 291 : 994-997
2. Sutow WW, Sullivan MP, Fernbach DJ et al (1975) Adjuvant chemotherapy in primary treatment of osteogenic sarcoma. Cancer 36 : 1598-1602
3. Taylor WF, Ivins JC, Dahlin DC et al (1978) Trends and variability in survival from osteosarcoma. Mayo Clinic Proc 53 : 695-700
4. Eilber F, Giuliano A, Eckhardt J et al (1987) Adjuvant chemotherapy for osteosarcoma : A randomized prospective trial. J Clin Oncol 5 : 21-26
5. Link MP, Goorin AM, Miser AW et al (1986) The effect of Adjuvant chemotherapy on relapse-free survival in patients with osteosarcoma of the extremity. N Engl J Med 314 : 1600-1606
6. Rosen G, Marcove RC, Caparros B et al (1979) Primary osteogenic sarcoma. The rationale for preoperative chemotherapy and delayed surgery. Cancer 43 : 2163-2177
7. Winkler K, Beron G, Kotz R et al (1984) Neo-Adjuvant chemotherapy for osteogenic sarcoma : Results of a cooperative german/austrian group. J Clin Oncol 2 : 617-624
8. Benjamin RS, Chawla SP, Carrasco CH et al (1990) Primary chemotherapy for osteosarcoma with systemic Adriamycin and intra-arterial Cisplatin. Cancer Bull 42 : 314-317

The role of preoperative and Adjuvant chemotherapy in the treatment on non rhabdomyosarcoma soft tissue sarcoma in children and adolescents

U Gross-Wieltsch, M Morgan, E Koscielniak, J Treuner

Non-rhabdomyosarcoma soft tissue sarcomas (NRSTS) account for 3 % of all tumours in children [4]. The treatment of childhood rhabdomyosarcoma, extraosseous Ewing sarcoma, malignant peripheral neuroectodermal tumours and synovial sarcoma with chemotherapy and radiotherapy has been well established. However in contrast the management of the NRSTS, such as neurofibrosarcoma, fibrosarcoma, liposarcoma and malignant histicytoma remains controversal [1, 2, 3]. In the German soft tissue sarcoma studies, the main target group for analysis consists of patients with a chemotherapy sensitive sarcoma. It has been the policy to register in addition the patients with NRSTS and information has been collected and a data bank established. Not all patients with NRSTS were treated uniformally according to the protocol.

Patients

For the purpose of this analysis patients with a diagnosis of neurofibrosarcoma (30), fibrosarcoma (20, including 8 infantile), malignant fibrous histiocytoma (11) and liposarcoma (8) were reviewed. Patients with metastatic disease at diagnosis were excluded. A total of 74 patients less than 19 years of age were registered in the CWS 81 and 86 studies. Sixty-nine were eligible for assessment. The median follow up was 4 years (1-98 months). The site of the primary tumour is shown in Table 1. Patients were staged according to the modified postoperative staging system of IRS which is defined as follows :
  Stage I : Tumour completely resected, regional lymph nodes not involved.
  Stage II : Tumour macroscopically resected, microscopic residual disease.
  Stage III : Incomplete tumour resection with macroscopic residual disease or biopsy only performed.
  In patients with a primary resectable tumour (stage I and II), surgery was the first line treatment. Subsequently some of the patients received Adjuvant chemotherapy or radiotherapy (15-70 Gy) or both. Patients in whom the tumour was considered initially to be unresectable were treated with preoperative chemotherapy. The definitive local tumour control was accomplished by means of second look surgery and radiotherapy. The chemotherapy regimen consisted of a 4 drug combination of Vincristine, Dactinomycin, Doxorubicin and Cyclophosphamid (VACA) or Ifosfamid (VAIA) for all patients. The response to chemotherapy was evaluated clinically and radiologically after the first cy-

---

Report from the German Cooperative Soft Tissue Sarcoma Study CWS 81 and 86
Olga-Hospital, Department Oncology/Hematology, Stuttgart, FRG

Table 1. Site of primary tumour

Diagnosis	Patients	H/N	Tr	Ext	Abd
Neurofibrosarcoma	30	7	4	12	7
Fibrosarcoma	20 (8)*	4	4 (2)*	11 (6)*	1
Malignant fibrous histiocytoma	11	2	2	7	0
Liposarcoma	8	1	0	4	3
	68	14	10	34	11

H/N = Head/Neck, Tr = Trunk, Ext = Extremity, Abd = Abdomen
()* = infantile fibrosarcoma

Table 2. Outcome

Stage	n	Survivors	Disease free survivors
I	26	24 (4)*	24 (4)*
II	18	13 (3)*	7
III	25	11 (1)*	6
	69	48	37

()* = infantile fibrosarcoma

Table 3.

Stage I	n	Complete remission	local relapse
S	12	12 (3)*	0
S + C	9	7 (1)*	2
S + R	1	1	0
S + C + R	4	4	0
	26	24	2

S = Surgery, C = Chemotherapy, R = Radiotherapy
()* = infantile fibrosarcoma

cle of treatment (week 7 to 9). Complete response (CR) was defined as no detectable tumour present, partial response (PR) as more than 1/3 and non response (NR) as less than 1/3 reduction in tumour volume.

Results

The overall outcome according to stage is shown in Table. 2. Twelve of the 26 patients with stage I disease were treated with surgery alone (Table 3). There were no local relapses and all remain in continuous complete remission (CCR).

13 received Adjuvant chemotherapy. Two local relapses occured within the group of patients treated with primary surgery and chemotherapy and both patients died of tumour progression. Four cases received Adjuvant chemo/radiotherapy and all are in CCR.

Out of the total group there were 18 stage II patients (Table 4). 15 received Adjuvant chemotherapy with or without additional radiotherapy. Six patients relapsed locally, 7 remained in CCR and 2 developed a distant relapse. The 3 patients who did not receive Adjuvant chemotherapy relapsed locally.

Table 4

Stage II	Patients	Complete remission	Local relapse	Distant relapse
S	2	0	2 (1)*	0
S + C	7	2 (2)*	5	0
S + R	1	0	1	0
S + C + R	8	5	1	2
	18	7	9	2

S = Surgery, C = Chemotherapy, R = Radiotherapy
()* = infantile fibrosarcoma

Sixteen of the 25 patients with stage III disease showed either a complete (2) or partial (14) response to the first cycle of chemotherapy. Only 1 of the complete responders remains in CCR, the other having relapsed locally and died of tumour progression. In 10 of the 14 partial responders (Table 5) a complete remission could be achieved by means of additional chemotherapy in 2, surgery in 5 and radiotherapy in 3, but only 4 remained in CCR and 6 relapsed locally of whom 3 died of tumour progression. Four patients died of progressive disease without ever achieving a complete remission. There were 9 non responders. In 4 a complete remission was achieved by mutilating surgery. However only 1 patient remained in CCR and 3 had a local relapse. The other 5 patients in this group died of progressive disease.

Table 5. Partial response

	Patients	Complete remission	Local relapse	Tumour progression
C	1	1	0	0
C + S	3	2 (1)*	0	1
C + R	3	0	2	1
C + S + R	6	1	3	2
S	1	0	1	0
	14	4	6	4

S = Surgery, C = Chemotherapy, R = Radiotherapy
()* = infantile fibrosarcoma

An additional 5 patients were not eligible for assessment as 3 were lost to follow up and there were 2 therapy related deaths.

Discussion

The role of chemotherapy in the management of children and adolescents with neurofibrosarcoma, fibrosarcoma, malignant fibrous histiocytoma and liposarcoma remains controversial [1]. It is generally agreed that primary tumour resection is the recommended treatment for localized disease [2, 5, 6, 8, 10]. Although the number is too small to make definitive conclusions, a review of the patients in the 2 german studies would suggest that 1) a radical resection of the tumour without mutilation should be performed if possible ; 2) patients with marginally resected tumours benefit from Adjuvant chemotherapy and radiotherapy has a role in local tumour control and 3) preoperative chemotherapy can render the tumour resectable in some patients with primarly inoperable disease and hence avoid mutilating surgery with loss of function.

In our series Adjuvant chemotherapy gives no survival advantage in stage I patients. For this group of patients with adequately resected tumours no additional therapy is required. In marginally resected tumours radiotherapy has been effective in providing local tumour control at high-doses in excess of 60 Gy [9]. In contrast to adults children are more likely to experience serious complications following radiotherapy, so that such high-doses should be avoided. In our series the radiotherapy doses for stage II patients ranged from 32 to 54 Gy. We found less local relapses in the patients who were treated with Adjuvant chemotherapy and radiotherapy than in those treated with surgery and chemotherapy alone. One may speculate that a lower radiation dose can be given to patients who are also receiving chemotherapy. The effectiveness of preoperative chemotherapy in stage III patients with neurofibrosarcoma, fibrosarcoma, malignant fibrous histiocytoma and liposarcoma is not well established. The cytostatic agents used in this series of patients were those with proven activity in the management of rhabdomyosarcoma. A measureable response to chemotherapy was seen in 16 out of the total 25 patients. In patients who present initially with inoperable tumours, it is then possible in some cases to carry out a resection following a reduction in the tumour volume with chemotherapy. For this group of patients chemotherapy is recommended in an attempt to shrink the tumour.

Histological grading of the tumour was identified as a risk factor in a study of adult patients with a soft tissue sarcoma by Roeoser et al [8]. An analysis of the histological grading was not performed in this series. The place for a histological grading system in paediatric practice is by no means well defined. It may be that an initial assessment of the degree of malignancy of the tumour could provide additional information about the necessity for adjuvant therapy.

References

1. Elias AD, Antman KH (1989) Adjuvant chemotherapy for soft tissue sarcoma : An approach in search of an effective regimen. Sem Oncology 16 (4) : 305-311
2. Hayani A, Mahoney DH, Hawkins HK, Steuber CP, Hurwitz R, Fernbach D (1992) Soft tissue sarcoma other than rhabdomyosarcoma in children. Med Pediat Oncol 20 : 114-118
3. Koscielnak E, Jürgens H, Winkler K, Bürger D, Herbst M, Keim M, Bernhard G, Treuner J (1992) Treatment of soft tissue sarcoma in childhood and adolescence. Cancer 70 (10)
4. Pizzo PA, Poplack DG (1989) Principles and Practice of Pediatric Oncology. Lippincott, Philadelphia
5. Raney RB, Allen A, O'Neill J, Handler SD, Uri A, Littman P (1986) Malignant fibrous histiocytoma of soft tissue in childhood. Cancer 57 : 2198-2201
6. Raney B, Schauffer L, Ziegler M, Chatten J, Littman P, Jarret P (1987) Treatment of children with neurogenic sarcoma. Cancer 59 : 1-5
7. Roeoeser B, Attewell R, Berg NO, Rydholm A (1988) Prognostication in soft tissue sarcoma. Cancer 61 : 817-823
8. Salloum E, Caillaud JM, Flamant F, Landman J, Lemerle J (1990) Poor prognosis infantile fibrosarcoma with pathologic features of malignant fibrous histiocytoma after local recurrence. Med Pediat Oncol 18 : 295-298
9. Tepper JE, Suit DH (1985) Radiotherapy alone for sarcoma of soft tissue. Cancer 56 : 475-479
10. Witz M, Shapira Y, Dinbar A (1991) Diagnosis and treatment of primary and recurrent retroperitoneal liposarcoma. J Surg Oncol 47 (1) : 41-44

Escalating doses of Epirubicin in combination with Ifosfamide and GM-CSF in previously untreated soft tissue sarcoma patients ; a phase I-II study

S Frustaci, A Buonadonna, D Favaro, M Santarosa, F Latini*, S Lamon, E Galligioni, S Monfardini

Soft tissue sarcomas are rare, malignant mesenchimal tumors characterized by a natural history of prolonged local growth, frequent hematogenous spread, predominantly to the lungs, and by a primary resistance to cytostatic agents. Doxorubicin is the most active and employed drug, showing a clear dose/response relationship. Doses of 50 mg/m^2 or less are clearly not so active as higher-doses, whereas the cumulative response rate in more than 1,000 treated patients is 23 % [1]. Furthermore, the analogue Epirubicin in a randomized trial as shown equal efficacy and less cardio- and myelotoxicity than the parent compound at equimolar doses [2].

Ifosfamide in combination with the uroprotector Mesna recently achieved a defined role in the treatment of metastatic soft tissue sarcomas giving a response rate of up to 30 % with different schedules [3].

Furthermore, the combination of Ifosfamide and antracyclines is 1 of the most active and also in our hand the combination of Iphosphamide and Epirubicin showed a 31.4 % of objective response rate, even if Leucopenia of grade 3-4 was observed in 55.8 % of the patients [4].

Aims of the study were to evaluate the feasibility of increasing the Epirubicin doses, employing in the meantime full doses of Ifosfamide and trying to overcome the expected hematological toxicities with the concomitant use of GM-CSF ; furthermore, to evaluate the response rate of such a combination and the toxicity of GM-CSF in soft tissue sarcoma patients.

Materials and methods

Inclusion criteria were : Histologically verified soft tissue sarcomas of connective, subcutaneous and other soft tissues and parenchimatous organ or hollow viscera ; inoperable and/or metastatic disease either measurable or evaluable ; previously untreated patients ; performance status < 2 (WHO scale) and life expectancy > 3 months ; WBC > 4.000/μl, platelets > 100,000/μl ; age : 18-60 years ; adequate renal, hepatic and respiratory functions.

Treatment consisted of escalating doses of Epirubicin in combination with Ifosfamide and GM-CSF. The Epirubicin starting dose level was 50 mg/m^2 day 1-2 ; Ifosfamide was given at the dose of 1.8 g/m^2 day 1-5 ; Mesna, at the dose of 20 % of IFO dose, was given at hours 0, 4, 8, day 1 to 5 ; GM-

---

Division of Medical Oncology, Centro di Riferimento Oncologico, Aviano, Italy ; * Schering-Plough, Milan, Italy

CSF 5 µ/Kg × 14 days, from day 6, was given during the first cycles as a 6 hours-i.v. infusion, whereas for any further cycle as a subcutaneous administration.

Treatment was repeated every 21 days, or at complete hematological recovery (WBC > 4.000/µl and PLTS > 100.000/µl) for at least 3 cycles before clinical evaluation of response, whereas further treatment was planned individually according to the site of parameter lesion. Toxicity and efficacy were evaluated according to the WHO criteria [5].

Results

Twenty-three patients entered the study, the median age was 52 (range 26-69 years), the median PS was 90 (range 70-100) ; other characteristics of the patients are reported in Table 1.

Up to now 23 patients are evaluable for toxicity and 18 for response. Overall, 83 cycles have been administered and 3 escalating levels of Epirubicin have been evaluated (50 mg/m^2 × 2 days, 60 mg/m^2 × 2 days, 70 mg/m^2 × 2 days). Table 2 reports in details the number of accrued patients for level, the administered cycles and particularly the deescalated and delayed cycles. In fact, we were obliged to deescalate 4 and 7 cycles in the second and third Epirubicin levels. Due to hematological or subjective toxicities encountered in the previous administered cycles, the dose deescalation and/or delay of treatment determined a relative dose intensity of 100 %, 93.7 % and 82.6 % for the 3 Epirubicin levels respectively.

Hematological toxicities are reported in Table 3. These toxicities determined the need of transfusion of RBC in 2, 5, 2 patients for each Epirubicin level and platelets in 3 patients at 60 mg/m^2 × 2 days level. Nineteen fever episodes (> 38.5° C) were reported, hoewever equally distributed in the 3 EPI levels. The GM-CSF related toxicities were always mild or moderate (G1-G2), the predominant symptoms were headache, fatigue, change of the taste, myalgias.

An objective response was observed in 9/21 patients (42.8 %) whereas as far as parameter lesions are concerned, metastatic disease to the lung was the most responsive site (9/15 ; 60 %). Considering the 3 different Epirubicin levels, responses are as follows : 1/4 ; 4/13 ; 4/4 ; for the up to now evaluable patients.

Discussion

These preliminary results of Epiribicin escalating doses in 23 metastatic soft tissue sarcoma patients lead us to draw some conclusions and indications on how to proceed with this study. First of all, the GM-CSF at these doses and schedule showed to be safe, effective and relatively well tolerated. No G3-G4 adverse events directly related to the growth factors were noted during 83 cycles and 1.162 days of GM-CSF administration and a careful prospective evalua-

Table 1. Patients' characteristics

— Entered patients	23
— Median age	52
range	26-69
— Median P.S. (karnofski)	90
range	70-100
— Histology	
• Leiomiosarcoma	7
• M. fibrous histiocytoma	6
• Liposarcoma	2
• Synovial sarcoma	2
• Others	6
— Parameter lesions	
• Lung	15
• Limbs	5
• Liver	3
• Retroperitoneum	3
• Others	6

Table 2. Escalation of Epirubicin and dose intensity (D.I.)*

Chemotherapeutic dose levels		# entered patients	Standard D.I. mg/m^2/w	Received D.I. mg/m^2/w	Relative D.I. (%)
IFO g/m^2 × 5d	EPI mg/m^2 × 2d				
1.8	50	4	33.3	33.3	100
	60	13	40	37.5	93.7
	70	6	46.6	38.5	82.6

* Evaluated on the 3 administered cycles

Table 2. Hematological toxicity relative to the first cycle only

Chemotherapeutic dose levels		#WBC nadir (range)	PLTS nadir (range)	Hb nadir (range)
IFO g/m^2 × 5d	EPI mg/m^2 × 2d			
1.8	50	700 (200-2.470)	95,000 (21.000-120.000)	9.9 (8.6-10.2)
	60	750 (100-4.900)	120.000 (38.000-200.000)	9 (7-13)
	70	300 (180-700)	78.000 (30.000-100.000)	9.9 (7.4-13)

tion of the patients. Recovery of leucocytes was prompt after the nadir and several cases of leucocytosis led us to stop GM-CSF before the completion of all 14 scheduled days. We were not able to find any differences between the 6 hours daily infusion and the subcutaneous administration either for toxicity or effectiveness.

As far as the escalation of Epirubicin in concerned, we regard the 50 mg/m^2 × 2 days as the less active and probably feasible also without hematopoietic growth factors. On the other hand, the 70 mg/m^2 × 2 days level seems to be quite toxic and untolerable for more than 2-3 cycles, but extremely active, since we obtained 4 objective responses on 4 treated patients.

Such an effectiveness, particularly on lung metastases (60 % of response rate) could be exploited for a short, presurgical induction treatment for those patients eligible for pulmonary multiple metastasectomies.

The study is ongoing in order to better define tolerability, efficacy and capability of peripheral blood hematopoietic progenitors' mobilization of the 70 mg/m^2 × 2 days Epirubicin level.

References

1. Lucas P, Spielmann M (1985) Traitement médical des sarcomes des tissus mous de l'adulte. Bull Cancer 72 : 183
2. Mouridsen HT, Bastholt L, Somers R et al (1987) Adriamycin versus Epirubicin in advanced soft tissue sarcomas. A randomized Phase II/Phase II study of the EORTC Soft Tissue and Bone Sarcoma Group. Eu J Clin Oncol 23 : 1477
3. Antman KH, Elias A, Ryan L (1990) Ifosfamide and Mesna : Response and toxicity at standard and high-dose schedule. Seminars in Oncology 17(2)S4 : 68-73
4. Miller AB, Hoogstraten B, Staquet M et al (1981) Reporting results of cancer treatment. Cancer 47 : 207
5. Frustaci S, Foladore S, Lo Re G et al (1989) Full doses of Ifosfamide (IFO) and Epirubicin (EPI) in advanced soft tissue sarcomas. ASCO Annual Meeting, S. Francisco, May 21-23, Abs. n° 601

Primary chemotherapy in malignant fibrous histiocytoma of bone — Updated UTMD Anderson Cancer Center Experience

SR Patel, T Armen, CH Carrasco, AK Raymond, AG Ayala, JA Murray, SP Chawla, RS Benjamin

Malignant Fibrous Histiocytoma (MFH) of bone is a relatively recently recognized entity. After the initial reports in the early 70 s [1], this entity became well established in the pathology and clinical literature by the late 70 s [2-4]. The age distribution is variable, patients are generally older than those with osteosarcoma, and there seems to be a slight predilection for males [5]. The skeletal distribution is also variable, with a predilection for the metaphyses of long bones [6]. Radiologically, it manifests as an aggressive radiolucent defect with ill-defined margins and often, an associated soft-tissue mass. Histologically, it shows striking resemblance to MFH arising in soft tissues. Not infrequently, it constitutes the high grade component of a de-differentiated chondrosarcoma, which has a relatively poorer prognosis. It often is a component of osteosarcomas, and histologically, the only major difference between a fibroblastic osteosarcoma and an MFH is the presence or absence of osteoid. In our experience at the UT MD Anderson Cancer Center, we have seen 2 patients, 1 of them reported in this series, where the initial biopsy and the final surgical specimen diagnosis was felt to be an MFH, but the metastatic disease that developed at a later date unequivocally demonstrated osteoid, making us hypothesise, that MFH of bone may indeed be a variant of fibroblastic osteosarcoma with no demonstrable osteoid initially, however it can manifest at a later date. The biologic behavior of this tumor tends to be extremely aggressive as is the case with osteosarcoma and the preferred therapeutic strategy is therefore a combined approach with chemotherapy and surgery. Investigators from our institution have previously reported a statistically significant advantage in continuous disease free survival (CDFS) and overall survival (OS) with surgery plus Adjuvant chemotherapy compared to surgery alone [6]. This current report is an update on the subset of patients who received chemotherapy preoperatively.

Materials and method

Patient characteristics

Fifteen patients, 10 males and 5 females, with a median age of 39 years, ranging from 19-76 years were treated with primary chemotherapy. Twelve patients

Departments of Melanoma-Sarcoma, Radiology, Pathology and Orthopedic Surgery, University of Texas MD Anderson Cancer Center, 1515 Holcombe Boulevard, Houston, Texas 77030

had their primary tumor in an extremity while 3 had pelvic primaries. Eight patients received our current front-line regimen including Adriamycin administered at a starting dose of 90 mg/m^2 as a 4 days continuous infusion as an out-patient, followed by in-hospital, 24 hours infusion of Cisplatin at a starting dose of 160 mg/m^2 given intra arterially when possible. Three patients who initially received this same Adriamycin + Cisplatin regimen or single agent Cisplatin required to be switched over to alternative regimens of high-dose Ifosfamide (total dose of 14 gm/m^2, 74 hours continuous infusion) in one, and Adriamycin + DTIC in the other 2, due to a sub-optimal response based on sequential angiograms. Two other patients received single agent Cisplatin preoperatively. One patient received CyADIC and the remaining patient received a combination of Adriamycin, Cisplatin and Ifosfamide. These different regimens represent the evolution of preoperative chemotherapy for bone tumors at our institution over the last decade. All, except 1 patient who developed rapidly progressive disease immediately after surgery, received postoperative chemotherapy which was designed based on histologic response to preoperative chemotherapy. Patients with ≥ 90 % necrosis to preoperative chemotherapy were continued on similar regimens postoperatively, whereas others were crossed over to alternate regimens and treated until maximal tolerance for an average of 9-12 months. The median number of cycles of chemotherapy administered preoperatively was 4 ranging from 2-6. Seven out of 12 patients with extremity primaries underwent limb-sparing surgery, while the remainder underwent an amputation.

Results

Investigators from our institution have shown that percent necrosis as a result of preoperative chemotherapy is the single most important predictor of long-term survival in osteosarcoma [7]. This data is available in 14/15 patients from this current series. Seven patients achieved ≥ 90 % necrosis, 2 patients achieved 80 % necrosis and the remaining 5 had < 60 % necrosis (Fig. 1).

Survival data was computed based on Kaplan Meier Life Table analysis. The median CDFS for all patients was 19 months and the median survival was 23 months. The CDFS for patients achieving ≥ 90 % necrosis was superior with a median of 43 months compared to that of patients achieving < 90 % necrosis, whose median CDFS was only 7 months (Fig. 2). This difference is statistically significant with a p value < 0.05 (one sided logrank test). The corresponding overall survivals broken down according to precent necrosis are shown in Figure 3. The median survival for the group with ≥ 90 % necrosis was 66 months while that for the < 90 % necrosis group was 20 months. This difference did not attain statistical significance.

At the time of last follow-up, 5 patients are alive. Of the 10 patients who have expired, one died of prolonged myelosuppression and sepsis while all others died of progressive disease or related complications. Of the 5 patients alive, 4 are in complete remission and long-term survivors ranging 75-140 months, and 1 patient is alive with recurrent disease approximately 20 months

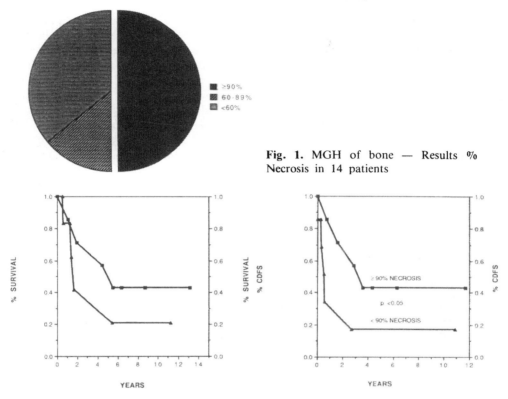

Fig. 1. MGH of bone — Results % Necrosis in 14 patients

Fig. 2. Continuous disease free survival by % necrosis
Fig. 3. Survival by % necrosis

since diagnosis. Three of the 4 patients had achieved ≥ 90 % necrosis while one long-term survivor had 80 % necrosis in the resected primary tumor. Two of these had extremity primaries with limb-sparing surgery while the other 2 had pelvic primaries that were resected.

Discussion

Primary MFH of bone is a very aggressive tumor with a high probability for the presence of microscopic metastatic disease at the time of diagnosis. Consequently, cure of a patient with this tumor depends more on the ability of the chemotherapy to control or eradicate this micrometastases, rather than expedient ablation of the primary tumor by surgery. The role of preoperative chemotherapy, as is the case with osteosarcomas, is to institute systemic therapy at the right earnest, to test the sensitivity of a patient's tumor *in vivo*, to enable identification of better prognosis based on histologic response, and hopefully enable less radical and less morbid surgery.

One patient in this group whose initial biopsy and subsequent resection diagnosis was MFH demonstrated osteoid in a resected lung metastasis at a later date. This supports our opinion that MFH of bone may indeed be a variant of fibroblastic osteosarcoma, where osteoid is not demonstrable at initial diagnosis but may become manifest at a later date.

In conclusion then, MFH of bone does respond to chemotherapy, chemotherapy response predicts for survival and we recommend the use of preoperative chemotherapy which helps identify patients with a better prognosis. Consequently, patients with a poor response to chemotherapy can be spared the toxicities of ineffective drugs and could be candidates for investigational studies.

References

1. Feldman F, Norman D (1972) Intra- and extraosseous malignant histiocytoma (malignant fibrous xanthoma). Radiology 104 : 497-508
2. Spanier SS, Enneking WF, Enriquez P (1975) Primary malignant fibrous histiocytoma of bone. Cancer 36 : 2084-2098
3. Huvos AG (1976) Primary malignant fibrous Histiocytoma of bone. Clinicopathologic study of 18 patients. NY State J Med 76 : 552-559
4. Dahlin DC, Unni KK, Matsuno T (1977) Malignant fibrous histiocytoma of bone. Fact or fancy. Cancer 39 : 1508-1516
5. Dahlin DC, Unni KK (1986) Malignant fibrous histiocytoma. In : Bone tumors. Charles C Thomas, Springfield, p 358
6. Chawla SP, Benjamin RS, Abdul-Karim FW, Ayala AG, Papadopoulos NEJ, Plager C, Romsdahl M, Jaffe N, Murray JA (1984) Adjuvant chemotherapy of primary malignant fibrous histiocytoma of bone-Prolongation of disease free and overall survival. In : Jones SE and Salmon SE (eds) Adjuvant Chemotherapy of Cancer IV. Grune and Stratton, New York, pp. 621-629
7. Raymond AK, Chawla SP, Carrasco CH, Ayala AG, Fanning CV, Grice B, Armen T, Plager C, Papadopoulos NEJ, Edeiken J, Wallace S, Jaffe N, Murray JA, Benjamin RS (1987) Osteosarcoma chemotherapy effect : a prognostic factor. Sem Diag Path 4 : 212-236

Concomitant radiation-Doxorubicin administration in locally advanced and/or metastatic soft tissue sarcomas

S Toma*,**, R Palumbo*, A Grimaldi***, S Barra*, G Canavese*, B Castagneto****, C Frola*****, E Aitini******, R Rosso*

In the last years, the use of concomitant continuous infusion chemotherapy and radiation therapy has been tested in a variety of solid tumors, with different concentrations and scheduling of drugs; effective improvements in objective responses and survival rates were found in relatively limited clinical experiences, such as advanced cancers of the anus, esophagus, bladder, head and neck, hepatic metastases of gastrointestinal and gynecologic tumors [1]. With regard to soft tissue sarcomas, both in vitro and in vivo studies support the possibility of a synergic activity of Doxorubicin, certainly the most active drug in advanced disease, when administered concomitantly with radiotherapy: Doxorubicin has shown a radiosensitizing effect [2, 3, 4, 5], while radiotherapy seems to be more effective after Doxorubicin administration [6]. By a clinical point of view, the possibility of obtaining objective responses by using doses lower than those usually necessary with radiotherapy alone or Doxorubicin alone, would lead to a lowering of toxicity, thus improving the therapeutic index and raising the number of eligible patients. In addition, previous studies had shown that when Doxorubicin is given by continuous infusion over 3 to 4 days is less cardiotoxic and as effective as bolus dosing [7, 8, 9]. Rosenthal and Rotman in a pilot study, while studying the kinetics of Doxorubicin, demonstrated the increased efficacy of radiation therapy in advanced sarcomas and hepatocarcinomas, by simultaneously administering the anthracycline in continuous infusion [10]. Based on these data, in October 1988 we began a phase II study to evaluate the effectiveness and toxicity of this combined regimen, using low doses of both Doxorubicin and radiotherapy, with the aim of improve the therapeutic index and reduce the cumulative toxicity. Up today, 31 patients affected with advanced and/or metastatic soft tissue sarcomas, 6 of which previously treated with chemotherapy, have entered the study. All patients were assessable for toxicity and 30 for response. Doxorubicin was administered by continuous infusion at dosage of 12 mg/m^2/day for 5 days, concomitantly with radiotherapy at fractionated doses (150 or 200 cGy/day for trunk or extremities lesions, respectively) for 5 days; cycles were repeated every 3 weeks. A total of 92 treatment courses were completed, with an average of 3 cycles per patient (range 1 to 5). The overall objective responses were 53 % (16/30) including 2 complete and 14 partial remissions; in addition,

---

* Istituto Nazionale per la Ricerca sul Cancro — IST- Genova, Italia
** Istituto di Oncologia Clinica e Sperimentale dell'Università di Genova, Italia
*** Divisione di Radioterapia Osp. Galliera — Genova, Italia
**** Osp. di Casale Monferrato (AL), Italia
*****Divisione di Radiologia Osp. S. Martino — Genova, Italia
****** Divisione di Oncologia Medica Osp. di Mantova, Italia

12 stable diseases were observed. Only irradiated lesions responded to the treatment, but 1 patient experienced a minor response in a non irradiated lesion, probably due to the systemic action of Doxorubicin. The pre-treated patients had the lower percentage of objective responses (33 % versus 58 % of non pre-treated patients). Additionally, we observed that patients with better performance status ($\leqslant$ 2) showed a response rate better than patients with performance status $\geqslant$ 2 (65 % v.s. 14 %). The duration of response ranged from 5 to 129 weeks, with a median value of 30 weeks. In all evaluable patients, the median survival time was 34 weeks (range 4-129), being 44 weeks in complete or partial responders (versus 24 weeks of non responders) ; pre-treated patients shown a median overall survival of 26 weeks. One of the 2 patients who achieved a complete remission (in a area previous irradiated 9 years early for breast carcinoma) is still alive and disease free after 129 weeks by treatment starting. Eleven of the evaluable patients (37 %) underwent radical surgical treatment, after 2 or 3 cycles of treatment, showing the longer median survival (74 weeks). It is to be underline that 90 % (10/11) of this subset of patients had primary, locally advanced, or relapsed disease, without metastases and that nobody of them was pre-treated with chemotherapy. Combined radio-chemotherapic treatment resulted very well tolerated and easily feasible in a day-hospital regimen ; neither delay of therapy or dose reduction was required because of toxicity. Dose-limiting myelosuppression was acceptable, even in pre-treated patients (no case of degree 3 or 4 leukopenia), and no sign of drug-induced hepatic or renal toxicity was observed. Expecially, cardiotoxicity, certainly the most important side effect of Doxorubicin administration, was nearly absent ; only 2 patients, 1 of which was previously treated with anthracyclines, experienced temporary and reversible tachycardia.

This study confirms our preliminary data on the effectiveness of a concomitant radiation-Doxorubicin administration in advanced and/or metastatic soft tissue sarcomas [11], and underline the possibility of achieving a good response rate (over 50 %), with low overall toxicity. In fact, in the whole group of 30 evaluable patients the higher response rate occurred in non pre-treated patients (58 % in the present study and 54 % in our previous report), and in who had a better performance status at the starting of treatment (65 %). Similarly, median survival time was confirmed to be positively influenced by the achievement of objective response : 44 weeks in the responder patients versus 34 weeks of the entire group and 24 weeks of non responders. Thus, the chance of using low doses of both Doxorubicin and radiotherapy seems to be effective in improving the therapeutic index of the treatment and in raising the number of eligible patients, as also reported by Rosenthal in a recent update of his pilot study [12]. In effect, in our experience objective responses (53 %) were obtained with median total doses of radiation of 3.000 cGy (range 1.500-5.000), very much lower than those usually necessary with radiotherapy alone (5.000-7.500 cGy), while Doxorubicin was delivered at the highest total dose of 300 mg/m^2. The median time of the achievement of objective response ranged from 6 to 9 weeks (2nd-3th cycle of treatment).

Based on these results, our future aim is to attempt an improvement of objective responses, by reducing the interval between 2 consecutive courses of therapy, thus producing a dose intensification of both Doxorubicin and radiotherapy. In view of this end-point, we are using granulocyte colony-stimulating factor and adequate cardioprotection, at each cycle of treatment. Additionally, we would to verify the importance of potential prognostic factors predicting the clinical response to the treatment (e.g. performance status, primary non-metastatic disease, no pre-treatment, etc), which in our experience seem to be related to an higher probability of response. We do feel that a better selection of patients who can benefit from this concomitant radiation-Doxorubicin treatment could consent to extent this therapeutic approach to patients in less advanced stage of disease, e.g. in a Neo-Adjuvant setting, in view of a radical surgery. In the last case, it is not yet known whether a similar combined regimen, shown efficacy in improving the control of local and regional disease, is also effective in precluding spreading metastases or needs to be associated with systemic effective chemotherapy. This and other aspects of the problem need to be further investigated through controlled randomized trials, such as the question of the long-term toxicity. Our study is continuing, and analysis is ongoing.

References

1. Rotman MZ (1992) Chemoirradiation : a new initiative in cancer treatment. Radiology 184 : 319-327
2. Phillips TL, Fu K (1976) Quantification of combined radiation therapy and chemotheraphy effects on critical normal tissues. Cancer 37 : 1186-1200
3. Durand R (1976) Adriamycin : a possible direct radiosensitizer of hypoxic cells. Radiology 119 : 217-222
4. Byfield JE, Watring WG, Lemkin SR et al (1975) Adriamycin : a useful adjuvant drug for combination radiation theraphy. Proc Am Assoc Cancer Res Am Soc Clin Oncol 16 : 253
5. Byfield JE, Lynch M, Kulhanian F, Chan PYM (1977) Cellular effects of combined Adriamycin and X-rays in human cells. Int J Cancer 19 : 194-204
6. Cassady JR, Richter MP, and Piro AJ (1975) Radiation-Adriamycin interaction : preliminary clinical observations. Cancer 36 : 946-950
7. Benjamin R, Yap B, Franzer Jr O (1981) Combination chemotherapy for sarcomas with Cyclophosphamide and continuous infusion Adriamycin and Dacarbazine (CyVADIC) with surgical intensification. Proceedings AACR and ASCO 22 : C756 ; 526
8. Legha S, Benjamin R, Mackay B et al (1982) Evaluation of cardiotoxicity by prolonged continuous intravenous infusion. Ann Intern Med 96 : 133-138
9. Baker L, Green S, Rykan J (1987) Combined modularity therapy for disseminated soft tissue sarcomas phase III. Proceedings ASCO 6 : 138
10. Rosenthal CJ, Rotman M (1988) Pilot study on interaction of radiation therapy with Doxorubicin by continuous infusion. NCI Monogr 6 : 285-290
11. Toma S, Palumbo R, Sogno G et al (1991) Concomitant radiation-Doxorubicin administration in locally advanced and/or metastatic soft tissue sarcomas : preliminary results. Anticancer Res 11 : 2085-2090
12. Rosenthal CJ, Rotman M (1991) Concomitant continuous infusion Adryamicin and radiation : evidence of synergistic effect in soft tissue sarcomas. In : Rotman M, Rosenthal CJ (eds), pp. 271-280

Malignant melanomas
and cerebral tumors

Chemotherapy as a first treatment for malignant primary CNS non-Hodgkin's lymphoma of the central nervous system (PCNSL)

A Boiardi, A Silvani, A Salmaggi, S Valentini, A Allegranza, G Broggi

Primary central nervous system lymphomas are a large group of neoplasms thought to account for about 1 % of primary brain tumors. Their incidence has increased rapidly in recent years notably in patients with acquired immunodeficiency syndrome (AIDS) and in immunocompetent and immunosuppressed subjects [1, 2]. Radiation therapy has mainly been applied to treat CNS-NHL, but low cure rate and lack of enduring response has stimulated the search for alternatives [3].

Taking a lead from published experience of high-dose Methotrexate [4] we used an intravenous M-BACOD scheme, after which radiotherapy was programmed. The aim was to determine whether M-BACOD was efficacious when administered immediately after histological diagnosis and prior to radiotherapy, and to test the feasibility of postponing subsequent radiotherapy until lymphoma recurrence.

Patients and methods

Fourteen consecutive immunocompetent patients, with primary CNS lymphoma had been treated from 1986 on, by the Milan Istituto Neurologico. Mean age was 44 years (range 34-67), and a Karnofsky performance status > 60. In all patients the diagnosis was confirmed by surgery. The patients were selected according to the following additional criteria: no clinical evidence of NHL localization other than CNS, normal chest and abdominal CT, normal bone marrow aspirates, normal liver and kidney biochemical tests. Immediately after histological diagnosis chemotherapy was begun for all patients according to a modified M-BACOD protocol (3 mg/m^2 Methotrexate). Cycles were repeated every 21 days up to five times prior to radiotherapy. Patients non-responsive after the second cycle were started on radiotherapy immediately. Radiotherapy was held up for some months in 6 patients after completing their chemotherapy cycles. Two patients were started on radiotherapy only when tumor relapsed at the 11th and 14th month respectively, in both cases complete response occurred. Two patients PR after chemotherapy became CR after TCT Whole-brain irradiation was at 1.8 to 2.0 Gy/day for 5 days/wk, to achieve a total whole-brain dose at least 50 Gy.

Istituto Nazionale Neurologico « C Besta », Milan, Italy

Results

The tumors found were of high or intermediate grade malignancy, according to the Kiel's classification. The effectiveness of treatment was assessed after 2 M-BACOD cycles. The median rate of Karnofky performance status of all our responder patients increased significantly after chemotherapy prior to radiotherapy. Radiotherapy was planned after chemotherapy or when M-BACOD scheme clearly seemed to become uneffective. In 2 patients irradiation began only when tumor relapse occurred at the 11th, and 14th month respectively. Two PR patients after 2 and 5 M-BACOD cycles had became CR after radiotherapy (Table 1). The disease free period could not be evaluated because the most of patients were not recurrent at the time of the study. No patients up to now had clinical evidence of systemic lymphoma. The toxicity of the M-BACOD program was generally acceptable.

Table 1. NHL-CNS : responses to M-Bacod before radiotherapy and outcome following radiotherapy

N.	Diagnosis	KPS	M-BACOD cycles	R**	KPS	TCT ***	R**	KPS	TTP mts
1	Cc-Cb	70	4	CR	90	6	CR	90	> 19
2	Cc-Cb	50	3	CR	80	6	CR	90	> 24
3	Cc-Cb	70	5	PR	90	6	CR	90	> 8
4	*Cb	70	5	CR	90	11	CR	90	> 13
5	*Cb	50	2	PR	70	3	CR	90	> 15
6	*Cb	40	2	NR	50	—			† 4
7	*Ib-B	40	2	PR	60	3	PR	80	11
8	Lpc	80	3	PR	80	5	PR	80	> 36
9	Cc-Cb	60	3	CR	90	7	CR	90	> 26
10	Cc-Cb	70	5	CR	90	14	CR	90	> 20
11	*Cb	60	4	CR	90	4	CR	80	14
12	Cc-Cb	60	3	PR	60	4	PR	60	12
13	*Ib-B	50	4	PR	80	—			> 6
14	*Cb	70	4	CR	90	8	CR	90	> 12

* High Grade KPS at T test P = 0.001 before TCT
** Response rates *** Radiotherapy
Cc-Cb = Centrocytic-centroblastic ; Cb = Centrobalistic ; Lpc = Lymphoplasmocytoid ; Ib-B = Immunoblastic ; CR = Complete Response ; PR = Partial Response ; NR = No Response ; The tumors found were of high or intermediate grade of malignancy, according to Kiel's classification. The median rate of Karnofky performance status of all our responder patients increased significantly after chemotherapy prior to radio therapy

Discussion

The optimum therapy for NHL-CNS has not been established [5]. Surgical biopsy or resection, with postoperative irradiation is the current standard therapy. Although CNS-NHL is considered radiosensitive and radiotherapy does achieve a high rate of initial remission, long-term results are disappointing [3]. The initial response to radiotherapy is good (70-80 %) but despite prolongation of survival compared to no treatment or surgery alone, the tumor eventually recurs [1, 2]. Chemotherapy has been mostly used.

A number of chemotherapeutic treatmen have been evaluated in NHL-CNS both in the adjuvant and recurrent setting with promising results as consolidative therapy [2]. Hochberg [6] also recommends that in immunocompetent patients intravenous or intra-arterial chemotherapy with MTX alone or in combination should be given prior to irradiation. We decided to administer the whole chemotherapy treatment prior to radiotherapy at least till M-BACOD schedule was effective. In 13/14 (93 %) the treament was useful and complete remission occurred in 7/14 (50 %) The median rate of Karnofky performance status of all our responder patients increased significantly after chemotherapy prior to radiotherapy (Table 1). The effectiveness of the M-BACOD scheme had produced impressive disease regression in NHL-CNS independently of the tumors' grade of malignancy, in advanced diffuse histiocytic or poorly differentiated lymphocytic lymphoma. Only for 2 patients the radiation was given when tumor relapsed, and in both cases a new resolution occurred. It should be emphasized that radiation given following chemotherapy appears to modify its failure, or to recover relapsed patients. It appears possible to achieve complete remission in a high proportion of patients with primary CNS lymphoma without resorting to radiotherapy. If in fact radiotherapy is relatively safe after chemotherapy, we asked ourselves when it should be given. Reserving radiotherapy until disease recurrence is an option worthy of continuing investigation to prolong pts survival.

References

1. De-Angelis LM (1991) Primary central nervous system lymphoma : A new challenge. Neurology 41 : 619-621
2. Hochberg FH, Loeffler JS, Prados M (1991) The therapy of primary brain lymphoma. J Neurooncol 10 : 191-201
3. Loffler JS, Ervin TJ, Mauch P (1985) Primary lymphomas of the central nervous system : patterns of failure and factors that influence survival. J Clin Oncol 3 : 490-494
4. Liang R, Chiu E, Chan TK, Todd D, Ho F (1991) M-BACOD chemotherapy for intermediate and high-grade non-Hodgkin's lymphoma. Cancer Chemother Pharmacol 28 : 135-138
5. Mackintosh FR, Colby TV, Podolsky WJ, Burke JS, Hoppe RT, Rosenfeld FP, Rosenberg SA, Kaplan HS (1982) Central nervous system involvement in non-Hodgkin's lymphoma : an analysis of 105 cases. Cancer 49 : 586-595
6. Hochberg FH, Miller DC (1988) Primary central nervous system lymphoma. J Neurosurg 68 : 835-853

Effect of six retinoids and retinoic acid catabolic inhibitor liarozole on two glioblastoma cell lines, and in-vivo experience in malignant brain tumor patients

ME Westarp*, MP Westarp*, W Bollag**, J Bruynseels***, H Biesalski****, N Grossmann*, HH Kornhuber*

Most adult brain malignancies, notably glioblastoma, astrocytoma and spongioblastoma, are of neuro-epithelial origin. Malignant glioma derive from glial cells that regularly express nuclear retinoic acid receptors of the beta type (RAR-β). Via these response elements, retinol derivatives seem to control target cell differentiation. In addition, sufficient retinol or retinoic acid concentrations are necessary for T-helper cell function [1], and cell mediated immunity in general [2, 3] and in brain tumor patients in particular [4]. Free retinol *in-vivo* circulates at more than a 100 times lower concentrations than RBP-bound retinol [5]. Unlike Vitamin-D and Vitamin-D binding protein, retinol carrier RBP is physiologically regulated by its ligand [6]. RBP binding sites have been demonstrated on choroidal epithelium, suggestive of a retinol transport across the blood brain barrier [7]. Intracellularly, retinol is irreversibly converted to retinoic acid [8], for which more than 20 nuclear receptors have been characterized [9]. Retinoic acid potently induces differentiation in human astrocytoma [10], neuroblastoma [11] and glioblastoma [12, 13]; in glioma cells, both the all-trans and the 13-cis stereoisomer upregulate cell adhesion [14]. While in retinoic acid-responsive acute promyelocytic leukemia, a (15 ; 17) (q 22 ; q 21) translocation has disrupted the retinoic acid receptor α gene located on chromosome 17q [15], neuro-ectodermal tumors harbour the potential to respond to retinoids by sharing embryonic origins with an established target of retinoic acid therapy, the skin.

The imidazole-derived steroid synthesis modulator liarozole (5-[(3-chlorophenyl)(1H-imidazol-1-yl) methyl]-1H-benzimidazole monohydrochloride ($C_{17}H_{13}ClN_4 \cdot HCl$, R75251) effectively inhibits retinoic acid degradation [16] and reaches brain tissue when given orally [17]. We compare 6 retinoic acid derivatives for effects on human glioblastoma nucleic acid turnover, and include the retinoic acid catabolic inhibitor liarozole as well as Interferon-α-2, which exerts an antiproliferative effect on human glioblastoma cells [18]. In a phase I and pharmacokinetic study we furthermore combine adjuvant 13-cis retinoic acid with liarozole (R75251) to increase the differentiation-inducing retinoid effect [19]. 13cRA has a longer plasma half life, additional metabolites and dramatically less effect on intracranial pressure compared to all-trans-RA [20].

---

* Universität Ulm, Abteilung Neurologie, RKU Oberer Eselsberg 45, W-7900 Ulm/Germany (Director Prof.Dr.Dr.h.c.H.H.Kornhuber),
** F Hoffmann-La Roche AG, Grenzacher Str. 124, CH-4002 Basel/Switzerland,
*** Janssen Research Foundation, B-2340 Beerse/Belgium,
**** Institut für Physiologische Chemie und Pathobiochemie der Universität, Duesbergweg 6, W-6500 Mainz/Germany

Methods

Human glioblastoma cells were cultured as described [21]. On 2 established cell line cultures (« M » and « N », kindly provided by Prof. Dr. D. Stavrou, Neuropathology UKE, Hamburg) we tested the following substances by quantitating β decay radioactivity of ^{3}H-thymidine one microcurie per well, added at 75 % confluence for 16-24 hours incubation : Nimustine (ACNU = [1-4-amino-2-methyl-5-pyrimidinyl]-methyl-3-[2-chloroethyl]-3-nitrosourea, mw 309.2) ; 13cRA = 13cRA = Ro4-3780 [(2Z,4E,6E,8E)-3,7-dimethyl-9-(2,6,6,-trimethyl-1-cyclohexen-1-y1)-2,4,6,8-nonatetraenoic acid] mw 300.4 ; Ro13-7410 [p-((E)-2-(5,6,7,8-Tetrahydro-5,5,8,8,-tetramethyl-2-naphthyl)-1-propenyl-benzoic acid] mw 348.5 ; acitretin = Ro10-1670 [all-trans-9-(4-methoxy-2,3,6-trimethylphenyl)-3,7-dimethyl-2,4,6,8-nonatetraenoic acid] mw 326.4 ; Ro13-6307 [(all-E)-3-methyl-7-(5,6,7,8-tetrahydro-5,5,8,8-tetramethyl-2-naphthyl)-2,4,5-octatrienoic acid] mw 338.5 ; Ro14-6113 [temarotene hydroxic metabolite] mw 320.5 ; and Ro22-6595 [13cis-4-oxo-retinoic acid] mw 314.4, alone and in combination with liarozole (R75251 and R85246, mw 345.2, see (Fig. 1) and interferon-α-2A at 10-7 to 10-9 final molar concentrations.

Total retinol and retinoid serum concentrations were measured by high pressure liquid chromatography (HPLC) after 5 minutes of hexane extraction [22], and retinol binding protein was measured by immuno nephelometry (Laser-nephelometer Behring Marburg, standard 1-20 ug/l). 13cRA, 4-oxo-13cRA and all-trans retinoic acid were kindly determined by Dr. U. Wiegand, Hoffmann-La Roche, Basel, from sera stored at $-85°$ C and protected from light and oxygen. Samples were sealed and covered by aluminum foil from bedside to HPLC to minimize oxidation and degradation. Patients with therapeutical retinol, estrogen, progesterone, tetracycline or iron application, malabsorption, maldigestion, cholestasis, cholestyramine medication, hepatic or renal insufficiency, chronic pancreatitis or pancreatic cancer, known skeletal hyperostosis [23] and patients with severe acute or subacute skin rashes were excluded unless otherwise indicated. Liarozole = 5-[(3-chlorophenyl)(1H-imidazol-1-yl)methyl]-1H-benzimidazole monohydrochloride ($C_{17}H_{13}Cl\ N_4$.HCl), registered under R75251 as hydrochloride (Fig. 1), and R85246 as fumarate, was kindly provided in 150 mg tablets (R75251) by Janssen Research Foundation. We have thus far treated 10 patients for more than 6 months or until death with 2.5 — 20 mg/d 13-Cis retinoic acid and 75 — 300 mg/d liarozole p.o., covered by liability agreements and the Ulm University Ethics Commission. Three elegible patients did not consent to enter the study, and 2 patients discontinued medication for mucocutaneous side effects. Toxicity was assessed by weekly monitoring of red and white blood cell count, hepatic transaminases, serum Bilirubin, Creatinine, Urea, Uric acid, Na, K, Cl, cholesterol, triglycerides, retinol, retinol-binding protein, erythrocyte sedimentation rate for the first 5 weeks, continuous documentation of any reported side effects, and followed by regular quarterly controls plus intermittent determinations as required by intercurrent disease, side-effects or course of the malignancy. Clinical assessment was done by monitoring of activities of daily living, Karnofsky index, regular outpatient reports from family and physicians, and quarterly neurological examinations.

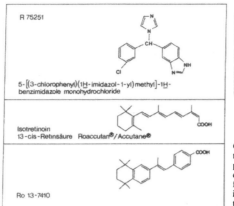
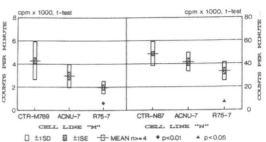

Fig. 1. Chemical structure of liarozole (R75251), 13-Cis-retinoic acid and arotinoid Ro13-7410

Fig. 2. Liarozole inhibits ³H-thymidine incorporation in 2 human glioblastoma cell lines (« M » and « N »)

Compared with media control essay (CTR), 10^{-7} molar concentrations of liarozole (R75-7) significantly reduced ³H-thymidine incorporation (cpm = counts per minute) in two human glioblastoma cell lines ["M" (p < 0.01) and "N" (p < 0.05), two-sided t-test for independent variables, mean of at least four cell cultures, 60 h incubation]. Both tumour cell lines were not particularly sensitive to the cytostatic nitroso-urea nimustine (ACNU 10^{-7} M).

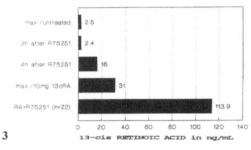
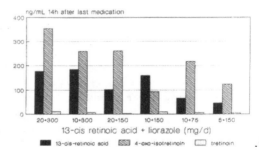

Fig. 3. Serum 13-Cis retinoic acid after oral administration of 13cRA and liarozole: Liarozole 50-100 mg/m² plus 13cRA 10 mg/m² lead to a mean 13cRA serum concentration (n = 22) more than 40 times the highest concentration in untreated patients

Fig. 4. Mean serum retinoids after combined oral therapy with 13-Cis retinoic acid plus its catabolic inhibitor liarozole: Steady-state serum concentrations after oral 13cRA (Roaccutan® in mg) plus oral liarozole (R75251, in mg) in 17 brain malignant tumor patients. Retinoic acids were undetectable in 16/17 patients prior to medication (physiological mean 2-4 ng/mL [23])

Results

In vitro results: ACNU, liarozole, 13cRA (13cRA) and interferon-α_2 reduced ³H-thymidine incorporation in glioblastoma cells in clinically relevant (10^{-7} molar) concentrations (Table 1). IFNα-2A decreased nucleoside incorporation down to 10^{-9} M on cell line « M » only (p < 0.001). Among 6 synthetic retinoic acids, only 13cRA plus Ro13-7410 demonstrated a synergistic effect at equimolar combined concentrations. On glioblastoma line « M », 13cRA plus

Ro13-7410 $[10^{-7}M]$ were more significantly active ($p < 0.001$) than 13cRA alone $[10^{-7}M]$. On cell line N, the arotinoid with a carboxylic acid end group Ro13-7410 combined with liarozole were more effective (Table 1) than liarozole alone or in combination with retinoids Ro14-6113 or Ro22-6595. Liarozole and 13cRA resulted in reproducible reduction of ^{3}H-thymidine incorporation.

Table 1. 13cRA and retinoid RO13-7410 on human glioblastoma cells

concentration	$10^{-6}M$		$10^{-7}M$	
cell line	« N »	« M »	« N »	« M »
ACNU	ns	ns	ns	ns
trifluoperazine	nma	ns	ns	ns
liarozole	ns	.01	ns	.05
13cRA	.001	.ns	.05	ns
13cRA + Ro13-7410	nma	ns	.001	.01

Reduction of ^{3}H-thymidine incorporation compared with controls, $p<0.01$, $p<0.05$. ns = not significant, nma = novalid measurement

Table 2. Plasma retinol and RBP in primary brain tumor patients

| | mean | ±SE | mean | ±SE | |
	Grade I-II (n = 6)		Grade III-IV (n = 7)		
RBP	48.3	± 3	60.9	±19.5	n.s.*
retinol	.825	±.098	.934	±.119	n.s.*
ratio	.92	±.06	1.04	±.10	n.s.*

values in µg/ml, *Fisher's exact test for untreated patients

In vivo results : Prior to surgical, radio- or chemotherapy 13 benign or malignant grade III-IV brain tumor patients did not differ significantly in plasma retinol, RBP or equimolar ratio (Table 2). Equimolar RBP-to-retinol ratios (EQ) on admission ranged from 0.66 to 1.36, and last measurements 1 to 4 weeks before death yielded ratios of EQ = 0.82, 0.84, 1.47 and 1.55. In 2 glioblastoma patients without radiotherapy or chemotherapy, EQ rose from 0.97 to 1.34 and 1.99, and from 0.66 to 1.55 2 weeks to 5 months post operatively on glucocorticoids only. Very low EQ values < 0.50 were regularly seen after radiotherapy without changes in renal retention or hepatic enzymes. In 16/17 untreated malignant brain tumor patients, retinoic acids were not quantitable in fasting serum ; in a single brain tumor patient we measured 2,5 ng/ml 13-cis-retinoic acid and 7,5 ng/ml 4-oxo-13-Cis-retinoic acid. 13cRA 10 mg/d given without liarozole did not result in serum levels beyond 31 ng/ml. Liarozole given without 13cRA did not yield measurable plasma concentrations in one patient examined. Two and 4 hours after having taken 300 mg of liarozole, a second patient measured 2.4 ng/ml and 16 ng/ml serum 13-cis-retinoic acid (Fig. 3). In 2 healthy controls, 600 mg/d liarozole lead to base-line liarozole concentrations of 1.4 ± .3 ng/ml, and peak serum concentrations of 2.8 ± .3 ng/ml measured 4 hours after intake (mean + SEM). In conjuction with 10 mg/m^2 13cRA, daily maintentance doses of 50 mg/m^2 liarozole p.o. were sufficient to regularly increase plasma 13cRA from traces ≤ 2.5 ng/ml to more than 70 ng/ml, and 4-oxo-13cRA from < 7.5 ng/ml to more than 150 ng/ml, while tretinoin remained below 10 % of 13cRA (Fig. 4). Combined with 20 mg retinoic acid, 150 mg liarozole was as effective as 300 mg in increasing and maintaining retinoid serum levels (mean retinoic acid 115 and 116 ng/ml, 4-oxo-13cRA 289 and 334 ng/ml, tretinoin 4.2 and 2.6 ng/ml). Cutaneous tolerance and pharmacologic concentrations came out best in patients with 75 to 150 mg/d liarozole plus 5 to 15 mg/d 13-cis retinoic acid p.o. (Fig. 4).

All patients treated developed slight cutaneous reactions, dry skin, mild cheilitis, and a temporary non-itching rash that promptly resolved upon dose reduction down to 5 mg/d. Leukocyte counts, liver enzymes did not change significantly, erythrocyte sedimentation rate remained unaffected, plasma retinyl esters measured in 6 tumor patients were not elevated, and even after 2 years of continuous combined adjuvant medication, plasma Vitamin-A and retinol-binding protein remained within normal ranges. In every case dry lips, peeling skin on upper arms and thighs, as well as an aseptic conjunctival injection corresponded to total plasma retinoic acid concentrations above 100 ng/ml. We adjusted dosages avoiding painful lips, generalized facial erythema or extensive livid dermal efflorescences, and neither observed fever as in typical « retinoic acid syndrome », nor musculoskeletal side-effects. As reported elsewhere [24] relapsed glioblastoma patients and 1 highly undifferentiated sarcomatous « malignant meningeoma » patient seemed to respond to additional retinoid therapy.

Discussion

Retinoic acid, Vitamin-A's main epidermal tissue derivative, is a potent differentiation inducer [25, 26]. Nuclear retinoic acid receptors RAR-α are found on hematopoietic cells, and RAR-β predominantly in spinal cord, cerebellum, brain cortex and glia cells [28]. 13-cis-retinoic acid (13cRA) reverses premalignant lesions in man [27], is being tested as adjuvant medication in a number of human cancers, and induces differentiation in a majority of human glioma cell culture subpopulations [12], while re-dedifferentiation occurs after termination of exposure [26]. Both cutaneous side effects and in-vitro proto-oncogene downregulation develop simultaneously within 1 week of exposure. Liarozole interferes with cytochrome P_{450} dependent degradation of retinoic acid, modulates human steroid synthesis, and in vitro both liarozole and 13cRA reduce glioblastoma thymidine incorporation ($p < 0.01$). At 10^{-7}M, 13cRA also demonstrates an in vitro synergism with both arotinoid Ro13-7410 and liarozole. Interferon-α-2A plus 13cRA have been successfully combined in squamous cell skin carcinoma [29]. In our dose range tested, both IFN-α-2A and IFN-α-2a plus 13cRA (10^{-7}M to 10^{-9}M) were equally effective in reducing glioblastoma nucleoside turnover.

In vivo 50 mg/m²/d liarozole and 10 mg/m²/d 13cRA given per os for up to 2 years increased and maintained high plasma concentrations of 13cRA and 4-oxo-13cRA, corresponding to a 10^{-7} molar steady state. Though liarozole upregulates progesterone and reduces testosterone, estradiol, aldosterone and to some extent plasma cortisol, patients did not show signs or symptoms of hormonal dysfunctions [30], despite the fact that 13cRA itself may decrease plasma testosterone by interfering with 5-α-reductase activity [31]. Cutaneous side effects occured after 1 to 2 weeks of retinoid therapy, and promptly responded to dosage adjustments. While successful differentiation therapy of acute promyelocytic leukemia with all-trans retinoic acid (> 45 mg/m²) has regularly been accompanied by headache and increased intracranial pressure, fatigue was the only central nervous side effect we have seen up-to-now in 10 patients treated with 13-Cis retinoic acid plus liarozole.

Measurements of retinol and its specific carrier RBP show drastic changes of retinol-to-RBP ratios in the course of grade III-IV primary brain tumors, yet adjuvant retinoic acid and/or liarozole did not lead to significant changes in retinol, RBP or their equimolar ratio — though retinoic acid potently induces cellular RBP mRNA [32]. Since hepatocytes react to increasing retinol demands by augmenting retinol-RBP secretion [33], stable plasma retinol/RBP and transaminases indicate a good hepatic tolerance of high 13cRA and 4-oxo-13cRA plasma concentrations. Further studies will see whether liarozole influences intracellular CRABP as a retinoic acid-absorbing « sink compartment » or alters retinoid glucuronidation. Unlike retinol, synthetic cis-retinoic acid does not accumulate in the liver [34]. Despite high protein binding, significant amounts of serum retinoic acids can be expected to cross the blood brain barrier [34], particularly in patients with an impaired barrier function. While oral Vitamin-A increases plasma 13cRA [35], oral 13cRA plus liarozole leave plasma retinol unaffected. This could be decisive for lymphocytic retinoid metabolism [36], potentially impaired by synthetic retinoids that downregulate plasma retinol [37, 38]. In human glioblastoma cell cultures, retinoic acid increases rather than diminishes γ-ray sensitivity [39]. Adjuvant retinoid therapy therefore has the potential to initiate cell re-differentiation at the invasion front and improve tumor defenses without contra-productive side-effects. 13cRA can be given orally as long-term adjuvant in synergy with an effective catabolic inhibitor, and plasma concentrations can be titrated by inspection. In malignant glioma RA modulates expression of growth signaling molecules such as EGFR [13]. Of particular interest will be whether glioma-associated oncogenes such as c-sis, HA/N-ras and c-myc [40] can be downregulated by long-term retinoid medication. Our more than 2 years' clinical experience [41, 24] with 13cRA and its catabolic inhibitor identifies the retinoid regimen as an encouraging oral and additional option to treat neuroepithelial malignancies.

Acknowledgements. We thank Prof. D Stavrou for glioblastoma cell line specimen, Prof. Hans-Peter Richter and Dr. Ulrich Kunz for serum specimen, Dr. Ulf Wiegand for skilful retinoic acid determinations, Prof. Otto Haferkamp for neuropathological support, the RKU laboratory for coding assistance, and Wolfgang Grundl, Heinz Zett-

lmeißl, Björn Welcker, Dr. Wolfgang Neis, and Dr. Eduard E. Holdener and Dr. Jan Bruynseels for constructive discussion.

References

1. Carman JA, Smith SM, Hayes CE (1989) Characterization of a helper T lymphocyte defect in Vitamin-A-deficient mice. J Immunol 142 : 388-393
2. Serrou B, Cupissol D (1980) A retinoic acid derivative can restore depressed immune function of patients with advanced solid tumors. Allergol Clin Immunol 8 : 373
3. Micksche M, Cerni C, Kokron O, Titscher R, Wrba H (1977) Stimulation of immune response in lung cancer patients by Vitamin-A therapy. Oncology 34 : 234-239
4. Stephanou A, Knight RA, Annicchiarico-Petruzzelli M, Finazzi-Agro A, Lightmann SL, Melino G (1991) Interleukin-1 β and interleukin-6 mRNA are expressed in human glioblastoma and neuroblastoma cells respectively. Funct Neurol 7 : 129-33
5. Creek KE, Silverman-Jones CS, DeLuca LM (1989) Comparison of the uptake and metabolism of retinol delivered to primary mouse keratinocytes either free or bound to rat serum retinol-binding protein. J Invest Dermatol 92 : 283-89
6. Cooke NE, Haddad JG (1989) Vitamin-D binding protein (Gc-Globulin). Endocrine Reviews 10 : 294-307
7. MacDonald PN, Bok D, Ong DE (1990) Localization of cellular retinol-binding protein and retinol-binding protein in cells comprising the blood-brain barrier of rat and human. Proc Natl Acad Sci USA 87 : 4265-69
8. Favennec L (1988) The biological effects of retinoids on cell differentiation and proliferation. J Clin Chem Clin Biochem 26 : 479-489
9. Mangelsdorf DJ, Ong ES, Dyck JA, Evans RM (1990) Nuclear receptor that identifies a novel retinoic acid response pathway. Nature 345 : 224-229
10. Rutka JT, De Armond SJ, Giblin J, McCulloch JR, Wilson CB, Rosenblum ML (1988) Effect of retinoids on the proliferation, morphology and expression of glial fibrillary acidic protein of an anaplastic astrocytoma cell line. Int J Cancer 42 : 419-27
11. Benjamin LA, McGarry RC, Hart DA (1989) Effect of retinoic acid on human neuroblastoma : correlation between morphological differentiation and changes in plasminogen activator and inhibitor activity. Cancer Chemother Pharmacol 25 : 25-31
12. Yung WKA (1989) In vitro chemosensitivity testing and its clinical application in human gliomas. Neurosurg Rev 12 : 197-203
13. Steck PA, Hadi A, Lotan R, Yung WK (1990) Inhibition of epidermal growth factor receptor activity by retinoic acid in glioma cells. J Cell Biochem 42 : 83-94
14. Reboul P, Broquet P, George P, Louisot P (1990) Effect of retinoic acid on two glycosyltransferase activities in C6 cultured glioma cells. Int J Biochem 22 : 889-893
15. Lo CF, Avvisati G, Diverio D, Biondi A, Pandolfi PP, Alcalay M, de Rossi G, Petti MC, Cantu-Rajnoldi, Pasqualetti D, Nanni M, Fenu S, Frontani S, Frontani M, Mandelli F (1991) Rearrangements of the RAR-α gene in acute promyelocytic leukaemia : correlations with morphology and immunophenotype. Br J Haematol 78 : 494-499
16. End DW, Wouters W, Van Ginckel R, Garrabant TA, Van Wauwe J, Coene MC, Bruynseels J, De Coster R, Bowden C (1991) R75251, an antitumoral agent which inhibits retinoic acid (RA) metabolism. Proc Am Assoc Canc Res 32 : 213
17. De Coster R, Van Ginckel R, van Moorselaar RJA, Schulken JA, Debruyne FMJ, Bruynseels J, Denis L (1991) Antitumoral effect of R75251 in prostatic carcinoma experimental and clinical studies. Proc Am Ass Canc Res 32 : 213

18. Hamada H, Asakura Y, Maeda Y, Yokoyama S, Niiro M (1986) A study of direct antitumor activity of α-Interferon against human glioma. Jpn J Cancer Chemother 13 : 464-471
19. Muindi J, Frankel SR, Miller WH, Jakubowski A, Scheinberg DA, Young CW, Dmitrovsky E, Warrell RP (1992) Continuous treatment with all-trans retinoic acid causes a progressive reduction in plasma drug concentrations : implications for relapse and retinoid « resistance » in patients with acute promyelocytic leukemia. Blood 79 : 299-303
20. McElwee NE, Schumacher MC, Johnson SC, Weir TW, Greene SL, Scotvold MJ, Hunter JR, Dinan BJ, Jick H (1991) An observational stuy of isotretinoin recipients treated for acne in a health maintenance organization. Arch Dermatol 127 : 341-346
21. Westarp ME, Westarp MP, Welcker B, Grossmànn N, Grundl W, Kornhuber HH (1991) Retinoic acid and its catabolic inhibitor, R75251, in human malignant glioma cells. Eur J Canc 27 (suppl 3) : 58
22. Biesalski HK, Weiser H (1990) Microdetermination of retinyl esters in guinea pig tissues under different Vitamin-A status conditions. J Micronut Analysis 7 : 97-116
23. Periquet B, Lambert W, Garcia J, Lecomte G, De Leenheer AP, Mazieres B, Thouvenot JP, Arlet J (1991) Increased concentrations of endogenous 13-cis — and all-trans-retinoic acids in diffuse idiopathic skeletal hyperostosis, as demonstrated by HPLC. Clin Chim Acta 203 : 57-65
24. Westarp ME, Westarp MP, Bruynseels J, Bollag W, Kornhuber HH (1993) Oral liarozole as a catabolic inhibitor potently increases retinoic acid in vivo : first experience from an ongoing therapeutic trial in highly malignant primary brain tumors, Onkologie 16 (in press)
25. Bollag W (1983) Vitamine-A and retinoids : from inhibition to pharmacotherapy in dermatology and oncology. Lancet i : 860-865
26. Fischer I, Nolan CE, Shea TB (1987) Effects of retinoic acid on expression of the transformed phenotype in C6 glioma cells. Life Sci 41 : 463-70
27. Meyskens FL, Gilmartin G, Alberts DS, Levine NS, Brooks R, Salmon SE, Surwit EA (1982) Activity of 13-Cis retinoic acid against squamous epithelial premalignancies and malignancies. Cancer Treat Rep 66 : 1315-19
28. De Thé H, Marchio A, Tiollais P, Dejean A (1989) Differential expression and ligand regulation of the retinoic acid receptor-α and β genes. EMBO J 8 : 429-433
29. Lippman S, Parkinson D, Itri L, Weber R, Schantz S, Ota D, Schusterman M, Krakoff I, Gutterman J, HOng W (1992) 13-Cis-retinoic-acid and Interferon-α-2A : effective combination therapy for advanced squamous-cell carcinoma of the skin. J Natl Cancer Inst 84 : 235-241
30. Westarp ME, Westarp MP, Bollag W, Kornhuler HH (1992) Hohe retinoid-Serumdauerspiegel bei primären ZNS-Tumoren durch orale kombination von 13cRA und Inhibitor R75251 (Permanently high serum retinoids in primary CNS tumors after oral 13cRA plus inhibitor R75251). Canc Res Clin Oncol 118 (suppl) : R122
31. Rademaker M, Wallace M, Cunliffe W, Simpson NB (1991) Isotretinoin treatment alters steroid metabolism in women with acne. Br J Dermatol 124 : 361-364
32. Okuno M, Chalala T, Caraveo V, Sasaki A, Goodman DS, Blaner WS (1992) Regulation of cellular retinol-binding protein (CRBP) and retinol-binding protein (RBP) expression in adipocytes : effects of retinoic acid (RA), Dexamethasone (DEX) and Triiodothyronine (T3). FASEB J 6 : A1782
33. Wolf G (1984) Multiple functions of Vitamine-A. Physiol Rev 64 : 873-937
34. Meyskens FL jr, Goodman GE, Alberts DS (1985) 13-Cis-retinoic acid pharmacology, toxicology, and clinical applications for the prevention and treatment of human cancer. CRC Critical Rev Oncol Hematol 3 : 75-101

35. Eckhoff C, Nau H (1990) Vitamin-A supplementation increases levels of retinoic acid coumpounds in human plasma : possible implications for teratogenesis. Arch Toxicol 64 : 502-503
36. Moriguchi S, Jackson JC, Watson RR (1985) Effects of retinoids on human lymphocyte function. Human Toxicol 4 : 365-378
37. Buck J, Derguini F, Levi E, Nakanishi K, Hammerling U (1991) Intracellular signaling by 14-hydroxy-4, 14, retro-retinol. Science 254 : 1654-56
38. Clerici E, De Palo G, Ferrario E, Trabattoni D, Villa ML (1992) Retinoids, breast cancer and NK cells. FASEB J 6 : A1433
39. Rutz HP, Little JB (1989) Modification of radiosensitivity and recovery from X-ray damage in vitro by retinoic acid. Int J Radiat Oncol Biol Phys 16 : 1285-88
40. Orian JM, Vasilopoulos K, Yoshida S, Kaye AH, Chow CW, Gonzales MF (1992) Overexpression of multiple oncogenes related to histological grade of astrocytic glioma. Br J Cancer 66 (1) : 106-112
41. Westarp MP, Westarp ME, Biesalski HK, Bollag W, Kornhuber HH (1992) 13-cis retinoic acid and R75251 in primary CNS tumors — Successful start of a clinical pilot study. J Neurol 239 (suppl 2) : 112

Abstract. Liarozole (5-[(3-chlorophenyl)(1H-imidazol-1-yl)methyl]-1H-benzimidazole monohydrochloride mw = 345, R75251/R85246 as fumarate) effectively inhibits cytochrome-P_{450} dependent 13-Cis-retinoic acid (13cRA) degradation. We have tested candidate compounds with molecular weight < 350, including the nitrosurea nimustine (ACNU), 13-Cis-retinoic acid (13cRA) (isotretinoin = Ro4-3780), arotinoid Ro13-7410, acitretin (Ro10-1670), Ro14-6113 (temarotene hydroxic metabolite), Ro22-6595 (13-Cis-4-oxo-retinoic acid) and retinoid Ro13-6307, alone and in combination with liarozole (R75251) in 2 human glioblastoma cell lines. At clinically obtainable concentrations, 13cRA, liarozole, and Interferon-α-2A significantly reduce ^{3}H-thymidine incorporation in the in-vitro assays, while the arotinoid Ro13-7410 synergizes with both 13cRA and liarozole in one glioblastoma line. Within the last 2 years 10 patients with primary malignant brain tumors have entered a first and open therapeutic pilot study with 13cRA plus liarozole. Cheilitis, conjunctivitis, and desquamation were frequent, while 50 mg/m²/d liarozole (R75251) combined with 10 mg 13cRA elevated total plasma retinoids more than 10-fold, increasing 13cRA and 4-oxo-13-Cis-RA more than all-trans-RA serum levels. Liver enzymes and plasma retinol and retinol binding protein did not change significantly, serum retinol palmitate was not elevated, and patients demonstrated no signs or symptoms of hormonal dysfunction. The combination in neuro-epithelial malignancies of 13-Cis-retinoic acid plus liarozole is well tolerated, affects intracranial pressure dramatically less than high-dose all-trans retinoic acid therapy, and due to a dose-dependent enhancement of ectodermal differentiation can be titrated by inspection.

Phase II trial with BCNU Plus α-2B-Interferon in patients with recurrent high-grade gliomas

A Brandes*, P Zampieri**, A Rigon***, E Scelzi*, PL Zorat***, A Rotilio**, P Amistà****, A Paccagnella*, MV Fiorentino*

Malignant gliomas are primary CNS tumors with a poor prognosis which has not improved recently.

The median survival of patients undergoing surgical resection is 17 weeks. Postoperative radiation therapy extends median survival to 37 weeks [1]. The optimal timing of chemotherapy in the treatment of gliomas is a question which has not been answered : in fact not all agree that adjuvant medical treatment can give a significantly prolonged survival or significant improvement in quality of life when compared to delayed chemotherapy after post radiation recurrence or progression [2].

In patients that recurred after surgery and radiotherapy Cloroethylnitrosoureas are the most active agents [3].

Although chemotherapy has prolonged survival of selected groups of patients, the majority are not cured and new modalities are needed to treat malignant gliomas. Interferon has been evaluated in clinical trials suggesting a definite activity [1]. There is *in vitro* support that BCNU can be synergistic with Interferon without significant toxicity enhancement [4].

Materials and methods

Patients eligibility

Eligibility criteria included 1) histologically proven anaplastic astrocytoma (AA) or multiform glioblastoma (GB) ; 2) evidence of tumor recurrence or progressive disease (PD) documented by contrast enhanced computed tomography (CT) ; 3) pts. who received and failed postoperative cranial radiotherapy (RT) ; 4) pretreated or non pretreated with nitrosoureas combinations ; 5) measurable disease on the brain CT scan ; 6) adequate bone marrow reserve (WBC count $\geq$ 3.000 and platelet count > 100.000) normal baseline liver (serum bilirubin level < 1.5 mg/dl) renal (serum creatinine level < 1.5 and cardiac function ; 7) no prior cytotoxic therapy within 4 weeks ; 8) age 18 to 70 ; 9) Karnofsky Performance Status (KPS) $\geq$ 50. Medical history and KPS score were recorded. Pretreatment laboratory data include complete blood cell count, platelet counts, SMA, ECG, brain CT scan.

---

* Oncology Unit
** Neurosurgery Unit
*** Radiotherapy Unit
**** Neuroradiology Unit Oncologic Center, Padova, Italy

Treatment plan

On day 1 Interferon-α-2B in a dosage of 6-MU is administered in a 2 hour-infusion, followed by BCNU 150 mg/m². IFN was repeated on alternating days for 3 times a week subcutaneously with recycling BCNU and IFN infusion on day 42. A minimum of 2 courses of therapy are required for evaluation, unless the patient has a rapid progression of disease. A CT scan of the brain was performed after 2 cycles, and 2 further cycles are given to stable or responding patients.

Time to tumor progression (TTP) was calculated from the beginning of treatment to tumor progression, and survival time (ST) from the beginning of treatment to death. World Health Organization toxicity criteria were used, based on the most severe degree per patient.

Response criteria

All evaluations were done by a multidisciplinary team including a neuroradiologist, oncologist, neurosurgeon, radiotherapist. Complete response (CR) : disappearance of all enhanced tumor on consecutive CT or magnetic resonance imaging (MRI) scans at least 1 month apart, off steroids and neurologically stable or improved

Partial response (PR) : ⩾ 50 % reduction in size of enhanced tumor on consecutive CT or MRI scans at least 1 month apart, steroids stable or reduced and neurologically stable or improved. Progressive disease (PD) : > 25 % increase in size of enhanced tumor or any new tumor on CT or MRI scans, or neurologically worse and steroids stable or increased.

Stable disease (SD) : all other situations [5].

Results

Patients characteristics are presented in Table 1. Fourteen pts. had GB and 10 had AA. Median age was 53 (26-70), Median KPS 60 (50-90). In Table 2 the results are summarized. We observed no CR in the 17 non pretreated patients (NCP) : 6 of them achieved PR (35 %) lasting 40, 76+, 16, 20, 22, 18 months ; and 4 SD (23 %) lasting 52, 32, 32, 28. The overall response rate (PR+SD) was 58 % ; 7 of 10 (70 %) patients with AA achieved PR or SD, whereas 4 of 7 (57 %) those with GB. The Kaplan Meier median Time To Progression (TTP) was 23.5 weeks (wks), the Median Survival Time (MST) was 42.71 wks, respectively 62.43 in AA and 32.86 in GB. In 7 chemotherapy pretreated patients (CP) we obtained only 2 SD (28 %) and MST was very poor.

Table 1. Patients' characteristics

Total	24
Male/female	17/7
Median age (range)	53 (26-70)
Median Karnofsky Index (range)	60 (40-90)
Histology (AA/GB)	10/14
Chemotherapy (untreated/treated)	17/7

Table 2. Results

Non Chemotherapy pretreated patients	
TOTAL	17
AA/GB	8/9
Partial remission (wks)	6 17 (35 %)
Stable disease	4/17 (23 %)
Median TTP (wks)	23
Median ST (wks)	40.7
AA	62
GB	32

Table 3. Results

Chematherapy pretreated patients	
TOTAL	7
AA/GB	1/6
Partial remission	0/7
Stable disease	2/7 (28 %)

Table 4.

	Toxicity			
	1	2	3	4
Haematologic				
WBC	2 (8 %)	8 (33 %)	1 (4 %)	0
PLT	6 (25 %)	1 (4 %)		
Neurological	3 (12 %)	2 (8 %)	3 (12 %)	0

Toxicity

The minority of patients experienced for some hours mild, non dose related, transient flu-like symptoms following Interferon i.v. infusion administration including fatigue, fever and chills. Premedication with Acetaminophen attenuated these symptoms and during subcutaneous administration these symptoms were not present.

Major toxicity is listed in Table 3.

Discussion

Nitrosoureas have been considered to be the standard chemotherapy and yielding response rates of approximately 20 to 30 % in relapsed patients. To date 2, 3 and 4 drug combinations have not significantly improved survival and only minimally changed the response rate [6].

Interferons *in vitro* inhibit human glioma cell growth [7]. Histological studies of the cells cultured with Interferon suggested maturation to more differentiated astrocytic cells containing increased amounts of glial fibrillary acidic protein [8] and this would be reflected on survival more than response rate.

In vivo it was demonstrated that intravenous IFNs reached the tumor in concentrations about 10 fold higher than in the normal brain [9] and with intramuscular injection a significant level was maintained [10] for a longer time.

In monochemotherapy [11] Yung had achieved with B interferon 23 % responses with a median time to progression of 23 weeks. Similar results were obtained from Mahaley [10] who treated 17 patients with Interferon-α and obtained 7 reductions. In non pretreated patients we obtained a high response rate according to Buckner [12] who used a similar regimen. Our median TTP is less than Yung but our patients had a very low KPS : 60 compared to Yung's 90.

The Kaplan Meier MST is rather satisfactory not only suggesting a cytotoxic activity of this combination but, also cell differentiation.

In chemotherapy pretreated patients we obtained only SD (28 %) according to the known chemoresistance pattern of these tumors and this regimen would not be advised for the pretreated patients.

References

1. Brandes A, Soesan M, Fiorentino M (1991) Medical Treatment in high grade malignant gliomas in adults : an overview. Anticancer Research 11 : 719-728
2. EORTC Brain Tumor Group (1978) Effect of CCNU on survival rate of objective remission and duration of free interval in patients with malignant brain glioma. Final evaluation. Eur J Cancer 14 : 851-856
3. Stewart DJ (1989) The role of chemotherapy in the treatment of gliomas in adults. Cancer Treatment Reviews 16 : 129-160
4. Creagan ET, Kovach JS, Long HJ et al (1986) Phase I study of Recombinant Leukocyte a human Interferon combined with BCNU in selected patients with advanced cancer. J Clin Oncol 4 : 408-413
5. McDonald DR, Cascino TL, Clifford S (1990) Response criteria for phase II studies of supratentorial malignant glioma. J Clin Oncol 8 : 1277-1280
6. Kornblith PL, Walker M (1988) Chemotherapy for malignant gliomas. J Neurosurg 68 : 1-17

7. Lundblad D, Lundgre E (1981) Block of a glioma cell line in S by Interferon. Int J Cancer 27 : 749-754
8. Korosue K, Takeshita I, Mannoji H et al (1983) Interferon effects on multiplication, cytoplasm protein and GFAP content, and morphology in human glioma cells. J Neuro-Oncology 1 : 69-76
9. Mihara Y, Kuratsu J, Takaki S et al (1991) Distribution of mouse Interferon-B in normal and brain tumour-bearing. Acta Neurochir 109 : 46-51
10. Mahaley MS, Jr, MD, Ph D et al (1985) Immunobiology of primary intracranial tumors. J Neurosurg 63 : 719-725
11. Yung WKA, Prodos M, Levin VA et al (1991) : Intravenous recombinant interferon-γ in Patients with recurrent malignant gliomas : a phase I/II Study. J Clin Oncol 9 : 1945-1949
12. Buckner JC, Brown LD, Cascino TL et al (1989) Recombinant Interferon-α (rIF-Nα) and BCNU in recurrent gliomas. J Biol Response Mod 8 : 332-333

Carboplatin combined with Carmustine and Etoposide in the treatment of glioblastoma (GBM) patients

A Boiardi, A Silvani, S Valentini, A Salmaggi*, M Botturi, M Farinotti, C Giorgi

Tumors of the CNS and specially the most frequently occurring glioblastoma mean a grim prognosis to patients with that presently incurable disease. Many authors [1-3] have expressed doubts about the advisability of chemotherapy in malignant glioblastomas. Cisplatinum coumpound has been evaluated in recurrent glial tumors and in the treatment of a variety of pediatric brain tumors [4] and some studies suggest efficacy and acceptable tolerance [2, 5]. Because Carboplatin-Etoposide combinations have proved synergistic against animal tumor models [6] we decided to try a combination of these drugs against primary glioblastoma. We were also seeking to determine the utility of continuing chemotherapy (PVC protocol) at time to tumor relapse at least for patients with good quality of life.

Patients and method

122 consecutive patients with histological diagnosis of GBM were considered for the study. Ninety-five glioblastoma patients were actually admitted (68 %) and divided into 4 omogeneous groups matched for histology, age (52 ± 12.3 years), Karnofsky status (70 ± 10.5) and life expectancy Group (A): 15 patients, treated with BCNU 80 mg/m^2 × 3 days every 6 weeks. Group (B): 27 patients, treated with CDDP 45 mg/m^2 + VP-16 120 mg/m^2 × 3 days every 4 weeks. Group (C): 14 patients treated with CBDCA 200 mg/m^2 + BCNU 60 mg/m^2 × 2 days every 5 weeks. Group (D): 39 patients, treated with CBDCA 200 mg/m^2 + BCNU 60mg/m^2 + VP-16 150 mg/m^2 × 2 days every 5 weeks. Courses were repeated every 4-6 week intervals for 5-8 cycles.Eligible patients were less than 65 years old and had: Karnofsky score of at least 70, normal peripheral blood count, normal kidney and liver function and no major organ system dysfunction. All patients received radiotherapy sandwiched between the second and third courses of chemotherapy. Doses ranged from 55 to 60 Gy.When the tumor relapse occurred patients belonging to the group (A) had been treated symptomatically with corticosteroids, but all other patients received another chemotherapeutic protocol (PVC: Procarbazine 75 mg/m^2 days 1-21, Vincristine 1.4 mg/m^2 days 1.15 and CCNU 60 mg/m^2 days 1.15.)

Istituto Nazionale Neurologico « C Besta » and *Divisione di Radioterapia, Ospedale Maggiore di Niguarda, Milan, Italy

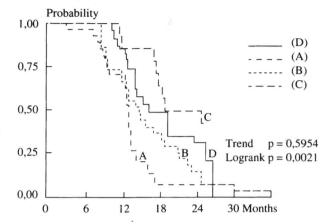

Fig. 1. The Kaplan-Meier graph concerning disparate group fo GBM patients, shows the effectiveness of the treatment according to ST C = CBDCA + BCNU ; D = CBDCA + BCNU + VP-16 ; B = CDDP + VP-16 ; A = BCNU

Results

Dose-limiting toxicity in our study was myelosuppression.

Leukopenia appeared more frequently than thrombocytopenia and was generally more severe. Cumulative toxicity was not observed.

The effectiveness of the protocols differed, but differences were not statistically significant, particularly when the PR and SD responses were considered together. There was also a statistically non significant difference between the treated patients as concern the time to tumor progression.

As concern the ST our data show that platinum based protocols have some activity against GBM. Differences of ST between the groups treated with carboplatinum as a main drug and those treated only with BCNU are statistically significant (Fig. 1).

Discussion

The chemotherapy protocols we employed were associated with acceptable toxicity and side effects with some positive response evaluated before radiotherapy Median TTP did not differ between the treatment groups, the median time to progression being 9-11 months from the operation ; nevertheless, TTP in the platinum-based protocols compares favourably with the best reported results using platinum [1, 2, 4, 5]. As concern the ST our data show that platinum based protocols have some activity against GBM, although other authors have reported little. At 18 months more than half the carboplatin-treated patients were alive, and the groups treated with platinum had a significantly longer ST than those treated with BCNU. Surprising results are those concerning carbo v.s. Cisplatin, although data express a borderline significance (p = 0.008). Carboplatin seems to be slightly more effective than Cisplatin, possibly because, as it as no significant cumulative toxicity, more carboplatin courses can be delivered. But mostly because the unbound plasma fraction of carboplatin has a longer half life than Cisplatin and the concentration gradient, driving it across the blood-brain barrier is therefore higher. It is thus safe to affirm the utility of continuing chemotherapy in recurrent GBM at least in patients enjoying a good quality of life. Our data support the idea that the currently widespread negative attitude towards chemotherapy for GBM should be abandoned. We conclude that platinum-based chemotherapy has a beneficial effect on glial tumors. Poor penetration to peritumoral brain tissue explains why postsurgery chemotherapy with these drugs does not achieve a lasting remission in most cases.

References

1. Kornblith P, Walker M (1988) Chemotherapy for malignant gliomas. J Neurosurg 68 : 1-17
2. Edwards MS, Levin VA, Wilson CB (1980) Brain tumor chemotherapy : an evaluation of agent use for phase II and III trials. Cancer Treat Rep 64 : 1179-1205
3. Levin VA, Sheline GE, Gutin PH. Neoplasms of the Central Nervous System : Cancer principles and practice in oncology. In : De Vita VT Jr, Hellman S, Rosenberg SA (eds). JB Lippincott Co, Philadelphia, p 1557
5. Steward DJ, O'Bryan RM, Al-Sarraf M (1983) Phase II study of Cisplatin in recurrent astrocytomas in adults : a Southwest Oncology Group Study. J Neurol Oncol 1 : 145-147
6. Stewart DJ, Richard MT, Hugenholtz H (1984) Penetration of VP-16 into human intracerebral and extracerebral tumors. J Neurol Oncol 2 : 133-139
7. Walker RW, Allen JC (1998) Cisplatin in the treatment in recurrent childhood primary brain tumors. J Clin Oncol 6 : 62-66

Phase II trial of Cystemustine, a new nitrosourea, as second-line treatment of malignant gliomas

A Tisserant*, R Plagne*, H Roché**, A Adenis***, P Fargeot****,
N Guiochet*****, P Cattan******, Y Krakowsky*******,
MA Lentz********, P Fumoleau*********,
B Chevallier**********, P Chollet*

Supratentorial malignant gliomas represent 50 % of the primary malignant brain tumors [1, 2].

Prognosis is always unfavourable with a median survival of about 1 year ; 25 % to 30 % of the patients are still alive at 18 months [3] with surgery and/or radiotherapy. These bad results have favoured attempts of combination with medical treatments.

Chemotherapy of malignant brain tumors has been mainly tried with cytostatics showing a good diffusion through the blood brain barrier, and as a chief of file, the nitrosoureas family.

Recently, new drugs have been put under study with this family, in pilot trials to achieve better results, at conventional doses, as well as in combined therapies associating surgery, radiotherapy and initial chemotherapy with very high-dose BCNU (800 mg/sq.m.) and bone marrow autograft ; however without resulting in a decisive prolongation of survival (for example : median survival of 12 months in [8], to 16.4 months in [9].

Cystemustine is a third generation 2 chloroethyl nitrosourea ($CMSO_2EN_2$) ; metabolite of the sulphur-containing nitrosourea CNCC. It has showed a high anti-tumour activity against a variety of murine tumors (i.p. or i.c. grafted L1210 leukemia, in ascitic form and solid tumor s.c. implanted in mice, such as well as B16 melanoma, glioma, Lewis lung, and colon carcinomas).

On the basis of its toxicological and pharmacological properties in various animal species, a phase I clinical trial was done in ICIG (Villejuif, France) [6].

During this phase I trial, two clinical responses were observed : one glioma and one soft tissue sarcoma. Since 1990, a phase II trial has been conducted by the Clinical Screening Group of the EORTC, to assess the antitumoral activity of Cystemustine in malignant gliomas and other tumoral localizations.

For the EORTC Cooperative Clinical Screening Group
From : Centre Jean Perrin*, F 63011 Clermont-Ferrand Cedex 1 ; Centre Claudius Regaud**, F 31052 Toulouse Cedex ; Centre Oscar Lambret***, F 59020 Lille Cedex ; Centre Georges-François Leclerc****, F 21034 Dijon Cedex ; Centre Hospitalier R.T. Laënnec*****, F 29107 Quimper ; Institut Jean Godinot******, F 51056 Reims Cedex ; Centre Alexis Vautrin*******, F 54511 Vandoeuvre-lès-Nancy Cedex ; EORTC Data Center********, B 12000 Bruxelles ; Centre René Gauducheau*********, F 44805 Saint-Herblain Cedex ; Centre Henri Becquerel**********, F 76038 Rouen Cedex

Patients and methods

Twenty patients with histologically confirmed and recurrent measurable malignant grade III or IV astrocytoma or glioma (WHO classification) were included in this trial at the time of recurrence.

Patients characteristics are summarized in Table 1. The therapeutic regimen consisted of an i.v. infusion of 60 mg/sq.m. every 2 weeks.

Table 1. Patient characteristics

	No of patients
Entered	20
Evaluted	15
Males/Feamles	14/6
OMS performance status : grade 0	6
grade 1	10
grade 2	4
Histology : glioblastoma	6
astrocytoma	12
oligodendroglioma	2
Previous radiotherapy	15
Previous chemotherapy	4
Previous nitrosoureas	1

Cystemustine was administered i.v. over 15 minutes in 5 per cent glucose. Prior to initial treatment and every 2 weeks, patients received a general medical assessment, and had routine hematological, hepatic and renal function tests. Measurement of appropriate targets was performed by CT scan before the third and fifth courses, then at least every 3 months.

Cortico steroid treatment was allowed when clinically necessary, but tumoral evaluation had to be done after onset of steroid administration. Assessment of responses has been submitted to external advice of 2 specialized experts [Pr Meder and Dr Borel].

Results

Fifteen of the 20 patients could be evaluated for response (5 too early).

Response rate according to the WHO classification was 4 objective responses (1 PR : 90 %, 2 PR > 50 per cent, 1 PR 40 %), 5 stabilizations $\geqslant$ 8 weeks (ST = 40 %) and 4 progressions (PD : 34 %) with 2 early progressions. Median duration of response was 19.5 weeks (4.8 months) (range 6-32). The > 50 % response rate was 20 % (confidence interval 3.8 − 43.4 %). The subcomplete response was delayed with regards to normal evaluation after 4 courses (2 months of treatment) and obtained after hematological toxicity indicating end of the protocol for this patient ; then treatment was resumed for a total duration of 12 Months and a cumulative dose of 1.735 mg of Cystemustine in 15 courses.

Toxic effects were fully evaluated in the 18 patients ; they were limited to hematological toxicity, consisting of cumulative thrombocytopenia (12.5 % grade 3 and 4) and neutropenia (25 % grade 3 and 4) (Table 2). Hematological toxicity was always reversible and no patient died of toxic effects ; no febrile aplasia did occur. Non-hematological toxicity (WHO grading) was mild : nausea and vomiting (2 grade 1, 2 grade 2) ; diarrhea (1 grade 1) ; alopecia (1 grade 1) ; hepatic toxicity (1 grade 1) ; neurotoxicity (1 grade 1) ; asthenia (2 grade 1). No grade 3 or 4 extra-hematological toxicity was observed. Nine patients left study for progression ; 3 for hematological toxicity and 3 for end of treatment period. Nine patients were responders or stabilized for at least 2 months (60 % of the evaluated patients). Four patients died after a survival greater than 12 months after onset of Cystemustine, and 5 are still alive as of February 1st, 1993.

Table 2. Nadir distribution in 20 glioma patients at 60 mg/sq.m

	WHO grading				
	0	1	2	3	4
Leukocytes (%)	8 (50.0)	2 (12.5)	5 (31.2)	1 (65.2)	—
Neutrophils (%)	10 (62.5)	1 (6.2)	1 (6.2)	3 (18.7)	1 (6.2)
Platelets (%)	11 (68.7)	1 (6.2)	2 (6.2)	1 (6.2)	1 (6.2)

Discussion

We report here the preliminary results of a phase II study of 18 patients with recurrent evaluable malignant gliomas who have been treated at the time of recurrence with a new nitrosourea : Cystemustine.

The objective response rate was 20 % and was very encouraging with regards to :

1. the comparable response rate of most employed nitrosoureas, to confirm in a greater number of patients [4, 5] ;

2. most of the patients (9 out of 15) were in response or at least objectively stable during this treatment period (60 %) ;

3. the best response (90 %) was obtained in a patient who had failed from a previous « adjuvant » chemotherapy with BCNU, showing an absence of cross resistance with Cystemustine ;

4. with its limited toxicity, easily controlled, Cystemustine seemed to have clinical activity and would be suitable for treatment of recurrent malignant gliomas ;

5. median survival of patients was greater than 12 months before Cystemustine ; at least some of them seemed to have a survival benefit with this well tolerated treatment.

References

1. Edwards MS, Levin VA, Wilson CB (1980) Brain tumor chemotherapy : an evaluation of agents in current use for phase II and III trials. Cancer Treat Rep 12 : 1179-1205
2. Poisson M, Pouillart P, Pertuiset BF (1927) La chimiothérapie des glioblastomes. Encyclopédie Médico-Chirurgicale — Neurologie, 17305, B10, 6
3. Malkin MG, Shapiro WR (1987) Brain tumors. In : Pinedo HM (ed) Cancer chemotherapy and biological response modifier annual 9. Elsevier Science Publishers, Chapter 25, p 377-389
4. Kornblith PL, Walker M (1988) Review article. Chemotherapy for malignant gliomas. J Neurosurg 68 : 1-17
5. Jelsma R, Bucy PC (1967) The treatment of glioblastoma of the brain. J Neurol Neurosurg Psychiatry 27 : 388-400
6. Mathé G, Misset JL, Triana K, Godeneche D, Madelmont JC, Meyniel G (1992) Phase I trial of Cystemustine, a new cysteamine (2 chloroethyl) nitrosourea : an intrapatient escalation schema. Drugs under Experimental and Clinical Research, XVIII (4) : 155-158
7. Biron P, Mornex F, Vial C, Chauvrin F, Philip I, Philip T (1987) Etude pilote associant chirurgie, BCNU haute dose, puis autogreffe de moelle et radiothérapie dans les gliomes. Bull Cancer 74 : 726
8. Veysseyre M (1990) Gliomes malins sus-tentoriels de l'adulte : association de la chirurgie, du BCNU haute dose suivi d'autogreffe de moelle osseuse, et de radiothérapie. A propos de 98 cas. Thèse de Médecine, Lyon, n° 65
9. Van Praagh I (1991) La chimiothérapie intensive des gliomes malins de haut grade de l'adulte. Thèse de Médecine, Clermont-Ferrand (7 juin)

Abstract. From January 1990 to November 1992, 20 patients with recurrent gliomas have been enrolled into a phase II trial testing a new nitrosourea : Cystemustine (CYST). The drug was given every 2 weeks at 60 mg/sq.m. as an I.V. 15 minutes infusion. All eligible patients were considered evaluable for response and toxicity (WHO criterias). Pathological diagnosis at inclusion were malignant gliomas and grade 3 or 4 astrocytomas (WHO classification). All patients had relapsed after radiotherapy ; 1 had also a high-dose « adjuvant » chemotherapy with BCNU and medullar autografting. Out of the 20 enrolled, 0 were ineligible and 5 too early, leaving 15 fully evaluable patients. One subcomplete and 3 partial responses have been obtained ; giving an overall greater than 50 % response rate of 20 % on evaluated patients (3 glioblastomas, 1 grade 3 astrocytoma) ; however this trial is still going on. Six patients were stable or had a minor response leaving only 6 progressions. It is interesting to make evident that the subcomplete response has been obtained in the patient previously irradiated and autografted after BCNU, showing an evident absence of cross resistance with this compound. The duration of the subcom-

plete response has been 8 months, and the overall survival of this patient with glioma is now 26+ months. Toxicity was mild and concerned mainly neutropenia (25 % grade 3 and 4) and thrombopenia (12.5 % grade 3 and 4). No other major toxicity was detected. Five patients are still under study, 13 have finished their treatment. In conclusion, Cystemustine seems to have clinical activity on recurrent gliomas, to confirm on a higher number of patients.

Age effect on the survival of patients with glioblastoma and anaplastic astrocytoma

J Hildebrand, The EORTC Brain Tumour Group

Several prognostic factors have emerged from number of phase-III-type studies testing various adjuvant treatments in adults with supratentorial malignant gliomas (SMG) [1, 2]. The most consistently found are : *pathology* (glioblastoma having the shortest survival), *age and neurological status*. Also important are extend of *tumour resection* [3, 4, 5], presence of *seizures* and *frontal* tumour location [7, 8, 9].

In this paper, we have analysed separately the survival curves in patients with glioblastoma (GB) or anaplastic astrocytoma (AA) enroled in 4 consecutive studies performed by the EORTC BTG [7, 8, 9, 10], in order to answer the following questions :
— How reproducible are the survival curves in consecutive studies for the 2 tumour types ?
— Is age an equally potent prognostic factor in GB and AA ?

Patients and treatments

Seven hundred eighty-three adults bearing SMG, included in 4 consecutive trials were analysed regardless to the adjuvant chemotherapy received since none affected the survival as compared to controls, treated by 60 Gy cranial irradiation. The adjuvant treatment consisted in :

a) VM-26, 60 mg/sqm on day 1 plus CCNU 130 mg/sqm on day 2, repeated every 6 weeks and initiated concomitantly to radiation therapy in the trial 26751 or,

b) the same treatment given in 3 courses before irradiation in trial 26841,

c) Misonidazole 1.3 g/sqm given during 9 first sessions of 350 cGy radiation therapy in trial 26801,

d) Cisplatin 60 mg given on days 1, 8, 15 and 22 of radiation therapy in trial 26851. 424 patients had GB (54 %) and 249 had AA (32 %).

The pathology of all tumours was based on the diagnosis of the same reviewer : Prof. JM Brucher.

Results

GB patients

The survival curves were almost identical in the 4 trials (Fig. 1a). The median survival for the whole group of 424 GB patients was 46 weeks with a 95 %

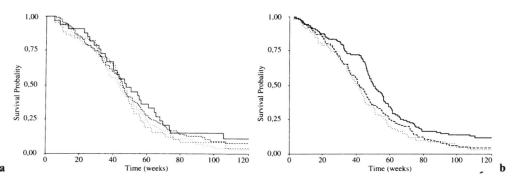

Fig. 1a. Survival curves for glioblastoma patients in four studies :
: trial 26751   : trial 26801   : trial 26841   : trial 26851

Fig. 1b. Survival curves for glioblastoma patients according to age :
: < 50 years   : 51 to 59 years   : > 60 years

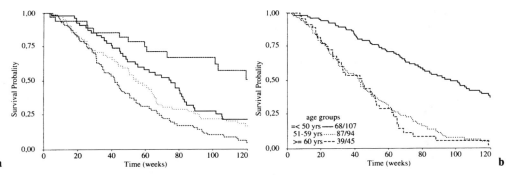

Fig. 2a. Survival curves for anaplastic astrocytoma patients in four studies :
: trial 26751   : trial 26801   : trial 26841   : trial 26851

Fig. 2b. Survival curves for anaplastic astrocytoma according to age :
: < 50 years   : 51 to 59 years   : > 60 years

confidence interval of 44 to 48 weeks. The median percentage of survivors for the whole group was 12 % at 18, and 7 % at 24 months, and it was fairly reproducible from 1 trial to another.

Patients under 50 years had longer median survival (Fig. 1b). However, although statistically significant, the difference as compared to the group aged 51 to 59 or over 60 years, was of only 8 and 9 weeks respectively.

AA patients

Unlike in GB patients the median survival and the survival curves (Fig. 2a) differed considerably from 1 trial to another.

The median survival for the whole group of 249 patients was 58 weeks with a 95 % confidence interval of 50 to 66 weeks. The median percentage of survivors for the whole group was 35 % at 18 and 25 % at 24 months, and likewise the survival curves, the median survival varied considerably from 1 study to another.

Patients aged 51 to 59 and over 60 years had similar survival curves but younger patients (Fig. 2b) had a considerably better prognosis since 61 % were alive at 18 months, and 47 % at 2 years.

Discussion

The present analysis shows that as a prognostic factor age does not affect equally GB and AA patients, although in both tumour types patients under 50 years survive statistically longer.

In GB group, however, the difference in median survival between younger and older patients was less than 20 %. The modest effect on survival of a very potent prognostic factor such as age possibly accounts for the remarkably stable survival curves, and percentage of survivor at 18 and 24 months, observed in 4 consecutive studies for patients with GB.

In contrast, in AA group, the median survival was more than twice longer in younger individuals as compared to patients aged 51 to 59 years or older. In patients with AA, survival curves observed in various trials, and percentage of long-term survivors correlated with the proportion of individuals under 50 years.

Thus AA patients under 50 have a much better prognosis as compared to other groups of patients with SMG.

Because of the growing concern raised by the increased number of dementia reported in long-term survivor after radiation therapy [11] and possibly concomitant chemotherapy, these findings may have implications in planning future trials, particularly those testing adjuvant therapies. One such a precaution could be the avoidance of concomitant use of adjuvant radiation and chemotherapy in younger patients with AA.

Another rationale for treating separately GB and AA is that the latter are possibly more sensitive to chemotherapy, notably to the combination of Procarbazine, CCNU, and Vincristine [12].

References

1. Byar DP, Breen SB, Strike TA (1983) Prognostic factors for malignant glioma. In : Walker MD (ed) Oncology of the Nervous System. Martinus Nyhoff, Boston, pp. 379-395
2. Hildebrand J, Delecluse F (1986) Malignant glioma in randomized trials in Cancer. In : Slavin ML and Staquet MJ (eds). Raven Press, New York, pp. 583-604
3. Ammirati M, Vick N, Liao YL, Ciric J, Mikhael M (1987) Effect of the extent of surgical resection on survival and quality of life in patients with supratentorial glioblastomas and anaplastic astrocytomas. Neurosurgery 21 : 201-206

4. Vecht CJ, Avezaat CJ, van Putten WLJ, Eijkenboom WMH, Stefanko SZ (1990) The influence of the extent of surgery on the neurological function and survival in malignant glioma. A retrospective analysis in 243 patients. J Neurol Neurosurg Psychiatry 53 : 466-471
5. Wood JR, Green SB, Shapiro WR (1988) The prognostic importance of tumour size in malignant gliomas : A computed tumographic scan study by the Brain Tumor Cooperative Group. J Clin Oncol 6 : 338-343
6. Smith DF, Hutton JL, Sanderman D, Foy PM, Shaw MDM, Williams IR, Chadwick DW (1991) The prognosis of primary intracerebral tumours presenting with epilepsy : The outcome of medical and surgical management. J Neurol Neurosurg Psy 54 : 915-920
7. EORTC Brain Tumour Group (1981) Evaluation of CCNU, VM-26, plus CCNU and procarbazine in supratentorial brain. J Neurosurg 55 : 27-31
8. EORTC Brain Tumour Group (1983) Misonidazole in radiotherapy of supratentorial malignant gliomas in adult patients : A randomized double-blind study. Eur J Cancer Clin Oncol 19 : 39-42
9. EORTC Brain Tumour Group (1991) Cisplatin does not enhance the effect of radiation therapy in malignant gliomas. Eur J Cancer 27 : 568-571
10. EORTC Brain Tumour Group (1987) Randomized comparison of radiotherapy versus VM-26 plus CCNU followed by radiotherapy in the treatment of supratentorial malignant brain gliomas in adult patients. Abstracts 15th International Congress of Chemotherapy, Istanbul
11. Imperato JP, Paleologos NA, Vick NA (1990) Effects of treatment on long-term survivors with malignant astrocytomas. Ann Neurol 28 : 818-822
12. Levin VA, Silver P, Hannigan J et al (1990) Superiority of post-radiotherapy adjuvant chemotherapy with CCNU, Procarbazine and Vincristine (PCV) and BCNU for anaplastic gliomas : NCOG 6G61. Final report. Int J Radiat Oncol Phys Biol 18 : 321-324

Concurrent radiochemotherapy in high-grade glioma

A Brandes*, P Zampieri**, A Rigon***, E Scelzi*, M Pignatarox***, F Berti***, A Rotilio**, A Padoan**, P Amistà****, A Paccagnella*, MV Fiorentino*

The prognosis of patients with malignant glioma is generally poor in spite of the progress that has been made in neurosurgery and radiotherapy of these tumors.

The average survival time after extensive resection of the tumor is 6-10 months, the 1 year survival rate is 30 %, while the 2 years rate is about 10 %. Complete remission or partial remission of the tumors is relatively rare after the exclusive application of radiation. Postoperative radiotherapy has increased the median survival from 6 months to 10 months and chemotherapy has improved these results which reached 12 to 14 months [1].

These disappointing results have induced us to explore a new combination. First : early use of a cytotoxic to favor log-kill during fast regrowth with the most active agent : BCNU. Second : concurrent radiochemotherapy. The rationale of this combination is that : 1) different cell lines are both attacked by radiation and chemotherapy ; 2) chemotherapy followed by radiation therapy decreases tumor cell regrowth ; 3) it increases G0 recruitment to a more susceptible cell cycle phase ; 4) repair inhibition due to sub-lethal radiation damage or recovery inhibition from potentially lethal radiation damage [2]. Cisplatin was useful in radiochemotherapy, but the use of Carboplatin carries the additional advantage of greater platinum concentration in free solution within cells at the time of irradiation, since Carboplatin is less toxic than Cisplatin, and thus has greater possibility for radiation potentiation [3]. Moreover, Carboplatin is synergistic with Epidophilotoxines [4] and among these the Teniposide (VM 26) is probably more active [5]. We decided not to deliver more than 2 cycles of BCNU because of the known phenomenon of early drug resistance.

Patients and methods

Eligibility

The characteristics of patients are summarised in Table 1. Twenty-one patients with high grade gliomas were entered into the study protocol. Patients were required to have 1) histologic diagnosis of AA or GB ; 2) Age 18 to 70 ; 3) Karnofsky Performance Status (KPS) ≥ 50 ; 4) adequate bone marrow

---

* Oncology Unit
** Neurosurgery Unit
*** Radiotherapy Unit
**** Neuroradiology Unit Oncology Center, Padua, Italy

reserve (WBC count ⩾ 3.000 and platelet count ⩾ 100.000) normal baseline liver (serum bilirubin level < 1.5 mg/dl) renal (serum creatinine level < 1.5), and cardiac function).

Table 1. Patients characteristics

Total	21 pts
Male/female	14/7
Median age (range)	49 (23-70)
Median Karnofsky Index (range)	70 (50-80)
Histologic Subtypes	
AA :	8 (38 %)
GB :	13 (61 %)

Response criteria

All evaluations were done by a multidisciplinary team including a neuroradiologist, oncologist, neurosurgeon, radiotherapist. Complete response (CR) : disappearance of all enhanced tumor on consecutive CT or magnetic resonance imaging (MRI) scans at least 1 month apart, off steroids and neurologically stable or improved. Partial response (PR) : ⩾ 50 % reduction in size of enhanced tumor on consecutive CT or MRI scans at least 1 month apart, steroids stable or reduced and neurologically stable or improved. Progressive disease (PD) : ⩾ 25 % increase in size of enhanced tumor or any new tumor on CT or MRI scans, or neurologically worse and stereoids stable or increased.

Stable disease (SD) : all other situations [5].

A CT scan was performed within 48 hours after surgery, before radiochemotherapy, 60 days later and after every 3 months or when clinical consideration required.

Study design

Surgery as extensive as possible.

BCNU 150 mg/m^2 9 days after surgery and 30 days later, radiotherapy 1.8 - 2 Gy/day for 5 days a week on limited fields is started up to 60 Gy with simultaneous chemotherapy with Carboplatin 200 mg/m^2 on days 1, 22, 43 and VM26 50 mg/m^2 days 1, 2, 3, 22, 23, 24, 43, 44, 45. BCNU 150 mg/m^2 is repeated for 2 cycles after 30 and 70 days from the end of the radiochemotherapy course. Dose reduction : on the recycling day the dose was reduced to 75 %, if wbc were 3.500-4.000 or platelets 100.000-140.000 ; the dose was reduced to 50 % if the wbc were 3.000-3.500 and platelets 80.000-100.000.

Results

Twenty-one patients completed the treatment and we obtained 8 PR (38 %)

(2 of these with more than 80 % reduction) and 10 SD (41 %). Three patients progressed. The Kaplan Meyer Median TTP was 37.4 wks for the entire group : 55.8 wks for AA and 30 wks for GB. Global MST was 59 wks : 55 wks for GB and 70 for AA. In AA 100 % were alive at 12 months and 60 % at 18 months ; in GB 63 % and 23 % were alive respectively at 12 and 18 months.

Table 2. Results

Entered	21
Partial Remission	8 (38 %)
Stable Disease	10 (47 %)
Median Time To Progression	37.4
AA :	55.8
GB :	30
Median Survival Tima (wks)	59
AA :	70
GB :	55
Alive at 18 months	30 %
AA :	60 %
GB :	23 %

Toxicity

We observed haematological toxicity WHO grade 1 in 5 patients ; grade 2 in 1 patient ; grade 3 in 1 patient. Neurological G3 toxicity in 1 patient. We did not observe gastrointestinal toxicity.

We reduced the BCNU dose to 75 % in 3 cycles and to 50 % in 3 other cycles ; Carboplatin was reduced to 75 % in 6 cycles and to 50 % in 4 other cycles.

Discussion

Yung et al [7] have reported a study with alternating BCNU and Cisplatin plus radiotherapy in malignant glioma. He obtained in 33 patients 82 % Global Response (33 % PR + 49 % SD), a TTP of 34.5 wks and a Global MST of 76 wks : 55 for GB and 110 for AA. In our study we obtained a similar rate of response and Kaplan Meyer Median TTP. Our Global MST is slightly lower for AA and similar for GB but at recurrence our behaviour was less aggressive.

Most patients tolerated the concurrent chemoradiotherapy well : no gastrointestinal complications were seen, haematological toxicity was mild. The superiority of the concurrent modality treatment can only be proven in a prospective randomized trial.

References

1. Brandes A, Soesan M, Fiorentino M (1991) Medical Treatment in high grade malignant gliomas in adults : an ovierview. Anticancer Res 11 : 719-728
2. Vokes EE, Wechselbaum R (1990) Concomitant chemoradiotherapy : rationale and clinical experience in patients with solid tumors. J Clin Oncol 8 : 911-934
3. Coughlin CT, Richmond RC (1989) Biologic and clinical developments of Cisplatin combined with radiation : concepts, utility, projections for new trials, and the emergence of Carboplatin. Sem in Oncol 16 : 31-43
4. Durand RE, Goldie JH (1987) Interaction of Etoposide and Cisplatin in an *in Vitro* Tumor Model. Cancer Treat Rep 71 : 673-679
5. Spremulli E, Schulz JJ, Speckart VJ (1980) Phase II study of VM-26 in adult malignancies. Cancer Treat Rep 64 : 147
6. McDonald DR, Cascino TL, Clifford S (1990) Response criteria for phase II studies of supratentorial malignant glioma. J Clin Oncol 8 : 1277-1280
7. Yung WKA, Janus TJ, Maor M et al (1992) Adjuvant chemotherapy with Carmustine and Cisplatin for patients with malignant gliomas. J Neuro Oncol 12 : 131-135

Interferon-α-2b + fotemustine in disseminated malignant melanoma

L Kowalzick*, P Mohr*, M Weichenthal*, H Langenbahn**, DK Hossfeld***, EW Breitbart*

Metastatic malignant melanoma has a poor prognosis with a median duration of survival of 1 to 14 months depending on the site of metastasis [1]. There is no established treatment for patient with disseminated malignant melanoma (DMM), the drug of reference is Dacarbazine with a response rate of 20 % [2]. In a study with 153 patients with DMM fotemustine was shown to be effective with an overall response rate of 24.2 %, including 25 % of cerebral lesions [3]. In our own hands, 33 patients with DMM showed an overall response of 27.3 % [4]. Interferon (IFN)-α was studied with various protocols in patients with DMM, the overall response rate ranging between 19 and 27 % [5, 6]. Because side effects of both therapies are comparable low and the mechanisms of action and the toxicities are different, we conducted a study with a combination of IFN-α-2b and fotemustine in patients with DMM in order to examine its possible additive or synergistic therapeutic effect.

Patients and methods

In this open phase II study 25 patients with DMM were included after informed consent. Included were only patients with an ECOG score ≤ 2, a life expectancy of ≥ 3 months, at least one measurable lesion, progression before less than 2 months, normal blood cell counts and normal liver and kidney values. Excluded were patients with pregnancy, other prior or concomitant malignancy except for basal cell carcinoma and *in situ* cervix carcinoma, uncontrolled infection or other severe condition e.g. autoimmune disease or recent myocardial infarction. We included 11 male and 14 female patients, the median age was 55 years (range 30 to 76), and with the following metastatic sites : 9 skin/soft tissue, 11 lymph node, 17 lung, 10 visceral, 1 bone and 2 brain. 15 patients had a limited (skin/soft tissue, lymph node or lung metastases only) and 10 an extended disease. After staging including chest X-ray, abdominal US-scan, abdominal and cerebral CT-scan, bone scintigraphy and skin/lymph node US-scan, treatment was begun as follows : IFN-α-2b (Intron-A®, Essex-Pharma, Munich, FRG) was given at a dose of 10 million international units (MU) by s.c. injection at days 1, 3, 5, 8, 10, 12, 15, 17 and 19. Fotemustine (Muphoran®, Servier, Courbevoie, France) was given at a dose of 100 mg/m² by i.v. infusion at days 8, 15 and 22. Under this regimen weekly controls of

---

Departments of Dermatology* and Hematology & Oncology***, University of Hamburg, D-2000 Hamburg 20, Martinistr. 52 and Servier Forschung und Pharma-Entwicklung GmbH Munich**, D-8000 München 21, Westendstr. 195, Germany

blood cell counts, liver enzymes and kidney values were performed. After a 5 week rest period, response evaluation was performed by another staging examination. If stabilization or response of the disease could be stated, patients received maintenance therapy consisting of 10 MU IFN 3 days a week for 1 week, followed by 1 administration of 100 mg/m^2 3 days later. This cycle was repeated every 4 weeks until progression or complete response ocurred, assesed by response evaluations every 2 months.

Toxicity and clinical responses were scored according to WHO criteria.

Results

Of the 25 patients with DMM treated 3 had complete responses (CR), 5 partial responses (PR), 4 a stable disease (SD) and 13 showed progressive disease. The overall response rate was 32 %. The 10 patients with extensive disease showed an overall response rate of 20 % (1 CR + 1 PR). The median duration of response is at least 6 months. Side effects were relatively low, all treatments could be performed on an outdoor basis : Anemia was observed in 22 %, leukopenia in 61 %, thrombopenia in 26 %, nausea in 39 %, liver-toxicity in 30 % and fever in 52 % of our patients. Toxicities were mostly WHO grade 1 and 2, only 1 event of WHO grade 4 (thrombopenia) was observed.

Discussion

Interferons have antiviral, antiproliferative and immunomodulating effects [7]. Several therapies combining IFN-α and cytostatic drugs have been performed in DMM with different clinical results ranging between 6 % and 39 % overall responses [8, 9]. In the present study IFN-α-2b was combined with fotemustine. Although the number of included patients is yet too low to declose significance, this regimen might be superior to fotemustine monotherapy (32 % v.s. 25 % overall response rate). This result is in contrast to that of a recent study [10] which combined fotemustine and IFN-α-2b in a different manner. In this protocol fotemustine was administered daily at a dose of 100 mg/m^2 on days 1 and 8, followed by 9 MU IFN-α-2a daily from day 9 to 22. The clinical outcome of this regimen was very disappointing with no observed responses, so that this study was discontinued after 10 included patients. This discrepance may be of importance in that the administration sequence of IFN and a chemotherapeutic agent might be crucial for the clinical efficacy for this and for other combined therapies. In conclusion, the combination of IFN-α-2b and fotemustine resulted in encouraging clinical response rates when the IFN is administered first. Further analysis of differentially sequenced treatment schemes combining IFN and cytostatic drugs seem requestable.

References

1. Amer MN, Al-Safaraf M, Vaitkevicus VK (1979) Clinical presentation, natural history and prognostic factors in advanced melanoma. Surg Gynecol Obstet 149 : 168
2. Luce JK, Thurman WG, Isaacs BL (1970) Clinical trials with the antitumor agent 5-(3.3-dimetyl-1-triazeno) imidazole-4-carboxamide. Cancer Chemother Rep 54 : 119-124
3. Jaquillat C, Khayat D, Banzet P (1989) Final report of the phase II study of the nitrosourea fotemustine in 153 evaluable patients with disseminated malignant melanoma including brain metastases. American Association for Cancer Research, San Francisco, Volume of Abstracts : 273
4. Mohr P, Weichenthal M, Altenhoff J (1992) Systemic chemotherapy with fotemustine in stage IV malignant melanoma. Arch Dermatol Res 284 : 19
5. Creagan ET, Ahmann DL, Frytak S (1987) Three consecutive phase II studies of recombinant Interferon-α-2a in advanced malignant melanoma : updated analyses. Cancer 59 : 638-646
6. Dorval T, Palangie T, Jouve M (1986) Clinical phase II trial of recombinant DNA Interferon-α-2b in patients with metastatic malignant melanoma. Cancer 58 : 215-218
7. Kirkwood JM, Ernstoff MS (1986) Potential applications of the interferons in oncology : lessons from the studies on malignant melanoma. Sem Oncol 13 (suppl 2) : 48-56
8. Kerr R, Pippen P, Mennel R (1989) Treatment of metastatic malignant melanoma with a combination of Interferon-α-2a and Dacarbazine. Proc Am Soc Clin Oncol 8 : 1122
9. Vorobiof DA, Falkson G, Voges CW (1989) DTIC versus DTIC and recombinant Interferon-α-2b in the treatment of patients with advanced malignant melanoma. Proc Am Soc Clin Oncol 8 : 1105
10. Civatte J, Avril MF, Bizarri JP (1991) Fotemustine, a new drug for metastatic malignant melanoma. III. International Dermatology Symposium, Berlin, 5-7 July

Tamoxifen-augmented biochemotherapy (Interferon-α-2b, Tamoxifen, BCNU, CDDP, DTIC) for malignant melanoma

H Voigt, R Claßen, J Ramaker

Depending on the metastatic pattern involved, therapeutic approaches in metastatic malignant melanoma are primarily focused on the surgical reduction of tumor masses (if solitary or operable) and palliation of disseminated disease. Despite major efforts to improve the efficacy of cytotoxic drug regimens, longterm survival or even cure is usually almost unfeasible once dissemination of disease has commenced. However, the administration of biomodulatory and/or immunomodulatory compounds has prompted broad investigational efforts since it had been demonstrated that neoplastic tumor growth can be modulated. Among others, the anti-hormonal agent Tamoxifen (TAM) has manifold biological properties that are approached to be exploited in cancer therapy [1]. Previous reports on combination therapy together with cytotoxic agents revealed promising palliative results exceeding those obtained by cytotoxic treatment only [8-12]. The investigational ITBCD protocol described here deals with sequential combination of TAM together with Interferon-α-2b preceding cytotoxic combination chemotherapy consisting of BCNU, DTIC, and Cisplatin. The modalities used are arranged sequentially (phase 1-3) and superimposed synergistically thus exerting overlapping biological effects (phase 1 : « Induction » ; phase 2 : « Priming » ; phase 3 : « Cytotoxic »). They are outlined to pharmacodynamically prime melanoma metastasis and thus augment the efficacy of cytotoxic compounds used.

Methods

The ITBCD treatment schedule is shown in Table 1. Pts were considered eligible if they had progressive, histologically proven advanced/metastatic malignant melanoma, measurable disease, expected life span > 3 m, and if they had given written informed consent.

Results

Since December 1991, a total number of 14 pts had been entered. Sex distribution M/F was 5/6, median age was 46 years. Four out of 14 pts had been pretreated with cytotoxic chemotherapy (DTIC n = 4, DTIC + Vindesine = 1). Eleven pts completed at least 2 cycles of ITBCD biochemotherapy and were

Melanoma Research Project, P.O. Box 1441, D-2358 Kaltenkirchen, Germany

Table 1.

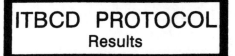

#	INITIALS	AGE	SEX	SITES	PRETREATMENT	RESPONSE	DURATION	STATUS
1	M.H.	70 yrs	M	Lungs, Skin, Nodes	NO	PR	11m+	ALIVE: WITH DISEASE (PD)
2	W.S.	36 yrs	W	Skin, Nodes, Skeleton	NO	MR	6m+	ALIVE: WITH DISEASE
3	H.A.	67 yrs	W	Lungs, Liver	NO	SD	4m+	ALIVE: WITH DISEASE
4	J.S.	21 yrs	M	Lungs, Skin	NO	CR	6m	DEAD: PD
5	L.R.	74 yrs	W	Lungs, Skin	NO	PR	9m+	ALIVE: WITH DISEASE (NC)
6	P.M.	46 yrs	W	Nodes, Mucous Membrane	YES: DTIC	PR	10m+	ALIVE: NED AFTER RE-SURGERY
7	P.H.	31 yrs	M	Skin, Skeleton, Spleen	YES: DTIC	PR	10m	DEAD: PD
8	W.K.	45 yrs	M	Lungs, Nodes	YES: DTIC	SD	4m+	ALIVE: WITH DISEASE
9	B.W.	53 yrs	M	Lungs, Skin, Liver	NO	PD	...	ALIVE: WITH DISEASE (PD)
10	P.I.	53 yrs	W	Skin, Nodes	NO	MR	10m+	ALIVE: NED AFTER RE-SURGERY
11	H.B.	30 yrs	W	Skin, Nodes, Brain	YES: DTIC+VDS	PD	...	DEAD: PD

Melanoma Research Project

Table 2.

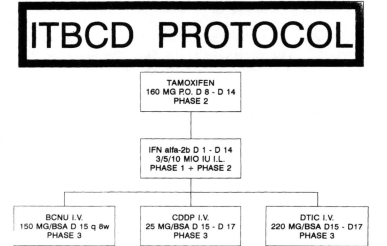

Melanoma Research Project

thus considered evaluable for response and toxicity. Preliminary response data are summarized in Table 2. Toxicity encountered was acceptable and mainly hematologic, but not exceeding WHO 2 except for thrombocytopenia. Neither bleeding nor thromboembolism occurred.

Discussion

On account of its anti-hormonal activity, Tamoxifen (TAM) has found its place within the adjuvant and palliative treatment setting for breast cancer. Recent preclinical research has additionally emerged data revealing that Tamoxifen exerts various biological effects on neoplastic tissues that can be utilized for chemosensitizing of resistant solid tumors other than breast cancer. TAM and its main metabolite, N-desmethyltamoxifen, are potent inhibitors of the protein kinase C (PKC). It binds to calmodulin thus inhibiting cell proliferation [1]. TAM was also found to have calcium-channel blocking properties thus providing higher target cell exposure to cytotoxic agents [2]. Similarly, high-dose levels of TAM are supposed to reverse multidrug resistance (MDR) through binding to membrane-bound p170 glycoprotein [3]. At the molecular level, further pharmacodynamic interactions have been identified, impacting on subcellular detoxification mediators (e.g. topoisomerase II, glutathione-S-transferase). Moreover, recent biopharmacologic investigations have demonstrated that the antiproliferative activity of TAM can be enhanced by Interferons, which might be attributed to its impact on cell surface marker expression, tumor cell immunogenicity, and NK cell activity [4-6].

Clinically, TAM has so far failed to demonstrate valuable activity in metastatic malignant melanoma [7]. When TAM had been given in combination with the cytotoxic agents BCNU, DTIC, and Cisplatin, 55 % of 20 pts initially treated were reported to respond, 20 % of them completely [8]. Later studies on this 4-drug regimen confirmed the efficacy of TBCD, but when TAM was omitted, which had been the case on account of its thrombogenic potential, response rates dropped to 10 % [9]. Interestingly, readministration of TAM to the same regimen resulted in increasing response figures as had been described previously, suggesting that TAM impacts essentially on tumor cell susceptibility towards cytotoxic agents [10]. In order to reduce its thrombogenic potential, which had repeatedly been reported to evoke severe thromboembolic complications, a high-dose regimen using daily doses of 160 mg TAM orally for only 1 week instead of 20 mg over 4-6 weeks was introduced. It could be demonstrated that thromboembolic complications can be effectively reduced or even prevented with this schedule of administration [11]. In addition, TAM tissue levels are substantially increased by high-dose loading (« priming »), thus making the metastatic tissue and especially the often-involved subcutaneous tissue layer an ideal target for the cytotoxic approach [12, 13]. In the study presented here, Interferon-α-2b was administered simultaneously. If subcutaneous metastases were present and accessible, Interferon was given intralesionally (I.L.) thus providing high metastatic tissue uptake of both agents. Since TAM and Interferons were reported to share several biomodulatory and immunomodulatory properties and thus might act synergistically [14], the administration of Interferon was commenced at low dose levels which are known to be most effective to mediate immunomodulatory effects [15, 16]. Intralesional administration of Interferon means that it is applied both intratumorally and intralymphatically. Therefore, the effects mediated by I.L. administration of Interferon are targeted to the functional metastatic microenvironment and thus focused also on the migrating immunological effector cells as well as the migrating tumor cells evading the morphologically confined metastatic tissue. Clinically, this may result in higher responses surpassing the effects of Interferons applied systemically [17,18].

Although the results presented here are preliminary, the response rate obtained even in pretreated pts is encouraging. Despite the fact that optimal sequencing of the modalities comprised in this protocol has yet to be elucidated, prolongation of survival even with « controlled » metastatic disease appears to be achievable. Except for thrombocytopenia, which has to be monitored carefully, overall tolerance of the regimen was acceptable.

References

1. Buckley MMT, Goa KL (1989) Tamoxifen : A reappraisal of its pharmacodynamic and pharmacokinetic properties, and therapeutic use. Drugs 37 : 451-490
2. Greenberg D, Carpenter C, Messing R (1987) Calcium channel antagonist properties of the antineoplastic antiestrogen Tamoxifen in the PC12 neurosecretory cell line. Cancer Res 47 : 70-74
3. Kaye SB (1990) Reversal of multidrug resistance. Cancer Treat Rev 17 (suppl A) : 37-43
4. Sica G, Iacopino F, Robustelli della Cuna G (1988) Recombinant α-2b Interferon (intron A) modifies steroid receptor level, inhibits cell proliferation and promotes the antiproliferative activity of Tamoxifen in a human breast cancer cell line. 6th Med Congr Chemother (MOC), Taormina, Italy 1988, May 22-27
5. Van den Berg HW, Leahey WJ, Lynch M, Clarke R, Nelson J (1987) Recombinant human Interferon-α increases oestrogen receptor expression in human breast cancer cells (ZR-75-1) and sensitizes them to the anti-proliferative effects of Tamoxifen. Br J Cancer 55 : 255-257
6. Josui K, Abe O, Kubota T, Koh J, Yamada Y, Asanuma F (1990) Interferon-α increases estrogen receptors of human breast carcinoma xenografts in nude mouse and enhances the antiproliferative activity of Tamoxifen. J Cancer Res Clin Oncol 116 (Suppl) : 456
7. Creagan ET, Ingle JN, Ahmann DL, Green SJ (1982) Phase II study of high-dose Tamoxifen (NSC-180973) in patients with disseminated malignant melanoma. Cancer 49 : 1353-1354
8. Del Prete SA, Maurer LH, O'Donnell J, Jackson Forcier R, Le Marbre P (1984) Combination chemotherapy with Cisplatin, Carmustine, Dacarbazine and Tamoxifen in metastatic melanoma. Cancer Treat Rep 68 : 1403-1405
9. McClay EF, Mastrangelo MJ, Bellet RE (1987) Combination chemotherapy and hormonal therapy in the treatment of malignant melanoma. Cancer Treat Rep 71 : 465-469
10. McClay EF, Mastrangelo MJ, Sprandio JD, Bellet RE, Berd D (1989) The importance of Tamoxifen to a cisplatin-containing regimen in the treatment of metastatic melanoma. Cancer 63 : 1292-1295
11. Berd D, McLaughlin CJ, Hart E, Wiebe VJ, Mastrangelo MJ, Bellet RE, De Gregorio MW (1991) Short course high-dose Tamoxifen (TAM) with cytotoxic chemotherapy for metastatic melanoma. Proc ASCO 10, 291 : 1016
12. McClay EF, Albright K, Jones J, Christen R, Howell SB (1991) Modulation of Cisplatin (DDP) sensitivity by Tamoxifen (TAM) in human malignant melanoma. Proc ASCO 10, 191 : 1017
13. Voigt H, Claβen R, Ramaker J, Rauschning W (1993) Tamoxifen plasma and tissue concentrations during ITBCD biochemotherapy for metastatic melanoma (in preparation)
14. Epstein L, Benz CC, Doty E (1987) Synergistic antiproliferative effects of Interferon-α and Tamoxifen on human breast cancer cells in vitro. J Clin Res 35, 1 : P 196A

15. Edwards BS, Merritt JA, Fuhlbrigge RC, Borden EC (1985) Low doses of Interferon-α result in more effective clinical natural killer cell activation. J Clin Invest 75 : 1908-1913
16. Kirkwood JM (1991) Studies of Interferons in the therapy of melanoma. Sem Oncol 18 (suppl 7) : 83-90
17. Von Wussow P, Block B, Hartmann F, Deicher H (1988) Intralesional Interferon-α in advanced malignant melanoma. Cancer 61 : 1071-1074
18. Voigt H, Bassermann R (1991) Intralesional (I.L.) Interferon-α-2b (rIFN-α-2b) as adjunct to the palliative management for advanced malignant melanoma. 35th Ann Clin Conf & 24th Ann Spec Pathol Progr « Advances in the biology and clinical management of melanoma », Houston, Texas 1991, November 20-23

Abstract. Tamoxifen has been shown to exert various biological effects on neoplastic tissues (antiproliferative, anti-hormonal, calcium-channel blocking, MDR-modulation, receptor expression, etc.) utilizable in biologically targeted cancer therapy. Together with cytotoxic drugs, Tamoxifen essentially enhances primary tumor responses in melanoma therapy as had been originally demonstrated by DEL PRETE et al in 1984. Although the pharmacodynamic mechanisms involved have ot yet been clarified thus far, subsequent controlled trials on larger scales have meanwhile confirmed the high overall and complete response rates achievable thus underlining the essential contribution of Tamoxifen to the efficacy of cytotoxic regimens employed. The phase-oriented addition of intra-/perilesionally administered Interferon-α-2b at immunomodulatory doses (3-5 Mio IU/1w) preceding combined administration of antiproliferative doses (10 MIO IU/1w) together with HD-TAM (160 MG P.O.(1w) prior to cytotoxic chemotherapy (BCNU 150 MG/BSA I.V. D15 q 8w, CDDP 25 MG/BSA I.V. D15-D17 q 4w, DTIC 220 MG/BSA I.V. D15-D17 q 4w) has been piloted in a consecutive series of melanoma patients with measurable metastatic or inoperable melanoma. Tamoxifen pharmocokinetics both in the serum and tissue revealed enhanced accumulation of Tamoxifen and its main active metabolite desmethyltamoxifen in metastatic tissues (« priming »), thus providing effective biomodulation in view of the subsequent administration of cytotoxic chemotherapy. Preliminary results indicate a 60 % ORR with durable responses in median excess of 6 m even in heavily pretreated pts. Toxicity assessed in this preliminary series consisted of pronounced thrombocytopenia, but being manageable without bleeding events. Responses could be documented likewise in visceral and non-visceral sites, and even in pts with stable disease continuation of protocol treatment was feasible for > + 9 m still providing control of disease progression without critical toxicity. Median survival has not yet been reached so far, since continuation of protocol treatment is currently employed in responding/stabilized pts.

Locoregional treatment

Chemofiltration for locally advanced cancer

M Inbar*, M Gutman, S Chaitchik*, JM Klausner

Regionally advanced cancer (RAC) represents a common problem, especially when metastases are confined to the liver or pelvic area. Since most regionally advanced cancer are not usually amenable to surgical resection, attempts at local control include irradiation or chemotherapy. Systemic chemotherapy has a low therapeutic index, since dosage is limited by toxicity to normal tissues. To increase the therapeutic index of cytotoxic drugs (CD), loco-regional techniques were developed. Intra-arterial treatment with CD have only slightly increased the response rate, since the drug is still distributed systemically from the infused organ. Attempts to limit systemic toxicity by means of vascular isolation during intra-arterial delivery of CD led to the development of isolated limb perfusion. Obviously, it is difficult to implement this technique of isolation perfusion in the trunk or abdominal viscera due to the complexity of their blood supply.

Recently a method has been developed which enables the delivery of high-dose CD to organs such as the liver or pelvis, while reducing systemic toxicity by concomitant detoxification of the venous effluent of the infused organ by hemofiltration [1, 2].

Materials and methods

During the past 2 years, 25 patients (pts) underwent chemofiltration (CF). There were 14 females and 11 males. The average age was 64.5 years. Eleven pts had metastatic cancer confined to the liver, originating in the colon (5), rectum (2), breast (2), pancreas (1) and ovary (1). Fourteen pts had RAC confined to the pelvis : rectum (5), lymph node metastases of malignant melanoma (5), ovary (1), uterine cervix (1), vulva (1) and anus (1). Sixteen out of the 25 pts (65 %) had received previous systemic chemotherapy and had tumor progression.

Treatment protocol

Liver chemofiltration

An hepatic arterial catheter was placed angiographically (8 pts) or during laparotomy (3 pts). The tip of the arterial catheter was situated distal to the bifurcation of the gastroduodenal artery. A large bore (16 F) catheter was in-

---

Departments of Oncology* and Surgery « B », Tel Aviv Sourasky Medical Center, 6 Weizmann Street, Tel Aviv 64239, and the Faculty of Medicine, Tel Aviv University, Israel

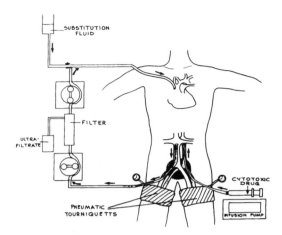

Fig. 1.

serted into the inferior *vena cava* via a cutdown in the saphenous vein (9 pts), femoral vein (1) or directly during laparotomy (1). Using fluoroscopic guidance, the tip of the catheter was positioned at the level of the diaphragm distal to the entrance of the hepatic veins. The venous catheter was then connected to a Gambro hemofiltration unit (Gambro, Lund, Sweden) using a 1.2 m^2 hollow tube filter. Blood was pumped out into the hemofiltration unit until a balanced hemofiltration was established. The filtered blood was returned to the superior *vena cava* via a large bore venous catheter. It was supplemented by preheated Ringers lactate solution infused at the same rate as the efflux of the ultrafiltrate. The anesthetized, fully heparinized pts were carefully monitored, and further fluid replacement was given to maintain normal hemodynamics. The CD was infused into the arterial catheter using an automatic infusion pump over 10-30 min, depending on the drug. After CD administration, CF was continued for an additional 30 min to ascertain further CD clearance.

Pelvic chemofiltration

An arterial catheter was angiographically placed in the aorta just distal to the renal arteries. The venous large bore catheter was inserted into the inferior *vena cava* via a saphenous cutdown (12 pts) or femoral venotomy (2 pts), its tip reaching the same level as the arterial catheter. Blood flow to both lower limbs was occluded using a pneumatic tourniquet (Fig. 1).

CD used included Mitomycine-C 30mg/m^2 and 5-FU 1 gr/m^2 for cancer of the colon, rectum, breast, pancreas and ovary ; Melphalanum 1.2 mg/kg or Cis-platinum 200 mg/m^2 for malignant melanoma, ovarian and uterine-cervix cancer ; and a combination of Bleomycin 50 mg/m^2, Cisplatinum 200 mg/m^2 and Mitomycine-C 20 mg/m^2 for vulvar cancer. Response rates were evaluated according to the UICC.

Results

All pts successfully completed CF of the liver (11) or pelvis (14). Two pts underwent a second CF of the liver (1) and pelvis (1). The average ultrafiltration was 11.500 ml. Despite the extensive fluid exchange, all pts but 1 were hemodynamically stable. One pt developed extreme bradycardia (20/min) and hypotension. The procedure was suspended and reperformed 48 h later.

Complications attributed to the surgical procedure were observed in 6/27 CF (21 %) and included wound hematoma (3), infection (2) and deep vein thrombosis (1). Two pts died 28 and 40 days following CF due to respiratory insufficiency.

Complications attributed to CD were observed in 14/25 CF (52 %) and included leukopenia, mild ($> 1\ 000\ mm^3$) in 5 pts and severe ($< 1\ 000\ mm^3$) in another 5. Of these 10 pts, 8 had received previous systemic CD. Two pts developed a prolonged paralytic ileus after liver CF. Partial hair loss was seen in another 2 pts and 1 pt who received Cisplatinum in 2 sequential pelvic CF developed moderate renal failure.

Twenty-two out of 25 pts had measurable disease. Two of the remaining 3 pts died and another had his entire tumor mass resected. A partial response (PR) was seen in 11/22 pts (50 %). Time to progression in this group was 5.4 months (4 weeks-20 months). Eight pts (36 %) showed stabilization of their disease (SD). three pts (14 %) experienced disease progression (PD). A decrease in CEA levels occurred in 8/12 (67 %) pts. Marked symptomatic relief occurred in 6/8 (75 %) of highly symptomatic pts.

Discussion

CF has the advantage of delivering 2 to 4 fold the systemic dose of CD directly to the cancer site. The close relationship between CD dosage and response has long been established, and even a slight increment may result in a marked increase in the drug's efficacy [3, 4]. This fact is attributed to the development of drug resistance and DNA repair that are allowed to occur when low doses of CD are administered. This drug resistance in previously CD treated pts may also have hindered the efficacy of the CF in the presented series. The dose dependency has recently been reinforced by the use of autologous bone marrow transplantation as a means of overcoming its suppression and thus achieving higher response rates [5].

The high-doses of CD delivered in CF led, in our opinion, to the relatively high response rates (50 % PR, and if SD are included — 85 %) in pts with advanced RAC, many of whom (67 %) had failed previous treatment modalities. It has also been demonstrated as a palliative treatment in symptomatic pts.

CF has several disadvantages : it is an invasive procedure, associated with general anesthesia, angiography, heparinization. Since CF is a semi-closed technique, one cannot expect to pump out all the venous effluent of area, which results in « leakage » of CD into the systemic circulation. This, coupled with the significant rate of CD binding to protein (5-10 %), and the late return of CD from the infused tissues, contributes to systemic leakage of 15-50 %. Considering the fact that the dose is higher than usual, this can result in systemic toxicity. This systemic leakage also prevents the use of higher doses of CD.

It is possible, however, that CF may prove to be more effective in pts with less bulky cancers, especially when applied as a first-line treatment.

References

1. Aigner KR, Muller H, Walther H, Lurk KH (1988) Drug filtration in high-dose regional chemotherapy. Contr Oncol 29 : 261-280
2. Muchmore JH, Krementz ET, Carter D, Preslan JG, George WJ (1991) Treatment of abdominal malignant neoplasms using regional chemotherapy with hemofiltration. Arch Surg 126 : 1390-1396
3. Frei E III, Canellos GP (1980) Dose : A critical factor in cancer chemotherapy. Am J Med 69 : 585-594
4. De vita VT (1986) Dose-response is alive and well. J Clin Oncol 4 : 1157-1159
5. Lazarus HM, Herzig RH, Wolff SN et al (1985) Treatment of metastatic melanoma with intensive Melphalan and autologous bone marrow transplantation. Cancer Treat Rep 69 : 473-477

Treatment optimization guidelines for hyperthermic antiblastic limb perfusion

M Pace*, L Millanta**, A Galli*, A Bellacci*

In our experience, consisting of 175 hyperthermic antiblastic regional perfusions in extracorporeal circulation (ECC) for limb malignancies, a primary objective has been the improvement of the technical aspects that constitute the basis of the method [1-3, 7]. Our interest has been therefore devoted to verifying and optimizing the following main points.

The vascular isolation optimization responds to the requirement of maximizing the extension of the treated area to cover the entire region of interest while, at the same time, minimizing the leakage (containment of the systemic toxic effects).

The ECC system is to be modified to be best suited to hyperthermal operation. A truly hyperthermic treatment must aim at obtaining high temperatures, close to the physiological tolerance limit. This in turn requires strict tolerances in the temperature distribution, i.e. high uniformity in space and time and high measurement accuracy. The target temperature is to be maintained for an extended time duration which also reflects on the need for a closely controlled procedure.

The purpose of this paper is to show the obtainable results in terms of reproducibility of the physical and clinical parameters of the method. A synthesis of the basic data is offered with reference to 9 consecutive treatments all based upon a protocol requiring high hyperthermia and long hyperthermal phase duration (WHO Melanoma Programme Trial 17, activated in October 1991). All 9 cases refer to lower limb melanoma.

Materials and methods

The fundamental aspects of the vascular isolation technique are described in [5]. We point out here in synthesis the opportunity offered by the blockage of the venous flow at the common iliac vein level, which permits to reduce the leakage to the system, the amount of leakage being mainly connected to possible pelvic venous variances. Improvement of the surface isolation also has been obtained by fastening the Esmarch belt to a pair of modified Steinmann nails inserted into the lower abdominal wall.

Heat to the limb is delivered both by means of the heated perfusate and of a circulating warm-water blanket entirely surrounding the limb, to obtain best temperature uniformity and stability [4]. The high operating temperatures with respect to the room temperature suggest special care for the thermal iso-

---

* 1st Surgical Clinic, University of Florence, Viale Morgagni 85, Florence, Italy
** Electronic Engineering Department, University of Florence, Italy

lation from the extracorporeal circuit and the blanket to the surroundings. In particular, the extracorporeal circuit tubing is kept as short as feasible in length and is protected by metallized plastic sleeves (emergency blanket). The essential role of the water blanket is to be pointed out. The water blanket represents with very good approximation a constant and uniform temperature ambient entirely surrounding the limb. This is an essential requirement in order to obtain temperature uniformity.

The accuracy and reliability required for the limb temperature measurements and for the temperature controlling sources are obtained by frequent calibration (accuracy) and by duplication (reliability). Calibration is performed after each treatment for each probe, by comparison against an accurate mercury thermometer in a constant and uniform temperature environment (warm water in Dewar vessel). Residual uncertainty after calibration is better than 0.05° C. The more critical temperatures (with respect to treatment effectiveness and risk of damage) are the perfusate input temperature (arterial cannula, the highest temperature in intimate contact to the patient) and the water blanket input temperature (the highest temperature available for contact to the patient). Special care is devoted to the control and surveillance of these 2 temperatures. Strict requirements of accuracy demand that these temperatures be measured in intimate contact to the fluids (needle probes inserted into the tubing). Six probes measure the temperature distribution at the limb. These 6 readings are not considered critical and are essentially taken into account only to determine the starting time of the hyperthermal phase. This is defined as the time when all 6 readings fall within − 0.5° C of the hyperthermal (steady-state) target temperature (41 to 41.8° C). The drug is administered at this time as a single bolus. The hyperthermal phase duration is 90 minutes.

Results

Direct fluorescence observations show that the limb root is well included in the perfused region. Leakage is 1.4 % at 10 min and 9 % at 30 min (average of samples from each patient). This particular result refers to a group of patients larger than the one considered in this paper (31 patients).

A large dispersion in the initial temperatures of the limb is observed from patient to patient and particularly for the various districts of the limb. A minimum temperature of 30.5° C was observed (cutis) and a maximum of 36.8° C (muscle). The average over all patients, all districts is 34.3° C. This gives the initial thermal situation prior to the activation of the water blanket. After a time delay of approximately 80 min (average) the ECC is activated. At this time the temperature dispersion is considerably reduced (35.8 to 38.2° C) and the average temperature is significantly increased (36.7° C average ± 0.7° C std. dev.). The time required to reach the hyperthermal-phase starting time is 67 min (from 45 to 90 min). The average temperature at this time is 41.1° C ± 0.4° C std. dev. The steady-state average temperature is 41.4° C ± 0.34° C std. dev. The averages are over all patients, all districts, all times.

The temperature at the oxygenator never exceeded 42.1° C. The temperature at the arterial cannula was a few tenths of a degree centigrade lower. The temperature difference between oxygenator and arterial input is obviously dependent upon the perfusate flow rate, higher differences corresponding to lower flow rates, which therefore represent the more critical situation. The inlet temperature of the water blanket never exceeded 42.7° C.

The flow rate was between 600 and 1.050 ml/min, with an average of 870 ml/min.

Local toxicity response during the post-operative period was between grade 2 and 3 according to Wieberdink and coll. [8]. Systemic acute toxicity was absent in all patients. Two patients developed complications : a bilateral pleuric effusion and a pulmonary microembolism and both patients recovered through standard medical therapy.

Discussion and conclusions

Our approach for vascular isolation allows us to include nodal districts of limb root in the hyperthermic treatment and to include patients with primary melanoma located at upper third of the thigh.

The large initial-temperature variability observed is of significant importance in the general planning of the treatment. The use of the uniform-temperature external heat source (blanket) helps overcome the above difficulty, reducing the time needed to reach the target temperature and is determinant to obtain a high temperature uniformity, with time stability. Comparable uniformity results cannot be obtained when heat dispersion to the surroundings is present.

The obtained results show the reproducibility and safety of the procedure along with expectations of increased clinical efficacy of the treatment.

References

1. Cavaliere R, Moricca G, Di Filippo F, Caputo A, Monticelli G, Santori FS (1980) Heat transfer problems during local perfusion in cancer treatment. Ann New York Acad Sciences 47 : 311-326
2. Di Filippo F, Cavaliere R, Carlini S, Calabro AM, Piarulli L, Moscarelli F, Cavaliere F, Zupi G, Greco G (1987) The role of hyperthermic perfusion in treating limb tumors : our experience at Regina Elena Institute. In : Field SB and Franconi C (eds) Physics and Technology of Hyperthermia. NATO ASI Series
3. Hahn GM (1987) Blood flow. In : Physics and Technology of Hyperthermia. NATO ASI Series E. N' 127 Kluwer Academic Publisher Group
4. S. Lazzerini, L. Millanta, R. Olmi, M. Pace (1991) An analysis of heat supply and temperature distribution in isolated hyperthermic perfusion of the limbs. Phys Med 4 : 135-143
5. M. Pace (1990) Optimization of the vascular isolation in isolated regional perfusion of the limbs. Reg Cancer Treat 3 : 90-97
6. M. Pace, L. Millanta, A. Bellacci, A. Galli, S. Lazzerini (1992) Heat administra-

tion, temperature monitoring and control in hyperthermic antiblastic perfusion of the limbs. Reg Cancer Treat (in press)
7. Stehlin JS, Giovannella BC, De Ipolyi PD, Muenz LR, Anderson RF, Gutierrez AA (1977) Hyperthermic perfusion of extremities for melanoma and soft tissue sarcomas. In Rossi-Fanelli A, Cavaliere R, Mondovi' B, Moricca G, Eds. Selective heat sensitivity of cancer cells. Springer-Verlag, Berlin pp. 171-185
8. Wieberdink J, Benkhuisen C, Braat RP, Van Slooten EA, Olthius GAA (1982) Dosimetry in isolated perfusion of the limbs by assessment of perfused tissue volume and grading of toxic tissue reaction. Eur J Cancer Clin Oncol 18 : 905-950

5-FU + Folinic Acid (FA, Rescuvolin®) i.a., 5-FU + FA i.v., 5-FUDR i.a., or 5-FUDR i.a. + i.v. for treatment of non-resectable colorectal liver metastases ?

KH Link*, ED Kreuser**, F Safi*, A Schalhorn***, E Schmoll****, J Pillasch*, HG Beger*

The treatment of nonresectable colorectal liver metastases (CRLM) remains an unresolved challenge. Besides systemic (i.v.) therapy with 5-FU or 5-FU + Folnic acid (5-FU + FA), regional intra-arterial (i.a.) chemotherapy is feasible, since CRLM may be biologically confined to the liver. Five-year survival rates up to 52 % after resection [19] and the fact, that CRLM receive their blood supply up to 95 % by the liver artery [1, 4] justify the i.a. treatment approach. With i.a. infusion of 5-FU or 5-FUDR, the arterial plasma concentrations exceed the drug levels achievable by systemic therapy and allow increases of drug exposure by factors of 50-100 for 5-FU and 100-400 for 5-FUDR [10]. The rationale to aim at highest concentrations at the tumor site is based on the fact that chemotherapeutic effectivity clearly depends on the drug concentration at the tumor cells [23]. In randomized studies, hepatic artery infusion with 5-FUDR produced significantly higher response rates when compared with 5-FUDR or 5-FU i.a. [5, 17, 20, 24], and a recent study demonstrated a significant survival advantage in CRLM patients treated with 5-FUDR i.a. v.s. a group receiving 5-FU or symptomatic therapy only [28]. These advantages of i.a. treatment with 5-FUDR are diminished by severe regional 5-FUDR specific toxic side effects, such as sclerosing cholangitis and gastritis or ulcer disease [16, 28, 29]. The lack of systemic 5-FUDR drug levels due to the up to 99 % hepatic extraction rate [11] may also be considered as a major disadvantage of its continous i.a. infusion, since the combination 5-FUDR i.a. + i.v. delays the extrahepatic disease progression when compared to 5-FUDR i.a. [30, 31]. With the alternative treatment option, 5-FU + FA i.v., response rates range betweeen 16-45 % [3], and thus are lower than the 8-83 % [6, 12, 14, 27] reported from regional chemotherapeutic studies. The higher i.a. response rates justify the search for more effective but less toxic i.a. protocols. Intra-arterial infusion of 5-FU + FA seems to be an attractive option for CRLM treatment, that might induce higher response rates than 5-FU + FA i.v. [3] with lower toxicity than 5-FUDR i.a. [28, 29].

In 1988, we started to treat CRLM patients with 5-FU + FA i.a. We were highly interested in the effectivity and toxicity of this protocol. We additionally measured systemic 5-FU levels during i.a. infusion to confirm, that with hepatic i.a. infusion not only regional high concentration — but also potential systemic standard treatment is performed. In parallel to our phase I/II study with 5-FU + FA i.a., a patient group with isolated CRLM was treated

---

* Dept.General Surgery, Univ.of Ulm, D-7900 Ulm, Germany ; ** Dept.Hematology/Oncology, FU Berlin Steglitz, D-1000 Berlin ; *** Dept.Hematology/Oncology, LMU Großhadern, D-8000 Munich ; **** Dept.Hematology/Oncology, MHH, D-3000 Hanover

with a phase III protocol, comparing 5-FUDR i.a. v.s. 5-FUDR i.a. + i.v., and this work has been already published seperately in detail [30]. Patients with metastatic colorectal cancer, including CRLM, who were not referred to our regional treatment programs, received 5-FU + FA i.v., with a standard systemic dosage and the same timing as with 5-FU + FA i.a. Since these i.a. and i.v. treatment regimens were run in parallel at our hospital, we are in the unique situation to compare the prospectively documented effectivities and toxicities in an observation study to find out, what chemotherapeutic approach could be optimal for CRLM-treatment. Though the results obtained seem to be conclusive, a definitive answer to our question can only be given in a prospective randomized trial.

Patients

Group A : 5-FU + FA i.a.

Twenty-six pts with CRLM received an intra-arterial port catheter (Implantofix®, B. Braun, Melsungen or Jet Port Plus Arterial II®, pfm, Cologne, Germany) via the gastroduodenal artery for hepatic infusion with 5-FU + FA. Vascular abnormalities were surgically respected. 6/26 pts (23 %) had extrahepatic metastases (CRM) at the time of surgery. Liver replacement was < 25 % in 12 pts, > 25 % ≤ 50 % in 3 pts, > 50 % ≤ 75 % in 9 pts an > 75 % in 2 pts. The primary tumors (20 colon, 7 rectum, including 1 double carcinoma of the colon and rectum), were lymph node positive in 17 pts. All pts had a life expectancy of more than 6 months, and none had received prior systemic therapy.

Group B : 5-FU + FA i.v.

34 pts receiving 5-FU + FA i.v. had metastatic disease of colon (26 pts) or rectal (8 pts) cancer. 18/34 pts (53 %) had isolated liver metastases (CRLM), 4/34 pts isolated lung metastases, while 12/34 pts had metastases at multiple sites. 7 pts had a history of at least one course of prior 5-FU i.v. monotherapy.

Group C and group D : 5-FUDR i.a. and 5-FUDR i.a. + i.v.

23 pts were randomized into group C, 21 in group D. The pts in group C received a continous i.a. infusion pump (Infusaid®, Infusaid Corporation, Norwood, MA, USA) with the catheter most frequently placed into the gastroduodenal artery. In case of a dual hepatic blood supply, the pts received a dual i.a. + i.a. pump. Group D received a dual i.a + i.v. infusion pump with the arterial arm infusing the hepatic artery and the i.v. line implanted into the inferior vena cava via the right testicular or ovarian vein. 66 % of the pump contents are infused via the i.a., and 33 % via the i.v. lines. Variations of the hepatic artery anatomy were surgically respected, and all pts, like with

port implantation, had prophylactic cholecystectomy. In group C, 87 % of the pts had a metastasis-volume not exceeding 50 % of the whole liver. In group D, 76 % of the pts had less than 50 % of the liver volume replaced by metastases. In group C there were 11 pts with cancer of the rectum and 12 of the colon. In group D 8 pts had rectal and 13 pts colon cancer. 43 % of the pts in group C had a primary tumor stage UICC II (no lymph node involvement), in group D 52 % of the pts had no lymph node metastases at the time of primary tumor removal. None of the pts had evidence of extrahepatic disease or received prior systemic chemotherapy. The preoperative Karnofsky status was $\geq$ 60 %.

Treatments and follow up

The pts of groups A and B were treated according to a protocol of the German Association for Regional Cancer Treatment (ART) with the first author as the surgical principle investigator. Group A received FA (Rescuvolin®, medac, Hamburg) 170 mg/m² for 10 min. i.a., followed by 5-FU (Fluoroblastin®, Farmitalia, Freiburg) 600 mg/m² for 120 min. i.a. from d1-d5 at 4-week intervals. Since hepatic extraction rates are individually different, we adjusted the i.a. dose levels according to systemic toxicities, that should not exceed WHO II°. The treatment was continued up to intra — or extrahepatic progression. Systemic 5-FU + FA treatment in group B was performed with the same timing at doses of 170 mg/m² of FA (Rescuvolin®) over 10 min., immediately followed by 400 mg/m² 5-FU (Fluooblastin®) over 120 min. d1-d5.

In both groups, the responses were prospectively evaluated by CT-scans, X-rays of the lungs, and abdominal ultrasound examinations at 2-4 month intervals. Toxic side effects were monitored with clinical and extensive laboratory examinations at each treatment cycle. Both, responses and toxicities were graded according to WHO-criteria [25]. The patients had a complete remission (CR) if all measurable disease disappeared and the tumor markers CEA/CA 19-9 turned normal. A partial response (PR) was defined as a $\geq$ 50 % reduction of the sum of the products from the largest perpendicular diameters of all measurable metastases. If this sum did not decrease by $\geq$ 50 % or increase by $\geq$ 25 %, the response was « NC ». A progression by > 25 % or the appearance of new metastases was evaluated as « PD ». CR, PR, or NC had to last for at least 2 months.

The pts in group C were treated for 2 weeks by continous infusion with 5-FUDR i.a. at 0.2 mg/kg/d, group D received 0.3 mg/kg/d (66 % i.a. and 33 % i.v.). This treatment was followed by a 2 week drug — free interval and continued thereafter with the same schedule, if no regional toxicity occured. Responses were estimated by i.a. — contrasted CT tumor volume changes. For CR, all tumor signs had to disappear, while a volume reduction by > 25 % was called a « PR » and an increase > 25 % « PD ». Every 2 weeks, the liver enzymes, cholestatic parameters, and blood counts were evaluated. If typical clinical symptoms occured, the pts had endoscopy to monitor chemical gastritis or ulcer disease. An elevation of the transaminases by >

100 % was the laboratory symptom for a « chemical hepatitis ». A rise in serum Bilirubin and clinical or ultrasound signs of cholestasis was checked by an ERCP to rule out or to confirm sclerosing cholangitis.

Measurements of 5-FU i.v. plasma levels during hepatic i.a. infusions of 5-FU

Systemic 5-FU levels were measured in peripheral venous plasma samples taken during the 120 min. 5-FU infusions and 3h thereafter. The drug concentrations were determined in the laboratory of A.Sch. according to a method extensively described by Schalhorn et al. [33] and the areas under the curve (AUC's) calculated by planimetry.

Results

Responses

The reponse rates of the 4 treatment modalities are summarized in Table 1. The response rate (CR + PR [WHO]) of 5-FU + FA i.a. in 25 evaluable pts was 48 % and of 5-FU + FA i.v. 29 %. The group receiving 5-FUDR i.a. had a response rate (CT-volume change) of 52 %, and the pts treated with 5-FUDR i.a. + i.v. responded in 48 %. Intra-arterially treated pts had a higher probability of CR's and were less likely to progress when compared to the systemic therapy group. Within the 5-FU + FA i.v. group, the pts with prior 5-FU i.v. did not response worse than the whole group (43 % v.s. 29 %, respectively).

Table 1. Response rates (%) in regional v.s. systemic treatment modalities for CRLM

Group	Therapy	Pts. (N)	Tumor[3]	CR	PR	NC	PD	CR+PR
A	5-FU/FA i.a.[1]	25	CRLM+CRM	12	36	40	12	48
B	5-FU/FA i.v.[1]	34	CRM+CRLM	3	27	35	35	29
C	5-FUDR i.a.[2]	23	CRLM	26	26	26	22	52
D	5-FUDR i.a.+i.v.[2]	21	CRLM	29	19	29	24	48

1 Who (i.v.CT)
2 Tumor volume change by 25 % (i.a.CT) from safi (30)
3 CRLM : isolated colorectal metastases, CRM : Extrahepatic colorectal metastases

Toxicities

Since toxicities WHO I and II were the limits of dose escalations in group A, this type of side effect was frequent, with GI-problems (diarrhoea) being the leading event in 75 % of the pts (Table 2). Unexpected toxicities grades WHO III and IV were noted in up to 10 %. One 75-years-old male pt with a history of splenectomy and amputation of the upper left arm developed irreversible bone-marrow toxicity and diarrhoea and died in spite of intensive care. There was no regional toxicity such as sclerosing cholangitis or chemotoxic ulcer disease. In 1 pt, chemical arteritis led to stenosis of the hepatic artery without any clinical symptoms.

Table 2. Toxicities according to WHO in regional v.s. systemic treatment for CRLM[1]

Type[2]/Grade	5-FU/FA i.v.	5-FU/FA i.a.	5-FUDR i.a.	5-FUDR i.a. + i.v.
GI 1+2	9 %	75 %	1-4 : 4 %	1-4 : 10 %
GI 3+4	1 %	8 %		
Stom 1+2	1 %	30 %	1-4 : 17 %	1-4 : 19 %
Stom 3+4	0 %	8 %		
BM 1+2	3 %	30 %	1-4 : 0 %	1-4 : 0 %
BM 3+4	0 %	10 %		
Alo 1+2	2 %	35 %	1-4 : 0 %	1-4 : 0 %
Alo 3+4	0 %	0 %		
Derm 1+2	0 %	10 %	1-4 : 0 %	1-4 : 0 %
Derm 3+4	0 %	0 %		
SC	0 %	0 %	26 %	24 %
Gastr./Ulc.	0 %	0 %	26 %	24 %
Other	0 %	15 %	65 %	43 %

1 FUDR toxicities from Safi [30]
2 Gi = Gastrointestinal, Stom = Stomatis, BM = Bone marrow, Alo = Alopecia, Derm = Skin, SC = Sclerosing cholangitis, Gast./Ulc. = Gastritis or Ulcer.

Systemic therapy with 5-FU + FA i.v. (Group B) was tolerated well and severe side effects grades WHO III or IV were induced in only 1 % (Table 2).

5-FUDR i.a. and 5-FUDR i.a. + i.v. (Groups C and D) had low systemic toxicity with mild forms (WHO I/II) of GI-toxicity or stomatitis in up to 19 % (Table 2). However, sclerosing cholangitis and gastritis or ulcer disease occured each in 24-26 % of the pts. One pt died as a consequence of sclerosing cholangitis in group C. Clinically less or nonrelevant side effects, such as chemical hepatitis were seen in 43 %.

5-FU pharmacokinetics

5-FU appeared in the systemic circulation during the 120 min. i.a. hepatic infusion and rapidly declined after the end of infusion. The AUC's in the 4 pts ranged between 528-4283 μMxmin (544, 820, 1683, 4283 μMxmin). The pt with the highest AUC had the highest infusion rate and a tumor load > 75 %.

Discussion

The spontaneous course of pts with nonresected liver metastases of colorectal cancer is dismal, depends on the stage of intrahepatic tumor involvement, and is limited to survival times between 1-24 months [7, 19, 35] ; long term survivors were reported in only 1-2 % of CRLM-pts [18, 19]. Systemic chemotherapy with 5-FU seems to contribute only little to a gain in life-expectancy [28] and the median survival times in studies with systemic 5-FU treatment of pts with metastatic colorectal carcinoma is 11-14.6 months [3]. When compared to 5-FU monotherapy, modulation of 5-FU with Folinic acid has produced higher response rates than with 5-FU (15 %-44 % v.s. 7-17 %) that translated to significant survival advantages of 19-23 weeks only in 2/9 phase III studies [3], so that the possibilities of systemic chemotherapy with the best drug, 5-FU, either modulated or unmodulated, must be still regarded as very limited [9]. Resection of CRLM with 5-year-survival rates of 20-52 % [19] demonstrate, that metastatic disease of colorectal cancer may be biologically limited to the liver for prolonged time periods. This behaviour is also documented pathologically [8]. Therefore, local control of isolated nonresectable CRLM may lead to better results than in systemic chemotherapy and to prolongation of life in these pts

To achieve that goal, treatment methods with higher complete or at least overall response rates than those known from systemic chemotherapy are required to keep intrahepatic tumor growth, eventually leading to the death of the pts, under control. Since tumor response clearly depends on drug concentration [22, 23], the application of regional instead of systemic drug infusion should gain a respectable therapeutic improvement. The response rates with 5-FU or 5-FUDR infused into the hepatic artery range between 8-83 % [12, 14] or 22-83 % [6, 27], respectively. Randomized trials comparing 5-FUDR i.a. vs. 5-FUDR i.v. [5, 17, 20] or 5-FU i.v. [24] have significantly demonstrated higher response rates with the i.a. treatment, that, however were not translated into survival advantages. This may be explained by the study designs and also by pharmacokinetic facts. Not all pts randomized into the i.a. study arms received 5-FUDR i.a., but all were evaluated according to the principle « intention to treat ». Pts who developed progressive intrahepatic disease during the i.v. treatment were shifted to the i.a. arm and fully evaluated as i.a. pts. Due to the > 95 % hepatic extraction rate of 5-FUDR, no systemically relevant drug levels are present during hepatic artery infusion [11]. Systemic drug levels, however, should be present during i.a. infusion to treat the portally supplied margins of the CRLM and the potentially existing extrahepatic microskopic disease [8, 36]. With the combination of i.a. and i.v. treatment either higher response rates are possible in liver tumors [21] or the extrahepatic disease progression could be extended significantly without, however, influencing survival [30, 31]. In spite of missing systemic levels of either 5-FUDR or, potentially more effective, 5-FU + FA, the study of Rougier et al [28] demonstrated a survival advantage of 5-FUDR i.a. v.s. symptomatically or 5-FU i.v. treated pts, however, at a cost of high regional 5-FUDR toxicity.

Since 5-FUDR i.a., 5-FUDR i.a. + i.v. or 5-FU + FA i.v. do not seem to prolong survival in pts with CRLM at an acceptable ratio of effect v.s. toxicity, and regarding the fact, that 5-FUDR i.a. specifically is associated with the not calculable and from our experience in 36 % of the pts nonreversible and potentially lethal toxic side effect of sclerosing cholangitis [16, 28-30] it has been suggested to try 5-FU + FA i.a. for treatment of CRLM [3, 28]. Using this regimen, lower regional toxicity should occur and sufficient systemic drug levels can be expected. Up to now, it has been unclear what regional and systemic toxicitites could appear and which response could be achieved with 5-FU + FA i.a., compared to 5-FU + FA i.v., and 5-FUDR i.a. or 5-FUDR i.a. + i.v. We compared these currently possible treatment options with Fluoropyrimidines for CRLM in an observation study using response and toxicity rates as parameters. Survival times were not related to each other, since the treatment protocols were nonrandomized and had different inclusion criteria. The initially planned randomized study between 5-FU + FA i.a. v.s. 5-FU + FA i.v. could not be activated, since the pts or referring collegues did not agree to randomization. However, our results clearly demonstrate, that 5-FU + FA i.a. produces response rates similar to 5-FUDR i.a. or 5-FUDR i.a. + i.v. (48 % v.s. 52 % or 48 %), but higher than 5-FU + FA i.v. The 29 % CR + PR with 5-FU + FA i.v. is in good coincidence with the response rates reported from similar systemic protocols [3, 9]. Regarding toxicity, 5-FU + FA i.a. was regionally far less toxic than 5-FUDR i.a. or i.a. + i.v. with rates of sclerosing cholangitis in 0 % (5-FU + FA) v.s. 24-26 %. (5-FUDR i.a. or i.a. + i.v.) and gastritis or ulcer disease in 0 % v.s. 24-26 %. Rougier et al compared 5-FU + Mitomycine C v.s. 5-FUDR i.a. treatments and observed the same 5-FUDR-specific toxicities without notifying sclerosing cholangitis in the 5-FU + MMC protocol [29].

We chose the infusion rate of 120 min., as *in vitro* experiments have shown, that this time range is appropriate for 5-FU [23]. The hepatic extraction rate of 5-FU varies with infusion time [34], dose rate [33] and hepatic tumor load [13]. Our starting dose of 600 mg/m^2 exceeded the systemic dose by 50 %. This dose was further escalated up to systemic toxicity WHO I or II, so that it could be assumed, that effective systemic 5-FU levels are present. The systemic AUC's of 5-FU measured in 4 pts during our 5-FU i.a. infusions were within the values achievable during 2 h infusions of 350-500 mg/m^2 5-FU i.v. [32]. As Folinic acid is not extracted by the liver during i.a. infusion [2], our choice of dosing and timing allows effective nontoxic regional high concentration therapy of CRLM with concomitant systemic treatment. We hope, that this systemic therapy will effect on the growth of extrahepatic micrometastases, since systemic 5-FU + FA seems to be most effective in microscopic disease [26]. These systemic levels in 1 75-years-old pt caused severe and irreversible toxicity to the bone marrow and large bowel. Similar events have been reported for old pts from systemic 5-FU + FA studies [15], so that in future, we will follow the suggestion to reduce the starting dose in pts more than 70-years-old and to stop treatment at the first signs of toxicity [3, 15]. Overall, the 120 min. i.a. and i.v. infusions with 5-FU have been well tolerated.

In conclusion, 5-FU + FA i.a. should be the solid base for further improvements and randomized studies in regional chemotherapy of colorectal liver metastases.

References

1. Ackerman NB, Lien WM, Kondi ES et al (1969) The blood supply in experimental liver metastases. I. The distribution of hepatic artery and portal vein to « small » and « large » tumors. Surgery 66 : 1067-1072
2. Anderson JH, Kerr DJ, Setanoians A et al (1992) A pharmacokinetic comparison of intravenous versus intra-arterial Folnic Acid. Br J Cancer 65 : 133-135
3. Arbuck SG (1989) Overview of clinical trials using 5-Fluorouracil and Leucovorin for the treatment of colorectal cancer. Cancer 63 : 1036-1044
4. Bassermann R (1986) Changes of vascular pattern of tumors and surrounding tissue during different phases of metastatic growth. In : Herfarth Ch et al (eds) Therapeutic strategies in primary and metastatic liver cancer. Springer-Verlag, Berlin-New York, p 256
5. Chang AE, Schneider PD, Sugarbaker PH et al (1987) A prospective randomized trial of regional versus systemic contiuous 5-Fluorodeoxyuridine chemotherapy in the treatment of colorectal liver metastases. Ann Surg 206 (6) : 685-693
6. Cohen AM, Kaufmann SD, Wood WC (1985) Treatment of colorectal cancer hepatic metastases by hepatic artery chemotherapy. Dis Col Rec 28 (6) : 389-391
7. Daly JM, Kemeny N (1986) therapy of colorectal hepatic metastases. In : DeVita V et al (eds) Important advances in oncology 1986. Lippincott, Philadelphia, p 251
8. Eder M, Weiss M (1991) Hämatogene Lebermetastasen — Humanpathologische Grundlagen. Chirurg 62 : 705-709
9. Einhorn LH (1989) Improvements in Fluorouracil chemotherapy ? J Clin Oncol 7 : 1377-1379
10. Ensminger WD, Gyves JW (1984) Regional cancer chemotherapy. Cancer Treat Rep 68 : 101-115
11. Ensminger WD, Rosowsky A, Raso V et al (1978) A clinical-pharmacological evaluation of hepatic arterial infusions of 5-Fluoro-2-Deoxyuridine and 5-Fluorouracil. Cancer Res 38 : 3784-3792
12. Fortuny IE, Theologides A, Kennedy BJ (1975) hepatic arterial infusion for liver metastases from colon cancer : Comparison of Mitomycine C (NSC-26980) and 5-Fluorouracil (NSC-19893). Cancer Chemother Rep 59 : 401-404
13. Goldberg JA, Kerr DJ, Willmott N et al (1988) pharmacokinetics and pharmacodynamics of loco-regional 5-Fluorouracil in advanced colorectal liver metastases. Br J Cancer 57 (2) : 186-189
14. Goldberg JA, Kerr DJ, Wilmott N et al (1990) Regional chemotherapy for colorectal liver metastases : a Phase II Evaluation of targeted hepatic arterial 5-Fluorouracil for colorectal liver metastases. Br J Surg 77 : 1238-1240
15. Grem JL, Shoemaker DD, Petrelli NJ et al (1987) Severe life-threatening toxicities observed in study using Leucovorin with 5-Fluorouracil. J Clin Oncol 5 : 1704

16. Hohn DC, Shea WJ, Gemlo BT et al (1988) Complications and toxicities of hepatic arterial chemotherapy. Contr Oncol 29 : 169-180
17. Hohn DC, Stagg RJ, Friedman MA et al (1989) A randomized trial of continous intravenous versus hepatic intra-arterial Floxuridine in patients with colorectal cancer metastases to the liver : The Northern California Oncology Group Trial. J Clin Oncol 7 (11) : 1646-1654
18. Hughes KS, Rosenstein RB, Songhorabodi S et al (1988) Resection of the liver for colorectal carcinoma metastases. Dis Col Rec 31 : 1-4
19. Hughes KS, Sugarbaker PH (1987) Resection of the liver for metastatic solid tumors. In : Rosenberg SA (ed) Surgical Treatment of Metastatic Cancer. Lippincott Company, Philadelphia, p 125
20. Kemeny N, Daly JM, Reichman B et al (1987) Intrahepatic or systemic infusion of Fluorodeoxyuridine in patients with liver metastases from colorectal cancer. Ann Int Med 107 (4) : 459-465
21. Khayat D, LeCesne A, Weil M et al (1988) Intra-arterial treatment of hepatic metastases using the 5-Fluorouracil, Adriamycin, Mitomycine C (FAM) chemotherapeutic Regimen. Reg Cancer Treat 1 : 62-64
22. Link KH, Aigner KR, Kessler D (1988) In vitro chemosensitivity profiles of human malignancies for high-dose (regional) chemotherapy. Contr Oncol 29 : 28-42
23. Link KH, Staib L, Beger HG (1989) Influence of exposure concentration and exposure time cxt on toxicity of Cytostatic drugs to HT29 human colorectal carcinoma cells. Reg Cancer Treat 2 : 189-197
24. Martin KJ, O'Connell MJ, Wieand HS et al (1990) Intra-arterial Floxuridine v.s. systemic Fluorouracil for hepatic metastases from colorectal Cancer. Arch Surg 125 : 1022-1027
25. Miller AB, Hoogstraten B, Staquet M et al (1981) Reporting results of cancer treatment. Cancer 47 : 207-214
26. Poon MA, O'Connell MJ, Moertel CG et al (1989) Biochemical modulation of Fluorouracil : Evidence of significant improvement of survival and quality of life in patients with advanced colorectal carcinoma. J Clin Oncol 7 : 1407-1418
27. Reed ML, Vaitkevicius VK, Al-Sarraf M et al (1981) The practicality of chronic hepatic artery infusion therapy of primary and metastatic hepatic malignancies. Cancer 47 : 402-409
28. Rougier Ph, Laplanche A, Huguier M et al (1992) Hepatic arterial infusion of Floxuridine in patients with liver metastases from colorectal carcinoma : long-term results of a prospective randomized trial. J Clin Oncol 10 : 1112-1118
29. Rougier Ph, Lasser PH, Elias D et al (1989) Intra-arterial hepatic chemotherapy for metastatic liver from colorectal carcinoma origin. Selective Cancer Therapeutics 5 : 47-54
30. Safi F, Bittner R, Roscher R et al (1989) Regional chemotherapy for hepatic metastases of colorectal carcinoma. Cancer 64 : 379-387
31. Safi F, Link KH, Beger HG (1993) Continuous simultaneous intra-arterial (IA) and intravenous (IV) Therapy of liver metastases of colorectal carcinoma. Results of a prospective randomized trial. 4th ICACC, Paris, France, 2-5 February
32. Schalhorn A (1988) Clinical pharmacology of Folnic Acid and 5-Fluorouracil. In : Erlichman C (ed) Leucovorin : An expanding role in chemotherapy. Pharm Libri, Montreal, p 33
33. Schalhorn A, Peyerl G, Heinlein W et al (1990) Regional therapy with 5-Fluorouracil : Dependence of systemic concentrations on the infusion Rate. In : Jakesz R et al (eds) Progress in Regional Cancer Therapy. Springer-Verlag, Berlin p 470

34. Wagner JG, Gyves JW, Stetson P et al (1986) Steady-state nonlinear pharmacokinetics of 5-Fluorouracil during hepatic arterial and intravenous infusion in cancer patients. Cancer Res 46 : 1499-1506
35. Weh HJ, Steiner P, Crone-Münzebrock W et al (1991) Diagnostik und spontanverlauf von Lebermetastasen. Chirurg 62 : 710-714
36. Weiss L (1989) Metastatic inefficiency and regional therapy for liver metastases from colorectal carcinoma. Reg Cancer Treat 2 : 77-81

Hepatic arterial chemotherapy (HAI) for unresectable liver metastases from gastrointestinal cancer

F Musca, R Esposito*, G Toma

The gastrointestinal carcinomas are second in the causes of cancer death. Liver metastases are present at diagnosis in 25 % of patients, and will occur in 60 % of patients who subsequently develop advanced disease. The value of hepatical resection has been proven with a 5 years survival rate of 25 %, but only 10-20 % of patients with liver metastases from gastrointestinal carcinomas will benefit from such surgery. When the metastases are unresectable, systemic chemotherapy is marginally active in palliation and survival prolongation.

Rationale

The rationale for hepatic arterial infusion is supported by the arterial supply of hepatic liver metastases, increased drug concentrations at tumor sites, and lowered systemic drug concentrations. Fluorouracil (FU) as a single agent has provided an overall reponse rate of 2O % in metastatic gastrointestinal cancer with an average reponse duration of 6 months. The administration method of FU may also influence the reponse rate. 44 % reponse rate was reported with infusion. The infusional form offers the advantage of being less myelosuppressive. The heavy metal Cisplatin (CDDP) has shown to have significant antitumor activity in a variety of solid tumors. Previous experiences have demonstrated synergistic interaction by enhancement of antineoplastic activity with CDDP and FU in phase II trials, suggesting activity of this combination in gastrointestinal carcinoma and the studies of phase III between 1987 and 1991 have confirmed the superiority of the association of FU and AF as compared to FU alone. This potential advantage of intra-arterial infusion and the synergy between l-Leucovorin (LAF) FU and CDDP, has induced us to treat patients with liver metastases of gastrointestinal cancer.

Patients and methods

Between March 1988 and July 1992, 18 patients with non resectable liver metastases from gastrointestinal cancer have been studied. Charateristics : 12 males, median age 65 (range 45-70) ; 6 females, median age 62 (range 58-69). Primitive disease : 16 with colorectal cancer, 1 gallbladder cancer, 1 pancreatic cancer. Perfomance status was 0-1 s. ECOG. 15 % of metastases were synchronous and 85 % were metachronous. No primary chemoterapy were administered. Sugarbaker stages of liver metastases were I-II.

F Pisico Hospital, Poggiardo (Italy) Department of Oncology. * M Tamborino Hospital, Maglie (Italy) Department of Surgery

Treatment

A hepatic arteriogram was done before catheter placement to define the arterial blood supply of the liver. The catheter was placed by laparatomy into the gastroduodenal artery and positioned at the junction of the proper common hepatic artery and gastroduodenal artery. A cholecystectomy was performed. Fluorescein dye was injected into the catheter to estimate the uptake in the liver and the absence of extrahepatic perfusion.

Chemotherapy

HAI was initiated postoperatively. Patients received 120 mg mq of l-AF and 1.000 mg mq of 5-FU coinfused continously for 5 days. CDDP (25 mg mq) was infused in 1 h for 4 days. The cycles were repeated every 4 weeks. Fifty-nine treatment cycles were administered to 16 patients. Doses administered were 92 %.

Follow up

During the infusion interval, patients were examined every 4 weeks. Complete blood counts, WBC differential counts, platelets counts, liver function tests, CEA and CA 19-9 were performed. Tumor evaluation was performed with ultrasonography /or CT scan, after the initiation of therapy, every 2 months until the demonstration of progression disease. Chest X-ray was repeated every 4 months.

Results

2/18 patients died too early : (motive : intestinal haemorrhage and cardiac infarctus). 7/16 (44 %) patients shawed a partial reponse. 4/16 (19 %) patients had no change. 5/16 (37 %) patients had hepatic progression. Median reponse duration was 7 months (range 3-11). The site of progression was 56 % (9/16) liver, 19 % (3/16) lung, 6 % (1/16) bones, 13 % (2/16) intra-abdominal Lymph nodes, 6 % (1/16) pelvis.

Complications and toxicity

Immediate complications were observed in 2 patients : 1 catheter pocket seroma, 1 fever. Secondary complications were observed in 3 patients : catheter trombosis. The obstruction was dissolved by urokynase. HAI was well tolerated. Mucositis grade 3 was observed in 7/16 pts (44 %). Granulocitopenia

< 1.500 µ/l occurred in 5/16 pts (31 %). Five patients developed gastrointestinal toxicity : 4/16 (25 %) diarrhea grade 2, 1/16 (6 %) grade 3. No renal, oto or neuro toxicity was observed.

Conclusion

This regimen may induce durable reponse and has moderate toxicity. We consider it necessary to carry on with the study for better evaluation.

References

1. Collins JM (1984) Pharmacologic rationale for regional drug delivery. J Clin Oncol 2 : 498-504
2. Cosimelli M, Anza M, Giannaffelli D, Sega FM, Tedesco M, Tjra P (1991) Bolus v.s. chronic hepatic arterial infusion of Cisplatin plus I.A. 5-FU chemotherapy for unresectable colorectal liver metastases : a RNSI phase II — randomized trial. Reg Cancer Treat 4 : 9
3. Diaz Rubio E, Milla A, Jimeno J (1988) Lack of clinical synergism between Cisplatin (CDDP) and 5-Fluoruracil (5-FU) in advanced colorectal cancer (CRC). Results of a randomized study. Proceedings Am Soc Clin Oncol 7 : 110
4. Kemeny N, Israel K, Niedzwiecky D, Chapman D, Botet J, Minsky B (1990) Randomized study of continuous infusion Fluorouracil versus Fluorouracil plus Cislpatin in patients with metastatic colorectal cancer. J of Clin Oncol 8 : 313-318
5. Poon MA, O'Connel MJ, Moertel CG (1989) Biochemical modulation of Fluorouracil : Evidence of significant improvement of survival and quality of life in patients with advanced colorectal carcinoma. J Clin Oncol 7 : 1407-1417
6. Rougier P, Laplanche A, Hugier M, Olliveier JM (1992) Hepatic arterial infusion of Fluoxuridine in patients with liver metastases from colorectal carcinoma : Longterm results of a prospective randmized trial. J Clin Oncol 10 : 1112-1118

Abstract. *Multidrug hepatic artery chemotherapy is superior to single agent therapy. The combined continuous infusion (CI) of Fluorouracil (FU) Folnic acid (AF) with Cisplatinum (CDDP) is a synergic association which had been tested in liver metastases from gastrointestinal cancer. Treatment consisted in HAI (CI), 5-FU 1.000 mg mq plus AF 120 mg mq coinfused for 5 days and CDDP 25 mg mq bolus for 4 days repeated every 4 weeks. We have treated 18 patients with liver metastases (Sugarbaker stages I-II) from gastrointestinal cancer. We obtained 44 % objective responses. The toxicity consisting mainly in mucositis, diarrhea and granulocitopenia. We conclude this regimen may induce durable reponse and has moderate toxicity, but we wish to continue the study with more patients for a better evaluation.*

The treatment of presacral recurrences of rectal cancer by the use of loco-regional pelvic chemotherapy. A discussion of these methods as a Neo-Adjuvant time in locally advanced rectal tumors

P Manivit, R Polo, D Tabary, M Nabet, M Polo, B Rubini, PN Chipponi, JM Fromaget, M Untereiner

We used a loco-regional chemotherapy in some cases of rectal cancer :
— as a salvage method in presacral recurrences, in combination with radiotherapy boost and/or surgical excision of a residual mass as possible, in cases previously treated by primary radiotherapy and surgery at the time of the primary tumor ;
— and sometimes, because of the results on the recurrences as a primary (Neo-Adjuvant) method before the classical strategy i.e. radiotherapy then surgery, in bulky rectal or anal tumors, and because of the proximity of the sphincter.

The patients are too few to allow a definitive conclusion to be drawn, but the effect of such a loco-regional chemotherapy is often conclusive :
— in the relief of pain ;
— in the decreasing of tumour volume ;
— and sometimes, in the « sterilization », from a pathological point of view, of the malignants cells.

What can this method bring among the usual strategy ?

I. Method

1. Introduction way : a catheter is inserted into each internal iliac artery by seldinger way. Serum, drugs and heparin are pushed by 2 arterial infusion pumps (Ivac 531 or Abott Life Care Mod 4), 1 on each side.

2. Duration : The cycle is 40 to 48 hours of continuous infusion, during which the legs, above all the knee, should remain still. Heaprin is administered by arterial route. Antiemetics, diuresis control and diet without risiduum are necessary.

3. Drugs : The cycle is 2 days long ; the dose per day is :
— in *adenocarcinomas :*
- MIC 6 to 8 mg. sq. m.,
- 5-FU 1.000 mg. sq. m. after CV administered by venous route,
- CDDP 30 to 50 mg. sq. m.,
— in *squamous epitheliomas :* the same schedule with BLM 20 to 25 mg/j.

Hôpital-Clinique Claude-Bernard, 57070 Metz, France

3. **Number of cycles :** 2 to 4.
4. **Intervals :** 4 to 5 weeks according to clinical and haematological status.

II. Material : 19 observations were made, which fit into 2 categories

A) Pelvic recurrences

Fourteen observations : 6 women, 8 men.
1. **Age** from 37 to 70 years, median 56.
2. **The primary tumors were :**
— 8 limited to the rectum,
— 1 extended to the recto-sigmoid junction,
— 2 extended to the anal canal,
— 3 on the recto-sigmoid junction, extended to the rectum.
Nine times bulky tumor.
3. **The treatment of the initial tumor** was always by surgery.
Radiotherapy was performed in 7 cases, most often before surgery.
For 7 other cases, radiotherapy was not performed (especially in recto-sigmoid localizations).
Adjuvant chemotherapy was performed only twice, and was, in 1 case, immediately stopped.
4. **The time before appearance of recurrence was :**
— nul for 1 patient treated with loco-regional chemotherapy as an immediate adjuvant ;
— of 44 and 139 months for 2 patients ;
— for the other 11 patients, the average time was 21 months.
5. **The symptoms of the recurrence :**
— sacral or perineal pain : 12 ;
— hydronephrosis : 3 ;
— rectal ulcer : 1 ;
— rectal bleeding : 1 ;
— vaginal discharge : 1 ;
— rectal dyschesis : 1.
6. **The treatment of the recurrence :**
— 3 courses of intra-arterial chemotherapy on average.
Once, only 1 course.
Once, 5 courses.
Twice, 4 courses.
Then, radiotherapy :
— For 3 patients having never been treated by radiotherapy.
— For 4 patients having been treated by surgery.
— Cases without added therapy : 4.
— Cases of chemotherapy :
• 1 alternating pelvic and hepatic chemotherapy.
• 4 systemic adjuvant chemotherapy.

— IA pelvic chemotherapy was performed twice ; once after radiotherapy. 20 Gy, and once after pelvic surgery.

B) As Neo-Adjuvant procedure, at the time of the primary tumor, IA chemotherapy was performed in 5 observations

1. First case : An 8 cm long anal canal coming out of the anus, like a clapper-bell, the recto-vaginal well being invaded, with pararectal nodes and external iliac nodes.
Treatment : 2 IA courses, 1 preoperative radiotherapy 32 Gy on the pelvis, and 1 15 Gy on the perineum, before abdomino-perineal amputation.

2. Three cases of rectal cancer, among patients from 44 to 62 years old.
— 1 lower rectum tumor (3 cm in diameter). 5.5-6 cm from the margin, the whole parietal thickness being invaded.
— 1 lower rectum tumor extended to the anal canal.
— 1 bulky tumor of the upper rectum.
Treatment :
The first case received 2 IA sequences before surgery : conservative surgery in the first and third cases, amputation in the second one.

3. One rectal tumor : 18 cm high, the pelvis being occupied by this unfixed mass.
Treatment :
The IA chemotherapy was performed only once, by inferior mesenteric artery, pushing during 30 mn 5-FU and CDDP, because of a major arteriosclerosis of 1 external iliac artery. Then, radiotherapy was performed, and then, the surgical amputation.

III. Follow up and results

A) Concerning the 14 recurrences observations

1. The relief of sacral pain is effective in 3 cases, after the first IA chemo course, and in 8 cases, after 2 courses.
But the pain returns after 1 month in 1 patient whose pelvic recurrence was primarily treated by initial surgery, in another patient who received previously 65 Gy external radiotherapy.
In 2 other cases, the pain returned after 5 months, and 19 months.
We could observe therefore 4 cases out of 14 without control of pain.
In the other cases pain did not return :
— up to death, happening for each case after 3, 6, 10, 11, 14, 14 and 29 months ;
— up to December 92, with NED living patients, after 5, 7, 14 and 14 months.

2. Local evolution of the recurrence.

— In 1 case, the presacral mass became totally calcified, without any pelvic symptom.

— In 1 case, we saw the disappearance and negative biopsy of an intravesical spot primarily biopsied, and the presacral mass was reduced but it persisted on the scanner without pain.

— Reduction of the tumor volume : no evidence in 2 cases, moderate in 8 cases, important reduction in 6 cases.

3. Survival.

Out of 10 deaths after 2 to 29 months (average : 10 months).

Four deaths occurred without total pelvic pain control ; the pelvic pain reappeared, for each case, after 1, 1, 5 and 15 months.

The other 4 deaths occured with good pelvic pain control, and other localizations (brain, bronchus, liver, abdominal wall).

Details :

— 2 iatrogen deaths :
— 1 death by chemotherapy toxicity, after 2 months.
— 1 death by pulmonary insufficiency after Kraske surgery, without pain, after 3 months.

Surgery after IA chemotherapy was performed 4 times.

— Once with this death after Kraske process after 3 months.
— Once after 4 IA courses and Kraske process after 2 months.
— Once after 3 IA courses and Kraske process : NED after 6 months.
— Once with the excision of the recurrence on the colorectal anastomosis, after IA courses and 48 Gy in the pelvis : NED after 13 months).

The limits of these excisions were pathologically normal, without any malignant cell, but the central parts of the pieces were not sterilized : the patient with bladder extension as a spot is alive NED after 14 months, without surgery.

B) *The 5 Neo-Adjuvant IA chemotherapy observations*

1. The anal tumor could be amputated : there was no malignant cell in it. After 7 months, inguinal nodes and hepatic localizations appeared.

Death after 12 months.

2. The rectal cancer which was infused by the inferior mesenteric artery presented no malignant cell at the pathological examination. NED after 36 months.

3. For the other 3 patients :

— One hepatic and peritoneal evolution was observed, with death after 14 months.

— One bulky tumor of the upper rectum had a good result on the periphery of the tumor. The centre was not sterilized on a pathological point of view. NED at 60 months.

— One of these patients could keep his sphincter without malignant cell on the section, and he is receiving systemic chemotherapy.

IV. Discussion

1. As initial treatment of pelvic recurrences, IA chemotherapy appears to have a good impact on pain.

— Two immediate failures with 2 patients whom vascularization was disturbed either after initial surgery or after initial radiotherapy.

— Good control of pain in 10 observations out of 14.

2. Pathological sterilization is uncommon : once on a spot invading the bladder after IA chemotherapy, twice after conjunction of IA chemoradiotherapy.

— IA chemotherapy is to be associated with other procedures.

3. The reduction of the volume of the tumor was observed at an important rate with 6 patients, less important with 6 others.

It was not obtained with 2 patients whose pain did not disappear, the recurrence having been previously treated with initial surgery or radiotherapy.

IA chemotherapy can clean the periphery of the masses, and reduce the tumor cells in the anatomical planes through which the surgeon has to pass, in order to pull out a reduced tumor with the minimum risk.

The importance of an intact vascular bed is obvious, in order to bring up the drugs to the tumor masses with an optimum blood flow.

4. IA chemotherapy is not a « PER SE » procedure, but must be associated, as the first step of the strategy, with other methods :

— radiotherapy : if it has not been employed previously because of intestinal and fibrous risk of overdosage ;

— surgery.

5. Another relevance of primary chemotherapy is that drugs do not remain in the pelvis, but are carried towards any site where metastasic colonies could develop, especially the liver. It may be like Taylor's procedure, before surgery.

6. After this chemo-radio-surgical association, the treatment has to be carried on with systemic intravenous chemotherapy, as 5-FU reinforced by citrovorum factor as often as possible.

7. Side effects of the procedure ;

— in this study, there were no cases of thrombosis ;

— side effects in relation with drugs :
  — here no buttock exudative erythema ;
  — peripheral neuropathy : 4 times grade 3.

8. To be discussed :

Is IA Chemo, used as a Neo-Adjuvant procedure in the treatment of primary tumor, able to reduce the rate of amputations when the limit of the tumor is closed to the sphincter ?

Has IA Chemo a more preventive impact on delated complications than the usual strategy using radiotherapy and surgery ?

9. One can argue about the number of cycles, the use of other drugs, Carboplatin instead of Cisplatin ? Other new drugs ?

The duration of a cycle can be discussed too, but 48 hours seems to be « acceptable ».

A simultaneous radiotherapy does not permit the use of full drug doses.

Is it better to obtain the major effect of drugs before radiotherapy and surgery ? Is it better to associate such an intra-arterial technic with short radiotherapy applications ?

Conclusion

Two indications have been discussed.

First of all, we discussed of the use of IA Chemotherapy, because of the lack of another active drug by systemic route, and because of inefficacy of using the classical method to treat pelvic recurrences.

IA Chemo was used in initial step as an antalgic procedure and as a reducing agent of the volume of the tumor. Then radiotherapy was performed especially if not previously used, and at least surgery, in hope to eradicate all tumor cells.

The second point of our discussion was of using IA Chemotherapy as a Neo-Adjuvant method in rectal or anal tumors, in order to prepare the other treatment steps. The intact vascular bed is, at that time, the best way to bring up drugs and optmise their impact.

This method could be indicated :
— for bulky masses ;
— in case of proximity of the sphincter, in order to reduce the rate of amputations ;
— to prepare the cleavage planes by chemotherapy.

We have recorded too few observations to talk about results. We only can say that the method is feasible. It set up a good response to pain, and contributed to decrease the volume of the tumor.

It sometimes allows a surgical eradication of recurrences.

In a Neo-Adjuvant use, it could be shown that previous IA chemotherapy in addition with radiotherapy and surgery has better results than the usual methods.

Repeated chemo-occlusion with Degradable Starch Microspheres (DSM)-Enhanced drug uptake and regional efficacy in the treatment of primary and secondary liver tumors

B Nilsson*, CJ Johansson*, B Bunke*, T Taguchi**

Only a minority of patients with primary hepatocellular carcinoma present with a resectable tumor. Following resection, recurrence within the remaining liver tissue is frequent because of local spread of the tumor cells within the liver [1, 2].

Therefore treatment modalities other than surgery have to be added in a multimodal management of hepatocellular carcinoma. Since the disease is in general confined to the liver, such treatment modalities should ideally be directed towards this organ.

Liver metastases from a primary tumor at another site is in general a sign of systemic spread of malignant cells. A number of patients will have liver metastases as the dominant manifestation of their disease. For such patients, regional chemotherapy directed at liver metastases could be a useful adjunct to systemically delivered therapies.

The concentration of cytostatic drugs in tumor cells is of importance for their therapeutic efficacy. In regional chemotherary, malignant cells are exposed to increased concentrations of cytotoxic drug without increased systemic toxicity. Vascular occlusion may enhance the therapeutic efficacy of regional chemotherapy due to increases in local drug concentration above that achieved by regional chemotherapy alone.

Degradable starch microspheres (DSM, Sphere®) are prepared from partially hydrolyzed starch and have a mean diameter of 45 μm (size range of 95 % of Spherex is 20-70 μm).

DSM are degraded in the blood stream and the rate of degradation is dependent on the degree of cross-linking of the sphere and the amount of α-analyse present in the blood stream. The dissolved microsphere material consists of substituted, unsubstituted and cross-linked glucose units [3].

Temporary vascular occlusion by DSM

After injection into the hepatic artery of DSM blood flow is reduced or temporarily blocked [4, 6], inducing a transient hypoxia. After 15 to 30 minutes blood flow is restored [7, 8].

Intra-arterial administration of DSM can redirect arterial blood flow to hypovascular areas of the tumor [9, 10]. The vascular occlusion increases ar-

---

* Kabi Pharmacia Oncology, S-25109 Helsingborg, Sweden, ** Department of Oncological Surgery, Osaka University, Japan

terial back pressure which can forceably redirect hepatic arterial flow into areas with previously low perfusion. As a consequence of this redistribution, an anticancer drug if co-administered with DSM would gain access to otherwise unresponsive tumor regions [11]. Since the anatomy of the vascular tree in the liver varies widely between different individuals it is necessary to give DSM at an individual dosage. If a too low amount is given, vascular occlusion will be less than optimal but on the other hand, a too high amount may give rise to safety problems. The individual dose can be determined in a number of ways such as angiography or by use of a γ camera [12, 13].

Enhanced drug uptake by DSM

Secondary to the increase in time when a given drug is lodged in liver vasculature due to blockage of blood flow by DSM, the uptake of such a drug in the tumor area is enhanced. Increased uptake of Doxorubin in the VX-2 tumor in the liver in rabbits was demonstrated when co-administered with DSM [14, 15]. In this study it was also demonstrated that the tumor to normal liver ratio of drug concentration increased from 0.25 to 1.24 which possibly was due to redistribution of liver blood flow.

Reduced systemic exposure to a drug given in regional chemotherapy may constitute indirect evidence of enhanced regional uptake of that drug as compared with systemic administration. Reduced systemic exposure to Mitomycin-C has been demonstrated when co-administered with DSM. This was manifested not only in pharmacokinetic parameters, but also in reduced hematologic toxicity [16, 17].

Cisplatin is being used for colorectal as well as hepatocellular cancer [18, 19]. When co-administered with DSM, a 4 to 6 fold increase in Cisplatin concentration in liver tumor regions has been shown as compared to intra-arterial administration of Cisplatin alone [20], which has been further corroborated in a study of intra-operatively administered platinum with or without DSM [11].

A 90 % decrease in the peripheral blood concentration AUC has also been reported for BCNU [21] when given with DSM.

Increased hepatic uptake of FUdR has been reported in patients treated with this agent co-administered with DSM for liver metastases from primary colorectal cancer [22].

In summary, DSM increases the uptake in the tumor area of a number of cytotoxic drugs. This is also seen as a decreased systemic exposure which has been documented as a decrease in plasma AUC of at least 25 % for hepatic low clearance drugs, such as Mitomycin-C. For drugs with a high vascular clearance, such as BCNU, systemic exposure will show a further decrease.

Enhanced cytotoxic efficacy

Different nitrosourea drugs have been given with or without DSM into the hepatic artery of rats with a transplantable colon adenocarcinoma implanted into the liver. In that study DSM significantly augmented the antitumor effect of nitrosourea although an increase in liver toxicity was noted [23] suggesting a too high dosage of DSM in this experimental model.

In clinical phase II studies of primary liver cancer treated with intra-arterial chemotherapy plus DSM, objective response rates of 25 % [with Mitomycin-C, 24] and 41 % [Adriamicyn, 25] have been reported (Table 1). In colorectal cancer, Lawrence et al [26] reported 4 responses of 11 patients with liver metastases from colorectal cancer treated with Mitomycin-C plus DSM. In other studies Mitomycin and other agents have been used for treatment of liver metastases from a variety of primary sites with regional response rates between 25 ans 59 % [25, 27].

Table 1. Regional response rates with a cytotoxic agent + DSM of liver tumors after hepatic artery infusion

Ref.	n	CR	PR	% CR + PR	Drug	Primary tumor
26	24	0	6	25	MMC	liver
27	39	2	14	41	ADR	liver
27	46	1	26	59	MMC	various
28	11	1	3	36	MMC	colorectal
29	12	1	2	25	various	various

In a comparative study 20 patients with liver metastases from colorectal cancer received no active treatment, 22 received hepatic artery embolization with lyophilized duramater (Lyo Dura®) and Gelfoam, and 19 patients were treated with intra-arterial 5-FU plus DSM.

The median survival time was 10.7 months for the DSM plus 5-FU group versus 7.9 for controls and 7 months for the embolization group, respectively. The difference was, however, not statistically significant due to the small number of patients [28].

In another randomized study 43 evaluable patients with primary liver cancer were randomized to receive Doxorubicin with and without DSM. The response rate was 36 % with DSM and 10 % without [17].

In the same study 42 evaluable patients with liver metastases from various primaries received Mitomycin-C with or without DSM. Objective response was recorded in 55 % of patients treated with DSM plus drug and 20 % in patients treated with Mitomycin-C only. The differences in response rates in this study were significant both for patients with liver cancer and liver metastases [29].

In patients treated with regional chemotherapy a number of extra hepatic recurrences have been recorded. In this context it is necessary to keep in mind that regional chemotherapy mainly addresses the regional problem of cancer and should be regarded as 1 treatment modality among others. If systemic spread of cancer has been documented or can be suspected, optimal systemic therapy should be considered as a complement even in patients where hepatic manifestations are dominating. Treatment results obtained so far indicate that the sensitivity of the cancer cells to chemotherapeutic as well as embolizating agents is at best moderate, and therefore optimal management should include repeated treatment sessions. Regional chemotherapy may be employed in a Neo-Adjuvant setting to improve resectability of an otherwise unresectable tumor, in adjuvant treatment to prevent recurrence of liver metastases, or in advanced disease with unresectable lesion.

Safety

Because of the large variation between individuals regarding vascular anatomy, individual adjustment of the DSM dose is necessary. DSM should only be administered to patients with a suitable vascular anatomy. As a consequence of the temporary vascular occlusion provided by DSM, ischemic epigastric pain, nausea and vomiting can ensue. These reactions are transient and disappear in general within 2-4 hours. Severe liver toxicity may arise if hepatotoxic drugs are given at high-doses together with DSM and therefore liver function tests should be monitored closely in order to avoid liver damage. Such toxicity has been reported in clinical as well as pre-clinical studies [24, 17]. Since occasional instances of cholecystitis have been reported [29], prophylactic cholecystectomy may be considered.

If an amount of DSM is given that exceeds what is needed for complete obstruction of the hepatic vessels, backflow into arteries supplying the gastroduodenal area may occur [4, 6].

In such instances, a co-administered cytotoxic drug may become lodged within the gastro duodenal mucosa, together with DSM and consequently, the cytotoxic drug may cause tissue damage. Gastritis and duodenitis from such a cause may be treated medically, but in the case of very severe organ damage with bleeding or perforation surgery may become necessary [22]. Arteriovenous shunting may result in DSM being passed through the liver with following occlusion of pulmonary blood flow. Such adverse events have been reported after DSM treatment [30, 31]. Thus, the administration of DSM needs to be monitored closely for symptoms indicating backflow, aberrant blood vessels, or arteriovenous shunting to the lungs or other sites.

Conclusion

When regional chemotherapy is combined with DSM the result is repeatable vascular occlusion, and a contributing redistribution of blood flow that lead to an increased drug uptake in the tumor area (Fig. 1). It has been shown that DSM when given at individual doses and closely monitored are reasonably safe to use. Currently available results from clinical studies suggest that repeated chemo-occlusion with DSM and a cytotoxic agent improves regional therapeutic efficacy as compared with regional chemotherapy without temporary administred-vascular occlusion. Therefore, repeated courses of DSM and a co-adminstered cytotoxic agent seems to be a reasonable modality for treatment of regional manifestations of a malignant disease.

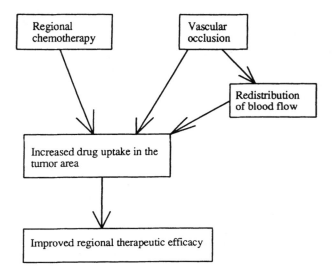

Fig. 1. The concept of chemo-occlusion

References

1. Lin TY, Lee CS, Chen KM, Chen CC (1987) Role of surgery in the treatment of primary carcinoma of the liver : A thirty-one year experience. Br J Surg 74 : 839-42
2. Ong GB, Chan PKW (1976) Primary carcinoma of the liver. Surg Gynecol Obstet 143 : 31-8
3. Edman P (1992) Rationale for the use starch as a vascular occlusive agent. In : Kemeny N et al (eds) An update on regional treatment of liver cancer : role of vascular occlusion. Wells Medical, pp. 35-38
4. Thulin L, Tydén G, Nyberg B, Calissendorff B, Hultcrantz R (1986) Reduction of hepatic arterial flow by degradable microspheres in patients with liver tumors. Acta Chir Scand 152 : 447-51
5. Starkhammar H et al (1983) Effect of microspheres (Spherex) on the arterial liver blood flow studied in tumor patients and in an experimental model. Acta Chir Scand 516 (suppl) : 67
6. Hakansson L, Starkhammar H (1990) Degradable starch microspheres in intra-arterial tumor treatment : An overview. In : Jakesz R, Rainer H (eds) Progress in Regional Cancer Therapy. Springer, Berlin, Heidelberg, pp. 89-97
7. Ensmiger WD, Gyves JW, Stetson P, Walker-Andrews S (1985) Phase I study of hepatic arterial degradable starch microspheres and Mitomycin. Cancer Research 45 : 4464-7
8. Lindell B, Aronsen KF, Nosslin B, Rothman U (1978) Studies in pharmacokinetics and tolerance of substances temporarily retained in the liver by microspheres embolisation. Ann Surg 187 : 95-9
9. Civalleri D, Scopinaro G, Balleto N et al (1989) Changes in the vascularity of liver tumours after hepatic arterial embolization with degradable microspheres. Br J Surg 76 : 699-703
10. Civalleri D, Rollandi G, Simoni G et al (1985) Redistribution of arterial blood flow in metastases-bearing livers after infusion of degradable starch microspheres. Acta Chir Scand 151 : 613-617

11. Civalleri D, Esposito M, Fulco R, Vannozzi M, Balletto N, DeCian F (1991) Liver and tumor uptake and plasma pharmacokinetics of arterial Cisplatin administratered with and without starch microspheres in patients with liver metastases. Cancer 68 : 988-994
12. Rauber K, Lorenz M, Kirkowa-Reimann M, Reimann H (1987) Digitale Subtraktionsangiographie zur Kontrolle subkutaner implantierter Katheter zur regionalen Chemotherapie von isolierten Lebermetastasen. Tumordiagnostik u. Therapy 8 : 11-15
13. Britten AJ, Flowerdew ADS, Hunt TM, Taylor I, Ackery DM, Flemming JS (1989) A γ camera method to monitor the use of degradable starch microspheres in hepatic arterial chemotherapy. Eur J Nucl Med 15 : 649-54
14. Sigurdsson ER, Ridge JA, Daly JM (1986) Intra-arterial infusion of Doxorubicin with degradable starch microspheres ; improvement of hepatic tumor drug uptake. Arch Surg 121 : 1277-1281
15. Thom AK, Zhang S, Deveny C, Daly JM (1990) Effects of Verapamil and degradable starch microspheres during hepatic artery infusion of Doxorubicin. Surgery 107 : 552-9
16. Andersson M, Aronson KF, Balch C et al (1989) Pharmacokinetics of intra-arterial Mitomycin-C with or without degradable starch microspheres (DSM) in the treatment of non-resectable liver cancer. Acta Oncol 28 : 219-222
17. Taguchi T, Ogawa N, Bunke B, Nilsson B, DSM study group (Japan) (1992) The use of degradable starch microspheres (Spherex) with intra-arterial chemotherapy for the treatment of primary and secondary liver tumors — results of a phase III clinical trial Reg. Cancer 4 : 161-165
18. Kemeny N, Niedzwiecki D, Riechmann B et al (1989) Cisplatin and 5-Fluorouracil infusion for metastatic colorectal carcinoma : Differences in survival in 2 patient groups with similar response rates. Cancer 63 : 1065-69
19. Carr BI (1992) High objective response rates in advanced hepatocellular carcinoma to intra-arterial chemotherapy. Proc ASCO 11 : 470
20. Aigner K, Müller H (1990) Time dependent Cisplatinum (CDDP) tissue concentrations after hepatic artery infusion of CDDP with (HAI-Spherex®) and without (HAI) starch microspheres. In Spherex® in loco-regional cancer treatment. Excerpt from a workshop (Eds : C. Hottenrott and L. Quick). Bergstens Grafiska AB, pp 9-11
21. Dakhil S, Ensminger W, Kyung C et al (1982) Improved regional selectivity of hepatic arterial BCNU with degradable microspheres. Cancer 50 : 631-35
22. Thom AK, Sigurdsson ER, Bitar M, Daly JM (1989) Regional hepatic arterial infusion of degradable starch microspheres increases Fluorodeoxyuridine (FUdR) tumor uptake. Surgery 105 : 383-92
23. Roos G, Abdien El Hag I, Teder H, Stenram U (1991) Improved antitumor effect of the nitrosourea drugs tauromustine (TCNU) and Carmustine (BCNU) on a rat liver adenocarcinoma after hepatic arterial administration with degradable starch microspheres. Anticancer Research 11 : 13-16
24. Wollner IS, Walker-Andrews SC, Smith JE (1986) Phase II study of hepatic arterial degradable starch microspheres and Mitomycine-C. Cancer Drug Deliver 3 : 279-284
25. Taguchi T, the DSM study group Japan (1990) Clinical results of chemotherapy combined with degradable starch microspheres. In : Hottenrot C, Quick L (eds) Spherex® in loco-regional cancer treatment. Bergstns Grafiska AB, pp 27-28
26. Lorenz M, Hermann G, Kirkowa-Reimann M et al (1989) Temporary chemoembolization of colorectal metastases with degradable starch microspheres. Eur J Surgical Oncol 15 : 453-62
27. Aronsen K, Hellekant C, Holmberg J et al (1979) Controlled blocking of hepatic

artery flow with enzymatically degradable microspheres combined with oncoloytic drugs. Eur Surg Res 11 : 99-106
28. Hunt TM, Flowerdew ADS, Birch SJ, Williams JD, Mullee MA, Taylor L (1990) Prospective randomized controlled trial of hepatic arterial embolization or infusion chemotherapy with 5-Fluorouracil and degradable starch microspheres for colorectal liver metastases. Br J Surg 77 : 779-782
29. Venook AP, Stag RL, Lewis BJ et al (1990) Chemoembolization of hepatocellular carcinoma. J Clin Oncol 77 : 779-782
30. Starkhammar H et al (1987) Effect of microspheres in intra-arterial chemotherapy. A study of arterio-venous shunting and pasage of a labelled marker. Med Oncol Tumor Pharmacotherap 4 (2) : 87-96
31. Zeissman H, Thrall J, Gyves J et al (1983) Quantative hepatic arterial infusion scintigraphy and starch microspheres in cancer chemotherapy. J Nuclear Med 24 : 871-875

Abstract : Liver tumors need multimodal therapy if cure is to be realistically hoped for. Systemic and loco-regional chemotherapy should often be combined in order to achieve high loco-regional drug concentrations as well as to obtain a meaningful cytotoxic activity at distant disease sites. Cytotoxic agents can kill only a fraction of malignant cells in primary or secondary liver tumors at each exposure, and therefore multiple treatment sessions need to be employed. Degradable starch microspheres (DSM, Spherex ®) can be coinjected into the hepatic artery with cytotoxic agent. DSM have a mean diameter of 45 µm an and intra-arterial injection occludes the arteries for about 25 minutes. During this time blood flow is gradually restored, and ischemic liver damage does not occur. Systemic exposure to coinjected drugs is decreased by 20-90 % when measured as area under the plasma concentration v.s. time curve by the use of DSM. As a consequence, systemic toxicity is reduced. Co-injection of DSM enhances uptake of Doxorubucin, Mitomycin-C and other agents in the tumor area. Comparative clinical studies in primary and secondary liver tumors have shown significantly improved loco-regional antitumor efficacy by use of DSM. Side effects of DSM include liver pain, nausea, cholecystitis, and enhanced toxicity of hepatotoxic compounds. Individual dosage is required. A too high amount of DSM may lead to backflow and subsequent damage to the gastroinstestinal mucosa. Moreover, DSM should not be used in patients with extensive arteriovenous shunting because of the risk of occlusion of pulmonary blood flow in such cases. In conclusion, DSM is an useful adjunct to regional chemotherapy for enhancement of regional efficacy of the treatment.

Antitumor efficacy of intraperitoneal hyperthermochemotherapy combined with aggressive surgery for patients with advanced gastric cancer

S Fujimoto, M Takahashi, K Kobayashi, T Mutou, M Kure, H Masaoka, H Ohkubo

Peritoneal metastasis is the most frequent site of a dismal failure after surgical treatment for an abdominal malignancy. There is no available curative treatment for disseminating peritoneal metastasis and survival time is limited to within one year [1]. Intraperitoneal chemotherapy is a potentially effective treatment for special types of malignancy occuring intraperitoneally [2]. The benefits of this treatment were noted in cases of gastro-intestinal and ovarian cancers [1, 2, 3, 4]. We report herein the results of intraperitoneal chemotherapy combined with hyperthermic perfusion (IPHP) with Mitomycin-C (MMC) for patients with advanced gastric cancer.

Patients and methods

From 1986 till 1992, 60 Japanese patients with advanced gastric cancer but no apparent hepatic metastasis were included in a comparative study concerning peritoneal metastasis and prevention of peritoneal recurrence (IPHP group). Within the same period of time, 52 patients were surgically treated for an advanced gastric cancer without IPHP (control group). Clinical characteristics are shown in Table 1.

Table 1. Clinicopathologic data on 112 patients

Factors	IPHP groupe (n = 60)	Control group (n = 52)
Age (years)	54.9 ± 10.3	60.3 ± 10.5
Sex (male/female)	27/33	31/21
TNM classification		
T3	25	30
T4	35	22
Peritoneal seeding		
p (−)	26	35
p (+)	34	17
Type of histology		
Differentiated	21	27
Undifferentiated	39	25

Social Insurance Funabashi Central Hospital, 6-13-10, Kaijin, Funabashi 273, Japan

Intraperitoneal hyperthermic perfusion (IPHP) and antitumor treatment for the control group.

IPHP using 10 μg/ml of MMC was given just after surgical operation. Details of the IPHP have been presented elsewhere [1, 4]. In brief, under hypothermic general anesthesia at about 31° C, IPHP was performed using IPHP equipment with a closed peritoneal perfusion (Fig. 1). The equipment for IPHP was inserted into Douglas' pouch (outflow tube) and the upper abdominal cavity (inflow tube) just before temporary closure of the abdominal wall. In advance of IPHP, the prehyperthermic hypothermia (31 to 32° C) was induced by means of a cooling mat and ice-bags. The perfusate 3.000 to 5.000 ml containing MMC circulates for about 120 min.

During the IPHP treatment, temperature monitoring was performed with 4 to 6 thermometer probes and temperatures at the inflow and outflow points were 45.5-46.0° C and 43.5-44.5° C, respectively. Temperature in the pulmonary artery was measured by means of Swan-Ganz catheter (Fig. 1) and did not exceed 40° C during the IPHP.

For 52 patients in the control group, 32.4 ± 8.7 mg of MMC was given intravenously and/or intraperitoneally. There was no statistical difference in doses of MMC between these 2 groups. Student's t-test and chi-square test were used for statistical analysis.

Results

Comparison of background factors

The mean age of the IPHP group was younger by 5.4 years compared with the control group, but the difference was not significant ($p = 0.100$). As shown in Table 1, the male to female ratio did not differ between the 2 groups ($p = 0.124$).

With respect to stage of the disease, the incidence of peritoneal seeding was more frequent in the IPHP group ($p = 0.0111$) than that of the control group. However, stage and histologic pattern of the primary tumor did not differ between the 2 groups ($p = 0.0919$ and 0.0717, respectively). Sixty patients in the IPHP group underwent surgical excision of multiple organs ($p = 0.0122$), compared with the 52 in the control group (Table 1).

Survival rates

Overall survival rates for the IPHP group were much superior to those for the controls. The 5-year survival rate was 40 % in the IPHP group and the 3-year survival rate for the control group was 15 % (Fig. 2). Twelve of 34 patients with peritoneal seeding in the IPHP group survived for 5 years but 17 with peritoneal seeding in the control group died within one year (Fig. 3). The 5-year survival rate of patients without peritoneal seeding was 53 % in the IPHP group, while the 3-year survival rate for the control group was 13 % (Fig. 4).

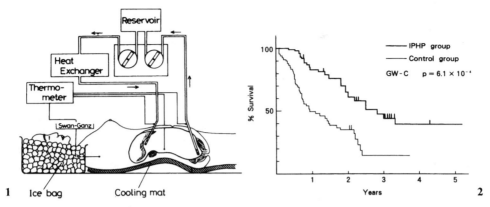

Fig. 1. Set-up of the IPHP. Arrows show flow direction of the perfusate

Fig. 2. Overall surival curves for IPHP and control groups

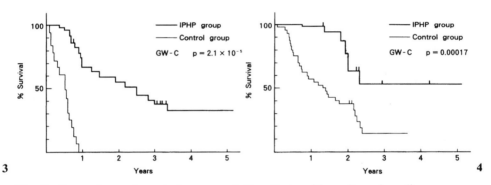

Fig. 3. Comparison of survival curves of 51 patients with peritoneal seeding

Fig. 4. Survival curves of 61 patients without peritoneal seeding

Cause of death

In the control group, all 17 patients with peritoneal seeding as well as 23 of 35 patients without peritoneal seeding died of peritoneal disseminating metastasis or intra-abdominal tumors. In the IPHP group, 11 of 34 patients with preoperative peritoneal metastasis died of recurrence of the cancer in the abdominal cavity and only 2 of 26 patients without peritoneal seeding died of the same cause.

Discussion and conclusion

Intraperitoneal hyperthermic perfusion (IPHP) is one alternative method for preventing or treating peritoneal metastasis. Anatomical sites with a high risk of postoperative recurrence, as well as the peritoneal surface, can be exposed to a high temperature with a high concentration of drugs that facilitates cytocidal effects. Again, as reported in previous study [5], MMC concentrations in the portal blood were 0.3-0.4 µg/ml all through the IPHP treatments. However, despite these levels, the incidence of hepatic metastasis was the same in the IPHP and control groups [6].

MMC is one of the most effective drugs for patients with gastric cancer, when given as an adjuvant treatement for curatively resectable gastric cancer rather than for far-advanced stage [7]. However, if we think out some device to maintain high concentrations of MMC in the target area for a long period, clinically positive results were obtained for tumors that are known not to respond to chemotherapy and/or surgery.

A larger number of patients and a longer follow-up period are required to validate the effectiveness of IPHP treatement. Post-IPHP adjuvant immunochemotherapy and/or chemotherapy will decrease intra-abdominal, pleural or liver recurrence in some patients.

References

1. Fujimoto S, Shrestha RD, Kokubun M, Kobayashi K, Kiuchi S, Konno C, Ohta M, Takahashi M, Kitsukawa Y, Mizutani M, Chikenji T, Okui K (1990) Positive results of combined therapy of surgery and intraperitoneal hyperthermic perfusion for far-advanced gastric cancer. Ann Surg 212 : 592-596
2. Sugarbaker PH, Landy D, Jaffe G, Pascal R (1990) Histologic changes induced by intraperitoneal chemotherapy with 5-Fluorouracil and Mitomycin-C in patients with peritoneal carcinomatosis from cytoadenocarcinoma of the colon and appendix. Cancer 65 : 1495-1501
3. Cunliffe Wj, Sugarbaker PH (1989) Gastrointestinal malignancy : rationale for adjuvant therapy using early postoperative intraperitoneal chemotherapy. Br J Surg 76 : 1082-1090
4. Fujimoto S, Shrestha RD, Kokubun M, Kobayashi K, Kiuchi S, Takahashi M, Konno C, Ohta M, Koike S, Kitsukawa Y, Mizutani M, Okui K (1989) Clinical trial with surgery and intraperitoneal hyperthermic perfusion for peritoneal reccurence of gastrointestinal cancer. Cancer 64 : 154-160
5. Fujimoto S, Shrestha RD, Kokubun M, Kobayashi K, Kiuchi S, Konno C, Takahashi M, Okui K (1989) Pharmacokinetic analysis of Mitomycin-C for intraperitoneal hyperthermic perfusion in patients with far-advanced or recurrent gastric cancer. Reg Cancer Treat 2 : 198-202
6. Fujimoto S, Takahashi M, Kiuchi S, Shrestha RD, Kokubun M, Kobayashi K, Konno C (1992) Relationship between histopathological findings and recurrent pattern or prognosis after combined treatement with surgery and intraperitoneal hyperthermic chemotherapy for patients with an advanced gastric cancer. Reg Cancer Treat 4 : 175-179
7. Fujimoto S, Akao T, Itoh B, Koshizuka I, Koyano K, Kitsukawa Y, Takahashi M, Minami T, Ishigami H, Itoh K (1976) A study of survival in patients with stomach cancer treated by a combination of preoperative intra-arterial infusion therapy and surgergy. Cancer 37 : 1648-1653

Intraperitoneal hyperthermic chemoperfusion in patients with peritoneal carcinomatosis and malignant ascites

F Kober, B Neugebauer, A Heiss, R Roka

Peritoneal carcinomatosis arising from ovarian or gastrointestinal cancer changes patients quality of life in a critical manner. Malignant ascites causes pain, immobilisation and pulmonary disorders, chronic bowel obstruction leads to nausea, recurrent vomiting, fistulas and a quick deterioration of general conditions. Therefore a therapy avoiding the manifestation or progression of peritoneal carcinomatosis is of special interest. While systemic chemotherapy is of low value intraperitoneal chemotherapy has been proved to be an effective treatment to reduce malignant ascites and to stop peritoneal carcinomatosis. Fujimoto and al [1] have shown that intraperitoneal chemotherapy combined with intraperitoneal hyperthermia is able not only to eradicate peritoneal carcinomatosis but also to improve recurrence free survival and overall survival in patients with advanced gastric cancer. The superior effect of hyperthermic chemoperfusion of the peritoneal cavity is due to :

1) Cytotoxic activity of temperatures above 42° C.
2) Increased uptake of cytostatic drugs into the tumor.
3) Widely unknown « biomodifying » effects of heat on drugs and tumorcells.

Encouraged by those observations shortly described above we have performed hyperthermic intraperitoneal chemoperfusion on patients suffering from peritoneal carcinomatosis of different origin since 1992.

Patients and therapy

Nine patients (pts), 7 of them female and 2 male, underwent 11 intraperitoneal hyperthermic chemoperfusions (IHPC) (Table 1). All had a histologically proved peritoneal carcinomatosis, 6 of them suffered seriously from malignant ascites. The site of primary tumor, clinical tumor stage, extent of ascites (0 — + + +) and Karnovsky — index at the time of IHCP are shown in Table 1. In the used TNM classification peritoneal carcinomatosis was not defined as M1, but was classified as P1-P3 according to the clinical stage outlined by the Japanese Research Society for Gastric Cancer.

On 3 patients a resection of the intra-abdominal primary tumor could be performed, on the other patients only a debulking procedure could be carried out. Normally IHCP was performed simultanously with the first operation. Three pts underwent IHCP 1 to 3 months after the first (abdominal) surgical intervention. Four patients had prior systemic and/or regional chemotherapy (ChTX).

Department of surgery, Kaiserin Elisabeth Spital, Huglgasse 1-3, A-1150 Vienna, Austria

Table 1. Characteristics of patients, K.I. = Karnovsky-index

Pat	Sex	Age	Diagnosis	Stage	Ascites	K.I.
B.T.	f	64	ovarian cancer	FIGO III	+ + +	50 %
H.I.	f	25	ovarian cancer	FIGO III	+	90 %
R.M.	f	46	ovarian cancer	FIGO III	+ + +	30 %
F.W.	m	74	gastric cancer	T4N3M0P3	+ + +	70 %
H.H.	f	66	gastric cancer	T4N2M0P3	+ +	70 %
F.L.	f	56	bilateral breast cancer	T4N1M1P3 M : liver	0	60 %
S.M.	f	60	ovarian cancer	FIGO III	+ + +	70 %
N.B.	f	62	ovarian cancer	FIGO IV M : liver, pulm	+ + +	40 %
S.E	m	78	recurrent rectal cancer	T4N3M0P3	+	70 %

Intraperitoneal hyperthermic chemoperfusion was carried out with a closed peritoneal perfusion system containing a roller pump and a heatexchanger. The volume of perfusate was determined with 2.000-2.500 ml/m^2 BSA. After a « preheating » period of 20-40 min reaching 42° C intra-abdominally 20 mg/m^2 BSA Mitomycin-C or 150 mg/m^2 BSA Cisplatin had been added. From that point on perfusion time was exactly 1 hour. Throughout the IHCP temperature was measured at the inflow and outflow line, the right subphrenic region, the left lower paracolic region or at the primary tumor. Systemic temperature was controlled by pulmonary catheter and rectal thermocable. Cooling mats or icebags had only been used if systemic temperature exceeded 38.5° C, we renounced pretherapeutic systemic hypothermia.

Up to now 2 patients underwent 2 IHCPs. Following IHCP all pts but 1 received systemic or intra-arterial ChTX.

Side effects

No intra-operative cardiopulmonary disturbances have been observed. The early postoperative period was remarkable uneventful, especially abdominal pain and postoperative bowel paralysis did not differ from pts with laparotomy but without IHCP. GOT/GPT levels had been uneffected. Repeated counts of leucocytes and thrombocytes did not reveale any haematological toxicity of IHCP.

In 2 pts treated with Cisplatin containing intraperitoneal and systemic ChTX for ovarian cancer we found increasing levels of serum creatinine (highest values : 7.1 mg/100 ml and 10.2 mg/100 ml). One pt returned promptly to normal values, the other pt developed chronic renal insufficiency with a serum creatinine about 8 mg/100 ml. Spontaneous perforation of the colon of a pt suffering from unresectable ovarian cancer was the only surgical complication which was observed.

Results

Only in 1 pt there was no measurable effect of the therapy. This pt suffering from ovarian cancer stage FIGO IV died as a result of progression of liver and pulmonary metastases as well as progression of the peritoneal carcinomatosis within 2 months. All others responded to IHCP. Malignant ascites which was detected in 8 pts before therapy, disappeared completely in 7 pts as demonstrated by ultrasound. As a consequence Karnovsky index increased in 6 pts (range 10 %-30 %).

Tumormarkers which had been elevated in 6 pts before therapy decreased to normal values in 5 pts, e.g. 1 female pt showed a dramatical decrease of CA 125 from 12.800 to 18.7 a few weeks after ICHP. The overall clinical response determined by clinical examination, tumormarkers, ultrasound and CT was as follows : Clinical complete remission was achieved in 3 pts, partial response in 4 pts, 1 pt developed progressive disease and 1 pt could not be evaluated because of too short follow-up. On 3 patients with ovarian cancer second look operations had been performed, 2 of them had histologically confirmed complete remissions.

Reference

1. Fujimoto S, Takahashi M, Kiuchi S, Shrestha RD, Kokobun M, Kobayashi K, Konno Ch (1992) Relationship between histopatological findings and recurrent pattern or prognosis after combined treatment with surgery and intraperitoneal hyperthermic chemotherapy for patients with an advanced gastric cancer. Reg Cancer 4 : 175-179

Intra-aortic infusion chemotherapy in advanced penile carcinoma

MC Sheen, HM Sheu, CY CHai, CH Huang, YW Wang

Penis is small in proportion to the rest of the body, however, it has a great deal of important functions and bears the symbol of man. For penile carcinoma the treatment most commonly employed is amputation, which is not acceptable for many patients. Intra-aortic infusion chemotherapy has been clinically introduced as an effective palliative treatment for locally advanced penile squamous cell carcinoma and has the unique advantage of preserving structure and function of the external genitals [1, 2]. For further evaluation of the effect of aortic infusion to the reproductive organs, a serial examinations including semen analysis, rigiscan for erectile function and duplex sonography for penile blood flow were performed for young patient.

Patients and methods

From November 1985 to December 1992, 9 cases of penile squamous cell carcinoma were refered for intra-aortic infusion therapy. Age ranged from 27 to 76 with the average of 51 years old. All received no prior therapy except forlk measures. Seven cases were exophytic and papillary the other 2 flat and ulcerative. The size varied for 2 to 15 cm in diameter. All lesions were solitary and first noted on glans penis except the oldest one whose lesion developed on proximal shaft and progressed to scrotum and pubic area. The duration of symptoms varied from 1 month to 3 years. Five cases were well differentiated the other 2 poor differentiated.

Jet Port Plus Allround made by PFM which has a long catheter (90 cm) was used for catheterization. A 5-cm incision was made over the inguinal area. The catheter was inserted through the lateral circumflex branch of profrund femoral artery retrogradely into abdominal aorta. The tip of the catheter was placed at about the level of third lumber vetebra. The proper location of the catheter was determined by X-ray and patent blue dye test. After the catheter was properly placed and fixed, the distal end was connected to the port. The port was implanted subcutaneously lateral and inferior to the umbilicus.

Initially, the patient was infusion continuously with 50 mg Methotrexate every 24 h using a portable pump (CADD-1 Pharmacia, USA). Citrovorum factor (6 mg) was given intramuscularly every 6 h during the period of Methotrexate infusion. The mean continuous infusion period was 9 days. Then all the patients were followed at out patient clinic regularly. From December 1988 no further anticancer therapy was given to the complete responder. The

---

Departments of Surgery*, Dematology**, Pathology*** and Urology****, Kaohsiung Medical College Hospital, 100 Shih Chuan 1st Road Kaoshiung 80708, Taiwan

partial responder subsequently received long-term, intermittent, intra-aortic single doses of various combinations including Pharmorubicin, Mitomycin-C, Cisplatin, etc.

Results

After treatment 8 cases were evaluable. Five patients (63 %) had complete remission. They were living disease-free 7 years, 6 years 4 months, 4 years, 2 years 7 months and 1 year 2 months respectively after initial therapy at the time of follow-up (Dec. 1992). Partial responses were not good enough, they were of short duration in spite of follow-up treatment [1, 2]. The most common side-effects were skin rash, leukopenia and anorexia. They were mild and tolerable. However, 1 case died suddenly and unexpectedly 3 days after stop of 8 days continuous infusion because of severe bone marrow suppression. For patient with poor general condition, MTX should be administered with caution.

Case report : A 27-years-old single young adult was admitted in August 1991 with a foul order cauliflower mass (5 × 5 cm) over glans penis which had been growing slowly for about 1 year. The lesion was obscured by phimosis until May 1992, when circumcision was carried out and biopsy of the mass was made. He was the only son and engaged. He has the duty to hand on generation. Of course, amputation of penis was refused by himself and all his family. He was seeking for any measure to preserve his penis. After port catheter implantation, continuous infusion was given through the CADD-1 pump for 10 days and stopped due to skin rash and itching. Then no further anticancer therapy was given. After treatment the tumor regressed draumatically. All tumor disappeared 2 wks after therapy. Epithelialization was first noted on 3rd wk. Two months after treatment, all wound healed. Post-infusion evaluations including : semen analysis, rigiscan for erectile function and duplex sonography for penile blood flow all revealed no abnormal change. Obviously, not only the external genitals but also the reproductive organs are not influenced by aortic infusion therapy. He is now living without evidence of disease for 14 months.

Before and during the treatment serial biopsies were taken every day for light — and electron-microscopic examinations until all the cancer cells disappeared microscopically. Under the light microscope, it showed a case of well differentiated squamous cell carcinoma. One day and 2 days after initiation of therapy cytoplasmic eosinophilic changes and disappearance of the cell boundary could be observed. Nuclear clearing and peripheral margination of chromatin were also found. Three and 4 days after initiation of therapy, the cytoplasmic eosinophilic change with loss of cell boundary became more obvious. Pyknotic nucleus and inflammatory cells were also seen. Eight days after therapy, all nuclear detail of tumor cells were lost and the cells became amorphous eosinophilic mass. Electron microscopy examination, before therapy revealed prominent nucleoli, well-formed tonofilaments, desmosomes and mitochondria. One day and 2 days after initiation of therapy, it showed obvious mitochondria swelling with rupture of mitochondria internal cristae. Six days after therapy, fragmented necrotic tissue became infiltrated with mixed inflammatory cells.

Discussion

Intra-aortic infusion therapy is a simple and effective regional treatment for advanced penile carcinoma with the unique advantage of preservation of structure and function not only of the external genitals but also the reproductive organs. Because of high complete response rate, it should be considered as a first line treatment before amputation is carried out. From previous [2] and these studies of the serial light and electron microscopic changes, it showed that the changes occurred early in the first day and was most obviously in the first week after initiation of therapy. Toxicity to the mitochondria plays an important role in the early stage of tumor necrosis.

References

1. Sheen MC (1988) Intra-aortic infusion chemotherapy in previously untreated squamous cell carcinoma of the penis. Reg Cancer Treat 1 : 12-125
2. Sheen MC, Sheu HM, Huang SL, Huang CH, Wang YW (1990) Serial clinical, light — and electron-microscopic changes of penile squamous cell carcinoma after intra-aortic infusion chemotherapy. Reg Cancer Treat 3 : 185-191

Abstract. From 1985 to 1992, 9 patients with advanced squamous cell carcinoma of the penis were treated by intra-aortic infusion chemotherapy. The age ranged from 27 to 76 years old. The catheter (Jet Port Plus Allround) was insered retrogradely through the lateral circumflex artery into the abdominal aorta. The catheter tip was placed at about the level of third lumber vertebra. Treatment consisting of continuous intra-aortic infusion with Methotrexate 50 mg/24 h using a portable pump and simultaneous intramuscular injection of citrovorum factor 6 mg/6 h was given for a mean of 9 days. Five patients achieved complete remission. They are living disease-free 84, 78, 48, 31, 14 months after initial therapy at the time of follow-up (Dec. 1992). For young patient, post-infusion evaluations including semen analysis, rigiscan for erectile function and duplex sonography for penile blood flow all revealed no abnormal changes. This therapeutic modality is a simple and effective method for advanced penile carcinoma with the unique advantages of anatomical and functional preservation not only of the external genitals but also the reproductive organs.

Psychosocial issues
in cancer

The influence of both surgery and Adjuvant chemotherapy on breast cancer women quality of life

O Caffo*, G Ambrosini*, S Agugiaro**, C Eccher***, S Maluta*

The primary targets of the physicians are usually the patient curing or other biological outcomes. While the practical meaning of a therapeutic success is strictly related to the functional, psychological and social aspects associated with the disease and its treatment. The quality of life (QL) represents this field of interest and its idea play a growing role in the management of the neoplastic diseases. So the QL is a multidimensional idea including the functional status, the patient well-being, the health perceptions and the disease — and treatement — related symptoms [1]. After reviewing the scientific literature about this topic, we assessed the QL by a purpose-made questionnaire. We particularly aimed our study at the influence of both surgical treatment (ST) and after surgical managment (ASM) on the QL of the breast cancer women.

Questionnaire

We made an 11-items questionnaire and tested its psychometric properties, assessing the reliability and the validity. Each question concerned a different QL aspect, expressed as surgery outcomes (Table 1). We assigned 5 possible categorical answers rated by a differential score ranging from 1 = the better status to 5 = the worse. We mailed the self-compilative questionnaire, including an explanation letter.

Table 1. Questionnaire items

- Had the surgical treatment make you anxious ?
- Had the surgical treatment make you nervous ?
- Had the surgical treatment make you depressed ?
- Had the surgical treatment make concentration failure ?
- Had the surgical treatment influenced the relationship with your partner ?
- Had the surgical treatment influenced the relationship with your sons ?
- Had the surgical treatment influenced the relationship with other people ?
- Had the surgical treatment influenced your work ?
- Have you discomfort seeing surgical scar ?
- Had the surgical treatment influenced your sexual life ?
- Had the surgical treatment influenced your quality of life on the whole ?

* All the questions had five categorical answers :
Not at all-Little-Somewhat-Much-Very much

St. Chiara Hospt, Trento, Italy, Unit of Oncology*, Unit of Surgery A**, Unit of Surgery B***

Patients

We mailed the questionnaire to a consecutive series of 661 patients underwent surgery for breast cancer from 1980 to 1991. All the patients had an ASM in the Unit of Oncology of St. Chiara Hospital, in Trento (Italy). Five hundreds and fifty-one patients (83.5 %) returned the questionnaire, in a short time of 2 weeks. Next we separated the 551 answering patients into 4 groups according to the ST (conservative or radical) and the ASM (Adjuvant chemotherapy — CMF — or none). We matched each patient included in a single group to 1 patient included in each other group. When it was possible, we based the matching on different variables as age at surgery, follow-up duration, work and marital status. So the study sample included 220 patients grouped into 4 55-patients exactly sized groups, differing for the ST and ASM. The main characteristics of final sample patients are listed in the Table 2.

Table 2. Main patients' characteristics

Age	average : 47 ys	range : 26-65 ys	
Follow-up	average : 44 ms	range : 6-10 m	
Work	houseworker : 125	retired : 14	worker : 81
Marital status	married : 189	widow : 15	single : 16
Disease status	RC : 212	PD : 8	
Surgical treatment	mastectomy : 4	quadrantectomy : 9	lumpectomy : 2
After-surgery Management	CMF : 4	none : 4	

Statistical assessment

At first step we performed a variance analysis for evaluating the influence of several factors (age at surgery, follow-up duration, ST, ASM, marital status, patient work) on the QL of the whole breast cancer women sample. Next we find out by a T-test whether all groups differed on any of the variables used for the matching. Finally we did a variance analysis for assessing ;
— the difference in QL of the patients sample stratified by the surgery and the ASM ;
— the influence of the local and sistemic treatment on the QL ;
— the influence of the matching variables on the QL.
We based all statistical assessments on the NCSS program for statistical analysis.

Results

At the firt step variance report, the QL was influenced mainly by the age. The ST had a significant influence only for the discomfort seeing surgical scar, while the ASM did not influence all QL aspects. We tried to increase the study specificity for the ST and ASM influence on the QL of the breast cancer women. So we stated to do the match described above for excluding as much as possible the influence of the matching variables and amounting the study sensibility. The matching efficacy was improved by the randomized choice between the stratified patients with the same characteristics. If 1 patient had 2 or several possible matchings in an other group, the correspondents were chosen by a randomized system. The variance analysis at the second step showed clearly that the ASM did never influence the QL of the breast cancer women while the ST is a highly significant variable (Table 3).

Table 3. Results of the statistical assessment by variance analysis

	Surgery univariate	Surgery multivariate	Adjuvant univariate	Adjuvant multivariate
Anxiety	0.3521	0.3221	0.9851	0.9481
Nervousness	0.1551	0.1943	0.4138	0.3986
Depression	0.0698	0.90	0.8617	0.8440
Concentration failure	0.6099	0.5440	0.5224	0.5778
Sexual life	0.0133	0.0310	0.4758	0.5328
Relationship partner	0.0567	0.0644	0.9239	0.9686
Relationship sons	0.3786	0.1914	0.7501	0.6445
Relat. acquaintances	0.0683	0.0850	0.5334	0.5277
Work	0.2848	0.1320	0.9598	0.9652
Discomfort seeing scar	0.0000	0.0000	0.5300	0.5394
QL on the whole	0.0375	0.0691	0.7232	0.7509

Discussion

Many authors had developed different methods to quantify the QL, now the most largely diffuse methods obtain a QL assessment by a questionnaire. We used a made-purpose questionnaire, including few and simple items. The patients' compliance to the questionnaire was very high, as showed by the high percentage of answering patients. Even the patients did a check on our method quality during the routine clinical control of the follow-up and at the questionnaire end, adding free words. Our study can add other data to the debate about both the appropriate surgery for breast cancer and the influence of Adjuvant chemotherapy on breast cancer and the influence of adjuvant chemotherapy on breast cancer QL. When it is possible, the surgeons choose the conservative technique (quadrantectomy or lumpectomy) thinking to a less disfiguring procedure with smaller body image damages and smaller psychological impact of the surgery. Now this aspect of the conservative surgery is unclear. Some authors showed no difference or worse QL aspects for the conservative surgery patients [8] while others proved the contrary [2, 3, 5, 6, 7, 9, 10]. These studies rarely concerned all QL domains but related to single aspects as psychological or sexual.

Our results agree with the conclusion of the review published by Kiebert [4] in the 1991 on this topic. The conservative technique does not improve the psychological distress after surgery for breast cancer, but the sexual life and the body image of the patients are better than mastectomy patients. About the effects of the chemotherapy on QL of the breast cancer women, we found few studies. These studies concerned mainly the QL difference between the patients undergone Adjuvant chemotherapy v.s. after-surgical radiotherapy. Anyhow the use of Adjuvant chemotherapy does not seem to influence the QL in the breast cancer women. We did this study as preliminar for assessing the patients' compliance to the items and the questionnaire power. The questionnaire proved to be feasible, easy, clear, powerful and useful. So we stated to start with a prospective study based on a multiple administration of this mean.

References

1. Aaronson Nk et al (1991) Quality of life research in oncology : past achievements and future priorities. Cancer 67 : 839-843
2. Bartelnik H et al (1985) Psychological effects of breast conserving therapy in comparison with radical mastectomy. J Rad Onc Biol Phys 11 : 381-385
3. Holmberg L et al (1989) Psychosocial adjustment after mastectomy and breast conserving treatment. Cancer 64 : 969-974
4. Kiebert GM et al (1991) The impact of breast-conserving treatment and mastectomy on the quality of life of early-stage breast cancer patients : a review. J Clin Oncol 9 : 8-30
5. Lasry JCM et al (1987) Depression and body image following mastectomy and lumpectomy. J Chron Dis 40 : 529-534
6. Lee MS et al (1992) Mastectomy or conservation for early breast cancer : psychological morbidity. Eur J Cancer 28A : 1340-1344
7. Margolis G et al (1990) Psychological effects of breast conserving cancer treatment and mastectomy. Psychosomatics 31 : 33-39
8. Maunsell E et al (1989) Psychological distress after initial treatment for breast cancer : a comparison of partial and total mastectomy. J Clin Epidem 42 : 765-771
9. Mc Ardle JM et al (1990) Reduced psychological morbidity after breast conservation. Br J Surg 77 : 1221-1223
10. Steimberg MD et al (1985) Psychological outcome of lumpectomy versus mastectomy in the treatment of breast cancer. Am J Psych 142 : 34-39

Psychological side effects induced by Interleukin-2/α-Interferon : clinical observations, biological correlations

MJ Smith, R Mouawad, E Vuillemin, A Benhammouda, C Soubrane, D Khayat

Psychoneuroimmunology is a fast-growing field that explores the relationship of psychological factors and the immune system. In particular, much research has focussed on the impact of psychological events on immune parameters. An equally interesting but less studied situation, however, is the occurrence of psychological side effects after administration of immune substances in humans. In this regard, lymphokines could be of particular interest, since they are regularly used to treat certain cancers. One such substance is Interleukin-2 (IL-2), which is often infused in metastatic cancer patients at substantial doses over several days. Such infusions represent a unique, « quasi-experimental » opportunity to study the psychological side effects accompanying the lymphokine. However, IL-2 is rarely the sole therapeutic agent used in the cancer setting (Siegel & Puri, 1991). In particular, α-Interferon (INF) is often co-administered.

Psychiatric effects of lymphokines have been repeatedly cited in anecdotal fashion, often without thorough symptom description and evaluation. α-Interferon used alone has been shown to cause fatigue, malaise, depressive feelings, and even confusion (Johnson et al 1983 ; Rosenberg et al 1989). Neuropsychiatric complications frequently reported during intravenous Interleukin-2 infusions include agitation, disorientation, mood disorders and impairments in vigilance or even coma (Adams et al 1984 ; Fisher et al 1988 ; Sculier et al 1988 ; Bender & Dudjak, 1990). Denikoff et al (1987) systematically screened a group of patients before and after undergoing IL-2 infusions with cognitive tests and found that half the patients had signs of cognitive impairment and a third showed signs of delirium, usually towards the end of the infusion.

A major question remains as to whether the neuropsychiatric symptoms are due to a direct Central Nervous System (CNS) effect of IL-2 and INF or whether they are caused indirectly by systemic complications, which are constant for both lymphokines and severe in the case of IL-2 infusions. For example, clouding of consciousness can be a indirect consequence of high fever or severe hypotension or alternatively a direct effect of IL-2 or another lymphokine on the CNS. Unequivocal evidence of a direct CNS effect would be interesting from a research point of view, since it would imply that IL-2, INF, or substances liberated by them have CNS effects. Finally, besides their interest for research, psychological side effects of IL-2/INF are an important clinical problem, since some side effects can be treatment-limiting. We thus

---

Department of Medical Oncology (SOMPS), Salpêtrière Hospital, 47 bd de l'Hôpital, 75651 Paris Cedex 13, France

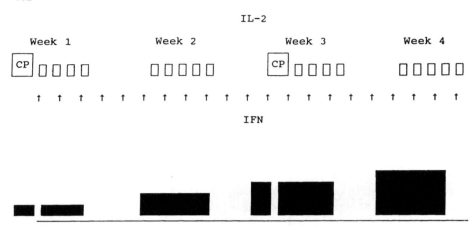

Fig. 1a. IL-2/IFN treatment

thought it important to closely monitor the occurrence of psychiatric side-effects in cancer patients with IL-2/INF therapies and analyze their pathophysiology in terms of concurrent systematic effects and biological changes. The main hypothesis was that it would be possible to show some sort of direct CNS effects of the lymphokines not due to concomittant somatic effects, as shown by the absence of strong correlations with physical symptoms.

Methods

Patients

Patients were hospitalized for a treatment protocol for metastatic melanoma or renal cancer including cis platinum, intravenous IL-2 infusions, and subcutaneous INF injections at Salpêtrière Hospital. This protocol has been amply described and yields a high response rate of over 50 % (Khayat et al this volume). Patients were usually started on the IL-2/INF protocol early in their disease, and they therefore were often in relatively good health, except for a few patients who had recently undergone cytoxic chemotherapies. Brain metastasis was an exclusion criterion. Briefly, the protocol included 2 series of two 1-week cycles of IL-2/INF/Cisplatin combination. Week 1 began with a single infusion of Cisplatin 100 mg/m². Two days later, IL-2 infusions at the dose of $18IU/m^2/day$ were given for 4 days. After a 1-week rest period, patients received the second week of treatment involving IL-2 infusions for 5 days. After a 1-week rest period the entire month-long cycle was repeated. Throughout the whole 8-week period subcutaneous INF injections were given at the dose of 9 MIU 3 times/week (Fig. 1a). Fifty-two patients (31M, 21W) with a mean age of 41 years (20-66) were evaluated at the beginning, in the middle and at the end of the intravenous IL-2 infusions by one of five investigators, either one of 4 psychologists or a psychiatrist. Due to patient fatigue, evaluations had to be kept to a minimum and took no longer than 15' per patient per evaluation except for the initial one.

Instruments

Evaluations were made using a standardized, in-house checklist rating degrees of various symptoms on 3-point scales (Table 1a). Near-perfect inter-rater reliablity was obtained easily after a few trials due to the simplicity of the ratings. When ratings could not be done at the proper time because of patient unavailability (approximately 30 % of evaluations, usually because of sleeping or absent patients), whenever possible, ratings were inferred from nurse accounts in addition to retroactive patient accounts from a later evaluation or occasionally left blank. Psychological side effect evaluation included ratings of depression, anxiety, fatigue, and delirium. For depression and anxiety, somatic signs were not taken into account when making the rating (due to the confounding effects of the somatic symptoms). In cases of delirium, careful description of symptomatology was made, including the evaluation of the following items : orientation, hallucinations, inappropriate behavior, incoherent reasoning or speech. Several of such symptoms were required for the rating of delirium ; in particular, simple somnolence was not considered delirium.

Table 1a. Checklist of psysical and psychological side effects and medecines

Psychological	Physical	Medicine
Apprehension	Insomnia	Anti-allergic
Anxiety	Nausea	Antinausseous
Dysphoria	Vomiting	Vasopressor
Depression	Anorexia	Antalgic
Disorientation	Fatigue	Transfusions
Hallucinations	Pain	Corticosteroids
Inappropriate behavior	Hypotension	Other somatic
Delusions	Erythema	Antidepressant
Incoherence	Fever	Anxiolytic
	Edema	Other psychopharmacological
	Renal failure	
	Trembling	
	Hiccups	
	Local infection	
	General infection	

Physical symptoms evaluated on the checklist included pain, nausea, etc. Somatic (blood transfusions, antinausea drugs, antalgic drugs, etc) and psychopharmacological (sleeping pills, tranquilizers, etc) medicines taken by the patients during the treatment period were recorded form chart review and patient and nurse accounts. One hundred and sixty-four treatment weeks were evaluated in this manner. Thirteen patients also filled out, before and after each week of infusions, a French adaptation of the Fatigue Severity Scale (FSS) self-report scale (Krupp et al 1989) as well as a visual analog scale for fatigue (VAS).

A subset of thirty-one patients with metastatic malignant melanoma underwent a full battery of blood tests measuring immunological parameters. Leukocyte counts were made of total lymphocytes, total polymorphonuclear leukocytes (PMN), phenotypic lymphocytes subsets were mead by flow cytometry : CD4, CD8, CD3, HLADR (stimulated T&B cells), CD25 (Tac, membrane IL-2 receptors), CD56 (Natural Killer cells), CD56+CD16+cells, a subset of NK (CD56−CD16+) cells, and Fc gamma receptor (PMN cells). An ELISA assay was made for soluble IL-2 receptors, alfa interferon, GM-CSF, and Tumor Necrosis Factor (TNF) (Soubrane et al, this volume).

Table 1b. Correlations between psychological side effects, physical symptoms, psychopharmalogical and somatic treatments

	Depression	Anxiety	Fatigue	Delirium	Anxiolytics	Antidepressants	Somatic Drugs
Anxiety	.62 **						
Fatigue	.57 **	.56 *					
Delirium	—	—	—				
Anxiolytics	.35	.50 *	.34	.34			
Antidepressant	.61 **	—	—	—	.38 *		
Somatic drug	—	—	—	—	41 *	—	
Physical symptoms	—	—	.55 **	—	.33	—	.84 ****

Only correlations > .30 are reported ; p<.05 * ; p<.01 ** ; p<.0001 ****

Results

Intense physical symptoms were constantly present during infusions and got worse from week 1 to week 4, but usually regressed completely at the end of each infusion (Fig. 1a). Observer ratings of fatigue correlated with observer ratings of physical symptoms ($r = .55$) (Table 1b). Observer evaluation revealed that all patients complained of intense fatigue by the end of week 4, even though only 30 % showed such signs at treatment onset. Observer evaluation of fatigue correlated well with results of the FSS self-report scale ($r = .73$; $p < .05$). Patients had higher mean fatigue (3.90 ; sd = 1.72) than unmatched controls (2.63 ; sd = .97) ($p < .05$). This probably reflects the effects of recent cytotoxic treatments in some of the patients. The FSS scale showed that patient fatigue increased progressively over the 4 weeks of infusion to a mean of 6.07 (sd = 1.14). This increase in fatigue was not uniform, since patients recuperated during the weeks of rest, although not completely (their following week's pre-infusion scores were higher than the pre-infusion scores of the preceeding week). When compared to a comparable group of cancer patients hospitalized for iterative chemotherapies in the same depart-

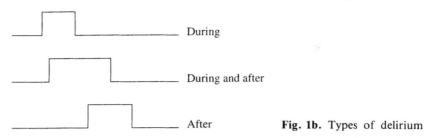

Fig. 1b. Types of delirium

ment, the IL-2 patients, although initially less fatigued than the chemotherapy patients, became more fatigued by the end of week 2. These results are presented graphically for the first 2 weeks in Fig. 2. In terms of the VAS, patients had higher mean fatigue rating of .43 (sd = .28) than unmatched controls, who had a mean rating of .30 (sd = .17), although this difference failed to reach significance. On this scale fatigue also increased significantly to .88 (sd = .16) by the end of week 4 ($p < .0005$).

76 % of patients showed severe depressive symptomatology (which would probably qualify them for DSM-III R diagnoses except for the duration criteria) by the end of week 4 compared to 12 % at treatment outset. Given the results of the fatigue ratings and scales, it seems probable that reported depressive signs (sadness, feelings of hopelessness, worthlessness, etc) were in large part due to the coexisting fatigue. Indeed, ratings of fatigue were significantly correlated with depression as well as with anxiety. Anxiety and depression were highly correlated with each other (Table 1b).

Thirty-five episodes of noticeable delirium signs (21 %) occurred, that, qualitively speaking, could be roughly broken up into 2 types. Some states were essentially somnolent or even stuporous, usually observed at the height of the physical symptoms during the week of infusion. In such cases hypoalertness was prominent, patients were usually able to orient themselves and tended to daydream rather than hallucinate. These states were considered a predictable consequence of the somatic insults, and correlated significantly with physical symptoms ($r = .87$), numbers of somatic drugs taken ($r = .67$), and IL-2 doses ($r = .54$), but not with age, sex, outcome or INF doses. The other type of delirium involved preferentially visual hallucinations with little disorder of alertness, but notable disorientation. Clinically this latter type of delirium was somewhat remarkable in that imaginary themes were observed (music, travel, eroticism, machines). This type of delirium occurred either exclusively after the end of the infusions or began just before and continued after the end of treatment and the resolution of somatic symptoms.

The most useful way of distinguishing the 2 types of delirious symptoms was by chronology, i.e., the former occurred « during » infusions and the latter « during and after » or « after » (diagram in Fig. 1b). The latter type, which can be called the « hallucinatory » type, was considered at least a priori not to be due to somatic effects. We specially analyzed this latter type of hallucination since it seemed the better candidate for a direct CNS effect of IL-2, and most likely to meet the objective of this study. Although 27 such cases occurred, only 24 (15 %) were considered adequate for further analysis. These cases of delirium occurred preferentially at the end of the first week, although

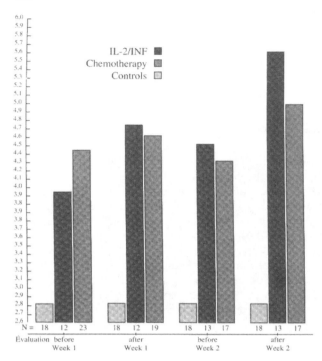

Fig. 2. Fatigue severity scale

they could be found all throughout the 4 infusion weeks. For this type of delirium there were no correlations with physical symptoms, disease outcome, depression, age, or sex. A non-significant trends were found for anxiolytic treatment, which usually consisted of benzodiazepine hypnotics (Table 1b).

The absence of significant correlation with physical symptoms and somatic treatments, along with the chronology and clinical presentation of these episodes suggests a direct CNS effect of the IL-2/INF combination. Curiously enough, two of the episodes involved auditory hallucinations only. Most resolved spontaneously within several days ; the others were successfully treated by small doses of Haloperidol so that duration was rarely exceeded 7-10 days.

The immune measurements made on a subset of 31 patients have been reported elsewhere (Soubrane et al this volume) ; basically in response to the infusions, certain phenotypic leukocyte parameters progressively increased, but the only predictive factor of clinical response might be levels of soluble IL-2 receptors, that were higher in responder than non-responder patients during the first two courses. None or very small amounts of TNF, INF, and GMCSF were detected. Correlations between observer ratings of psychological symptoms (depression, anxiety, fatigue, hallucinatory delirium) and immune parameters for the end of the first week are shown in Table 2. Briefly, depression, anxiety, and fatigue correlated negatively with lymphocyte counts, although fatigue correlated more with PMN values. Delirium did not correlate with most of these parameters, although trends for positive correlations were seen for a few. On subjective evaluation of individual lymphocyte profiles, most patients who developed delirium showed inversions of the T4/T8 ratio, although this could

Table 2. Correlations at the end of the first week of IL-2 treatment

	Lymp	Poly	T4 tot	T8 tot	T3 tot	T & 3 sit (HLA dr)	T sti	T non stim	B sti	R-IL2 mb	NK CD56	NK sub set	Fcg R PMN	sol IL2 R
Depression	−.63**	−.44	−.44*	−.80****	−.65***	−.44	−.60**	−.60**	−.31		−.44			
Anxiety	−.28	***	−.63	−.41	−.40			−.47						
Fatigue	−.39	−.64	−.30	−.38	−.32			−.38		−.29	−.33		−.24	
Delirium				.28								−.44*		.24

Correlations > .25 are reported; $p < .05$ *; $p < .01$ **; $p < .005$ ***; $p < .0001$ ****

be coincidental. The correlation patterns shown here were largely reproduced when the same analyses were done for end of weeks 2, 3 and 4, and when all 12 measurements are taken together, although the validity of grouping all measurement times has been questioned.

Discussion

Psychological side effects of IL-2/INF treatment consist essentially of a block of intercorrelated symptoms involving fatigue, depression, and anxiety that correlates with physical distress. Separate from these, episodes of clinically atypical hallucinatory delirium showed little relation to physical symptomatology and its chronology and clinical characteristics suggest that it was due to a different mechanism. Somnolent, non-hallucinatory delirium seemed to belong more to the first block and was related to physical symptoms. Likewise, results from the immune parameter analysis tend to show different patterns of correlation for the fatigue-depression-anxiety block and hallucinatory delirium. The former correlates negatively with several phenotypic parameters (T4, T8, T3) whereas the latter is not well correlated and its correlations tend to be positive.

We therefore believe that Il-2/INF induced hallucinatory symptoms in these patients that cannot be considered due to intense somatic distress. Although confusion and hallucinations have been often reported during IL-2/INF treatment, it has not been possible to attribute them to a direct action of the lymphokines. At lower doses fatigue and somatic effects have been observed, but delirium is rarer (Fenner et al this volume). We have previously presented clinical evidence that some hallucinatory symptoms linked to IL-2/INF treatment are due to a direct CNS effect (Smith & Khayat, 1992). In the present, more systematic study, the chronology and the correlation pattern again suggests that direct CNS effects of the lymphokines were responsable. There are no arguments for incriminating Cisplatin in this type of side effect (Chabner & Myers, 1989), nor the accompanying drugs except for a possible contributory effect of anxiolytics. Further, not all hallucinatory phenomena occurring in our patients were included in this analysis. Several patients reported minimal hallucinatory activity of a similar nature such as strange and unpleasant imagery when going to sleep after the end of treatment and frequent nightmares were reported during and after IL-2/INF infusions.

The mechanism of such hallucinatory activity is totally unknown, as is whether or not such effects are observable only in certain predisposed subjects or with certain concomitant pharmacological treatments such as benzodiazepines. Some interesting possible explanations that have been suggested are cerebral edema (Saris et al, 1989), liberation of neurœndocrine hormones (Denicoff et al, 1989), and direct action on neurotransmitters (Johnson et al, 1983). Animal studies have shown neuronal degeneration in response to IL-2 (Nemni et al, 1992), and in patients focalized neurological deficits suggesting ischemia have been observed (Bernard et al, 1990). Action of other cytokines such as TNF, IL-1, or other Interleukins is possible, although in this study there was no change in peripheral blood levels of some of them (INF, GMCSF,

TNF). Finally, IL-2 might have anticholinergic activity, a known cause of many types of delirium.

Fatigue and depressive mood can be important to recognize because they can cause unwillingness to continue treatment and even withdrawal. Although hallucinatory delirium's main interest is pathophysiological, it can be bothersome as a side effect. Benzodiazepine tranquilizers do not seem to prevent such syndromes and may even be contributing factors when given with IL-2/INF. Neuroleptics on the other hand seemed effective in cases of frank delirium occurring after the end of treatment, and clinical observation suggests that given at minimal doses as a hypnotic during the infusions they could have a preventive effect. In as much as IL-2/INF treatments will be increasingly used for research and therapy in humans, psychological side effects should be carefully watched for so that causal factors and better preventive or curative measures can be identified.

References

1. Adams F, Quesada J, Gutterman J (1984) Neuropsychiatric manifestations of human leukocyte Interferon therapy in patients with cancer. JAMA 252 (7) : 938-941
2. Bender CM, Dudjak LA (1990) Neurological/psychological alterations. In : Biological Response Modifier Therapy. Cetus Corporation, pp. 53-61
3. Bernard J, Ameriso S, Kempf M et al (1990) Transient focal neurologic deficits complicating Interleukin-2 therapy. Neurology 40 : 154-5
4. Chabner BA, Myers CE (1989) Clinical pharmacology of cancer chemotherapy. In : Devita VT, Hellman S, Rosenberg SA (eds) Cancer : principles & practice of oncology, 3rd ed, JB Lippincot, Philadelphia
5. Denicoff KD, Durkin TM, Lotze MT et al (1989) The neuroendocrine effects of IL-2 treatment. J Clin Endocrin Metab 69 (2) : 402-10
6. Denicoff KD, Rubinow DR, Papa MZ et al (1987) The neuropsychiatric effects of treatment with Interleukin-2 and lymphokine-activated killer cells. Ann Intern Med 107 : 293-300
7. Fisher RI, Coltman CA, Doroshow JH et al (1988) Metastatic renal cancer treated with Interleukin-2 bolus priming followed by continuous infusion with lymphokine activated killer cells. A phase II clinical trial. Ann Intern Med 108 : 518-523
8. Johnson D, Hande KR, Hainsworth JD et al (1983) Neurotoxicity of Interferon. Cancer Treat Rep 67(10) : 958-941
9. Krupp LB, LaRocca NG, Muir-Nash J et al (1989) The fatigue severity scale. Arch Neurol 46 : 1121-1123
10. Nemni R, Iannaccone S, Quattrini A et al (1992) Effect of chronic treatment with recombinant Interleukin-2 on the central nervous system of adult and old mice. Brain Res 591 (2) : 248-52
11. Rosenberg SA, Longo DL, Lotze MT (1989) Principles and applications of biologic therapy. In : Devita VT, Hellman S, Rosenberg SA (eds) Cancer : principles and practice of oncology. 3rd edition, JB Lippincot, Philadelphia
12. Saris SC, Patronas NJ, Rosenberg SA et al (1989) The effect of intravenous IL-2 on brain water content. J Neurosurg 71 : 169-74
13. Sculier JP, Bron D, Verboven N et al (1988) Multiple organ failure during Interleukin-2 administration and LAK cells infusion. Intensive Care Med 14 : 666-667

14. Siegel JP, Puri RK (1991) Interleukin-2 Toxicity. J Clin Oncol 9 (4) : 694-704
15. Smith MJ, Khayat D (1992) Residual acute confusional and hallucinatory syndromes induced by IL-2/INF treatment. Psychooncology 1 : 115-8
16. Spiegel RJ (1986) Intron A (Interferon α-2b) : Clinical overview and future directions. Seminars in Oncology XIII 3 (suppl 2) : 89-101

Abstract. Fifty-two patients undergoing a protocol of cisplatinum, intravenous Interleukin-2 infusions and subcutaneous α-interferon injections for metastatic melanoma and renal cancer were systematically screened for psychiatric disorders before, during and after each of 4 infusions. Fatigue was constant and treatment-limiting in some cases, and was highly correlated with depressive symptoms, which were frequent at the end of the treatment cycle. Some patients showed transient, predominantly hallucinatory delirium occurring or persisting several days after the termination of the infusions. Many cases of delirium occurred after complete resolution of concurrent somatic distress, making it likely that in these cases delirium was due to direct action of the lymphokines on the brain. Neuroleptics were the preferred treatment and benzodiazepines may be counterproductive. Certain lymphocyte phenotype counts correlated negatively with depressive symptomatology whereas fatigue tended to correlate negatively with polymorphonuclear leukocyte counts. Delirium somewhat correlated positively with certain lymphocyte parameters and negatively with others. Hallucinatory delirium, but not depressive disorders, seems to be a direct cerebral effect of the Interleukin-2/α-Interferon combination that is not a consequence of the somatic effects. Patients undergoing lymphokine treatments should be carefully screened for psychological side effects and preventive or curative treatments should be given.

Quality of life in advanced colorectal cancer

G Francini, R Petrioli, A Aquino, S Marsili, S Bruni ; L Lorenzini*, S Mancini*, M Lorenzi*, G Marzocca*, F Tani* ; S Armenio**, G Tanzini**, F Cetta**, F Silvetrini**, C Stacci** ; M Nardini***, I d'Errico***

Colorectal carcinoma is a knowingly chemoresistant neoplasia. Fluorouracil (5-FU) is considered the standard drug for the treatment of advanced colorectal cancer and it is known that the action of 5-FU is potentiated by Folinic-acid (FA).

Our initial results, using the classic outline for combined FA/5-FU (for 5 days every 3 weeks), reported a slight advantage over 5-FU alone, with the improvement of some tumor related symptoms [1]. However, many side effects such as diarrhea, stomatitis and nausea usually occurred with the use of 5-FU and above all, with the combined FA/5-FU with a progressive worsening of quality of life [2]. Thus, we decided to administer supportive care before and during chemotherapy in order to reduce or prevent these side effects. At the same time, to achieve a better response rate and survival, we increased the dose intensity of FA/5-FU by reducing the interval between cycles, rather than using ultrahigh-dose chemotherapy [1].

However, quality of life assessment is known to be an important endpoint in treating advanced cancer patients and a higher tumor response does not necessarily indicate an improvement in palliation [3].

The aim of the study was to evaluate the quality of life on the patients participant in a trial comparing 5-FU alone v.s. FA/5-FU in untreated advanced colorectal cancer.

Patients and methods

From January 1985 to December 1990, 185 patients entered in the study : 91 were randomized to receive 5-FU 400/mg m^{-2} i.v. for 5 days every 4 weeks, and 94 were randomized to receive FA 200 mg/m^{-2} + 5-FU 400 mg/m^{-2} i.v. for 5 days every 3 weeks. Together with tumor related symptoms, the characteristics were similarly distributed in both treatment groups. All patients, 5 days before and then during chemotherapy, received daily supportive care consisting of hydration with normal saline i.v. plus Vitamin-C, carnitine derivatives and ademetionine. Antimycotics and spore suspension of *Bacillus subtilis* were administered × os. Performance status was performed using the ECOG scale and toxicity using the WHO guidelines.

Quality of life was evaluated by a questionnaire consisting of tumor relat-

---

Medical Oncology : * Clinical Surgery ; ** General Surgery ; *** Clinical psychiatry, University of Siena, Italy ed symptoms and toxicity to treatment. The interview occurred by randomization and then continued every week. The questionnaire consisted of 5 major areas of interest ; physical symptoms, functional conditions, psychological conditions, family and social relationships and adverse effects to treatment.

Physical symptoms consisted of : weakness, dry mouth, sweating, constipation, loss of appetite, drowsiness, headache, tremors, confusion, dizziness, hiccups, insomnia, itching, pain, nausea and the overall feeling of not being well. Functional conditions consisted of : difficulties at daily activities or at work.

Psychological and social relationships consisted of : depression, anxiety, nervousness, difficulties in concentration, isolation and difficulties in social relationships with family members. Adverse effects to treatment were : stomatitis, diarrhea, nausea, vomiting, conjunctivitis, leukopenia, anemia, hair loss. Most patients of both treatment groups reported pain, constipation, anorexia, weakness, psychological symptoms and difficulties with daily activities.

The judgment of whether a patient had an improvement in quality of life was performed by a referee without knowledge of whether the patient belonged to the 5-FU group or the FA/5-FU group. Answers on physical symptoms were indicated by the patients on a 0-10 scale. Toxic effects were expressed as : none, slight, moderate, severe. The data on quality of life was analyzed only if patients had undergone at least 6 cycles of chemotherapy or delayed treatment no more than 14 days. The responses given on the questionnaire during the sample week were compared to those given by the same patients at randomization.

Patients were categorized according to whether they had improved their quality of life or whether it remained unchanged or worsened. The judgment on quality of life was based upon the answers reported by the patients in the interview. The information, provided from the patients, determined the mean scores in the 5 issues of the questionnaire.

Differences between groups were analyzed by independent 2 sided t tests.

Results

The group of patients receiving 5-FU alone achieved a response rate of 18.5 % (95 % confidence limit : 10 % to 27 %) with a median survival of 7.5 months. The group receiving FA/5-FU achieved a response rate of 33.7 % (95 % conficence limit : 23 % to 43 %) with a median survival of 13 months. The differences were significant in response rate (p = 0.04 : x^2-test) and survival (p = 0.041 : log-rank test).

Performance status showed a significant improvement for patients receiving FA/5-FU over 5-FU alone. Side effects were well tolerated and consisted mainly of stomatitis, diarrhea, dermatosis and conjunctivitis. There was no significant difference between the 2 treatments (p = 0.078). Data on quality of life, evaluated after 6 cycles of chemotherapy in 64 patients treated with 5-FU and in 58 treated with FA/5-FU, showed that 11 patients (17 %) and 24 patients (41 %) improved, respectively. In the 5-FU group, 22 (34 %) and

31 (49 %) patients were considered unchanged and worsened. In the FA/5-FU group, 19 (32 %) and 15 (27 %) patients appeared unchanged and worsened (Table 1). The median duration of the improvement in « quality of life » was 2.0 months in the 5-FU group and 4.5 months in the FA/5-FU group. In the 5-FU group only 5 patients were considered free from any tumor related symtoms, while in ghe FA/5-FU group 13 patients became free of these symtoms. A good correlation was noted between the improved and free-symptom patients with objective response to treatment (Table 2).

Table 1. Changes in quality of life in advanced colorectal cancer patients treated with 5-FU or FA/5-FU.

Judgment	5-FU (n = 64)	FA/5-FU (n = 58)	p value
Improved	11 (17 %)	24 (41 %)	<0.005
Unchanged	22 (34 %)	19 (32 %)	n.s.
Worsened	31 (49 %)	15 (27 %)	< 0.001

Table 2. Number of improved and symptoms-free patients according to objective response to treatment

		Objective response	Improved	Symptom-free
5-FU	CR	3	3	3
	PR	13	7	2
	SD	41	1	0
	PD	29	0	0
FA/5-FU	CR	4	4	4
	PR	23	17	9
	SD	35	3	0
	PD	19	0	0

Pain, depression and capacity of daily activity were the items which showed the most significant improvement in FA/5-FU group over the 5-FU group. Pain had the closest correlation with the global judgment of not feeling well among all psychical symptoms. However, functional and psychological conditions seemed to have a major role in the evaluation of quality of life. In fact, isolation, depression and anxiety may usually produce more discomfort for the patient than the pain itself [4, 5].

Conclusions

This study indicates the importance of supportive care in advanced colorectal cancer, simultaneoulsy with chemotherapy, which allows the administration of an accelerated FA/5-FU without major side effects. This accelerated chemotherapy achieved a better response rate and survival over 5-FU alone. At the 6th cycle of chemotherapy, 41 % of FA/5-FU group showed an improvement in the score related to the quality of life.

References

1. Francini G, Lorenzini L, Armenio S, Gennari C (1987) Palliative chemotherapy for relief of subocclusive symptoms, Lancet ii : 578
2. Machover D, Goldschmidt E, Chollet P, Metzger G, Zitoun J, Marquet J, Vandenbulcke JM, Misset JL. Schwarzenberg L (1986) Treatment of advanced colorectal and gastric adenocarcinoma with 5-Fluorouracil and high-dose Folinic acid. J Clin Oncol 4 : 685-696
3. Watson JW (1981) What does « response » in cancer chemotherapy really mean ? Br Med J 283 : 34-37
4. Cassileth BR, Lusk EJ, Strousse TB, Miller DS, Brown LL, Cross PA (1985) A psychological analysis of cancer patients and their next-of-kin. Cancer 55 : 72-76
5. Ventafridda V, De Conno F, Ripamonti C, Gamba A, Tamburini M (1990) Quality-of-life assessment during a palliative care programme. Ann Oncol 1 : 415-420

Advance directives in the intensive care unit of a tertiary cancer center

MS Ewer, J Taubert, MK Ali

Living will legislation was placed in effect in the United States on November 1, 1991. The purpose of this legislation was to ensure that the health care desires of patients who had become ill to the extent that they could no longer express their wishes would be respected [1]. It had been hoped that through living will legislation patients who had little chance of surviving their critical illness, and who had executed an advance directive stipulating that they did not wish to be kept alive in the event of medical futility, would be spared the burden of life support systems. Families or other decision makers of such patients would not have to face the difficult and often recurrent decisions of whether or not, and to what extent, to continue therapy as a meaningful recovery became progressively unlikely. Society as a whole would be better able to channel limited health care resources towards patients for whom recovery was more likely and to those patients who desired such measures.

There are 2 advance directives in common use in the United States [2]. The first, the *Living*, will stipulates that in the event of a medical condition where there is no chance of recovery, as determined by 2 physicians, and where continued treatment would only delay the moment of death, the patient instructs the health care team not to initiate or, if already initiated, to discontinue therapy that would interfere with the natural process of death. Comfort measures are authorized, and the wording may additionally stipulate that such measures may be generously used even if there is concern that vital life functions might be suppressed. The second directive, commonly referred to as a *durable power of attorney for health care decisions*, authorizes a specified individual to make decisions in the event that a patient no longer is able to do so.

When the conditions implied in an advance directive are clearly met, i.e., when the futility of continued life support is obvious, and, when all parties are in agreement (patient, family, or other designee named in the durable power of attorney, as well as the physician), and when these facts are clear prior to a life-threatening deterioration, patients are generally not transferred to an intensive care unit. Patient care is then focused on comfort measures rather than towards a therapeutic-goal of reversing a progressively life-threatening condition. Even though most people would prefer not to be kept alive on life-support systems in the event of medical futility, there is still considerable controversy as to when, in the course of a deteriorating medical condition, the conditions stipulated in an advance directive are satisfied. Even the definition of « meaningful life » differs among patients and among the various physicians caring for them [3].

In order to evaluate problems with advance directives in the intensive care unit of a tertiary cancer center, and the outcomes for patients who had executed such documents who were admitted to the intensive care unit, a study of all patients with advance directives who were admitted to the intensive care unit was undertaken.

Materials and methods

During a fourteen month period, from November 1, 1991 until December 31, 1992, the records of all patients who were admitted to the intensive care unit were reviewed. In all 26 patients with living wills were identified, which accounted for 16 % of all critically ill patients admitted to the facility's intensive care unit. There were 17 male and 9 female patients. Fifteen of these had hematologic malignancies and 11 had solid tumors. Patients were admitted to the intensive care unit with sepsis (16 patients), hematological complications (6 patients), congestive heart failure (2 patients), exacerbation of chronic pulmonary disease (1 patient), and drug overdose, (1 patient).

Results

Of the 26 patients transferred to the Intensive care unit, 24 were placed on mechanical ventilators ; 1 refused to be placed on the ventilator, and 1 recovered to the extent that she could be discharged to a regular hospital unit without requiring mechanical ventilation. Of the 24 patients who were placed on mechanical ventilators, 8 died while on the ventilator, and 9 had life-support systems including their ventilators removed and were allowed to die, i.e., were terminally weaned after it was recognized that further support would only delay the moment of death. The remaining 7 were weaned from the ventilator. All of the weaned patients lived for at least 24 hours, but 6 of the 7 experienced a recurrence of critical illness, were not re-intubated and expired before leaving the hospital. In all of these cases death occurred within 3 weeks of extubation. One patient was discharged home in stable condition.

The length of time on the mechanical ventilator for the above-noted subgroups was 3-35 days for those that expired on the ventilator, 1-25 days for patients who were terminally weaned, and 2-28 days for the group that was weaned and who later expired. The lone survivor was intubated for 42 days.

Several problems related to the advance directive were identified. Nine cases were transferred to the intensive care unit and only after being placed on life support systems was the fact made known that an advance directive existed. In all 9 of these cases the delay in presenting the documents rested with the patient or his or her family ; the family either feared that notifying the physician of the advance directive might influence care in a detrimental way, or they felt that there was no need to present the documents before the onset of critical illness. In at least 5 of these cases the patient might not have been transferred to the intensive care unit had the presence of the advance directive been known. In 2 cases there was conflict between the dictates of the living will and the desires of the individual designated in the durable power of attorney. In both instances the patient was considered moribund by the attending physician who sought to terminate life support according to the provisions of the living will. In each case the implementation of this decision was delayed for several days because the designee would not agree with termination of life-support. In 1 of these cases the refusal to agree with the withdrawal was based on a religious belief, the designee asking that we not « play God » but allow the patient, who was already on life-support systems, to die naturally.

There were 9 instances where controversy between various physicians caring for these critically ill patients surrounded the decision to continue or discontinue life support. While there was concurrence among attending and consulting physicians as to poor prognosis, some physicians were willing to terminate life support earlier than others. The point at which a particular patient became « hopelessly ill without realistic chance of recovery » meeting the criteria for withdrawal of support systems according to the advance directive was not clearly defined. In 1 instance a physician agreed to withdraw all treatment including pressor agents, antibiotics, and nutrition in accordance with the advance directive, but could not bring himself to withdraw the mechanical ventilator. In 1 instance a patient's family demanded removal from life support systems despite objections of the attending physician.

Discussion

Patients who present advance directives to their physicians wish to minimize the likelihood of prolonged biological survival in cases where recovery is impossible, i.e., in cases of medical futility. Patients often express the opinion that life-support systems are acceptable if there is at least some chance of a meaningful recovery. The dilemma for most health-care professionals who must deal with advance directives is arriving at some estimation of at what probability of a successful outcome an individual patient would wish to have treatment stopped [4].

For the present, some problems with advance directives have been identified among this group of patients, and can be minimized. Patients should be encouraged to present their advance directives early during the course of their disease, thereby reducing the likelihood of being placed on support systems against their wishes, and reducing the likelihood of family being asked to decide issues which have already been adequately addressed by the patient him or herself. Physicians must keep patients informed as to changes in prognosis so that an appropriate level of care can be agreed upon, but also can be modified as the likelihood of success increases or decreases. Finally, in order to improve the impact of advance directive on health care, additional data must be sought regarding specific desires of patients, and costs of critical care, both financial as well as social and emotional. Perhaps only with greatly improved prognostication will the dilemmas of advance directives be ultimately resolved [5].

References

1. Emanuel LL, Emanuel EJ (1989) The medical directive : a new comprehensive advance care document. JAMA 261 : 3288-3293
2. Ewer MS (1991) Ethical issues confronting today's physician : Perspective on directives to physicians. Intern Med World Report 6 : 3-4
3. Ewer MS (1991) Decision-making in critical care oncology. The Cancer Bulletin 43 : 298-302
4. Danis M, Southerland LI, Garrett JM et al (1991) A prospective study of advance directives for medical care : a case for greater use. N Eng J Med 324 : 882-888
5. Ewer MS, Gibbs HR, Swafford J, Ali MK (1992) Appropriate use of intensive care facilities in a cancer hospital. The Cancer Bulletin 44 : 168-172

Do cancer related pain problems exist in France ?

L Brasseur*, F Larue*, M Dubiez*, S Colleau**, C Cleeland**

It has already been shown that 70 % of patients with advanced cancer suffer significant pain (Bonica, 1985). Similarly, surveys have suggested that adequate pain relief can be provided to more than 3/4 ou three quarters patients, if optimal administration of opioids and adjuvant drugs is prescribed (WHO 1986 ; Ventafridda 1985). In developed countries, little improvement in therapeutic outcome is probably due to a lack of understanding of the use of analgesic drugs and especially morphine and also factors due to patients' attitudes (Baines 1989 ; Portenoy R 1993).

Cancer is the second cause of dying in France. Its incidence was 227/100,000 inhabitants (1989) ; there is approximately 200,000 new cases a year (Ministère des Affaires Sociales et de la Solidarité 1990).The situation of cancer pain in France over a short period of time was surveyed through 3 studies :
— prevalence and severity of cancer pain in patients,
— Physicians' attitude,
— Public's attitude.

Assessing the prevalence and severity of cancer pain in France

This study was overtaken using the Brief Pain Inventory (BPI) as a tool. This questionnaire was designed as an evaluation instrument by the Pain Research Group, University of Wisconsin Medical School, Madison, WI, USA : it can index the degree of pain that patients experience and also the impact of pain on various aspects of patients' life. BPI was translated into French and cross-translated by bilingual speakers to insure compability of meaning between the 2 languages. The French version was then validated in a preliminary sample in 2 hospitals in Paris. Following validation, a representative sample of 605 cancer patients (breast, prostate, lung, colorectal, gynecological cancers at any stage of the disease) was drawn from 20 randomly selected treatment settings in the country. Sample institutions included anti cancer centers, university hospitals, general hospitals, private clinics and 1 home care setting.

Of the 605 patients who were included in the study, 329 were in pain (56,6 %) : 69 % rated their worst pain 5 or above and 53,8 % rated their average pain 5 or above on a 0 to 10 scale. As expected, pain interfers with additional dimensions of a patients' life in a similar way that pain increases. Of the 329 patients in pain, physicians reported that 45,5 % were not getting any pain medications : only 27 % of patients with pain claimed to receive satisfactory pain relief from analgesic medications.

---

* GERD Action Douleur, 80 avenue de l'épi d'or, 91400 Orsay, France
** Pain Research Group, University of Wisconsin, 1900 University avenue, Madison, WI 53705, USA

Physicians' attitudes

In order to evaluate physicians' attitude toward cancer pain, a survey was performed in the whole country : a representative sample of 300 oncologists (ONC) and 600 general practitionners (GP) were interviewed by telephon call according to a structured questionnaire.

ONC were difficult to get in touch and a majority seemed to be interested by more « scientific » subjects. Physicians underestimate the prevalence of severe cancer pain (less than 20 % according to a majority). 90 % of physicians evaluate patients' pain according to their own statement. 40 % of GP prefers « on demand » administration of analgesics. In case of severe pain, 83 % of physicians say they will prescribe sustained release morphine tablets as first choice drug ; however, 6 % say they will never prescribe morphine. 55 % of ONC say they will give morphine to less than 1/5 patients and only 46 % of GP say that they will prescribe morphine by themselves. 50 % of ONC and 25 % of GP are unwilling prescribing morphine, mainly because of the fear of side effects : ONC have concerns about « tolerance » (53,6 %) and constipation ; GP have concerns about respiratory depression. Narcotic regulation is said to be an impediment (ONC = 33 % ; GP = 26 %). 22 % of physicians say they need informations on how to use morphine : 61 % of ONC and 73 % of GP say they never had any specific pain management teaching.

50 % of ONC and 40 % of GP think that cancer pain is properly managed in France ; 93 % of ONC and 85 % say that they personally manage cancer pain adequately.

Public attitude

An opinion poll was used to survey French population. Basic informations were collected through INSEE (National Institute for Statistics) : the sample had the feature of the French population of 18 years old and above. One thousand persons were interviewed by telephon call : a small minority (less than 1 %) did not want to answer.

Nearly 50 % were emotionally concerned. 44 % do not know the impact of cancer pain at an early stage of the disease, but a vast majority (72,4 %) think it is very frequent at terminal stage. Public underestimate the efficacy of pain treatment : only 26 % think it may give pain relief. They have little knowledge of pain treatement modalities since less than 33 % of the persons advocate the « round the clock » administration of analgesic medication. 44 % associate morphine to pain relief, 14 % to euthanasia, 24 % to near death and 26 % to toxicomania. 55 % will be afraid to get addicted if they have to receive morphine.

Conclusion

These results are part of bigger investigation intended to evaluate the statement of cancer pain management in France : 2 studies on nurses and pharmacists need to be completed. Other points would need to be investigate as the role of French narcotic regulations on physicians' prescriptions. However, we can say now that according to the supra results, there is a need to establish a national program to improve the quality of cancer pain management in France.

Acknowledgements. Those surveys were supported by La Direction Générale de la Santé (French Ministry of Health), Professeur Schwartzenberg, La Section Départementale du Val de Marne de la Ligue Nationale contre le Cancer, Les laboratoires Baxter et Sarget and we would like to express our thanks.

References

1. Bonica JJ (1985) Treatment of cancer pain : current status and future needs. In : Fields HL et al (eds) Advances in pain research and therapy, vol 9. Raven Press New York, p 589
2. World Health Organisation (1986) Cancer Pain Relief. World Health Organisation, Geneva
3. Ventafridda V, Tamburini M, DeConno F (1985) Comprehensive treatement in cancer pain. In : Fields HL et al (eds) Advances in pain research and therapy, vol 9. Raven Press, New York, p 617
4. Baines M, Kirkham SR (1989) In : Wall et al (eds) Textbook of Pain. Churchill Livingstone, Edinburgh, p 590
5. Portenoy RK (1993) In : Patt RB (ed) Cancer Pain. Lippincott, Philadelphia, p 119
6. Ministère des Affaires Sociales et de la Solidarité (1990) Annuaire des Statistiques Sanitaires et Sociales. SESI, Paris

Intravenous granisetron-simple, safe and effective single-dose. Administration for control of chemotherapy induced nausea and vomiting

SG Dilly

There is no evidence that nausea and vomiting are necessary for the antitumour efficacy of cytotoxic drugs. Nausea and vomiting are merely an unfortunate side-effect of cancer chemotherapy. However, the severity of the symptoms and the complexity of « conventional » antiemetic regimens has led to antiemetic therapy becoming a significant issue in patient care. The new 5-HT$_3$ antagonists, such as granisetron, offer the possibility that antiemetic therapy can be so simple and effective that nausea and vomiting are no longer a significant issue in determining treatment regimens.

Simple single-dose administration

High-dose Metoclopramide regimens, the most efficacious conventional antiemetic, are cumbersome to administer involving intermittent bolus dosing or 8 hour continuous infusions ; these regimens are clearly incompatible with out patient usage. Thus, an agent which provides 24 hour antiemetic cover following a single dose will minimise nursing intervention, need for hospitalisation and disruption to patients'lives. Examination of the granisetron database shows that 76 % of patients (527/697) required only a single prophylactic dose (40 µg/kg) to provide control of nausea and vomiting for 24 hours, demonstrating the compound's long duration of action. When examined according to the chemotherapy regimen administered, 69 % (217/313) of patients exposed to Cisplatin ($\geqslant$ 50 mg/m^2) and 81 % (310/384) of those receiving other emetogenic therapies, attained adequate 24 hour symptom control with a only single prophylactic dose (40 µg/kg) of granisetron (Fig. 1).

Same dose — All patients

It is usual practice to tailor the antiemetic dose to the patients requirements, taking account of the chemotherapy regimen and patient characteristics. However, granisetron has a wide therapeutic index and relatively shallow dose response curve, allowing the same dose to be administered to all patients.

The relationship between IV granisetron dose (over the range of 2 and 160 µg/kg) and therapeutic effect was studied in 4 double-blind studies involving a total of 1,349 patients receiving their first course of chemotherapy. The

---

SmithKline Beecham Pharmaceuticals, Reigate, UK

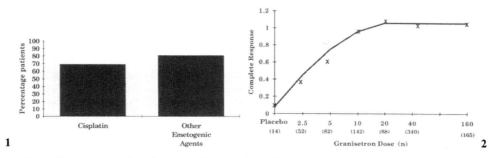

Fig. 1. Percentage of patients requiring only a single prophylactic dose of granisetron (40 mcg/kg)

Fig. 2. Complete response in granisetron dose-ranging studies : results expressed as response relative to 40 mcg/kg dose

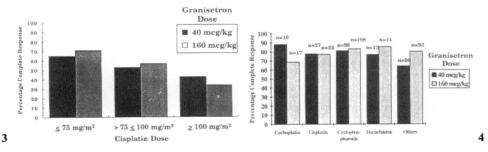

Fig. 3. Response to Granisetron According to Cisplatin

Fig. 4. Percentage complete response following administration of each primary cytostatic therapy in patients receiving granisetron (40 or 60 mcg/kg)

pooled findings of the 4 studies are presented in Figure 2. The dose response curve showed a predictable rise in response with increasing dose, approaching a plateau at doses above 30 μg/kg. No dose related toxicity was observed. Therefore, a fixed 3 mg IV dose can safely be recommended for all patients, equivalent to 40 μg/kg for an average 75 kg person but ranging from 30 μg/kg for a heavy patient (100 kg) up to 100 μg/kg for a lightweight patient (30 kg) ; these doses lie on the plateau of the dose response curve, ensuring optimal antiemetic cover for all patients across the weight range.

Although granisetron is associated with a small reduction in the complete response rate in patients exposed to very high dose Cisplatin regimens (> 100 mg/m^2), no additional benefit is conferred by a 4 fold dose increase from 40 to 160 μg/kg (Fig. 3). Moreover, doses of 40 and 160 μg/kg provided similarly effective antiemetic cover against a range of cytotoxic therapies (Fig. 4) lending further support to the use of a fixed 3 mg IV dose for all patients.

No special precautions

Antiemetic therapy is frequently associated with certain prescribing precautions. Studies with granisetron have not identified any special precautions associated with its use in patient subgroups, nor a potential for drug interactions. Granisetron was equally well tolerated by elderly as by younger patients and by hepatically and non-hepatically impaired patients. There are no special concerns associated with its use in patients with cardiac disease or renal impairment. Moreover, the absence of drug interactions is consistent with its highly selective pharmacological action, high potency and wide therapeutic index. The safety profile of granisetron is similar in males and females, although headache occurs with a higher incidence in females.

Conclusion

Granisetron 3 mg IV is recommended for all patients. This simple, versatile regimen meets the needs of patients with differing characteristics without requirement for dose adjustment. The compound's long duration of action permits single dose administration for the majority of patients, offering benefits to both patients and medical care staff.

Control of refractory nausea and vomiting with adjuvant propofol during cancer chemotherapy

A Borgeat, OHG Wilder-Smith, K Rifat, M Forni

Nausea and vomiting remain one of the most distressing and unpleasant side-effects of cancer chemotherapy [1, 2]. These symptoms cause significant delayed psychological morbidity such as anticipatory nausea/vomiting or depression [3] and are the most frequently cited reasons patients give for not wanting to continue chemotherapy or even start treatment. Recently, selective serotonin antagonists (5HT3-antagonists) have shown considerable antiemetic potency during highly emetogenic therapies with fewer side-effects [4, 5]. Despite these improvements, 20-30 % of patients undergoing Cisplatin chemotherapy still remain unresponsive to the most efficient antiemetic regimens available i.e. 5HT3-antagonists plus Dexamethasone [6].

A new agent for inducing and maintaining anesthesia, propofol (2,6 Di-isopropylphenol), has been demonstrated to result in less post-operative nausea and vomiting [7, 8]. Subhypnotic doses of propofol have recently been shown to possess direct antiemetic properties [9]. Propofol was also associated at the same dosage with significant anxiolytic effects [10]. The observation of these properties led us to investigate the efficacy of adjuvant subhypnotic doses of propofol for the management of chemotherapy-associated nausea and emesis inadequately controlled by 5HT3-antagonists and Dexamethasone.

Forty patients who suffered during their first chemotherapy cycle from more than 5 emetic episodes in the first 24 hours despite antiemetic prophylaxis with 5HT3-antagonists and Dexamethasone were prospectively included in the present investigation. For the 2 subsequent chemotherapy cycle propofol was added to the usual antiemetic prophylaxis at a rate of $1 \text{ mg.kg}^{-1}.\text{hr}^{-1}$ starting 4 hours prior induction of chemotherapy up to the end of the study period (24 hours). Twenty patients had Cisplatin $> 80 \text{ mg/m}^2$ (CIS-PT group) and 20 had Cyclophosphamide 600 mg/m2 or Epirubicin 120 mg/m^2 (NON CIS-PT group).

The number of emetic episodes during the first 24 hours, appetite, defined as present if patients asked for and ate a complete standard hospital breakfast the following morning, and activity defined, as present if patients ambulated spontaneously, initiated conversation or asked for entertainment material (e.g. television, newspapers, games), were assessed.

In the NON CIS-PT group total control of nausea and vomiting was observed in all patients. Appetite and activity as well were present in all patients. Increase in sedation was not seen. In the CIS-PT group the addition of propofol increases the number of patients free of vomiting from 0 % to 90 %. Appetite was present in 45 % and activity in 50 %. Slight increase in sedation was observed in 1 patient (5 %). All 40 patients preferred propofol-supplemented antiemesis for future chemotherapy.

Departments of Anesthesia and Oncogynecology, University Hospital of Geneva, Switzerland

In this preliminary study the addition of subhypnotic doses of Propofol to 5HT3-antagonists and Dexamethasone in these previously refractory patients resulted in total control of emesis in the NON CIS-PT group and a marked improvement in the CIS-PT group during the first 24 hours. Improvement of patient's well-being assessed by appetite and activity was noted in all patients in the NON CIS-PT group and in 50 % in the CIS-PT group. All patients expressed a preference for Propofol-assisted regimen for subsequent chemotherapy treatment.

References

1. Coates A, Abraham S, Kaye SB, Sowerbutts T et al (1983) On the receiving end-patient perception of the side effects of cancer chemotherapy. Eur J Cancer Clin 19 : 203-208
2. Gralla RJ, Tyson LB, Kris MG, Clark RA (1987) The management of chemotherapy-induced nausea and vomiting. Med Clin North Am 71 : 289-301
3. Chin SBY, Kucuk O, Peterson R, Ezdinli EZ (1992) Variables contributing to anticipatory nausea and vomiting in cancer chemotherapy. Am J Clin Oncol (CCT) 15 : 262-267
4. Marty M, Pouillart P, Scholl S, Oroz JP, Azab M, Brian N, Pujade-Hauraine E, Paule B, Paes D, Boris J (1990) Comparison of the 5HT3 antagonist ondansetron with high-dose Metoclopramide in the control of Cisplatin-induced emesis. N Engl J Med 322 : 816-822
5. Stables R, Andrews PLR, Bailey HE, Costall B, Gunning GJ, Hawthorn J, Naylor RJ, Tyers MB (1987) Antiemetic properties of the 5HT3-receptor antagonist, GR 38032F. Cancer Treat Rev 14 : 333-336
6. Roila F, Tonato M, Cognetti F et al (1991) Prevention of Cisplatin-induced emesis : A double-blind multicenter randomized crossover study comparing ondansetron and ondansetron plus Dexamethasone. J Clin Oncol 9 : 675-678
7. Fahy LT, Van Mourick GA, Utting JE (1985) A comparison of the induction characteristics of Thiopentone and Propofol. Anaesthesia 40 : 939-944
8. Mc Collum JS, Milligan KR, Dundee JW (1988) The antiemetic action of Propofol. Anaesthesia 43 : 239-240
9. Borgeat A, Wilder-Smith OHG, Saiah M, Rifat K (1992) Subhypnotic doses of Propofol possess direct antiemetic properties. Anesth Analg 74 : 539-541
10. Ure RW, Dwyer SJ, Blogg CE, White AP (1991) Patient-controlled anxiolysis with Propofol. Br J Anaesth 67 : 657P-658P

Liposomal Daunorubicin treatment increases quality of life in HIV-associated Kaposi's Sarcoma

CA Presant, M Scolaro, P Kennedy, DW Blayney, B Flanagan, J Lisak, J Presant

Kaposi's Sarcoma has become a common tumor, which occurs in AIDS patients [1, 2]. The quality of life in these patients is almost universally adversely impacted by the chemotherapy treatment and/or opportunistic infections.

Since liposomes specifically target to Kaposi's Sarcoma lesions [3], and can be loaded with chemotherapy to treat mice with transplanted tumors [4, 5], we reasoned that liposomal chemotherapy could successfully manage HIV associated Kaposi's Sarcoma [3].

Method

Liposomal Daunorubicin (DaunoXome, Vestar, Inc., San Dimas, California) was administered at 40 mg per meter square every 2 weeks, to patients with biopsy proven Kaposi's Sarcoma, with HIV antibodies by elisa test. AZT was continued.

The doses of liposomal Daunorubucin and AZT were modified according to granulocyte count and platelet counts on the day of therapy.

Prior to therapy, and at each subsequent treatment, patients evaluated their quality of life. The instrument used consisted of 7 linear analog scales assessing level of physical performance, emotional state, nausea, emesis, stomatitis, fatigue, change in tumor size and swelling, and alopecia. Of these, 3 questions dealing with level of physical performance, fatigue and emotional state were evaluated in detail to determine the general quality of life of the patients.

The questionnaire was administered to 10 « normal » individuals to determine the normative range of data for these questions [6]. Patients scores were compared to the normative data in order to generate comparative response data.

Tumor response was defined as follows : complete response was absence of any detectable residual disease persisting for at least 4 weeks (patients with laryngeal lesions had repeat endoscopic procedures to document response).

Partial response was a 50 % or greater decrease in the sum of the products of the largest perpendicular diameters of marker lesions, or a complete flattening of at least 50 % of all previously raised nodular or plaque-like lesions. In addition, no new lesions or new visceral sites of involvement must have occurred, and there must have been no worsening of tumor associated edema of pleural effusion.

Los Angeles Oncologic Institute, St. Vincent Medical Center, Los Angeles, CA, USA

Results

Tumor response

Twenty-four patients were evaluable. Complete responses were observed in 2/24 (8.3 %), and partial responses were seen in 13/24 (54.2 %). The overall response rate was 62.5 %.

Quality of life response

The result of the patient-measured quality of life assessments indicated a high frequency of palliative responses (Table 1). Twenty-one patients completed the quality of life diaries and were evaluable. Normal individuals evaluated their « performance » at a median of 80 (based on the best score of 100). Patients with Kaposi's Sarcoma had a median pretreatment score of only 57. The median best sustained post treatment score was 69. Complete palliative response (post treatment score > 80 [6]) was observed in 7 and partial palliative response (increase in score greater than 10 [6]) was seen in 8, for a total response rate of 71 %. Of the 16 patients with pretreatment scores less than 80, 4 (25 %) had improvement to greater than 80.

Table 1. Quality of life assessments

Scores (0-100) :	Performance	Emotion
Pretreatment (median)	57	49
Post-treatment sustained Maximum (median)	69	76
Response :		
Complete response	7 33 %	10 48 %
Partial response	8 38 %	6 29 %
No response	6 29 %	5 24 %

The median length of treatment until at least a partial palliative response was observed was 2 weeks median (range 2 to 8 weeks) and the median duration of palliative response until worsening (fall of greater than 10 units) on 2 successive evaluations was 9 weeks (range 2 to 24 weeks). Patients also rated their « emotional » quality of life.

Compared to a normal median of 78, patients had a median score before therapy of 49. Therapy produced a median maximum score post therapy of 76. There were 10 complete palliative responses, and 6 partial palliative responses [6] for a total response rate of 77 %. In 15 patients with pretreatment scores less than 78, 5 had sustained improvement to normal (33 %). The median time to at least a partial response was 2 weeks (range 2-4 weeks) and the median duration of response was 6 weeks (range 2 to 23 weeks).

Patients also evaluated their own tumor responses. When asked to grade the reduction in size of their tumors, 12 of 21 patients scored their lesions as significantly smaller on at least 2 successive measurements. When asked to grade the reduction in swelling, 15 of 21 patients scored the swelling as significantly less.

The patient-scored tumor response was compared to the physician-evaluated tumor therapy response. Of the 13 patients with measured tumor complete response or partial responses, patients evaluated their own tumor sizes as smaller in 10 patients and not improved in 3 patients. Of the 8 patients without measured tumor response, patients evaluated their tumors as smaller in 2 patients and not improved in 6 patients.

Discussion

The high objective response rate (64 %), and the high frequency of improvement in quality of life (71-77 %) indicate considerable anti-tumor activity and clinical efficacy of this treatment. Furthermore, toxicity was mild with this regimen.

The quality of life responses were similar in frequency to the objective responses. Since patients with HIV-associated Kaposi's Sarcoma are also receiving other therapy for other complications of HIV, it is difficult to conclude unequivocally that the measured improvement in quality of life was due solely to liposomal Daunorubicin. However, the high frequency of subjective response evaluated by accepted and standardized criteria, and close correlation of time of response with objective tumor remission, strongly suggest a cause-and-effect relationship between liposomal Daunorubicin and improvement in quality of life.

We conclude that liposomal Daunorubicin is associated with a high frequency of objective tumor regression, as well as with a high frequency of improvement in quality of life (as measured by patients). Therefore, it may be the treatment of choice in many patients with HIV-associated Kaposi's Sarcoma.

References

1. Friedman-Kien AE, Laubenstein LJ, Rubinstein P et al (1982) Disseminated Kaposi's Sarcoma in homosexual men. Ann Internal Med 96 : 693-700
2. Gill PS, Rarick M, McCutchan JA et al (1991) Systemic treatment of AIDS-related Kaposi's Sarcoma : results of a randomized trial. Am J Med 90 : 427-443
3. Presant CA, Blayney DW, Proffitt RJ (1988) Preliminary report : imaging of Kaposi's Sarcoma and lymphoma in AIDS with Indium-III-Labeled liposomes. Lancet 335 : 1307-1309
4. Forssen EA, Coulter DM, Proffitt RJ (1992) Selective in vivo localization of small unilameller vesicles in solid tumors. Cancer Res 51 : 3255-3261
5. Forssen EA (1988) Chemotherapy with Anthracycline Liposomes. In : Gregoriadis G (ed) Liposomes as Drug Carriers. John Wiley and Sons, pp 335-364
6. Presant CA, Wiseman C, Blayney DW et al (1990) Proposed criteria for serial evaluation of quality of life in cancer patients. J National Cancer Inst 82 : 322-323, 796

Biology and clinical pharmacology

Comparison of 12 multidrug-resistance modulating agents in a model of doxorubicin-resistant rat glioblastoma cells in vitro

J Robert, S Huet, S Bennis, C Chapey

Since the original discovery by Tsuruo et al [1] that Verapamil and other calcium channel blockers were able to reverse multidrug resistance, a great variety of compounds have been shown to possess this property [2]. The compounds able to reverse multidrug resistance share some physical-chemical properties, all of them being lipophilic cations [3]. The structural requirements are not very strict, and about 1 % of organic compounds display this property (Lavelle, personal communication).

Several of these agents are able to compete with the « natural substrates » of P-glycoprotein and inhibit its photoaffinity labeling by Azidopine or Vinblastine analogues [4]. This is especially the case for Verapamil, and it has been thought that all multidrug resistance reversing agents directly interfered with P-glycoprotein [5]. The restoration of intracellular drug accumulation to the level obtained in sensitive cells has been observed for most modulators and is generally associated to restoration of cytotoxicity [6, 7]. However, it is not clear at present time if all the agents able to reverse multidrug resistance can act by the same mechanism. Using photoaffinity labelling with Azidopine, and its displacement, it has been shown that several independent sites may exist on P-glycoprotein, and that other proteins could be involved [8].

There is a challenge toward the identification of multidrug resistance-reversing agents devoid of pharmacologic effects other than their action on P-glycoprotein, in order to avoid any supplementary toxicity. In the course of the preclinical development of a new MDR-modulating agent, S9788, a Triazineaminopiperidine derivative, originating from the Institut de Recherche International Servier [9], we have compared its reversing properties to those of eleven other compounds already known to reverse multidrug-resistance and belonging to various classes of MDR modulators. This study was performed on a single model of sensitive and multidrug resistant cells that we had already studied [10, 11]. The C6 0.5 line, which is 400-fold resistant to Doxorubicin, obviously displays a multifactorial resistance, associating a classical MDR phenotype and a non-MDR phenotype which is presently under investigation.

Materials and methods

Drugs and products

Doxorubicin was a generous gift from Laboratoire Roger Bellon. Verapamil and Amiodarone were clinical formulation (respectively Isoptine® and Cordar-

---

Fondation Bergonié, 180, rue de Saint-Genès, 33076 Bordeaux, France

one®) ; Tamoxifen, Nifedipine, Nicardipine, Trifluoperazine, Quinine, Quinidine and Dipyridamole were purchased from Sigma ; Cyclosporine A was obtained from Sandoz, and diltiazem from Synthelabo. S9788 (6-{4[2,2-di(4-Fluorophenyl) Ethylamino] Piperidin 1-yl} N,N'-Dipropen-2-yl 1,3,5-Triazine 2,4-Diamine, Bimethanesulfonate) was obtained from Laboratoires Servier (Courbevoie, France). Some drugs had to be first dissolved in absolute Ethanol : Cyclosporine A, Dipyridamole, Tamoxifen, Nifedipin, Nicardipin, and Trifluoperazine. The amount of Ethanol thus introduced during cell incubations had no effect on cell growth and Doxorubicin cytotoxicity.

Cell culture and Doxorubicin accumulation

The C6 rat glioblastoma clone [18] and its Doxorubicin resistant counterpart C6 0.5 [19] were routinely cultivated in Petri dishes (Nunc) with Dulbecco's modified Eagle medium supplemented with 10 % fetal calf serum (Seromed) as already described [10].

Appropriate numbers of cells were seeded in 20 cm² Petri dishes with 5 ml of medium without drug. The effect of the various multidrug resistance reversing agents was then tested on Doxorubicin accumulation at several concentrations of the modulator between 0.1 and 100 μM. The concentration of Doxorubicin was set at 17.2 μM in a first series of experiments, then it was equaled to the IC_{50} of the drug as evaluated in the presence of the modulator. Incubations were performed for 2 hours in the presence of both Doxorubicin and the modulator. At the end of this incubation, the monolayers were washed with 0.15 M NaCl, harvested, and pelleted at 3,000 rpm for 5 min. This was rapidly done in order to avoid any significant drug efflux during these steps. 0.5 ml of water and 0.5 ml of 40 % trichloroacetic acid were then added and the samples were kept at 4 °C overnight, then centrifuged for 30 min at 3,000 rpm. The acid-soluble fraction was used to evaluate the intracellular concentrations of non-covalently bound drug by fluorometry with a Kontron spectrofluorometer, model SFM 25.

The acid-insoluble pellet was solubilized with 1M NaOH and used to evaluate the protein content. All incubations were performed in triplicate and at least two independent experiments were performed for each drug.

Doxorubicin cytotoxicity

A colorimetric assay using the tetrazolium salt MTT [13] was used to assess cytotoxicity of a 2-h exposure to Doxorubicin in the presence or absence of the various multidrug resistance modulators. Appropriate numbers of cells were plated in 96-well plates (Nunc) in a volume of 200 μl of culture medium. The cells were then exposed for 2 hours to the appropriate concentrations of Doxorubicin and the modulator. Culture medium was removed, the cell layers were rinsed twice ; fresh tissue culture medium was added, and the cells allowed to grow further. The cells were kept in the logarithmic phase of growth all along the experiment. At the end of the incubation, MTT assay for cell number was performed in triplicate. Cytotoxicity was expressed as IC_{50}, i.e. the concentration of Doxorubicin causing 50 % decrease of absorbance as compared to controls.

Results

The C6 0.5 line has been already characterized in our laboratory [10, 11, 14]. The resistance factor to Doxorubicin is around 400 (IC_{50} = 62 µM vs 0.155 µM in the sensitive line). Doxorubicin accumulation for a 2-hour exposure at 17.2 µM is reduced by a factor of 14 in this resistant line (0.205 nmole/10^6 cells vs 2.95 in the sensitive line). This line is however able to incorporate nearly 20 times more Doxorubicin than the sensitive line when exposed at doses giving the IC_{50} (« intracellular IC_{50} ») : 0.495 nmol/10^6 cells vs 0.029 in the sensitive line).

The effect of the modulators on Doxorubicin accumulation after a 2-hour exposure at the dose of 17.2 µM is presented in the Figure 1 ; most of them were able to restore, in the resistant cells, the intracellular Doxorubicin concentration measured in the sensitive cells, but with very different efficiencies : complete restoration occurred with 3 µM of Cyclosporine A, 6 µM of Verapamil and Nicardipine, 10 µM of S9788, 20 µM of Amiodarone, Trifluoperazine and Dipyridamole, 40 µM of Diltiazem and Tamoxifen ; complete restoration did not occur at the tested concentrations (up to 100 µM) for Nifedipine, Quinine and Quinidine.

The effect of the multidrug resistance modulators on Doxorubicin cytotoxicity is presented in the Figure 2. For each compound, we have plotted the Doxorubicin IC_{50} of the C6 0.5 line as a function of the concentration of modulator. Only one compound, Amiodarone, was able to completely reverse the doxorubicin IC_{50} value of the resistant C6 0.5 line to that observed in the sensitive line ; this occurred at a concentration of 20 µM. None of the other compounds was able to completely reverse Doxorubicin resistance. For Cyclosporine-A and S9788, a residual resistance factor of 4 could not be overcome, even at high-concentrations. The compounds which completely restored Doxorubicin accumulation did not completely reversed resistance to the drug, and a residual resistance factor of 10-20 was never overcome for Verapamil, Nicardipine, Dipyridamole, Diltiazem, Trifluoperazine and Tamoxifen. When considering the dose-effect relationship, it appeared that this maximal effect was obtained at lower doses for Verapamil and Nicardipine (around 1-3 µM) than for Trifluoperazine and Tamoxifen (around 10-30 µM) and was reached only at higher dose (30-50 µM) for Dipyridamole and Diltiazem. The three compounds not able to completely restore drug incorporation in the resistant line were however able to reverse Doxorubicin resistance in the same proportions as others (about 20 fold), and only at high concentrations (40-60 µM). We have also measured Doxorubicin accumulation in C6 0.5 cells for exposures corresponding to the IC_{50} values obtained at each concentration of the modulator (« intracellular IC_{50} », Figure 2). Amiodarone was the only modulator able to decrease efficiently this parameter low enough to reach the values ob-

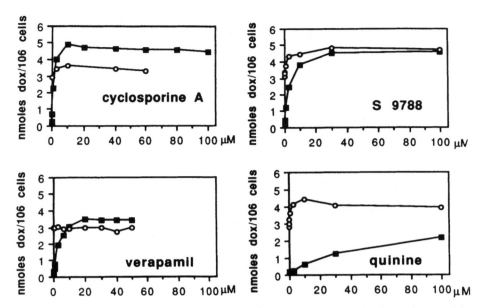

Fig. 1. Examples of incorporation of Doxorubicin in C6 sensitive cells (—O—) and in C6 0.5 cells (—■—) in the presence of various concentrations of 4 different modulators

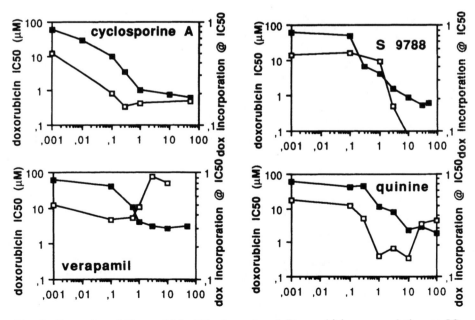

Fig. 2. Examples of Doxorubicin IC_{50} (—■—) and Doxorubicin accumulation at IC_{50} exposure « intracellular IC_{50} » (—□—) in C6 0.5 cells for various concentrations of 4 different modulators.

served in sensitive C6 cells. Some compounds were able to decrease this intracellular IC_{50} in important proportions : Cyclosporine-A, S9788, Trifluoperazine, Tamoxifen, Quinine, and Nifedipine. In marked contrast, Verapamil and Nicardipine, although very efficient in drug resistance reversal, were unable to decrease significantly the amount of drug incorporated in C6 0.5 cells for an IC_{50} exposure ; this was also the case for Dipyridamole, Diltiazem, and Quinidine.

Discussion

We have shown that the various drugs tested on this model differ qualitatively and quantitatively in their ability to reverse multidrug resistance. This may have consequences in the choice of the best candidate for clinical studies, and provides guidelines for the screening of multidrug resistance reversing agents. We have especially tested a new compound S9788, a triazine derivative not belonging to a family known to reverse multidrug resistance, and which has been proven to be active in vitro and in vivo [9].

The reversal of resistance itself does not appear to directly depend on the level of accumulation : several compounds are able to potentiate 2-fold the cytotoxicity of Doxorubicin without any change in Doxorubicin accumulation : Cyclosporine-A, Amiodarone, Trifluoperazine, Tamoxifen, Quinine and Quinidine. These observations clearly dissociate Doxorubicin activity from its intracellular accumulation.

The modulators tested can be divided in two categories : those able to decrease the intracellular IC_{50} (Cyclosporine-A, S9788, Amiodarone, Trifluoperazine, Tamoxifen, Quinine and Nifedipine) and those which do not decrease this parameter, or even increase it when used at higher concentrations (Verapamil, Nicardipine, Dipyridamole, Diltiazem and Quinidine). This property of decreasing intracellular IC_{50} appears independent from the efficacy of the modulator to reverse Doxorubicin resistance on a molar basis. We had hypothesized [10] that a mechanism of Doxorubicin tolerance to high intracellular concentrations was operating in our C6 0.5 cells and was added to the classical MDR P-glycoprotein-mediated drug extrusion. It appears that the modulators able to increase the intracellular IC_{50} can reverse the phenomenon of tolerance, whereas the other compounds cannot do so, and only reverse classical MDR resistance. This interpretation would suggest that there are intracellular targets only to the first class of modulators, those of the second class being either unable to reach them, or devoid of activity on these targets. It is tempting to assimilate these intracellular targets to transport proteins analogous or identical to P-glycoprotein, located in subcellular membrane systems and devoted to the segregation of the drugs in compartments from where it cannot reach its usual nuclear targets. The effect observed on Doxorubicin accumulation and cytotoxicity with these modulators would therefore be the result of 2 distinct phenomena : an effect on plasma membrane P-glycoprotein, modulating the intracellular content of the drug ; and an effect on another intracellular target, modulating drug distribution within the cell.

From a clinical point of view, it appears difficult to choose the better MDR modulator only from in vitro preclinical studies, since the problem of the individual toxic properties of the drugs are not taken into account. Several clinical studies have been undertaken, mostly in hemalogical malignancies with Verapamil [15], Quinine [16] and Cyclosporine A [17], but definitive results showing a clinical reversal of resistance of solid tumors are still lacking. In view of the possible existence of two distinct types of targets of these modulators, it could be interesting to try to associate the best compounds acting on drug accumulation (Verapamil type) to the best compounds acting on intracellular tolerance (Quinine type). This could allow to use smaller doses of each instead of the optimal dose of compounds acting on both targets. On the other hand, S9788 appears as a promising agent in view of its major efficiency on both processes.

References

1. Tsuruo T, Iida H, Tsukagoshi S, Sakurai Y (1981) Overcoming of Vincristine resistance in P388 leukemia in vivo and in vitro through enhanced cytotoxicity of Vincristine and Vinblastine by Verapamil. Cancer Res 41 : 1697-1672
2. Ford JM, Hait WN (1990) Pharmacology of drugs that alter multidrug resistance in cancer. Pharmacol Rev 42 : 155-199
3. Zamora JM, Pearce HL, Beck WT (1988) Physical-chemical properties shared by compounds that modulate multidrug resistance in human leukemic cells. Mol Pharmacol 33 : 454-462
4. Safa AR, Glover CJ, Sewell JL, Meyers MB, Biedler JL, Felsted RL (1987) Identification of the multidrug resistance-related membrane glycoprotein as an acceptor for calcium channel blockers. J Biol Chem 262 : 7884-7888
5. George E, Sharom FJ, Ling V (1990) Multidrug resistance and chemosensitization. Therapeutic implications for cancer chemotherapy. Adv Pharmacol 21 : 185-220
6. Ganapathi R, Grabowski D, Rouse W, Riegler F (1984) Differential effect of the Calmodulin inhibitor Trifluoperazine in cellular accumulation, retention and cytotoxicity of anthracyclines in Doxorubicin-resistant P388 mouse leukemia cells. Cancer Res 44 : 5056-5061
7. Schuurhuis GJ, Broxterman HJ, Cervantes A, van Heijningen THM, de Lange JHM, Baak JPA, Pinedo HM, Lankelma J (1989) Quantitative determination of factors contributing to Doxorubicin resistance in multidrug resistant cells. J Nat Cancer Inst 81 : 1887-1892
8. Jaffrézou JP, Herbert JM, Levade T, Gau MN, Chatelain P, Laurent G (1991) Reversal of multidrug resistance by calcium channel blocker SR 33557 without photoaffinity labelling of P-glycoprotein. J Biol Chem 266 : 19858-19864
9. Régnier G, Dhainaut A, Atassi G, Pierré A, Léonce S, Kraus-Berthier L (1992) New triazine derivatives as potent modulators of multidrug resistance. J Med Chem 35 : 2481-2496
10. Huet S, Schott B, Robert J (1992) P-glycoprotein overexpression cannot explain the complete Doxorubicin-resistance phenotype in rat glioblastoma cell lines. Br J Cancer 65 : 538-544
11. Schott B, Londos-Gagliardi D, Ries C, Huet S, Robert J (1993) Pharmacological and molecular characterization of intrinsic and acquired Doxorubicin resistance in murine tumoral cell lines. J Cancer Res Clin Oncol (in press)

12. Benda P, Lightbody J, Sato G, Levine L, Sweet W (1968) Differentiation of rat glial cell strain in tissue culture. Science 161 : 370-371
13. Carmichael J, Degraff WG, Gazdar AF, Minna JD, Mitchell JB (1987) Evaluation of a Tetrazolium-based semi-automated colorimetric assay : assessment of chemosensitivity testing. Cancer Res 47 : 936-942
14. Schott B, Robert J (1989) Comparative cytotoxicity, DNA synthesis inhibition and drug incorporation in a model of Doxorubicin-sensitive and -resistant rat glioblastoma cells. Biochem Pharmacol 38 : 167-172
15. Dalton WS, Grogan JM, Meltzer PS, Scheper RJ, Durie BGM, Taylor CW, Miller TP, Salmon SE (1989) Drug resistance in multiple myeloma and non-Hodgkin's lymphoma : detection of P-glycoprotein and potential circumvention by addition of Verapamil to chemotherapy. J Clin Oncol 7 : 415-424
16. Chauffert B, Pelletier H, Corda C, Solary E, Bedenne L, Caillot D, Martin F (1990) Potential usefulness of quinine to circumvent the anthracycline resistance in clinical practice. Br J Cancer 62 : 395-397
17. Sonneveld P, Durie BGM, Lokhorst HM, Marie JP, Solbu G, Suciu S, Zittoun R, Lövenberg B, Nooter (1992) Modulation of multidrug-resistant multiple myeloma by Cyclosporine. Lancet 340 : 255-259

Differential formation, repair and tolerance of Cisplatin-induced DNA damage in two human small cell lung carcinoma cell lines

BT Hill, SA Shellard

Chemotherapy unequivocally improves survival in small cell carcinoma (SCLC), even curing a small fraction of patients with limited disease, although drug refractory distant metastases are the most common cause of treatment failure [1]. The effectiveness of Cisplatin in treating SCLC is often limited by the development of drug resistance. Laboratory-based investigations of mechanisms associated with the expression of resistance to Cisplatin [2] have implicated various factors including: reduced drug accumulation; enhanced drug inactivation involving glutathione (GSH) or the metallothioneins (MT); differential DNA damage and repair; increased DNA damage tolerance. In this study our objective was to characterise the parameters associated with inherent differential Cisplatin sensitivities identified in 2 human SCLC cell lines, both established from patients not previously treated with Cisplatin, so as to determine whether the mechanisms operating in the more resistant subline were similar to or different from those associated with Cisplatin resistance expressed by *in vitro* drug-selected sublines.

Materials and methods

The 2 SCLC cell lines, SW900 and SW1271, were maintained in McCoys 5A medium plus 10 % foetal calf serum [3]. Drug sensitivities were evaluated by colony forming assay (CFA) after a 1-hour to Cisplatin or a 24-hour exposure to cadmium chloride, plating cells directly onto plastic. For drug cytotoxicity potentiation, cells were exposed to 20 μM buthionine sulphoximine (BSO) for 24-hour with Cisplatin addition for the last hour [4]. GSH content was measured by the method of Griffith [5] and that of MT by Eaton and Toal [6]. Immunochemical quantitation of Platinum (Pt)-DNA adducts and Pt uptake were determined as detailed earlier [4, 5].

Results

SW1271 cells proved 5-fold more resistant to Cisplatin than the SW900 cells, as judged by a comparison of IC_{50} values (drug concentration required to reduce cell survival by 50 %) from CFAs.

Pt-uptake, normalised for extracellular drug concentration and for the

Laboratory of Cellular Chemotherapy, Imperial Cancer Research Fund, London, WC2A 3PX, UK

1.4-fold differing cell volumes of these 2 cell lines was significantly higher in the more sensitive SW900 cells (1.33 ± 0.18 versus 0.81 ± 0.13 pmol Pt 10^6 cells/μg/ml Cisplatin/unit cell volume, $p < 0.001$). However, the extent of this difference (1.6-fold) appears unlikely to explain their 5-fold difference in Cisplatin sensitivities.

Total cellular GSH was 6-fold higher in the more resistant SW1271 cells. In both cell lines preincubation with 20 μM BSO depleted their GSH levels by 80 % and this resulted in a 2.5-fold increased sensitivity to Cisplatin only in the more resistant SW1271 cells. These SW1271 cells also proved resistant to cadmium chloride and this was associated with a 3.5-fold higher MT content.

The most Cisplatin sensitive SW900 cells had a 2.8-fold higher level of total platination immediately after drug treatment, much greater than could be accounted for by their higher Pt-uptake. During an 18-hour post-treatment incubation, these SW900 cells removed only 24 % of this platination, indicative of some repair of drug-induced damage, but less proficiently than the 50-60 % rate of removal identified in other tumour cells studied, within this time period [5, 7]. Evaluation of specific adduct formation and removal (Table 1) shows that SW900 cells only appeared to repair the major Pt-GG adduct, suggesting that Pt-AG and Pt-(GMP)$_2$ adducts are likely to constitute the lethal lesions in these cells. In contrast, however, the more resistant SW1271 cells appeared unable to remove most of the DNA platination, proving deficient in repair of Pt-AG, Pt-GG and Pt-(GMP)$_2$ adducts, suggesting that these cells are able to tolerate these lesions and replicate on a damaged template.

Table 1. Induction and removal of Pt-DNA adducts

Cell line	Adduct	n mole adduct/gDNA*		% Removal
		0 – hour ± SD	18 – hour ± SD	
SW900	Pt-GMP	11.1 ± 0.9	6.0 ± 0.9	46 %
	Pt-AG	5.3 ± 0.4	4.7 ± 0.6	11.4 %
	Pt-GG	20.2 ± 1.0	14.9 ± 1.1	26.3 %
	Pt-(GMP)$_2$	4.3 ± 0.1	5.7 ± 0.4	0 %
	Total	40.9 ± 2.4	31.3 ± 3.0	24 %
SW1271	Pt-GMP	4.7 ± 0.4	2.4 ± 0.2	49 %
	Pt-AG	2.2 ± 0.2	2.4 ± 0.2	0 %
	Pt-GG	5.9 ± 1.5	9.9 ± 1.1	0 %
	Pt-(GMP)$_2$	1.7 ± 0.3	2.3 ± 0.1	0 %
	Total	14.5 ± 2.4	17.5 ± 1.6	0 %

* The number of adducts were determined immediately after a 1-hour exposure to 10 μg/ml (33 μM) Cisplatin and following an 18-hour posttreatment incubation period. Values at 18-hour were corrected for dilution by DNA synthesis as described earlier [7]

Discussion and conclusions

These results indicate that inherent resistance to Cisplatin in SW1271 cells, relative to the more sensitive SW900 cells, was characterised by : (i) decreased Pt uptake ; (ii) cross resistance to cadmium chloride associated with increased MT content ; (iii) elevated levels of GSH ; (iv) significantly reduced total DNA platination level ; (v) deficient removal of the major Pt-GG, Pt-AG and Pt(GMP)$_2$ adducts, indicative of increased tolerance of drug-induced DNA damage.

A comparison of these findings with published data relating to drug-selected Cisplatin resistant SCLC cell lines reveals that consistent alterations in drug uptake, increased GSH and MT content were not consistently observed. One group reporting analyses of the formation and removal of specific Pt-adducts [8] found lower total DNA platination in their GLC$_4$-CDDP resistant cells, but concluded that altered repair was not implicated, consistent with our findings in these inherently resistant SW1271 cells. The apparent lack of repair of the major Pt-GG adduct by these more resistant cells was also noted earlier in investigations relating to inherent Cisplatin resistance in an ovarian carcinoma SKOV-3 cell line [5]. These data generally would be consistent with the proposal that this major Pt-GG adduct is not responsible for cytotoxicity in these various tumour cell types.

Acknowledgements. The MT data were kindly provided by Dr. John Lazo, Pittsburgh, PA, USA and Dr. AMJ Fichtinger-Schepman, Rijswijk, Netherlands, helped by advising on Pt-adduct quantitation.

References

1. Ihde DC (1992) Chemotherapy of lung cancer. N Engl J Med 327 : 1434-1441
2. Scanlon KJ, Kashani-Sabet M, Tone T et al (1991) Cisplatin resistance in human cancers. Pharmac Ther 52 : 385-406
3. Long BH, Musial ST, Brattain MG (1986) DNA breakage in human lung carcinoma cells and nuclei that are naturally sensitive or resistant to Etoposide and Teniposide. Cancer Res 46 : 3809-3816
4. Dempke WCM, Shellard SA, Hosking LK et al (1992) Mechanisms associated with the expression of Cisplatin resistance in a human ovarian tumor cell line following exposure to fractionated X-irradiation in vitro. Carcinogenesis 13 : 1209-1215
5. Shellard SA, Hosking LK, Hill BT (1991) An anomalous relationship between Cisplatin sensitivity and the formation and removal of platinum-DNA adducts in two human ovarian carcinoma cell lines in vitro. Cancer Res 51 : 4557-4564
6. Eaton DL, Toal BF (1982) Evaluation of the Cd/hemoglobin affinity assay for the rapid determination of metallothionein in biological tissues. Toxicol & Applied Pharmacol 66 : 134-142
7. Bedford P, Fichtinger-Schepman AMJ, Shellard SA et al (1988) Differential repair of platinum-DNA adducts in human bladder and testicular tumor continuous cell lines. Cancer Res 48 : 3019-3024
8. Hospers GAP, de Vries EGE, Mulder NH (1990) The formation and removal of Cisplatin (CDDP) induced DNA adducts in a CDDP sensitive and resistant human small cell lung carcinoma (HSCLC) cell line. Br J Cancer 61 : 79-82

Identification of a distinctive multiple drug resistance phenotype in tumour cells following in vitro exposure to X-irradiation

BT Hill, RDH Whelan, S McClean

The clinical observation that reduced response rates to chemotherapy appear characteristic of certain subsets of patients whose tumours have been previously irradiated, prompted our investigations aimed at determining whether we could identify a biological basis for this phenomenon [1]. Using Chinese hamster ovary (CHO) cells as an in vitro model system, we showed that their exposure to fractionated X-irradiation resulted in the expression of drug resistance [2]. Our investigations of the cause of this resistance revealed that these irradiated cells had increased levels of P-glycoprotein (Pgp), the « classic » multidrug-resistance (MDR)-associated membrane glycoprotein. These irradiated cells exhibited resistance to multiple drugs, including the Vinca alkaloids and epipodophyllotoxins, as well as sensitivity to reversal of Vincristine resistance by Verapamil. However, unlike « classic » MDR cells, they showed no change in their sensitivity to anthracyclines. Furthermore, Pgp overexpression occurred in these irradiated cells despite a lack of Pgp gene amplification or of significant alteration in Pgp messenger RNA (mRNA) levels. These initial studies, therefore, suggested that the multiple drug resistance phenotype expressed by these tumour cells following their exposure to fractionated X-irradiation, appeared distinctive from the « classic » MDR phenotype identified in drug resistant tumour cells selected for resistance after exposure to drugs.

Recent studies have now further clarified the distinctive phenotype of these irradiated CHO cells and identified a similar resistance phenotype in two irradiated human ovarian tumour cell lines.

Materials and methods

The AuxB1 CHO cell line received ten 9Gy fractions of X-rays (a dose resulting in 2 logs of cell kill) and were maintained as detailed earlier [2], to yield sublines designated CHO/DXR-10I and DXR-10II, or a single dose of 30Gy, resulting in approximately 7 logs of cell kill, providing a subline designated DXR-30. Derivation and maintenance of the irradiated sublines of the human ovarian lines SK-OV-3 and JA-T, have been published [3]. Methods used to evaluate drug and X-ray cytotoxicity by colony forming assays, drug uptake, and techniques used for Western and Northern blot analysis of Pgp expression and Pgp turnover are detailed in earlier publications [2-4]. The construction and characterisation of intraspecific CHO hybrids has been described recently [5].

Laboratory of Cellular Chemotherapy, Imperial Cancer Research Fund, London, WC2A 3PX, UK

Results

Studies with Chinese hamster ovary cell lines

Confirmation that the Pgp overexpressed by CHO/DXR-10I and DXR-10II cells is a functional molecule, was obtained by monitoring Rhodamine 123 (Rh123) accumulation and efflux. Both CHO/DXR-10 sublines showed reduced Rh123 accumulation, relative to the parental AuxB1 cells and enhanced efflux, which was significantly reduced by the addition of Verapamil.

The construction of intraspecific hybrids provided evidence of a genetic alteration in these irradiated sublines since the distinctive resistance phenotype is dominantly expressed [5]. Additionally, as summarised in Table 1, this multiple drug resistance phenotype can also be identified in the CHO/DXR-30 subline. The expression of this distinctive phenotype associated with overexpression of functional Pgp following a single supra-lethal X-ray dose is significant since it implies that X-irradiation, irrespective of frequency of exposure, can generate multiple drug resistance.

Table 1. Characteristics of the irradiated drug resistant sublines

	CHO cell lines			Human cell lines	
	DXR-10	DXR-30	CHRC-5	SK-OV-3 DXR-10	JA-T DXR-10
In vitro resistance to* :					
Vincristine	+ +	+ +	+ + + +	+	+
Etoposide	+	+	+ + +	+	+
Adriamycin	–	–	+ + + +	–	–
Pgp overexpression** :					
protein	+	+	+ + +	+	+
mRNA	–	ne	+ + +	–	ne
Pgp half-life (hour)	≥ 40	ne	17	39	ne

* As judged by comparing IC_{50} values derived by colony forming assays [2, 3]. + = 2-3 ; + + = 6-8 ; + + + = 30-50 ; + + + + > 100
** Using western or Northern blotting as described earlier [2, 5]

One of the most distinctive characteristics of the CHO/DXR-10 cells was their overexpression of Pgp without any concomitant elevation of Pgp mRNA, implicating altered translational and/or post-translational regulation of Pgp. Evaluation of the turnover of Pgp in these irradiated sublines has now revealed a significantly longer half-life, compared with that identified in the « classic » MDR drug-selected CHRC-5 subline (see Table 1) [4]. These data provide one of the first detailed examples of Pgp regulation by a post-translational increased stability.

Studies with human ovarian tumour cell lines

Data summarised in Table 1 indicate that the distinctive multiple drug resistance phenotype resulting from in vitro exposure to fractionated X-irradiation can also be identified in human tumour cell lines [3, 4, 6]. Furthermore, recent studies suggest that this post-translational regulation of Pgp may represent a unique and specific effect of X-irradiation on this particular protein, since SK-OV-3/DXR-10 cells also overexpressed the heat-shock protein HSP-27, recently implicated in drug-selected drug resistant tumour cells, but this is associated with increased HSP-27 mRNA, indicative of transcriptional regulation.

Conclusions

Exposure of tumour cells in vitro to fractionated X-irradiation results in specific genetic alterations which are responsible, directly or indirectly, for the dominantly expressed distinctive multiple drug resistance phenotype and post-translational stabilisation of Pgp. These studies, therefore, provide an explanation for the expression of clinical drug resistance in certain patients whose tumours have been previously irradiated and may have clinical significance in the design and optimisation of combined modality treatment protocols.

References

1. Hill BT (1991) Interactions between antitumour agents and radiation and the expression of resistance. Cancer Treat Rev 18 : 149-190
2. Hill BT, Deuchars K, Hosking LK et al (1990) Overexpression of P-glycoprotein in mammalian tumour cell lines after fractionated X-irradiation in vitro. J Natl Cancer Inst 82 : 607-612
3. Dempke WCM, Whelan RDH, Hill BT (1992) Expression of resistance to Etoposide and Vincristine in vitro and in vivo after X-irradiation of ovarian tumor cells. Anti-Cancer Drugs 3 : 395-399
4. Hill B, McClean S, Hosking LK et al (1992) Identification of a distinctive multidrug resistance phenotype expressed by tumour cells following exposure to fractionated X-irradiation. Clin Exptl Metastases 10 (suppl 1) : 84
5. McClean S, Hosking LK, Hill BT (1993) Dominant expression of multiple drug resistance after in vitro X-irradiation exposure to intraspecific Chinese hamster ovary hybrid cells. J Natl Cancer Inst 85 : 48-53
6. McClean S, Dempke WCM, Whelan RDH et al (1992) Overexpression of P-glycoprotein in human ovarian carcinoma cells following exposure to fractionated X-irradiation in vitro. Proc Am Assoc Cancer Res 33 : 470

Functional activity of P-glycoprotein localized in subcellular structures and reversal of multidrug resistance (MDR)

G Toffoli, L Tumiotto, MG Dall'Arche, C Cernigoi, M Boiocchi

The multidrug resistant (MDR) phenotype in human cells is thought to be primarily consequent to the increased expression of the mdr1 gene which encodes for a glycoprotein of 170 KD (P-gp) [1]. P-gp causes a reduced intracellular drug accumulation through an energy-dependent active drug efflux [1]. However variations in drug-transmembrane equilibria due to P-gp activity cannot completely explain the MDR phenotype since MDR cells can tolerate intracellular drug concentrations higher than those tolerated by their drug-sensitive parent cells [2].

The biochemical basis of intracellular drug resistance in MDR cells has not been completely identified yet. It might be due to intracytoplasmic membrane-bound P-gp molecules, which may compartment drugs in cytoplasmic vacuole-like structures, thus preventing drugs from reaching the target sites of their cytotoxic effect [3-5].

In this study 4 human colon carcinoma (HCC) cell lines exhibiting the classical MDR phenotype [6] were analyzed. In every MDR subline, the intracellular Doxorubicin (DOX) concentration required to inhibit cell growth by 50 % (IC_{50} int DOX) was higher compared to that of parent sensitive cells (Table 1). This increased intracellular drug resistance was due to an impaired subcellular drug distribution. Metabolically active MDR cells incubated for 1 h with DOX at the extracellular drug concentration inhibiting cell growth by 50 % (IC_{50} ext) showed intracytoplasmic but not nuclear drug accumulation. Intracytoplasmic DOX compartmentation was not observed in drug sensitive cells since DOX achieved a nuclear location in these cells (Fig. 1).

Treatment of MDR cells with subcytotoxic concentrations of P-gp-activity inhibitors (PAIs) [racemic Verapamil (VER) ; Amiodarone (AMD) ; Cyclosporin A (CPA) ; Trifluoperazine (TFP) ; and Nifedipine (NFD)] was associated with a rapid intracellular DOX redistribution — disappearance of DOX cytoplasmic localization and DOX compartmentation in the nucleus, where the DOX target macromolecules are located (Fig. 1). This phenomenon was rapidly and completely reversible since disappearance of DOX nuclear accumulation occurred after removal of the PAIs from the culture medium. DOX nuclear accumulation was also achieved by lowering the culture temperature to 4 °C, and was reverted by restoring the physiological temperature. Finally, no reversion of DOX nuclear accumulation was observed after continuous exposure to sodium azide/deoxyglucose. Therefore DOX distribution into intracytoplasmic organelles and DOX removal from the nuclear space are energy-dependent

---

Division of Experimental Oncology 1, Centro di Riferimento Oncologico, via Pedemontana Occidentale 12, 33081 Aviano (PN), Italy

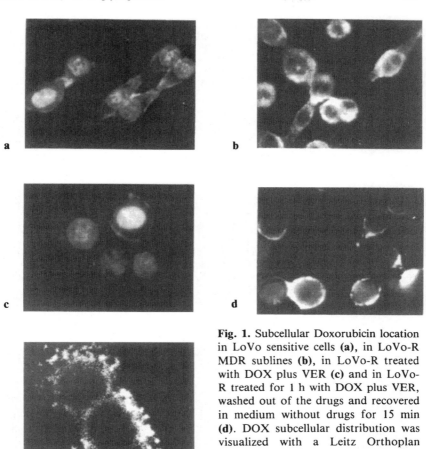

Fig. 1. Subcellular Doxorubicin location in LoVo sensitive cells (**a**), in LoVo-R MDR sublines (**b**), in LoVo-R treated with DOX plus VER (**c**) and in LoVo-R treated for 1 h with DOX plus VER, washed out of the drugs and recovered in medium without drugs for 15 min (**d**). DOX subcellular distribution was visualized with a Leitz Orthoplan Fluorescence microscope. At the bottom of the figure (**e**) P-gp distribution in LoVo-R cells as shown by confocal microscopy (Sarastro, CA). Immunostaining was performed on adherent cells fixed with methanol-acetone (3 : 7). The JSB-1 monoclonal antibody was used

processes, possibly related to the drug-transporting ability of the P-gp. This hypothesis was supported by the evaluation of P-gp intracellular distribution by immunofluorescence and immunocytochemistry. In all cell lines, high definition confocal microscopy identified P-glycoprotein molecules within the cytoplasm, particularly around the nucleus (Fig. 1).

Removal of antineoplastic drug from macromolecular complexes originated by the interaction of drugs with their intracellular macromolecule targets is a major biochemical phenomenon that must be considered in treatments with the P-gp-activity inhibitors, the so called « resistance modifying agents ». In cells which are not irreversibly injured, restablishment of the P-gp activity by removing P-gp inhibitory factors from the culture medium allowed DOX, complexed with its target cellular macromolecules (DNA), to be rapidly displaced, recomparted in cytoplasmic membraneous structures and finally extruded

Table 1. Intracellular Doxorubicin concentrations inhibiting cell growth by 50 % (IC_{50} int) in sensitive (LoVo, DLD 1, SW948 and SW1116) and in MDR (LoVo-R, DLD 1-R, SW948-R and SW1116-R) HCC cells

Cell line	RI[a]	IC_{50} int[b] (pmols DOX 10^6 cells)	Res/sens[c]
LoVo	1	171 (18)	
LoVo-R	23	625 (18)	3.7
DLD1	1	160 (16)	
DLD1-R	11	554 (95)	3.5
SW948	1	147 (21)	
SW948-R	6	548 (55)	3.7
SW1116	1	134 (17)	
SW1116-R	4	349 (22)	2.6

[a] RI, resistance index to DOX obtained by the ratios between extracellular DOX concentration inhibiting cell growth by 50 % (IC_{50} ext) in resistant and sensitive cells,
[b] IC_{50} int, intracellular DOX concentration (SD),
[c] Res/sens, ratios between IC_{50} int in resistant and sensitive cells. IC_{50} int DOX was determined after exposing cells for 1 h to the IC_{50} ext DOX. For this purpose radioactive ^{14}C DOX was used

Table 2. Effect of different modalities of treatment with resistance modifying agents (RMAs) on DOX cytotoxicity in MDR LoVo-R cells

	IC_{50} ext DOX (ng/ml)[a]		
RMAs (conc)	A	B	C
No RMA	3727 (369) [273 (32)]	—	—
Verapamil (8 μM)	—	1430 (307)	201 (35)
Amidarone (5 μM)	—	1246 (178)	220 (51)
Cyclosporin (2 μM)	—	2342 (151)	358 (62)
Trifluoperazine (8 μM)	—	3647 (531)	1283 (107)
Nifedipine (4 μM)	—	3118 (423)	1472 (302)

[a] Extracellular Doxorubicin (DOX) concentration inhibiting cell growth by 50 % after : 1-h exposure of LoVo-R cells to DOX in absence of RMA ; B, 1-h cell co-incubation with DOX plus RMA ; and C, 1-h co-incubation with DOX plus RMA, wash out of DOX and culturing in medium containing RMA. [ ] In brackets the IC_{50} ext of LoVo sensitive cells. Data were obtained from at least triplicate experiments (SD). Drug cytotoxic effects were determined by cell counting 72 h since the beginning of pharmacological treatment by a Coulter Counter ZM C256 (Coulter, England). Drug cytotoxicity was calculated as the percentage of cell survival in drug-treated cultures compared with that in untreated controls. IC_{50} ext was extrapolated by linear regression of experimental data

through the plasma membrane. Therefore, to prevent DOX nuclear clearance and to have the maximum cytotoxic effect, P-gp inhibiting pressure must be maintained uninterruptedly for a time sufficient to allow drug to exert its cytotoxic effect.

By treating the LoVo-R MDR subline with VER, AMD and CPA, cells completely reverted their DOX resistance if the PAIs were maintained in the culture medium uninterruptedly. Conversely, when the cells were exposed to these PAIs only during a 1-h treatment with the antineoplastic drug a partial reversion was obtained (Table 2). Continuous inhibition of P-gp activity by VER, but not a temporary inhibition (1 h) performed only during the chemotherapeutic treatment, reversed also drug resistance of LoVo-R cells to actinomycin-D and vincristine (data not shown). This suggests that to overcome MDR a protracted P-gp inhibition activity is required. Even though protracted treatments with NFD and TFP were more effective than a temporary inhibition of P-gp, there was not a complete reversion of MDR, probably because the inhibitory effect of these two compounds on P-gp activity is lower than that of VER, AMD and CPA.

In conclusion our studies contributed to a better understanding of the biochemical mechanisms activated by MDR cells to prevent drug cytotoxicity. This permitted us to develop pharmacologic treatments based on the continuous inhibition of the drug-transporting activity of P-gp which, in vitro, proved to be extremely effective in reverting the MDR phenotype.

References

1. Endicott JA, Ling V (1989) The biochemistry of P-glycoprotein-mediated multidrug resistance. Ann Rev Biochem 58 : 137-171
2. Toffoli G, Viel A, Tumiotto L, Biscontin G, Rossi C, Boiocchi M (1991) Pleiotropic-resistant phenotype is a multi-factorial phenomenon in human colon carcinoma cell lines. Br J Cancer 63 : 51-56
3. Willingham MC, Richter ND, Cornwell MM, Tsuruo T, Hamada H, Gottesman MM, Pastan IH (1987) Immunocytochemical localization of P-170 at the plasma membrane of multidrug-resistant human cells. J Histochem Cytochem 35 : 1451-1456
4. Gervasoni JE Jr, Fields SZ, Krushua S, Baker MA, Rosado M, Thuraisamy K, Hindenburg AA, Taub RN (1991) Subcellular distribution of Daunorubicin in P-glycoprotein-positive and — negative drug-resistant cell lines using laser — assisted confocal microscopy. Cancer Res 51 : 4955-4963
5. Boiocchi M, Toffoli G (1992) Mechanism of multidrug resistance in human tumour cell lines and complete reversion of cellular resistance. Eur J Cancer 28 : 1099-1105
6. Toffoli G, Viel A, Tumiotto L, Maestro R, Biscontin G, Boiocchi M (1992) Expression of the mdr1 gene in human colorectal carcinomas : relationship with multidrug resistance inferred from analysis of human colorectal carcinoma cell lines. Cancer Chemother Pharmacol 29 : 283-289

New strategy for the production of monoclonal antibodies to external portion of the P-glycoprotein

M Pagé, X Yang, P Roby, R Paradis, N Berkova

As early as 1970, Biedler and Riehm have described the MDR phenotype [1]. They characterized Chinese hamster cell lines that showed a high level of resistance to Actinomycin D or Daunorubicin. These cells showed crossresistance to various structurally unrelated natural products such as Vinblastin, Vincristin, Puromycin and Mitomycin C. Some years later, Ling and co-workers reported a similar phenotype in Chinese hamster ovary cell lines [2]. Although the relative resistance may vary quantitatively between different MDR cell lines, the pattern of crossresistance is qualitatively uniform regardless of the selecting drug. The net cellular accumulation of drugs involved in resistance is usually reduced and this presumably accounts, in part, for the decreased cytotoxicity [3]. Although the entry of these drugs appears to occur by simple diffusion, there seems to be an energy dependent drug efflux system. This enhanced efflux appears to be the major determinant of reduced drug accumulation in MDR cell lines.

Juliano and Ling [4] have shown that there was an overexpression of a 170 kd membrane glycoprotein associated with the MDR in resistant Chinese hamster cell lines. This protein, or family of proteins, was found to be expressed in most highly resistant MDR cell lines as well as in many human tumors [5, 6, 7]. These proteins were later referred as the P170, GP-140 and 180 or the P-glycoproteins. Studies done on genes referred the gene as the MDR gene family encoding the P-glycoproteins. Later studies have shown that there were some specific DNA sequences that were amplified in MDR cell lines. Gene transfer experiments have proved that these genes encode for the gene product involved in the multidrug resistance phenotype. Also, a strong relationship was found between the level of drug resistance and the level of MDR gene expression in cells as measured by specific messenger RNA levels [8, 9, 10]. Analyses of the nucleotide and the amino acid sequence of the P-glycoprotein reveal that some regions of the P-glycoprotein show striking similarities to some regions of transmembranous, bacterial transport proteins. The protein contains twelve hydrophobic transmembrane domains for a strong binding to the membrane and two sequences with an ATPase activity. Although the exact mechanism of transport and the normal function of P-glycoproteins remains speculative, it seems generally recognized that they work alone in binding the drug and in the efflux through channels created by their transmembrane domains.

Although various molecular biology techniques such as in situ hybridization or Northern or Western Blot have been used to detect the P-glycoprotein, immunohistochemistry and cytofluorometry seem to be more appropriate for routine clinical analysis of tissue specimens. These techniques allow visualisa-

---

Department of Biochemistry, Faculty of Medicine, Université Laval, Ste-Foy, Québec, Canada, GlK 7P4

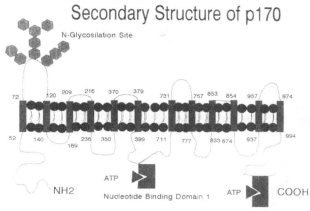

Fig. 1. Structure of P-glycoprotein

tion of microanatomic features of a tissue and can identify the degree of heterogeneity and the intensity of expression within a tumor. However the precise knowledge of antibody specificities is necessary for achieving accurate results. Monoclonal antibody such as C-219, that is commercially available, recognizes the internal portion of the P-glycoprotein and thus requires membrane permeabilization. Epitope analysis on C-219 has showed that it recognized a highly conserved amino acid sequence found in MDR1 and MDR-2 gene products. Also, it was found by various authors that antibody C-219 recognize non-P-glycoprotein molecules in cardiac and skeletal muscle. Among the antibodies that recognize the external portion of P-170 protein, MRK-16 seems to be unique even though the exact epitope mapping has not been determined.

In order to develop a useful antibody for clinical specimens, we have used a different approach for the production of monoclonal antibodies against a P-glycoprotein in which mice were stimulated with a synthetic peptide of the external portion of the P-glycoprotein conjugated to keyhole limpet hemocyanin (KLH) (Fig. 1) and the screening was performed with sensitive and resistant cells. Mice were also stimulated with resistant cells and the screening was performed with sensitive and resistant cells as well as the peptides. We describe below this new approach for the production of monoclonal antibodies against the external portion of P-glycoprotein.

Materials and methods

Peptide synthesis. Specific peptides of the external portion of the P-glycoprotein were synthetized by the Fmoc method. Synthesis of the following sequences of the P-glycoprotein was performed : peptide A (residues 73-93) ; peptide B (residues 97-119) ; peptide C (residues 85-103) ; peptide D (residues 367-387) ; peptide E (residues 732-756) ; peptide F (residues 950-973) and peptide G which comprises the loop formed by peptides A, B, C (residues 73-120).

After the synthesis, the peptide was cleaved from the resin with trifluoroacetic acid containing anisole and ethyl methyl sulfide and ethanethiol as scavengers. The peptides were then filtered and evaporated to dryness. They were then dissolved in acetic acid and lyophilized.

The crude peptides were purified on the FPLC with a reverse-phase Bakerbond C18 column with a H_2O : acetonitrile gradient (10 : 100) (0,1 %/TFA). The pure peptides were analyzed by capillary electrophoresis, mass spectrometry and amino acid analysis.

Peptides were activated by SPDP and conjugated to KLH by the method we have already described.

Cells

Cells SKOV-3 and SKVLB and culture conditions were obtained originally from Dr V. Ling in Toronto, Canada. These cells were regularly passaged once a week at 1/10 dilution and SKOV-3 and SKVLB maintained in 100 nanograms/ml of vinblastin.

Immunization

BALB/c mice were injected weekly intraperitonealy with intact SKVLB cells for ten weeks or with three injections of KLH peptide conjugate in complete Freund adjuvant. Blood tests were performed and after the final boosters, spleens from the immunized mice were used for fusion with SP-2 myeloma cells. Hybridomas obtained from splenocytes stimulated with resistant cells were screened by Elisa using either the intact cells fixed on 96 well microtitration plates or with the four synthetic peptides fragments of the P-glycoprotein coated on the 96 well microtitration plates. Twenty thousand SKVLB or SKOV-3 cells were seeded per well and grown for twenty-four hours. They were then washed and fixed with 0.5 % glutaraldehyde in phosphate buffer saline. After washing, the plates were filled with one percent bovine serum albumin to block excess glutaraldehyde. After washing, 50 µl of spent medium was added for two hours to each well, washed with PBS and 50 µl of the peroxidase labelled goat antimouse IgG was reacted for one hour at 37 °C. The presence of antibody was revealed with Orthophenylendiamine (OPD). Hybridomas was also screened with synthetic peptides coated on microtitration plates by overnight incubation at 4 °C. Plates were washed with PBS and blocked with 1 % gelatin in phosphate buffer saline. The remaining steps of the assay were the same as described above.

Indirect immunofluorescence

Air dry cell smears were fixed with 3.7 % formaldehyde for ten minutes and washed with PBS ; 0.1 ml of supernatant was used to cover the smear and reacted for twenty minutes at room temperature. After washing with PBS, the cells were incubated with fluorescein conjugated goat antimouse IgG and cells were examined under the microscope.

Cytofluorometry

Antibodies were also tested with FACS system (Becton Dickinson, Mississauga, Canada). For the analysis, cells were treated with purified antibodies or supernatant as described for the immunofluorescence. They were then analyzed on the FACS system.

Results

Production of monoclonal antibodies

Three fusions were performed using spleens stimulated from KLH-peptide conjugates or from resistant cells. Out of these three fusions, we obtained the results described on the following table.

Table 1. Summary of fusions

Fusion	No of wells with hybridomas	No of anti-P-glycoprotein wells	Saved
1	480	19	3
2	403	39 (anti-SKVLB)	2
3	470	20 (anti-SKVLB)	2
Total	1,353	78	7

These results show that the fusion rate was normal but one may notice that the screening procedure permits to eliminate a large number of non specific antibodies. The antibodies that were saved reacted by Elisa with the resistant cells while being negative with the parent sensitive cells. The respective antibodies were then screened with the peptide fragments of the external portion of the P-glycoprotein and only these antibodies which reacted were saved as P-glycoprotein positive.

Immunofluorescence

We found a very strong membrane reaction when XY-5 antibody was reacted with resistant SKVLB cells, very low levels were found on sensitive SKOV-3 cells. The antibody did not react with resistant cells preincubated with the external peptide fragment thus showing its specificity for the P-glycoprotein.

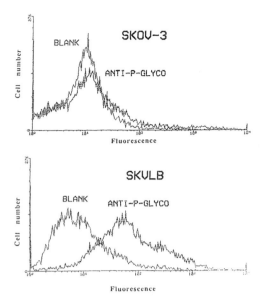

Fig. 2. Analysis of sensitive SKOV-3 and resistant SKVLB cells by cytofluorometry. Cells were scraped from the culture dish and treated with 10 µg of purified XY-5 antibody in phosphate buffer saline, washed and reacted with FITC labelled goat antimouse antibody

Cytofluorometry

The following figure (Fig. 2) shows the results obtained when SKOV-3 and SKVLB cells were reacted with antibody XY-5. We noticed that when the cells are not fixed before the reaction with the antibody, the reaction was weaker for unknown reasons (results not shown).

Discussion

A consistent finding of in vitro studies of MDR cell lines has been the overexpression of P-glycoprotein. In order to study the problem of MDR, several laboratories have produced MAbs against this protein. At present there are several MAbs that react specifically with this high-molecular weight glycoprotein. MAb MRK-16 detects an external epitope of the P-170, which corresponds to one of our synthetic peptides, designed peptide E. It is an extracellular loop that links transmembrane segments 7 and 8, located in the C-terminal half of the P-170. MAb C-219 is directed against peptide epitopes in positions 568-574 and 1213-1219 in the amino acid sequence of P-170, which are the internal cytoplasmic determinants. JSB-1 also recognizes internal cytoplasmic determinants, a region located in the C-terminal fragment of the P-170. Using human MDR ovary cells, SKVLB, we obtained the MAb, XY-5, which reacted with the 170 kD membrane glycoprotein that is specifically expressed in multidrug-resistant human cell lines. Our MAb, XY-5, recognizes the synthetic peptide G, which corresponds to an external segment in the N-terminal part of Pgp. Using human MDR ovary cells, SKVLB, we obtained the MAb, XY-5, which reacted with the 170 kD membrane glycoprotein that is specifically expressed in multidrug-resistant human cell lines. This external epitope may be a good target for immunotherapy as well as for the diagnosis of the refractory stage of malignancy.

References

1. Biedler JL, Riehm H (1970) Cancer Research 30 : 1174-1184
2. Beck-Hansen NT, Till JE, Ling V (1976) J Cell Physiol 88 : 23-32
3. Riordan JR, Ling V (1985) Pharmac Therapeutics 28 : 51-75
4. Juliano RL, Ling V (1976) Biochemical Biophysical Acta, 455 : 152-162
5. Kartner N, Riordan JR, Ling V (1983) Cancer Research 43 : 4413-4419
6. Beck WT, Muller TJ, Tanzer LR (1979) Cancer Research 39 : 2070-2076
7. Shen D, Cardarelli C, Whang J et al (1986) Mol Cell Biol 6 : 4039-4044
8. Fairchild CR, Ivy SP, Kaoo-Shan CS et al (1987) Cancer Research, 47 : 5141-5148
9. Shen DW, Fojo A, Robinson IB (1986) Science 232 : 643-646
10. Riordan JR, Deushars K, Kartener L (1985) Nature 316 : 817-819

Supported in part by the UICC for a fellowship to X. Yang, the FCAR for a fellowship to P. Roby and the Cancer Research Society for a research grant.

Abstract. Multidrug resistance of cancer cells is very often related to the presence of P-glycoprotein on the membrane. This protein is involved in the energy dependent efflux of cytotoxic agents. We have developed a peptide approach for the production of monoclonal antibodies specific for the external portions. From the known aminoacid sequence, the following external segments were synthetized by the Fmoc method : peptide A (residues 73-93) ; peptide B (residues 97-119) ; peptide C (residues 85-103) ; peptide D (residues 367-387) ; peptide E (residues 732-756) ; peptide F (residues 950-973) ; and peptide G which comprises the loop formed by peptides A,B,C (residues 73-120). Peptides were linked to keyhole limpet hemocyanin (KLH) as a carrier ; the conjugate was then used for mouse immunostimulation. Screening of monoclonal antibodies was performed with the various peptides and selectivity for resistant cells was tested on sensitive (SKOV-3) and resistant (SKVLB) human ovarian cancer cells both by immunohistology and by cytofluorometry. This specific approach allows the development of monoclonal antibodies specific for the desired segments and facilitates the screening procedure.

Myeloperoxidase is involved in Vincristine resistance in human myeloblastic leukemia

D Schlaifer, MR Cooper, M Attal, AO Sartor, JB Trepel, C Muller, G Laurent, CE Myers

Horseradish peroxidase (HRP) has been shown to destroy Vincristine (VCR) by oxidation [1]. HRP is a member of the heme peroxidase family of enzymes, all of which share similar substrate specificities. Myeloperoxidase (MPO) is a heme peroxidase expressed in AML, but not in ALL. We have investigated the hypothesis that oxidative destruction of VCR by MPO determines VCR resistance in AML. We were able to show that : (1) VCR was more cytotoxic in a subcloned MPO-negative HL-60 cell line (IC_{50} : 3.5 nM) than in the MPO-positive HL-60 cell line (IC_{50} : 13 nM). (2) 100 μM of VCR were almost completely degraded by 0.1 mg (2-U) of MPO plus H_2O_2 in a cell-free system monitored by HPLC analysis. (3) VCR was more completely degraded by the MPO-positive HL-60 cell line than by the MPO-negative HL-60 cell line. (3) The differential resistance to VCR observed between the cell lines could be increased by increasing the concentration of H_2O_2 available to the enzyme. (4) VCR was more efficiently degraded in MPO-positive cells from AML patients in comparison with the MPO-negative cell lines KG-1a and U-937. These data support the hypothesis that MPO could be responsible, at least in part, for the VCR resistance of some AMLs.

Materials and methods

Cell culture

The cell lines were supplied from the American Type Culture Collection, and were grown in standard conditions.

High performance liquid chromatography (HPLC) of VCR : HPLC was performed with a Gilson HPLC system, and a Knauer 8700 variable wavelength ultraviolet-visible absorbance detector. [^{3}H]VCR was detected by a Flo-One beta radioactive flow detector (Radiomatic Instruments & Chemical Co, Inc, CT). Samples were analysed on a Waters Nova-Pak C18 Cartridge column. Elution was effected by an isocratic mobile phase of acetonitrile and water (5 : 5, v : v) with 0.005 M dibasic ammonium phosphate and 0.005 M 1-pentanesulfonic acid. Absorbance was monitored at 220 nm.

From the Service d'Hématologie, Hôpital de Purpan, Toulouse, France and Clinical Pharmacology Branch, Clinical Oncology Program, Division of Cancer Treatment, National Cancer Institute, National Institutes of Health, Bethesda, MD, USA

In vitro degradation of VCR by MPO

Incubations of VCR and MPO were performed in 100 mM acetate buffer pH 6, 250 µM of H_2O_2, 2-U of MPO, and 100 µM of VCR. The mixtures were incubated at 37 °C for 3 h in the dark.

Degradation of VCR by the cell lines

[^{3}H]VCR (20 nM) was added to exponentially growing MPO-positive and -negative HL-60 cells and incubated 3 h at 37 °C in the dark. The supernatant was then extracted with a C-18 Sep-Pak cartridge and analyzed by HPLC. The cell pellets were extracted and analyzed by HPLC. To address the possibility that hydrogen peroxide could be a limiting factor in our cell experiments, we used in some experiments an enzyme system, the glucose oxidase-mediated oxidation of glucose to gluconic acid, which reduces molecular oxygen directly to hydrogen peroxide. 2 mU/ml and 11 mM of respectively glucose oxidase and glucose were used. We then processed the supernatants and the cell pellets as above.

Cytotoxicity assays

Cells were adjusted to a concentration of 200,000 cells/ml in complete growth medium and continuously exposed to VCR at different concentrations (0.1 to 10,000 nM). Cell number was determined after 72 h with an electronic particle counter (model ZBI; Coulter Electronics, Hialeah, FL).

Cytotoxicity assays in the presence of a hydrogen peroxide-generating system

We investigated the effects of 2 mU/ml glucose oxidase (a non-cytotoxic concentration) on the survival of MPO-positive and -negative HL-60 cell lines treated with increasing concentrations of VCR. The concentration of glucose was initially 11 mM in all experiments. Glucose oxidase and glucose were added daily during all experiments.

Degradation of VCR by cells from AML patients

Bone marrow samples of four patients suffering from AML were collected before treatment in RPMI 1640 with 100 U/ml Heparin and separated by Ficoll-Hypaque density centrifugation. The cells were then incubated with 20 nM of [^{3}H]VCR. HPLC analysis was performed in the same conditions as for the HL-60 cells. The MPO-negative myeloid cell lines KG-1a and U-937 were used as negative controls.

Results

VCR degradation in a cell-free system

100 μM of VCR were almost completely degraded by 0.1 mg of MPO plus H_2O_2. Degradation of VCR was not seen when VCR was incubated with H_2O_2 in the absence of enzyme or when VCR was incubated with the enzyme in the absence of H_2O_2. These results document that VCR can act as an electron-donating substrate for MPO.

VCR degradation in tissue culture

VCR degradation by MPO-positive and -negative cell lines was assessed by HPLC. Although 75 % + 2 % of the [^{3}H]VCR was still present in the supernatant of the MPO-negative HL-60 cell line, only 58 % + 5 % of the [^{3}H]VCR was found in the supernatant of the MPO-positive HL-60 cell line (p = 0.006). When the cell pellets were analysed, 78 % + 3 % of the [^{3}H]VCR was present in the MPO-negative HL-60 cells compared to 55 % + 5 % in the MPO-positive HL-60 cells (p = 0.002). Glucose oxidase dependent H_2O_2 generation clearly increased the degradation of [^{3}H]VCR by the MPO-positive HL-60 cell line, suggesting that hydrogen peroxide availability was a limiting factor in the [^{3}H]VCR degradation.

Cytotoxicity of VCR on the MPO-negative and -positive cell lines

The cytotoxicity curves showed that the MPO-positive HL-60 cell line was more resistant than was the 5-10 % MPO-positive HL-60 cell line or its MPO-negative HL-60 subclone. The IC_{50} values show a significant 3-4-fold increase for the MPO-positive HL-60 cell line compared to the MPO-negative HL-60 subclone.

P-170-glycoprotein expression by FACS analysis

All the HL-60 clones were negative for P170-glycoprotein expression as detected by the MRK-16 antibody.

Effect of the hydrogen peroxide-generating system on the cytotoxicity of VCR

A hydrogen peroxide-generating system, using the reduction of glucose by glucose oxidase, was used to overcome any limitation of the availability of hydrogen peroxide in the cytotoxicity experiments. The result was an increase in the difference between the sensitivity to VCR seen in the MPO-positive HL-60 cells as compared to MPO-negative HL-60 cells.

VCR degradation by cells from AML patients

[^{3}H]VCR was more efficiently degraded in MPO-positive cells from AML patients in comparison with the MPO-negative AML cell lines KG-1a and U-937.

Discussion

We first confirmed that MPO, like HRP [1], is capable of mediating the oxidative destruction of VCR in the presence of hydrogen peroxide in a cell-free system.

HL-60 is a myeloblastic cell line that is usually strongly MPO-positive. We were fortunate in observing the spontaneous development of an HL-60 clone that had weak (5-10 % of cells positive) expression of MPO, allowing for the further development of subclones with no detectable MPO.

As expected, degradation of VCR occurred more rapidly in tissue culture when the drug was added to MPO-positive HL-60 cells than when it was added to the MPO-negative HL-60 cell line. Of interest, this occurred when no hydrogen peroxide was added to the medium, suggesting that HL-60 cells must produce hydrogen peroxide, as has been recently reported for other cell lines [2]. This degradation was sufficient to deplete VCR from both supernatant and cell pellet, and interestingly enough, it was significantly increased by increasing hydrogen peroxide availability, suggesting that hydrogen peroxide is a limiting factor for this degradation.

Malignant cells from four MPO-positive AML patients were able to degrade VCR without the addition of hydrogen peroxide, suggesting that this VCR degradation may occur in patients. Further studies with a larger number of MPO-positive and -negative AML patients are needed to correlate the MPO content of the malignant blasts and the VCR degradation.

Moreover, since VCR degradation occurred at clinically relevant concentrations for VCR in the HL-60 cell lines (i.e., 1 to 1,000 nM), this phenomenon might provide an explanation for the poor prognosis of adult [3] or childhood [4] ALL in which MPO activity or mRNA has been detected.

Acknowledgement. We thank Professor J. Pris and Drs J. Breton-Gorius, C. Demur, E. Duchayne, C. Payen, and B. Sinha for critical guidance and support.

References

1. Rosazza JPN, Duffel MW, Elmarakby S, Ahn SH (1992) Metabolism of the Catharanthus alkaloids : from Streptomyces griseus to monoamine oxidase-B. J Nat Prod 55 : 269
2. Szatrowski TP, Nathan CF (1991) Production of large amounts of hydrogen peroxide by human tumor cells. Cancer Res 51 : 794
3. Reiffers J, Darmendrail V, Larrue J, Villenave I, Bernard P, Boisseau M, Broustet A (1981) Ultrastructural cytochemical prospective study of adult acute lymphoblastic leukemia : detection of peroxidase activity in patients failing to respond to treatment. Cancer 48 : 927
4. Zhou M, Little F, Findley HW, Zaki S, Ragab AH (1991) Prognostic importance of myeloperoxidase gene expression in acute lymphoblastic leukemia of childhood. Blood 78 : 39 (abstr)

A new multidrug resistance modulating agent S 9788 : preliminary report of the phase clinical trial in combination with Vincristine

D Khayat*, A Benhammouda*, M Weil*, E Vuillemin*,
G Bastian*, E Antoine*, O Rixe*, G Auclerc*, C Lucas**,
M Sarkany**, JP Bizzari**

S 9788 is a novel triazinoaminopiperidine derivative which does not belong to any of the classes of compounds known to reverse multidrug resistance (MDR) [1]. This compound showed to be particulary active in overcoming MDR both *in vitro* on 48 murine and human tumor cell lines (1 to 300 times more potent than Verapamil and 0.6 to 119 times more potent than Cyclosporin) and *in vivo* [2].

Based on these results, various phase I studies have been conducted in Europe (Switzerland, Belgium, France) according to different protocols. We report herewith the preliminary data of the phase I clinical trial combining S 9788 with Vincristine.

Clinical phase I study : methods and patients

The aims of this phase I study were to define :
— the maximal tolerated dose of S 9788 and of the combination S 9788 + Vincristine,
— the toxicity of S 9788 and of the combination and to determine whether any potentiation occurred,
— the pharmacokinetic parameters of S 9788 and the combination S 9788 + Vincristine and to appreciate any interaction. The question was also to see if an active *in vitro* concentration could be reached,
— the activity whenever possible.

S 9788 was administered alone on day 1 (30 mimutes, IV infusion) and on day 8, S 9788 administration was followed by an IV bolus of Vincristine at the dose of 1 mg/m^2. This latter therapeutic regimen was performed every 2 weeks until severe toxicity or progression of the disease.

Toxicity was scored according to WHO criteria.

This clinical trial was based on standard phase I methods : starting dose of S 9788 was equal to 1/10 lethal dose 10 (LD_{10}) in mice, i.e. 8 mg/m^2. Dose escalation was performed according to a modified Fibonacci scheme. Intermediate dose levels were also studied.

Thirty patients with various tumors have been included. Main characteristics of these patients are presented in Table 1.

Dose levels and corresponding numbers of patients are presented in Table 2.

---

* Hôpital Pitié-Salpêtrière, Paris, ** IRI Servier, Courbevoie, France

Table 1. Characteristics of the patients

	Number of patients
Entered	30
Evaluable	28
Male/female	17/11
Age	58 (29-74)
Prior chemotherapy	15
Prior hormono- or immunotherapy	10
Tumor type :	
• Colorectal	7
• renal	15
• NHL	2
• Melanoma	1
• cardia	1
• pancreas	1
• breast	1

Table 2. Dose levels and number of patients

Dose level (mg/m^2)	Number of patients
8	3
16	3
26	3
40	3
48*	1
56	3
64*	1
72	3
80*	1
88*	2
96	6
104	1

* intermediate dose level

AUC 0 - 24 h at D1 versus total dose

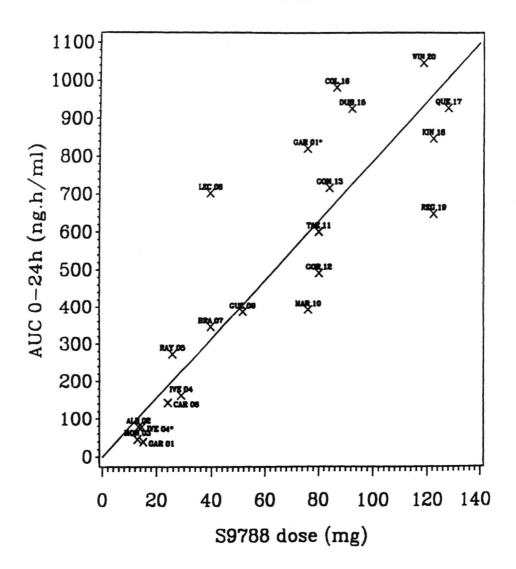

(*) Patient IVE 04 included by error at the 8 mg/m2 level
Patient GAR 01 also included at the 40 mg/m2 level

Fig. 1. Phase I study : S 9788 + VCR - Pr Khayat

Results

From 8 to 88 mg/m², no major toxicity was reported :

— pain at the site of administration : 1 patient,
— bitter taste in the mouth : 3 patients,
— dryness of the mouth : 1 patient.

At 96 mg/m², a vaso-vagal syncope occurred in 1 of the 6 patients treated at this dose level.

The patient treated at 104 mg/m² presented the same vaso-vagal syncope. This symptomatology was characterised by :
— faintness (pre-syncope),
— bradycardia : 30/min,
— hypotension, nausea, pallor, cold perspiration,
— loss of consciousness.

These symptoms occurred respectively 28 and 32 minutes after the beginning of the infusion of S 9788 in the two previously described patients. The signs persisted 10 and 18 minutes, respectively.

The pharmacokinetic parameters showed :
— a 3 compartment model (127 pharmacokinetic profiles analysed) with $t\ 1/2\alpha < 5$ minutes, $t\ 1/2\beta = 2\text{-}8$ hours and $t\ 1/2\gamma$ greater than 30 hours ;
— a linearity of the concentration at the end of infusion (C_{max}) versus dose :
• at 96 mg/m² : 1.82 ± 0.82 μ,
• at 104 mg/m² : 2.10 μM,
— a linearity of AUC (0-24 h) versus dose (Fig. 1) ;
— no modification of the pharmacokinetics of Vincristine by the co-administration of S 9788.

Among the 30 patients entered in the study, 23 were evaluable for response : 1 minor response has been documented in a pancreatic tumor mass and 4 stabilisations (1 colonic, 3 renal carcinomas) have been observed.

Conclusion

Based on these data, we can conclude that :
— the maximal tolerated dose (MDT) of S 9788 is 104 mg/m²,
— the dose limiting toxicity is cardiotoxicity (bradycardia, hypotension),
— the recommended dose of S 9788 is 96 mg/m²,
— no potentiation of Vincristine toxicity by S 9788 has been observed (either hematoxicity or neurotoxicity),
— pharmacokinetic parameters show a good linearity of C_{max} and AUC versus dose. An active *in vitro* concentration (1.82 ± 0.82 μM) can be reached with 96 mg/m²,
— early proof of activity has been noted.

Optimisation of the therapeutic regimen is being investigated in various indications (colon, kidney, hematological malignancies).

References

1. Pierre A, Dunn TA, Kraus-Berthier L, Leonce S, Saint-Dizier D, Regnier G, Dhainaut A, Berlion M, Bizzari JP, Atassi G (1992) In vitro and in vivo circumvention of multidrug resistance by Servier 9788, a novel triazinoaminopiperidine derivative. Inv New Drugs 10 : 137-148
2. Cros S, Guilbaud N, Berlion M, Dunn TA, Regnier G, Dhainaut A, Atassi G, Bizzari JP (1992) In vivo evidence of complete circumvention of Vincristine resistance by a new triazinoaminopiperidine derivative S 9788 in P 388/VCR leukemia model. Cancer Chemother Pharmacol 30 : 491-494

Effect of Pentoxifylline, ethacrynic acid and O⁶-benzyl-guanine as resistance modifiers to alkylating agents in haematological malignancies

MR Müller, L Schlenger, Chr Boogen, MR Nowrousian, S Seeber

Cellular resistance to alkylating agents is probably a multifactorial event including several detoxification pathways. In cell lines, the principal cellular non-protein thiol glutathione (GSH) reacts with several cytotoxic agents by conjugation reaction catalysed by Glutathione-S-transferases (GST). Circumvention of GSH-mediated resistance may thus be achieved by blocking of GSTs. EA has been shown to inhibit GSTs and to enhance chemosensitivity to alkylating agents in cell lines.

Also, increased capacity to repair DNA lesions has been linked to cellular resistance to cytotoxic drugs. Enzymatic DNA repair includes the removal of alkyl-adducts at the O^6-position of Guanine by the enzyme AGT. O^6-BG was shown to inhibit AGT thus increasing the cytotoxicity of BCNU in cell lines.

Furthermore, modulation of resistance to alkylating agents has been reported for methylxanthines such as caffeine and PTX. Various mechanisms for this enhancement have been proposed including inhibition of postreplication repair of DNA and inhibition of poly(ADP-ribose)-polymerase.

We were interested to study the effect of these putative RMs on the cytotoxicity of MAF and BCNU in isolated lymphocytes from CLL patients or healthy donors and in leukaemic blasts from patients with AML.

Methods

Drugs

PTX and EA were supplied by Sigma (Deisenhofen, Germany) and BCNU by Bristol-Myers (Bergisch Gladbach, Germany). MAF was provided by ASTA (Bielefeld, Germany). O^6-BG was kindly supplied by Jürgen Thomale (Institute of Cell Biology (IFZ), University of Essen Medical School, Essen, Germany).

Isolation of leukaemic cells from patients with CLL or AML and healthy donors

Blood samples obtained from patients with CLL or AML and healthy donors were taken before treatment. Heparinized blood (10 ml) was layered onto 10 ml

---

Innere Klinik und Poliklinik (Tumorforschung), West German Cancer Centre, University of Essen Medical School, Hufelandstr. 55, 4300 Essen, FRG

Ficoll-Hypaque and centrifuged for 25 min at 200 × g at room temperature. Cells at the interface were removed, washed twice and resuspended in PBS. After counting, cell numbers were adjusted for the MTT assay.

MTT assay

The tetrazolium dye (MTT) assay was carried out in wells on 96-well microtitre plates. Cells were seeded into 96-well microtitre plates using 200 µl per well of a cell suspension containing 10^6 cells/ml RPMI medium with 10 % fetal calf serum. 20 µl of drugs dissolved in PBS were added. On day 4, 20 µl of a solution of 5 mg MTT/ml PBS were added to each well, and the plates were returned to the incubator for a period of 5 hours. Thereafter, the plates were centrifuged for 10 min at 100 x g. The medium was then removed from each well, 200 µl of dimethyl sulphoxide were added to dissolve the crystals and the plates were shaken for 10 min on a plate shaker. The absorbance at 540 nm and 690 nm in the wells was read on a dual wavelength Dynatech MR 7,000 plate-reader. In all experiments, four replicate wells were used for each concentration. The concentration of drug required to reduce the absorbance at 540 nm to 50 % of control was taken to be the ID_{50} of the sample.

Results

The table displays the means and standard deviations of sensitisation ratios (ie. ratios of cytotoxic drug ID_{50}s in the absence or presence of resistance modifiers). The ID_{50} values of leukaemic blast cells for MAF in the presence or absence of 1 mM PTX are shown in the figure. Identical ID_{50} values lie on the line as shown in the figure. Points in the lower field of the plot represent samples sensitised by PTX.

Table 1. Sensitisation ratios

Type	Mafosfamide			BCNU		
	PTX	O^6-BG	EA	PTX	O^6-BG	EA
NL (n = 8)	1.7 ± 0.6	1.3 ± 0.2	1.1 ± 0.1	0.9 ± 0.5	1.3 ± 0.3	1.5 ± 0.5
CLL (n = 12)	1.1 ± 0.2	1.3 ± 0.3	1.7 ± 0.6	1.2 ± 0.3	1.0 ± 0.1	1.3 ± 0.3
AML (n = 26)	1.3 ± 0.8	1.6 ± 0.8	1.1 ± 0.1	1.0 ± 0.2	1.0 ± 0.3	1.1 ± 0.2

Mean ± standard deviation

Conclusions

In cell lines, all of the examined RMs have been reported to enhance the cytotoxicity of DNA-affine substances. However, this situation maybe differ-

EFFECT OF PENTOXIFYLLINE ON CYTOTOXICITY OF MAFOSFAMIDE IN ISOLATED LEUKAEMIC BLASTS

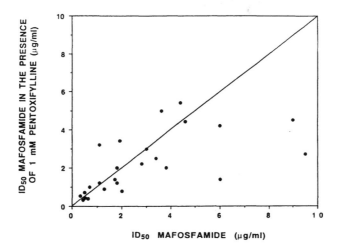

ent in tumour cells derived from patients whereby a small but clinically significant degree of resistance may occur. Therefore, we evaluated the properties of EA, O^6-BG and PTX to sensitise lymphocytes or blasts derived from patients with CLL or AML as well as healthy donors. EA did not influence the cytotoxicity to MAF and BCNU neither in lymphocytes from healthy donors or CLL patients nor in leukaemic blasts from AML patients. This observation may indicate that the activity of GSTs is not an important determinant of cellular resistance to alkylating agents in CLL and AML patients.

BCNU-induced DNA lesions are at least partly repaired by AGT in cell lines. In the present study, the presumed inhibition of AGT by O^6-BG failed to sensitize lymphocytes and leukaemic blasts to BCNU and MAF. This observation suggests that AGT-mediated DNA repair is not a major determinant for drug resistance to alkylating agents in haematological malignancies.

Furthermore, the overall data did not show any significant sensitisation effect of PTX. In single cases, however, a striking sensitisation was observed in leukaemic blast cells with increased *in vitro* resistance to MAF. At present, we can only assume that PTX-mediated inhibition of DNA repair pathways may account for this observation. Future studies should relate the observed chemosensitising effect of PTX to the capacity to repair induced DNA lesions.

References

Lambert E, Rees JH, Twentyman PR (1992) Resistance circumvention strategies tested in clinical leukaemia specimens using the MTT colorimetric assay. Leukaemia 6 : 1063-1071

Walker MC, Masters JRW, Margison GP (1992) O^6-alkylguanine-DNA-alkyltransferase activity and nitrosourea sensitivity in human cancer cell lines. Br J Cancer 66 : 840-843

Petru E, Boike G, Sevin BU (1990) Potentiation of Cisplatin cytotoxicity by methylxanthines in vitro. J Cancer Res Clin Oncol 116 : 431-433

Abstract. Using the MTT assay, the effects of putative resistance modifiers (RM) on the cytotoxicity of Mafosfamide (MAF) and bis-chloroethylnitrosourea (BCNU) were evaluated in isolated blood cells derived from patients with chronic lymphatic leukaemia (CLL ; n = 12) and acute myeloid leukaemia (AML ; n = 26) or healthy donors (NL ; n = 8). Ethacrynic acid (EA) enhances the cytotoxicity of alkylating agents by inhibiting Glutathione-S-transferases (GST) in cell lines. Pentoxifylline (PTX) has also been shown to restore sensitivity to alkylating drugs by interfering with DNA repair pathways. O^6-benzyl-guanine (O^6-BG) inhibits the DNA repair enzyme O^6-alkylguanine-DNA alkyltransferase (AGT). The overall data showed no significant sensitisation effect of EA (1 μM), PTX (1 mM) and O^6-BG (50 μM) in clinically achievable concentrations. However, in 5 out of 26 AML samples we observed a striking sensitisation to MAF up to a factor of five by PTX with in vitro resistance to MAF. In this group of patients, the observed chemosensitising effect should be related to the expression of mechanisms of resistance such as DNA repair capacity.

Structural alterations of human topoisomerase IIα responsible for drug-resistance, DNA-binding and nuclear localization

F Boege, F Gieseler, P Meyer

Topo(isomerase) II is the subcellular target of many potent cytostatic drugs. It is known to be susceptible to epigenetic structural modifications, which drastically alter its catalytic properties [1-9]. Charge heterogeneity has been demonstrated for the α-isoenzyme in human cancer cells [10, 11]. Appearently, structural modifications are not homogenously distributed in the enzyme pool. Here, we separated functionally different subforms of human HL-60 topo IIα by virtue of their charge heterogeneity. These subforms coexist in sensitive and resistant human promyelocytic HL-60 cells.Changes in their relative distribution affects drug-sensitivity of these cells.

Results and discussion

Structural variants of topo IIα coexisting in HL-60 cells can be separated by virtue of different charge (Fig. 1) : We purified nuclear topo II from HL-60 cells [12] and fractionated the enzyme preparation by anion-exchange chromatography [11] : α-, and β-forms of 170 and180 kDa respectively were eluted in close sequence by 150-200 mM NaCl. This has also been described by others [17, 18]. In addition we observed a peak of topo II specific DNA-decatenation activity, which bound more tightly to the anion-exchanger and accordingly was eluted by higher ion concentrations (> 300 mM NaCl). This second form, which has not been described before, exhibited the same molecular weight as the early eluting a-form (170 kDa) and cross-reacted with anti-peptide antibodies specific for the carboxyterminal 18 amino acid residues of human topo IIα [19]. We concluded, that this second activity peak consists of a structural variant of topo IIα.

Table 1. Functional differences between early and late-eluding topoisomerase II variants

Chromatographic fraction No (see : Fig. 1)	4	6	9
Isoenzyme (judged by immunoreactivity)	IIα	IIβ	IIα (late)
Catalytic pH-optimum	8.5	7.5	> 9.3
Orthovanadate sensitivity (IC$_{50}$, μM)	30	30	> 1,000
Amsacrine sensitivity (IC$_{50}$, nM)	10	10	10,000
Etoposide sensitivity (IC$_{50}$, nM)	3	10	10,000
Covalently DNA-bound fraction (%)	15	—	80

— Not determined

Medizinische Poliklinik, University of Würzburg, Medical School, Klinikstraβe 6-8, 8700 Würzburg, Germany

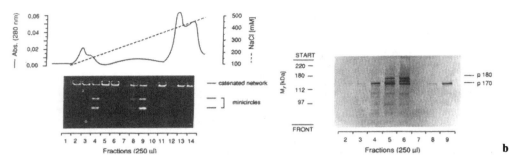

Fig. 1. Fractionation of subforms of HL-60 topoisomerase II by anion-exchange chromatography : partially purified HL-60 topoisomerase II was adsorbed to a Mono Q HR5/5 column and eluted by a NaCl gradient. Fractions were analyzed for DNA-decatenation activity and immunoblot using rabbit-anti-human topoisomerase II antibodies crossreacting with α- and β-isoenzymes

Functional differences between early and late-eluting topo IIα variants (Table 1) : From the fractionation depicted in Fig. 1 we selected fractions No 4 (only early-eluting topo IIα), 6 (mainly topo IIβ), and 9 (only late-eluting topo IIa) for further functional studies. These data are summarized in Table 1.

Catalytic pH-optimum : topo IIβ was most active at pH 7.3-7.6. The early eluting form of topo IIα was maximally active at pH 8.3-8.6. In contrast activity of the late eluting variant of topo IIa peaked at pH > 9.3. Similar catalytic pH-optima have been observed in crude nuclear extracts [20]. The three pH-intervals of maximal activity do not significantely overlap. The different forms of topo II are probably not simultaneously active.

Orthovanadate is known to inhibit topo IIα- and β with similar efficiency [17]. Here, topo IIβ and the early eluting variant of topo IIα exhibited a similar sensitivities, the EC_{50}— values beeing in good aggreement with previous observations [17]. In contrast, the late eluting topo IIα variant was highly resistant to ortovanadate.

Sensitivity to amsacrine and etoposide : It has previously been described [17] that topo IIα and β differ 7-fold with respect to etoposide sensitivity. Here, we failed to detect such a difference but we found pronounced differences between early and late eluting forms of topo IIα. The early eluting topo IIα is highly drug-sensitive : In the presence of this enzyme form both topo II inhibitors induced linearization of pBR322 DNA with EC_{50} values of 3-10 nM. Similar values were also obtained with topo IIβ. In comparison, the late eluting form of topo IIα is ≈ 1000-fold resistant (EC_{50} ≈ 10μM for both drugs) This resistance of the late eluting topo IIα could be due to its shifted catalytic pH-maximum to pH > 9.0. Even with the sensitive enzyme form, drug-induced DNA-cleavage was only observed between pH 7.0 and 7.5 but not in alkaline milieu.

DNA-binding : to further characterize the drug-DNA-enzyme interaction for both forms of topo IIα, we studied depletion of the immuno-reactive protein-band by Western-blot analysis after incubating enzyme fractions 4 or 9 with calf-thymus DNA (1 mg) in the presence or absence of etoposide (100 nM). In the case of the early eluting topo IIα, the result was as expected : in the absence of etoposide an immunoreactive band of 170 kDa was stained by topo IIα specific antibodies. In the presence of etoposide this band dissappeared, because etoposide induces a covalent high-molecular DNA-enzyme complex, which is unable to penetrate the polyacrylamide-matrix. Digestion of the calf-thymus DNA (with detergent resistant endonuclease Benzonase) prior to electrophoresis restored the signal. Unexpectedly, with the late-eluting topo IIα SDS alone induced an almost complete disappearance of the 170 kDa band in the presence of calf thymus DNA. Accordingly, a further « band-depletion » effect by etoposide could not be detected. After DNA-digestion the 170 kDA band re-appeared. From these observations we concluded, that the two forms of topo IIα transgress the catalytic cycle in different ways : in the case of the early-eluting topo IIα, the covalent DNA-enzyme complex is a transient stage, which can be stabilized by etoposide, cleaved by SDS and then detected by the « band-depletion » phenomenon. In contrast, the late eluting topo IIα binds tightly to DNA. It predominantely forms a SDS-cleavable complex, which is stable without drug. Accordingly, it can be detected by the « band-depletion » phenomenon in the absence of drug.

Sensitive and resistant HL-60 cells differ in DNA-binding, nuclear localization of topo IIα and in the relative distribution of topo IIα variants : we previously reported [14, 16] of a HL-60 subclone (HL-60R), which is 1000-fold resistant to several topo II inhibitors, although it had not been selected for resistance. These cells are sensitive to a variety of cytostatic agents, which do not target topo II. P-glycoprotein expression (as determined by specific antibody staining of the cells and quantification of cellular m-RNA levels) is not increased and sensitivity of HL-60R cells to topoisomerase II inhibitors can not be restored by verapamil or other p-glycoprotein inhibitors. We assumed, that cytostatic drug-resistance of HL-60R cells is caused by an altered response of the cellular drug-target topo II.

The late eluting topo IIα variant is predominant in drug-resistant HL-60 R cells (Fig. 2) : Drug-sensitive wild type HL-60 (WT) cells contain 15-20 % of the late eluting topo IIα variant. In contrast, in the resistant HL-60R cells more than 80 % of nuclear topo IIα (as detected by carboxy-terminus specific antibodies) eluted from anion-exchangers by more than 300 mM NaCl (Fig. 2, right). This predominance of late eluting topo IIα coincides with a strong decatenation activity at pH > 9 in nuclear extracts from these cells . Unlike in HL-60 wild type cells, relatively little decatenation activity was observed between pH 8-8.5 (Fig. 2, left). This agrees with the low level of early eluting topo IIα (Fig. 2, right). Nuclear extracts from both cell lines show similar decatenation activity at pH 7.5 (Fig. 2, left), indicating similar levels of topo IIβ. The total amount of decatenation activity extractable per nucleus was similar in HL-60 WT and HL-60 R cells. Western-blot analysis (Fig. 3) indicates, that HL-60WT and HL-60R cells contain similar amounts of topo IIα and β and that both iso-enzymes are present in similar proportions. Appeerently, in HL-60 R cells the late-eluting topo IIα variant is increased on the expense of the early eluting form.

Covalent DNA-binding of topo II is increased in HL-60R cells (Fig. 3) : we previously observed [15] that the background level of protein-DNA complex formation is increased in HL-60 R cells. More than 80 % of cellular DNA

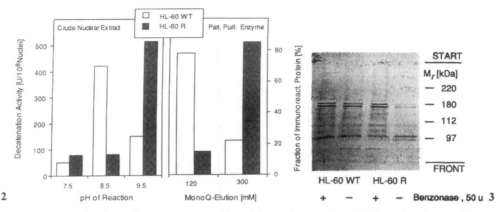

Fig. 2. Distribution of topoisomerase IIα subforms in sensitive (WT) and resistant (R) HL-60 cells. Left : topoisomerase II was extracted from nuclei of sensitive and resistant HL-60 cells Decatenation activity was quantified under the pH — conditions indicated by serial dilution of the sample. Right : Fractionation was carried out as described in legend to Fig. 1 and the relative amount of early and late eluting topoisomerase IIα was measured by densitometry of the Western blots

Fig. 3. Increased covalent DNA binding of topoisomerase II α and β in resistant (R) HL-60 cells : 10^7 sensitive (WT) or resistant (R) HL-60 cells were lysed with SDS, optionally treated with detergent resistant endonuclease (+ Benzonase) and subjected to electrophoresis and Western-blotting. Blots were probed with antibodies cross-reacting with both isoenzymes of human topoisomerase II

can be trapped as covalent protein complexes after SDS-lysis of HL-60R cells. The DNA-bound enzyme does not migrate in gel-electrophoresis and can only be detected in Western-blots after DNAse treatment (Fig. 3). In sensitive HL-60 WT cells less than 20 % of cellular DNA can be trapped as protein-complexes. Accordingly in these cells the DNAse treatment is not necessary for Western-blot visualization of topo II in the absence of drug (Fig. 3). It has been reported that resistant mutants of topo II also exhibit an unusually high level of DNA-linking activity, when challenged with SDS in the absence of drug [21]. These observations support our notion that increases in covalent DNA attachment may be a feature specific for resistant topo II variants.

The nuclear distribution of topo IIα is altered in HL-60 R (Fig. 4) : After sorting cells according to cell cycle, we used confocal laser immuno-fluorescence microscopy and a double-staining technique in order to analyze sub-cellular distribution of topo II α and β between normal and resistant HL-60 cells in a single cell-orientated manner. The quantitative analysis of the data (not shown) is in good agreement with the results from immunoblot analysis (Fig. 2). Although, the absolute amounts of both enzymes (per cell) are similar in HL-60 and HL-60R, the nuclear concentrations are lower in HL-60R. This is mostly due to the increased nuclear size of these cells. Unexpectedly, we failed to observe significant changes in expression of the two isoenzymes during cell cycle, which have been previously reported from NIH-3T3 cells [18]. The absolute and relative levels of topo IIα and β isoforms did not significante-

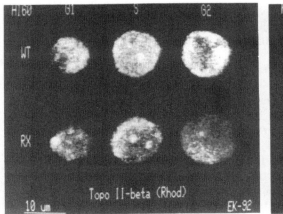 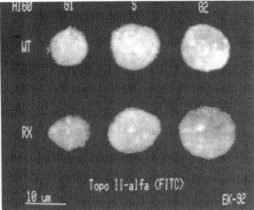

Fig. 4. Nuclear distribution of topoisomerase IIα and β in sensitive (WT) and resistant (RX) HL-60 cells: Fixed cells were sorted according to cell cycle (G1, S, G2) and then simulataneously stained with antibodies against human topoisomerase IIα (rabbit-antipeptide, secondary antibody FITC-labelled) and topoisomerase IIβ (monoclonal mouse-anti-human, secondary antibody rhodamin-labelled). Nuclear distribution of topoiosmerase II isoenzymes was visualized by scanning confocal laser fluorescence microscopy. Photographs were taken directly from the computer screen

ly change during the cell cycle of both resistant and sensitive HL-60 cells. On the basis of these data, it can be excluded that differences on the expression levels of topo II account for the altered topo II function in the resistant subclone HL-60R. Looking, however, at the nucle(ol)ar staining pattern (Fig. 4) a morphological difference between resistant and sensitive cells becomes apparent: In normal sensitive HL-60 cells the nuclear distribution is in good aggreement with previous observations [22, 23]: topo IIα is diffusely distributed in the whole nucleus and the nucleoplasm while the β-isoenzyme shows a nucleolar localization. In contrast, in the resistant cells (RX) both isoforms appear to be predominantely localized in the nucleoli. In the nuceloplasm of these cells levels of both topo II isoforms are very low as compared to those in sensitive cells.

Concluding remarks

An as yet unidentified structural alteration of human topo IIα increases negative surface charge of the enzyme molecule. This allows for chromatographic separation of two enzyme variants. Appearently, the structural change is part of a complex regulatory mechanism, which simultaneously changes catalytical properties, increases DNA-binding and directs the enzyme to the nucleoli. As a crucial consequence, the enzyme becomes resistant to clinically relevant topoisomerase inhibitors. On a molecular basis, this lack of drug-sensitivity could be achieved by two mechanisms: (i) the late eluting enzyme variant is preferentially active under alkaline conditions, which do not favor cleavable complex formation ; (ii) it is predominantly bound to DNA in a covalent manner. One should assume, that in this DNA-bound state the enzyme would be inaccessible to ternary complex- forming topoisomerase II inhibitors, such as amsacrine and etoposide.

We observed low levels of the resistant enzyme form in drug-sensitive HL-60 cells, directely subcultered from the ATCC cell sample. Levels where significantely increased in a drug-resistant HL-60 subclone [14] As both sensitive and resistant HL-60 cell lines had not been exposed to topo II inhibitors prior to the experiments, it seems unlikely that the structural heterogeneity of topo IIα is due to one of the mutations known to develope in cell lines selected for resistance by stepwise increasing the drug concentration in the propagation medium over a long period of time [13, 24, 25]. It rather seems, that we are observing a mechanism, which allows sensitive tumor cells to acquire tolerance to cytotoxic topo II inhibitors, without undergoing mutations or changes at the expression level of topo II.

Acknowledgements. We are grateful for exellent technical assistance to Michaela Müller und Michael Clark. We would like to thank Dr. Eigil Kjeldsen for carrying out the confocal immunofluorescent microscopy. We are grateful to Prof. Ole Westergaard, Prof. Yves Pommier and Prof. Leonhard Zwelling for discussing the data and giving helpful advice. The rabbit-anti-human topoisomerase II antibody was a generous gift by Prof. Leroy F. Liu. The monoclonal mouse-anti-human topoisomerase IIβ antibody was gifted by Dr Astaldi-Ricotti.

References

1. Darby M, Schmitt B, Jonstra-Bilen J, Vosberg HP (1985) Inhibition of calf thymus type II DNA topoisomerase by poly ADP-ribosylation. Embo J 4 : 2129-2134
2. Ackermann P, Glover CVC, Osheroff N (1985) Phosphorylation of DNA topoisomerase II by casein kinase II : Modulation of eukariotic topoisomerase II activity in vitro. Proc Natl Acad Sci (USA) 82 : 3164-3168
3. Saijo M, Enomoto T, Hanaoka F, Ui M (1991) Purification and characterization of type II DNA topoisomerase from mouse FM3A cells : phosphorylation of topoisomerase II and modification of its activity. Biochemistry 29 : 583-590
4. Saijo M, Ui M, Enomoto T (1992) Growth state and cell cycle dependent phosphorylation of DNA topoisomerase II in Swiss 3T3 cells. Biochemistry 31 : 359-363
5. Cardenas ME, Dang Q, Glover CV, Gasser SM (1992) Casein kinase II phosphorylates the eukaryote-specific C-terminal domain of topoisomerase II in vivo. EMBO J 11 : 1785-1796
6. DeVore RF, Corbett AH, Osheroff N (1992) Phosphorylation of topoisomerase II by casein kinase II and protein kinase C : effects on enzyme-mediated DNA cleavage/religation and sensitivity to the antineoplastic drugs etoposide and 4'-(9-acridinylamino)methane-sulfon-m-anisidide. Cancer Res 52 : 2156-2161
7. Takano H, Kohno K, Ono M, Uchida Y, Kuwano M. (1991) Increased phosphorylation of DNA topoisomerase II in etoposide-resistant mutants of human cancer B cells. Cancer Res 51 : 3951-3957
8. Darkin-Rattray SJ, Ralph R (1991) Evidence that a protein kinase enhances am-

sacrine mediated formation of topoisomerase II-DNA complexes in murine mastocytoma cell nuclei. Biochim Biophys Acta 1088 : 285-291
9. Kroll DJ, Rowe TC (1991) Phosphorylation of DNA topoisomerase II in a human tumor cell line. J Biol Chem 266 : 7957-7961
10. Wright WD, Roti Roti JL (1992) Resolution of DNA topoisomerase II by two-dimensional polyacrylamiude gel electrophoresis and western blotting. Ann Biochem 204 : 124-130
11. Boege F, Gieseler F, Biersack H, Clark M (1991) Use of anion-exchange chromatography and chromatofocussing to reveal the structural and functional heterogeneity of topoisomerase II in a HL-60 cell line resistant to multi-drug treatment. J Chromatogr 587 : 3-9
12. Boege F, Gieseler F, Müller M, Biersack H, Meyer P (1992) Topoisomerase II is activated during partial Purification by Heparin-Sepharose Chromatography. J Chromatogr 625 : 67-71
13. Zwelling LA, Hinds M, Chan D, Mayes J, Sie L, Parker E, Silberman L, Radcliffe A, Beran M, Blick M (1989) Characterization of an Amsacrine-resistant Line of Human Leukemia Cells. J Biol Chem 264 : 16411-16420
14. Gieseler F, Boege F, Erttmann R, Tony HP, Biersack H, Spohn B, Clark M (1992) Characterization of Human Leukemic HL-60 Cell Sublines as a Model for primary and secondary Resistance against Cytostatics. In : Hiddemann (ed) Hematology and Blood Transfusion 34. Springer Verlag, Berlin-Heidelberg, pp 44-48
15. Meyer P, Boege F, Gieseler F (in press) Topoisomerase II function detected as protein-DNA complexes in two sublines of HL-60 cells. Toxicol (Lett)
16. Boege F, Gieseler F, Biersack H, Meyer P (1992) The Assessment of nuclear topoisomerase II inhibition in vitro : a possible tool to detect resistance on a subcellular level in haematopoietic malignancies. Eur J Clin Chem Clin Biochem 30 : 63-68
17. Drake FH, Hofmann GA, Bartus HF, Mattern MR, Crooke ST, Mirabelli C (1989) Biochemical and pharmacological properties of p 170 and p 180 forms of topoisomerase II. Biochemistry 28 : 8154-8160
18. Woessner RD, Mattern MR, Mirabelli C, Johnson R, Drake FH (1992) Proliferation- and cell cycle-dependent differences in expression of the 170 kilodalton and 180 kilodalton forms of topoisomerase II in NIH-3T3 cells. Cell Growth Differ 2 : 209-214
19. Smith PJ, Makinson TA (1989) Cellular Consequences of Overproduction of DNA Topoisomerase II in an Ataxia-Teleangiectasia Cell Line. Cancer Res 49 : 1118-1124
20. Gieseler F, Boege F, Clark M, Meyer P (in press) Correlation between the DNA-binding affinity of topoisomerase inhibiting drugs and their capacity to induce hematopoetic cell differentiation. Toxicol Lett
21. Pommier Y, Kerrigan D, Schwartz RE, Swack JA, McCurdy A (1986) Altered DNA Topoisomerase II Activity in Chinese Hamster Cells Resistant to Topoisomerase II Inhibitors. Cancer Res 46 : 3075-3081
22. Zini N, Martelli AM, Sabatelli P, Santi S, Negri C, Astaldi Ricotti GC, Maraldi NM (1992) The 180-kDa isoform of topoisomerase II is localized in the nucleolus and belongs to the structural elements of the nucleolar remnant. Exp Cell Res 200 : 460-466
23. Negri C, Chiesa R, Cerino A, Bestagno M, Sala C, Zini N, Maraldi NM, Astaldi Ricotti GC (1992) Monoclonal antibodies to human DNA topoisomerase I and the two isoforms of DNA topoisomerase II : 170- and 180-kDa isozymes. Exp Cell Res 200 : 452-459
24. Hinds M, Deisseroth , Mayes J, Altschuler E, Jansen R, Ledley FD, Zwelling

LA (1991) Identification of a point mutation in the topoisomerase II gene from a human leukemia cell line containing an amsacrine-resistant form of topoisomerase II. Cancer Res 51 : 4729-4731

25. Bugg BY, Danks M, Beck WT, Suttle DP (1991) Expression of a mutant DNA topoisomerase II in CCRF-CEM human leukemic cells selected for resistance to teniposide. Proc Natl Acad Sci USA 88 : 7654-7658

Measurement of human tumor pharmacokinetics in vivo noninvasively by 19-F magnetic resonance spectroscopy predicts clinical 5-FU sensitivity and resistance

CA Presant, W Wolf, V Waluch, R Brechner, C Wiseman, DW Blayney, P Kennedy

5-Fluorouracil is one of the most widely-used chemotherapeutic drugs. However, it is impossible at present to determine which patients are destined to respond to 5-FU, and which patients will be unresponsive to that treatment.

We have previously used nuclear magnetic resonance spectroscopy (NMRS) to identify 5-FU in the liver and tumors of mice and humans with tumors [1, 2, 3]. In order to determine if the identification of 5-FU in tumors was able to predict clinical tumor sensitivity, we initiated this trial.

Methods

Patients were eligible if they had a solid tumor of greater than 2 cm diameter within 8 cm of the skin surface. Patients were positioned in an MRI (Siemens 2T Helicon) equipped with 19-F surface coils and appropriate spectroscopy software. The patients received 5-FU 600 mg per meter square as an intravenous bolus. Spectra were acquired every 4.17 minutes for one hour. The data collected were evaluated, and the disappearance of the 5-FU peak in the spectra was calculated. A T1/2 of less than 20 minutes was defined as absence of trapping, and a T1/2 of greater than 20 minutes was defined as trapping of 5-FU in the tumor. Responses of the tumors to subsequent chemotherapy were determined objectively from serial tumor measurements, using standard response criteria.

Results

Forty-three patients were studied in this trial. The patients had colorectal cancer [16], pancreatic cancer [7], breast cancer [7], as well as gastric, esophageal, head and neck, lung, kidney, bladder, endometrial and cervical cancer. After NMRS, 20 patients received chemotherapy with 5-FU post-leucovorin, and 5 with 5-FU alone. Other patients received combinations of chemotherapeutic agents with 5-FU, which included Interferon, Doxorubicin, Mitomycin, Cyclophosphamide, Cis-platinum, and VP-16. The most commonly studied site was a metastasis in liver, followed by lung metastases, breast

---

Los Angeles Oncologic Institute, St Vincent Medical Center, Los Angeles, CA, USA

metastases, retroperitoneal metastases, and a variety of othersites. The only intratumoral signals detected in these studies were due to 5-FU. Of the 43 patients, 35 showed uptake of 5-FU. In these 35, 23 showed no trapping, and 12 showed trapping. Thirty-five patients were evaluable for tumor response.

Of 25 patients treated with 5-FU alone or 5-FU plus Leucovorin, 5 of 6 patients who had demonstrated trapping had a partial response to chemotherapy. Of the 19 patients demonstrating no trapping, none showed a partial response (P = 0.0001). Of 10 patients receiving 5-FU plus other chemotherapy, 3 of 3 patients with trapping showed partial response, and 2 of 5 patients without trapping had a partial response. However, it was impossible to know whether those responses were due to the 5-FU, the other chemotherapy, or an interaction between the 5-FU and the other chemotherapy.

In addition, we have been able to utilize chemical-shift imaging in order to determine the 5-FU clearance rate in different areas of tumors. We have been able to use this technique to identify a T1/2 for 5-FU in the peripheral areas of the tumor, closest to the coil, the central areas of the tumor, and the distal areas of the tumor, most distant from the surface coil. In 12 patients, we have evaluated the subtumoral pharmacokinetics. In 9 patients, the overall clearance of 5-FU in the entire tumor was similar to the clearances in each of the subtumoral regions, indicating homogeneity of clearance rate. However, 3 patients exhibited different clearances in different portions of the tumor. We have termed this heterogeneous trapping of 5-FU. In these 3 patients, the response to 5-FU chemotherapy indicated a mixed response. Some areas of the tumor were found to have tumor regression, but other areas showed either tumor progression, or the appearance of new tumors.

We conclude that the presence of tumor heterogeneity by 19-F MRS may be capable of identifying areas of the tumor which consist of different vascularity, different tumor clones, or different tissue characteristics such as pH, oxygen tension, or other characteristics. The clinical significance of tumor heterogeneity, as revealed by subtumoral pharmacokinetic assessment, needs to be studied further in order to determine implications for therapy and research.

Overall the close correlation between the presence or absence of tumor trapping of 5-FU and subsequent response to 5-FU-containing chemotherapy indicates a potential clinical usefulness of magnetic resonance spectroscopy and is worthy of further confirmatory testing.

References

1. Wolf W, Albright MJ, Silver M et al (1987) Fluorine 19-NMR spectroscopic studies of metabolism of 5-Fluorouracil in the liver of patients undergoing chemotherapy. Res Imaging 5 : 165-169
2. Wolf W, Presant CA, Servis L et al (199?) In vivo 19-F Spectroscopic pharmacokinetics in tumor-bearing hormones. Proc Nat Acad Sci 87 : 492-496
3. Presant CA, Wolf W, Albright MJ et al (1990) Human tumor clinical correlations of in vivo 19-F Nuclear Magnetic Resonance Spectroscopy Pharmacokinetics. J Clin Oncol 8 : 1868-1873

Immunoregulation by tumor necrosis factor α (TNF): an opportunity for therapeutic intervention ?

E Mihich, D Maccubbin, S Pocchiari, S Ujházy, S Verstovsek, MJ Ehrke

Tumor necrosis factor α (TNF), a protein cytokine, is an endogenous pleiotropic mediator of inflammatory, immune and host defense functions. It is extremely potent, acting either alone or in combination with other cytokines or factors. It acts both as an autocrine and a paracrine mediator of a wide variety of localized responses as well as in a more generalized fashion. Based on current knowledge, its critical roles as local mediator of homeostasis and host defense are considered advantageous and those on systemic metabolic responses are not. In fact, systemic TNF has been demonstrated to be a/the causative agent in septic shock, in cachexia and in certain autoimmune diseases. TNF was so named because of its extremely potent anti-tumor (hemorrhagic necrosis) activity observed following systemic administration [1]. As the understanding of the molecular and cellular mechanisms of action of this cytokine is improved, opportunities for therapeutic intervention based on this knowledge are increased and should be given further consideration.

Coley [2] may well have been the first to induce hemorrahagic necrosis of tumors with therapeutic intent while investigating this phenomenon which was known to occur occasionally in cancer patients with an infectious disease. Studies by Shear and coworkers [3] designed to identify the therapeutic moiety in Coley's toxins led to the isolation of a moiety now known as lipopolysaccharide (LPS). Then they reported that serum from animals treated with LPS could induce hemorrhagic necrosis of tumors grown in animals that had not been exposed to LPS [4]. Subsequently Old and coworkers described essentially the same phenomenon and named the serum factor « tumor necrosis factor » [1]. The isolation of TNF in pure form and the molecular cloning of the recombinant molecule were accomplished nearly simultaneously by a number of different workers about 10 years later [5]. During this period of time, studies of cachexia led to the isolation of a factor termed « cachectin » and, once purified products became available, the chemical identity of cachectin and TNF was established [6, 7]. Thus, the complex and contradictory nature of this cytokine was better defined. Once an adequate supply of pure TNF became available, further advances were made in knowledge about the pleiotropic effects of this molecule.

The severe toxicity of TNF in early clinical trials [5] demonstrated that at the pharmacological doses tested this agent cannot be tolerated and spurred attempts to find ways to reduce toxicity while retaining therapeutic effectiveness. Many of these studies have attempted to derive TNF antagonists or mimetics through molecular modifications. The very recent report of the characterization of a human TNF mutant (a change of arginine to tryptophan at

Grace Cancer Drug Center, Roswell Park Cancer Institute, Buffalo, NY 14263, USA position 32) indicates the promise of such approaches [8]. Herein, an alternative approach is proposed for consideration ; that of using TNF, at doses well below those inducing toxicity, as an immunomodulating agent, given alone or in combination with other agents to stimulate the host anti-tumor response.

Material and methods

Animals : Female C57B1/6NCr mice six weeks old were obtained through the National Cancer Institue, USA and used between eight and twelve weeks of age.
Reagents : TNF [recombinant human (rHu, 2900 units/μg protein) and murine (rMu, 3,100 units/μg protein)] were gifts from Asahi Chemical Industry Co., Tokyo, Japan. Adriamycin (ADM) was a gift from Adria Laboratories, Columbus, OH. RHu Interleukin 2 (IL-2, 3700 BRMP units/μg protein) was a gift from E.I. DuPont de Nemours & Co., Inc., Glenolden, PA. Cyclophosphamide was purchased from Sigma Chemical Co., St Louis, MO. RPMI 1640 tissue culture medium supplemented with 10 % fetal calf serum (Hyclone, Logan, UT), 25 mM HEPES buffer (Research Organics, Cleveland, OH) and 50 μg/ml gentamycin was used with and without further supplementation with 1 mM sodium pyruvate, 0.1 mM nonesential amino acids, 2 mM glutamine and 50 μM 2-mercaptoethanol (GIBCO Labs, Grand Island, NY). Endotoxin levels were < 0.001 ng/ng protein for each of the cytokines and < 0.05 ng/ml for the culture medium and the fetal calf serum. Cell Lines : The tumor cell lines used in these studies were : EL-4 lymphoma and C1498 myeloid leukemia (syngeneic to C57B1/6 mice) ; YAC-1 lymphoma (syngeneic to A/Sn mice) ; P-815 mastocytoma (syngeneic to DBA-2 mice) ; and the murine D10.G4.1 cloned T-helper cell line. All these cells grow in suspension culture and in addition EL-4 was maintained by weekly i.p. passage in syngeneic mice.
Survival studies and effector function assays : All the techniques used in obtaining the data described herein have been fully described in previous publications from this laboratory [9-13].

Results and discussion

This laboratory became interested quite early in understanding the regulatory roles TNF plays in host defense responses [14]. It was thought that it must be these functions and not those mediating the pathophysiological manifestations of acute toxicity that were the biological reason not only for its conservation through evolution but also for the extreme redundancy of functions mediated by TNF, IL-1 and lymphotoxin. These cytokines serve as priming and activating signals for all the various classes of leukocytes. The examples of monocytes/macrophages and lymphocytes are given herein.
Monocytes/macrophages : TNF in combination with a number of other factors has been shown to induce tumoricidal macrophage activation. The other factors include a lymphokine rich supernatant [15], Interferon-γ (IFN-γ) [16],

LPS [10], and IL-2 [12]. Although TNF + IFN-γ can induce the production of IL-1 and IFN-γ + IL-1 can induce macrophage activation it was shown that TNF-mediated macrophage activation was not dependent upon endogenous IL-1 [11]. Furthermore, even though endogenous TNF produced by these activated macrophages may be the mechanism by which certain TNF-sensitive tumor target cells are lysed, these macrophages have the capacity to lyse TNF insensitive targets by other mechanisms [10]. These effects were obtained, in general, with concentrations of TNF in the range of 0.1 to 100 units/ml; concentrations one would expect to be easily reached in an area of localized response. Furthermore, concentrations higher than 1,000 units/ml were far less effective in inducing these effects.

Lymphocytes: TNF, in a strictly species-specific manner, can regulate murine thymocyte proliferation independently of IL-1 [9]. A similar species specificity requirement is not seen with human thymocytes with which both murine and human TNF induces an increase in proliferation in the comitogen assay [17]. The generation of cytotoxic T cells was augmented by the addition of TNF to the stimulation cultures [14]. There are a few reports of TNF modulation of NK activity, but in most cases, cytokines such as IL-2 or IFN-γ were also added [18]. In the absence of such factors no effect on NK activity were seen in a murine system [14]. In the presence of low concentrations of IL-2, TNF induces increased LAK generation with both murine splenocytes and thymocytes [19, 20]. Again, as seen with the monocytes/macrophages, the effective concentration of TNF was ⩽ 100 units/ml and at higher concentrations less activity was induced.

The results from these studies indicated that TNF, at relatively low concentrations, in combination with appropriate second signals, often other cytokines, caused upregulation of many host defense effector functions having anti-tumor activity. Of equal importance is the fact that, in general, TNF at concentrations > 1,000 units/ml was less effective than at lower concentrations. These results suggested that low dose TNF might have therapeutic potential if combined with a second agent which also would provide host response boosting signals. One such approach is to combine TNF with other cytokines and, as recently reviewed [5, 18], this has been tried with mixed success. A second approach would be to combine low dose TNF with anti-cancer chemotherapeutic agents known to have immunomodulating potential. Two agents which have been extensively characterized for immunomodulating properties are Adriamycin (ADM, Doxorubicin) and Cyclophosphamide (CY) (see [21] for a recent review). ADM, at doses within its reported therapeutic range, has been shown to upregulate many of the same effector functions stimulated by TNF and to induce increased production of TNF and IL-2. CY, at low doses, has been shown to selectively eliminate the generation of T suppressor cells, through effects either on the precursor of that cell or on an inducer (helper) cell critical to its development. The consequence of ablated T suppressor cell development is that a number of effector functions remain augmented under conditions where otherwise they would be suppressed (e.g. in the face of progressively growing tumor).

As this laboratory had considerable experience with those two agents [21], related combination treatment experiments were carried out. The syngeneic

EL4-C57B1/6 tumor mouse model with 5×10^4 lymphoma cells inoculated on Day 0 was used. It should be noted that, with the exception of CY, no long term survivors (LTS, surviving ≥ 60 days) resulted from the use of any of the treatments singly and that the inoculation of only 10-100 EL-4 cells resulted in the death of all the animals.

ADM plus TNF combined treatment : ADM was used at 4 or 5 mg/kg and was injected i.v. on Day 8. The experience gained in other studies [13, 22] had indicated that : 1) ADM at these doses was immunomodulatory ; 2) ADM on Day 8 only vs on Day 1 + 8 ; *a)* was equally effective in combination with IL-2 as a therapeutic treatment in this syngeneic tumor model, *b)* caused little or no tumor debulking although the Day 1 + 8 did, and *c)* was equally immunomodulatory. In combination with ADM, various doses and schedules of TNF, also administered i.v., were evaluated and it was found that the administration of 1,000 to 2,000 units per 20 g mouse starting on Day 13 and continuing on an alternating every second day or every third day schedule for 5 to 7 injections, but not exceeding a total of 10,000 units per mouse, resulted in the greatest numbers of LTS. Using this protocol, up to 80 % of the combination treated mice were LTS. A panel of assays for host anti-tumor effector functions including those for NK, LAK, tumoricidal macrophages (TMΦ) and specific anti-EL-4 CTLs were carried out using cells from various lymphoid tissues including spleen, thymus and peritoneal exudate. It was found that most host anti-tumor effector functions were up-modulated and/or sustained in the face of immunosuppressive progressive disease. Comparisons between the effects seen with cells from the combination treated mice and those receiving either agent singly or those not treated indicated that the effects most clearly associated with the propensity to survive > 60 days were : 1) the recovery of thymic cellularity following treatment induced hypocellularity ; 2) the development of specific anti-EL-4 CTLs and TMΦ in the spleen ; 3) the development of specific anti-EL-4 T-memory in the thymus and spleen. The evidence for the establishment of anti-EL-4 memory was two fold, 1) LTS reinjected with EL-4 (5×10^4 cells) 80 days after the initial inoculation rejected the tumor and 2) spleen and thymus cells obtained from LTS up to 445 days after initial tumor inoculation developed specific anti-EL-4 CTLs when challenged with x-irradiated EL-4 in culture. The development of specific CTLs was abrogated by preincubation of the lymphoid cells with anti-CD-44 + complement and the activity of the effectors was ablated by treatment with anti-CD-8 + complement.

CY plus TNF combined treatment : The day and the dose of CY administration were varied in combination with five injections of TNF (2,000 or 1,000 units per injection) on various schedules. The results of these studies indicated that : 1) CY administration on Day 12 was much more effective than that on Day 2 or Days 2 and 12 ; 2) up to 50 % of the mice receiving a dose of 150 or 250 mg/kg of CY alone on Day 12 became LTS ; 3) 80 to 100 % of the mice receiving 150 mg/kg CY on Day 12 plus 1,000 units TNF per injection on an every second day and every third day alternating schedule starting on either Day 8 or Day 13 became LTS ; 4) in comparison to the LTS which had received CY alone those which had received the combination treatment developed markedly more anti-EL-4 memory as determined by rejection of reimplanted EL-4 tumor and generation of specific anti-EL-4 activity with both spleen and thymus cells.

These combination treatment studies demonstrated that when low dose TNF was administered in conjunction with an immunomodulating/immunopermissive dose of either chemotherapeutic agent, considerable therapeutic advantage over that with any of the agents alone was seen. Under the conditions yielding the highest percentage LTS no toxicity was detected. In fact these animals survived for a further $1^1/_2$ year and at that point were still able to reject reimplanted EL-4, suggesting that a recurrence of primary tumor following such therapy would be unlikely. These findings are encouraging and support the need to consider approaches other than those defining the maximally tolerated dose when attempting to determine the optimal clinical dose for an agent whose mechanism of action is expected to involve the host defenses. Although the difficulties in doing so are recognized, the potential benefits of minimal toxicity and maximal long term anti-primary tumor immunity would seem to justify efforts in this regard.

References

1. Carswell EA, Old LJ, Kassel RL, Green S, Flore N, Williamson B (1975) An endotoxin-induced serum factor that causes necrosis of tumors. Proc Natl Acad Sci USA 72 : 3666-3670
2. Coley WB (1896) The therapeutic value of the mixed toxins of the streptococcus of erysipelas in the treatment of inoperable malignant tumors, with a report of 100 cases. Am J Med Sci 112 : 251-281
3. Shear MJ, Turner FC, Perrault A, Shovelton J (1943) Chemical treatment of tumors. V. Isolation of the hemorrhage-producing fraction from *Serratia marcesens (Bacillus prodigiosus)* culture filtrate. J Natl Cancer Inst 4 : 81-97
4. O'Malley WE, Achinstein B, Shear MJ (1962) Action of bacterial polysaccharide on tumors. II. Damage of sarcoma 37 by serum of mice treated with *Serratia marcesens* polysaccharide, and induced tolerance. J Natl Cancer Inst 29 : 1169-1175
5. Alexander RD, Rosenberg SA (1992) Tumor necrosis factor : clinical applications. In : DeVita VT Jr, Hellman S, Rosenberg SA (eds) Biologic Therapy of Cancer. JB Lippincott, Philadelphia, p 378
6. Kawakami M, Cerami A (1981) Studies of endotoxin-induced decrease in lipoprotein lipase activity. J Exp Med 154 : 631-639
7. Beutler B, Greenwald D, Hulmes JD, Chang M, Pan YC, Mathison J, Ulevitch R, Cermi A (1985) Identity of tumour necrosis factor and the macrophage-secreted factor cachectin. Nature 316 : 552-554
8. Van Ostade X, Vandenabeele P, Everaerdt B, Loetscher H, Gentz R, Brockhaus M, Lesslauer W, Tavernier J, Brouckaert P, Fiers W (1993) Human TNF mutants with selective activity on the p55 receptor. Nature 361 : 266-269
9. Ehrke MJ, Ho RLX, Hori K (1988) Species-specific TNF induction of thymocyte proliferation Cancer Immunol Immunother 27 : 103-108
10. Mace KF, Ehrke MJ, Hori K, Maccubbin DL, Mihich E (1988) Role of tumor necrosis factor in macrophage activation and tumoricidal activity. Cancer Res 48 : 5427-5432
11. Hori K, Mihich E, Ehrke MJ (1989) Role of tumor necrosis factor and Interleukin 1 in γ-Interferon-promoted activation of mouse tumoricidal macrophages. Cancer Res 49 : 2606-2614

12. Verstovšek S, Maccubbin D, Ehrke MJ, Mihich E (1992) Tumoricidal activation of murine resident peritoneal macrophages by Interleukin-2 and tumor necrosis factor α. Cancer Res 52 : 3880-3885
13. Maccubbin DL, Wing KR, Mace KF, Ho RLX, Ehrke MJ, Mihich E (1992) Adriamycin-induced modulation of host defenses in tumor-bearing mice. Cancer Res 52 : 3572-3576
14. Ehrke MJ, Mace K, Maccubbin D, Mihich E (1986) Regulatory role of human recombinant tumor necrosis factor on murine, control and Adriamycin modified, host defense functions. Abstr XIVth Intl Cancer Congress 3 : 916
15. Hori K, Ehrke MJ, Mace K, Maccubbin D, Doyle M, Otsuka Y, Mihich E (1987) Effect of tumor necrosis factor on the induction of macrophage tumoricidal activity. Cancer Res 47 : 2793-2798
16. Hori K, Ehrke MJ, Mace K, Mihich E (1987) Effect of tumor necrosis factor on tumoricidal activation of macrophages : synergism between tumor necrosis factor and Interferon-γ. Cancer Res 47 : 5868-5874
17. Pocchiari S, Krawczyk C, Ho R, Mihich E, Ehrke MJ (1991) Stimulation of thymocyte proliferation by Interleukin-1, tumor necrosis factor, and a synthetic tumor necrosis factor peptide. Abstr Soc Biol Therapy 4 : 17
18. Spriggs DR (1992) Tumor necrosis factor : basic principles and preclinical studies. In : DeVita VT Jr, Hellman S, Rosenberg SA (eds) Biologic Therapy of Cancer. JB Lippincott, Philadelphia, p 354
19. Ujházy P, Maccubbin DL, Eppolito C, Ehrke MJ, Mihich E (1992) Kinetic and phenotypic studies of Interleukin-2 ± tumor necrosis factor generated lymphokine activated killer cells from murine thymus and spleen. Proc AACR 33 : 324
20. Ujházy P, Maccubbin DL, Eppolito C, Mihich E, Ehrke MJ (submitted for publication 1993) TNF potentiation of the lymphokine activated killer response in murine spleen and thymus
21. Mihich E, Ehrke MJ (1992) Immunomodulation by anticancer drugs. In : DeVita VT Jr, Hellman S, Rosenberg SA (eds) Biologic Therapy of Cancer. JB Lippincott, Philadelphia, p 776
22. Ho LXR, Maccubbin D, Zaleskis G, Krawczyk C, Wing K, Mihich E, Ehrke MJ (submitted for publication 1993) Development of a non-toxic Adriamycin plus Interleukin-2 therapy effective against both Adriamycin sensitive and resistant lymphomas

Tumor necrosis factor alpha: its relationship with clinical data

JJ Bosco Lopez, M Escobar*, P Gallurt, P Rodriguez, A Lorenzo, A Morán*, A Senra, J Millán

A large number of highly potent peptide factors, such us the various interleukins, interferons, colony stimulating factors (CSF) and Tumor Necrosis Factor (TNF), all of them referred as cytokines, have been discovered in the past 10-20 years. Cytokines regulate or modify cellular responses in inflammatory and immune reactions, and this feature is particularly important in cancer patients. Cytokines elicit biological responses upon binding to specific cell surface receptors of sensitive cells. Many of these receptors are expressed by more than one cell type and so, pleiotropism of action is a common property of cytokines [1]. TNF was first discovered by its capacity to induce hemorrhagic necrosis of certain transplantable tumors in mice. The term TNF is used to refer collectively to the two related factors: TNF-α or cachectin and TNF-β or lymphotoxin.

Degradation by proteolysis, modulation of cellular receptors, and inhibition of the signal transduction downstream from the receptor all may limit the action of cytokines and indeed of TNF. Recently, further mechanisms which control cytokine activities have been discovered. First, receptor antagonists which are structural homologues of a cytokine and bind to the receptor molecule but are unable to elicit signal transduction were found to compete with the cytokine. Second, soluble receptor molecules which bind cytokines compete with the cellular receptors and now are thought to act as neutralizing buffers which limit systemic action [2]. These latter two inhibitory reactions could be relevant features in pathophysiological mechanisms.

The production and biological properties of TNF may be specially considered in tumor patients because of their pathogenic, physiopathological, and therapeutic implications. TNF may be a useful cytokine because it can induce the regression of tumors (both, endogenous and exogenous TNF). Otherwise, TNF production in cancer patients is generally considered as a host reaction against cancer and this feature could be evaluated as a biological marker of a central host response [3].

TNF has been identified as a tumor marker in malignancies. TNF-α may be specially important as a tumor marker in hepatocellular carcinoma and metastatic liver carcinoma [4], in head and neck carcinoma [5], in genitourinary cancer [6], in lung cancer [7] and in breast cancer [8]. In some of these tumors it is possible to find that patients with progressive disease had higher levels than patients without recurrences [8]. The role of increased concentrations of plasma TNF in the development of cancer cachexia appears very clear and those patients who had developed weight loss show TNF-α concentrations

---

Department of Medicine and Central Laboratory*, University Hospital School of Medicine, Cádiz, Spain

significatively higher than those in patients with similar stage but with not developed weight loss [9]. TNF-α has been investigated also in pleural effusion in cancer and non-cancer patients, with high TNF activity in both sera and pleural fluid levels of cancer patients in contrast with both sera and pleural fluid of patients with benign pleural effusions [10]. Pleural effusion from lung cancer patients could appear with cytotoxic activity against the patient's cancer cells, mainly due to local TNF activity [11].

In this work our purpose has been to evaluate the usefulness of quantification of serum immunoreactive Tumor Necrosis Factor (TNF-α) in cancer patients in order to stablish its role as biological marker according to anatomoclinical diagnosis of cancer, stage of disease and progression/response under chemotherapy treatment.

Material and methods

We have studied 53 tumor patients with diagnosis histologically verified. According with sex they were : 22 male (41.5 %) and 31 female (58.5 %). The localization of tumors was : breast cancer [28], lung cancer [18], head and neck carcinoma [3], digestive tract cancer [3] and gynecological cancer [1].

TNF-α in sera was quantified by a immunoenzymetric assay (Medgenix Diag. Brussels) with a coeficient of variation of 1.4 % intra-assay and 8.0 % inter-assay. Results are expressed in pg/ml and differences were evaluated by Student's t test.

Results

We have not found any difference by comparing TNF-α concentrations in male (89.45 $\pm$ 23.44 pg/ml ; SD : 109.96 ; range : 6.25-306.46) and female (81.13 $\pm$ 17.73 pg/ml ; SD : 98.73 ; range : 5-364.85) (Fig. 1).

TNF-α in sera of cancer patients was 84.58 $\pm$ 14.09 pg/ml (x + SEM) with SD : 102.58 and range : 5-364.85. Patients with breast cancer has a mean level of 86.10 $\pm$ 19.41 pg/ml. with SD : 102.74 and range : 5-364.85. In patients with lung cancer mean level was 106.72 $\pm$ 27.07. with SD : 114.86 and range : 6.94-306.46. There were not found differences between these tumors or with overall group of cancer patients (Fig. 2).

Fig. 3 show the differences according to clinical stage. Patients with local disease has serum TNF-α (34.06 $\pm$ 21.85 pg/ml) that differs (p < 0.01) of that one found in loco-regional disease (92.92 $\pm$ 23.68 pg/ml) and in metastatic disease (91.53 $\pm$ 20.64 pg/ml). Loco-regional or extended disease do not show significatively differences.

In relation with chemotherapy treatment, 22 patients were in complete remission and 31 has active disease. TNF-α in active disease patients was higher (90.5 $\pm$ 17.51 pg/ml ; SD : 97.49) — but not significatively — than that one found in patients with complete remission after treatment (76.1 $\pm$ 23.6 pg/ml ; SD : 111.14) (Fig. 4).

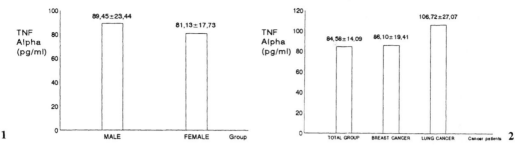

Fig. 1. TNF-alpha ($\overline{X} \pm$ sem) in relation with sex

Fig. 2. TNF-alpha ($\overline{X} \pm$ sem) in relation with anatomoclinical localization

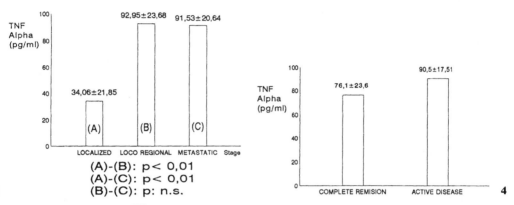

Fig. 3. TNF-alpha ($\overline{X} \pm$ sem) and standing

Fig. 4. TNF-alpha ($\overline{X} \pm$ sem) according response to chemotherapy

Discussion

The Tumor Necrosis Factor, preliminary identified because of its antitumor properties, refers to two kinds of similar polypeptides (TNF-α or cachectin and TNF-β or lymphotoxin). Mature cachectin share a 28 % amino acid sequence homology with lymphotoxin ; it is produced by a wide variety of cells, phagocytic and non-phagocytic, mainly by activated macrophages and monocytes. The biological effects mediate by cachectin may be beneficial or deleterious to the body, in part depending on the quantity produced [12]. Physiological or therapeutic level of TNF could play a role in restriction of tumor growth, but TNF overproduction may be involved in human cancer cachexia, and probably in experimental tumor growth progression as a promoter [13].

High levels of endogenous TNF-α in cancer patients should be the expression of either TNF produced or induced in human tumors, although tumor cells may also lead to TNF induction in normal cells [14, 15]. It is demonstrated the local expression of TNF mRNA in human tumors and this knowledge led to the conclusion of evidence in the production of TNF protein by tumor cells ; this production may influence the cachexia and tumor progression, and alter the response to therapy [16].

A high endogenous production of TNF is very important in cancer patients because of the findings indicate that endogenous TNF is one of the protective factors against the cytotoxic activity of TNF [17]. So, based on the finding that expression of endogenous TNF is not detected in TNF-susceptible cells but observed in TNF-resistant cells, the assumption was made that endogenous TNF may be a protective protein against cytotoxic activity of TNF [17]. In fact, sera of the cancer patients frequently had a marked inhibitory effect on the *in vitro* cytocidal activity of TNF [18] and simultaneously a high level of TNF and TNF receptors. This feature is probably related with two inhibitory reactions [1] : the presence of blockadge by an antagonist for TNF receptor and the presence of soluble receptors which bind TNF. In these cases, soluble forms of the cell surface receptors for TNF have been detected in urine [18]. Cancer patients appears as a situation with high levels of TNF but not necessary with increase of TNF activity.

High concentrations of both soluble receptors for TNF and immunoreactive TNF protein have been detected in cancer patients and the incidence and extent of the increase correlated with the staging of disease. So, the receptors and the immunoprotein could be an useful diagnostic tests as a biological marker in malignancies, but only in relation with progressive disease or response to treatment. Otherwise, this immunoprotein could be a potential therapeutic agent because of the relative biological inactivity of endogenous TNF.

References

1. Lesslauer W (1992) TNF, TNF receptors and recombinant inhibitors. Cytokine Congress Reports 1 : 8-10
2. Tartaglia LA, Weber RF, Figari IS, Reynolds C, Palladino MA, Goeddel DV (1991) The two different receptors for tumor necrosis factor mediate distinct cellular responses. Proc Natl Acad Sci USA 88 : 9292-9296
3. McCall JL, Funamoto S, Yun K, Parky BR (1991) Tumour necrosis factors-α immunodetection in blood monocytes and serum : preliminary findings in weight-losing cancer patients. Aust NZJ Surg 61 : 141-146
4. Nakazaki H (1992) Preoperative and postoperative cytokines in patients with cancer. Cancer 70 : 709-713
5. Gallo O, Pinto S, Boccuzi S, Dilaghi M, Gallina E, Attanasio M, Gori AM, Martini F, Abbate R (1992) Monocyte tumor necrosis factor production in head and neck squamous cell carcinoma. Laryngoscope 102 : 447-450
6. Akdas A, Turkeri L, Akoglu T (1990) Serum and urine levels of tumour necrosis factor in patients with genitourinary cancer and their relevance to disease status. Int Urol Nephrol 22 : 501-506
7. Theilmann L, Meyer U, Kommerell B, Dierkesmann R, Moller A (1990) Tumor-Nekrose-Faktor-α im Serum von Patienten mit Sarkoidose, Tuberkulose oder Bronchialkarzinom. Pneumologie 44 : 735-738
8. Mallmann P, Diedrich K, Mallmann R, Koenig UD, Krebs D (1991) Determination of TNF-α, Interferon-α, Interleukin-2 and reactivity in the leucocyte migration inhibition test in breast cancer. Anticancer Res 11 : 1509-1515

9. Knapp ML, Al-Sheibani S, Riches PG, Hanham IW, Phillips RH (1991) Hormonal factors associated with weight loss in patients with advanced breast cancer. Ann Clin Biochem Pt 5 : 480-486
10. Martinet N, Charles T, Vaillant P, Vignaud JM, Lambert J, Martinet Y (1992) Characterization of a tumor necrosis factor-α inhibitor activity in cancer patients. Am J Resp Cell Mol Biol 6 : 510-515
11. Ishii Y, Uchiyama Y, Hasegawa S, Kinoshita T, Mitsui K, Kojima H, Fujita T (1990) Detection of tumour necrosis factor/cachectin in pleural effusion of patients with lung cancer. Clin Esp Immunol 80 : 350-353
12. Martins e Silva J (1991) Caracterizacao bioquimica e efeitos metabolicos do factor de necrose tumoral. Acta Med Port 4 (suppl 1) : 20S-27S
13. Gelin J, Moldawer LL, Lonnroth C, Sherry B, Chizzonite R, Lundholm K (1991) Role of endogenous tumor necrosis factor α and Interleukin-1 for experimental tumor growth and the development of cancer cachexia. Cancer Res 51 : 415-421
14. Malik ST (1992) Tumour necrosis factor : roles in cancer pathophysiology. Sem Cancer Biol 3 : 27-33
15. Zielinski CC, Mueller C, Tyl E, Tichatschek E, Kubista E, Spona J (1990) Impaired production of tumour necrosis factor in breast cancer. Cancer 60 : 1944-1948
16. Naylor MS, Malik ST, Stamp GW, Jobling T, Balkwill FR (1990) In situ detection of tumour necrosis factor in human ovarian cancer specimens. Eur J Cancer 26 : 1027-1030
17. Himeno T, Watanabe N, Yamauchi N, Maeda M, Tsuji Y, Okamoto T, Neda H, Niitsu Y (1990) Expression of endogenous tumor necrosis factor as a protective protein against the cytotoxicity of exogenous tumor necrosis factor. Cancer Res 50 : 4941-4945
18. Aderka D, Englemann H, Hornik V, Skornick Y, Levo Y, Wallach D, Kushtai G (1991) Increased serum levels of soluble receptors for tumor necrosis factor in cancer patients. Cancer Res 51 : 5602-5607

The antiproliferative effect of lymphoblastoid α interferon and its ability to re-induce or amplify major histocompatibility complex antigen expression on human renal carcinoma cells in culture

RL Angus, CMP Collins*, MO Symes

Expression of Major Histocompatibility Complex (MHC) antigens by renal carcinoma cells declined as the period of culture increased. Exposure to α-IFN produced a dose dependant induction or increase in Class I MHC Ag expression by cells, growing *in vitro*, from half of the tumours studied (MS in preparation). The present experiments examine the relationship between the effect of α-IFN on cell proliferation and MHC Ag expression in individual tumours.

Materials and methods

Tumour cells from 11 renal carcinomas were established in culture. Within the first 14 days of *in vitro* growth and a variable time thereafter, the antiproliferative action of α-IFN on the cells of each tumour was measured in terms of inhibition of protein synthesis reflected by a reduction in the uptake of [^{75}Se]selenomethionine. At the same time intervals for each tumour expression of Class I and Class II Ag by the tumour cells, and the effect thereon of *in vitro* exposure to α-IFN was estimated. Class I and Class II Ag expression was recognised by exposure to appropriate monoclonal antibodies followed by indirect immunoperoxidase staining.

Interferon α-NI (Wellferon) was used throughout. The separation of tumour cells [1] and their culture [2] have previously been described.

Cells from each tumour were cultured in medium alone or in the presence of 100, 500 or 1,000 IU/ml of α-IFN for 48 hours. Thereafter the cells were cultured for 48 hours in methionine free medium to increase the uptake of [^{75}Se]selenomethionine added to the culture. Inhibition of isotope uptake by cells exposed to each concentration of α-IFN, with reference to cells maintained in medium alone, was calculated.

Class I MHC Ag was recognised by exposure to MoAb M736 (Dako) derived from clone w 6/32 and Class II Ag by exposure to MoAb M704 (Dako) from clone DK22 as previously described.

Tumour cells were harvested from cultures after the periods of *in vitro* growth detailed belowand plated on 3 well slides in medium alone or in medium containing 100, 500 or 1,000 IU/ml α-IFN. After 3 days cells in the first well were exposed to M736, in the second well to M704 and in the third well to TBS as a negative control. The cells in each well were then stained by the indirect immunoperoxidase technique using 3-amino 9-ethylcarbazole as chro-

---

University Departments of Surgery and Pathology*, Bristol Royal Infirmary, Bristol BS2 8HW, UK

The antiproliferative effect of lymphoblastoid α interferon

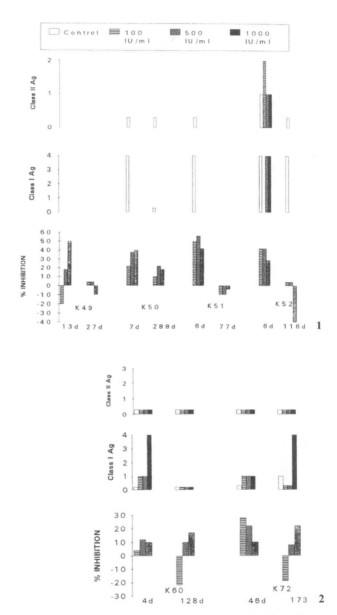

Fig. 1. In 4 RCC the signifiant antiproliferative effect of α-IFN was lost as the culture period increased. In K50 this was accompanied by a loss of Class I MHC Ag expression. In K52 Class II expression was lost

Fig. 2. In K60 & K72 there was no signifiant change in sensitivity to the antiproliferative action of α-IFN or in MHC Ag expression in the absence of α-IFN

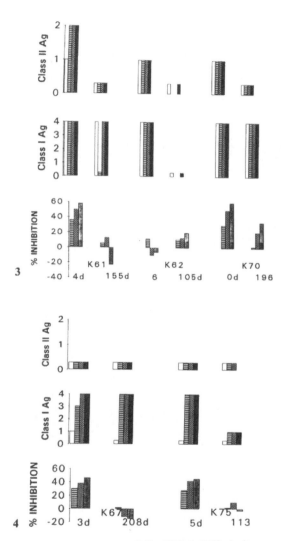

Fig. 3. Three tumours, K61, K62 & K70, lost expression of Class II Ag as the culture period increased. This could not be re-induced by exposure to α-IFN. Two of these tumours which were initially sensitive to the antiproliferative effect of α-IFN showed reduced sensitivity on prolonged culture

Fig. 4. In two tumours, K67 & K75, the ability of α-IFN to induce or increase Class I Ag expression was maintained as the culture period increased. However the antiproliferative action of α-IFN was lost

mogen. The expression of Ag was graded as nil or 1 to 4 in increments of 25 % of the total number of stained cells present in the well.

Results

The inhibition of protein synthesis by renal carcinoma cells following exposure to increasing concentrations of α-IFN, together with effect of IFN on the MHC Ag expression, are detailed for individual tumours in Figures 1-4.

In 8 of 11 tumours (K49, K50, K51, K52, K61, K67, K70 & K75) an increasing period of *in vitro* growth resulted in loss of the inhibitory action of α-IFN on protein synthesis. In 2 of these tumours (K50 & K67) the reduction of the antiproliferative action of α-IFN was associated with a reduction or loss of Class I Ag expression by tumour cells maintained in medium alone. Tumours K52, K61, K62 & K70 showed a similar loss of Class II Ag.

Discussion

Two main conclusions seem to emerge from these results. First MHC Ag expression, on which depends the host immune response to the tumour, and susceptibility to the antiproliferative action of α-IFN, decline on prolonged culture of renal carcinoma cells. Second, in 3 tumours Class II Ag expression could not be reinduced by exposure to α-IFN.

Tumour growth *in vitro* is associated with cell cloning which may be similar to that which accompanies the formation of metastases *in vivo* [3]. This together with loss of MHC Class I Ag expression by cells of metastatic compared to primary renal carcinomas suggests that α-IFN may be less effective in the treatment of metastases than would be the case if the cells had retained the characteristics of the primary lesion.

References

1. Ford TC, Lai T, Symes MO (1987) Morphological and functional characteristics of mouse mammary carcinoma separated on Nycodenz columns. Br J Exp Path 68 : 453-60
2. Lai T, Collins CMP, Hall P, Morgan AP, Smith PJB, Stonebridge BR Symes MO (1993) Verapamil enhances Doxorubicin activity in cultured human renal carcinoma cells. Eur J Cancer 29A : 378-83
3. Alam SM, Whitford P, Cushley W, George WD, Campbell AM (1992) Aneuploid subpopulations in tumour invaded lymph nodes from breast cancer patients. Eur J Cancer 28A : 357-62

Is there any predictive factor of the clinical response to IL-2 therapy in metastatic malignant melanoma?

Cl Soubrane, R Mouawad, M Ichen, J Suissa, E Vuillemin, Ch Borel, A Benhammouda, M Weil, D Khayat

The ominous prognosis of metastatic malignant melanoma has led to a large number of clinical treatment trials [1, 2]. Some improvement in terms of response rate seems to have been achieved, but the main question asked by clinicians remains: is there a biological predictive factor for the therapeutic response to IL-2 therapy? It is now well established that IL-2 plays a pivotal role in the immune response, both in its own receptor expression and other cytokine release. To exert its biological effect, IL-2 interacts with specific membrane receptors. Three types of IL-2 binding sites have been described: a 55 kD protein (α-chain, TAC) low-affinity receptor unable to deliver a signal to the cell, a 70 kD (β-chain) intermediate-affinity receptor which can transduce a signal and a high-affinity receptor made up of both the p 55 and p 70 molecules. More recently a third receptor has been cloned: γ-chain. Moreover, activated T cells release a truncated form of the α-chain molecule as a soluble Interleukin-2 receptor (sIL-2R) [3, 4]. We report here the study of immunological events both cellular and humoral following CDDP, IL-2 and Interferon-α in 31 patients treated for malignant metastatic melanoma.

Materials and methods

Patients

Thirty-one patients (16 male/15 female) with metastatic malignant melanoma were included in this study. Median age was 44 years (range: 21-68) and median ECOG performance status was 0 (range: 0-2) [Khayat and al, in this volume]. A group of 20 healthy donors was also evaluated: they included 12 women and 8 men with an age range (25-55 years).

Protocol

Patients received 100 mg/m^2 of Cisplatin (CDDP) over 4 hours on days 1 and 28, followed by 18 MUI/m^2/day of Interleukin-2 (rIL-2-Eurocetus©) in continuous intravenous infusion from days 3 to 6, 17 to 21, 31 to 34 and 45 to 49. α-Interferon (IFN, Roche©) 9 MUI was given subcutaneously three times weekly.

Oncology Medical Laboratory, Salpêtrière Hospital, 75013 Paris, France

Cytofluorometric analysis

Using flow cytometry, phenotypic lymphocyte subsets were determined : CD3, CD4, CD8, activated B and T cells (HLA-Dr), CD56 and CD25 (low affinity receptor of IL-2). Results are expressed as percentage of fluorescent cells.

Cytokine assays

Cytokine release was determined by ELISA technic using different appropriate kits : GM-CSF, IFN-gamma, TNF-α and soluble IL-2 receptor. Results are expressed in pg/ml for the most of cytokines except for the soluble IL-2 receptor expressed in pM.

Statistical analysis

Statistical significance of the differences between the two groups of patients responder (R) and non responder (NR) was determined by the non-parametric Mann-Whitney test. Differences were considered as significant at $p \leqslant 0.05$. Correlation coefficients were determined by the Spearman rank test. Data processing was carried out using the PCSM statistical package (Deltasoft, 1988).

Results

Clinical response

All patients received the two induction cycles and were fully evaluable (Table 1).

Table 1.

	No pts	%
Complete remission	4/31	13
Partial response	15/31	48
Stabilization	5/31	16
Progressive disease	7/31	23

Phenotypic lymphocyte subsets

CD4/CD8 ratio did not show any change between responder and non responder patients, both at onset or during treatment. However, at the end of the treatment (after the fourth course of IL-2), a generalized increase in CD8 cells was observed in all patients.

NK cells (CD56+) increased throughout the entire cycle with no difference between responder and non-responder patients. However, we found a significant difference (p = 0.03) between R and NR in cells expressing exclusive CD56+ CD16+ phenotype at the end of day 35.

Cytokine release

TNF α and GMCSF were not detected at any time for either group of patients.

IFN-γ was detected in all patients, but the release was variable among patients and not correlated with treatment response.

IL-2 receptors

Concerning the percentage of cells expressing TAC receptor before any therapy, neither significant change was observed in healthy volunteers (21.7 ± 6) and patients (24.6 ± 9.8) or between responder (23.3 ± 6.5) and non responder (26.4 ± 8.3) patients, even during treatment. However, after each IL-2 infusion, lymphocytes expressing CD25+ decreased concurrently with the lymphopenia observed.

Before any therapy, we observed a significant increase (p = 0.001) in soluble IL-2R shedding (PM) in patients (79.04 ± 40) compared to healthy volunteers (30.6 ± 15). In contrast, no significant variation (p = 0.1) was seen between R (57 ± 29) and NR (79 ± 38) patients.

During treatment, the sIL-2R ratio increased in both groups but, interestingly, a significant difference was found between responder and non-responder patients from day 7 (p < 0.05) to day 21 (p ≤ 0.01) (Fig. 1).

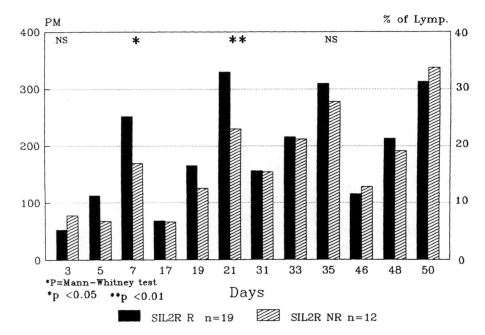

Fig. 1.

Since sIL-2R level seems to play an important role, we tried to determine how much sIL-2R is linked to the clinical response. For this study, we used logistic regression using different parameters (age, sex, metastatic site and soluble IL-2R) on clinical response (complete, partial, stabilization versus progressive disease). We found that, at day 21, sIL-2R is significantly linked to the clinical response ($p = 0.0063$). Therefore a patient with sIL-2R level greater than 250 pM at day 21 has twelve fold more chances to present a clinical response.

Discussion

In this study we tried to answer one of the question asked by clinicians : is there any early predictive factor for the clinical response to chemo-immunotherapy ? We reported here the results of different immunological parameters following CDDP, IL-2, IFN-α combination in 31 patients with metastatic malignant melanoma. Taken together, these data suggest that soluble IL-2 receptor level is significantly correlated to the clinical response during the first two courses of therapy and might be an early predictive factor.

In contrast with most of the published data, we found a significant difference in the s-IL-2R levels between responder and non responder patients during the first two induction courses, suggesting that the non-responder lymphocytes may be slower in becoming stimulated as appreciated through CD25 shedding. It might be the most striking point of our study since, at our knowlewdge, no one to date has mentioned this type of variation. Indeed, Lissoni et al [5] reported opposite results regarding soluble IL-2R release between responder and non responder patients. However their study used low dose subcutaneous Interleukin-2 alone in advanced renal cancer. Moreover the small number of patients ($n = 13$; $R = 4$; $NR = 9$) did not allow them to draw definite conclusions about the relationship between immune changes and clinical response.

It is known that sIL-2R serum concentrations rapidly increase in response to IL-2 infusion and remain high until the end of IL-2 cycle. Furthermore we obtained a significant dissociation in soluble IL-2R release between R and NR patients and this only up to day 21 suggesting that sIL-2R might be an early predictive factor of the clinical response. Indeed the statistical analysis based on logistic regression using different factors (sex, age, metastatic site and sIL-2R level) on clinical response, concerns this assumption.

Although the above results must be interpreted with caution, given the risk inherent in multiple subset analyses, we therefore speculate from this study that soluble IL-2R level may be of potential value in the follow-up of patients with metastatic malignant melanoma. However we need further investigation which are on-going in our department.

References

1. Legha SS (1989) Current therapy for melanoma. Sem Oncol 16 : 34-44
2. Rosenberg SA, Mullé JJ, Spiess PJ, Reichert CM, Schwarz SL (1985) Regression of established pulmonary metastases and subcutaneous tumor mediated by the systemic administration of high-dose recombinant Interleukin-2. J Exp Med 161 : 1169-1188
3. Rubin L, Jay G, Nelson D (1986) The released Interleukin-2 receptor binds Interleukin-2 efficiently. J Immunol 137 : 3841-3845
4. Voss SD, Hank JA, Nobis C, Fisch P, Sosman JA, Sondel PM (1989) Serum Interleukin-2 receptor levels during IL-2 therapy reflect systemic lymphoid mass activation. Cancer Immunol Immunother 29 : 261-265
5. Lissoni P, Barni S, Ardizzoia A, Crispino S, Paolorossi F, Archili C, Vaghi M, Tancini G (1992) Second line therapy with low-dose subcutaneous Interleukin-2 alone in advanced renal cancer patients resistant to Interferon-α. Eur J Cancer 28 : 92-96

How IL-2 can affect melanoma cells

S Plaisance, A Alileche, E Rubinstein, D Han, B Azzarone, C Jasmin

Interleukin-2 (IL-2) is a T cell derived lymphokine strictly required for T lymphocytes proliferation. In T cells, it delivers a growth signal through a specific receptor (IL-2-R$\alpha\beta$) which binds IL-2 with high affinity (Kd 10-50 pM). IL-2-R is composed of at least two distinct IL-2 binding molecules : the α chain (IL-2-Rα) and the β chain (IL-2-Rβ) displaying low (Kd 10 nM) and intermediate affinity (Kd 1-2 nM) respectively [1]. Recently, a third chain IL-2-Rc (p64) which confers the functionality to the IL-2-R has been described [2]. *In vivo* infusion of IL-2 and Lymphokine Activated Killer cels (LAK) has been shown to induce tumor regression in 10-20 % of patients with metastatic melanomas [3]. IL-2 displays several other effects on lymphoid cells including B lymphocytes and NK cells[1], as well as on non-lymphoid cells of mesenchymal origin such as myelomonocytic cells[1], endothelial cells [4] fibroblasts and fibrosarcomas [5, 6]. In addition, IL-2 is active on cells derived from the neural crest such as oligodendrocytes precursors [7]. Here we show that other cells of neuro-ectodermal origin are sensitive to IL-2.

Result and discussion

In Figure 1A, a flow cytometric analysis with monoclonal antibodies (mAbs) specific for the IL-2 binding site of the α (IOT-14) and β-chain [8] (MIKβ1) shows the co-expression of the two chains of the IL-2-R on five human melanoma cell lines (M14, GLL19, IGR3, ME1477, MEL-JUSO) derived from different body sites and exhibiting heterogeneous pattern of differentiation.

Membrane expression of the IL-2-R was confirmed by the detection, in Northern blot assays, of specific mRNAs for the IL-2-Rα gene (Fig. 1B) [9]. Southern blot on PCR products using cDNA probes specific for the IL-2-Rβ gene [10] and for the IL-2-R gene [2] shows the presence of specific transcripts for the IL-2-Rβ chain (1C) and for the IL-2-R chain in 3 out of 5 melanoma cell lines (1D). As positive controls, we used PHA blasts, YT and IARC 305 T cell lines which express the different subunits of the IL-2-R. We also studied the expression of the IL-2 gene in the five melanoma cell lines using the cDNA probe plW55 specific for the human IL-2 gene (ATCC Rockville, MD). In M14 cells, but not in the other melanoma lines, we found the typical transcript of 0.9 kb (Fig. 2A). By using a Radio Immuno Assay for human IL-2, we could detect the presence of about 200 IU/ml of IL-2 in the supernatant of M14 cells (control PHA-blasts produced 8 folds more IL-2, Fig. 2B). The IL-2 secreted by M14 cells induced the proliferation of the murine IL-2-dependent lym-

---

INSERM Unité 268, Hôpital Paul-Brousse, 94800 Villejuif

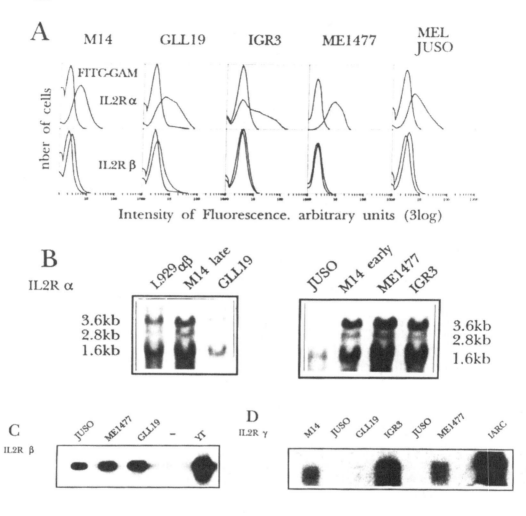

Fig. 1. A Quantitative flow cytometric analysis of 5 human melanoma cell lines incubated with anti IL-2-Rα (10T14 Immunotech, Luminy, France) or with anti IL-2-Rβ (MIKβ1) mAb. Viable cells were analyzed after combination of FS-SS gating and propidium iodide exclusion. The left curve of each panel represents the profile of cells stained with Fab[1] fluorescein conjugated goat anti mouse antibodies clone. **B** Northern blot analysis of IL-2-Ra (3-6 and 1-4 Kb) transcripts in human melanoma cells with the specific cDNA probe pIL-2-R2 using 5 **mg** of Poly (A) + RNA. **C** PCR analysis of IL-2-Rb gene expression in melanoma cells. Southern blot on the PCR products with a specific cDNA probe [10]. As positive control, we used the YT T cell line. **D** PCR analysis of IL-2-Rc gene expression in melanoma cells. Southern blot of the PCR products with a specific cDNA probe [2]. As positive control, we used the T cell line IARC 305

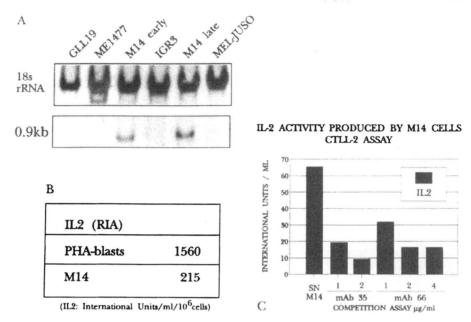

Fig. 2 A-C. IL-2 production in human melanoma cells. **A** Northern blot analysis of the IL-2 gene was performed with the specific cDNA probe pLW55 (ATCC) using 30 μg of total RNA. The typical 0.9 Kb transcript was only found in M14 cells either at early or late passage level. **B** IL-2 analysis in the supernatant of melanoma cells and PHA-blasts by RIA specific for the human IL-2 (RIA KIT IM-1971, Amersham, France). **C** Detection of biologically active IL-2 in the supernatant of M14 cells was performed using the mouse IL-2 dependent CTLL-2 cell line and the standard IL-2 reference reagent provided by the Biological Response Modifier Program (BRMP) of the NCI. Dose dependent inhibition of the IL-2 activity produced by M14 cells was obtained preincubating their supernatant with two different anti-IL-2 blocking mAbs (mAb 35 and mAb 66, Immunotech, Luminy, France)

phoid cell line CTLL-2 and inhibition of proliferation was obtained by preincubating M14 supernatants with two different IL-2 blocking mAbs (Fig. 2C). However, IL-2 could not modify the growth rate of M14 cells.

We finally investigated the role of IL-2 on the surface expression of several molecules which are modulated by IL-2 in human embryonic fibroblasts [6, 11]. As shown in Fig. 3A hu rIL-2 down modulates the expression of ICAM-1 protein, whereas alone or in combination with IFN gamma. IL-2 causes the up-regulation of CD44 surface expression (two fold and eight fold increase of the basal level respectively). By contrast, IL-2 inhibits the stimulation by IFN gamma of the surface expression of hystocompatibility antigens class I and class II. IL-2 also decreases their spontaneous expression. The specificity of these results is shown by the fact that overnight incubation of the IL-2 secreting M14 melanoma cells with polyclonal anti-IL-2 antibodies and anti IL-2-Rα mAbs induces the up-regulation of ICAM-1, HLA class I and HLA class II (fig. 3B).

In conclusion, the expression of a functional IL-2-R in human melanoma

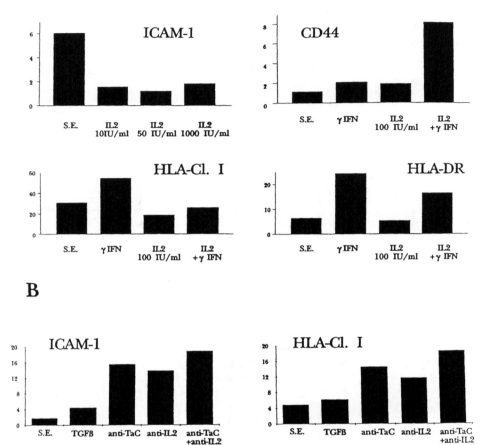

Fig. 3 A, B. ICAM-1, CD44, HLA class II expression and effect of IL-2 and IFN gamma. Flow cytometric analysis of spontaneous expression (S.E.) of ICAM-1, CD44, HLA class I and HLA class II and modulation by r-IL-2 and/or IFN gamma (Roussel-Uclaf, France) **(A)**. Overnight incubation with EP-100 polyclonal rabbit anti human IL-2 antibodies (Genzyme, Boston) and/or anti IL-2-Rα mAb 10T14 (Immunotech, Luminy, France) causes the up-regulation of ICAM-1, HLA class I and HLA class II in M14 melanoma cells **(B)**

cell lines and the modulation by recombinant or endogenous IL-2 of surface antigens involved in the interactions with immunocompetent cells (ICAM-1, HLA class I and class II) and in tumour progression (CD44, ICAM-1) may be important events in the course of IL-2 treatment of these tumours.

References

1. Waldmann TA (1991) The Interleukin-2 receptor. J Biol Chem 266 : 2681-2684
2. Takeshita T, Asao H, Ohtani K, Ishii N, Kumaki S, Tanaka T, Munaka H, Nakamura M, Sugamura K (1992) Cloning of the c chain of the human IL-2 receptor. Science 257 : 379-182
3. Rosenberg SA (1988) Immunotherapy of cancer using Interleukin-2 : current status and future prospects. Immunol Today 9 : 58-62
4. Frazier SK, Hatzakis H, Seong D, Jones CM, Wu KK (1988) Influence of natural and recombinant Interleukin-2 on endothelial Cell metabolism. J Clin Invest 82 : 1877-1883
5. Carloni G, Paterson H, Aygery-Bourget Y, Sahraoui Y, Rubinstein E, Suarez H, Azzarone B (1989) N-ras dependent revertant phenotype in human HT1080 fibrosarcoma cells is associated with loss of proliferation within normal tissues and expression of adult membrane antigenic phenotype. Oncogene 4 : 873-880
6. Plaisance S, Rubinstein E, Alileche A, Krief P, Augery-Bourget Y, Sahraoui Y, Jasmin C, Suarez C, Azzarone B (1992) Expression of the Interleukin-2 receptor on human fibroblasts and its biological significance. Int Immunol 4 : 739-746
7. Saneto RP, Altman A, Knobler RL, Johnson HM, De Vellis (1986) Interleukin-2 mediates the inhibition of oligodendrocyte progenitor cell proliferation *in vitro*. Proc Natl Acad Sci USA 83 : 9221-9225
8. Tsudo M, Kinamura F, Miyasaka M (1989) Characterisation of the Interleukin-2 receptor β-chain using three distinct monoclonal antibodies. Proc Natl Acad Sci USA 86 : 1982-1986
9. Leonard WJ, Depper JM, Crabtree GR, Rudikoff S, Pumphrey J, Robb RJ, Kronke M, Svetlik PB, Peffer NJ, Waldmann TA, Green WC (1984) Molecular cloning and expression of cDNAs for the human Interleukin-2 receptor. Nature 311 : 626-631
10. Hatakeyama M, Tsudo M, Minamoto S, Kono T, Miyata T, Miyasaka M, Taniguchi T (1989) Interleukin-2 receptor β-chain gene : generation of three receptor forms by cloned human α- and β-chain cDNA's. Science 244 : 551-556
11. Plaisance S, Alileche A, Han D, Rubinstein E, Sahraoui Y, Jasmin C, Azzarone B (1992) Expression and role of surface markers of immunocompetent cells in non lymphoid systems. In : Jacquemin-Sablon (ed) New Developments in flow cytometry. NATO ASI Series, Villejuif

Abstract. Human melanoma cell lines are sensitive to IL-2. Indeed, they express an Rαβ IL-2 binding heterodimer and three out of six present a specific transcript for the IL-2-Rc. One of these cell lines (M14) also secretes a biologically active IL-2. IL-2 modulates the surface expression of adhesion molecules such as ICAM-1 and CD44 as well as of histocompatibility antigens

(HLA class I and HLA class II). Moreover, in M14 cells overnight incubation with anti IL-2-Rα and anti IL-2 mAbs, causes the up-regulation of ICAM-1, HLA class I and HLA class II molecules showing the existence of an autocrine-paracrine loop, controlling the surface level of molecules important in the immuno recognition.

Human solid tumors which express the IL-2-R may be expected to directly respond to exogenously supplied IL-2, and this mechanism in addition to immuno-modulatory effects could contribute to therapeutic effects if IL-2 administrated locally or systematically to patients with cancer.

Potentiation of 5-Fluorouracil-[6RS]leucovorin cytotoxicity by recombinant human Interferon-α2A in colon carcinoma cells

JA Houghton, DA Adkins, PJ Houghton

In Phase III randomized clinical trials in adults presenting with colorectal carcinoma, response rates to FUra-[6RS]LV in comparison to FUra administered alone are 33-48 % vs 7-15 %, respectively [1-4], with significant increases in time to disease progression [1, 2, 4] and increased patient survival [2, 4] reported. Although the use of FUra with [6RS]LV has improved response rates, there is a need to build upon this combination to develop more efficacious therapy for colorectal carcinoma. Recently, there has been an interest in the clinical utility of FUra in combination with interferons (IFN's), specifically rIFN-α-2A. Single institutional trials utilizing 9×10^6 IU of rIFN-α-2Aa three times weekly and FUra (750 mg/m²/day × 5) given by infusion i.v. in previously untreated patients report response rates as high as 76 % [5], or lower, in the range of 26-35 % [6, 7]. These trials had been initiated from reports of studies conducted in cultured colon adenocarcinoma cells that had shown potentiation of the growth inhibitory or cytotoxic activity of FUra by IFN's [8-11].

These studies suggested that IFN effects are dependent on initial inhibition of thymidylate synthase by the Fluoropyrimidine. The study of Chu et al [9] suggested that rIFN-γ abrogates the FUra-induced increase in total thymidylate synthase that may be responsible for reducing cellular sensitivity to FUra. As [6RS]LV enhances the inhibition of thymidylate synthase by FdUMP [12, 13], the combination of FUra, [6RS]LV, and rIFN-α-2A may be more effective that FUra combined with each modulator independently. We subsequently examined the interaction of rIFN-α-2A as a direct modulator of the cytotoxic activity of FUra combined with [6RS]LV.

Results

GC_3/cl cells were exposed to various concentrations of FUra alone or in combination with [6RS]LV (1 μM), rIFN-α-2A (5,000 IU/mL) or both modulators either in the absence or in the presence of dThd (20 μM) for 72 hrs Cytotoxicity was determined by clonogenic assay (Fig. 1).

At 5,000 IU/mL, rIFN-α-2A was not cytotoxic. The IC_{50} for FUra was 2.46 μM and was decreased by 3.7-fold in combination with [6RS]LV, by 3.4-fold with rIFN-α-2A, and by 13-fold in the presence of both [6RS]LV and rIFN-α-2A. The activity of FUra-[6RS]LV or FUra-rIFN-α-2A was potentiated a further 3.5-to 3.8-fold by the addition of the second modulator. Potenti-

---

Department of Biochemical and Clinical Pharmacology, St Jude Children's Research Hospital, Memphis, TN 38101, USA

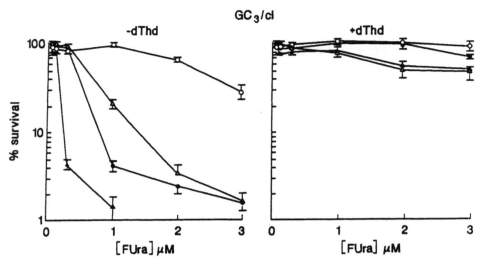

Fig. 1. Effects of rIFN-α-2A (5,000 IU/mL) or [6RS]LV (1 μM) used as single modulators or combined with various concentrations of FUra in GC$_3$/cl cells. Cells were treated in the absence of dThd with (○) FUra alone, or FUra combined with (●) [6RS]LV, (○) [6RS]LV + rIFN-α-2A, or in the presence of dThd (20 μM) with (○) FUra alone, or FUra combined with (●) [6RS]LV, (▲) rIFN-α-2A, or ( ) [6RS]LV + rIFN-α-2A. Each point is the mean ± SD of triplicate wells per group. The number of colonies per control well was 340 ± 9. Data show a representative experiment from three separate experiments

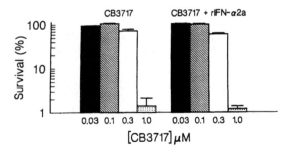

Fig. 2. Clonogenic survival of GC$_3$/cl cells following a 72 hour exposure to CB3717 either (○) alone or (●) in combination with rIFN-α-2A (500 IU/mL). Each point represents the mean ± SD of three wells

ation observed in these groups was significant (P < 0.001). Only small differences were observed between FUra-[6RS]LV and FUra-rIFN-α-2A groups that were significant at 1 μM FUra (P < 0.0001). When cells were exposed in the presence of dThd (20 μM), FUra ± [6RS]LV cytotoxicity was completely reversed, although cytotoxicity obtained in the presence of rIFN-α-2A ± [6RS]LV was only partially reversed. Data obtained with 500 IU/ml rIFN-α-2A were similar (not shown).

To determine whether thymidylate synthase inhibition *per se* was a requirement for initiation of a cellular response to rIFN-α-2A, the activity of various concentrations of the quinazoline-based thymidylate synthase inhibitor CB3717 was examined either alone or combined with rIFN-α-2A (500 IU/mL, Fig. 2).

The IC_{50} value for CB3717 was 0.34 μM and was similar when CB3717 was combined with rIFN-α-2A (0.32 μM).

Discussion

In GC_3/cl colon adenocarcinoma cells, rIFN-α-2A was not cytotoxic when administered alone at concentrations as high as 5,000 IU/mL and yet it was capable of increasing the cytotoxic activity of FUra. Of particular interest was the influence of rIFN-α-2A on the cytotoxicity of FUra combined with [6RS]LV. rIFN-α-2A and [6RS]LV administered as single modulators were approximately equivalent in their degree of potentiation of FUra cytotoxicity (3.2-to 3.4-fold). When combined, however, these agents further potentiated FUra efficacy an additional 4-fold beyond that observed with either agent alone. These results suggest that the effect of [6RS]LV and rIFN-α-2A in potentiating FUra cytotoxicity are at least additive and potentially act at independent loci. Studies by Wadler et al [10] suggest that although non-cytotoxic concentrations of rIFN-α-2A or rIFN-β can potentiate the cytotoxicity activity of FUra in two human colon cancer cell lines, it is necessary to expose cells to concentrations of FUra alone that cause some degree of cytotoxicity to mediate this effect. In GC_3/cl cells, however, rIFN-α-2A decreased clonogenic survival at non-cytotoxic concentrations of FUra or FUra combined with [6RS]LV.

With regard to the mechanism of interaction between FUra, rIFN-α-2A, and [6RS]LV, there have been reports suggesting that IFN's may influence dThd salvage by inhibition of the uptake of dThd [14] or may act at the level of thymidine kinase [15]. In the experiments presented, however, studies were conducted in dialyzed serum lacking dThd, where dThd salvage would be minimal. The cytotoxicity of FUra and potentiation of FUra or FUra-[6RS]LV cytotoxicity by rIFN-α-2A and reversibility of the effects by dThd does suggest, however, that modulation by rIFN-α-2A occurs only after some level of inhibition of thymidylate synthase. Only partial reversal of the cytotoxic action of FUra-rIFN-α-2A ± [6RS]LV by dThd in GC_3/cl suggests that part of the modulating action of rIFN-α-2A may be due to a dThd-independent or even thymidylate synthase-independent mechanism. Lack of potentiation by rIFN-α-2A of the cytotoxic action of CB3717, a specific quinazoline-based inhibitor of thymidylate synthase, suggests that thymine-less stress *per se* does not increase cell sensitivity to rIFN-α-2A. Data thus suggest that a Fluoropyrimidine rather than purely thymidylate synthase inhibition is required in the interaction mechanism but that potentiation of enzyme inhibition increases the extent of the interaction. Interaction either at the level of the enzyme or DNA following the action of the Fluoropyrimidine is thus indicated in colon adenocarcinoma cells.

Acknowledgements. Supported by National Cancer Institue grants CA-32613, CA-23099, and CA-21765, and by the American Lebanese Syrian Associated Charities (ALSAC).

References

1. Doroshow JH, Multhauf P, Leong L et al (1990) Prospective randomized comparison of Fluorouracil versus Fluorouracil and high-dose continuous infusion leucovorin calcium for the treatment of advanced measurable colorectal cancer in patients previously unexposed to chemotherapy. J Clin Oncol 8 : 491
2. Erlichman C, Fine S, Wong A, Elhakim T (1988) A randomized trial of Fluorouracil and folinic acid in patients with metastatic colorectal carcinoma. J Clin Oncol 6 : 469
3. Petrelli N, Herrera L, Rustum Y et al (1987) A prospective randomized trial of 5-Fluorouracil versus 5-Fluorouracil and high-dose Leucovorin versus 5-Fluorouracil and Methotrexate in previously untreated patients with advanced colorectal carcinoma. J Clin Oncol 5 : 1559
4. Poon MA, O'Connell MJ, Moertel CG et al (1989) Biochemical modulation of Fluorouracil : evidence of significant improvement of survival and quality of life in patients with advanced colorectal carcinoma. J Clin Oncol 7 : 1407
5. Wadler S, Schwartz EL, Goldman M et al (1989) 5-Fluorouracil and recombinant Interferon-α-2A : an active regimen against colorectal carcinoma. J Clin Oncol 7 : 1769
6. Kemeny N, Younes A, Seiter K et al (1990) Interferon-α-2A and 5-Fluorouracil for advanced colorectal carcinoma. Cancer 66 : 2470
7. Pazdur R, Ajani JA, Patt YZ et al (1990) Phase II study of Fluorouracil and recombinant Interferon-α-2A in previously untreated advanced colorectal carcinoma. J Clin Oncol 8 : 2027
8. Elias L, Crissman JA (1988) Interferon effects upon the adenocarcinoma 38 and HL-60 cell lines : antiproliferative responses and synergistic interactions with halogenated Pyrimidine antimetabolites. Cancer Res 48 : 4868
9. Chu E, Zinn S, Boarman D, Allegra CJ (1990) Interaction of γ-Interferon and 5-Fluorouracil in the H630 human colon carcinoma cell line. Cancer Res 50 : 5834
10. Wadler S, Wersto R, Weinberg V et al (1990) Interaction of Fluorouracil and interferon in human colon cancer cell lines : cytotoxic and cytokinetic effects. Cancer Res 50 : 5735
11. Wadler S, Schwartz EL (1990) Antineoplastic activity of the combination of interferon and cytotoxic agents against experimental and human malignancies : a review. Cancer Res 50 : 3473
12. Houghton JA, Williams LG, Cheshire PJ et al (1990) Influence of dose of [6RS]Leucovorin on reduced folate pools and 5-Fluorouracil-mediated thymidylate synthase inhibition in human colon adenocarcinoma xenografts. Cancer Res 50 : 3940
13. Keyomarsi K, Moran RG (1988) Mechanism of the cytotoxic synergism of fluoropyrimidines and folinic acid in mouse leukemic cells. J Biol Chem 263 : 14402
14. Brouty-Boye D, Tovey MG (1978) Inhibition by interferon of thymidine uptake in chemostat cultures of L1210 cells. Intervirology 9 : 243
15. Divizia M, Baglioni C (1984) Lack of correlation between thymidine kinase activity and the antiviral or antiproliferative response to interferon. Virology 133 : 216

Evidence for a role of immunosuppression in the pathogenesis of small cell lung cancer

JR Fischer, M Schindel, N Stein, H Lahm*, H Gallati**, P Drings, PH Krammer***

To understand the biology of malignant growth, the interactions between tumor cells and the immune system on a molecular level have to be understood. Therefore, we investigated the effects of soluble mediators secreted by Small cell lung cancer (SCLC) lines on modulation of cytokine-induced growth of lymphocytes. We found that IL-2 mediated T cell growth is inhibited by a cytokine secreted by the SCLC line NCI-N417. This cytokine is serologically identical to TGF β1. To approach the possible clinical relevance of these findings, we tried to establish a cytokine secretion profile in patients with the clinical diagnosis of Small cell lung cancer. For this purpose we tested whether lymphocytes and macrophages of patients with Small cell lung cancer show an impaired capacity to produce different cytokines after *in vitro* stimulation. We measured cytokine concentrations of IL-1α, IL-1β, IL-2, IFN-α, IFN-γ, TNF-α in the supernatant (SN) of lymphocytes from healthy donors and from patients with Small cell lung cancer by use of an enzyme-linked immunosorbent assay (ELISA).

Materials and methods

Cell lines and culture conditions. The small cell lung cancer cell line NCI-N417 was cultured in RPMI 1640 medium (GIBCO Laboratories, Grand Island, NY) supplemented with HEPES (10 mM final concentration), L-Glutamine (2 mM final concentration), Penicillin (100 U/ml), Streptomycin (100 μg/ml) and 10 % fetal calf serum. This line was routinely reidentified cytologically as SCLC.

Cytokine preparations. NCI-N417-SN was produced by incubating 5×10^5 cells/ml in serumfree medium at 37 °C and 5 % CO_2 in air for 72 h. The SN was harvested and stored a 4 °C until further use. Highly purified human TGF-β1, anti-TGF β1 antibody and TGF β-probe were purchased from Hermann Biermann (Bad Nauheim, Germany).

SN-Concentration. SN from NCI-N417 was concentrated 100 fold by Amicon filtration using an YM-10 membrane (Amicon Corporation, Scientific Division, Danvers, MA).

Interleukin-2 Assay. The IL-2 dependent T cell line W2 was used for the detection of factors inhibitory to IL-2 induced T cell growth. In addition to an IL-2 standard, different concentrations of NCI-N417-SN were added to the

---

Thorax Hospital, Dept of Medical Oncology, Amalienstraβe 5, 6900 Heidelberg, FRG, *Swiss Institute for Experimental Cancer Research, Dept of Cellular Biology, Ch. des Boveresses 155, 1066 Epalinges, Switzerland, **Hoffmann-La Roche, Basel and ***Institute for Immunology and Genetics, German Cancer Research Center, 6900 Heidelberg, FRG

cells. Proliferation was measured by ^{3}H-TdR incorporation after pulsing the cells with 0.5 µCi ^{3}H-TdR for the last 4 h of a 24 h culture period.

Blood samples. 10 ml of heparinized blood were taken from healthy adults and from patients with SCLC during the initial staging and diagnosis, prior to any treatment.

Whole blood cell culture. Whole blood was diluted 1 : 5 with RPMI 1640-medium containing 10 % FCS.

Stimulation of cytokine production. Cells were incubated in 96 well plates in a final volume of 200 µl at 37 °C and 5 % CO_2 in humified air and stimulated for 24 h in the presence of 10 µg/ml PHA (Welcome) for the secretion of TNF-α and IL-1β, for 48 h in the presence of 10 µg/ml PHA for the secretion of IL-2, for 24 h in the presence of NDV 1 : 100 for the secretion of IFN-α, for 72 h in the presence of 10 µg/ml PHA for the secretion of IL-1α and IFN-γ.

Determination of cytokine concentrations. Supernatants were tested for the presence of cytokines by using an enzyme-linked-immunosorbent-assay (ELISA). ELISA for determination of IL-1α, IL-1β, IL-2, IFN-α, IFN-γ, TNF-α was established by Gallati at Hoffmann, La Roche, Basel. Cytokine of the standard and the cell supernatants were bound to a murine monoclonal antibody that previously has been absorbed to the bottom of a microtiter plate. A second murine monoclonal antibody against the cytokine conjugated with peroxidase was added. After an incubation time of 16-24 h the immunologically bound peroxidase was determined by means of a redox indicator. The intensity of the color measured with a multichannel photometer is directly proportional to the cytokine concentration.

Statistical analysis. The difference of the results between the test groups and controls was tested for a possible significance by using the Wilcoxon Rank Sum Test.

Results

Conditioned medium of NCI-N417 but not of H69 was found to contain a cytokine that inhibited IL-2 mediated growth of the T cell line W2 in a dose dependent way. To further characterize this immunosuppressive activity, we tested a variety of mediators known to be secreted by solid tumor cell lines, including transforming growth factor α (TGF-α), TGF-$β_1$, adrenocorticotropic hormone (ACTH), bombesin, insulin like growth factor I (IGF-I). We found, that TGF-$β_1$ inhibited IL-2 mediated growth of the T cell line W2 in a dose dependent way. Thus, IL-2 mediated growth of the T cell line W2 was blocked by NCI-N417 derived factor and TGF-$β_1$ in a similar manner. Since TGF-$β_1$ was the only of the factors tested blocking growth of W2 in a way similar to the effect exerted by the factor secreted by NCI-N417, we tested whether NCI-N417 secreted TGF-$β_1$ or a TGF-$β_1$-like activity. For this purpose, we used an antibody directed against highly purified human TGF-$β_1$. The immunosuppression mediated by highly purified human TGF-$β_1$ was overcome by the addition of anti-TGF-$β_1$ antibody. More important, the antibody

Evidence for a role of immunosuppression

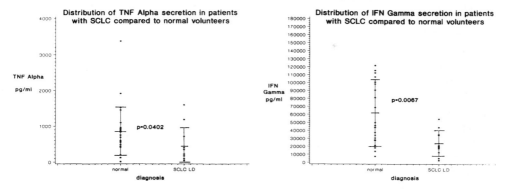

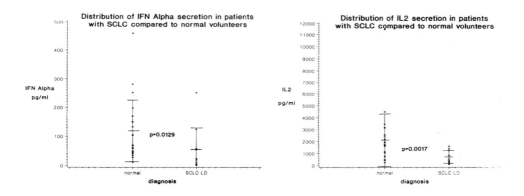

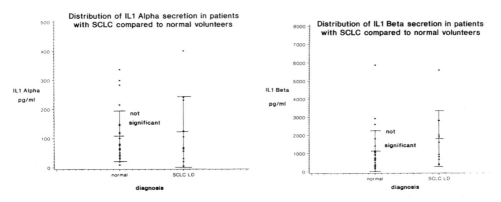

Fig. 1. Study of different cytokines concentration in the SN of lymphocytes from healthy donors and from patients with SCLC

directed against TGF-β_1 also neutralized the immunosuppressive activity mediated by NCI-N417 derived factor. Thus, the IL-2 mediated growth of W2, that was inhibited by the addition of NCI-N417 SN, was reconstituted after addition of anti-TGF-β_1 antibody. This suggests, that the NCI-N417 derived immunosuppressive cytokine is serologically related or identical to TGF-β_1. In addition, mRNA fot TGF β was expressed in NCI-N417 but not in H69.

To test the clinical relevance of these findings, we asked whether lymphocytes and macrophages of patients with SCLC show an impaired capacity to produce different cytokines after *in vitro* stimulation. Therefore, lymphocytes were taken from these patients during the initial diagnosis and mitogen-stimulated *in vitro*. After a defined incubation time, we tested cytokine concentrations of IL-1α, IL-1β, IL-2, IFN-α, IFN-γ, TNF-α in the SN of lymphocytes from healthy donors and from patients with SCLC by ELISA. We used this test system to evaluate the actual status of immunity in patients with SCLC. Compared to healthy individuals SCLC patients showed a significantly reduced capacity to produce IL-2, IFN-α, IFN-γ and TNF-α. In contrast, the capacity to secrete IL-1α and IL-1β was not reduced (Fig. 1). Furthermore, in some SCLC patients an overall suppression of cytokine secretion was observed (not shown).

Discussion

We investigated effects of soluble mediators secreted by SCLC lines on modulation of cytokine-induced growth of lymphocytes. We found that IL-2 mediated T cell growth is inhibited by a cytokine secreted by the SCLC line NCI-N417. This immunosuppressive cytokine secreted by NCI-N417 is serologically identical or related to TGF-β1. Immunosuppression may be crucial for *in vivo* growth of SCLC. To test the clinical relevance of these findings, we tested whether lymphocytes and macrophages from patients with SCLC show an impaired capacity to produce different cytokines after *in vitro* stimulation. We tested cytokine concentrations of IL-1α, IL-1β, IL-2, IFN-α, IFN-γ, TNF-α in the supernatant (SN) of lymphocytes from healthy donors and from patients with SCLC by ELISA. We used this test system to evaluate the actual status of immunity in patients with SCLC. Compared to healthy individuals SCLC patients showed a significantly reduced capacity to produce IL-2, IFN-α, IFN-γ and TNF-α. Furthermore, in some SCLC patients an overall suppression of cytokine secretion was observed. Further studies will elucidate, whether the clinical immunosuppression is in some way related to the immunosuppressive activity of TGF-β_1 secreted by SCLC tumor cells. In addition, it remains to be established, whether survival of these patients may be related to the cytokine secretion profile assessed during diagnosis.

In recent years, knowledge about growth control of solid tumors as well as lymphoid malignancies by soluble growth factors has considerably increased. Experimental evidence accumulates indicating that Autocrine growth stimulation or impaired Autocrine growth inhibition might represent one mechanism that enables malignant cells to escape from normal growth control [1-3]. On the other hand, a detailed insight into the control mechanisms that regulate activation, proliferation and differentiation of normal lymphocytes by cytokines has been obtained. In contrast, the mechanisms leading to downregulation of immune functions are largely unknown. Interestingly, TGF-β_1, that has been identified as an inhibitor of immune functions is not only released by lymphocytes but also by a variety of tumor cells [4-6]. Whether or not malignant outgrowth is influenced by inhibition of an intact immune system, is an open question. It has been speculated that the release of immunosuppressive factors might be another important step in malignant evolution [4, 5]. Thus, tumor cells may not only escape from growth control by secretion of Autocrine growth factors but may in addition escape from immune surveillance by secretion of factors inhibitory to the immune system.

SCLC is rapidly destroyed by cytotoxic drugs leading to complete clinical remission in a high-percentage of cases. Nevertheless, most patients relapse within a rather short period of time. Thus, it is clear, that despite this complete remission some residual tumor cells are likely to survive chemotherapy and remain intact in the body giving rise to repeated tumor outgrowth that in most cases is deleterious to the patient.

It is tempting to speculate that these residual tumor cells after chemotherapy might effectively be eliminated by the immune system if the immune system was not again inhibited by immunosuppressive factors released by these residual tumor cells. Future modalities for the treatment of SCLC might include antibodies against immunosuppressive factors as adjuvant therapy after chemotherapy and radiation. Alternatively, cytokines might be used as a therapeutic possibility to restore selective immunocompromised conditions. Furthermore, certain drugs might demonstrate an immunostimulating activity. At the present time, we are investigating a number of agents for such immunostimulating effects.

References

1. Sporn M, Roberts A (1985) Autocrine growth factors and cancer. Nature 313 : 745
2. Fischer JR, Lahm H, Debatin KM, Falk W, Krammer PH (1986) Malignant B cells secrete cytokines with Autocrine and IL-1 like activities. Immunobiology 173 : 151
3. Lahm H, Fischer JR, Reichert Y, Hederer R, Falk W, Debatin KM, Krammer PH (1989) Autocrine growth factors secreted by the malignant human B cell line BJAB are distinct from other known cytokines. Eur Cytokine Network 1 : 41
4. Bodmer S, Strommer K, Frei K, Siepl C, De Tribolet N, Heid I, Fontana H (1989) Immunosuppression and Transforming growth factor β in glioblastoma. J Immunol 143 : 3222
5. Coffey RJ, Shipley GD, Moses HL (1986) Production of Transforming growth factors by human colon cancer lines. Cancer Research 46 : 1164
6. Fisher JR, Stehr S, Lahm H, Falk W, Drings P, Krammer PH (1992) Different cytokines with autocrine and immunosuppressive activities are secreted by a small cell lung cancer cell line. In : Freund (ed) Cytokines in Hemopoiesis, Oncology and AIDS. Springer-Verlag, Berlin, Heidelberg, p. 107

p53 expression in human soft tissue sarcomas. Correlation with biological aggressiveness

G Toffoli*, T Perin*, C Doglioni*, S Frustaci*, A Buonadonna**, A de Paoli***, C Cernigoi*, L Tumiotto*, MG Dall'Arche*, M Boiocchi*

The p53 gene located at chromosome 17 p13 encodes a MW 53,000 nuclear phosphoprotein which is frequently mutated in many human cancers [1]. The mutant p53 protein has a much longer half-life than the wild-type protein; the result is a large amount of mutant proteins in transformed cells and tumours. The exact function of p53 protein expression abnormalities in tumour cells has not been completely clarified yet. Several studies have shown that reintroduction of a wild-type p53 gene into p53 deficient cells leads to suppression of the neoplastic phenotype [2]. This suppressor activity may be exerted through the transcriptional control of the proliferation-related genes [3] and/or regulation of DNA replication through wild-type p53 association with DNA replication complexes [4, 5]. It has been supposed that p53 mutations might have a predisposing effect in carcinogenesis and be a favourable event in progression of human tumours. Abnormalities of p53 have been related to the development of various cancers including bladder [6], lung [7], breast [8], colorectal [9] and brain [10] cancer. In this study we investigated p53 expression in human soft tissue sarcomas [HSTS]. The aim was to compare p53 expression with the tumour behaviour of HSTS.

Materials and methods

Sixty-one patients with HSTS (diagnosed and surgically treated from 1988 to 1991) were included in this study. Tumoral tissue samples were obtained from surgical specimens, cleared of necrotic and haemorrhagic tissue, quick-frozen in liquid nitrogen and stored at −80 °C until use. A fragment of each specimen was analysed histopathologically. Tumours were classified according to the WHO criteria and histologic grading was based on the criteria of Enzynger and Weiss.

p53 staining was performed on frozen sections fixed in acetone using the monoclonal antibody PAb 1801 (Oncogene, Science) as previously described [11]. Negative controls were included by running parallel HSTS sections with the primary antibody replaced by a non specific IgG. Positive controls consisted of sections from colonic adenocarcinoma previously shown to express high-levels of p53.

Flow cytometry DNA analysis was performed on frozen samples as

* Division of Experimental Oncology 1, ** Division of Medical Oncology, *** Division of Radiotherapy, Centro di Riferimento Oncologico, Aviano 33081, Italy

described [12] using a Becton-Dickinson FACS IV cytometer. Normal human periferal blood lymphocytes were used to determine the G 1/0 diploid peak. Data were collected for 10,000 cells per sample and analysed for coefficient of variation (CV) and integration of the modal DNA peak. A CV value of the diploid peak lower than 7.5 was accepted. Tumours with DNA index greater than 1.2 were considered aneuploid.

Statistics

p53 positivity was compared to the following variables : sex, hystogenetic type, size of the gross lesion, tumour location, stage, hystological grading, chemotherapeutic treatment, local and distal relapse and ploidy. For statistic analysis the chi-square or Fisher exact test was used.

Table 1. Relationship between p53 expression and various parameters in HSTS

	p53 pos.	neg.	
Sex male	8	14	
female	23	16	p NS
Tumour location			
trunk and extremities	23	20	
visceral	8	10	p NS
Tumour size <5 cm	11	13	
>5 cm < 10 cm	5	1	
≥ 10 cm	10	11	p NS
Stage I A-B	2	7	
II A	1	—	
II B	1	7	
III A	6	5	
III B	21	11	$p < 0.01$
Hystogenetic type			
malignant firous hystiocytoma	13	6	
liposarcoma	2	7	
fibrosarcoma	1	3	
synovial sarcoma	3	1	
leiomyosarcoma	6	5	
schwannoma	3	3	
miscellaneous sarcomas	3	5	p NS
Tumour type primary	16	14	
recurrenced	15	16	p NS
Chemotherapy yes	11	10	
no	19	21	
Histologic grade G1	2	8	
G2	2	6	
G3	28	15	$p < 0.01$
Ploidy aneuploid	24	11	
diploid	7	18	$p < 0.01$

Results

In all positive cases p53 overexpression was confined to the tumour cell population. Inflammatory cells and blood vessels present in the positive specimens were negative. No anti-p53 immunoreactivity was noted in any of the 4 benign tumours analysed (2 rabdomyomas and 2 fibromas). Nuclear staining of tumour cells was considered a positive p53 expression. In few cases nuclear staining was associated with a cytoplasmic staining and these tumours were considered positive.

Positive staining was seen in 31 of the 61 HSTS analysed (51 %). The proportion of the cells showing p53 overexpression varied among the tumours. Intra- and inter-tumour variation in nuclear staining intensity was also observed in about 25 % of the positive samples which were considered to show strong staining.

Among the various parameters analysed a significant association was observed between p53 overexpression and aggressive biological parameters — aneuploid, high hystological grades ($p < 0.01$) and more aggressive tumour stages ($p < 0.01$) (Table 1).

Discussion

A relatively high-level of p53 positive staining is seen to occur in the HSTS analysed (51 %). This is consistent with the findings of similar studies on other malignancies [13] and suggests that the role of p53 in HSTS may be similar to that exerted in other cancers. Moreover the data presented here, in accordance with previously published data, support the hypothesis that positive p53 immunostaining is restricted to malignant tumours cells and thus it may be of potential diagnostic significance.

The exact significance of p53 overexpression in human tumours is not well known up to now. It is thought to represent an early event which allows cells to acquire the transformed phenotype [11]. Alternatively, p53 overexpression could be a biochemical phenomenon related to tumour progression. In the HSTS we analysed p53 overexpression appears to be related to this latter phenomenon since p53 overexpression was associated ($p < 0.01$) with aggressive biological parameters (aneuploidy, high-histological grades and more aggressive stages).

The significance of HSTS lacking immunohistochemically detectable p53 is uncertain. They might represent tumours with normal levels of wild-type p53 or tumours that have deleted both alleles, resulting in no p53 protein expression. HSTS unexpressing p53 but exhibiting biological aggressiveness parameters might be included in this latter subset of tumours. More appropriated molecular biological techniques could be useful in addressing this issue. The different patterns of p53 overexpression noted in our study, too, may be a function of malignant progression, resulting in allelic loss in a subpopulation of tumour cells.

In conclusion our study suggests that overexpression of p53 is present mainly in the most biologically aggressive forms of HSTS and therefore it may represent a neoplastic progression index that can be used for prognostic purposes.

References

1. Levine AJ, Momand J, Finlay CA (1991) The p53 tumour suppressor gene. Nature 351 : 453-456
2. Finaly C, Hinds P, Levine A (1989) The p53 proto-oncogene can act as a suppressor of transformation. Cell 57 : 1083-1093
3. Raycroft L, Wu H, Lozano G (1990) Transcriptional activation by wild-type but not transforming mutants of the p53 anti-oncogene. Science 249 : 1049-1051
4. Braithwaite A, Sturzbecher HW, Addison C, Palmer C, Rudge K, Jenkins J (1987) Mouse p53 inhibits SV 40 origin-dependent DNA replication. Nature 329 : 458-460
5. Kern S, Kinzler K, Bruskin A, Jarosz D, Friedman P, Prives C, Vogelstein B (1991) Identification of p53 as a sequence-specific DNA-binding protein. Science 252 : 1708-1711
6. Fujimoto K, Yamada Y, Okajima E, Kakizoe T, Sasaki H, Sugimura T, Tereda M (1992) Frequent association of p53 gene mutation in invasive bladder cancer. Cancer Res 52 : 1393-1398
7. Takahashi T, Nau MM, Chiba I, Birrer MJ, Rosemberg RR, Vinocur M, Levitt M, Pas M, Gazdar AF, Minna JD (1989) p53 : a frequent target for genetic abnormalities in lung cancer. Science 246 : 491-494
8. Mazars R, Spinardi L, Ben Cheikh M, Simony-La Fontaine J, Jeanteur P, Theillet C (1992) p53 mutations occur in aggressive breast cancer. Cancer Res 52 : 3918-3923
9. Remvikos Y, Laurent-Puig P, Salmon RJ, Frelat G, Dutrillaux B, Thomas G (1990) Simultaneous monitoring of p53 protein and DNA content of colorectal adenocarcinoma by flow cytometry. Int J Cancer 45 : 450-456
10. Sidransky D, Mikkelsen T, Schwechheimer K, Rosenblum ML, Cavancee W, Vogelstein B (1992) Clonal expansion of p53 mutant cells is associated with brain tumour progression. Nature 355 : 846-847
11. Maestro R, Dolcetti R, Gasparotto D, Doglioni C, Pelucchi S, Barzan L, Grandi E, Boiocchi M (1992) High-frequency of p53 gene alterations associated with protein overexpression in human squamous cell carcinoma of the larynx. Oncogene 7 : 1159-1166
12. Toffoli G, Frustaci S, Tumiotto L, Talamini R, Gherlinzoni F, Picci P, Boiocchi M (1992) Expression of MDR1 and GST-π in human soft tissue sarcomas : relation to drug resistance and biological aggressiveness. Ann Oncol 3 : 63-69
13. Porter PL, Gown AM, Kramp SG, Coltrera M (1992) Widespread p53 overexpression in human malignant tumours. Am J Pathol 140 : 145-153

Synergistic cytotoxicity as an endpoint for the development of rational chemotherapeutic. Drug combinations

JL Abbruzzese, P Frost

Combination chemotherapy remains the principle approach to the treatment of disseminated human malignancies and evolved from the observation that single agents were ineffective against most metastatic cancers. Combination drug treatment was based on the premise that each agent, acting independently, would eradicate a unique population of cells sensitive to that agent, but possibly resistant to a second or third agent. The cumulative effect of all the drugs used would then translate into clinically detectable tumor regression. The agents used for the combination were selected on the basis of single-agent activity against the malignancy in question, often with the additional criterium that anticipated toxicities would not overlap [1].

This empiric approach has resulted in considerable success with specific malignancies typified by Hodgkin's disease and testicular cancer. However, the results have been marginal for the more common malignancies of adulthood, such as carcinomas of the lung and gastrointestinal tract. There is little evidence that combination chemotherapy prolongs survival for patients with these diseases, once the neoplasm has metastasized. These facts, in conjunction with the proliferation of available antineoplastic agents, now including genetically engineered molecules, necessitates a reassessment of the empiric approach to combination therapy.

One alternative is to develop combination regimens that rely on established interactions between agents. The goal of this « biochemical » approach to combination chemotherapy would be to develop drug combinations in which the individual agents interact to potentiate cytotoxicity in a supra-additive or synergistic manner.

With this background we will describe some of our efforts to develop synergistic chemotherapeutic combinations for solid tumors. In the context of this discussion we will specifically address four questions.

1. What is drug synergy and why use it as an endpoint for the development of drug combinations ?

2. Can synergy provide any information regarding the mechanism of drug interactions ?

3. Will combinations with synergistic cytotoxicity be complicated by excessive toxicity ?

4. Do the results of clinical trials validate the selection of combinations based on *in vitro* synergy ?

The University of Texas M.D. Anderson Cancer Center Department of Gastrointestinal Oncology, Houston, TX 77030 (JLA) and the Sandoz Research Institute, East Hanover, NJ 07936 (PF)

Synergistic cytotoxicity

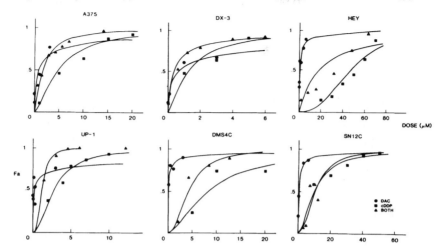

Fig. 1. Concentration-response curves for DAC and cDDP, alone or in combination. These computer generated curves are based on the colony forming ability of each cell line at the doses indicated. The concentration values when both drugs were used were derived by adding the individual drug concentrations used in the combination experiments and plotting these values vs Fa

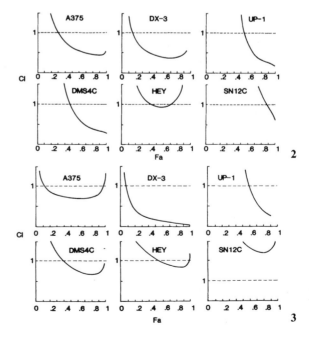

Fig. 2. Computer generated curves describing the interaction between DAC and Cisplatin, the combination index (CI). Drug interactions are as follows: All points above a CI of 1 are antagonistic; those below are synergistic, and those at 1 are additive. Fa = Fraction of cells affected

Fig. 3. Computer generated curves describing the interaction between DAC and 4-HC, the combination index (CI). Drug interactions are as follows: All points above a CI of 1 are antagonistic; those below are synergistic, and those at 1 are additive. Fa = Fraction of cells affected

Methodology

Quantitation of cytotoxicity was determined following single or combination drug exposure using a colony-forming assay previously described [2]. With this technique concentration-effect curves are generated for single and two-drug exposures which allows calculation of the 50 % effective dose or ED50.

The cell lines chosen for study represented a spectrum of human neoplasms generally resistant to combination chemotherapy. These included the A375 and DX-3 melanomas, DMS4C, a lung adenocarcinoma, UP-1, an unknown primary adenocarcinoma, HEY, a cisplatinum resistant ovarian carcinoma and SN12C, a sarcomatoid renal carcinoma.

Synergy was quantitated using the median effect principle to determine the concentration ratio of one agent to the other that would allow calculation of the interaction between both drugs. For the experiments to be described the ratio of one agent to the other was always: ED50. Additionally linear correlation coefficients (r) were calculated to determine the applicability of the data to this method of analysis. In all cases the r-values for all synergy experiments was ≥ 0.9. Synergism, summation, or antagonism of drug effects were assessed using the analysis developed by Chou and Talalay [3]. This analysis calculates the combination index (CI) which measures the degree of drug interaction and plots the data as CI vs the fraction of cells affected (Fa).

Results

In these studies we have used the investigational antimetabolite 2'-deoxy-5-azacytidine (DAC). DAC is metabolized to the triphosphate and incorporated into DNA. While the mechanism of its cytotoxicity is unknown, DAC has been shown to induce hypomethylation of genomic DNA through inhibition of the enzyme DNA methyl-transferase [4]. DAC has also been shown to induce alkali-labile sites in DNA [5]. Our interest in DAC evolved from preliminary experiments with the potent alkylating agent MNNG and DAC's interesting biochemical properties outlined above.

Based on these observations our initial studies focused on the interaction between DAC and the alkylating agents cyclophosphamide and Cisplatin. Fig. 1 shows the concentration-effect curves for DAC, Cisplatin and the combination. Similar data was generated for DAC, 4-hydroperoxycyclophosphamide (4-HC) and the combination (data not shown). The interaction of these two-drug combinations is summarized in Fig. 2 and 3. Evident from these curves is the variability in the effects of each combination across the various cell lines. Clearly, however a synergistic *in vitro* interaction between DAC and Cisplatin is evident for the A375, DX-3, UP-1 and DMS4C lines and between DAC and 4-HC for the DX-3, UP-1 and DMS4C lines [2].

This data can also analyzed quantitatively to indicate whether the drug concentrations required to achieve a synergistic interaction are achievable in patient plasma. Table 1 shows this data for the DAC/Cisplatin interaction. If

Table 1. Comparison of the effect of DAC or cDDP as single agents to the concentration of each drug when used in combination*

Cell line	Ratio DAC : cDDP	ED	Concentration of single agent DAC	Concentration of single agent cDDP	Drug concentration for combination DAC	Drug concentration for combination cDDP
A375	1 : 6	50	0.89	4.92	0.24	1.44
		70	3.80	8.64	0.47	2.83
		90	37.90	21.20	1.37	8.20
DX-3	1 : 1	50	0.71	1.29	0.18	0.18
		70	3.74	2.46	0.53	0.53
		90	52.60	6.83	2.92	2.92
UP-1	0.36 : 2.7	50	0.36	2.78	0.43	0.77
		70	1.86	4.30	0.59	1.04
		90	76.80	8.60	0.94	1.68
DMS4C	0.04 : 8.3	50	.04	8.3	0.17	4.13
		70	.24	14.3	0.26	6.14
		90	4.40	33.5	0.48	11.62
HEY	0.30 : 47	50	0.29	46.7	0.56	17.9
		70	1.23	64.2	1.27	40.9
		90	13.40	106.4	4.71	152.0
SN12C	0.30 : 10	50	0.31	10.2	0.32	10.4
		70	1.16	16.5	4.71	11.0
		90	9.80	35.7	8.73	20.4

* All drug doses are in uM. The concentrations of DAC and cDDP needed to achieve an ED50, 70, or 90 is shown for each drug used alone or when the drugs were used in combination

we focus on the data for A375, the concentrations of DAC or Cisplatin necessary to achieve a 90 % cell kill are 37.9 and 21.2 micromolar, respectively. However, in sequential combination the concentrations are reduced to 1.4 and 8.2 micromolar for DAC and Cisplatin respectively. Both values are achievable plasma concentrations.

Based on these data we then developed an approach to try to exploit these observations. First, we began to explore possible mechanisms for the synergy between DAC and Cisplatin with the goal of developing strategies to augment the DAC/Cisplatin interaction. Second we developed two phase I trials to evaluate the DAC/Cisplatin and DAC/Cyclophosphamide toxicity profiles. Specifically, since synergy does not guarantee specificity we were concerned that the synergistic cytotoxicity observed *in vitro* could be manifested in patients through excessive toxicity.

Our approach to explore the synergistic interaction between DAC and Cisplatin involved two sets of experiments. In the first experiments we used plasmid DNA to evaluate the effects of methylation on plasmid replication and Cisplatin binding. The amount of Cisplatin bound to plasmid DNA varied inversely with the methylation status of the plasmid as assessed by restriction enzyme analysis and direct measurement using flameless atomic absorption spectrophotometry [6]. The second series of experiments explored the degree of synergy observed using alternative antimetabolites with defined biochemical properties and DAC-sensitive and resistant cell lines [7]. To summarize, these experiments showed that :

1. Hypomethylation of DNA was not sufficient to produce synergy or enhance Cisplatin binding.
2. DAC must be incorporated into DNA for synergy to occur.
3. Incorporation of DAC into DNA resulted in increased Cisplatin binding.

Our current data therefore supports the view that incorporation of DAC into cellular DNA leads to stearic alterations in DNA structure which allows increased Cisplatin binding and may then lead to the increased cytotoxicity documented in many of the cell lines studied. Thus, strategies to increase the amount of DAC incorporated into DNA, such as use of inhibitors of ribonucleotide reductase, may further potentiate the DAC/Cisplatin interaction. Preliminary studies with hydroxyurea support this hypothesis [8].

The initial clinical studies exploring this combination have been completed through a phase I clinical trial of DAC and Cisplatin. The schedule of drug administration involved a rapid intravenous infusion of DAC on days 1-3 followed by Cisplatin over 1-hour on day four. We have documented the MTDs to be DAC 50 mg/m^2 and Cisplatin 75 mg/m^2 [9]. For Cisplatin the single agent MTD would be approximately 100-120 mg/m^2 suggesting that the combination did result in mild but manageable additive or synergistic host toxicity. Antitumor activity was documented in one patient with metastatic unknown primary adenocarcinoma. The phase I trial of DAC and cyclophosphamide is on-going.

Discussion

Using synergistic cytotoxicity as an endpoint to develop drug combinations has allowed the exploration of novel drug combinations, formed the basis for studies of mechanism and facilitated generation of new clinical trials for solid tumors. More recently we have extended this approach to explore interactions between DAC and the new topoisomerase-1 inhibitor topotecan, and between combinations of topoisomerase I and topoisomerase II inhibitors-topotecan and VP-16. This technique may also provide an endpoint for *in vitro* studies of drug scheduling and sequencing prior to clinical testing. The promise held by this approach is currently being validated in Phase I and Phase II clinical trials.

References

1. DeVita VT, Schein PS (1973) The use of drugs in combination for the treatment of cancer : rationale and results. N Engl J Med 288 : 998-1006
2. Frost P, Abbruzzese JL, Hunt B et al (1990) Synergistic cytotoxicity using 2'-deoxy-5-azacytidine and Cisplatin or 4-hydroperoxycyclophosphamide with human tumor cells. Cancer Res 50 : 4572-4577
3. Chou TC, Talaley P (1984) Quantitative analysis of dose effect relationships : the combined effects of multiple drugs on enzyme inhibitors. Adv Enzyme Regul 22 : 27-55
4. Jones PA, Taylor SM (1980) Cellular differentiation, Cytidine analogs and DNA methylation. Cell 20 : 85-93
5. D'Incalci M, Covey JM, Zaharko DS et al (1985) DNA alkali-labile sites induced by incorporation of 5-aza-2'-deoxycytidine into DNA of mouse leukemia L1210 cells. Cancer Res 45 : 3197-3202
6. Ellerhorst JA, Frost P, Abbruzzese JL et al (1993) 2'-deoxy-5-azacytidine increases binding of Cisplatin to DNA by a mechanism independent of DNA hypomethylation. Br J Cancer (in press)
7. Abbruzzese JL, Frost P (1992) Studies on the mechanism of the synergistic interaction between 2'-deoxy-5-azacytidine and Cisplatin. Cancer Chemother Pharmacol 30 : 31-36
8. Abbruzzese JL, Hunt B, Frost P (1990) Potentiation of the synergistic cytotoxicity between 2'-deoxy-5-azacytidine and Cisplatin with hydroxyurea. Proc Am Assn Cancer Res 31 : 408
9. Abbruzzese J, Raber M, Vrijhof W et al (1991) A phase I trial of a laboratory derived synergistic chemotherapeutic combination : 2'-deoxy-5-azacytidine and Cisplatin. Proc Am Assn Cancer Res 32 : 204

5-Fluorouracil may have different mechanisms of action depending on the dose schedule: clinical implications

C Aschele, A Sobrero, A Guglielmi, A Mori, L Tixi, E Bolli, R Rosso, JR Bertino

Chemotherapy of colorectal cancer has improved over the last several years thanks to both biochemical modulation of 5-Fluorouracil (FUra) [1] and attempts to optimize its schedule of administration [2]. However, resistance, either intrinsic or acquired, continues to be the major cause of treatment failure, and the use of multiple agents in combination or high-dose chemotherapy seems to offer no advantage over FUra alone. The outcome of FUra therapy may be improved if the biochemical basis for FUra resistance in tumors is identified and strategies are designed to overcome resistance to this agent.

Both experimental and clinical data suggest that pulse FUra and continuous infusion (CI) FUra might have different mechanisms of cytotoxicity. In the clinic, the maximum tolerated dose, the spectrum of toxicity and the dose-limiting toxicity of FUra depend upon the schedule of administration [3]. Moreover, the slopes of the dose-response curve to FUra, both in experimental systems and in the clinic [4], are different, depending on the schedule of drug administration.

Based on these observations, we investigated the possibility that different schedules of FUra produce resistance via different mechanisms. By using a clinically relevant dose schedule (repeated exposures to fixed doses of drug), human colon carcinoma (HCT-8) cells resistant to short pulses FUra, were obtained that maintained sensitivity to the Fluoropyrimidine given by CI. This observation was extended to the clinics where a phase II trial was conducted to test the efficacy of CI FUra on advanced colorectal cancer patients, progressing after failing bolus FUra. A second phase II study has been initiated in untreated patients with colorectal cancer using sequential treatment with pulse FUra followed by CI FUra.

Materials and methods

In vitro studies

Resistant cell lines were selected, starting from a clone of sensitive HCT-8 cells, with a low selection pressure technique as previously described for antifolates [5]. The resulting FUra-resistant sublines were designated 4 hR for the one ob-

---

Departments Medical Oncology National Cancer Institute, Genova, Italy and Memorial Sloan Kettering Cancer Center, New York, USA

tained with 4-h exposure to FUra, and 7dR, for the one obtained with 7-day exposure to FUra, and were maintained as described for the parental cell line.

In order to quantitate the degree of resistance to Fura and cross-resistance of the cell lines to other drugs, a monolayer clonogenic assay was used [5].

The time course of thymidylate synthase (TS) inhibition and recovery following FUra exposure in intact cells was studied with an *in situ* assay as previously described [6].

Incorporation of FUra into nucleic acids was measured on cells cultured for 12-24 h in 150 mm dishes (approximately 10^7 cells/dish). Old medium was replaced with complete medium containing a range of concentrations of [6-$_3$H]-FUra. At the end of the desired incubation time (4 or 24 h), cultures were washed 3 times with saline and either incubated for 24 h in drug-free medium or immediately harvested. Samples were then processed as described [6].

Clinical studies

The preliminary results of two phase II studies are summarized in this paper. The first regards the activity of CI FUra (300 mg/sqm daily) in patients with advanced colorectal cancer, in progression after failing FUra alone (500 mg/sqm daily bolus × 5 q 4 weeks), 3 patients, or FUra + high-dose LV (370 mg/sqm FUra preceeded by 100 mg/sqm LV given as daily boluses × 5 q 4 weeks), 12 patients.

The second is an ongoing phase II study on previously untreated advanced colorectal cancer patients. In this study patients receive alternating 2 biweekly cycles of FUra bolus (600 mg/sqm), preceeded by (24 h interval) MTX, 200 mg/sqm (in order to maximize the RNA effect of the drug) and FUra CI, 200 mg/sqm qd for 3 weeks, modulated by LV, 20 mg/sqm weekly bolus (in order to maximize the DNA effect).

Results

Development of resistance and cytotoxicity studies : the concentration of FUra used in the selection of resistance were 1,000 μM (4-h exposure) and 15 μM (7-d exposure), i.e. approximately 3 and 7 fold the ED_{50} values measured by inhibition of HCT-8 colony growth. These experimental conditions represent the highest drug concentration that allowed minimal clonogenic survival (5-20 clones), thus reflecting approximately 4 logs of cell kill. The time to reach confluence after the first drug treatment illustrates this high degree of cell kill : 33 and 35 days. At the end of the selection process (6 cycles) a low degree of resistance was obtained in the 4hR cells (3.3-fold increase in ED_{50} values). In contrast, a higher level of resistance was achieved in 7dR cells (15-fold increase in ED_{50} values). More importantly, 4hR cells displayed full sensitivity to FUra when challenged with a 7-d exposure of this drug.

In situ TS activity : when the *in situ* assay for thymidylate synthesis was used to follow the time course of TS inhibition after FUra exposure in intact cells, only slight differences in the degree of thymidylate synthesis inhibition between sensitive and resistant cells were shown at the end of a 4-h exposure to either 10 or 30 μM FUra. However, a marked recovery of thymidylate synthesis activity occurred in 7dR cells when FUra was removed and the cells were incubated in drug-free-medium for 24 and 48 hours. In particular, at 48 hours both HCT-8 and 4hR cells previously exposed to 100 μM FUra, still showed greater than 90 % inhibition of thymidylate synthesis activity, while under the same conditions thymidylate synthesis in 7dR cells recovered to 80 % of untreated controls.

Incorporation of FUra into RNA : in parental sensitive HCT-8 cells, FUra incorporation into RNA increased linearly with increasing concentration of the Fluoropyrimidine. The amount of drug incorporated into RNA after a 4-h exposure to 300 μM was approximately 6-fold greater than that obtained with 30 μM. The same relationship between the concentration of FUra and its incorporation into RNA was observed in the 2 resistant cell lines. However, in 4hR cells the amount of FUra incorporated into RNA after a 4-h exposure to this drug was significantly lower when compared to parental sensitive or 7dR cells, independently of the concentration of FUra used (30-300 μM). Incubation in drug free-medium after FUra removal resulted in increased drug accumulation into RNA in both sensitive and resistant cell lines. However, also in this condition, the total amount of FUra incorporated into RNA in 4hR cells was 3-fold lower as compared to both the parental sensitive and the continuous infusion resistant cell line.

Clinical activity of CI FUra in patients resistant to bolus FUra : continuous infusion FUra showed to be a feasible and well-tolerated treatment for patients progressing after failing FUra bolus. The median duration of treatment was 14 weeks (range 3-50) and the median delivered dose intensity during the first three months of treatment was 1 650 mg/sqm/week (79 % of planned). No myelotoxicity was observed. Mild diarrhoea, mucositis and vomiting occurred in 32, 26 and 19 % of patients, respectively, with no WHO grade III or IV episodes. Six out of 15 patients complained of hand-foot syndrome, that was severe in two instances, lasting approximately one week. One partial response of 7-month duration (indicator lesion in the liver and lung) was obtained in a patient previously treated with 3 monthly cycles of FUra plus LV. In addition, 6 disease stabilizations were observed, lasting 3, 4, 5, 8, and 9 months ; 3 of these were minor responses, defined as more than 25 % but less than 50 % decrease in tumor mass. Finally, 8 patients failed CI FUra.

Alternated bolus FUra and CI FUra in untreated advanced colon cancer patients : this schedule was based on the results of our *in vitro* studies, and using biochemical modulation was used to maximize RNA effects of FUra, i.e., MTX, and DNA effects of FUra, i.e. LV. So far, the dose of FUra has been reduced in 25 out of 109 courses of bolus treatment and in 21 out of 102 weeks of infusion, indicating that the degree of toxicity is comparable between the two schedules. Only three episodes of WHO grade III toxicity have been observed (2 mucositis and 1 vomiting). A higher incidence of mucositis and hand-foot syndrome was observed during CI treatment, while bolus treatment resulted in a higher occurrence of nausea/vomiting and conjunctivitis. No myelotoxicity was reported following treatment with MTX → bolus FUra. Among the first 12 patients completing at least one cycle of treatment

(2 months), we observed 4 PR, 5 MR 2 SD and 1 failure. No data on duration of response are available yet.

Discussion

This experimental and clinical project was based on the hypothesis that pulse FUra and CI FUra might have different mechanisms of cytotoxicity and resistance. The first piece of evidence, from our work, supporting this hypothesis, comes from cytotoxicity studies, showing that cells resistant to pulse FUra still retain full sensitivity to the Fluoropyrimidine given as a 7-d exposure. This finding provided the rationale for a phase II clinical trial of CI FUra in advanced colon cancer patients resistant to bolus FUra. Only one partial response was observed. However, three minor responses and three disease stabilizations were obtained and the median duration of response, in these progressing patients, was six months. These encouraging results support the clinical relevance of our *in vitro* model and confirm a recent anecdotal report [7] on the lack of clinical cross-resistance between the two schedules of FUra administration. A further improvement in this strategy might be obtained if appropriate agents were identified to specifically modulate CI FUra. In fact, evidence is building up that FUra alone, no matter whether given by bolus or CI, is only partially effective against colorectal cancer.

When the mechanisms of resistance were investigated in the two resistant sublines, a reduced RNA uptake was detected in pulse resistant cells, while prolonged exposures to low-dose FUra resulted in ineffective TS inhibition. This result has important clinical implications. The addition of LV may not enhance the clinical activity of pulse FUra, because this effect is mediated via TS inhibition. Channeling FUra into RNA, using other modulating agents like MTX, may improve results when high-dose short-term administration is used. On the other hand, enhancement of FUra cytotoxicity with LV may be greater when the Fluoropyrimidine is administered as a continuous infusion.

We are currently testing this hypothesis in the clinic studying a regimen of alternating bolus FUra, modulated by MTX and CI FUra modulated by LV. The preliminary results of this study support the hypothesis that the outcome of FUra therapy may be improved with a careful selection of modulating agents as a function of the schedule of FUra administration. In addition, our study support the proposal that bolus and CI FUra may be considered as two different drugs, with different biochemical targets as well as pharmacological properties. This hypotesis deserves further investigation and, if confirmed, may offer the possibility to double the therapeutic armamentarium against colorectal cancer.

References

1. Poon MA, O'Connell MJ, Moertel CG et al (1989) Biochemical Modulation of Fluorouracil : evidence of significant improvement of survival and quality of life in patients with advanced colorectal carcinoma. J Clin Oncol 7 : 1407-1417

2. Lokich JJ, Ahlgren JD, Gullo JJ et al (1989) A prospective randomized comparison of continuous infusion Fluorouracil with a conventional bolus schedule in metastatic colorectal carcinoma : a Mid Atlantic Oncology Program study. J Clin Oncol 7 : 425-432
3. Shaah A, Mac Donald W, Goldie J et al (1985) 5-FU infusion in advanced colorectal cancer : a comparison of three dose schedules. Cancer Treat Rep 69 : 739-742
4. Seifert P, Baker LH, Reed ML et al (1975) Comparison of continuously infused 5-Fluorouracil with bolus injection in treatment of patients with colorectal adenocarcinoma. Cancer 36 : 123-128
5. Sobrero A, Aschele C, Rosso R et al (1991) Rapid development of resistance to antifolates in vitro : possible clinical implications. J Nat Cancer Inst 83 : 24-28
6. Aschele C, Sobrero A, Faderan MA et al (1992) Novel mechanism(s) of resistance to 5-Fluorouracil in human colon cancer (HCT-8) sublines following exposure to two different clinically relevant dose-schedules. Cancer Res 52 : 1855-1864
7. Izzo J, Zarba J, Rougier PH et al (1992) Low dose of 5-FU continuous infusion (FUCI) in advanced colorectal cancer (ACC) : clinical evidence for reversal of acquired/intrinsic resistance to 5-FU or 5-FU Folinic (FUFO). Proceedings American Society Clinical Oncology, San Diego, California, 19-24 May

Clinical studies of CPT-11 in Japan

T Taguchi

CPT-11, Irinotecan hydrochloride, is a new antitumor agent developed in Japan [1]. CPT-11 is synthesized from Camptothecin, a plant alkaloid originally isolated from *Camptotheca acuminata* [2].

Based on the preclinical information, we conducted phase I studies of CPT-11 by single and weekly schedules [3, 4]. In the single administration schedule, the dose limiting factor (DLF) was leukopenia and the recommended dose for phase II study was 200 mg/m^2, and in weekly schedule leukopenia and diarrhea, and 100 mg/m^2, respectively. From 1989, we have been conducting disease oriented phase II studies.

Methods

Patients were selected according to the inclusion criteria of the each studies. CPT-11 was administered by intravenous drip infusion for 90 minutes at a dose of 100 mg/m^2 weekly (methods A), 150 mg/m^2 biweekly (method B) or 40 mg/m^2 for 3 consecutive days weekly (method C). The patients with non-small cell lung cancer (NSCLC) and small cell lung cancer (SCLC) were treated by method A, uterine cervical, ovarian and colorectal cancers by method A and B, and malignant lymphoma by method C.

Clinical responses were reviewed by extramural committees.

Results and discussions

Response in late phase II studies

Response in late phase II studies were summarized in Table 1. Among 67 evaluable patients with previously untreated NSCLC, 23 partial responses (PRs) were observed (response rate 34.3 %) with various histological types [5].

Out of 27 patients with SCLC received prior chemotherapy, 2 complete responses (CRs) and 7 PRs were observed (33.3 %), while 4 PRs were observed in 8 cases with no prior chemotherapy (50 %). The overall response rate for SCLC was 37.1 % [6].

Out of 55 patients with uterine cervical cancer, 5 CRs and 8 PRs were observed (response rate 23.6 %). CPT-11 was effective for the patients with prior radiotherapy or chemotherapy, and for distant metastatic lesions including the lung and the lymph nodes as well as the primary lesion [7].

Director, Cooperative Study Group of CPT-11. Research Institute for Microbial Diseases, Osaka University, 3-1, Yamadaoka, Suita-shi, Osaka, Japan

Table 1. Summary of response

	Prior Therapy	No of pts*	CR	PR	MR	NC	PD	Response Rate (%)
NSCLC	No	67		23	7	33	4	34.3
SCLC	No	8		4		2	2	50.0
	Yes	27	2	7		13	5	33.3
	Total	35	2	11		15	7	37.1
Cervical ca.								
Chemotherapy	No	19	2	4		8	5	31.6
	Tes	36	3	4	7	7	15	19.4
	(with pt)	(21)	(1)	(3)	(3)	(3)	(11)	(19.0)
Radiotherapy	No	14		2	3	5	4	14.3
	Yes	41	5	6	4	10	16	26.8
	Total	55	5	8	7	15	20	23.6
Ovarian ca.								
Chemotherapy	No	3		1		1	1	33.3
	Yes	52		12	4	17	19	23.1
	(with pt)	(52)		(12)	(4)	(17)	(19)	(23.1)
	Total	55		13	4	18	20	23.6
Colorectal ca.		53		17	2	17	17	32.1
NHL		47	8	15	5	11	7	48.9

* Evaluable for efficacy

Table 2. Main adverse reactions

	WBC ↓	Hb ↓	Plt ↓	Diarrhea	N/V
NSCLC	18/72 (25.3 %)	11/72 (15.2 %)	0/72 (0 %)	15/72 (20.8 %)	16/72 (22.2 %)
Gynecological ca.	72/126 (57.1 %)	33/126 (26.2 %)	10/126 (7.9 %)	24/125 (19.2 %)	20/126 (15.9 %)
Colorectal ca.	10/62 (16.1 %)	9/62 (14.5 %)	3/62 (4.8 %)	8/62 (12.9 %)	8/63 (12.7 %)

(≧ Grade 3)

Fifty-five ovarian cancer patients were evaluable for efficacy and 13 patients achieved PR (23.6 %). These responses were showed on patients with prior chemotherapy including platinum compounds. CPT-11 was effective for not only primary lesion but also distant metastatic lesions such as the lung and the liver [7].

Out of 53 patients with metastatic colorectal cancer, 17 PRs were observed (32.1 %). CPT-11 was effective on the lung and liver metastases as well [8].

According to interim result of late phase II study on malignant lymphoma, 8 CRs and 15 PRs were observed in non-Hodgkin's lymphoma (NHL) (response rate 48.9 %). It was noteworthy that all 8 CRs patients had suffered from relapsed and/or refractory lymphomas [9].

Adverse reactions

Major adverse reactions were leukopenia and gastrointestinal (GI) toxicities (Table 2). The incidence of grade 3 or higher toxicity was 16.1-57.1 % for leukopenia, 13-20.8 % for diarrhea and 12.7-22.2 % for nausea/vomiting. Thrombopenia was in low incidence (0-7.9 %).

Conclusion

CPT-11, a novel topoisomerase I inhibitor, showed response on various malignant tumors such as NSCLC, SCLC, uterine cervical, ovarian, colorectal cancers and NHL, being effective against tumors refractory to conventional chemotherapies and distant metastatic lesions.

Major adverse reactions were leukopenia and GI toxicities, however, those were reversible and clinically tolerable.

CPT-11 is suggested to be useful for treatment of patients with tumors. Further studies including combination therapies and control of adverse reactions were warranted in order to provide our patients with more useful therapies.

References

1. Kunimoto T, Nitta K et al (1987) Antitumor activity of 7-ethyl-10-(4-1-piperidino)-1-piperidino carbonyloxy camptothecin, a novel water soluble derivative of camptothecin, against murine tumors. Cancer Res 47 : 5944-5947
2. Wall ME, Wani MC et al (1966) Plant antitumor agents 1. The isolation and structure of camptothecin, a novel alkaloidal leukemia and tumor inhibitor from *Camptotheca acuminata*. J Am Chem Soc 88 : 3883-3890
3. Taguchi T, Wakui A et al (1990) Phase I study of CPT-11. Jp J Cancer Chem 17 : 115-120
4. Negoro S, Fukuoka M et al (1991) Phase I study of weekly administration of CPT-11. J Natl Cancer Inst 83 : 1164-1168
5. Fukuoka M, Niitani H et al (1992) A phase II study of CPT-11, a new derivative of camptothecin, for previously untreated non-small cell lung cancer. J Clin Oncology 10 : 16-20
6. Negoro S, Fukuoka M et al (1991) Phase II study of CPT-11, new camptothecin derivative, in small cell lung cancer (SCLC). Am Soc Clin Onc Houston, 19-21, May
7. Umesaki N, Takeuchi S et al (1993) Clinical Studies of DNA topoisomerase I inhibitor (CPT-11) on gynecological cancers. In : Andoh T et al (ed) Molecular biology of DNA topoisomerases and its application to chemotherapy. CRC press, p 337-344
8. Shimada Y, Wakui A et al(1991) A phase II study of CPT-11, a new camptothecin derivative, in patient with metastatic colorectal cancer. In : Andoh T et al (eds)

Molecular biology of DNA topoisomerases and its application to chemotherapy. CRC press, pp 345-349
9. Tsuda H, Ohta K et al (1992) A late phase II trial of a potent topoisomerase I inhibitor, CPT-11, in malignant lymphoma. Am Soc Clin Onc San Diego, 17-19, May

Evaluation of CPT-11 against human xenografts of colon adenocarcinoma and childhood sarcomas

PJ Houghton, JA Hougthon

We have used human tumors maintained in immune-deprived mice as a model for evaluating new agents that may have utility against frequently occurring cancers such as colorectal adenocarcinoma and rare tumors such as rhabdomyosarcoma of childhood. The predictive value of these models appears excellent, with intrinsic chemorefractoriness of colon cancers, and high-sensitivity of rhabdomyosarcomas being retained in mice [1]. In the current study, the topoisomerase I inhibitor, CPT-11, has been evaluated against colon tumors and rhabdomyosarcomas. We have examined the schedule dependency, and cross-resistance to Vincristine, Melphalan (LPAM), and the camptothecin analogue 9-diemethylaminomethyl-10-hydroxycamptothecin (topotecan) in tumors selected for resistance *in situ*.

Materials and methods

Human colon tumors and childhood rhabdomyosarcomas have been described previously [1-4]. Tumors were propagated in the subcutaneous space of immune-deprived CBA/CaJ mice, and treatment was started when tumors were 0.5 to 1 cm diameter. CPT-11 was administered i.v. daily for 5 days for two consecutive weeks ([dx5]2) defined as 1 cycle of therapy. For each dose level, 12-14 tumors were evaluated for each tumor line. Tumor responses were graded as: $-$, no growth inhibition; $+$, growth inhibition $\geq$ 1 tumor volume doubling time (TD_2); $++$, inhibition $\geq 2 \times TD_2$; $+++$, inhibition $\geq 3 \times TD_2$; $++++$ 50 % regression (PR); $+++++$ complete regression (CR) with regrowth; $++++++$, CR without subsequent regrowth.

Results

Colon adenocarcinomas: The maximal tolerated dose of CPT-11 was 40 mg/kg/administration on the [dx5]2 i.v. schedule (4 % mortality). Responses of 8 lines of colon adenocarcinoma are shown in Table 1. One cycle of CPT-11 caused PR or CR or HC_1, and SJC_3A and B xenografts, and inhibited growth significantly in 6/8 tumor lines. Dose response curves for moderately well differentiated HC_1, xenografts are shown in Figure 1.

Childhood rhabdomyosarcomas: One cycle of CPT-11 treatment caused CR without regrowth in 5/6 tumor lines. In addition CR were obtained at 20 and 10 mg/kg/dose in these lines.

Dept. Biochemical and Clinical Pharmacology, St. Jude Children's Research Hospital, Memphis, TN 38101, USA

Table 1. Responses of colon adenocarcinoma xenografts to CPT-11

Tumor	Response
HC_1	+ + + +
GC_3	+ + +
VRC_5	+ + +
ELC_2	+ +
SJC_2	+ + +
SJC_3A	+ + + + + +
SJC_3B	+ + + +
SJC_8	+ + + +

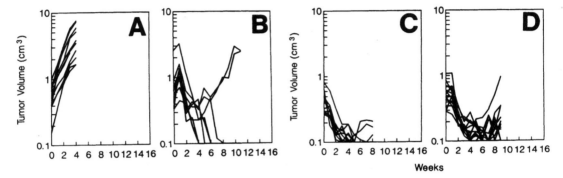

Fig. 1. Responses of HC_1 colon adenocarcinoma xenografts to CPT-11. Mice bearing advanced s.c. tumors were treated i.v. with CPT-11 [dx5]2 (1 cycle). *A :* controls (vehicle treated), *B :* CPT-11 40, *C :* 20, and *D :* 10 mg/kg/dose. Each curve represents growth of an individual tumor

Cross-resistance to CPT-11 : We next examined the cross-resistance profile of CPT-11 in a spectrum of tumors selected *in vivo* for resistance to Vincristine (rhabdomyosarcomas Rh12/VCR, Rh18/VCR), Melphalan (rhabdomyosarcoma Rh28/LPAM) and the topoisosemrase I inhibitor Topotecan (Rh18/TOPO and colon tumor VRC_5/TOPO). Results are presented in Table 2.

Efficacy of prolonged schedules of CPT-11 administration : We have shown previously that low dose prolonged schedules of Topotecan had high-efficacy against tumor with intermediate sensitivity to this topoisomerase I inhibitor [8]. To determine if this was similar for other agents acting at this locus, we have evaluated CPT-11 given at 10 or 5 mg/kg/dose i.v., for 3 cycles, each separated by 1 week. Results for two tumors of intermediate sensitivity, VRC_5 and rhabdomyosarcoma Rh12, are shown in Figure 2.

Discussion

The inhibitor of topoisomerase I, CPT-11, demonstrates significant activity against a panel of human tumor xenografts. Of note is that this agent is the

Table 2

Tumor	Response
Rh12	+ +
Rh12/VCR	+ + + +
Rh18	+ + + + +
Rh18/VCR	+ + + + + +
Rh18/TOPO	+ + + + + +
Rh28	+ + + + + +
Rh28/LPAM	+ + + + +
VRC_5	+ + +
VRC_5/TOPO	+ + +

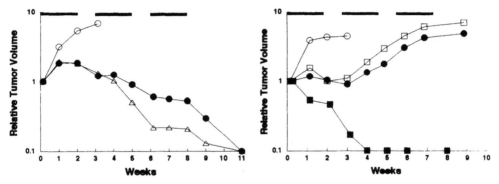

Fig. 2. Responses of VRC_5 colon adenocarcinoma and Rh12 rhabdomyosarcoma to single or repeated cycles of CPT-11. Mice bearing advanced tumors were treated [dx5]2 i.v. for a single cycle or repeated every 21 days for 3 cycles (designated as blocks). Each curve demonstrates the relative tumor volume of 12 or 14 tumors per group. *Left :* VRC_5 (○) control, 3 cycles at (●) 10 and (△) 5 mg/kg/dose. *Right :* Rh12, (○) control, 1 cycle at 40 (●) and 10 (□) mg/kg/dose ; (■) 3 cycles at 10 mg/kg/dose

most active against a series of colon adenocarcinoma models that have proven refractory to most other agents examined [1]. CPT-11 demonstrated « curative » activity against 5/6 xenografts of childhood rhabdomyosarcoma, even at relatively non-toxic dose levels. As with Topotecan, the efficacy of CPT-11 appears to be determined by the duration of therapy rather than the intensity of treatment. Thus, 3 cycles of low dose therapy were more effective than 1 cycle of intensive therapy, even though the total dose delivered was lower. Of particular note is that there was no cross resistance with tumors selected for Vincristine resistance, and only slight cross-resistance in Rh28/LPAM, a line selected for Melphalan resistance [6]. Rh28/LPAM is cross-resistant to Vincristine and completely resistant to Topotecan [8]. Significant also, is the observation that CPT-11 retained essentially complete activity against two tumor lines selected for primary resistance to Topotecan.

Supported by PHS awards CA23099 and CA21765 and by American, Lebanese, Syrian Associated Charities (ALSAC).

References

1. Houghton PJ, Horton JK, Houghton JA (1991) Drug sensitivity and resistance in the xenograft model. In : Rhabdomyosarcoma and related tumors in children and adolescents. CRC Press, pp 187-202
2. Houghton JA, Houghton PJ (1990) On the mechanism of cytotoxicity of fluorinated pyrimidines in four human colon adenocarcinoma xenografts maintained in immune-deprived mice. Cancer 45 : 1159-1167
3. Houghton JA, Taylor DM (1978) Growth characteristics of human colorectal tumours during serial passage in immune-deprived mice. Br J Cancer 37 : 213-219
4. Houghton JA, Houghton PJ, Webber BL (1982) Growth and characterization of childhood rhabdomyosarcomas as xenografts. J Natl Cancer Inst 68 : 437-443
5. Houghton PJ, Houghton JA, Myers L, Cheshire PJ, Howbert JJ, Grindey GB (1989) Evaluation of N-(5-indanylsulfony)-N'-4-chlorophenyl) urea against xenografts of pediatric rhabdomyosarcoma. Cancer Chemother Pharmacol 25 : 84-88
6. Houghton JA, Houghton PJ (1987) The suitability and use of human tumor xenografts. In : Rodent tumor models in experimental cancer therapy. Pergamen Press, New York, pp 199-204
7. Horton JK, Houghton PJ, Houghton JA (1987) Reciprocal cross-resistance in human rhabdomyosarcomas selected in vivo for primary resistance to Vincristine and L-phenylalanine mustard. Cancer Res 47 : 6288-6293
8. Houghton PJ, Cheshire PJ, Myers L, Stewart CF, Synold TW, Houghton JA (1992) Evaluation of 9-dymethylaminomethyl-10-hydroxycamptothecin against xenografts derived from adult and childhood solid tumors. Cancer Chemother Pharmacol 31 : 229-239

Microencapsulation, Tamoxifen analogues, and in vivo microscopy for tumor targeting

D Yang, S Wallace, L-R Kuang, C Li, A Cherif, Z Kan, P McCuskey, KC Wright

The potential of sustained release microcapsulated cytotoxic agents (1 μm or less) with surface characteristics for tumor targeting is explored in real time by *in vivo* microscopy of hepatic metastases in an animal model.

Microencapsulation is the use of a matrix or encapsulating material to enclose gases, liquids, or solids into particles. The size, charge, and composition of the capsular material are selected according to the intended use of the particles. Microcapsules have been prepared by coacervation, interfacial polymerization, polymer dispersion, matrix encapsulation and mechanical methods among others. The method used in this study, solvent evaporation, has yielded consistent particles of 0.5 μm to 500 μm as a sustained release drug delivery system for diagnostic imaging, chemoembolization and tumor targeting.

Contrast or therapeutic agents encapsulated into particles of 1 μm or less provide an ideal size for intravascular delivery for bioimaging studies or tumor management particularly if combined with capsular material selected to concentrate in the organ of interest. When delivered intravenously approximately 50 % of the 1 μm particles accumulate in the liver, primarily in the Kupffer cells, compared to 70 % when injected intra-arterially. The 100 μm particles injected intra-arterially for chemoembolization of neoplasms occlude the peripheral vessels, slow blood flow and increase contact time between an effective chemotherapeutic agent and a sensitive tumor. Theoretically, the ischemia of the neoplasm would be associated with a decrease in pO_2 and pH with a concomitant increase in pCO_2 and lactic acid resulting in dilatation of the capillary bed and enhanced transport across the endothelial lining into the interstitial space. Similar results might be possible by the intra-arterial infusion of a reducing agent like Vitamin C, Ascorbic acid.

There in an infinite number of capsular materials available, both degradable (polymers, cholesterol, monodiglycerides, alginates, etc.) and non-degradable (polymers, cellulose, wax, etc.). Degradable capsules would release the payload after erosion of dissociation while diffusion, through « pores », might be the mechanism operative with the non-degradable. The composition would depend on the intended purpose and the proposed speed of delivery. The size of the particle should influence transit and site of deposition. Most encapsulated particles greater than 1 μm are phagocytosed by the Kupffer cells while nanoparticles seem to elude their tentacles. The charge of the particle in also significant — positively charged materials are usually thrombogenic ; negatively charged, non-thrombogenic ; most blood components are negatively charged. The charge may also influence Kupffer cell and hepatocyte activity as well as the transit across the endothelial lining of the sinusoids or through the fenestrae. Previous studies from our laboratory have shown the biodistribution and

Kupffer cell uptake can be altered by changing the surface hydrophilicity. In addition, the interaction of the plasma proteins, enzymes, electrolytes and cellular elements may be an essential ingredient. The ultimate fate of the capsular materials is yet to be defined, i.e., as a foreign body, excreted or metabolized.

When phagocytosed by the Kupffer cells, what are the precautions and limitation to be considered ? It is possible to saturate these cells ? Will the release of a cytotoxic agent in the Kupffer cell jeopardize its status ? With death or saturation, what are the consequences ? Will the phagocytic or therapeutic function of the Kupffer cells be altered by saturation ? Will additional particles therefore circulate in the vascular pool with greater opportunities for targeting ? Kupffer cell function can be suppressed, e.g., Dextran. What are the potential advantages and disadvantages ? Will that offer greater possibilities to increase contact with the target cell ? Can we « fool » the Kupffer cell ? These aspects demand further exploration !

The ability to deliver the payload to a chosen site, « targeting », has great appeal. This may entail diverting the particle from its ultimate fate, i.e., phagocytosis by the Kupffer cells. An attractive alternative is altering the surface of the particle. Conjugation to the capsular coat has considerable potential. This can be accomplished by a chemical interaction physical adherence or mechanical alteration. Estrone has been conjugated to a polymer resulting in targeting to estrogen receptor sites because of its strong binding affinity.

Tamoxifen, an estrogen antagonist, has been widely used in the treatment of post-menopausal patients with breast cancer. Radioisotopic ligands of halogenated Tamoxifen have been developed for positron emission tomography (PET) and single photon emission computed tomography (SPECT) which may predict response to Tamoxifen therapy. In addition, surface modified microcapsules with these Tamoxifen ligands (1 μm) could be formulated for breast tumor targeting. ^{18}F and ^{131}I Tamoxifen analogs were synthesized and estrone was conjugated to polymer microcapsules. *In vitro* pharmacologic characterization of Tamoxifen analogs and conjugated microcapsules were followed in estrogen receptor assays for their relative binding affinity (IC_{50}). A human breast tumor cell line (MCF7) was studied for the antitumor potency of these ligands.

In rats primed with Estradiol (60 μg × 3 days), the biodistribution of ^{18}F Tamoxifen at 2 h revealed the uterus to blood ratio of 11 to 16 : 1 ; when blocked by pretreatment with estradiol (30 μg) the ratios then ranged from 5 to 8 : 1.

Biodistribution of estrone — polymer microcapsules loaded with ^{131}I ethyl iopanoate revealed the uterus to muscle ratios were higher than non-conjugated microcapsules. PET imaging of pigs after injection of ^{18}F Tamoxifen (10mCi) showed increased uptake in the uterus and fallopian tubes — ovarian complex, which could be blocked by Diethyl stilbesterol (DES), Tamoxifen or Estrone-polymer microcapsules. The results indicate that Estrone-polymer microcapsules or Tamoxifen analogs uptake in the uterus is via an estrogen receptor process and that these agents have some potential for use in the diagnosis and treatment of ER (+) breast cancer patients. Even more attractive would be the use of halogenated Tamoxifen conjugated to the microcapsular surface as a targeting agent for ER (+) tumor cells because of the killing power of halogenated Tamoxifen in addition to its significant binding affinity. Other surface targeting agents include monoclonal antibodies antibody fragments, peptide, e.g. CD4, etc.

The need for a better understanding of microanatomy and microcirculation in both health and disease has prompted improvements in microscopic methodologies. *In vivo* microscopy is a unique technique which permits real-time observation of dynamic physiologic and pathologic events occurring at the cellular level in the intact living animal. Selected organs or tissues are trans-or epi-illuminated with specific wave lengths of light and observed using water immersion objectives for optimum contrast and resolution. When used in combination with the administration of vital dyes or fluorescent tracers, *in vivo* microscopy can provide additional information about structural functional relationships.

In vivo microscopy allows the visualization of hepatic blood flow through the vascular network-hepatic artery, portal vein and hepatic vein the sinusoids and its cellular components. After surgical exposure, the liver of a living small animal (mouse or rat) is placed on the stage of a microscope to which is attached a video camera. The hepatocytes, bile canaliculi, portal and hepatic veins are readily appreciated. The Kupffer cells are identified with the assistance of ultraviolet light by the uptake of Fluorescein impregnated latex particles.

We are currently using *in vivo* microscopy in four separate research projects. These include : Study of hepatic tumor vascularization, development of small ($\leqslant 1$ μm) microcapsules for targeted delivery of diagnostic and therapeutic agents, evaluation of Tamoxifen analogs for use in the diagnosis and treatment of estrogen receptor positive tumors, and the investigation of the behavior of Lipiodol in the hepatic circulation when injected intra-arterially. A videotape containing segments from each of these studies will be shown and discussed.

The various radiopaque contrast agents have been delivered via the hepatic artery by direct cannulation or the portal vein through a mesenteric branch. Ionic contrast materials (Meglumine diatrizoate) resulted in subtle slowing of flow in the sinusoids. The non-ionic agents (Ioxilan) yielded no significant alterations. Lipiodol (Ethiodol), an oil based material, acts as an embolic agent after injection into the hepatic artery dramatically affecting the hepatic circulation, the Kupffer cells and the other cellular components. Lipiodol passes through the sinusoids to the hepatic veins and then to the systemic circulation. The Lipiodol also enters the portal vein especially through the peribiliary plexus which offers the potential for a combined embolic approach via the hepatic arterial and portal venous circulation. Hepatic arterial flow is restored as the Lipiodol is washed out of the normal elements. The use of particulate material (Gelfoam, Ivalon, etc.) with Lipiodol prolongs the deposition of Lipiodol during chemoembolization. Activated Kupffer cells assist in clearing the Lipiodol as well as participating in the host defense to tumor invasion and probably the release of toxic mediators.

Microencapsulated contrast materials (particle approximately 1 μm) containing Ionic (Diatrizoate), non-Ionic (Ioxilan), Iopanoic acid (Telepaque) and Lipiodol (Ethiodol) were well tolerated and accumulated in the Kupffer cells.

Because of its unique capabilities, utilization of *in vivo* microscopy is expected to expand significantly in the future.

A new generation of Doxorubicin-loaded liposomes with improved localization in tumors: preclinical and clinical studies

A Gabizon, B Uziely, B Kaufman, T Safra, R Catane, Y Barenholz

In most instances, liposomes have been used as carriers of cytotoxic drugs with a strategy based on reduction of toxicity and/or passive delivery to liver-infiltrating tumors. The fast and dominant uptake of most types of liposomes by the reticulo-endothelial system (RES) has prevented so far the adoption of a more direct strategy based on selective homing of liposomes to tumors. Recent developments [1] have shown that the inclusion of some negatively-charged glycolipids in the liposome bilayer coupled with phospholipids of high-phase-transition temperature, cholesterol, and careful size control result in: 1) inhibition of RES uptake, 2) prolonged circulation half-life, 3) minimal leakage of liposome contents during circulation, and 4) concomitant enhancement of tumor uptake. We refer to these liposomes with prolonged circulation time as Stealth liposomes to indicate that they are not recognized by the RES and to differentiate them from conventional liposomes.

Although the pharmacological importance of many of the above mentioned liposome attributes (high-phase-transition phospholipids, cholesterol, and small particle size) was identified more than ten years ago by several groups of investigators, it was not until recently that the contribution of molecules, such as monosialoganglioside and phosphatidylinositol, to liposome circulation half-life and liposome localization in tumors was recognized. A further refinement of the Stealth technology is the use of a polyethylene-glycol derivatized phosphatidylethanolamine which has been shown to confer optimal prolongation of vesicle circulation time in animal models [2]. Although these molecules confer to the vesicles a net negative charge, the uptake by the RES is actually decreased, in contrast to the acceleration of RES uptake commonly observed with the inclusion of other negatively-charged lipids, such as Phosphatidic acid, Phosphatidylserine, and Phosphatidylglycerol [3].

Preclinical studies with Doxorubicin Stealth liposomes

The development of these new formulations of long-circulating liposomes, with reduced uptake by the RES and enhanced accumulation in tumors, has broadened the potential applications of these carriers in cancer drug delivery. In pharmacological studies in rodents and dogs, DOX encapsulated in Stealth liposomes has been shown to circulate in liposome-associated form with very long half-lives in the range of 15 to 30 hours [4, 5]. We have investigated the tissue distribution, anti-tumor activity, and toxicity of Stealth liposomal Dox-

---

Sharett Institute of Oncology, Hadassah University Hospital, and Department of Membrane Biochemistry, Hebrew University School of Medicine, Jerusalem, Israel

orubicin (S-DOX) in tumor-bearing mice. The liposome formulations tested consisted of 70-90 nm mean diameter vesicles composed of hydrogenated phosphatidylcholine, cholesterol, and a polyethylene-glycol derivative of distearoyl-phosphatidyl-ethanolamine. DOX was present in the vesicle aqueous interior. When S-DOX was injected IV into BALB/c mice bearing an ascitic tumor (J6456 lymphoma), 10-20 % of the injected dose was recovered in the ascitic fluid in liposome-associated form, 24 to 48 hours after injection. No significant accumulation of S-DOX was observed in peritoneal washes from tumor-free mice. S-DOX was significantly more effective than free Doxorubicin in the ascitic J6456 tumor model at all dose levels tested. Larger vesicles of the same composition were less effective. The reduced toxicity of S-DOX enabled an additional twofold increase of the therapeutic index. These studies provide evidence that S-DOX extravasates with relative selectivity in tumor areas, resulting in an improved therapeutic activity [6]. S-DOX shows a superior therapeutic antitumor activity and decreased toxicity when compared to free DOX in a variety of mouse models [2, 7, 8]. Thus, long-circulating liposomes appear to offer a double advantage as an anticancer drug delivery system : toxicity buffering as with other previous liposome formulations, and selective tumor accumulation. We have proposed [6] that the latter phenomenon is the result of the long circulation pattern of Stealth liposomes on one hand, and the increased microvascular permeability of tumors [9] on the other.

Regarding methodology, two important aspects should be mentioned :

1) DOX is loaded into preformed liposomes by a proton gradient generated by liposome-encapsulated ammonium sulfate. This method enabled us to obtain a high-drug encapsulation efficiency in small vesicles of < 100 nm mean diameter. Also, the drug is entrapped in the liposome water phase thus avoiding phenomena such as drug exchange and partitioning which cause leakage problems when drug is entrapped in the lipid bilayer.

2) The use of a Dowex cation-exchange resin enabled us to separate liposome-associated DOX from protein-bound and free DOX circulating in plasma. Thus, we could separately analyze the pharmacokinetics of the fraction of drug circulating in association with liposomes. Pharmacokinetic analysis is of limited value without precise knowledge on the pool where the drug is located and its bioavailability.

Clinical studies with Doxorubicin Stealth liposomes
Preliminary results

The specific aims of this pilot clinical study were to describe the pharmacokinetics of S-DOX in humans at two dose levels (25 and 50 mg/m^2), compare the pharmacokinetics of S-DOX and free DOX in the same patients, and examine the drug levels in malignant effusions after S-DOX or free DOX in an attempt to estimate the putative drug levels in the tumor interstitial fluid. The S-DOX formulation used in this study, referred to as Doxil^{tm}[1] contains a polyethylene-glycol derivatized phospholipid. Treatments were given by IV bolus injection at three-week intervals. Doxil was cleared very slowly with a distri-

---

[1] Doxil is a registered trademark name of Liposome Technology Inc.

bution phase median half-life of 42-46 hours, as opposed to the rapid distribution of free DOX ($t_{1/2} \approx 5$ min). With Doxil, $\approx 100\%$ of the injected dose was recovered in the patient's plasma volume, 5 min after injection, and nearly all the drug measured in plasma was accounted for by liposome-associated drug through 7 days after injection. There was a linear increase in plasma drug concentration when the dose of Doxil was raised from 25 to 50 mg/m^2, with no major effect on the pharmacokinetic parameters. Significant drug concentrations (10^{-6} M) were detected in malignant effusions of patients receiving Doxil, as well as in cells from the effusions. After Doxil treatment, the drug levels in malignant effusions were four to ten-fold greater than after free DOX treatment. In a total of 15 patients receiving 53 courses, Doxil was generally well tolerated, stomatitis being the most significant side-effect in three heavily-pretreated patients. In 6 patients receiving Doxil only who were evaluable for hair toxicity, moderate hairloss was seen in one case only. Antitumor effects ranging from stabilization to partial response were observed in patients with ovarian cancer, mesothelioma, and breast cancer.

These results are consistent with preclinical observations and indicate that Doxil pharmacokinetics are controlled by the liposome carrier and differ substantially from free DOX pharmacokinetics. These drastic changes in the drug pharmacokinetic pattern raise the possibility of a change in the drug biodistribution and pharmacodynamics. Dose escalation studies of Doxil are currently ongoing.

References

1. Woodle MC, Lasic DD (1992) Sterically stabilized liposomes. Biochim Biophys Acta 1113 : 171-199
2. Papahadjopoulos D, Allen TM, Gabizon A, Mayhew E, Matthay K, Huang SK, Lee KD, Woodle MC, Lasic DD, Redemann C, Martin FJ (1991) Sterically stabilized liposomes : improvements in pharmacokinetics and antitumor therapeutic efficacy. Proc Natl Acad Sci USA 88 : 11460-11464
3. Gabizon A, Papahadjopoulos D (1988) Liposome formulations with prolonged circulation time in blood and enhanced uptake by tumors. Proc Natl Acad Sci USA 85 : 6949-6953
4. Gabizon A, Shiota R, Papahadjopoulos D (1989) Pharmacokinetics and tissue distribution of Doxorubicin encapsulated in stable liposomes with long circulation times. J Natl Cancer Inst 81 : 1484-1488
5. Gabizon A, Barenholz Y, Bialer M (1993) Prolongation of the circulation time of Doxorubicin encapsulated in liposomes containing a polyethyleneglycol-derivatized phospholipid : Pharmacokinetic studies in rodents and dogs. Pharm Res (in press)
6. Gabizon A (1992) Selective tumor localization and improved therapeutic index of anthracyclines encapsulated in long-circulating liposomes. Cancer Res 52 : 891-896
7. Vaage J, Mayhew E, Lasic D, Martin FJ (1992) Therapy of primary and metastatic mouse mammary carcinomas with Doxorubicin encapsulated in long-circulating liposomes. Int J Cancer 51 : 942-948
8. Mayhew EG, Lasic DD, Barvar S, Martin FJ (1992) Pharmacokinetics and antitumor activity of epirubicin encapsulated in long-circulating liposomes. Int J Cancer 51 : 302-309
9. Jain RK (1990) Vascular and interstitial barriers to delivery of therapeutic agents in tumors. Cancer Metastasis Rev 9 : 253-266

Degradable starch microspheres increase the cytostatic effect of the bioreductive drug RSU-1069 (aziridine 2-nitroimidazole) at arterial administration in rats with a liver carcinoma

U Stenram, G Roos

DSM are prepared for intraarterial use in a size of as a rule 45 μm with the intention to temporarily block the blood flow for about 30 min [3]. Thereby coinjected drugs remain in the target area for a longer time and hypoxia is produced. Systemic exposure decreases. The DSM are degraded by serum amylase.

At hepatic arterial administration in rats with a carcinoma implanted into the liver, DSM increased the effect of the cytostatic agents TCNU, BCNU [4] and Doxorubicin [1]. Side effects were seen, viz. liver necroses, and, with Doxorubicin, also body weight loss and gastric necroses or ulcerations [2]. It was therefore considered to be of interest to examine the effect of DSM at coinjection of the bioreductive drug RSU-1069 in this tumor model.

Material and methods

A dimethylhydrazine-induced adenocarcinoma of the colon (generation 162) was inoculated in the liver of 18 male Wistar Fu rats. After 10 days, RSU-1069 (aziridine 2-nitroimidazole, a gift from MRC, Chilton, UK) 50 mg kg^{-1} with or without DSM (Spherex®, a gift from Kabi Pharmacia Ther, Helsingborg, Sweden) 60 mg kg^{-1}, or saline was given over 60 s via a catheter. This was placed in the gastroduodenal artery with the tip at the origin of the proper hepatic artery. Retrograde flow was prevented during infusion with a loop around the common hepatic artery. Tumor size and body weight were recorded. There were no differences between the groups in body weight or tumor size at treatment. The rats were killed after one week. Tumor growth was determined as the volume at sacrifice over the volume at treatment (V_7/V_0). One of the rats given the combined treatment died after 3 days. This animal had a temporary apnoe at treatment and bled from the liver afterwards. This rat was not included in the table and the statistical analyses.

Statistical analysis was performed using the Mann-Whitney U-test and with all p-values two-tailed. Number of rats with liver necrosis was analysed with Fisher's exact test (two-tailed).

Details of methods and experimental design are published [1, 4].

Department of Pathology, Lund University, S-221 85 Lund, Sweden

Results

The tumor growth decreased significantly at treatment with RSU-1069 and furthermore at the combined treatment, RSU-1069 + DSM, also compared to RSU-1069 only (table). All rats had pulmonary metastases and all, with the possible exception of one control and one RSU-1069 treated, small abdominal metastases.

Large coagulation necroses in the liver (> 0.4 cm^2) and gastric necroses or ulcerations appeared only in rats given the combined treatment (table). Heavy weight loss, 89 and 86 g, occurred in the two rats with gastric necroses. The tumor volume decreased in these two rats. One of them had aspiration pneumonia.

There was a significant difference in body weight change between the saline and the combined treatment groups (table). Two rats given combined treatment increased in weight, one of them in spite of liver necroses with a cross section area of 1.33 cm^2.

Treatment	V_7/V_0	Body weight changes in g	Number of rats with large liver necroses	gastric ulcerations	n
Saline	6.8 ± 1.1[a]	+12 ± 4[c]	0	0	6
RSU-1069	3.6 ± 0.7[b]	+3 ± 3	0	0	6
RSU-1069 + DSM	1.3 ± 0.5	−42 ± 20	4[d]	2	5

[a] p = 0.0250 compared to RSU-1069 ; p = 0.0062 compared to RSU-1069 + DSM
[b] p = 0.0446 compared to RSU-1069 + DSM
[c] p = 0.0174 compared to RSU-1069 + DSM
[d] p = 0.015 compared to each of the other groups

A small liver abscess, cross section are of 0.26 cm^2, was encountered in one of the control livers, and a bigger one, 1.5 cm^2, in one of the rats given the combined treatment.

Discussion

RSU-1069 alone decreased tumor growth. Addition of DSM to RSU-1069 further decreased tumor growth significantly. The same principal results have been obtained with the nitrosourea drugs TCNU and BCNU [4] and with Doxorubicin [1]. DSM alone have no effect on tumor growth, nor on survival of the rats [4]. It appears safe to conclude that addition of DSM can increase the effect of several cytostatic drugs on tumor growth, perhaps especially those acting under hypoxia.

However, the side effects are important. In the present study, addition of DSM to RSU-1069 gave liver and gastric necroses. Combination with body weight loss was found at gastric necroses, arguing for a relationship between these two findings. A similar result was obtained when Doxorubicin was combined with DSM [2], but the changes were not so conclusive as with RSU-1069.

Rather extensive liver necroses of coagulation type has been encountered at combination of DSM also with Doxorubicin [1, 2] or TCNU or BCNU [4] but not with either of these drugs alone.

It must be considered that the antitumor effect of RSU-1069 + DSM might be partly related to the gastric ulcerations, probably giving decreased food intake, and body weight loss. The possible effect of the liver necroses on tumor growth is also unknown.

Side effects must be reduced. The drug or DSM dose can be decreased. A third way is to give all drug with a small part of the DSM, for example 10 %, and then give pure DSM. A fourth way is to infuse the drug-DSM combination slowly just to match the degradation of DSM to avoid backflow.

Finally we want to suggest the use of DSM with drugs via the portal vein in adjuvant treatment of liver metastases.

References

1. El Hag IA, Teder H, Roos G, Christensson PI and Stenram U (1990) Enhanced effect of adriamycin on a rat liver adenocarcinoma after hepatic artery injection with degradable starch microspheres. Select Cancer Ther 6 : 23-34
2. Jakobsson B, Teder H, Roos G, Stenram U (1991) Reduction by norepinephrine of the side effects induced by combined hepatic arterial administration of degradable starch microspheres and Adriamycin in rats with a liver adenocarcinoma. Select Cancer Ther 7 : 93-101
3. Lindberg B, Lote K, Teder H (1984) Biodegradable starch microspheres — A new medical tool. In : Davis SS, Illum L, McVie JG and Tomlinson E (eds) Microspheres and drug therapy. Pharmaceutical, immunological and medical aspects. Elsevier Science Publishers BV, pp. 153-188
4. Roos G, El Hag IA, Teder H, Stenram U (1991) Improved antitumor effect of the nitrosourea drugs Tauromustine (TCNU) and Carmustine (BCNU) on a rat liver adenocarcinoma after hepatic arterial administration with degradable starch microspheres. Anticancer Res 11 : 13-16

Abstract. Degradable starch microspheres (DSM) have a size of 45 μm and are dissolved by amylase. Given intravascularly they retard blood flow, expose infused tissue for a longer time to coinjected drugs and induce hypoxia. In rats with a cancer implanted into the liver, the bioreductive drug RSU-1069 decreased tumor growth as measured one week after a single treatment via the hepatic artery. Coinjection of DSM further decreased tumor growth, but side effects also apperared, body weight loss and, in some rats, liver and/or gastric necroses. DSM alone have no effect.

Therapeutic use of polyspecific mab-labelled liposomes as carriers for radioisotopes and drugs

G Rombi*, F Cossu*, G Melis**, V Anedda***, A Facchini**

The authors use from several years monoclonal antibodies labelled liposomes as selective artificial carriers for radioisotopes and drugs (radiosensitizer, 131-I, Fe_3O_4, etc.) (Fig. 1). This technique has been used during radiobiology studies on experimental *in vitro* patterns, which confirmed the internalization of the liposomes and their content into target cells. The use of liposomes for immunoscintigraphy, never reported in international literature, making possible to enhance the amount of entrapped radiotracer molecules or to achieve a local circulating carriers concentration and a plasmatic perfusion slowing down after exposure to a magnetic field (Fig. 2), shows the premises to improve the ratio signal/noise and consequently a good imaging of the lesions. The authors have successfully demonstrated the ability of mab-labelled and iron charged liposomes to reach the target area and present the preliminary results of the artificial carriers use in Cancer therapy.

Materials and methods

This study has been made on 14 patients ; 3 affected by different metastatic localizations of breast cancer (1 case of liver localisation, 1 of brain localisation and 1 of lung localisation), 6 affected by liver localisation of colorectal cancer, 3 affected by lung cancer, 1 affected by medulloblastoma and 1 affected by glioblastoma. All patients have an high plasmatic level of at least one tumor antigen which has been used to label the liposomes. Immunoscintigraphy has been carried out using unilayer 131-I charged liposomes (or Fe_3O_4 and Tc99 in the case of brain localisation submitted to a magnetic field) and labelled with specific monoclonal antibodies. In 3 cases, afterwards undergone to surgery, has been executed surgical and bioptic drawing for the necessary hystological confirmation with a determination of the markers by immunoperoxydase and measurement of the residual radioactivity.

Liposomes composition and preparation

Unilayer liposomes 0.05 μ in diameter have been obtained by dipalmitoyl-phosfaditil-choline (DPC), dipalmitoyl-phosfatidil-ethanolamine (DPE), GM1 or Sulphatides (in the case of brain localisation) and cholesterol.

1 — Incubation of DPE (10 μM) for 2 hours at 25° C in a solution of chloroform/methanol 9:1, containing SPDP (12 μM) and triethylamine (20 μM).

---

* Istituto Radiologia, Universita'di Cagliari, Italy,
** Medicina Nucleare, Ospedale "G Brotzu", Cagliari, Italy,
*** Laboratorio Centrale, Ospedale "G Brotzu", Cagliari, Italy

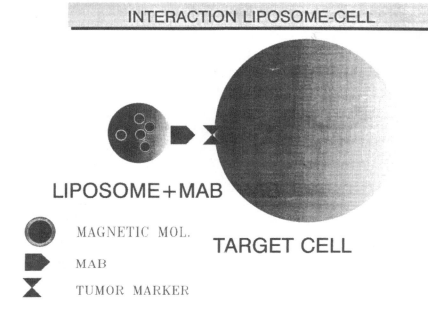

LIPOSOME-CELL INTERACTION
125-I UPTAKE IN FUNCTION OF FLOW SPEED

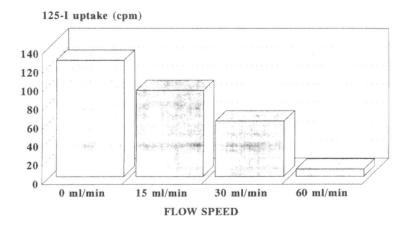

DYNAMIC SHORT-TIME MICROCARRIER CELL CULTURE

2 — Drawing of the organic phase into water, evaporation in chloroform with a final concentration of 5 μM/ml.

3 — Preparation of a solution containing DPC 10 μM, GM1 or Sulphatides 1 μM, cholesterol 5 μM and DPE modified with SPDP 0.6 μM.

4 — Incubation of the DTT treated (Fab')2 monoclonal antibodies and removal of the solvent.

5 — Addition of a solution containing the radioisotopes or drugs and preparation of unilayer liposomes after the detergent removal by a dyalitical membrane.

Anti Ca 15.3 , anti TAG 72 , anti CEA, anti Ca 19.9 and anti Tenascine (Primitive brain localisation) (Fab') 2 activated, at the concentration of 200 μg/ml, resulted to be linked at the rate of 6-10 molecules per liposomes with a labelling efficiency of 75 %.

Preparation of patients

The patients receiving 131-Iodine liposomes have been treated by KI (40 mg/die) three days before the administration of the tracer and until the end of the search, in order to avoid 131-I concentration in the thyroid. Besides, one hour before administering the labelled liposomes, they have been perfused with a suspension of cold liposomes in order to obtain saturation of the R.E.S.

The total liposome entrapped dose was of 50 mCi for one administration. The patients receiving drugs have been perfused with liposome containing different antiblastic compounds according to the different hystological type of tumors at the following concentrations : 5-FU 500 mg, BCNU 200 mg, Cis-Pt 50 mg, ADM 40 mg, MYTO-C 2 mg, MTX 25 mg, VCR 1 mg, EDX 250 mg and Fe_3O_4 when submitted to a magnetic field. All patients have been treated weekly for at least 8 courses.

Results

In the first 3 studied cases, patients afterwards undergone to surgery, it has been revealed in the bioptycal specimens the presence of the used tumor markers by immunoperoxydase and the measurement of the residual radioactivity. The results of this study confirmed the uptake of liposomes and their contents in the tumoral tissues. The scintigraphic images have been carried out on the first patients at 12-24-48-96 hours. The early images showed a diffused radioactivity determined by the persistence of the liposomes injected in the blood stream. In the scansions at 48 and 96 hours the diffused radioactivity decreases and it can be noted an higher localization in the areas with the metastatic localizations.

The scansions in earlier times often show an important uptake of liver and spleen determined at one side by the circulating radioactivity and on the other side by a non specific uptake of liposomes in the R.E.S. The previous injection of "cold" liposomes reduces the phenomenon. In many cases it may be useful to use electronic techniques of images subtraction connecting an hepatosplenic scintigraphy contemporaneously with the immunoscintigraphy and obtained by 99m-Tc. The hepatic or the R.E.S. radioactivity decreases rather quickly and in the later scansions (96 hours and more) generally the radioactive background of the liver does not interfere with the showing of hepatic images. The clinical results show 6 C.R., 3 P.R. and 2 progression after 3 months demonstrated by C.T. and N.M.R means as shown in (Figs. 3 and 4).

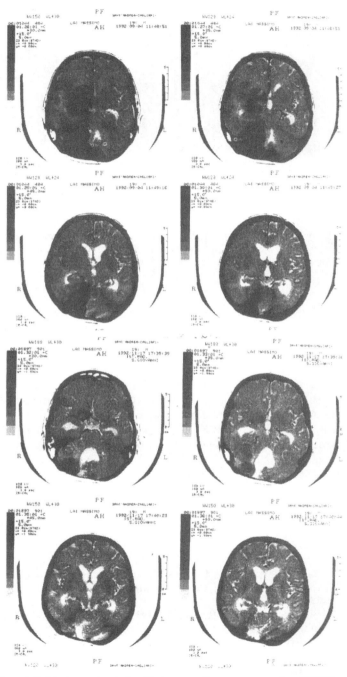

Fig. 3. C.T. control of medulloblastoma treated with immunoliposomes carrying BCNU, MTX and VCR before and after 8 courses. Imaging showing a dramatic reduction of the lesions

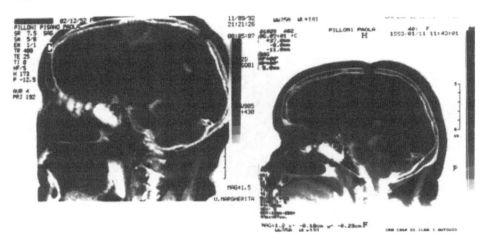

Fig. 4. M.N.R. of brain localisation of metastatic breast cancer. The patient has been treated with immunoliposomes containing ADM, EDX and 5-FU. Complete response after two months

Conclusions

This work is a preliminary about the possibility of using unilayer liposomes as carriers for radioisotopes or drugs in therapy. Some problems are still to be solved such as the removal of the free Iodine during the liposomes preparation in order to avoid an high concentration in the thyroid, the partial lekeage of some hydrophilic drugs or the non-selective targeting on R.E.S. and bone marrow (this phenomenon can be avoided using iron-charged liposomes). Finally, the authors think that this method is one of most promising technique for selective carrying of radioisotopes, drugs and other non-specific substances in cancer therapy.

References

1. Bast CR, Feeney M, Lazarus H, Nadler LM, Colvin RB, Knapp RC (1981) Reactivity of a monoclonal antibody with human ovarian carcinoma. J Clin Invest 68 : 1331-1337
2. Bistolfi F, Olzi E, Asdente M (1985) Targeting magnetotassico di farmaci e radiofarmaci in terapia oncologica. In : Bistolfi F (ed) Campi magnetici e cancro. Ed. Minerva Medica, Torino, pp. 57-86
3. Bloomer WD, Lipsztein R, Dalton JF (1985) Antibody-mediated radiotherapy. Cancer 55 : 2229-2233
4. Dabrowska W (1984) Liposomes and lymphoscintigraphy. Br J Radiol 57 : 545-546
5. Deland FH, Kim EE, Simmons G, Goldenberg DM (1980) Immaging approach in radioimmunodetection. Cancer Reasearch 40 : 3046-3049

6. Green AJ, Begent RHJ, Keep PA, Bagshawe KD (1984) Analysis of radioimmunodetection of tumours by the subtraction technique. J Nuclear Med 25 : 96-100
7. Gregoriadis G, Neerunjun ED (1975) Homing of liposomes to target cells. Biochem Biophys Res Commun 65 : 537-544
8. Groyer A, Robel P (1980) DNA measurement by mitramycin fluorescence in chromatin solubilized by heparin. Analytical Biochemistry 106 : 262-268
9. Imai K, Nakanishi T, Noguchi T, Yachi A, Ferrone S (1983) Selective in vitro toxicity of purothionin conjugated to monoclonal antibody 225.28S to a human high-molecular-weight melanoma-associated antigen. Cancer Immunol Immunother 15 : 206-209
10. Johansson A, Nielsen V (1980) Biosilon a new microcarrier. 3rd General Meeting of ESACT, Oxford 1979. Develop Biol Standard 46 : 125-129 (S. Karger, Basel)
11. Kabawat SE, Bast RC, Welch WR, Knapp RC, Colvin RB (1983) Immunopathologic characterization of a monoclonal antibody that recognize common surface antigens of human ovarian tumors of serous, endometrioid and clear cell types. Am J Clin Path 79 : 98-104
12. Kelleher PJ, Mathews HL, Woods LK, Far RS, Minden P (1983) A solid-phase radioimmunoassay to detect antibodies produced by hybridomas to antigens derived from human melanoma cells. Cancer Immunol Immunother 14 : 185-190
13. Kishida K, Masuho Y, Saito M, Hara T, Fuji H (1983) Ricin A-chain conjugated with monoclonal anti-L1210 antibody. In vitro and in vivo antitumor activity. Cancer Immunol Immunother 16 : 93-97
14. Leserman LD, Weinstein JN, Blumenthal R, Terry WD (1980) Receptors-mediated endocytosis of antibody-opsonized liposomes by tumor cells. Proc Natl Acad Sci USA 77 : 4089-4093
15. Leserman LD, Barbet J, Kourilsky F (1980) Targeting to fluorescent liposomes covalently coupled with monoclonal antibody or protein A. Nature 288 : 602-604
16. Leserman LD, Macky P, Barbet J (1981) Cell-specific drug transfer from liposomes bearing monoclonal antibodies. Nature 293 : 226-228
17. Machy P, Barbet J, Leserman LD (1982) Differential endocytosis of T and B lynphocyte surface molecules evaluated with anibody-bearing fluorescent liposomes containing methotrexate. Proc Natl Acad Sci USA 79 : 4148-4152
18. Morimoto Y, Sugibayashi K, Okumura M, Kato Y (1981) Biomedical applications of magnetic fluid. Preparation and magnetic guidance of magnetic albumine microspheres for site specific drug delivery in vivo. J Phar Dyn 4 : 624-631
19. Ott RJ, McCready VR, Slack N (1984) Visualisation of tumours using labelled antibodies (letter). Br J Radiol 56 : 353
20. Ott R, Gray LJ, Zivanovich MA, Flower MA, Trott NG, Moshakis V, Coombes RC, Neville AM, Ormerod MG, Weestwood JH (1983) The limitations of the dual radionuclide substraction technique for the external detection on tumours by radioiodine-labelled antibodies. Br J Radiol 56 : 101-108
21. Pelham JM, Gray JD, Flannery GR, Pimm MV, Baldwin RW (1983) Interferon-alfa conjugation to human osteogenic sarcoma monoclonal antibody 791T/36. Cancer Immunol Immunother 15 : 210-216
22. Perkins AC, Pimm MV, Armitage NC (1984) Imaging the tumour uptake of radiolabelled antibodies. Br J Radiol 57 : 652-653
23. Perkins AC, Hardy JG, Herdcastle JD (1983) The optimization of dual isotope imaging techniques in immunoscintigraphy. J Nuclear Med 24 : 15
24. Rombi GP, Cossu F, Carboni G (1987) Selectivity and effectiveness of Nitroimidazolic Radiosensitizers encapsulated in liposomes marked with monoclonal antibodies. 6th Annual Meeting ESTRO (European Society for Therapeutic Radiology and Oncology), Lisbona 25-28 maggio (p. 297, abstr.)

25. Rombi G, Cossu F, Onorato D, Tuveri V (1987) Liposomi marcati con anticorpi monoclonali e/o incorporanti molecole ferromagnetiche : possibilità di un loro uso come veicoli artificiali di radioisotopi e farmaci. Suppl Tumori, 73 (suppl. 4) : 197
26. Senyei A, Widder K, Czerlinski G (1978) Magnetic guidance of drug-carrying microspheres. J Appl Phys 49 : 3578-3583
27. Uadia P, Blair AH, Ghose T (1983) Uptake of methotrexate linked to an anti-EL4-lymphoma antibody by EL4 cells. Cancer Immunol Immunother 16 : 127-129
28. Van Dalen A, Favier J, Eastham WN (1984) Preliminary observations with New Monoclonal Antibody in Ovarian Carcinoma. Tumor Diag Ther 5 : 67-69
29. Webb KS, Ware JL, Parks SF, Briner WH, Paulson DF (1983) Monoclonal antibodies to different epitopes on a prostate tumor-associated antigen. Implications for immunotherapy. Cancer Immunol Immunother 14 : 155-166
30. Widder KJ, Senyei A, Sears B (1982) Experimental methods in cancer therapeutics. J Phar Sci 71 : 379-387

An in vitro model for neutrophil-mediated damage to tumour vasculature : effects of a novel anti-cancer agent

JC Murray, KA Smith, M Bastaki, KB Wilson

Vascular occlusion due to endothelial damage may occur in a number of pathological situations. It has only recently been recognised that such damage may also occur in tumours in response to a variety of anti-cancer agents including several chemotherapeutic drugs [1]. In these instances, it appears that vascular damage contributes to the overall effectiveness of the anti-cancer therapy, bringing about oxygen and nutrient deprivation which in turn leads to further tumour cell death.

Flavone acetic acid (FAA) is a novel anti-cancer agent which is highly effective against murine solid tumours [2]. Although its mechanism of action is poorly understood, damage to tumour vasculature is presumed by several groups to play an important role [3, 4]. We previously demonstrated that FAA induces changes in vessel permeability and neutrophil (PMN) margination *in vivo* [5], and endothelial monolayer permeability *in vitro* [6]. PMN, with appropriate activation, may become cytotoxic toward endothelial cells [7], as well as tumour cells [8]. We reasoned that PMN might therefore play an active role in bringing about vascular damage within tumours in response to FAA, and have established an *in vitro* model to test this hypothesis.

Materials and methods

Microvascular endothelial cells : Murine endothelial cells were isolated from epididymal fat essentially by the method of Madri and Williams [9]. Briefly, freshly excised fat is digested with collagenase at 37° C for 30 min. The resulting suspension is centrifuged through a Percoll gradient to isolate microvessels, which are then washed and cultured on collagen-coated multi-well plates in complete growth medium. After several days endothelial cells have migrated out of the microvessel fragments to form small colonies. These colonies are isolated by trypsinisation and grown to confluence. The cells were characterised as endothelial based upon « cobblestone » morphology, uptake of acetylated low density lipoprotein labelled with an indocarbocyanine dye, and positive staining with Banderaea simplicifolia lectin and antibodies to von Willebrand factor.

Polymorphonuclear granulocyte neutrophils : PMN were isolated from freshly collected, anti-coagulated mouse blood by centrifugation through a Histopaque gradient (Sigma). Populations of greater than 90 % purity were routinely obtained.

Endothelial Biology Group, CRC Gray Laboratory, PO Box 100, Mt Vernon Hospital, Northwood Mddx HA6 2JR, UK

Tumour-conditioned medium : TCM was obtained from confluent cultures of P479 murine astrocytoma cells (a kind gift of Dr J Darling, Institute of Neurology, London), by incubating monolayers in complete growth medium, then harvesting the medium after 48 h, and filtering to remove floating cells and debris.

PMN adhesion assay : Adhesion of PMN to the endothelial cell monolayers under different conditions was assessed using a novel adhesion assay which relies upon the presence of high levels of myeloperoxidase in PMN [10]. After incubating PMN with endothelial cells for appropriate periods under various conditions, plates were washed twice with warm phosphate-buffered saline (PBS) to remove non-adherent cells. Cells were lysed with 50 μl 0.5 % hexadecyltrimethyl ammonium bromide for 30 min prior to the addition of 250 μl dianisidine hydrochloride (0.2 mg ml^{-1} containing 0.4 mM H_2O_2). The optical density of each well was read 15 min later at 450 nm with a Titertek Multiscan. Percent PMN binding was calculated by dividing myeloperoxidase activity in washed wells by total available activity in control wells before washing.

Cytotoxicity assay : PMN-dependent cytotoxicity was assessed using a simple ^{51}Chromium release assay. Briefly, confluent endothelial cell monolayers grown in 96-well dishes were incubated overnight in complete medium supplemented with sodium ^{51}chromate (0.1 MBq per well). Excess radioactive label was removed by washing twice with warm medium. In some instances radioactive label was added with TCM for the overnight incubation, in which case appropriate controls were included. Freshly isolated PMN were added directly to wells at different effector : target ratios, and in some cases with differing doses of flavone acetic acid (FAA ; LIPHA Pharmaceuticals, Lyon). After 4 h or 24 h samples of supernatants containing released ^{51}Cr, indicating cytotoxicity, were carefully removed and counted in a gamma-counter. Specific cytotoxicity was calculated taking into consideration spontaneous release of label, and relating counts released to total incorporation.

Results

The results of adhesion assays carried out at 30 min and 3 h after the addition of PMN to the endothelial monolayers are shown in (Fig. 1). FAA was added simultaneously with the PMN. In every case adhesion was greater at 30 min than at 3 h. TCM reduced adhesion slightly at 30 min, but seemed to have no effect at 3 h. FAA produced a small (but not statistically significant) increase in adhesion at 30 min in the control cultures.

The results of cytotoxicity assays at 24 h are summarised in (Fig. 2) PMN alone produced a slight increase in ^{51}Chromium release at 24 h, which appeared to be reversed in the presence of TCM. Low levels (0.2 and 0.4 mg ml^{-1}) of FAA inhibited this effect, release remaining below control levels. At 0.8 mg ml^{-1} FAA in the presence of PMN there was a significant increase in cytotoxicity, up to 20 %. In the presence of TCM and PMN, cytotoxicity reached its highest levels, at approximately 40 %. This was clearly PMN-dependent, and nearly twice that seen with control medium.

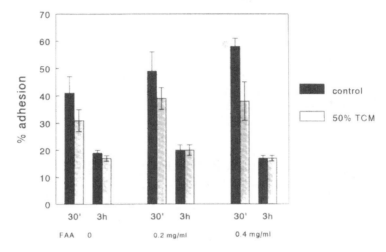

Fig. 1. The effects of flavone acetic acid and tumour-conditioned medium on the adhesion of murine PMN to endothelial cells. Adhesion was measured by assaying myeloperoxidase activity of bound PMN. Data represent the means of at least 6 replicates

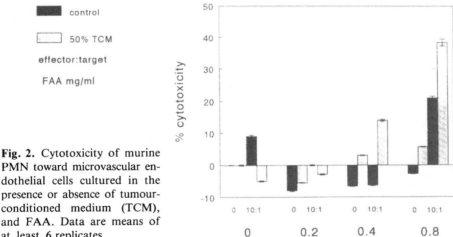

Fig. 2. Cytotoxicity of murine PMN toward microvascular endothelial cells cultured in the presence or absence of tumour-conditioned medium (TCM), and FAA. Data are means of at least 6 replicates

Discussion

While the mechanism of action of flavone acetic acid is far from clear, it is generally thought to be indirect; FAA is barely cytotoxic to cultured tumour cells or any other type of cell studied, but induces rapid and dramatic regression of solid murine tumours. It appears to behave as a biological response modifier, mimicking many effects of the cytokine TNFα [11]. Although the data are somewhat confusing and contradictory, much consideration has also been given to the possibility that FAA induces cytotoxic activity in normal host effector cells, in particular macrophages [12].

While studying the effects of FAA on vascular permeability of murine tumours and normal tissues, we observed enhanced margination of PMN in blood vessels of the liver of tumour-bearing mice treated with FAA, but not in their normal counterparts [5]. This was in accord with changes in vascular permeability observed in the livers of these same mice. We therefore hypothesised that the PMN is a potential mediator of vascular damage associated with FAA treatment of tumour-bearing animals.

The results described in this paper suggest that PMNs are capable of cytotoxicity toward endothelial cells under very specific conditions. It is already known that certain cytokines, such as TNFα, can induce PMN-dependent endothelial cytotoxicity *in vitro* [7]. Little is known about the role of PMNs in tumours, although one recent paper suggests that interactions between PMN and tumour-associated endothelial cells are likely to be less frequent than in normal tissues, possibly due to the down-regulation of endothelial adhesion molecules within tumours [13]. Our adhesion data are consistent with this, in that TCM appears to reduce adhesion ; however, the cytotoxicity data suggest that pretreatment of endothelial cells with TCM renders them sensitive to PMN. Furthermore, this effect is potentiated by FAA. This leads us to speculate that endothelial cells within tumours are "primed" to respond to cytotoxic PMN, and that drugs such as FAA can exploit this sensitivity, producing selective damage to tumour vasculature.

Acknowledgements. This work was entirely supported by the Cancer Research Campaign (UK).

References

1. Murray JC (1992) Vascular damage and tumour response. Eur J Cancer 28 : 1593-1594
2. Plowman J, Narayanan VL, Dykes D, Szarvasi E, Briet P, Yoder OC, Paull KD (1986) Flavone acetic acid : a novel agent with preclinical anti-tumour activity against colon adenocarcinoma 38 in mice. Cancer Treat Rep 70 : 631-635
3. Zwi LJ, Baguley BC, Gavin JB, and Wilson WR (1989) Blood flow failure as a major determinant in the antitumor action of flavone acetic acid. J Natl Cancer Inst 81 : 1005-1013
4. Hill SA, Williams KB, and Denekamp J (1989) Vascular collapse after flavone acetic acid : a possible mechanism of its anti-tumour action. Eur J Cancer Clin Oncol 25 : 1419-1424
5. Smith KA, Thurston G, and Murray JC (1991) Systemic effects of FAA are enhanced by implanted tumours. Int J Radiat Biol 60 : 389-393
6. Watts ME, Murray JC, Smith KA, Woodcock M (1992) Flavone acetic acid as a modifier of endothelial cell function. Int J Radiat Oncol Biol Phys 22 : 431-435
7. Ward PA (1991) Mechanisms of endothelial cell injury. J Lab Clin Med 118 : 421-426
8. Clark RA and Klebanoff SJ (1975) Neutrophil-mediated tumor cell cytotoxicity : role of the peroxidase system. J Exp Med 141 : 1442-1447

9. Madri JA, and Williams SK (1983) Capillary cell culture : phenotypic modulation by matrix components. J Cell Biol 106 : 153-165
10. Bath PMW, Booth RFG, Hassall DG (1989) Monocyte-lymphocyte discrimination in a new microtitre-based adhesion assay. J Immunol Meth 118 : 59-65
11. Smith GP, Calveley SB, Smith MJ, Baguley BC (1987) Flavone acetic acid (NSC 347512) induces haemorrhagic necrosis of mouse colon 26 and 38 tumours. Eur J Cancer Clin Oncol 23 : 1209-1211
12. Ching LM, Baguley BS (1988) Enhancement of *in vitro* cytotoxicity of mouse peritoneal exudate by flavone acetic acid (NSC 347512). Eur J Cancer Clin Oncol 24 : 1521-1525
13. Wu NZ, Klitzman B, Dodge R, Dewhirst MW (1992) Diminished leukocyte-endothelium interaction in tumor microvessels. Cancer Res 52 : 4265-4268

Abstract. Polymorphonuclear granulocyte neutrophils (PMN) can kill endothelial cells as well as tumour cells under appropriate conditions. We have developed an in vitro model for examining the potential role of PMN as damaging agents in tumour vasculature. The model comprises murine microvascular endothelial cells grown in multi-well plates in the presence of tumour-conditioned medium (TCM) to simulate a tumour environment. Murine PMN are added to the plates after pre-labelling the endothelial cells with ^{51}Chromium. Release of radioactive label is taken as evidence of PMN-mediated cytotoxicity. We found that TCM alone did not stimulate cytotoxicity, while the anti-cancer agent flavone acetic acid (FAA) did stimulate some PMN-dependent release of ^{51}Cr. In the presence of TCM, FAA induced greater PMN-dependent cytotoxicity. There was no relationship between PMN adhesion to endothelial cells, and cytotoxicity.

Stimulation of tumor growth in vitro and in vivo by Suramin in an experimental model

M Julieron, L Ramirez, M Bonnay, G Vassal, A Gavoille, D Piron, D Gandia, L Mir, JN Munck

Suramin has been used for decades in the treatment of trypanosomiasis, and only recently it has been tested for its antitumor activity [1]. The precise mechanism(s) of action is still unknown, and Suramin probably exerts its inhibitory effects by impairing growth factors mediated cell proliferation [2]. Moreover suramin may interfere with intracellular signal transduction by inactivating protein kinase C and certain G proteins [3], and also probably modifies growth factor binding by accumulating glycosaminglycans [4]. An inhibition of tumor angiogenesis has been reported [5, 6].

The cytostatic effect of Suramin has been tested against a lot of different cell lines, including squamous cell carcinomas, with a variable sensitivity. The best antiproliferative effects were obtained with Suramin concentration over 150 µg/ml [1, 7, 8]. Some clinical trials have shown a therapeutic activity of Suramin against adrenocortical [9], prostatic [10] and renal carcinomas [11], and lymphomas [12]. The responses were seen with a therapeutic threshold of 150 µg/ml and side effects are limiting at concentrations superior to 300 µg/ml. No trial have been reported on squamous cell carcinomas.

The present study was conducted to evaluate the action of Suramin on an experimental squamous cell carcinoma : the VX2 tumor implanted in the liver of new Zealand rabbits. We studied and compared the effects of Suramin on *in vivo* and *in vitro* tumor growth and on tumoral neoangiogenesis.

Materials and methods

The VX2 tumor model. Experiments were performed on New Zealand female rabbits. The VX2 tumor is a papillomavirus induced fast growing squamous cell carcinoma of the rabbit. The tumor was maintained by serial passages in the liver.

Drugs and chemicals. Suramin was purchased from Bayer Laboratories and AntiAlpha smooth muscle Acyine antibody (cat A 9172) from Sigma laboratories.

In vivo evaluation of Suramin. Fresh tumoral cell suspensions were prepared from anecrotic and aseptically prepared tumor specimens. Tumor tissues were minced in NCTC 109 medium, and filtered through a layer of cotton gauze. After centrifugation (5 mn at 1500 rpm) simple cell suspensions were adjusted at a concentration of 10^6 cells/ml. One ml per rabbit was injected through the portal vein after laparotomy under anaesthesia. Twenty-four rabbits were used in a block-design experiment. Groups were individualised (group 1-2-3-4) as blocks, and within each group all rabbits were grafted the same

---

Institut Gustave-Roussy, 94800 Villejuif, France

day with the same cell suspension in order to avoid grafting variations between experiments. In each experiment, rabbits were randomly assigned to a control and a suramin group. The treatment started 3 days before the tumor graft.

Suramin doses and schedule of administration were based on previous pharmacokinetic. Suramin blood levels were measured by reverse-phase high-performance liquid chromatography with ion pairing [13]. A computerised analysis with simulation (Apis : MIIPS France) allowed the determination of a scheme of treatment maintaining Suramin plasma level between 150 and 300 µg/ml.

Intravenous injections of Suramin (40 mg/kg) were accordingly administered every 3 days during 3 weeks.

Twenty-one days after, rabbits were sacrificed and the livers and lungs were removed from each animal and analysed histologically. The liver tumor involvement was evaluated by computerised image analysis (percentage of liver involvement/total liver area). Lungs were analysed systematically and the number of microscopic lung metastasis was recorded.

Angiogenesis evaluation in tumors. Tumor vessels within tumors were investigated by immunostaining with anti-α smooth muscle actine antibody, and the number of vessels was scored by two independent observers (mean number count in 10 fields).

In vitro study. Tumor cell suspensions were prepared as for the in study. VX2 cells were grown in MEM containing 10 % FBS and incubated in a humidified incubator at 37° C in 5 % CO_2 in air. Cells were cultured in 96 well-plates with 25 000 cells per well. Suramin was added for continuous exposure at concentrations of 10, 50, 100, 200, 300 µg/ml and none for control groups. After 3 days of proliferation, cells were washed, and a crystal violet incorporation test was performed. The difference of absorbency of control and incubated groups was recorded. Each experiment was done four times.

Statistical analysis. Comparisons were made by analysis of variance. For *in vivo* study variance was studied in each group of experience (1-2-3-4).

Results

In vivo, Suramin was found to lead to an unexpected stimulation of tumor growth. In the treated group the liver involvement was significantly ($p < 0,05$) greater than in control rabbits (Fig. 1).

In lungs, a trend for increased metastatic dissemination was found in Suramin treated rabbits but the difference was not statistically significant (Fig. 2).

As Suramin has been reported to exert antiangiogenic effects, the tumoral neovascularisation was also analysed in this study. In this experimental model no difference in vascular score in tumor was found between the Suramin and the control group (Table 1).

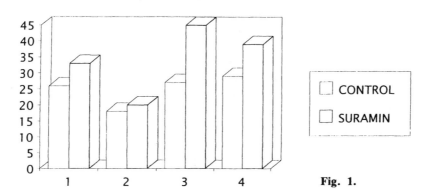

Fig. 1.

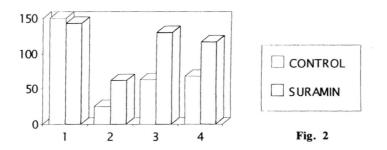

Fig. 2

Table 1.

	Control	Suramin	P
Count of vessels	12.64 +4.43	15.19 +5.2	0.22

The *in vitro* study correlated with the *in vivo* results. Suramin concentration from 50 µg/ml to 300 µg/ml led to a significant growth stimulation of the VX2 cells ($p < 0,02$) (Table 2).

Table 2.

Suramin concentration	0	10	50	100	200	300
D.O.	0.128 ±0.064	0.105 ±0.049	0.122 ±0.069	0.129 ±0.054	0.134 ±0.044	0.172 ±0.055

Discussion

Suramin is an original compound that has been found to exert anti cancer effects on various cell lines *in vitro*[1, 8]. Few studies have reported suramin effects on squamous cell carcinoma : low IC 50 have been found on 2 head and neck cancer lines 7 and among 21 fresh tumor specimen of non small lung cancer 80 % were found to be sensitive at concentration of 200 µg/ml [8].

The drug is also active in patients and is currently be tested in phase II trials in various type of cancer, but no clinical data of suramin efficiency on squamous cell cancers have been reported.

We tested Suramin on a squamous cell cancer as preclinical investigation preliminary to clinical studies on patients with squamous cell cancer. Our results show that Suramin may have paradoxical effects on tumor growth *in vivo* and *in vitro*. The original and probably very different mechanism of action of Suramin as compared to the common anticancer agents that act through non specific cytotoxic effects may explain such results. It can be postulated that, if Suramin acts by interference with growth factors and growth factors receptors, imbalance in autocrine loops of tumor cells could lead to growth stimulation as well as to antiproliferative effects, depending on the cellular type. Others *in vitro* studies have indeed demonstrated that under certain conditions Suramin can act as a growth promoting agent. These effects have been described at low doses [7, 12]. However at supposedly antiproliferative concentrations, on two squamous cell carcinoma cell lines, opposite effects have been reported depending on the expression of TGFα and R-EGF by the cells [14]. *In vivo*, an immunosuppressive effect mediated by antiproliferative action on lymphoid cells [15] could be an additional factor for tumor growth facilitation.

These results suggest a cautious use of Suramin in clinical phase II studies.

References

1. La Rocca RV, Stein AC, Myers CE (1990) Suramin : Prototype of a new generation of antitumor compounds. Cancer Cells 2 : 106-115
2. Coffey RJ, Leof EB, Shipley GD, Moses HL (1987) Suramin inhibition of growth factor receptor binding and mitogenicity in AKR2B cells. J Cell Physiol 132 : 143-148
3. Hensey CE, Boskoboinik D, Azzi A (1989) Suramin, an anti-cancer drug inhibits protein kinase C and induces differentiation in neuroblastoma cell clone NB2A. FEBS Lett 258 : 156-158
4. Constantopoulos G, Rees S, Cragg BG, Barranger JA, Brady R (1980) Experimental model for mucopolysaccharidosis : Suramin-induced glycosaminoglycan and sphingolipid accumulation in the rat. Proc Natl Acad Sci USA 77 : 3700-3704
5. Wilks JW, Scott PS, Vrba LK, Cocuzza JM (1991) Inhibition of angiogenesis with combination treatments of angiostatic steroids and Suramin. Int J Radiat Biol 60 : 73-77
6. Pesenti E, Sola F, Mongelli N, Grandi M, Spreafico F (1992) Suramin prevents neovascularisation and tumour growth through blocking of basic fibroblast growth factor activity. Br J Cancer 66 : 367-372

7. Olivier S, Formento P, Fischel JL, Etienne MC, Milano G (1990) Epidermal Growth factor receptor expression and Suramin cytotoxicity *in vitro*. Eur J Cancer 26 : 867-871
8. Taylor CW, Lui R, Fanta P, Salmon SE (1992) Effects of Suramin on *in vitro* growth of fresh human tumors. J Natl Cancer Inst 84 : 489-494
9. Stein CA., La Rocca RV, Thomas R, McAtee N, Myers E (1989) Suramin : An anticancer drug with a unique mechanism of action. J Clin Oncol 7 : 499-508
10. Myers CE, Cooper M, Stein C, La Rocca R, McClellan M, Walther M, Weiss G, Choyke P, Dawson N, Steinberg S, Uhrich M, Cassidy J, Kolher DR, Trepel J, Linehan WM (1992) Suramin : a novel growth factor antagonist with activity in hormone-refractory metastatic prostate cancer. J Clin Oncol 10 : 881-889
11. La Rocca RV, Stein CA, Danesi R, Cooper MR, Uhrich M (1991) A Pilot study of Suramin in the Treatment of Metastatic Renal Cell Carcinoma. Cancer 67 : 1509-1513
12. La Rocca RV, Cooper MR, Stein CA, Kolher D, Uhrich M, Myers CE (1992) A pilot study of Suramin in the treatment of progressive refractory follicular lymphomas. Ann Oncol 3 : 571-573
13. Klecker R, Collins J (1985) Quantification of Suramin by reverse — phase ion-pairing high-performance liquid chromatography. J Liqu Chromatogr 8 : 1685-1696
14. Cardinali M, Sartor O, Robbins KC (1992) Suramin, an experimental chemotherapeutic drug, activates the receptor for epidermal growth factor and promotes growth of certain malignant cells. J Clin Invest 89 : 1242-1247
15. Spigelman Z, Dowers A, Kennedy S, Disorbo D, O'brien M, Barr R (1987) Antiproliverative effects of Suramin on lymphoid cells. Cancer Res 47 : 4694-4698

Phase I-II trial of Seraspenide (AcSDKP) : a supressor of myelopoiesis protects against chemotherapy myelotoxicity (version 10 february 1993)

P Carde, E Gonçalves, F Isnard, E Deschamps de Paillette,
C Chastang, N Mathieu-Tubiana, E Vuillemin, V Delwail,
O Corbion, A Vekhoff, J-M Ferrero, E Garcia-Giralt, J-F Gimonet,
AM Stoppa, E Leger-Picherit, J-P Monpezat, E Fadel, C Domenge,
F Guilhot, F Thomas, D Khayat, A Monnier, R Zittoun, B Brun,
D Maraninchi, J-N Munck, F Beaujan, M Guigon, E Frindel,
A Najman, M Tubiana

The Colony Forming Units in the Spleen (CFU-S), pluripotent stem cells in mice, are normally quiescent and it has been demonstrated that they are therefore relatively protected from the toxicity of drugs until they are triggered into cycle through a feed-back mechanism [1]. The existence of low molecular weight endogenous negative regulators was demonstrated using dialysable fetal calf bone marrow extracts that are able to inhibit the entry into cell cycle of the CFU-S pluripotent stem-cells challenged by Cytarabine & varied stimulations [2]. Fetal calf bone marrow and liver extracts were proved, through multistep purification, to contain the tetrapeptide acetyl-SDKP. A myeloprotection from myelotoxic drugs was anticipated to occur, using acetyl-SDKP as preventing a proportion of the stem cell pool to be prompted into cycle and therefore to be destroyed by the next application of the cytotoxic drug [3, 4]. Acetyl-SDKP (INN = Seraspenide) has been identified as a small peptide (4 amino-acids = Acetyl-Ser-Asp-Lys-Pro = Acetyl SDKP) and synthesized [5]. It plays a physiological hemoregulatory role in mice as suggested for instance by the observation that the CFU-S are induced into cycle when mice are given anti-acSDKP monoclonal antibodies [6, 7, 8]. It has been isolated from human placenta and it is found in man, where it is particularly aboundant in lymphopoietic and hemopoietic organs [9]. It has been possible to quantify the concentration of acetyl-SDKP in the blood of normal volunteers and of patients with varied malignancies : myeloproliferative disorders appear to demonstrate high circulating levels of acetyl-SDKP. Acetyl-SDKP is synthetized in long-term marrow cultures (Charbord, personal communication) and it inhibits in a reversible way the proliferation of human progenitors [10, 11]. The potential for inhibiting hemopoietic stem cells in human beings appear to be more pronounced for the more primitive stem cells (CD 34/DR low progenitors rather than CD 34/DR high or later progenitors). The mechanism of action of AcetylSDKP may call for intermediary cells [12, 13] but there is also evidence for a direct action on stem cells.

Institut Gustave Roussy, 39 rue Camille Desmoulins, 94805, Villejuif, France

Patients and methods

A phase I-II study was undertaken in 1991 in cancer patients (Table I), mostly heavily pretreated, undergoing 2 consecutive cycles of monochemotherapy (cytarabine or ifosfamide).

Table 1. Cancer type distribution in Seraspenide phase I-II study (n = 53)

Hematological tumors n = 14	Solid tumors n = 39	
6 non Hodgkin lymphoma	10 metastatic breast ca.	3 metastatic hepatic ca.
3 acute lymphoid leukaemia	5 sarcoma	2 rhino-pharyngeal ca.
2 acute myeloid leukaemia	4 HEENT	2 endometrial ca.
3 misceallenous	3 ovarian ca.	1 colon ca.
	3 esofagus ca.	6 misceallenous

The Phase I-II study has been designed so as to combine Seraspenide to chemotherapy at the 1st or the 2d cycle with a double-blind cross-over :
1st cycle : chemotherapy + Seraspenide or placebo
2d cycle : chemotherapy + reverse order

Assessment of the protective activity of Seraspenide against myelotoxicity : on the comparison of 6 parameters concerning the blood leukocytes and neutrophils : the integration of their area under the curve (AUC) from day 8 to day 22, the depth of their nadir and the durations of hypoplasia < 1000 leukocytes /mm^3 and < 500 neutrophils /mm^3. The demonstration of a statistical difference providing evidence for a protective effect of Seraspenide has been performed using the Wilcoxon matched-paired rank test.

Thirty-one patients had unevaluable data for myelotoxicity assessment : 27 of them had only 1 cycle of monochemotherapy in combination with placebo (18 patients) or Seraspenide (9 patients), mostly due to tumor progression prior to the initiation of cycle 2. Four patients had major protocol violations.

Treatment groups were :
— Cytarabine 0.75 to 2 g/m^2 i.v. 1 hour infusion q. 12 hours x 4 (= 2 days) + Seraspenide 0.5 to 62.5 mg/kg i.v. 12 hours perfusion for 48 hours (4 dose levels : 0.5 to 62.5 mg/kg/administration of chemotherapy). Seraspenide infusion was initiated 2 hours prior cytarabine and continued 10 hours after the ending of the last cytarabine infusion.
— Ifosfamide 1.5 to 3.0 g/m^2/d i.v. 1 hour infusion x 4 days + Seraspenide i.v. continuous infusion for 96 hours (4 dose levels : 2.5 to 156.25 mg/kg/administration). Seraspenide infusion was initiated simultaneously with ifosfamide and continued 23 hours after the ending of the last ifosfamide infusion.

Results

The tolerance of Seraspenide either alone (n = 13 patients) or combined with monochemotherapy (n = 53 patients) has been so far excellent. The maximal tolerated dose has not been reached.

The myeloprotective effect was apparent in the series of the first 53 evaluable patients. In the overall series (n = 53) as judged on the AUC, depth of the nadir of leukocytes (p < 007) and neutrophils and duration of neutropenia (5.7 vs 7.1 days, p < 0.04). The results were more impressive at the Seraspenide doses of 2.5 and 12.5 mg/kg (levels 2 and 3) overall (n = 30) : when the Seraspenide was associated with the chemotherapy the nadirs were less profound for the leukocytes (p < 0.004) as well as for the neutrophils (p < 0.008). The AUC for the leukocytes as well as for the neutrophils were greater in combination with the Seraspenide (p < 0.04 et < 0.01, respectively). Finally, the duration of the neutropenia was 1.8 days shorter in combination with Seraspenide (5.9 vs 7.7 days, p < 0.05) (Table 2).

Table 2. Results : myeloprotection against both monochemotherapies on the comparison of the hematological data in the 30 patients at the 2.5 & 12.5 µg/kg Seraspenide dose levels

Patient groups & end-points		Placebo		Seraspenide		
		mean	st error	mean	st error	p*
Leucocytes	AUC	44,111	3,734	47,561	3,842	0.038
	Nadir/mm^3	1,622	187	2,078	256	0.004
	Duration < 1,000/mm^3	3.8	0.9	3.9	0.9	ns
Neutrophils	AUC	23,623	2,234	27,757	2,752	0.01
	Nadir/mm^3	518	97	796	145	0.008
	Duration < 500/mm^3**	7.7	1.2	5.9	1.3	< 0.05

* Wilcoxon matched-paired rank test
** 1.8 day shorter in the cycle with Seraspenide

These results reflect the advantage that has observed individually in the Seraspenide arm for each chemotherapy :
— in patients treated with cytarabine (n = 17) as judged on the nadir of the leukocytes and neutrophils (Table 3) :

Table 3. Myeloprotection against Cytarabine assessed on the comparison of the hematological data in all the 17 patients & in 11 patients at the 2.5 et 12.5 µg/kg Seraspenide dose levels

Patient groups & end-points		Placebo		Seraspenide		
		mean	st error	mean	st error	p*
Cytarabine (n = 17) Nadir leucocytes/mm^3	All dose levels	1,540	242	2,062	345	< 0.05
Cytarabine Nadir leucocytes (n = 11)	Dose levels 2.5 & 12.5 µg/kg	1,453	274	2,173	484	< 0.05
Nadir neutrophils/mm^3		81	53	504	220	< 0.01

* Wilcoxon matched-paired rank test

The impact on peripheral blood for the Cytarabine patients is translated in an improvement of the WHO index of toxicity for leukocytes and neutrophils (also perhaps with a trend for platelets) as suggested by the comparison of the grade 3 & 4 toxicity levels (Table 4).

Table 4. WHO index for hematological toxicities in the 2.5 & 12.5 dose levels (n = 17)

Parameters			Grade WHO*	Placebo (n)	Seraspenide (n)
Erythrocytes ($\times 10^3/mm^3$)	<	2.5	4	4	4
	2.5 à <	3.0	3	6	8
	3.0 à <	3.5	2	5	3
	3.5 à <	4.0	1	2	1
	> =	4.0	0	0	1
Leukocytes ($\times 10^3/mm^3$)	<	1.0	4	8	5
	1.0 à <	2.0	3	3	4
	2.0 à <	3.0	2	3	3
	3.0 à <	4.0	1	3	3
	> =	4.0	0	0	2
Neutrophils ($\times 10^3/mm^3$)	<	.5	4	14	12
	5 à <	1.0	3	2	1
	10 à <	1.5	2	1	2
	15 à <	2.0	1	0	1
	> =	2.0	0	0	1
Platelets ($\times 10^3/mm^3$)	<	25.0	4	9	8
	25.0 à <	50.0	3	7	4
	50.0 à <	75.0	2	1	1
	75.0 à <	100.0	1	0	4
	> =	100.0	0	0	0

* WHO index except for erythrocytes

— in patients treated with ifosfamide (n = 36), as judged on the AUC of the leucocytes and neutrophils (Table 5) :

Table 5. Myeloprotection against Ifosfamide assessed on the comparison of hematological data in all the 36 patients and in the 19 patients at the 2.5 & 12.5 μg/kg Seraspenide dose levels

Patient groups & end-points		Placebo		Seraspenide		
		mean	st error	mean	st error	p*
Ifosfamide (n = 36)	All dose levels					
AUC leucocytes/mm³		43,864	3,223	46,505	3,060	< 0.07
AUC neutrophils/mm³		27,755	2,640	29,585	2,343	< 0.06
Ifosfamide (n = 19)	Dose levels 2.5					
AUC leucocytes (n = 19)	& 12.5 μg/kg	41,271	4,046	47,145	4,603	< 0.05
AUC neutrophils/mm³	& 12.5 μg/kg	23,622	2,516	29,710	3,623	< 0.01

* Wilcoxon matched-paired rank test

Discussion

Seraspenide is the first isolated and characterized inhibitor that inhibits the entry of stem cells into cycle [2] and protects from cytotoxic drugs *in vivo* [3, 4]. Unlike growth factors it may preserve the stem cell pool [14]. At the difference of TGFb or TNFa, the Seraspenide is remarkably well tolerated, but no comparison is possible with other inhibitors, such as the MIP-1a [15] and the pentapeptide pEEDCK [16], which have not been tested in the clinic. Up to now Seraspenide appears to inhibit reversibly and specifically the normal progenitors [10, 11], thus Seraspenide should enhance the therapeutic index.

Conclusion

Seraspenide is non-toxic in patients undergoing chemotherapy. Preliminary data in the first 53 patients who undergone chemotherapy with and without Seraspenide suggest that it protects from drug-induced hemopoietic damage. Only one modality of administration and few dose levels have been explored till now. The optimal chronology of administration in relation to chemotherapy initiation and discontinuation is yet to be explored. The potential for hemoprotection has only been tested over 1 cycle of chemotherapy; it may be improved with the repetition of the cycles. Further clinical investigations are required to assess for long term protection, which is not warranted by current methods, specially positive growth factors, except for bone marrow transplants. In this setting the potential benefits from negative bone marrow regulators like the Seraspenide may be even greater than anticipated.

Aknowledgements. Our gratitude to Emilia Frindel, Martine Guigon & Maurice Tubiana, who conceived the role of negative regulators of hemopoiesis and searched for the substance, to Maryse Lenfant et Johanna Wdzieczak-Bakala who pioneered the search for the active peptide and its mechanism of action, to our co-workers and clincian colleagues, to Arthur Bogden, François Thomas for stimulating discussions. Funds Suzanne Axel, Jacques et Monique Roboh contributed to the realisation of preclinical & clinical studies (Drs Elie Fadel, Emmanuel Gonçalvès, chercheurs & techniciens U250 (Dr E. Frindel) and unité CNRS ICSN (Mme M. Lenfant).
Seraspenide (INN) = manufactured by Ipsen-Biotech/Beaufour (Paris). Patent = Institut Gustave Roussy/INSERM/CNRS. Granted by the ANVAR.

References

1. Vassort F, Frindel E, Tubiana M (1971) Effect of hydroxyurea on the kinetics of colony forming units of bone marrow in the mouse. Cell Tissue Kinet 4 : 423-431
2. Frindel E, Guigon M (1977) Inhibition of CFU entry into cycle by a bone marrow extract. Exp Hematol 5 : 74-76
3. Guigon M, Mary JY, Enouf J, Frindel E (1982) Protection of mice against lethal

doses of 1b-D-arabinofuranosylcytosine by pluripotent stem cell inhibitors. Cancer Res 42 : 638-641
4. Bogden Ae, Carde P, Deschamps De Paillette E, Moreau JP, Tubiana M, Frindel E (1991) Amelioration of chemotherapy induced toxicity by co-treatment with AcSDKP, a tetrapeptide inhibitor of hematopoietic stem cell proliferation. Ann NY Acad Sci 628 : 126-139
5. Lenfant M, Wdzieczak-Bakala J, Guittet E, Prome JC, Sotty D, Frindel E (1989) Isolation and structure determination of an inhibitor of hematopoietic pluripotent stem cell proliferation. Proc Natl Acad Sci USA 86 : 779-782
6. Volkov L, Pradelles P, Conte L, Frindel E (1992) L'étude du rôle d'un régulateur négatif (Ac-Ser-Asp-Lys-Pro) dans les phénomènes de prolifération cellulaire. CR Acad Sci Paris 315, série III : 499-504
7. Frindel E, Monpezat JP (1989) The physiological role of the endogenous colony forming units-spleen (CFU-S) inhibitor Acetyl-N-Ser-Asp-Lys-Pro (AcSDKP). Leukemia 3 : 753-754
8. Frindel E, Masse A, Pradelles P, Volkov L, Rigaud M (1992) The correlation of endogenous plasma levels in mice and the kinetics of CFU-S entry into cycle after ARA-C treatment : fundamental and clinical aspects. Leukemia 6 : 579-601
9. Pradelles P, Frobert Y, Creminon C, Liozon E, Masse A, Frindel E (1990) Negative regulator of pluripotent hematopoietic stem cell proliferation in human white blood cells and plasma as analysed by enzyme immunoassay. Biochem Biophys Res Com 170 : 986-993
10. Guigon M, Bonnet D, Lemoine F, Kobari L, Parmentier C, Mary J-Y, Najman A (1990) Inhibition of human bone marrow progenitors by the synthetic tetrapeptide AcSDKP. Exp Hematol 18 : 1112-1115
11. Bonnet D, Lemoine F, Khoury E, Pradelles P, Najman A, Guigon M (1992) Reversible inhibitory effects and absence of toxicity of the tetrapeptide Acetyl N — Ser-Asp-Lys-Pro (AcSDKP) in human long-term bone marrow culture. Exp Hematol 20 : 1165-1169
12. Cashman JD, Eaves AC, Eaves CJ (1992) Evidence for an indirect mechanism mediating the inhibitory effect of the tetrapeptide AcSDKP primitive human hematopoietic cell proliferation. J Cell Biochem (suppl) 16C
13. Robinson S, Lenfant M, Wdzieczack-Bakala J, Melville J, Riches A (1992) The mechanism of action pf the tetrapeptide Acetyl-N-Ser-Asp-Lys-Pro (AcSDKP) in the control of haematopoietic stem cell proliferation. Cell Prolif 25 : 623-632
14. Hornung RL, Longo DL (1992) Hematopoietic stem cell depletion by restorative growth factor regimens during repeated high dose cyclophosphamide therapy. Blood 80 : 77-83
15. Dunlop DJ, Wright EG, Larimore S, Graham GJ, Holycake T, Kerr DJ, Wolpe SD, Pragnell IB (1992) Demonstration of stem cell inhibitor and myeloprotective effects of SCI/rh MIP 1 a in vivo. Blood 79 : 2221-2225
16. Paukovits WR, Moser MH, Binder KA, Paukovits JB (1991) Protection from arabinofuranosyl cytosine and N-mustard induced myelotoxicity using hemoregulatory peptide p-Glu-Glu-Asp-Lys-Lys monomer and dimer. Blood 77 : 1313-1319

Abstract. Seraspenide, a synthetic tetrapeptide, inhibits cell cycle entry of normal hematopoietic stem cells. In mice it protects hemopoiesis against the damage caused by cytarabine, cyclophophamide and carboplatin. Seraspenide has been given to 53 cancer patients undergoing monochemotherapy. Patients underwent 2 consecutive cycles of monochemotherapy (cytarabine or ifosfamide) in a double-blind cross-over randomized study : first cycle : chemotherapy +

Seraspenide or placebo ; second cycle : chemotherapy + reverse order. Treatment groups were : Cytarabine 0.75 to 2 g/m² i.v. q. 12 h. x 4 or Ifosfamide 1.5 to 3.0 g/m²/d i.v. 1 h x 4 d. + Seraspenide (or placebo) 0.5 to 156.25 mg/kg continuous i.v. infusion. A protective effect of Seraspenide has been demonstrated (Wilcoxon matched-paired rank test) on the comparison of 6 parameters concerning the blood leucocytes and neutrophils during the 2 cycles : area under the curve (AUC) from day 8 to day 22 & depth of the nadir of leucocytes ($p < 0.07$) and neutrophils and duration of leucopenia & neutropenia < 500/ml (5.7 vs 7.1 days, $p < 0.04$). Seraspenide has been devoided of toxicity. These results reflect the advantage observed in the Seraspenide arm for each individual chemotherapy. Seraspenide, as an inhibitor of cell cycle entry of hemopoietic cells, protects from drug-induced hemopoietic damage. Its assessment for long term protection is underway.

Résumé. Le Séraspénide est un tétrapeptide présent chez l'homme (acétyl-Ser-Asp-Lys-Pro), initialement isolé de la moelle de fœtus de veau. Il inhibe l'entrée en synthèse d'ADN des cellules souches hématopoïétiques pluripotentes chez la souris qu'il protège de la toxicité de l'aracytine in vitro et in vivo. Il inhibe in vitro de façon réversible la prolifération des progéniteurs chez l'homme. Dans un essai clinique, de phase I-II, le Séraspénide seul a été administré et très bien toléré c/o 13 patients ; 53 patients ont reçu 2 cycles successifs d'une monochimiothérapie aracytine ou ifosfamide (respectivement 17 et 36 patients), l'un avec, l'autre sans Séraspénide. La comparaison des leucocytes et des polynucléaires aux 2 cycles montre une réduction de la toxicité avec le Séraspénide.

A review on the use of sheep epidermal squamous cell carcinoma to evaluate intra-arterial infusion chemotherapy

GJS Harker, FO Stephens

Epidermal squamous carcinoma in sheep

The primary purpose of on experimental tumour is to serve as a model for human cancer, to be used in experiments which provide information concerning both the biology of neoplasia, and techniques, agents and regimens which might improve the clinical process of cancer therapy. However, the original characteristics of a neoplastic clone maintained through many generations of serially transplanted animals, or passaged *in vitro*, may change· appreciably [Leibovici and Wolman, 1984]. Whilst extremely useful, experimental models can have their cost, and they should not abstract so far from reality that relevance to the ultimate goals of being better able to prevent disease, or improve treatment is lost. Therefore, a naturally occurring epidermal squamous cell carcinoma in sheep warrants investigation.

The reported similarities of this neoplastic condition is sheep and man, living in similar environments in Australia, are remarkable. As in man, solar radiation plays an important part in the genesis of sheep tumours. There is an increase in tumour incidence with decrease in latitude, reflecting a recognised geographic pattern [Harker, 1991]. The incidence of solar related epidermal carcinoma in sheep increases with animal age, indicating that development of skin cancer is related to the duration of UV radiation exposure. Lesions are uncommon in sheep aged less than 4 years [Ladds and Daniels, 1982 ; Harker, 1991] ; however, Ladds and Entwhistle [1976] reported that a sheep tumour incidence of 0.95 %, on a northern Australian farm, increased dramatically to 12 % if only the number of tumours in 12-year-old sheep was evaluated. Similarly, anatomical areas in the head and neck region of sheep most exposed to ultraviolet radiation are the most common tumour sites. The outer aspect and anterior edge of the ear suffer a great exposure than the inner aspect and posterior edge. The same applies to the more distal part of the ear compared to the proximal portion which is protected by neck wool. The muzzle area is always exposed [Lloyd 1961, Harker 1991]. Where an episode of photosensitisation has occurred, an infrequent interaction in exposed sheep skin between plant formed pigment and sunlight, unusually high numbers of epidermal carcinomas ultimately develop [March, 1965].

On a pathological basis, development of squamous carcinoma in sheep is associated with pre-existing lesions associated with sunlight exposure such as solar keratosis and cutaneous horns [Lloyd, 1961 ; Harker, 1991]. Such hyperkeratotic lesions, similar to premalignant lesions seen in man, are prone to occur on the sunlight exposed aspect of sheep's ears. The neoplastic process

---

Department of Surgery, The University of Sydney, Sydney, Australia

usually produces a unilateral tumour mass which, once established, becomes either a cauliflower-like lesion with circumscribed nodules or an ulcerated lesion invading cartilage. Sheep tumours may also develop in association with identifying ear tag marks or « punch holes » supporting the hypothesis that trauma, scarring and chronic irritation might play a part in tumour development [Lloyd, 1961 ; Harker, 1991]. However, the fact that solar hyperkeratotic skin is also seen adjacent to such sites of irritation perhaps suggests that the two aetiological factors may augment the incidence of tumour development. Histologically, epidermal carcinoma of sheep skin is equivalent to squamous cell carcinoma of the skin in man, lesions being classified as well, moderately or poorly differentiated [Lloyd, 1961 ; Harker, 1991]. In terms of metastatic behaviour, sheep epidermal carcinomas have a reported rate of 12 %, involving spread to the pre-auricular, parotid, mandibular, retropharyngeal and prescapular lymph nodes [Harker, 1991].

Intra-arterial (IA) induction chemotherapy in sheep

Of particular importance is that the sheep carcinoma under study occurs on the body surface, is usually large enough to afford ease of access for clinical observation and biopsy, and behaves essentially as a regional disease. For IA drug delivery a catheter is inserted, under general anaesthesia, into the external carotid artery on the tumour affected side, via either the superficial temporal or the cranial thyroid artery [Harker, 1991]. Catheter position is checked by blue dye injection into the regional arterial network to ensure that an infused drug will access the target tumour. In randomised studies, similar catheters are inserted into the jugular vein of tumour bearing sheep to be infused IV [Harker, 1991].

Bleomycin : The reported objective response rate for 18 sheep epidermal carcinomas infused IA with Bleomycin (0.2 units/kg/24 h × 21 days) was 61 %, with a mean tumour volume reduction of 57 % ± 26(sem) [Harker, 1991 ; Harker and Stephens, 1991]. Comparative IV therapy (n = 18) resulted in an objective response of 22 %, and a mean response of 30 % ± 26(sem). The difference for the two modes of Bleomycin administration was significantly in favour of IA infusion for both parameters (P < 0.05 and P < 0.01, respectively). This was supported by the tissue distribution of Indium ^{111} labelled bleomycin in one sheep after completion of a 24-hour IA infusion of the tagged drug. There was an obviously greater drug concentration on the IA infused side [Harker, 1991 ; Harker and Stephens, 1991]. Toxicity with IA Bleomycin was limited to mild regional erythema, with negligible systemic effects : during IV therapy 2 sheep developed loss of appetite.

Methotrexate : For IA Methotrexate administration (0.25 mg/kg/24 h × 21 days, n = 18), 56 % of sheep tumours have demonstrated an objective reponse, with a mean response of 50 % ± 25(sem) [Harker, 1991 ; Harker and Stephens, 1992a]. In contrast, only 22 % of 18 tumours treated IV showed an objective response, the mean reduction in volume being 28 % ± 27(sem). The difference was significant for both parameters (P < 0.05). In one animal with bilateral auricular carcinomas, of similar histological differentiation, the larger lesion was infused IA with a 76 % tumour volume reduction. By comparison the smaller contralateral tumour received the equivalent of systemic therapy, due to Methotrexate passing into the venous circulation after traversing the arterial vascular bed in the head and neck region, and only regressed by 20 %. With IA Methotrexate mild regional erythema and ease of depilation was seen in 50 % of cases with no significant system toxicity. In the case if IV therapy 4 sheep developed gastrointestinal tract symptoms, 3 of these showing a decrease in the white cell count to 3,000 u/l.

5-Fluorouracil (5-Fu) : For 5-FU (7 mg/kg/24 h, n = 18 for both groups), the observed difference in the numbers of sheep carcinomas exhibiting a greater than 40 % reduction in volume, over a designated 2 week treatment period, was significantly in favour of IA infusion (50 %) compared with IV therapy (11 %) (P < 0.05) [Harker, 1991 ; Harker and Sthephens, 1992a]. Similarly, analysis of the mean tumour volume reduction was significantly in support of IA (37 % ± 23 sem) compared with IV treatment (11 % ± 22 sem) (P < 0.05). With the dosage of 5-FU used, regional and systemic toxicity was minimal for both treatment groups.

Cisplatin : Preliminary results in the study of cisplatin (0.35 mg/kg/24 hr × 12 days) suggest a response advantage with IA administration [Harker and Stephens, unpublished data]. Seven of 10 sheep tumours have demonstrated an objective response compared with 3 of 10 tumours treated with an equivalent dose IV. Of particular significance is that one animal with histologically similar bilateral tumours was treated IA : the IA infused lesion regressed by 80 % compared with a 15 % regression of the contralateral carcinoma.

Cyclophosphamide : The four agents mentioned above are biologically active in their stable state. However, an agent such as cyclophosphamide is not though to be biologically effective until it has been metabolised, initially in the liver. In a study by Harker and Stephens [1992c], the difference in the response patterns for IA and IV cyclophosphamide delivery (2.5 mg/kg/24 h × 21 days) in the sheep model was not significant. The objective response rates were 50 % (IA) and 63 % (IV) (P > 0.05), with mean tumour volume reductions of 42 % ± 19(sem) (IA) and 50 % ± 13(sem) (IV) (P > 0.05), respectively. One IA treated lesion, a nasal carcinoma, extended equally on either side of the nasal midline. The 96 % tumour reduction was uniform and not predominantly confined to the side infused IA. In terms of toxicity, 5 sheep (3 IA and 2 IV) demonstrated loss of appetite, with 3 animals (1 IA and 2 IV) showing a moderate decrease in leukocyte count.

Discussion

The sheep epidermal squamous cell carcinoma model, discussed in this review, has proven to be the first experimental design in which long term IA cytotoxic drug infusion has been maintained via the external carotid artery of a large animal, bearing a spontaneous carcinoma, comparable to the human situation. Previous small animal models involved artificially induced transplanted tumours, and experienced technical difficulties due to the arterial dimensions in the head and neck region [Sindram, 1974 ; Schouwenber, 1980 ; Karafilian, 1983]. The origins and behaviour of these models do not compare to sheep epidermal carcinoma which is virutally analogous to the human condition in terms of aetiology, histology, local behaviour and regional lymphatic/metastatic spread [Lloyd, 1961 ; Harker, 1991].

IA induction chemotherapy has the potential advantage of achieving higher regional tissue and tumour drug concentrations, and total dosage, than are attainable by equivalent dose systemic drug delivery, without an attendant increase in systemic toxicity. On this basis, sheep epidermal carcinoma has been shown to have the necessary attributes for appropriate, randomised IA and IV chemotherapeutic studies including : (i) a natural history demonstrating primarily regional disease ; (ii) a definable and accessible regional arterial supply ; (iii) tolerance of a delivery system that permits safe, continuous long term infusion ; (iv) sensitivity to commonly used antineoplastic agents with appropriate pharmacokinetic properties [Harker, 1991 ; Harker and Stephens, 1991, 1992a, 1992b, 1992c].

The reported studies of sheep head and neck squamous carcinoma to evaluation Bleomycin, Methotrexate, 5-FU and Cisplatin administration indicate that IA infusion produces a greater tumour response than equivalent dose IV drug delivery. The difference in numbers of tumors attaining an objective response in the case of Bleomycin and Methotrexate, and a greater than 40 % regression for 5-FU, was significantly in favour of IA delivery statistically, as was the difference in the mean reduction in tumour volume. Preliminary data in the case of comparative IA and IV Cisplatin infusion supports these findings. In order to obtain a response equivalent to the IA route, a greater systemic dosage of each drug would be required with, however, an attendant increase in general toxicity. The experimental evidence lends strong support to the need for continuing study, in appropriate centres, of the clinical application on intra-arterial induction chemotherapy.

The above agents are all known to exhibit antineoplastic activity in their natural state. The results in the sheep model further indicate that the entire advantage of regional IA delivery is accrued the first time such drugs reach the target tumour tissue within the regional arterial blood supply. Having traversed the tissues supplied by the discrete regional arterial network, in the head and neck region, most of the drug enters the systemic circulation and behaves as though it had been administered IV [Stephens, 1983 ; 1988]. Conversely, there are theoretical reasons for believing that there should be no such advantage in delivering an agent such as Cyclophosphamide by direct regional IA infusion, as opposed to systemic administration. This is based on the hypothesis that the drug may not be biologically effective until it has been activated by a multistep process that intially requires metabolism in the liver. Observations in the sheep carcinoma model regarding Cyclophosphamide reflect an equivalent tumour response irrespective of the mode of administration. The data support the hypothesis that, in contrast to Bleomycin, Methotrexate, 5-FU and apparently Cisplatin, such an agent infused IA is inactive regionally before reaching the systemic circulation.

References

1. Harker GJS (1991) Intra-arterial infusion chemotherapy in a sheep carcinoma model. PhD thesis, University of Sydney, 2-98
2. Harker GJS, Stephens FO (1991) The use of sheep epidermal squamous cell carcinoma to evaluate intra-arterial Bleomycin infusion chemotherapy. Reg Cancer Treat 4 : 121-126
3. Harker GJS, Stephens FO (1992a) Sheep epidermal squamous cell carcinoma as a solid tumour model in the comparative evaluation of intra-arterial and intravenous Methotrexate administration. Reg Cancer Treat (in press)
4. Harker GJS, Stephens FO (1992b) Comparison of intra-arterial versus intravenous 5-Fluorouracil administration on epidermal squamous cell carcinoma in sheep. Eur J Cancer 28 : 1437-1441
5. Harker GJS, Stephens FO (1992c) A report on the efficacy of Cyclophosphamide administered intra-arterially in sheep bearing epidermal squamous carcinoma. Reg Cancer Treat 4 : 170-174
6. Karanfilian RG, Rush BF, Murphy T (1983) Regional versus systemic effect of cis-dichlorodiamine platinum on squamous cell carcinoma in rats. Am Surg 3 : 353-360
7. Ladds PW, Daniels PW (1982) Animal model of human disease : ovine squamous cell carcinoma. Am J Path 107 : 122-123
8. Ladds PW, Entwhistle KW (1977) Observations on squamous cell carcinoma of sheep in Queensland, Australia. Br J Cancer 35 : 110-114
9. Leibovici J, Wolman M (1984) Models for tumour progression. Anticancer Res 4 : 165-168
10. Lloyd LC (1961) Epithetial tumours of the skin in sheep. Br J Cancer 15 : 780-789
11. March H (1965) Diseases caused by poisonous plants, in Newson's sheep diseases, The Williams and Wilkins Company, Baltimore, pp. 425-428
12. Schouwenberg PF, Van Putten LM, Snow GB (1980) External carotid artery infusion with single and multiple drug regimens in the rat. Cancer 45 : 2258-2264
13. Sindram PJ, Snow GB, Van Putten LM (1974) Intra-arterial infusion with Methotrexate in the rat. Br J Cancer 30 : 349-354
14. Stephens FO (1983) Pharmacokinetics of intra-arterial chemotherapy. Recent Results Cancer 86 : 1-12
15. Stephens FO (1988) Why use regional chemotherapy ? Principles and pharmacokinetics. Reg Cancer Treat 1 : 4-10

Cellular and pharmacokinetic factors which influence genotoxicity of topoisomerase II inhibiting drugs in human leukemia cells

F Gieseler, V Nüßler *, F Boege, D Biller, P Meyer, W Willmanns *, K Wilms

Background

Multidrug resistance (MDR) is a cellular phenomenon which is defined by simultaneous development of resistance against cytostatic drugs from different chemical classes. The cells might even develop cross-resistance against drugs which they did not get entouched with. The molecular alterations of resistant cells can be located on every subcellular level, but only two of them are able to explain MDR. The overexpression of the membrane-bound P170 glycoprotein (PGly) results in MDR which includes vinca-alcaloids and can be affected by modulators such as Verapamil [1]. Alterations of DNA-topoisomerases (Topo) can lead to MDR with low resistance against vinca-alcaloids [2]. A number of clinically most important cytostatics, such as anthracyclines, podophyllotoxins, mAMSA and mitoxantrone are both, inhibitors of Topo II and substrate of PGly. Here, we present data regarding intracellular factors which influence the cytotoxicity of these drugs.

Anthracyclines exhibit multiple intracellular effects such as DNA-intercalation, the liberation of free oxygen-radicals and direct membrane toxicity but the inhibition of the life-important enzyme Topo II seems to be the final molecular event leading to cell death. The inhibition of the religation-step of Topo II results in protein-associated DNA-double strand breaks (the « cleavable complex ») which correlate directly with cell death [3]. The cleavable complex is a ternary complex between the DNA, the drug and Topo II and its formation depends on the affinity of the drug and Topo II to the DNA and the affinity between the drug and Topo II (Fig. 1). Modulating factors are the amount, activity and sensitivity of Topo II, drug uptake and efflux and the DNA sequence and structure as well as DNA-binding proteins, such as histones.

Material and methods

HL-60 cell are commercially available (ATCC = CCL240). Gastric carcinoma cell line EPG85-257 and resistant subline had been described before [4]. AlHi cells had been derived from a patient with AML FAB M2 in first relaps after

Medizinische Poliklinik, University Hospital, Würzburg, Germany
* Klinikum Großhadern, Med Klinik III, University of Munich, Germany

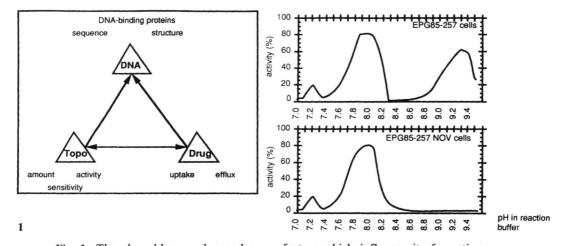

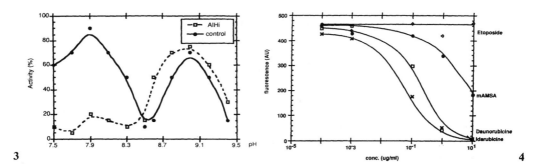

Fig. 1. The cleavable complex and some factors which influence its formation

Fig. 2. Topo II characteristics of EPG85-257 cells and resistant subline (EPG85-257 NOV)

Fig. 3. Topo II characteristics of AlHi patient cells

Fig. 4. DNA-binding affinity of Topo II inhibitors

DAV-polychemotherapy. The following patients relapsed after first-line therapy and had been treated with idarubicine monotherapy : Pat. 1 (WW, T-ALL) was sensitive, pat. 2 (AML FAB M4) showed no change. These cells had been used as control : HL-60 cells (sensitive to Idarubicin), DMSO-differentiated HL-60 cells (resistant) and normal leukocytes (resistant). Topo II activity had been determined by DNA-relaxation and DNA-decatenation as described before [5]. Sensitivity of cells had been measured by the ability of the cells to reduce MTT after four days incubation in increasing drug doses (0-10 μg/ml). Cellular drug uptake had been determined by measurement of drug-fluorescence in a FACscan (Beckton-Dickensen), the concentration of Idarubicin in these experiments was 10 μg/ml which resembles plasma concentrations after treatment as the patients shown here have been treated with a single dose of 12 mg Idarubicin per m^2 every week for three weeks. It had been shown, that after 7-9 mg Idarubicin per m^2 in five consecutive doses, the plasma peak concentration was 40 ng/ml, nadir 2 ng/ml [6]. DNA-binding affinity of drugs had been measured by the ability of the drugs to remove the AT-binder Hoechst dye from pBR322.

Results

Alterations of Topo II and cellular resistance

Two different isoenzymes of Topo II, called Topo I-alpha and Topo II-beta, and posttranslational modifications, such as phosphorylation, result in a functional heterogeneity with several pH- and salt-dependent isoactivities which also exhibit different sensitivity to cytostatic drugs [7]. The loss of isoactivities might lead to decreased cellular sensitivity to specific drugs. In the Figs. 2 and 3, two examples of this mechanism are shown. In Fig. 2, the Topo II activity of a sensitive and resistant gastric-carcinoma cell line EPG85-257 NOV is shown. In contrast to the sensitive cells, the resistant cells have lost the isoactivity at pH 9.2-9.4. These cells additionally display the phenomenon of vesicular drug-trapping which had been described before [4]. In Fig. 3, Topo II activity of normal leukocytes in comparison to multidrug-resistant patient cells (AlHi) is shown. The patient cells were derived from a acute myeloid leukemia (FAB M2) in first relaps after treatment with DAV. These cells have lost their isoactivity at pH 7.4-7.8.

DNA-binding affinity of Topo II inhibitors

In Fig. 4, the ability of different drugs to remove the AT-binder Hoechst dye from pBR322 is shown. Etoposide which also inhibits Topo II, but does not intercalate served as a internal control and shows no replacement. The DNA-binding affinity of mAMSA is significantly lower, than the one of Daunorubicine and Idarubicin. The DNA-affinity of its first derevate Idarubicinole is as high, as the one of Idarubicin (not shown).

DNA-binding and cell death

In the following, we show experiments with patient cells, human promyelocytic HL-60 cells and control leukocytes. Patient 1 (WW, T-ALL) was sensitive, patient 2 (RH, AML, FAB M4) showed no change, HL-60 cells are sensitive and control leukocytes are resistant to single-drug treatment with Idarubicin.

In Fig. 5, the correlation between the amount of drug bound to the DNA, and cell-viability is shown for sensitive HL-60 cells (upper graph), and resistant leukocytes (lower graph) is shown. The correlation between these two parameters is linear.

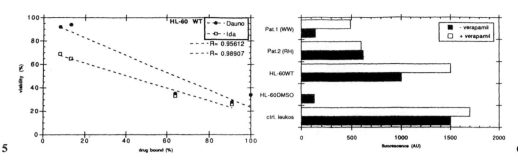

Fig. 5. Correlation between the DNA-binding of drugs and cell viability

Fig. 6. Cellular uptake of Idarubicin

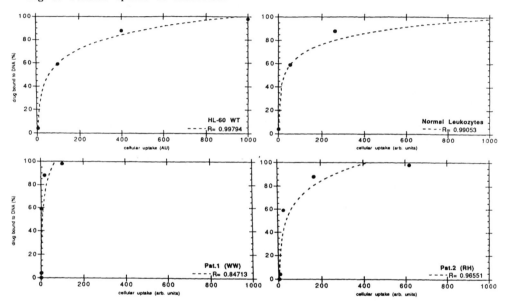

Fig. 7. Correlation between the cellular drug uptake and DNA-binding rate

Cellular drug uptake and clinical outcome

In Fig. 6, the netto drug uptake and the influence of Verapamil had been measured by scanning the cellular fluorescence after 30 min. incubation in 10 μg Idarubicin per ml +/− Verapamil in a FACscan. Patient 1 (WW), sensitive to Idarubicin, had a low drug uptake which could be slightly increased by Verapamil. Patient 2 (RH), who showed no change after treatment, had a higher uptake and no change with Verapamil. Undifferent HL-60 cells (sensitive) had a high drug uptake, increasing with Verapamil, comparable to the uptake of leukocytes. The fluorescence had been measured after 30 minutes and reflects the netto uptake. The fluorescence after inhibition of pGly by Verapamil indicates the true uptake. In these experiments, we found no correlation between cellular drug uptake and sensitivity or clinical outcome.

Cellular drug uptake and DNA-binding

In Fig. 7, the celluar drug uptake and the DNA-binding rate of Topo II-inhibiting drugs is shown. The correlation between these two parameters follows a logarithmic function as well for the sensitive cells, as for the resistant cells. Even the leukemic cells derived from patient 1 (WW) with a low uptake for Idarubicin exhibit a high DNA-binding rate of the drug, which might be the reason for sensitivity of these cells to Idarubicin.

Conclusions

Alterations of Topo II resulting in lower activity (not shown) or loss of isoactivity are intranuclear factors affecting drug resistance. These modifications might be due to different expression of Topo II-isoenzymes, posttranscriptional modifications or changes is regularly proteins. We found no correlation between the cellular drug uptake and the sensitivity of the cells which indicates the importance of intracellular factors. The correlation between the DNA-binding affinity of Topo II inhibiting drugs and viability was linear which points to the importance of Topo II inhibition for cell death. The correlation between drug uptake and cell death is logarithmic which means that even low drug-uptake rates might result in high DNA-binding rates and subsequently cell death.

Acknowledgement. Technical assistance by M Müller and M Clark ?

References

1. Boiocchi M, Toffoli G (1992) Mechanisms of multidrug resistance in human tumour cell lines and complete reversion of cellular resistance Eur J Cancer 28 : 1099-1105
2. Wolverton JS, Danks MK, Schmidt CA, Beck WT (1989) Genetic characterization of the multidrug-resistant phenotype of VM-26-resistant human leukemic cells. Cancer Res 49 : 2422-2426
3. Liu LF (1989) DNA Topoisomerase poisons as antitumior drugs. Ann Rev Biochem 58 : 351-375
4. Dietel M, Arps H, Lage H, Niendorf A (1990) Membrane Vesicle formation due to Acquired Mitoxantrone Resistance in Human Gastric Carcinoma Cell Line EPG85-257. Cancer Res 50 : 6100-6106
5. Gieseler F, Boege F, Ruf B, Meyer P, Wilms K (in press 1993) Molecular pathways of topoisomerase II regulation and consequences for chemotherapy. In : Hiddemann W et al Leukemia IV (eds). Springer-Verlag, Heidelberg
6. Robert J, Rigal-Huguet F, Harousseau JH, Pris J, Huet S, Reiffers J, Hurteloup P, Tamassia V (1987) Pharmacokinetics of Idarubicin After Daily Intravenous Administration in Leukemic Patients. Leuk Res 11 : 961-966
7. Gieseler F, Boege F, Clark M, Meyer P (in press 1992) A model of the molecular mechanism how DNA-topoisomerase inhibiting drugs influence hematopoetic cell differentiation. Toxicol Lett 60

Abstract. *The stabilization of a ternary complex between DNA, drug and topoisomerase II (Topo II) is the genotoxic event leading to cell death in chemotherapy with anthracyclines, podophyllotoxines, mAMSA and mitoxantrone. Its formation is determined by the affinity of the drug and Topo II to the DNA, and the affinity between the drug and Topo II. Some factors affecting the cleavable complex are amount, activity and sensitivity of Topo II, drug uptake and efflux, the DNA sequence and structure, and other DNA-binding proteins. Two different isoenzymes of Topo II (alpha and beta) and posttranscriptional alterations have been described. These Topo II isoforms can be destiguished functionally by Ph and anion alterations in the reaction buffer. In sensitive cells, we detected all isoforms, but in resistant cells, the loss of Topo II isoforms results in decreased sensitivity to Topo II inhibiting drugs. This is shown by funcional analysis of Topo II activity in a resistant akute myeloid leukemia and a resistant gastric carcinoma celle line. The DNA affinity of anthracyclines is higher, than the one of mAMSA, idarubicine and idarubicinole have higher affinities than doxorubicine. The correlation between the amount of drugs bound to the DNA and cytotoxicity is linear, whereas the correlation between drug uptake and DNA binding of drugs is logarithmic. This indicates the importance of Topo II inhibition for cell death and develuates the factor of drug uptake for cell death, as low uptake rates are sufficient for high DNA binding rates.*

Clinical application of gene transfer in oncology : preliminary results of a French study

Y Merrouche, C Bain, G Clapisson, S Negrier, B Coronel,
A Mercatello, JF Moskovtchenko, B Mœn*, T Philip, MC Favrot

Biotherapy represents a new field of investigation and treatment in oncology. In parallel with the treatment of patients with conventional radiochemotherapy or surgery, the aim of our institution is to develop new therapeutic approaches in oncology, using in particular biological modifiers. In this field, *in vitro* or *in vivo* modifications of immunocompetent and/or malignant cell functions by gene transfer are one of the major advances [1].

We initiated a gene marking study of patients with advanced cancer using tumor infiltrating lymphocytes (TIL) transduced with the gene of resistance to neomycin (NeoR). The first purpose of this protocol was to evaluate ethical, pratical and safety issues of long cultures of human cells and retroviral-mediated gene transduction using the marker gene NeoR [2]. Considering the results published by the group of Rosenberg and Anderson [3], this protocol had two other objectives : to define the toxicity and efficacy of IL2 and TIL injection in patients with melanoma or renal cell cancer, to better define the survival of TIL in blood and tumor sites after reinjection. The reinfusion of TIL transduced with the NeoR gene was accepted by the French Ethical Committee in January 1991 and by the Local Ethical Committee of our Institute in April 1991.

Methodology

Inclusion criteria

Patients over 18 years old with metastatic renal cell cancer or melanoma for whom standard curative or palliative measures did not exist or were no longer effective. Informed consent was obtained from each patient.

Exclusion criteria

Patients requiring steroid therapy ; or having cerebral metastasis ; or with a performance status less than 2 ; patients who have received therapy with cytotoxic agents, steroids, other biologics or radiotherapy in the 4 weeks prior to cell inoculation.

Centre Léon Bérard and Hôpital Edouard Herriot, Lyon, France and *Genetic Therapy Inc, Gaithersburg, USA

Treatment plan

Patients received a first 5-day cycle of Interleukin-2 given as continuous infusion (18×10^6 IU/m²/day) followed by 6 days of rest. On the 11th day, they received TIL infusion followed, 2 to 6 hours later, by a second 5-day cycle of Interleukin-2 at the same doses as above. After 2 days rest, patients underwent 6 successive cycles of subcutaneous Interleukin-2 given at 1.8×10^6 IU/m²/day, twice a day, 5 days a week, for 6 weeks, with 2 days rest between cycle.

TIL expansion

The tumor, taken surgically under local anesthesia when feasible, was transported in sterile conditions to the lab for enzymatic dilaceration. The cells were then expanded during 4 to 7 weeks, as previously described by Rosenberg [4, 5] in synthetic medium (X-Vivo 10) plus IL2. All cultures were started and expanded in polyolefin culture bags.

Protocol of NeoR gene transduction

The helper free LNL6 retroviral vector (packaging cell line PA317) was approved for use in man in 1989. The NeoR vector supernatant was provided by Genetic Therapy Inc., after safety and quality controls. The cells were transduced between day 8 and day 18, when reaching 2 to 4 fold expansion. The cells were incubated at 37°C for 2 hours at a multiplicity of infection of 2 (ratio virons/cells). The procedure was repeated after a 24 hours interval with extensive washing between the two.

Results and discussion

We received tumor samples from 15 patients for TIL expansion. In 6 cases, TIL obtained from 6 tumors under 10 g, taken on local anesthesia, did not grow. In three cases, TIL were grown but were not transduced nor reinjected because patients progressed rapidly. Currently, 6 patients have been included : 5 patients suffering from metastatic melanoma who all had been heavily pretreated (surgery plus 1 or 2 lines of systemic immunotherapy and/or chemotherapy) ; 1 patient with metastatic renal cell carcinoma who had been treated with TIL since diagnosis (compassionate case).

Tumor weights ranged from 10 to 80 g. At initiation of the culture, the total number of mononuclear cells ranged from 1 to 32×10^8. TIL were transduced 13 to 27 days after initiating the culture ; the number of transduced TIL ranged from 1.25 to 13.2×10^8. TIL were grown from 27 to 47 days.

In the first two cases, the growth of transduced TIL was very low, compared to non manipulated TIL cultures ; in the other four patients, the expansion was equal in both transduced and non transduced populations.

The total number of cells reinfused ranged from 4 to 92 × 10^9 with a percentage of transduced cells ranging from 0.7 to 26. Within the transduced cell population, the efficiency of infection with the NeoR vector, evaluated by semi-quantitative PCR analysis, ranged from 1 to 10 % without variation from the day of transduction to the end of the culture and reinjection.

Safety controls were performed before TIL reinjection. The cell viability was greater than 70 % ; no tumor cell was detected (double immunofluorescence, limit of detection 10^{-5}). IL2 was withdrawn from the culture medium of an aliquot for at least one week to assure that cells did not exhibit autonomous growth in the absence of IL2.

Sterility was assured by testing regularly along culture for aerobic and anaerobic bacteria, fungus and mycoplasma. In two cases, we observed a fungal contamination of half the culture bags which were not reinjected to the patient. The absence of replication competent retrovirus was asserted by reverse transcriptase assay after amplification on DUNNI cell line (permissive for all four classes of murine leukemia viruses).

Two patients did not receive transduced TIL : one because of fungal contamination, as mentionned above, and one because of a false positive Dunni test. In that case, the culture was frozen and checked for negativity but transduced cells could not be reinjected after control because of patient's clinical status.

After the reinjection, controls on blood samples were performed periodically during the follow up to detect replication-competent retrovirus. All tests performed until day 60 after reinjection were negative. The side effects of the treatment were similar to those observed in patients treated with IL2 plus LAK cells, without life-threatening toxicity. No additional toxicity due to the reinjection of transduced cells occured.

After reinjection, we have been able to demonstrate the presence of NeoR positive cells in the peripheral blood by semi-quantitative PCR. Analyses of tumor samples are ongoing.

Before reinjection, TIL were predominantly CD3+ CD8+ T cells ; the phenotype was not modified by transduction. A specific cytoxicity against autologous tumor cells was observed in one case (melanoma).

The clinical evaluation is as follows : 3 patients progressed on therapy and died, 1 progressed after 180 days, 1 remained in complete response after 200 days.

Conclusion

Long term culture of TIL is feasible although large tumor samples are necessary. Fungal contamination was the major technical problem. Our study confirmed the feasibility of *in vitro* gene transfer in cultured lymphocytes with retroviral vector [6] and the safety of the procedure (no detection of replication competent virus, no side effect after reinjection) [3]. The NeoR marker gene can be used to study the survival of hematopoietic human cells after reinjection [3].

Acknowledgement. We express our gratitude to A Duc for expert technical assistance, to F Lanier and MO Heilman, the research nurses in our institute, and to MD Reynaud for help in preparing the manuscript.

References

1. Merrouche Y, Favrot MC (1992) Retroviral gene therapy and its application in oncohematology. Hum Gen Ther 3 : 285-291
2. Favrot MC, Philip T, Merrouche Y et al (1992) Treatment of patients with advanced cancer using tumor infiltrating lymphocytes transduced with the gene of resistance to Neomycin. Hum Gen Ther 3 : 533-542
3. Rosenberg SA, Aebersold P, Cornetta K et al (1990) Gene transfer into humans. Immunotherapy of patients with advanced melanoma, using tumor infiltrating lymphocytes modified by retroviral gene transduction. N Engl J Med 323 : 570-578
4. Rosenberg SA, Spiess P, Lafreniere R (1986) A new approach to the adoptive immunotherapy of cancer with tumor infiltrating lymphocytes. Science 233 : 1318-1321
5. Rosenberg SA, Packard BS, Aebersold PM et al (1988) Use of tumor-infiltrating lymphocytes and Interleukin-2 in the immunotherapy of patients with metastatic melanoma : a preliminary report. N Engl J Med 319 :1676-1680
6. Kasid A, Morecki S, Aebersold P et al (1990) Human gene transfer : characterization of human tumor-infiltrating lymphocytes as vehicles for retroviral mediated gene transfer in man. Proc Natl Acad Sci USA 87 : 473-477

Effects of Vitamin-A on the oestrogen dependant breast carcinoma cell line ZR75-1

PG Horgan, J O'Donoghue, J Byrne, C Phelan, HF Given

ZR75-1 cells at a concentration of 2×10^5 cells/ml were placed in a 24 well tissue culture plate to which was added Tamoxifen, Megoestrol Acetate or Vitamin-A. The culture plates were then incubated at 37 degrees centigrade in 5 % carbon dioxide. Cell growth was monitored every 48 hours for fourteen days.

The anti-oestrogen agent Tamoxifen and the aromatase inhibitor Megoestrol Acetate were found to be cytostatic in inhibiting the growth of ZR75-1 cells when compared with control untreated cells. Vitamin-A in doses of 1 International Unit (IU), 2 IU, 5 IU, and 10 IU/well effected cell death in all treated ZR75-1 wells within the study period. On investigating the effect of these doses of Vitamin-A on normal healthy lymphocytes it was noted that cell toxicity was dose-dependant. 5 IU/well and 10 IU/well of Vitamin-A resulted in lymphocyte death but 1 IU/well and 2 IU/well had no effect on lymphocyte proliferation.

These data suggest a therapeutic role for low-dose Vitamin-A in breast carcinoma patients.

Lotan (1980) [1] has defined Vitamin-A and its related derivatives (retinoids) as a group of substances capable of restoring normal growth in retinol-deficient experimental animals. These substances have a central polygenic chain and a polar terminal group. Natural retinoids are ingested in food in the form of retinol, retinyl esters, retinoic acid and a pro-Vitamin B-Carotene. The latter follows a different metabolic pathway within the body than do the others. Retinoids are stored in the liver and released on demand. Specific membrane receptors have been described for retinol binding protein enabling the retinol to pass into the cell. Little is known on the trans-cellular transport of the other retinoids.

Retinol and the other retinoids have powerful hormone-like effects on cell growth and differentiation [2, 3]. Retinoids have been investigated as potential agents in cancer prevention in laboratory experiments, animal studies and in human populations. In addition, retinoid administration has been shown to effect the regression of induced tumours [4] and delay the appearance of transplanted tumours [5].

This laboratory has studied the biology of breast cancer for the past number of years with particular emphasis on immunology and the potential for immunotherapy as an adjunct to surgery. This study investigated the effect of the commonly employed endocrine agents Tamoxifen and Megoestrol Acetate, and Vitamin-A on an oestrogen dependant metastatic breast carcinoma cell line ZR75-1.

National Breast Cancer Institute, University College Hospital, Galway, Ireland

Materials and methods

Media and reagents

Dulbecco's Modified Eagles Medium (DMEM), RPMI 1640, Heat inactivated foetal calf Serum, Fungizone, and L-Glutamine were purchased from Gibco, UK. Penicillin, Streptomycin, B-Estradiol, Trypsin EDTA, phytohaemagglutinin (PHA) and Vitamin-A (all trans retinol) were purchased from Sigma UK. Lymphoprep was purchased from Novopath, Ireland.

ZR75-1 growth curve

ZR75-1 cells were obtained as a gift from the Department of Microbiology, University College Galway. Cells were cultured in 75cm^2 tissue culture flask with Complete Culture Medium (DMEM, 10 % heat inactivated foetal calf Serum, 1 % Penicillin/Streptomycin, 1 % L-Glutamine, 0.8 % Fungizone, and 10^{-8}M B-Estradiol) until growth was confluent. The adherent monolayer of ZR75-1 cells was removed from the bottom of the tissue culture flask by removing the culture medium, rinsing with DMEM, placing 5 ml Trypsin EDTA into the flask and incubating at 37°C for five minutes until the layer of cells had completely lifted. Trypsin EDTA was deactivated by the addition of Complete Culture Medium. The suspension was then centrifuged at 1,000 revolutions per minute (RPM) for 5 minutes at room temperature.

The supernatant was discarded and the cell pellet re-suspended in 10 ml of Complete Culture Medium by vortex agitation until a uniform cell suspension was achieved. Addition of Acridine Orange/Ethidium Bromide fluorescent stain enabled counting of viable cells in a hemocytometer and calculation of cell concentration. Serial dilution was used to achieve a cell concentration of 2×10^5 cells/ml in Complete Culture Medium. 2.0 ml of this cell suspension was placed into each well of a 24 well culture plate. Plates were then incubated at 37°C and 5 % CO_2. Growth of ZR75-1 was monitored at intervals of 48 hours. The culture plate was removed from the incubator and transferred to a laminar flow cabinet where the media was removed with care. Trypsin EDTA (0.5 ml) was added to each well and the plate re-incubated for a further 5 minutes. Addition of 1.5 ml of Complete Culture Medium is followed by agitation resulting in a single cell suspension. 100 ul of suspension is once again stained with Acridine Orange/Ethidium Bromide and counted in a hemocytometer. The mean value for six wells is then calculated and plotted against time.

The effect of addition of the substance under investigation (Tamoxifen, Megoestrol Acetate and Vitamin-A) was determined by the addition of the appropriate dose of the agent to six wells of the culture plate. Each time the plates are monitored the agent is re-added before further incubation.

Lymphocyte growth curve

Peripheral venous blood was drawn from healthy female controls. Peripheral blood mononuclear cells (PBMC's) were separated using Lymphoprep density gradient. Cells were washed three times in RPMI 1640, counted in a hemocytometer and diluted to achieve a standard cell concentration of 1.0×10^6 cells/ml. Cells were then incubated in tissue culture plates in triplicate with control wells, with 5 IU Vitamin-A, or with 10 IU Vitamin-A. Phytohaemagglutinin (0.1 ug) was added to all wells to induce blastogenesis. In addition 1.5ml of medium containing RPMI 1640, 10 % foetal calf Serum and 1 % Penicillin/Streptomycin was added to each well bringing the cell concentration to 2.5×10^5. Incubation was at 37°C in 5 % CO_2 as before. Four days later the cells were agitated and a 100ul sample taken, stained and counted as previously described.

Drug dosages

Tamoxifen was diluted to a concentration of 200 ng/ml and 200 ul of this solution was added to each well containing ZR75-1 cells. Megoestrol Acetate was made up to a solution of 2 ug/ml, 200 ul was added to each well. Vitamin-A was used in a concentration of 1IU/ml. This concentration is the equivalent of 0.3 ug retinol.

Results

The ZR75-1 cell line reproduced well in tissue culture. Six days into the experiment the cells consistently increased in concentration from 2×10^5 to almost 6×10^5/ml. The addition of the anti-oestrogen agent tamoxifen effected an immediate inhibition in the growth curve of the cancer cells. On the sixth day the cell concentration had decreased to 1.4×10^5 cells/ml. This effect was essentially cytostatic. The effect of adding the aromatase inhibitor Megoestrol Acetate to the ZR75-1 cells in culture was found to be similarly cytostatic.

The addition of 10IU Vitamin-A to the ZR75-1 cancer cells demonstrated a dramatic cytotoxic inhibition of cell proliferation. There was complete tumour cell death by day 9 of tissue culture (Fig. 1). Similarly a lower dose of Vitamin-A (5IU/well) was found to be cytotoxic with cell death observed by day 14 of culture (Fig. 1). When physiological doses of Vitamin-A were investigated the effect of addition of 3.66IU/well to the ZR75-1 cell line resulted in cell death by the fifteenth day of tissue culture (Fig. 2). A low dose of 1.23 IU/well was also used and the effects were similar to larger doses but delayed until the eighteenth day of tissue culture.

Normal lymphocytes were also subjected to Vitamin-A in cell culture. These studies confirmed the safety of the low doses of Vitamin-A used in the cancer cell cultures. There was no interference in the proliferation of normal lymphocytes when treated with Vitamin-A in doses of 5 IU/well and 10IU/well.

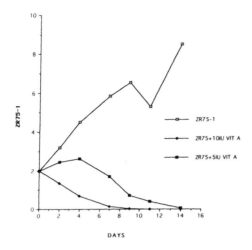

Fig. 1. The effect of addition of Vitamin-A (5IU/well, 10IU/well) to ZR75-1 cells in culture. ZR75-1 proliferation is expressed as number of cells × 10^5

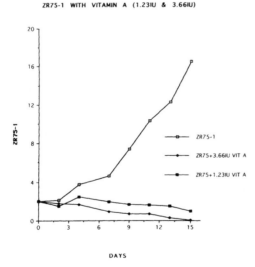

Fig. 2. The effect of physiological doses of Vitamin-A (1.23IU/well, 3.66IU/well). ZR75-1 proliferation expressed as number of cells × 10^5

Discussion

Woolbach & Howe (1925) [2] first noticed the neoplastic effect of deprivation of Vitamin-A and initiated research into the role of retinoids as preventative and therapeutic anti-neoplastic agents. Vitamin-A was first recognised by Stepp in 1909 [6] and named by Drummond three years later [7]. Naturally occurring Vitamin-A plays a central role in epithelial growth, reproduction and vision [8]. Many investigators have reported that retinoids block the phenotypic expression of cancer in animals and humans irrespective of the initiating or promoting factors involved [9, 10]. In most cells there exists a retinoic acid-sensitive G1 restriction or commitment point, but no link has been described between retinoid induced growth inhibition and the cell doubling time [11]. G1 growth arrest may in fact be regulated separately from differentiation as has been reported in studies on the HL-60 human promyelocytic cell line [12].

Moon et al [13] investigated the chemopreventative effects of retinoids in their chemical carcinogenesis studies of the mammary glands of rats. Following initiation of breast carcinoma by 7.12-Dimethylbenz(a)-Antracene (DMBA) and treatment with Vitamin-A, there was a 52 % reduction in cancer development compared to rodents on a placebo diet.

This work demonstrates that Vitamin-A has profound effects on the human metastatic breast carcinoma cell line ZR75-1. The cytostatic effects of Tamoxifen on the cell line is not unexpected as it's known anti-breast cancer action is by competitive inhibition at the oestrogen receptor level on the cancer cell. As ZR75-1 is an oestrogen dependant line the cells cannot proliferate with Tamoxifen present in culture. Similarly Megoestrol Acetate displays a cytostatic action in culture. This effect however is more difficult to explain given its known mode of action in breast cancer as an aromatase inhibitor but presumably is also capable of interfering with the growth enhancing effect of oestrogen already present in tissue culture.

Vitamin-A in doses of 5IU, 10IU and 15IU/well effected complete inhibition of ZR75-1 cells within the study period with complete death of breast cancer cells. The lower doses used in this work are calculated from the normal range of b-carotene found in normal individuals. This range when converted to equivalent doses of Vitamin-A are 1.23-3.66 IU/well. At 1.23IU/well there is complete death of cancer cells following eighteen days of incubation. It is of prime importance however to demonstrate that Vitamin-A in these concentrations do not have toxic effects on normal cells. In order to look at this possibility the study of the effect of Vitamin-A on normal peripheral lymphocytes was undertaken. At all doses of Vitamin-A used on the ZR75-1 cancer cell line there was no effect on the proliferation of normal lymphocytes in culture.

In conclusion therefore these data suggest a role for further research into the potential use of low doses of Vitamin-A as adjunctive therapy in breast cancer.

References

1. Lotan R (1980) Effects of Vitamin-A and its analogues (retinoids) on normal and neoplastic cells. Biochem Biophys Acta 605 : 33-91
2. Wolbach SB, Howe PR (1925) Tissue changes following deprivation of fat soluble A Vitamin. J Exp Med 42 : 735-777
3. Moore T (1967) Effects of Vitamin-A deficiency in animals. Pharmacology and toxicity of Vitamin-A. in : Sebrell WH, Harris RS (eds) The vitamins, 2nd ed, vol 1. Academic Press, New York, pp 245-266, pp 280-294
4. Mayer H, Bollag W, Hanni R, Ruegg R (1978) retinoids. A new class of compounds with prophylactic and therapeutic activities in oncology and dermatology. Experientia 34 : 1105-1119

5. Trown PW, Buck MJ, Hansen R (1976) Inhibition of growth and regression of transplantable rat chondrosarcoma by three retinoids. Cancer Treat Rep 60 : 1647-1653
6. Stepp W (1909) Versuche uber futterung mit lipoidfrier nahrung. Biochem Z 22 : 452-460
7. Drummond JC (1920) The nomenclature of the so-called accessory food factors (Vitamins). Biochem J 14 : 660
8. Bollag W (1983) Vitamin-A and retinoids : from nutrition to pharmacotherapy in dermatology and oncology. Lancet 1 : 860-863
9. Mayshens FL jr. Modulation of abnormal growth by retinoids : a clinical perspective of the biological phenomenon. Life Sci 28 : 2323-2327
10. Moon RC, McCormick DL, Mehta RG (1983) Inhibition of carcinogenesis by retinoids. Cancer Res 42 : 2469-2475
11. Lotan R, Nicolson GL (1977) Inhibitory effects of retinoic acid or retinyl acetate on the growth of untransformed, transformed and tumour cells in vitro. J Natl Cancer Inst 59 : 1717-1722
12. Vitale C, Rakowski I, Raza A (1986) (abstr). Number of DNA replication cycles completed by HL-60 cells during differentiation induced by 13 Cis-retinoic acid(RA). Blood 68 (Suppl) : 194a
13. Moon RC, Grubbs CJ, Sporn MB. Inhibition of 7,12, Dimethylbenz(a) Antracene-induced mammary carcinogenesis vy Retinyl Acetate. Cancer Res 36 : 2626-2630

Abstract. *Natural and synthetic analogues of Vitamin-A are involved in the modulation of differentiation and proliferation processes in many cell types. Vitamin-A has been under intense scrutiny by many investigators for the past decades. The aim of this study was to investigate the effects of Vitamin-A on a metastatic oestrogen dependant breast cancer cell line ZR75-1.*

Measurement of the early level of mdr1 gene expression is a predictive marker of tumour response in breast cancer patients treated by Neo-Adjuvant chemotherapy

JY Pierga, S Chevillard, P Pouillart, Ph Vielh

The development of resistance to Adriamycin (ADR) remains a major obstacle in the treatment of cancer patients [1]. The main mechanism of resistance termed multidrug resistance (MDR) has consistently been associated with an increased expression of the 170 Kd membrane glycoprotein (Gp170) [2]. Gp170 is encoded by the mdr1 gene [3] and functions as an energy-dependent drug efflux pump that reduces intracellular drug accumulation [4]. The overexpression of Gp170 and the increased mdr1 gene transcription found in *in vivo* and *in vitro* MDR cells correlate with the level of resistance [5, 6].

We have recently shown in the human A549 lung adenocarcinoma, cell line that : 1) three days after an ADR treatment, cells exhibit overexpression of Gp170, and ; 2) three months after the initial ADR treatment, cells cultivated in ADR free medium constitutively express Gp170 and are resistant to an ADR retreatment [7].

The purpose of our study was : 1) to test if these *in vitro* data were relevant in *in vivo* human cancer, and ; 2) to investigate whether an early mdr1 gene transcription was a reliable marker of the long term clinical response, in a prospective series of breast cancer patients treated by Neo-Adjuvant chemotherapy.

Material and methods

A prospective series of 38 consecutive patients with breast adenocarcinomas treated by Neo-Adjuvant chemotherapy was conducted at the Institut Curie. Patients with stages II or III breast cancer were treated by 4 cycles of 1 week consisting of either 5-Fluorouracil, Adriamycin and Cyclophosphamide (FAC) or 5-Fluorouracil, thiotepa and Cyclophosphamide (FTC). Sequential fine needle sampling without aspiration [8] were performed in all patients with a 23 gauge needle before treatment (day 0), at the end of the first cycle (day 8) and before the beginning of the second cycle of chemotherapy (day 28). RNA extraction was done using the RNAzol kit (Biotech). The study of mdr1 gene transcription was performed by reverse PCR [9]. cDNA obtained using random hexanucleotide primers were used for enzymatic amplification with specific primers, and the yield of the mdr1 gene transcription was normalized to the yield of the PCR product for an internal control sequence (β2 microglobulin). PCR products were analyzed after polyacrylamide gel electrophoresis, blotting,

---

Institut Curie, 26 rue d'Ulm, 75231 Paris Cedex 05, France

and hybridization with internal oligonucleotides to the amplified sequences. Clinical response was measured at the end of the four months of chemotherapy : complete response, partial response (> 50 %), and incomplete response (< 50 %) or progression.

Results and discussion

Typical examples of autoradiographies obtained from sequential fine needle samples of breast tumours are shown in Fig. 1. In each panel the upper bands (160 bp) and the lower bands (120 bp) correspond to the mdr1 and $\beta2$ microglobulin PCR products, respectively. The 3 lanes (1, 2, 3) of a given panel correspond to the sequential tumour samples obtained at day 0, day 8 and day 28 of a patient, respectively. The lower right panel corresponds to the controls. The KBA1 cell line overexpressing the mdr1 gene is on the left lane, the KB3.1 cell line which does not express the mdr1 gene is on the middle lane, and the right lane corresponds to the negative control without RNA. Patient A shows the absence of any detectable mdr1 gene expression before and after the first cycle of chemotherapy. Patient B shows no detectable mdr1 gene expression before the first cycle of chemotherapy and an increased expression after the first cycle of treatment. Patient C shows a detectable and constant mdr1 gene expression before and after the first cycle of chemotherapy.

Table 1 illustrates the number of patient's tumours in which a mdr1 gene overexpression was observed, according to the type of Neo-Adjuvant chemotherapy. Out of the 38 patients sequentially analyzed, 27 and 11 were treated by FAC and FTC, respectively. Out of these 38 tumours, 13 (34 %) exhibited a mdr1 gene overexpression during the first cycle of chemotherapy. This increased expression was more often observed following FAC (41 %) than FTC (18 %).

Table 2 summarizes data comparing mdr1 gene expression measured at the end of the first cycle, and clinical response evaluated at the end of the fourth cycle. Out of the 38 cases, 30 were found concordant and 8 discordant. Concordant results are shown in the upper part of the table showing that : 1) a low and constant level of mdr1 gene expression corresponds to a tumour size reduction of more than 50 % in 14 cases, and ; 2) a high or increased level of mdr1 gene expression corresponds to a non significant reduction or a progression of the tumour size in 16 cases. Discordant results (21 %) are depicted in the lower part of Table 2.

In summary, a correlation between measurement of mdr1 gene expression at the end of the first cycle of chemotherapy, and tumour response evaluated at the end of the fourth cycle of treatment is observed in 78.9 % of patients.

Determining mechanisms of drug resistance is critical to the development of rational therapeutic strategies in order to overcome or prevent drug resistance. The question of the relevance of the mdr1 gene transcription in the clinical situation is still opened. Our results obtained from this preliminary series of 38 breast cancer patients treated by Neo-Adjuvant chemotherapy show that : 1) an early increased expression of the mdr1 gene may be observed *in vivo* in one-third of patients, and ; 2) the analysis of this early mdr1 gene expression seems to be a reliable predictive marker of clinical response.

Measurement of the early level of mdr1 expression

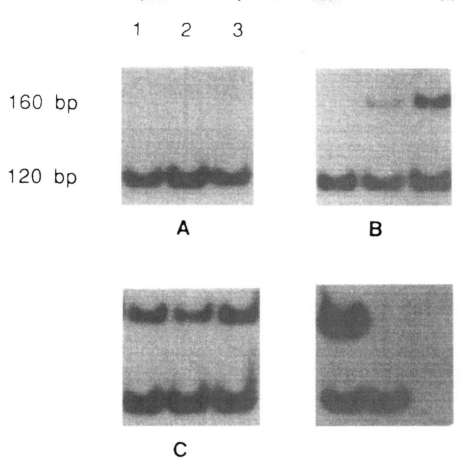

Fig. 1. Typical examples of autoradiographies showing mdr1 and β2 microglobulin expression in sequential fine needle samples obtained from breast cancer patients treated by Neo-Adjuvant chemotherapy

Table 1. Mdr1 gene overexpression according to the type of Neo-Adjuvant chemotherapy

Type of chemotherapy	Number of patients	mdr1 gene overexpression
FAC	27	11 (41 %)
FTC	11	2 (18 %)
Total	38	13 (34 %)

Table 2. Comparison of mdr1 gene expression (end of the 1st cycle) and clinical response (end of the 4th cycle)

mdr1 gene expression	clinical response	FAC	FTC	
low and constant	↓	10	4	14
high or increased	→ or ↑	12	4	16
		22 81.5 %	8 72.8 %	30 78.9 %
low and constant	→	2	1	3
high or increased	↓	3	2	5
		5 18.5 %	3 27.2 %	8 21.1 %

References

1. I Pastan, M Gottesman (1987) Multiple-drug resistance in human cancer. N Engl J Med 316 : 1388-1393
2. M Bradley, P Juranka, V Ling (1988) Mechanism of multidrug resistance. Biochim Biophys Acta 948 : 87-128
3. M Gottesman, I Pastan (1988) The multidrug transporter, a double-edged sword. J Biol Chem 263 : 12163-12166
4. J Endicott, V Ling (1989) The biochemistry of P-glycoprotein-mediated multidrug resistance. Ann Rev Biochem 58 : 137-171
5. D Shen, A Fojo, J Chin, I Roninson, N Richert, M Gottesman (1986) Human multidrug-resitant cell lines : increased mdr1 expression can preceed gene amplification. Science 232 : 643-645
6. G Goldstein, H Galski, A Fojo, M Willingham, S Lai, A Gazdar, R Pirker, A Green, W Crist, G Brodeur, M Lieber, J Cossman, M Gottesman, I Pastan (1989) Expression of multidrug resistance gene in human cancers. J Natl Cancer Inst 81 : 116-124
7. S Chevillard, Ph Vielh, G Bastian, J Coppey (1992) A single 24 h contact with Adriamycin provokes the emergence of resistant cells expressing the Gp170. Anticancer Res 12 : 495-500
8. A Zajdela, P Zillhardt, N Voillemot (1987) Cytological diagnosis by fine needle sampling without aspiration. Cancer 9 : 1201-1205
9. K Noonan, C Beck, T Holzmayer, J Chin, J Wunder, I Andrulis, A Gazdar, C Willman, B Griffith, D Von Hoff, I Roninson (1990) Quantitative analysis of mdr1 (multidrug resistance) gene expression in human tumors by polymerase chain reaction. Proc Natl Acad Sci 87 : 7160-7164

Hematologic effects of recombinant human Interleukin-6 (rhIL-6) in sarcoma patients receiving maid chemotherapy : phase I trial

RM Bukowski*, R Isaacs**, M Gordon***, GD Demetri****, B Amuels*****, DC Young**, S Samuel**, D McLain*, D Levitt**

Currently, standard therapy for unresectable sarcoma consists of cytotoxic chemotherapy. Overall, Doxorubicin has been the most effective single agent in the treatment of sarcoma, with response rates ranging from 15 % to 35 % [1]. Long-term survival, however, is ≤ 5 % following optimal Doxorubicin-based combination chemotherapy [2, 3]. These clinical results may be improved upon by increasing the dosages administered, and a correlation has been noted between the doses of Doxorubicin and tumor response rates in at least 3 randomized clinical studies [4-6]. One regimen utilized as current treatment for patients with unresectable sarcomas is the MAID chemotherapy regimen, consisting of Doxorubicin, Ifosfamide and DTIC with the uroprotective agent Mesna. This regimen has been reported to result in a 47 % overall response rate, with 10 % complete responders [7]. The primary dose limiting toxicity of this regimen, however, is myelosuppression, which results in a reduction of the Ifosfamide dosage in at least 40 % of the patients following the first cycle of chemotherapy [7]. The neutropenia associated with the MAID chemotherapy appears to be less severe and shorter in duration when agents such as rhGM-CSF or rhIL-3 are administered following the chemotherapy [8].

The biological and pharmacologic effects of IL-6 on hematopoiesis have been extensively examined in animal models. Originally characterized as Interferon-β-2, a B-cell stimulating factor [9], IL-6 has many pleiotropic effects, such as stimulation of T lymphocyte proliferation, and induction of differentiation of cytotoxic T lymphocytes [10]. Additionally, it has been found to enhance synthesis of acute phase proteins by hepatic cells [11]. IL-6 also elevates blood platelet counts in normal rodents and primates *in vivo* with concomitant increases in bone marrow cellularity and megakaryocyte size and ploidy [12-16]. More importantly, however, the hematopoietic activity of rhIL-6 has resulted in accelerated recovery from myelosuppression due to cytotoxic chemotherapy and radiation and following bone marrow transplantation in murine models [17-19]. The purpose of the present trial is to determine the toxicity of rhIL-6 and in a preliminary fashion its hematopoietic effects when given following MAID chemotherapy.

Cleveland Clinic Cancer Center*, Cytokine Development Unit, Sandoz Pharmaceuticals**, Indiana University School of Medicine***, Dana Farber Cancer Institute****, Lutheran General Hospital*****

Patients and methods

Patient eligibility

Patients ⩾ 16 years old, with previously untreated, histologically documented sarcoma were eligible for this trial. Patients were required to have a performance status of ⩾ 60 % (Karnofsky scale), a life expectancy of > 12 weeks, and adequate organ function characterized by WBC > 3.000/ul, platelets > 100,000/ul, bilirubin < 2.0 mg/dl, SGOT < 2x normal, serum creatinine < 1.8 mg/dl, BUN < 30 mg/dl and negative HIV antibody titer. Exclusion criteria included bone marrow or CNS metastases, significant cardiac disease or respiratory disorder, prior pelvic radiotherapy or radiotherapy within 3 weeks, any prior investigational agent within 4 weeks, or any other cytokine or biological agent within 8 weeks. Informed consent was obtained as required by Institutional and Food and Drug Administration guidelines.

Treatment plan

Cohorts of 4 to 6 patients are receiving rhIL-6 at planned dose levels of 1.0, 2.5, 5.0, 10.0 and 25.0 ug/kg/d S.Q. once daily for 10 days in cycle 0. This is followed by a 7 days rest, at which time MAID chemotherapy is initiated at the following dosages on days 1-3 : Mesna 500 mg/m^2 I.V. bolus (x4), Doxorubicin 20 mg/m^2 I.V., Ifosfamide 2500 mg/m^2 I.V., and DTIC 300 mg/m^2 given every 21 days. Patients are then randomized to receive the same rhIL-6 dose as in cycle 0 on days 5-14 in either the first cycle (treatment group I) or second cycle (treatment group II) of MAID. Patients are eligible for additional MAID + rhIL-6 cycles upon completion of cycles 0, 1, and 2 based upon clinical response or disease stabilization/improvement.

Evaluation criteria

Safety and tolerability parameters to be examined, in addition to spontaneous and solicited symptomatology and physical examination, included : hematologic variables, serum chemistries, serum and urine protein examinations, abdominal CT scan for liver and spleen size, and serum antibodies to IL-6. Pharmacodynamic parameters included WBC and differential, platelet count and size, bone marrow histology and CFU determinations, and serum levels of acute phase proteins. Assessments of tumor size and metastases are planned in all cycles to determine the possible adjuvant antineoplastic activity of rhIL-6. Serum pharmacokinetic specimens are being collected and will be later analyzed in an attempt to correlate rhIL-6 concentrations with the concentration of C-reactive protein and with the rate and extent of WBC and platelet count increases.

Results

Sixteen patients were entered into the study as of January 1993, with 1 patient ineligible and subsequently discontinued on day 2 due to positive Hepatitis B surface antigen. The median age of the patients was 57 years (range 29-78), with a male to female ratio of 6/9, and performance status distribution as follows: 100 % — 6; 90 % — 6; 80 % — 1; 70 % — 2. Leiomyosarcoma was the predominant diagnosis (40 %), with the remaining diagnoses consisting of fibrosarcoma (13 %), myxoid sarcoma (13 %), chondrosarcoma (7 %), and unclassified sarcoma (27 %). Patient enrollment has proceeded as follows (dose level — treatment group I/treatment group II): 1.0 ug/kg — 2/2, 2.5 ug/kg — 3/1, 5.0 ug/kg — 3/2, 10.0 ug/kg — 1/1. To date, 13 patients are evaluable.

Toxicity related to rhIL-6 has been mild to moderate, consisting of constitutional symptoms such as fever/chills, arthralgia/myalgia, nausea, vomiting, fatigue, diarrhea and headache. Elevations from baseline in hepatic enzymes have occurred, but were mild to moderate and did not appear dose related. Mild anemia has been observed in all patients and may, however, be related to increasing rhIL-6 dose.

All patients completed cycle 0, with corresponding increases in WBC, neutrophil and platelet counts. Eight of 13 patients completed treatment through cycle 2, with 3 of the patients discontinuing due to progressive disease. Of these 8 patients, 4 experienced an increase in platelet count, 1 a response based upon ANC, and 3 progressive disease or no hematological response. Although preliminary, both RBC and platelet transfusion requirements were decreased within the MAID + rhIL-6 cycle. Illustrated below are the mean hematologic values obtained within each cycle for WBC and platelet counts.

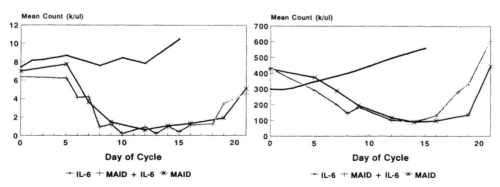

Fig. 1. Phase I Study of rhIL-6/MAID in sarcoma mean WBC count (n = 13)
Fig. 2. Mean platelet count (n = 13)

Discussion

To date, dose limiting toxicity of rhIL-6 has not been reached, and tolerance is good. The major toxicity is the occurrence of chills, fever, and a flu-like syndrome. The MTD will be $\geqslant$ 10 ug/kg/day. When cycles of chemotherapy followed by rhIL-6 are compared to those without concomitant growth factor, no difference in total white blood cell or absolute neutrophil counts were seen, but platelet recovery may occur earlier. The biologic effects noted during cycle 0 include thrombocytosis and increases in acute phase reactants. Preliminary results of this trial indicate rhIL-6 has moderate toxicity at the doses employed, and may have effects on thrombopoiesis.

References

1. Antman K, Elias A (1988) Chemotherapy of advanced soft tissue sarcomas. Semin Surg Oncol 4 : 53-58
2. Subramaniam S and Wiltshaw E (1978) Chemotherapy of sarcoma — A comparison of three regimens. Lancet 1 : 683-686
3. Yap BS, Sinkovics JG, Benjamin RS et al (1979) Survival and relapse patterns of complete responders in adults with advanced soft tissue sarcomas. Proc Am Assoc Cancer Res 20 : 352 (Abstr)
4. Schoenfeld D, Rosenbaum C, Horton J et al (1982) A comparison of Adriamycin v.s. Vincristine and Adriamycin and Cyclophosphamide for advanced sarcoma. Cancer 50 : 2757-2762
5. Bodey GP, Rodriguez V, Murphy WK et al (1981) Protected environment-prophylactic antibiotic program for malignant sarcoma : Randomized trial during remission induction chemotherapy. Cancer 47 : 2422-2429
6. Pinedo HM, Bramwell VHC, Mouridson MS et al (1984) CYVADIC in advanced soft tissue sarcoma : A randomized study comparing two schedules. A study of the EORTC soft tissue and bone sarcoma group. Cancer 53 : 1825-1832
7. Elias A, Ryan L, Smith A et al (1989) Response to Mesna, Doxorubicin, Ifosfamide and Dacarbazine in 108 patients with metastatic or unresectable sarcoma and no prior chemotherapy. J Clin Oncol 7 : 1208-1216
8. Antman KS, Griffin JD, Elias A et al (1988) Effect of recombinant granulocyte-macrophage colony-stimulating factor on chemotherapy-induced myelosuppression. N Engl J Med 319 : 593-598
9. Okada M, Sakaguchi N, Yoshimura N et al (1983) B cell growth factors and B cell differentiation factor from human T hybridomas. Two distinct kinds of B cell growth factor and their synergism in B cell proliferation. J Exp Med 157 (2) : 583-590
10. Okada M, Kitahara M, Kishimoto S et al (1988) IL-6/BSF-2 functions as a killer helper factor in the in vitro induction of cytotoxic T cells. J Immunol 141 (5) : 1543-1549
11. Gauldie J, Richards C, Harnish D et al (1987) Interferon $B_2$2/B-cell stimulatory factor type 2 shares identity with monocyte-derived hepatocyte-stimulating factor and regulates the major acute phase protein response in liver cells. Proc Natl Acad Sci 84 : 7251-7255
12. Ishibashi T, Kimura H, Shikama Y et al (1989) Interleukin-6 is a potent thrombopoietic factor in vivo in mice. Blood 74 : 1241-1244

13. Asano S, Okano A, Ozawa K et al (1990) In vivo effects of recombinant human interleukin-6 in primates : Stimulated production of platelets. Blood 75 : 1602-1605
14. Carrington PA, Hill RJ, Stenberg PE et al (1991) Multiple in vivo effects of Interleukin-3 and Interleukin-6 on murine megakaryocytopoiesis. Blood 77 : 34-41
15. Hill RJ, Warren MK, Stenberg P et al (1991) Stimulation of megakaryocytopoiesis in mice by human recombinant Interleukin-6. Blood 77 : 42-48
16. McDonald TP, Cottrell MB, Swearingen CJ, Clift R (1991) Comparative effects of thrombopoietin and Interleukin-6 on murine megakaryocytopoiesis and platelet production. Blood 77 : 735-740
17. Takatsuki F, Okano A, Suzuki C et al (1990) Interleukin-6 perfusion stimulates reconstitution of the immune and hematopoietic systems after 5-Fluorouracil treatment. Cancer Res 50 : 2885-2890
18. Patchen ML, MacVittie TJ, Williams JL et al (1991) Administration of Interleukin-6 stimulates multilineage hematopoiesis and accelerates recovery from radiation-induced hematopoietic depression. Blood 77 : 472-480
19. Okano A, Suzuki C, Takatsuki F, et al (1991) Effects of Interleukin-6 on hematopoiesis in bone marrow-transplanted mice. Transplantation 47 : 738-740.

Role of G-CSF and GM-CSF in the treatment of febrile neutropenia induced by chemotherapy; preliminary results of a randomized trial

F Rivera, JI Mayordomo, MT Díaz-Puente, MP Lianes, M López-Brea, E López, L Paz-Ares, S Alonso, H Cortés-Funes

Febrile neutropenia (FN) is the second most frequent cause of death in patients receiving chemotherapy [1]. Mortality of FN remains about 5-10 % in spite of modern antibiotic regimens, and moreover the human and financial cost are high [2, 3, 4]. Minor changes in antibiotic therapy are unlikely to result in substantial decrease of the mortality of FN and so new approaches are needed.

In previous studies [5, 2] it has been shown that neutrophil count and the duration of neutropenia, are the most important prognostic factors.

Two haematological colony-stimulating factors, G-CSF and GM-CSF have been shown to prevent chemotherapy-induced myelosupression and their value in the prophyilactic setting has been explored in several tumors and chemotherapic regimens, through randomized trials [6, 12]. However, in spite of their potential ability to reduce the duration of neutropenia, the role of these factors in the treatment of FN remains unexplored: there is no randomized trial in the medical literature testing the value of adding CSFs to standard antibiotic therapy in patients who have already developed neutropenia and fever [12].

Patients and methods

In patients with solid tumors or lymphoma on treatment with standard-dose chemotherapy who develop febrile neutropenia, we are testing if the addition of G-CSF or GM-CSF to standard antibiotic therapy can improve the following parameters:

• Major endpoints: 1) Duration of severe neutropenia ($< 500/mm^3$); 2) Duration of global neutropenia ($< 1,000/mm^3$); 3) Duration of fever; 4) Duration of hospital stay.

• Secondary endpoints: 1) Necessity to change antibiotic therapy; 2) Cost of therapy of FN; 3) Pharmacological toxicity in FN.

Patiens must fulfil all of the following inclusion criteria: 1) Histologicaly-proven neoplasm; 2) Being on chemotherapy at the Division of Medical Oncology of the « 12 de Octubre » Hospital of Madrid. 3) Neutrophil count $< 500/mm^3$; 4) Axilary temperature >38 °C and 5) Informed consent.

The exclusion criteria are: 1) Life expectancy less than 1 month; 2) History of hypersensitivity to G-CSF and/or GM-CSF; 3) Treatment with G-CSF

Sv. de Oncología Médica, Hospital « 12 de Octubre », Madrid, Spain. Ctra Andalucía, km 5.4. Madrid 28041, Spain

or GM-CSF in the previous 15 days ; 4) Previous or actual diagnosis of myeloid leukemia (AML or CML) ; 5) Non-fultfilment of any inclusion criteria.

Procedure of inclusion and randomization : Patients with FN are seen at the emergency room (or clinic) by the medical oncologist on duty. Vital signs, physical exploration, data of infectious focality are assesed. All these complementary explorations are performed : Blood counts, cultures (blood, orine...), blood and urine chemistries, chest X-ray and other if indicated.

With all these data a decision on antibiotic schedule is taken : in most cases Ceftazidime, plus Amikacin [3, 4, 13]. This antibiotic therapy is initiated immediately. Informed consent is obtained and randomization is done using closed envelopes : Arm A : G-CSF, 5 microgrames/Kg once a day, s.q. ; Arm B : GM-CSF, 5 microgrames/Kg once a day, s.q. and Arm C : Placebo, s.q. Treatment with CSFs or placebo is initiated immediatly after diagnosis of FN.

Criteria for discontinuation of therapy : Treatment with G-CSF, GM-CSF or placebo is stopped when neutrophils are above $1,000/mm^3$ for 2 consecutive days. For discontinuation of antibiotics all of the following requisites must be fulfilled : 1) Two days afebrile ; 2) ANC $>1,000/mm^2$ for 2 consecutive days and 3) At least 5 days on i.v. antibiotics (7 days for patients with clinically or microbiologically documented infection). The patient is to be discharged as soon as i.v. antibiotics are stopped.

Results

Between November of 1991 and January of 1993, 90 patients have been included in the study.

The most important prognostic factors for febrile neutropenia are well balanced in the 3 treatment arms : age, mean neutrophil count on admission, number of patients with ANC $<100/mm^3$, number of pts with microbiologically-documented infection and number of patients with criteria of severity on admission (hipotension, oliguria, metabolic acidosis). The initial antibiotic schedule in the 3 arms were similar too (in most patients Ceftazidime plus Amikacin).

Results are shown in Table 1. With the addition of G-CSF or GM-CSF we have found a reduction statistically significant in the following parameters : a) the median number of days with ANC $< 500/mm^3$ (Fig. 1) ; b) the median number of days with ANC $< 1,000/mm^3$ (Fig. 2) and c) the median number of days of hospital stay (Fig. 3). Difference was found between each of the CSFs-treatment arms and the placebo group ($p < 0.001$ in all cases). The number of patients with ANC $< 100/mm^3$ on admission falling later under $100/mm^3$, was significatively less in the group receiving CSFs than in the placebo group ($p < 0.05$).

We have found no difference in the median number of days with fever, nor in the number of patients requiring change of antibiotics.

We have found no difference between the G-CSF and the GM-CSF arms.

Seven patients included in this study died during the hospital stay for FN. Only 4 of them were infection-related deaths. One was in the GM-CSF arm

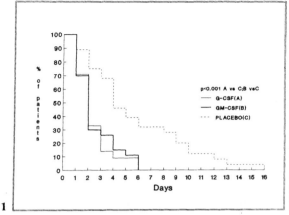
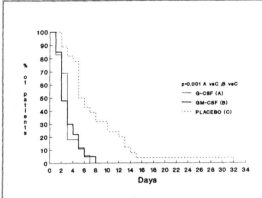
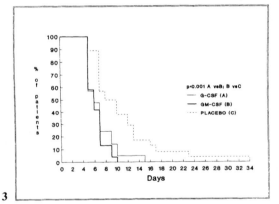

Fig. 1. Number of days with ANC < 500/mm^3
Fig. 2. Number of days with ANC < 1000/mm^3
Fig. 3. Number of days of hospital stay

Table 1. Treatment results

	G-CSF	GM-CSF	Placebo	p
Median number of days with ANC<100 (range)	2 (1-4)	2 (1-5)	4 (1-10)	<0.05 *
Median number of days with ANC<500 (range)	1 (1-6)	1 (1-6)	3 (1-16)	<0.001 *
Median number of days with ANC<1000 (range)	2 (1-7)	1 (1-8)	5 (2-32)	<0.001 *
Pts ANC>100 on admission falling <100 later	4/18	2/19	6/19	<0.05 *
Median number of days with fever (range)	1 (1-8)	2 (1-7)	2 (1-10)	NS
Medain number of days of hospital stay (range)	5 (5-15)	5 (5-10)	8 (5-34)	<0.001 *
Number of pts requiring change of antibiotics	5	12	10	NS
Infection-related deaths (+ other deaths)	2 (+1)	1 (+1)	1 (+1)	NS

* G-CSF v.s. placebo ; GM-CSF v.s. placebo. ** G-CSF + GM-CSF v.s. placebo

2 in the G-CSF arm and 1 in the placebo arm. All of them had an ANC < $100/mm^3$ on admission and in all cases there were a microbiologically documented infection (blood culture positive). The other 3 patients (1 in each arm) died because progressive disease. In terms of mortality we have found no significant difference between the 3 treatment arms. The only CSF-related toxicity observed has been fever related to GM-CSF in 4 patients and to G-CSF in 1 patient. Two patients developed asymptomatic neutropenia after withdrawal of the CSF (both in the GM-CSF arm). The ANC went down to 480 and 630 but it went up in 1 day and there were no problem.

The median number of days under CSFs treatment was 4 (range 2-8) in the G-CSF arm and 4 (range 2-8) in the GM-CSF arm. The median cost in thousands of US dollars was 2, 3 (range 2, 1-6, 3) in the G-CSF arm ; 2, 3 (2, 1-5, 5) in the GM-CSF arm and 3, 1 (2, 0-17) in the placebo group. The difference is significative between each of the CSFs arms and the placebo one ($p < 0.01$).

Discussion

These results are provisional and accrual of patients is continuing. In spite of this, with the data we already have conclude that : 1) the addition of G-CSF or GM-CSF to usual antibiotic therapy in patients with febrile neutropenia due to standard-dose chemotherapy results in a significant shortening of the period of neutropenia ; 2) this leads to a shorter duration of hospital stay ; 3) this approach is cost-effective ; 4) discontinuation of G-CSF or GM-CSF after ANC > 1,000 for 2 consecutive days is safe ; 5) toxicity of short-term G-CSF or GM-CSF is negligible, and it may be superseded by toxicity of long-term anti-infectious agents in cases of long-lasting febrile neutropenia and 6) the effect on mortality may be very difficult to quantify, given the low infection-related mortality (5 %).

A increasingly frequent practice is giving CSFs in a prophylactic setting to all patients after each course of standard-dose chemotherapy. Only less than 20 % of patients develop febrile neutropenia after a course of most of these regimens. We think it could be interesting to compare in a randomized trial this simple approach of giving G-CSF or GM-CSF to patients on standard-dose chemotherapy only when they develop febrile neutropenia with the systematic administration of CSFs to all patients after each course of chemotherapy.

References

1. Lieschke GM (1990) Infections in patients receiving chemotherapy. Focus on Growth Factors 1 : 6-9
2. Elliot CR, Patter JL (1988) The effect of different measures of outcome on the results of studies of antibiotic therapy in febrile neutropenic patients. Clin Invest Med 11 : 327-330

3. Wade JC (1989) Antibiotic therapy for the febrile granulocitopenic patient : Combination therapy v.s. monotherapy. J Infect Dis 11 (Suppl 7) : 1572-1581
4. Patter JL, Weir L (1986) Reporting the results of randomized trials of empiric antibiotics in febrile neutropenic patients : a critical survey. J Clin Oncol 4 : 346-352
5. Bodey GP, Buckley M, Sathe YS, Freireich EJ (1966) Quantitative relationships between circulating leukocytes and infection in patients with acute leukemia. Ann Intern Med 64 : 328-340
6. Bronchud MH, Scarffe JH, Tatcher N, Crowther D, Souza LM, Alton K, Testh NG, Dexter TM (1987) Phase I/II study of recombinant human granulocyte colony-stimulating factor in patients receiving intensive chemotherapy for small cell lung cancer. Br J Cancer 56 : 809-813
7. Morstyn G, Souza LM, Keech J et al (1988) Effect of granulocyte colony-stimulating factor on neutropenia induced by cytotoxic chemotherapy. Lancet 1 : 667-670
8. Gabrilove JL, Jakubowski A, Scher H et al (1988) Effect of granulocyte colony-stimulating factor on neutropenia and associated morbidity due to chemotherapy for transitional-cell carcinoma of the urothelium. N Engl J Med 318 : 1414-1422
9. Antman K, Griffin J, Elias A et al (1988) Effect of recombinant human granulocyte-macrophage colony stimulating factor on chemotherapy-induced myelosupression. N Engl J Med : 593-598
10. Herrmann F, Wieser M, Schulz G et al (1988) Single daily subcutaneous administration of rhGM-CSF ameliorates hematopoietic toxicity of chemotherapy in outpatients. Blood 72 (suppl) : 390 a (abstract)
11. Morstyn G, Stuart-Harris R, Bishop J et al (1989) Optimal scheduling of granulocyte-macrophage colony stimulating factor (GM-CSF) for the abrogation of chemotherapy induced neutropenia in small cell lung cancer. Proc Am Soc Clin Oncol 8 : 850 a (abstact)
12. Lieschke GJ, Burgess AW (1992) Granulocyte colony-stimulating factor and granulocyte-macrophage colony-stimulating factor. N Engl J Med 327 : 28-35 (1st part) ; 327 : 99-106 (2nd part)
13. EORTC International Antimicrobial Therapy Project Group (1978) Three antibiotic regimens in the treatment of infections in granulocytopenic patients with cancer. J Infect Dis 137 : 14-29

First line chemotherapy for patients with multiple myeloma with vad regimen followed by consolidation with high-dose chemoradiotherapy with peripheral stem cells autograft (PSCA): the experience of IGR center

P Brault*, E Gilles*, A Ibrahim*, F Beaujean**, S Jimenz*, G Tertian***, M Hayat*, JH Bourhis*, JL Pico*

No significant progress has been achieved in the treatment of multiple myeloma. Indeed, the reference combination Melphalan-Prednisone, introduced in 1970's by Alexanian affords a median survival of between 20 and 44 months and between 20 and 26 months, exclusively for stage III disease [1].

The use of more aggressive regimens with the adjunction of one or several alkylating agents yields better results in terms of response, but they are not significantly different in terms of survival [4, 5, 10].

A novel approach, developed since 1984, is based on the VAD protocol designed by Barlogie's team. This particular combination regimen consists in administering low doses of Adriamycin and Vincristine over 4 days in a continuous infusion. A corticoid (Dexamethasone) is given daily for 4 consecutive days every 5 days, in association at high-doses. Initially administered as second line therapy in refractory patients or those who relapsed early after standard treatment (Melphalan — Prednisone), the first documented series achieved 60 % of objective responses, albeit of relatively short duration (around 8 months) [2].

These promising results prompted certain teams to propose this regimen as first line treatment of bulky, poor prognosis myeloma (Stage III with a high ß-2-microglobulin level).

The aim of our study was to test the feasibility and efficiency of a conventional chemotherapy regimen comprising 3 cycles of VAD (Vincristine 0.4 mg/m^2/d in continuous infusion d1 to d4, Adriamycin, 9 mg/m^2/d in continuous infusion, d1 to d4, Dexamethasone, 40 mg total dosage, d1 to d4, d9 to d12 and d17 to d20) followed, in the event of response, by a cycle of high-dose Endoxan (120 mg/kg over 2 days). Endoxan is used to obtain a maximum reduction of the tumor load and, most of all, as the period of aplasia comes to an end, it permits the collection of circulating hematopoietic stem cells by cell separation. Patients then receive total body irradiation (TBI) as consolidation therapy, (if not contraindicated, according to their medical history) and high-dose Melphalan (140 mg/m^2) followed by an autograft of peripheral stem cells. Inclusion criteria are summarized in Table 1.

---

* Institut Gustave Roussy, rue Camille Desmoulins, 94805 Villejuif Cedex-France, ** Centre Départemental de Transfusion Sanguine, 94000 Créteil-France, *** Centre Hospitalier Universitaire, 94270 Le Kremlin Bicêtre, France

Table 1. Inclusion criterias

- Age < 65 years
- Stage ⩾ II
- Index OMS ⩽ 2
- Diagnosis of multiple myeloma according to the durie and salmon criterias

Materials and methods

From February 1989 to December 1992, 32 patients (20 males, 12 females, median age 48 (range 28-63) were included in this study. The type of paraprotein secreted by multiple myeloma was IgA, IgG and a light chain protein in 11, 10 and 8 cases respectively, in 2 patients, no paraprotein was secreted and 1 patient had plasma-cell leukemia. There were 31 cases of stage III and 1 case of stage II disease with a heavy tumor burden. Most patients had not been treated prior to inclusion in the protocol, 9 had already received a maximum of 6 cycles of the Alkeran-Prednisone combination, and 3 irradiation to isolated lytic lesion.

Results

One hundred and fourteen cycles of VAD were administered (median number of 3 cycles per patient, range 1-6). A 72 % response rate was observed after 3 courses of treatment (12.5 % were refractory primaries, 15.5 % exhibited progressive disease at 3 cycles of VAD). Twenty-five patients were given a course of high-dose Cyclophosphamide which allowed peripheral stem cells to be collected in 14 patients. The 9 others, for whom grafting was contraindicated, were treated by α-Interferon immunotherapy. Two patients had an allogeneic bone marrow transplant. Peripheral stem cells were collected as originally planned and growth factors were not used. The median number of times cell separation was performed per patient was 4 [3, 8]. The median number of mononuclear and CFU-GM harvested were respectively $5.2.10^8$/kg (2.4-6.0) and $42.5.10^4$/kg (2.5-84). To date 16 patients have had a graft, 14 of whom received an autograft of peripheral stem cells and 2 young patients (< 45 years), a bone marrow allograft from an HLA-matched sibling donor. The median age of autograft patients is 48 years (36 — 54) ; 13 patients had stage III disease and 1 stage II. The conditioning treatment comprised total body irradiation (TBI) and Melphalan (140 mg/m^2) in 11 cases and combination Busulfan (16 mg/kg) and Melphalan (140 mg/m^2) in 3 cases (for whom TBI was contraindicated due to a previous history of radiotherapy). Hematological toxicity and blood transfusion requirements are reported in Table 2. A single patient died of veno-occlusive disease of the liver and infectious complications were never the cause of a dismal outcome.

With an average post-graft follow-up of 18 months (1-40), relapse-free survival for autograft patients is 71 %. Three relapses occurred at a median post-graft period of 12 months (11-23). The patient who had plasma-cell leukemia relapsed 19 months after the diagnosis (12 months after the autograft) and died with progressive disease 24 months post-graft. The 2 patients who received an allogeneic graft died rapidly, at 4 and 5 months after the transplant due to graft-related complications. For the whole group, relapse-free survival is 50 % at 22 months whereas the relapse-free survival of non grafted patients is 21 % at 22 months.

Table 2. Autologous transplantation of peripheral hemotopoietic progenitors

*Hemotological Toxicity**	
• Days with anc < 500 :	9 (4-13)
• Days with anc < 100 :	9 (4-12)
• Days with platelets < 50,000 :	23 (2-94)
• Days with platelets < 20,000 :	16 (2-80)
Blood Transfusion support	
• Packed red cells :	4 units (0-16) in 2 episodes (0-8)
• Platelets :	50 units (6-210) in 5 episodes (1-18)

* 1 patient received G-CSF

It is obvious that the autograft recipients in this series were highly selected and therefore cannot be compared with the other patients, most of whom were refractory to therapy or treatment failures (9 patients) or cases whose general condition was poor (7 patients).

These results (71 % DFS at 18 months) are comparable to those published in the literature [6]. Intensified therapy with stem cell autografts as consolidation after conventional chemotherapy is a new, interesting approach to the management of this disease. The problem posed is that of the possible contamination of the stem cell graft with malignant plasma cells. Several studies conducted by Fermand at St Louis Hospital in Paris, have shown that the risk of contamination with this type of stem cell graft is mild. This risk could be probably eliminated by developing a more sophisticated procedure which consists in the positive selection of CD34+ stem cells and thus guaranteeing that there will be no likelihood of graft contamination.

Although *a prior* less satisfying, the use of bone marrow after *in vivo* and *in vitro* purging continues to be promoted by certain teams [3, 9]. Results are not very different with this method (estimated median duration of survival of the order of 70 % at 4 years).

The role of allogeneic bone marrow transplantation in the treatment of myeloma remains to be defined, since it has not been used extensively in this disease. According to the European Registry [7, 8] a median survival of 26 months has been achieved in a series of 90 patients (52 stage III, 38 stage I, 2 stage II, 9 CR, 41 PR, 40 PD at the time of graft). Deaths due to allograft-related complications were high (40 %). The likelihood of achieving cure or at least enhancing survival must be weighed against the potential risks of this type of graft.

Conclusion

Although highly selected, our 14 autograft patients enjoy a totally acceptable quality of life and the relapse-free survival rate is 71 % at 18 months. Even though the follow-up is short, this rate nonetheless demonstrates an improvement in the treatment of what was until now, constantly a fatal disease. The intensification of the treatment of multiple myeloma in patients below the age of 60 with stem cell autografts is a therapeutic strategy which ought to be developed in the years to come. This graft would not only permit an attenuation of the complications associated with myelosuppression, compared to other types of grafts. Safety against its possible contamination by neoplastic cells would also be ensured.

Another more sophisticated procedure, namely, that of blood grafts with the positive selection of CD34 + cells is in the process of being developed and deserves to be tested rapidly in this disease.

References

1. Alexanian R, Dreicer R (1984) Chemotherapy for multiple myeloma. Cancer 53 : 583-588
2. Barlogie B, Smith L, Alexanian R (1984) Effective treatment of advanced multiple myeloma refractory to alkylating agents. N Engl J Med 310 : 1353-1356
3. Barlogie B, Gharton G (1991) Bone marrow transplantation in multiple myeloma. Bone Marrow Transplant 7 : 71-79
4. Boccadoro M, Marmont F, Tribalto M et al (1991) Multiple Myeloma : VMCP/VBAP alternating combination chemotherapy is not superior to Melphalan and Prednisone even in high risk patients. J Clin Oncol 9 : 444-448
5. Cavagnaro F, Lein JM, Pavlosky S et al (1980) Comparison of two combination chemotherapy regimens for multiple myeloma : methyl CCNU, Cyclophosphamide and Prednisone versus Melphalan Prednisone. Cancer Treat Rep 64 : 73-79
6. Fermand JP, Levy Y, Gerota J et al (1989) Treatment of aggressive multiple myeloma by high-dose chemotherapy and total body irradiation followed by blood stem cells autologous graft. Blood 73 : 20-23
7. Gharton G, Tura S, Belanger C et al (1989) Allogeneic bone marrow transplantation in patients with multiple myeloma. Eur J Haematol 51, 43 : 182-185
8. Gahrton G, Tura S, Ljungman P et al (1991) Allogeneic bone marrow transplantation in multiple myeloma. N Engl J Med 325 : 1267-1273
9. Jagannath S, Barlogie B, Dicke K et al (1990) Autologous bone marrow transplantation in multiple myeloma : identification of prognostic factors. Blood 76 : 1860-1866
10. Pavlosky S, Saslavski J, Tezanos Pinio M et al (1984) A randomized trial of Melphalan and Prednisone versus Melphalan, Prednisone, Cyclophosphamide, Me CCNU and Vincristine in untreated multiple Myeloma. J Clin Oncol 2 : 836-840

Authors' index

A

Abbruzzese JL, 79
Abeler WM, 464
Adenis A, 607
Adkins DA, 785
Agugiaro S, 677
Ahmad K, 191
Aitini E, 558, 561, 581
Al-Sarraf M, 185, 191, 389
Alfeirán A, 565
Ali MK, 695
Alileche A, 779
Allegranza A, 587
Alonso S, 880
Amato R, 535
Ambrosini G, 677
Amistà P, 599, 616
Amuels B, 875
Andersen J, 196
Andry G, 291
Anedda V, 826
Angus RL, 770
Antoine E, 40, 70, 740
Antón A, 422
Anzai H, 411
Aquino A, 692
Aranda E, 422
Arbuck S, 172
Armand JP, 357
Armen T, 577
Armenio S, 692
Armes F, 105
Arthur Li KC, 179
Aschele C, 804
Asselain B, 131
Astre C, 396
Athanasiadis I, 207
Athannasiades A, 146
Atlan D, 135
Attal M, 736
Auclerc G, 40, 70, 740
Ayala AG, 577
Azli N, 357
Azzarone B, 779

B

Bacoyiannis H, 303
Bafaloukos D, 146
Bahmed Y, 243
Baillet F, 70, 516
Bain C, 861
Baiocchi C, 548
Ballatori E, 520
Banis C, 303
Banzet P, 40
Barak V, 315
Bardon M, 274
Barenholz Y, 820
Barra S, 581
Bassot V, 243
Bastaki M, 833
Bastian G, 740
Bastit P, 135
Battesti JP, 328
Beaujean F, 843, 885
Beer M, 146
Beerblock K, 488
Beger HG, 433, 639
Bélembaogo E, 127
Belivanis J, 523
Belón J, 422
Benasso M, 234, 307
Benhammouda A, 40, 681, 740, 774
Benjamin RS, 577
Benner SE, 298
Bennis S, 713
Berardi F, 150
Berghammer P, 311
Berkova N, 730
Bernard JP, 351
Berti F, 616
Bertino JR, 804
Besana C, 319, 548
Biesalski H, 590
Biller D, 855
Biron P, 551
Bitterman A, 315
Bizzari JP, 740
Blache JL, 476
Blayney DW, 757
Blengio F, 234
Blijham G, 155
Boaziz C, 328
Boccardo F, 527
Boege F, 749, 855
Bohas C, 351
Boiardi A, 587, 604
Boiocchi M, 726, 794
Bolla M, 291
Bollag W, 590
Bolli E, 804

Bonnay M, 838
Boogen CHr, 745
Booser D, 167
Borel Ch, 40, 70, 774
Borri A, 319, 548
Borsellino N, 257
Bosco López JJ, 765
Botturi M, 604
Bourhis JH, 885
Bouzy J, 551
Brachman D, 283
Brandes A, 599, 616
Brandi M, 150
Branscheid D, 362
Brasnu D, 243
Brasseur L, 699
Brault P, 885
Breau JL, 328
Brechner R, 757
Breitbart EW, 620
Breton JL, 354
Brette MD, 219
Brewer Y, 375
Brigham B, 331
Brindle JS, 389
Broggi G, 587
Bron H, 155
Brugger W, 24
Brugère J, 291
Brun B, 843
Bruni S, 692
Bruno M, 263
Bruynseels J, 590
Bucci E, 548
Budd GT, 428
Bukowski RM, 428, 875
Bunke B, 658
Buonadonna A, 573, 794
Busse P, 196
Bussi E, 319
Buzdar A, 163, 167
Buzdar AU, 105
Byhardt R, 389
Byrne J, 865

C

Cabane J, 288
Cabot GG, 237
Caffo O, 677
Campana F, 131

Camps C, 422
Canavese G, 561, 581
Cannata G, 257
Canobbio L, 527
Cantoni E, 561
Carde P, 843
Carrasco CH, 577
Carrato A, 422
Cartei G, 469
Cascinu S, 405
Casey D, 196
Castagneto B, 581
Castañeda N, 565
Castillo J, 248
Catalano G, 405
Catane R, 820
Catino A, 150
Cattan P, 607
Cavallari M, 234, 307
Cernigoi C, 726, 794
Cerrina J, 336, 503
Cervantes A, 422
Cervantes G, 485
Cetta F, 692
Chabner BA, 10
Chai CY, 672
Chaitchik S, 631
Chang HC, 479
Chang HK, 479
Chang TC, 479
Chapelier A, 336, 503
Chapey C, 713
Chastang C, 843
Chastang Cl, 354, 843
Chatikhine V, 135
Chauvel P, 251, 291
Chauvet B, 375
Chawla SP, 577
Cherif A, 817
Cheriff-Cheikh PY, 219
Cherqui D, 399
Chevallier B, 135, 551, 607
Chevillard S, 871
Chevreau C, 551
Chiostrini C, 260
Chipponi PN, 652
Chollet P, 127, 607
Chollet Ph, 473
Christopoulou A, 396
Chrétien Y, 516
Ciccarese G, 366
Citterio A, 548

Authors' index

Citterio G, 319
Claβen R, 623
Clapisson G, 861
Clark J, 196
Clavier J, 354
Cleeland C, 699
Clemm C, 499
Clocchiatti G, 469
Colardelle F, 516
Colleau S, 699
Collins CPM, 770
Colomb HM, 386
Contini L, 201
Cooper J, 389
Cooper MR, 736
Cope FO, 29
Corbion O, 843
Coronel B, 861
Cortesi E, 520
Cortés-Funes H, 880
Corvo R, 307
Cossu F, 201, 826
Cotti C, 319
Coudert B, 120
Couteau C, 135
Cremone L, 419
Cremoux H de, 357
Crinò L, 366
Crown J PA, 172
Cruz JJ, 211, 348
Cruz-Hernández JJ, 422
Cueto J, 248
Curotto A, 527
Curreli L, 201
Currie V, 172
Curé H, 127, 473, 551
Cussoto M, 527
Cvitkovic E, 357

D

D'Anjou J, 135
d'Ercole Cf, 476
d'Errico I, 692
Dall'Arche MG, 726, 794
Dalley D, 331
Dalton WS, 90
Danicot H, 354
Daniel Haraf J, 370
Daniilidis J, 303
Dao TH, 131

Dartevelle P, 336, 377, 503
Darwish S, 366
Dassonville O, 225, 251, 274
Dauplat J, 473
David Crawford E, 542
Davis L, 389
Déchaux M, 243
De Vos LN, 464
Del Giacco GS, 201
Delanian S, 516
Deloche C, 127
Delpero JR, 476
Delwail V, 843
Demard F, 225, 251, 274, 291
Demetri GD, 875
Demuynck B, 488
Denis L, 98
Depierre A, 354
Deschamps de Paillette E, 843
Dhumeaux D, 399
Di Lucca G, 319
Díaz-Puente MT, 880
Díaz-Rubio E, 422
Dilly SG, 702
Dimopoulous Th, 523
Dirix LY, 55
Dittrich C, 311
Dobrowsky W, 311
Doglioni C, 794
Domenge C, 843
Domínguez H, 495
Domínguez-Malagón H, 513
Dreyfuss A, 196
Drings P, 362, 789
Drinkard LC, 386
Droz JP, 551
Dubiez M, 699
Dufour B, 516
Dulmet E, 336, 503
Durán A, 328
Durán M, 565
Durst AL, 315
Duvoux C, 399

E

Eccher C, 677
Ehrke MJ, 759
Emami B, 389
Erazo A, 485
Escobar M, 765

Espie M, 219
Esposito R, 649
Etienne MC, 274
Everett Vokes E, 370
Ewer MS, 695

F

Facchini A, 826
Fadel E, 843
Fagniez PL, 399
Faiella F, 419
Falkson G, 160
Falkson HC, 160
Fallai C, 260
Fargeot P, 120, 551, 607
Farinotti M, 604
Favaro D, 573
Favrot MC, 861
Fedeli A, 405
Fedkovi Y, 396
Feillel V, 127
Felix Faure C, 375
Ferguson MK, 386
Fernández-Marto C, 422
Ferrero JM, 843
Fiaschini P, 366
Fickers M, 155
Fidler IJ, 3
Finn L, 535
Fiorentino MV, 599, 616
Firouz Daneshgari MD, 542
Fischer JR, 362, 789
Fleury J, 127, 473
Fliedner V von, 322
Flores G, 565
Folco U, 558, 561
Fonseca E, 211, 348
Fontanini G, 336
Formento JL, 225
Forscher C, 79
Forsythe P, 172
Fountzilas G, 146, 303
Fourquet A, 131
Francini G, 692
Francoual M, 225
Franks C, 40
Fraschini G, 163
Frasci G, 419
Frei III E, 196
Freireich EJ, 7

Frindel E, 843
Frola C, 581
Fromaget JM, 652
Frost P, 798
Frustaci S, 573, 794
Frye D, 105, 167
Fujii M, 411
Fujimoto S, 665
Fumoleau P, 607

G

Gabez P, 120
Gabizon A, 820
Gaimberti V, 123
Gallagher PJ, 414
Gallati H, 789
Galligioni E, 573
Gallurt P, 765
Ganavese G, 558
Gandia D, 838
Gaona R, 495, 513, 565
Garcia J, 211, 348
Garcia MJ, 211, 348
Garcia-Giralt E, 843
Garcia Puche JL, 248
Garciá-Paredes M, 422
Garin A, 510
Garton GR, 482
Garza-Salazar J de la, 557
Gavoille A, 838
Gebbia N, 257
Gebbia V, 257
Gerl A, 499
Ghislandi E, 548
Giaccone G, 19
Giannakakis T, 146
Gibbs H, 167
Gibson V, 428
Gieseler F, 749, 855
Gilewski TA, 172
Gilles E, 885
Gimmon Z, 315
Gimonet JF, 843
Gioacchini N, 520
Giorgi C, 604
Giovannoni M, 469
Gislain C De, 120
Giuliani L, 527
Given HF, 865
Globitz S, 441

Godeau P, 288
Gómez A, 211, 348
Gómez E, 513
Gómez F, 248
Gonçalves E, 843
Gordon M, 875
Gouyette A, 237
Graic Y, 135
Gramont A de, 488
Grange Cl, 288
Grasl M, 311
Gravis G, 476
Gray R, 160
Greco M, 123
Grever MR, 10
Grimaldi A, 581
Grob JPh, 322
Grogan TM, 90
Gross-Wieltsch U, 568
Grossmann N, 590
Guarneri D, 527
Guerrero R, 248
Guévin R, 114
Guglielmi A, 804
Guigon M, 843
Guilhot F, 843
Guillot T, 274
Guiochet N, 607
Gutierrez Delgado F, 510
Gutman M, 631

Herskovic A, 389
Hildebrand J, 612
Hill BT, 720, 723
Hoffmann PC, 386
Holmes F, 163
Holmes FA, 105, 167
Hong WK, 298
Honigman J, 315
Horgan PG, 865
Hortobagyi G, 62, 163, 167
Hortobagyi GN, 105
Hoshi M, 393
Hossfeld DK, 620
Houghton JA, 785, 813
Houghton PJ, 785, 813
Housset M, 70, 516
Houvenaeghel G, 476
Hrushesky WJM, 29
Hsueh S, 479
Huang CH, 672
Huang SF, 479
Hudis CA, 172
Huet J, 357
Huet S, 713
Hupperets P, 155

H

Hainz A, 311
Hakes TB, 172
Hallez JP, 516
Han D, 779
Haraf DJ, 207, 283, 386
Hardin JM, 343
Harker GJS, 850
Hartenstein R, 499
Hartmann LC, 482
Harvey Golomb M, 370
Hasumi K, 453
Hatzigiannis J, 523
Hayat M, 885
Heiss A, 295
Heiss A, 669
Hennequin C, 219
Hentrich M, 499
Héron JF, 551

I

Ibrahim A, 885
Ichen M, 774
Ihde DC, 50
Imbert JC, 288
Inbar M, 631
Ingria F, 257
Inuyama Y, 280
Inversi F, 319
Isaacs R, 875
Ishihara S, 411
Ishizuka K, 393
Isnard F, 843
Israel L, 328
Izard JPh, 383

J

Jacob JH, 383
Jacobs J, 191
Jacoulet P, 354
Jager J, 155
Janot F, 237

Jasmin C, 779
Jimenz S, 885
Johansson CJ, 658
Jong J de, 155
Julien JP, 135
Julien M, 399
Julieron M, 838

K

Kaern J, 464
Kan Z, 817
Kanamaru R, 393
Kantor G, 291
Kanz L, 24
Karstens JH, 444
Kato T, 453
Kau S, 163
Kaufman B, 820
Kautzky M, 311
Kennedy P, 757
Kerbrat P, 551
Ketterer N, 322
Khayat D, 40, 70, 681, 740, 774, 843
Khlebnov A, 510
Khoury MT el, 351
Kies MS, 207
Kindermans C, 243
Kitamura Y, 411
Klausner JM, 631
Kment G, 311
Kobayashi K, 665
Kober F, 295, 669
Köhne-Wömpner CH, 444
Kohl P, 499
Kohn KW, 85
Kornek G, 441
Kornhuber HH, 590
Koscielniak E, 568
Kosmidis P, 146, 303
Kowalzick L, 620
Kozloff M, 207
Krakowsky Y, 607
Kramar A, 551
Krammer PH, 789
Kreuser ED, 639
Krulik M, 488
Kuang L-R, 817
Kunlin A, 135
Kure M, 665

L

Laccourreye H, 243
Lahma H, 789
Lai CH, 479
Lam PK, 179
Lamaille C, 120
Lamas G, 288
Lamon S, 573
Landonio G, 548
Langenbahn H, 620
Laramore GE, 191
Larue F, 699
Latini F, 573
Latini P, 366
Laurent G, 736
Laurent M, 131
Le Bourgeois JP, 399
Le Roy Ladurie F, 336
Lebeau B, 354
Leblanc P, 219
Lee Drinkard C, 370
Lee JS, 298
Lefèbvre JL, 291
Legault S, 114
Leger-Picherit E, 843
Legros A, 473
Leichman L, 389
Lejeune F, 322
Lelièvre, 214
Lemarie E, 354
Lena M De, 150
Lenot B, 336, 503
Lentz MA, 607
Lepore J, 172
Levin L, 460
Levin V, 66
Levitt D, 875
Leyvraz S, 322
Li C, 817
Lianes MP, 880
Link KH, 433, 639
Linn SC, 19
Lippman SM, 298
List AF, 90
Littera S, 201
Livni N, 315
Logothetis C, 535
Lombard JN, 354
Long HJ, 482
Longo S, 150
López E, 880

López-Brea M, 880
Lorenzi M, 692
Lorenzini L, 692
Lorenzo A, 765
Lorusso V, 150
Louvet C, 488
Lowenbraun S, 79
Luboinski B, 237, 291
Lucarini J, 196
Lucas C, 740
Luckett P, 283
Luzi Fedeli S, 405

M

Maafs E, 565
Macchiarini P, 336, 343, 503
Maccubbin D, 759
Majeski A, 542
Makrantonakis P, 303
Malaurie E, 214
Maluta S, 677
Mancini S, 692
Manegold C, 362
Manivit P, 652
Manny J, 315
Mansutti M, 469
Mantovani G, 201
Maraninchi D, 843
Maranzano E, 366
Marcatti M, 319
Margarino G, 307
Mark Ferguson K, 370
Marks L, 172
Marpeau L, 488
Marsili S, 692
Martin G, 211, 348
Martin Lopez I, 248
Martin M, 214
Martineau N, 127
Martorana G, 527
Marty M, 219
Martz K, 389
Marzocca G, 692
Marzullo F, 150
Masaoka H, 665
Matai K, 411
Mathieu D, 399
Mathieu-Tubiana N, 843
Matteucci P, 548

Maublanc MA de, 110
Maulard C, 516
Mayer F, 120
Maylin C, 219
Mayordomo JI, 880
Mazeron JJ, 214
Mazumdar AT, 260
McClean S, 723
McCuskey P, 817
McEvilly J, 207
McEvilly JM, 283
McLain D, 428, 875
McNeese M, 163
McNeese MD, 105
Melis G, 826
Mendelsohn J, 7
Mendoza A, 495, 513
Mercatello A, 861
Mercati U, 366
Merlano M, 234, 307
Merrouche Y, 861
Mertelsmann R, 24
Métreau JM, 399
Meyer B, 288
Meyer P, 749, 855
Michaud E, 351
Michel-Langlet P, 214
Mick R, 207
Miech G, 354
Mihich E, 759
Milano G, 225, 274
Millán J, 765
Miller TP, 90
Milleron B, 354
Minotti V, 366
Mir L, 838
Mittal B, 207
Moen B, 861
Mohr P, 620
Monaco M, 419
Monfardini S, 573
Monnet I, 357
Monnier A, 843
Monpezat JP, 843
Monteil JP, 219
Montpreville V de, 336, 503
Morán A, 765
Morán W, 207, 283
Moreau S, 488
Morere JF, 328
Morgan M, 568
Mori A, 804

Moro D, 354
Moskovtchenko JF, 861
Motohashi H, 411
Mouawad R, 681, 774
Muller C, 736
Mulloy W, 540
Munck JN, 838, 843
Murray JA, 577
Murray JC, 833
Murthy S, 428
Musca F, 649
Mutou T, 665
Myers CE, 736
Müller CH, 441
Müller MR, 745

N

Nabet M, 652
Najman A, 843
Nakajima T, 411
Nakajima Y, 411
Nardini M, 692
Negrier S, 861
Neugebaeur B, 295, 669
Nicholas Vogelzang J, 370
Nicolaou A, 303
Nilsson B, 658
Nishi N, 411
Nizri D, 70
Noirclerc M, 476
Norris Jr C, 196
Norton L, 172
Nowrousian MR, 745
Nüßler V, 855

O

O'Connor PM, 85
O'Donoghue J, 865
Ocampo O, 495, 513
Ohkubo H, 665
Olencki T, 428
Ollivier JM, 383
Olmi P, 260
Onetto N, 172
Oosterom AT van, 54

Orsatti M, 527
Ortega B, 485

P

Paccagnella A, 599, 616
Pace M, 527
Padoan A, 616
Pagé M, 730
Pai VR, 260
Paillot N, 354
Palumbo R, 561, 581
Panadero A, 211, 348
Panje W, 207
Panje WR, 283
Pantelakos P, 303
Paoli A de, 794
Papaspyrou P, 303
Paradis R, 730
Parikh DM, 260
Parise Jr O, 237
Patel SR, 577
Paull KD, 10
Pavlidis N, 146
Paz-Ares L, 880
Pechikoff P, 476
Pegoraro C, 527
Pellegrini A, 520
Pelzer H, 207
Perin T, 794
Persico G, 419
Pessey JJ, 291
Petrioli R, 692
Pettersen EO, 464
Peynegre R, 214
Peytral C, 214
Phelan C, 865
Philip Hoffman C, 370
Philip T, 861
Pichlmayr R, 444
Pico JL, 551, 885
Piedbois P, 399
Pierga JY, 399, 871
Pignatarox M, 616
Pigné A, 488
Pillasch J, 639
Pinedo HM, 19
Piron D, 838
Plagne R, 127, 473, 607
Plaisance S, 779
Pocchiari S, 759
Podratz KC, 482

Poisson R, 114
Polo M, 652
Polo R, 652
Polyzonis M, 523
Pouillart P, 871
Praagh I Van, 127
Presant CA, 757
Proto E, 201
Protopsaltis J, 146
Pujol H, 396
Puxeddu P, 201

Rossi R, 196
Rosso R, 234, 307, 561, 581, 804
Rotilio A, 599, 616
Rouanet Ph, 396
Roussel A, 383
Rubagotti A, 527
Rubin S, 283
Rubini B, 652
Rubinstein E, 779
Ruffié P, 357
Rugarli C, 319, 548

Q

Quoix E, 354

R

Raab HR, 444
Racanelli A, 150
Raderer M, 441
Rahmouni A, 131
Ramaioli A, 225
Ramaker J, 623
Ramirez L, 838
Ramirez-Mendoza M, 510
Ramouni A, 399
Rao RS, 260
Ravoux MA, 127
Raymond AK, 577
Rebischung JL, 377
Reboul F, 375
Reichman BS, 172
Resbeut M, 476
Restivo S, 257
Reynoso-Gómez E, 557
Rigon A, 599, 616
Rivera F, 880
Rixe O, 40, 70, 740
Robert J, 713
Roby P, 730
Roché H, 607
Rodriguez P, 765
Roisman I, 315
Roka R, 295, 669
Rombi G, 826
Romestaing P, 351
Roos G, 823
Rosen G, 79
Rossetti R, 366

S

Sachs C, 243
Safi F, 433, 639
Safra T, 820
Saint-Aubert B, 396
Salmaggi A, 587, 604
Salmon SE, 90
Saltiel JC, 357
Salvia G, 527
Samantas E, 303
Samuel S, 875
Sánchez J, 422
Sánchez P, 211, 248, 348
Sanguineti G, 307
Santarosa M, 573
Santini J, 225, 251
Sapia MG, 150
Sapio U, 419
Sapir D, 315
Sarkany M, 740
Sartor AO, 736
Sato H, 393
Scelzi E, 599, 616
Schalhorn A, 639
Schappack O, 311
Scheithauer W, 441
Schenk T, 441
Schenone M, 527
Schindel M, 789
Schittulli F, 150
Schlaifer D, 736
Schlenger L, 745
Schmoll E, 639
Schmoll HJ, 444
Schneider M, 251
Schneider M, 274
Schneider Ph, 322
Schöffski P, 444

Schoenheit A, 548
Schouten H, 155
Schouten L, 155
Schuller D, 191
Schwade JG, 191
Scneider M, 225
Scott CB, 191
Seeber S, 745
Seidman AD, 172
Sella A, 535
Senra A, 765
Sheehan TD, 207
Sheen MC, 672
Shellard SA, 720
Sheu HM, 672
Shimizu Y, 453
Sibau A, 469
Signor M, 469
Silvani A, 587, 604
Silvetrini F, 692
Simone G, 150
Singh KP, 343
Singletary S, 163
Singletary SE, 105
Sinodinou M, 303
Skarlos D, 146, 303
Smeets J, 155
Smith KA, 833
Smith MJ, 681
Sobrero A, 804
Sobrevilla-Calvo P, 557
Soong YK, 479
Soria P, 348
Soubrane C, 681
Soubrane Cl, 40, 70, 774
Soubrane D, 488
Souhrada M, 172
Souquet PJ, 351
Stacci C, 692
Stein N, 789
Stenram U, 823
Stephens FO, 414, 840
Stoppa AM, 843
Storey BY DW, 414
Stravoravdi P, 523
Stupp R, 47
Sugiyama K, 393
Suissa J, 774
Suzan BA, 542
Suzanne F, 473
Symes MO, 770

T

Tabary D, 652
Taguchi T, 658, 809
Takahashi M, 665
Takeshima N, 453
Tani F, 692
Tanzini G, 692
Taubert J, 695
Taulelle M, 375
Tcherakian F, 328
Terrioux P, 354
Tertian G, 885
Testa A, 257
Tetezner CH, 441
Theriault R, 163, 167
Theriault RL, 105
Thill L, 40
Thomas A, 70
Thomas F, 843
Thyss A, 251, 274
Tisserant A, 607
Tixi L, 804
Tjulandin S, 510
Toffoli G, 726, 794
Tognella S, 319, 548
Tokunaga A, 411
Toma G, 649
Toma S, 234, 561, 581
Tonato M, 366
Tonkin K, 460
Torrecillas L, 485
Tourani JM, 40
Traverso GB, 527
Trepel JB, 736
Tres A, 422
Tresoldi M, 319
Treuner J, 568
Tropé CG, 464
Tubiana M, 843
Tumiotto L, 726
Tumiotto L, 794
Tzitzikas J, 303

U

Ujházy S, 759
Umezawa S, 453
Untereiner M, 652
Uryshiyama M, 393
Uziely P, 820

Authors' index

V

Vaitkevicius VK, 389
Valentini S, 587, 604
Valenza R, 257
Valero V, 167
Vallejo JC, 211, 348
Vannetzel JM, 377
Varette C, 488
Vassal G, 838
Vekhoff A, 843
Venturini M, 527
Vergnes L, 214, 357
Vergote IB, 464
Verjus M, 237
Vernhes JC, 383
Veronesi U, 123
Vertovšěh, 759
Veyret C, 135
Vicencio L, 495, 513, 565
Vielh Ph, 871
Viens P, 476
Vigevani E, 469
Vincent P, 375
Vincenti M, 561
Virdis RA, 520
Vitale V, 307, 527
Vogt-Moykopf I, 362
Voigt H, 623
Voisin S, 357
Vokes EE, 48, 207, 283, 386
Volovics L, 155
Vritsios A, 303
Vuichard P, 322
Vuillemin E, 40, 70, 681, 740, 774, 843

W

Walers R, 167
Wallace S, 817
Walter King WK, 179
Walter S, 219
Waluch V, 757
Wang YW, 672
Waugh RC, 414
Weichenthal M, 620
Weichselbaum R, 207
Weichselbaum RR, 283
Weil M, 40, 70, 740, 774
Weinstein JN, 10
Wenig B, 207, 283
Westarp ME, 590
Westarp MP, 590
Whelan RHD, 723
Wildfang I, 444
Willmanns W, 855
Wilmanns W, 499
Wilms K, 855
Wils J, 155
Wilson KB, 833
Wilson TO, 482
Winderen M, 464
Wiseman C, 757
Wolberg WH, 160
Wolf W, 757
Wright KC, 817

Y

Yang D, 817
Yang X, 730
Yao TJ, 172
Ychou M, 396
Young DC, 875
Young K, 167

Z

Zampieri P, 599, 616
Zenone T, 351
Zerrillo G, 257
Zinser JW, 495, 513, 565
Zittoun R, 843
Zorat PL, 599
Zurrida S, 123
Zylberait D, 488

Achevé d'imprimer par Corlet, Imprimeur, S.A.
14110 Condé-sur-Noireau (France)
N° d'Imprimeur : 9891 - Dépôt légal : janvier 1994

Imprimé en C.E.E.

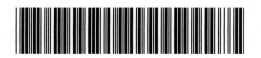